Evidence-based
Respiratory Medicine

Updates for *Evidence-based Respiratory Medicine* will be regularly posted to the following website. These updates give the latest trial data and recommendations for implementation in practice.

www.evidbasedrespiratorymed.com

Evidence-based Respiratory Medicine

Edited by

Peter G. Gibson

John Hunter Hospital, Newcastle, New South Wales, Australia

Section Editors

Michael Abramson

Monash University, Central & Eastern Clinical School, The Alfred, Melbourne, Victoria, Australia

Richard Wood-Baker

University of Tasmania, Hobart, Tasmania, Australia

Jimmy Volmink

University of Cape Town, Cape Town, South Africa

Michael Hensley

University of Newcastle, Newcastle, New South Wales, Australia

Ulrich Costabel

Ruhrlandklinik, Essen, Germany

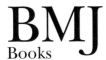 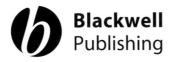

First published 2005
2   2006

Library of Congress Cataloging-in-Publication Data

Evidence-based respiratory medicine / edited by Peter G. Gibson / founding editor;
Section editors, Richard Wood-Baker, Michael Abramson, Jimmy Volmink, Michael
Hensley, Ulrich Costabel.
       p. ; cm.
   Includes bibliographical references and index.
   ISBN-13: 978-0-7279-1605-1 (hardback, cloth bound)
   ISBN-10: 0-7279-1605-X (hardback, cloth bound)
1. Lungs—Diseases. 2. Evidence-based medicine.
   [DNLM: 1. Respiratory Tract Diseases-therapy. 2. Evidence-Based Medicine. WF
145 E936 2005] I. Gibson, Peter, Dr. II. Wood-baker, Richard. III. Abramson,
Michael. IV. Volmink, Jimmy. V. Hensley, Michael. VI. Costabel, Ulrich.
   RC756.E954 2005
   616.2'0046—dc22

                                                   200505218

ISBN-13: 978-0-7279-1605-1
ISBN 10: 0 7279-1605-X

A catalogue record for this title is available from the British Library

Set in Minion 10 on 12pt by SNP Best-set Typesetter Ltd, Hong Kong
Printed and bound by Replika Press Pvt. Ltd, India

Commissioning Editor: Mary Banks
Development Editor: Veronica Pock
Production Controller: Debbie Wyer

www.evidbasedrespiratorymed.com

For further information on Blackwell Publishing, visit our website:
http://www.blackwellpublishing.com

The publisher's policy is to use permanent paper from mills that operate a sustainable
forestry policy, and which has been manufactured from pulp processed using acid-free and
elementary chlorine-free practices. Furthermore, the publisher ensures that the text paper
and cover board used have met acceptable environmental accreditation standards.

Contents

Contributors

Michael Abramson

Department of Epidemiology and Preventive Medicine, Monash University, Central and Eastern Clinical School, The Alfred, Melbourne, Victoria, Australia

Nick Adams

St Thomas's Hospital, London, UK

Robert P Baughman

University of Cincinnati Medical Center, Cincinnati, OH, USA

Scott C Bell

Adult CF Unit, Brisbane, Queensland, Australia

William C Black

Department of Radiology, Dartmouth-Hitchcock Medical Center, Lebanon, NH, USA

Michael L Burr

Department of Epidemiology, Statistics and Public Health, Wales College of Medicine, Cardiff University, Cardiff, UK

Yvon Cormier

Centre de Pneumologie, Hôpital Laval, Ste-Foy, Quebec, Canada

Ulrich Costabel

Ruhrlandklinik, Essen, Germany

Alan Joseph Crockett

Department of General Practice, University of Adelaide, Adelaide, South Australia, Australia

Juhi Dhar

Department of Medicine, Sitaram Bhartia Institute of Science and Research, New Delhi, India

Francine M Ducharme

Departments of Pediatrics and of Epidemiology & Biostatistics, McGill University Health Centre, Montreal, Quebec, Canada

Jim Egan

The Mater Misericordiae Hospital, University College Dublin, Dublin, Ireland

Richard M Fagerstrom

Biometry Research Group, National Cancer Institute, Bethesda, MD, USA

Tom Fahey

Tayside Centre for General Practice, University of Dundee, Dundee, UK

Duncan M Geddes

Department of Respiratory Medicine, Royal Brompton Hospital and Imperial College, London, UK

Peter G Gibson

John Hunter Hospital, Newcastle, New South Wales, Australia

John K Gohagan

Early Detection Research Group, National Cancer Institute, Bethesda, MD, USA

Roger S Goldstein

West Park Healthcare Centre, Respiratory Medicine, Toronto, Ontario, Canada

Michael J Hensley

The University of Newcastle, Newcastle, New South Wales, Australia

Michael E Hyland

Department of Psychology, University of Plymouth, Plymouth, UK

Philip Ind

Hammersmith Hospital, London, UK

John P A Ioannidis

Department of Hygiene and Epidemiology, University of Ioannina School of Medicine, Ioannina, Greece

Christine Jenkins

Woolcock Institute of Medical Research, Camperdown, New South Wales, Australia

David Peter Johns

Discipline of Medicine, University of Tasmania, Royal Hobart Hospital, Hobart, Tasmania, Australia

Paul W Jones

St George's Hospital Medical School, London, UK

Fotini B Karassa

Clinical and Molecular Epidemiology Unit and Clinical Trials and Evidence-Based Medicine Unit, Department of Hygiene and Epidemiology, University of Ioannina School of Medicine, Ioannina, Greece

Samuel T Kim

Department of Thoracic Medicine, The Prince Charles Hospital, Chermside, Australia

Terry P Klassen

Stollery Children's Hospital, Edmonton, Alberta, Canada

John Kolbe

Respiratory Services, Auckland City Hospital, Auckland, New Zealand

Barnett S Kramer

Disease Prevention, National Cancer Institute, Bethesda, MD, USA

Yves Lacasse

Centre de Pneumologie, Hôpital Laval, Ste-Foy, Quebec, Canada

Tim Lancaster

Department of Primary Health Care, Institute of Health Sciences, Oxford, UK

Richard Light

Saint Thomas Hospital, Nashville, TN, USA

François Maltais

Centre de Pneumologie, Hôpital Laval, Ste-Foy, Quebec, Canada

Pamela M Marcus

Biometry Research Group, National Cancer Institute, Bethesda, Maryland, USA

Guy B Marks

School of Public Health and Community Medicine, The University of New South Wales, Sydney, New South Wales, Australia

Nicola A Marks

Hammersmith Hospital, London, UK

Irvin Mayers

Division of Pulmonary Medicine, Walter C. Mackenzie Centre, Edmonton, Alberta, Canada

Colleen Murphy

Research & Analysis, Global Health Council, Washington, DC, USA

Horst Olschewski

Abteilung Pneumologie der Medizinische Klinik II, Universität Giessen Pulmonale Hypertonie, Giessen, Germany

Liesl M Osman

Chest Clinic, Aberdeen Royal Infirmary, Aberdeen, UK

Jihendra N Pande

All India Institute of Medical Sciences, New Delhi, India

Paul F Pinsky

Early Detection Research Group, National Cancer Institute, Bethesda, MD, USA

Barry Plant

The Mater Misericordiae Hospital, University College Dublin, Dublin, Ireland

Heather Powell

Hunter Medical Research Institute, Department of Respiratory and Sleep Medicine, John Hunter Hospital, Locked Bag 1, Hunter Region Mail Centre, New South Wales, Australia

Phillip C Prorok

Biometry Research Group, National Cancer Institute, Bethesda, MD, USA

Cheryl D Ray

Newcastle Sleep Disorders Centre, Newcastle, New South Wales, Australia

Martin Riedel

Deutsches Herzzentrum und I. Medizinische Klinik, Technische Universität München, München, Germany

Brian H Rowe

Division of Emergency Medicine, University of Alberta Hospital, Edmonton, Alberta, Canada

Cassandra A Slader

Faculty of Pharmacy, University of Sydney, Australia, and Pharmacy Department, St Vincent's Public Hospital, Darlinghurst, Australia

Olof Selroos

University of Helsinki, Helsinki, Finland

G Sowmya

Department of Medicine, Sitaram Bhartia Institute of Science and Research, New Delhi, India

Michael Stone

Llandough Hospital, Penarth, UK

Brett G Toelle

Royal Prince Alfred Hospital and the University of Sydney, Sydney, New South Wales, Australia

Tudor P Toma

National Heart & Lung Institute, London, UK

Johny A Verschakelen

Afdeling Rontgendiagnose, Katholieke Universiteit Leuven, Leuven, Belgium

Jimmy Volmink

Faculty of Health Sciences, University of Cape Town, Cape Town, South Africa

Haydn Walters

University of Tasmania, Tasmania, Australia

Julia Walters

Discipline of General Practice, Royal Hobart Hospital, Hobart, Tasmania, Australia

Peter A B Wark

Hunter Medical Research Institute, John Hunter Hospital, Newcastle, New South Wales, Australia

Peter J Wijkstra

Department of Pulmonary Diseases / Home Mechanical Ventilation, University Hospital Groningen, Groningen, The Netherlands

Richard Wood-Baker

University of Tasmania, Hobart, Tasmania, Australia

Ian A Yang

Human Genetics Division (Asthma Genetics), Southampton General Hospital, Southampton, UK

Alicia R ZuWallack

Kent County Memorial Hospital, Warwick, RI, USA

Richard L ZuWallack

St Francis Hospital and Medical Center, Hartford, CT, USA

Acknowledgement to Cochrane Library

The following metaviews that have been included in *Evidence-based Respiratory Medicine* are copyright of the Cochrane Library, and have been reproduced with permission.

Chapter, figure and page number in *Evidence-based Respiratory Medicine*	Cochrane review Title of review, year and issue number, and author(s)	Comments
Chapter 1.3.3, Fig. 1, 117	Silagy; CD000146 Nicotine replacement therapy for smoking cessation (2004, Issue 3) Silagy C, Lancaster T, Stead L, Mant D, Fowler G	Figure prepared based on data in tables
Chapter 2.1, Fig. 1, 125	Cates; CD000052 Holding chambers versus nebulisers for β- agonist treatment of acute asthma (2003, Issue 2) Cates CJ, Bara A, Crilly JA, Rowe BH	Comparison 01:01
Fig. 2, 127	Rowe; CD002178 Early emergency department treatment of acute asthma with systemic corticosteroids (2001, Issue 1) Rowe BH, Spooner C, Ducharme FM, Bretzlaff JA, Bota GW	Comparison 01:01
Fig. 3, 128	Rowe; CD001490 Magnesium sulfate for treating exacerbations of acute asthma in the emergency department (2000, Issue 1) Rowe BH, Bretzlaff JA, Bourdon C, Bota GW, Camargo CA Jr	Comparison 01:01
Fig. 4, 129	Rowe; CD000195 Corticosteroids for preventing relapse following acute exacerbations of asthma (2001, Issue 1) Rowe BH, Spooner CH, Ducharme FM, Bretzlaff JA, Bota GW	Comparison 01:01
Fig. 5, 130	Edmonds; CD002361 Inhaled steroids for acute asthma following emergency department discharge (2000, Issue 3) Edmonds ML, Camargo CA Jr, Brenner BE, Rowe BH	Comparison 01:01
Chapter 2.4, Fig. 5, 180	Ram; CD003137 Long-acting β_2-agonists versus anti-leukotrienes as add-on therapy to inhaled corticosteroids for chronic asthma (2005, Issue 1) Ram FSF, Cates CJ, Ducharme FM	Comparison 01:01
Chapter 2.5; Fig. 2, 185	Gibson; CD001005 Limited (information only) patient education programs for adults with asthma (2002, Issue 1) Gibson PG, Powell H, Coughlan J, Wilson AJ, Hensley MJ, Abramson M, Bauman A, Walters EH	Comparison 01:13
Fig. 3, 186	Gibson; CD001117 Self-management education and regular practitioner review for adults with asthma (2002, Issue 3) Gibson PG, Powell H, Coughlan J, Wilson AJ, Abramson M, Haywood P, Bauman A, Hensley MJ, Walters EH	Comparison 01:01
Fig. 6, 190	Gibson; CD001117 Self-management education and regular practitioner review for adults with asthma (2002, Issue 3) Gibson PG, Powell H, Coughlan J, Wilson AJ, Abramson M, Haywood P, Bauman A, Hensley MJ, Walters EH	Comparison 01:01

Chapter, figure and page number in *Evidence-based Respiratory Medicine*	Cochrane review Title of review, year and issue number, and author(s)	Comments
Fig. 7, 190	Gibson; CD001117 Self-management education and regular practitioner review for adults with asthma (2002, Issue 3) **Gibson PG, Powell H, Coughlan J, Wilson AJ, Abramson M, Haywood P, Bauman A, Hensley MJ, Walters EH**	Comparison 01:03
Chapter 2.6; Fig. 1, 195	Abramson; CD001186 Allergen immunotherapy for asthma (2003, Issue 4) **Abramson MJ, Puy RM, Weiner JM**	Comparison 01:01
Fig. 2, 196	Gotzsche; CD001187 House dust mite control measures for asthma (2004, Issue 4) **Gøtzsche PC, Johansen HK, Schmidt LM, Burr ML**	Comparison 01:02
Chapter 2.7; Fig. 1, 208	Davies; CD000391 Methotrexate as a steroid sparing agent for asthma in adults (1998, Issue 3) **Davies H, Olson L, Gibson P**	Comparison 01:01,02,07
Fig. 2, 209	Evans; CD002985 Gold as an oral corticosteroid sparing agent in stable asthma (2000, Issue 4) **Evans DJ, Cullinan P, Geddes DM, Walters EH, Milan SJ, Jones PW**	Comparison 01:02
Fig. 3, 209	Evans; CD002993 Cyclosporin as an oral corticosteroid sparing agent in stable asthma (2000, Issue 4) **Evans DJ, Cullinan P, Geddes DM, Walters EH, Milan SJ, Jones PW**	Comparison 01:02,05
Fig. 4, 212	Wark; CD001108 Azoles for allergic bronchopulmonary aspergillosis associated with asthma (2004, Issue 3) **Wark PAB, Gibson PG, Wilson AJ**	Comparison 01:01,02
Chapter 3.1, Fig. 1, 235	McCrory; CD003900 Anticholinergic bronchodilators versus β_2-sympathomimetic agents for acute exacerbations of chronic obstructive pulmonary disease (2002, Issue 3) **McCrory DC, Brown CD**	Comparison 01:01
Fig. 2, 236	McCrory; CD003900 Anticholinergic bronchodilators versus β_2-sympathomimetic agents for acute exacerbations of chronic obstructive pulmonary disease (2002, Issue 3) **McCrory DC, Brown CD**	Comparison 02:01
Fig. 3, 237	Barr; CD002168 Methylxanthines for exacerbations of chronic obstructive pulmonary disease (2003, Issue 2) **Barr RG, Rowe BH, Camargo CA Jr**	Comparison 04:01
Fig. 4, 238	Ram; CD004104 Non-invasive positive pressure ventilation for treatment of respiratory failure due to exacerbations of chronic obstructive pulmonary disease (2004, Issue 3) **Ram FSF, Picot J, Lightowler J, Wedzicha JA**	Comparison 01:01

Chapter, figure and page number in *Evidence-based Respiratory Medicine*	Cochrane review Title of review, year and issue number, and author(s)	Comments
Chapter 4.2, Fig. 3, 316	Dear; CD000422 Vaccines for preventing pneumococcal infection in adults (2003, Issue 4) Dear KB G, Andrews RR, Holden J, Tatham DP	Comparison 01:06
Fig. 4, 316	Dear; CD000422 Vaccines for preventing pneumococcal infection in adults (2003, Issue 4) Dear KB G, Andrews RR, Holden J, Tatham DP	Comparison 01:01
Fig. 5, 317	Dear; CD000422 Vaccines for preventing pneumococcal infection in adults (2003, Issue 4) Dear KB G, Andrews RR, Holden J, Tatham DP	Comparison 01:08
Fig. 6, 317	Dear; CD000422 Vaccines for preventing pneumococcal infection in adults (2003, Issue 4) Dear KB G, Andrews RR, Holden J, Tatham DP	Comparison 01:09
Chapter 4.3; Fig. 1, 326	Smeija; CD001363 Isoniazid for preventing tuberculosis in non-HIV infected persons (1999, Issue 1) Smieja MJ, Marchetti CA, Cook DJ, Smaill FM	Comparison 01:01
Fig. 2, 327	Woldehanna; CD000171 Treatment of latent tuberculosis infection in HIV infected persons (2004, Issue 1) Woldehanna S, Volmink J	Comparison 01:01
Chapter 4.7; Fig. 8, 403	Southern; CD002203 Macrolide antibiotics for cystic fibrosis (2004, Issue 2) Southern KW, Barker PM, Solis A	Comparison 01:01
Fig. 9, 407	Southern; CD002203 Macrolide antibiotics for cystic fibrosis (2004, Issue 2) Southern KW, Barker PM, Solis A	Comparison 01:02
Chapter 5.1; Fig. 1, 422	Lacasse; CD003793 Pulmonary rehabilitation for chronic obstructive pulmonary disease (2002, Issue 3) Lacasse Y, Brosseau L, Milne S, Martin S, Wong E, Guyatt GH, Goldstein RS	Comparison 03:04
Fig. 2, 423	Lacasse; CD003793 Pulmonary rehabilitation for chronic obstructive pulmonary disease (2002, Issue 3) Lacasse Y, Brosseau L, Milne S, Martin S, Wong E, Guyatt GH, Goldstein RS	Comparison 03:05
Chapter 5.2; Fig. 1, 431	Ram; CD004104 Non-invasive positive pressure ventilation for treatment of respiratory failure due to exacerbations of chronic obstructive pulmonary disease (2004, Issue 3) Ram FSF, Picot J, Lightowler J, Wedzicha JA	Comparison 01:01

Chapter, figure and page number in *Evidence-based Respiratory Medicine*	Cochrane review Title of review, year and issue number, and author(s)	Comments
Fig. 2, 431	Ram; CD004104 Non-invasive positive pressure ventilation for treatment of respiratory failure due to exacerbations of chronic obstructive pulmonary disease (2004, Issue 3) Ram FSF, Picot J, Lightowler J, Wedzicha JA	Comparison 01:02
Fig. 3, 432	Ram; CD004104 Non-invasive positive pressure ventilation for treatment of respiratory failure due to exacerbations of chronic obstructive pulmonary disease (2004, Issue 3) Ram FSF, Picot J, Lightowler J, Wedzicha JA	Comparison 01:03
Fig. 4, 432	Ram; CD004104 Non-invasive positive pressure ventilation for treatment of respiratory failure due to exacerbations of chronic obstructive pulmonary disease (2004, Issue 3) Ram FSF, Picot J, Lightowler J, Wedzicha JA	Comparison 01:04

PART 1

Practising evidence-based respiratory medicine

CHAPTER 1.1

Introduction

Brian H Rowe and Terry P Klassen

What is evidence-based respiratory medicine (EBRM) and why do we need it? The term evidence-based medicine (EBM) has a long history, and controversy exists regarding its components and value in decision making.[1,2] In most cases, however, it can be described as the combined use of experience, best evidence and patient's preference and values to develop an approach to a clinical problem, often referred to as evidence-based medical care.

An example may help readers understand the issue better. A 25-year-old woman presents to an emergency department with an exacerbation of her previously well-controlled asthma due to an upper respiratory tract infection. She improves slowly with inhaled β agonists and oral prednisone (pulmonary function tests improve from 55% to 75% predicted over 4 hours in the emergency department) and is ready for discharge home. From an evidence perspective, the clinician wishes to prescribe a short course of oral corticosteroids [best evidence based on systematic review (SR) of randomized controlled trials (RCT)].[3] Moreover, experience reminds the clinician that patients with moderate asthma can also deteriorate, require hospitalization and even die (clinical experience). The clinician is concerned and wishes to protect her from any and all of these events (and so does her lawyer). Unfortunately, the patient protests this decision because corticosteroids cause her to develop acne, retain fluids and have insomnia. She has a major weekend function and feels that these medications may create havoc with her social life. Despite the clinician's protestations, she refuses the oral corticosteroids (patient preference and values). Readers in clinical practice will be very familiar with this type of scenario.

What is the evidence-based decision in this case? Some traditionalists may suggest that their decision is final and the patient should accept the oral corticosteroid treatment. The EBM clinician might also use the evidence to clarify the benefits and risks of treatment options, in conjunction with the patient's preference and his/her experience. In the event that agreement cannot be achieved, the EBM clinician would propose an alternative 'next-best evidence' and similarly reasonable approach. For example, the clinician may recognize that very short courses of corticosteroids (1–2 days) are less likely to create side-effects. Moreover, the addition of inhaled corti-

costeroids,[4] asthma education[5] and very close follow-up may be safe in such patients.

Why EBM?

This approach may seem intuitive to many practitioners, which begs the question why is this being proposed in respiratory medicine? In a therapy issue, clinicians must ultimately decide whether the benefits of treatment are worth the costs, inconvenience and harms associated with the care. This is often a difficult task; however, it is made more difficult by the exponentially increasing volume of literature and the lack of time to search and distil this evidence.[6] Although clinicians of the early twenty-first century have an urgent need for just-in-time, on-demand clinical information, their time to access such information has probably never been as compressed. Increases in patient volume and complexity, patient care demands and the lack of access to resources have exacerbated the work frustrations for many clinicians. These concerns often take precedence over seeking the most relevant, up-to-date and comprehensive evidence for patient problems.

Despite the fact that most patient problems presenting clinically may be seen by many clinicians daily around the world, the appropriate treatment approaches are often not fully employed and practice variation is impressive. For a variety of reasons, the results from high-level evidence such as RCTs are not readily available to busy clinicians and keeping up to date is becoming increasingly difficult. Moreover, a valid, reliable and up-to-date clinical bottom line to guide treatment decisions has been elusive.[6]

However, access to information is not the only barrier to practising 'best evidence medicine'. Clinicians also need rigorously produced, synthesized best evidence information to assist them at the point-of-care. As time is increasingly more precious, the need for this digestible information has never been greater.

Levels of evidence

Levels of evidence have been developed and employed in clinical medicine to reflect the degree of confidence with which results from research may be accepted as valid. From levels of evidence, strength of recommendations are generated that are graded according to the strength of the scientific evidence supporting them. The highest level of evidence (Level I) in therapy is based on RCTs [or meta-analysis (M-A) of such trials] of adequate size to ensure a low risk of incorporating false-positive or false-negative results.[7] Although Level I status is awarded to RCTs, many trials are not large enough to generate Level I evidence. While considerable debate exists regarding the relative merits of evidence derived from large individual trials versus systematic reviews,[8] owing to the costs associated with large, multicentred trials, they remain uncommon across many clinical specialties and topic areas. Consequently, it is likely that systematic reviews will play an increasingly important role in the future decisions made by patients, clinicians, administrators and society in all areas of health care.

Level II evidence is based on RCTs that are too small to provide level I evidence. They may show either positive trends that are not statistically significant or no trends and are associated with a high risk of false-negative results. Level III evidence is based on non-randomized controlled or cohort studies, case series, case–control studies or cross-sectional studies. Level IV evidence is based on the opinion of respected authorities or expert committees as indicated in published consensus conferences or guidelines. Level V evidence is based on the opinions of those who have written and reviewed the guidelines, based on their experience, knowledge of the relevant literature and discussion with their peers.

Levels of evidence and systematic reviews

One possible solution to the information dilemma for clinicians is to focus on evidence from SRs.[9] Systematic reviews address a focused clinical question, using comprehensive search strategies, assessing the quality of the evidence and, if appropriate, utilizing meta-analytic summary statistics, and synthesize the results from research on a particular topic with a defined protocol. They represent an important and rapidly expanding body of literature for the clinician dealing with respiratory complaints and are an integral component of EBM. Despite a recent increase in the production of diagnostic testing SRs, the most common application of SRs is in therapeutic interventions in clinical practice.

Despite publications illustrating the importance of methodological quality in conducting and reporting both RCTs[10] and SRs,[11] not all SRs are created using the same rigorous methods described above. Like most other research, there are shades of grey in methodological quality associated with research in this field. High-quality SRs of therapies attempt to identify the literature on a specific therapeutic intervention using a structured, a priori and well-defined methodology. Rigorously conducted SRs are recognizable by their avoidance of publication and selection bias. For example, they include foreign language, both published and unpublished, literature and employ well-described comprehensive search strategies to avoid publication bias. Their trial selection includes studies with similar populations, outcomes and methodologies and use of more than one 'reviewer'.

Systematic reviews regarding therapy would most commonly combine evidence from RCTs. In the event that statistical pooling is possible and clinically appropriate, the resultant statistic provides the best 'summary estimate' of the treatment effect. A SR with summary pooled statistics is referred to as a *meta-analysis*, while those without summary data are referred to as a *qualitative systematic review*. Both these options represent valid approaches to reporting SRs, and both are now increasingly commonly published in the medical literature.

Levels of evidence and the Cochrane Collaboration

The Cochrane Collaboration represents one source of high-quality SR information available to most clinicians with very little effort. By way of brief review, the Cochrane Collaboration is a multinational, volunteer, collaborative effort on the part of researchers, clinicians from all medical disciplines and consumers to produce, disseminate and update SRs on therapeutic interventions.[12] The Cochrane Collaboration takes its name from the British epidemiologist, Archie Cochrane, who drew attention to the overwhelming and seemingly unmanageable state of information pertaining to clinical medicine. A famous quote from Cochrane summarizes his thoughts on the topic:

> It is surely a great criticism of our profession that we have not organized a critical summary, by specialty or subspecialty, adapted periodically of all relevant randomized controlled trials.

The Cochrane Library is a compendium of databases and related instructional tools. As such, it is the principal product of the large international volunteer effort in the Cochrane Collaboration. The quality of SRs contained within the Cochrane Library has been shown to be consistently high for individual topic areas as well as throughout the Cochrane.[13,14] Within the Collaboration, the Cochrane Airway Group (CAG; www.cochrane-airways.ac.uk) is responsible for developing, completing and updating systematic reviews in 'airway' topics [e.g. asthma, chronic obstructive pulmonary disease (COPD), bronchiectasis, interstitial lung disease, sleep apnoea and pulmonary embolism]. Based at St George's Hospital Medical School in London, UK, the CAG editorial office co-ordinates this huge international respiratory effort. The Co-ordinating Editor (Professor Paul Jones: 1993–2003; Dr Christopher Cates: 2003–present) and the editorial team are responsible for the direction, quality and supervision of the reviews provided in the Cochrane Library. The CAG Review Group Co-ordinator (Mr Stephen Milan:

1995–2001; Mr Toby Lasserson: 2001–present) administratively co-ordinates this effort and assists reviewers in completing their reviews. Reviewers within the CAG represent consumers, researchers, physicians, nurses, physiotherapists, educators and others interested in the topic areas. Respiratory topics are particularly well covered by members of the Cochrane Airway Group.[15]

Systematic reviews produced by members of the Cochrane Collaboration are products of a priori research protocols, meet rigorous methodological standards and are peer reviewed for content and methods before dissemination. Specifically, this process of review production is designed to reduce bias and ensure validity, using criteria discussed in the *Journal of the American Medical Association*'s 'User's Guide' series.[16] This text will focus on evidence derived from SRs and, as often as possible, those contained within the Cochrane Library.

Cochrane Library

The Cochrane Library is composed of several databases, three of which require some description here. The Cochrane Central Register of Controlled Trials (CENTRAL) is an extensive bibliographic database of controlled trials that has been identified through structured searches of electronic databases and hand searching by Collaborative Review Groups (CRGs). Currently, it contains over 440 000 references (CL, Version 1, 2005) and can function as a primary literature searching approach with therapeutic topics. The Database of Abstracts of Reviews of Effects (DARE) consists of critically appraised structured abstracts of non-Cochrane published reviews that meet standards set by the Centre for Reviews and Dissemination at the University of York, UK. The last, and possibly most important, resource is the Cochrane Database of Systematic Reviews (CDSR), a compilation of regularly updated systematic reviews with meta-analytic summary statistics. Contents of the CDSR are contributed by CRGs, representing various medical topic areas (e.g. airways, stroke, heart, epilepsy, etc.). Within the CDSR, 'protocols' describe the objectives of SRs that are in the process of being completed; 'completed reviews' include the full text and usually present summary statistics. Both protocols and reviews are produced using a priori criteria, adhere to rigorous methodological standards and undergo peer review before publication. Regular 'updates' are required to capture new evidence and address criticisms and/or identified errors.

Reporting systematic reviews

There is a unique lexicon used in SRs, and it is helpful to describe several of the important terms here. This is especially true of the statistical issues reported in SRs.

For dichotomous variables (alive/dead; admit/discharge), individual statistics are usually calculated as odds ratios (OR) or relative risks (RR) with 95% confidence intervals (95% CI). Pooling of individual trials is accomplished using sophisticated techniques using either a fixed effects (FE) or a random effects (RE) model. The 'weight' of each trial's contribution to the overall pooled result is inversely related to the trial's variance. In practical terms, for dichotomous outcomes, this is largely a function of sample size; the larger the trial, the greater contribution it makes to the pooled estimate. The results of most efforts to pool data quantitatively are represented as Forrest plots, or 'blob-o-grams'; these figures will be used extensively by reviewers in this textbook. In such displays, the convention is that the effects favouring the treatment in question are located to the left of the line of unity (1.0), while those favouring the control or comparison arm are located to the right of the line of unity. When the 95% CI crosses the line of unity, the result is considered non-significant (Fig. 1).

For continuous outcomes, weighted mean differences (WMD) or standardized mean differences (SMD) and 95% CIs are usually reported. The use of WMD is common in many SRs and is the difference between the experimental and control group outcomes, when similar units of measure are used.[17] The SMD is used when different units of measure are used for the same outcome. For continuous variables with similar units (e.g. airflow measurements), a WMD or effect size (ES) is calculated. The 'weight' of each trial's contribution to the overall pooled result is based on the inverse of the trial's variance. In practical terms, for continuous outcomes, this is largely a function of the standard deviation and sample size: the smaller the SD and the larger the sample size, the greater contribution the study makes to the pooled estimate. For continuous measures with variable units (such as quality of life or other functional scales), the SMD is often used. For example, if quality of life was measured using the same instrument in all studies, a WMD would be performed; if the quality of life was measured using multiple methods, all producing some 'score', an SMD would be calculated. For both the SMD and a WMD, the convention is the opposite of that for dichotomous variables, that is effects favouring the treatment in question are located to the right of the line of unity (0), while those favouring the control or comparison arm are plotted to the left. Once again, when the 95% CI crosses the line of unity, the result is considered non-significant.

Number needed to treat (NNT) is another method of expressing a measure of effect.[18] In the Cochrane Library reviews, the absolute risk reduction (ARR) is represented by the risk reduction statistic, and the inverse of this (and its 95% CI) provides the NNT estimation. A less exact method is to examine the pooled percentages in each column. For example, in the meta-analysis on corticosteroid use in acute asthma to prevent admission, the OR was 0.75 (95% CI 0.63–0.86).[19] The RR was 0.13, resulting in an NNT of 8 (95% CI 5–20). By subtracting the approximate percentage admission in the control group (0.50) from the treatment group (0.37), one obtains an ARR of 0.13 and a similar NNT of 8. Caution is advised, as this

Comparison: 01 Corticosteroids vs control
Outcome: 01 Admissions to hospital

Study	Corticosteroids (n/N)	Control (n/N)	RR (95% CI fixed)	Weight (%)	RR (95% CI fixed)
Study 1 (2001)	11/157	21/144		39.9	0.48 (0.24, 0.96)
Study 2 (2000)	3/31	5/29		9.4	0.56 (0.15, 2.14)
Study 3 (1999)	2/18	4/16		7.7	0.44 (0.09, 2.11)
Study 4 (2000)	5/68	18/79		30.3	0.32 (0.13, 0.82)
Study 5 (2003)	2/25	7/25		12.7	0.29 (0.07, 1.24)
Total (95% CI)	23/299	55/293		100.0	0.41 (0.26, 0.65)

Test for heterogeneity chi-squared = 0.90 df = 4 P = 0.92
Test for overall effect z = −3.76 P = 0.0002

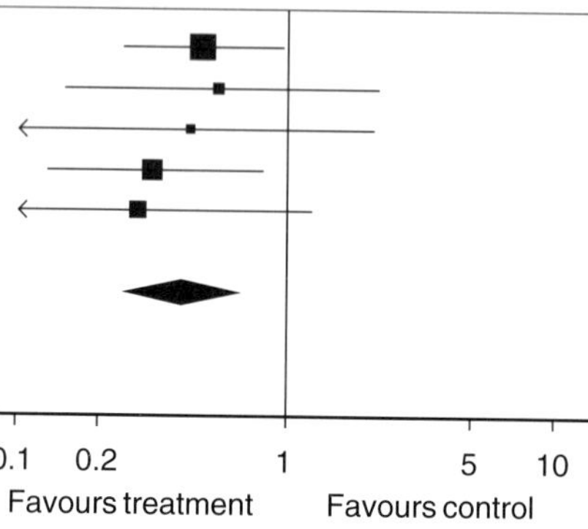

0.1 0.2   1   5   10
Favours treatment   Favours control

Figure 1. Hypothetical and typical Forrest plot of the effect of corticosteroids on admission to hospital in an illustrative respiratory disease.

approach is an approximation method for calculating NNT. Heterogeneity among pooled estimates is usually tested and reported.[20] Sensitivity and subgroup analyses are often performed to identify sources of heterogeneity, when indicated.

Question development

Patients presenting with many of the respiratory complaints presented in this book represent typical cases commonly encountered in clinical medicine. Many potentially important questions arise from these encounters; all these questions vary based on the perspective of the person asking the question (e.g. clinician, patient, administrators, primary care providers, public health officers and government policy makers). For example, using the previous example above, what is the *aetiology* of this patient's acute asthma problem? What *diagnostic tests* should be performed (if any) and which can the health care system afford? What additional *therapy* could be added in order to reduce the chances of an adverse outcome? What is her *prognosis* over the next 3 weeks with respect to her respiratory status? Would instituting a policy of closer follow-up provided by nurse clinicians improve the long-term *prognosis* for this woman? Finally, would influenza vaccination *prevent* further asthmatic exacerbations or reduce their severity?

The success of any search for answers is the development of a well-defined, clinically relevant and succinct question.[21] This approach is similar for the clinicians at the bedside, the policy maker in the office, the patient searching for options and the researcher performing a systematic review. Some have referred to this process as developing an 'answerable question', and this is a useful approach that will be used throughout this book. The rationale for developing a question is that the approach will save time and needless repetition throughout the complicated process of progressing from question to answer.

Components of a good question

Designing an appropriate clinical question includes consideration of the components of a good question (described below), compartmentalizing the topic area and describing the design of studies to be included. All questions should include focused details on the **p**opulation, **i**ntervention (and comparison treatment) and **o**utcomes associated with the question. This approach is often abbreviated as PICO, but these are only part of the components necessary for developing the question. Each component is described in further detail below, and examples are illustrated in Table 1.

Population
Clearly defining the population under consideration is the first step in developing a successful question; however, this can be a difficult task at times. The selection should be based on the interests and needs of the clinician and the patient's problem.

Intervention/exposure
Clearly defined interventions must be articulated before searching for answers. For example, corticosteroids may be a particularly problematic topic in question development. As corticosteroids can be administered via may routes (e.g. inhaled, intravenous, oral and intramuscular), using varying doses and over different durations, these must all be considered when searching for evidence. Moreover, the use of different agents is common (e.g. dexamethasone, prednisone, budesonide, fluticasone, methylprednisolone, etc.) and is clearly an important consideration in question development.

Outcome
There are a variety of outcomes reported in respiratory research studies. For example, in acute asthma studies, administrative designations (e.g. death, admission/discharge, obser-

Table 1. Example of PICO methodology for developing clinically appropriate questions (see text for details).

Population	Intervention	Outcome	Design	Topic
Children with asthma in ED	Ipratropium bromide versus standard care	Admissions to hospital	RCT	Therapy
Children < 18 years	Exposure to cigarette smoke	Development of asthma	Prospective cohort	Aetiology
Children in ED with acute asthma	Use of pulse oximetry versus clinical examination	Admissions to hospital	Prospective cohort	Diagnosis
Asthmatic children discharged	Corticosteroids versus control from the ED	Relapse to additional care	RCT	Therapy/prognosis
Children and adults in primary care practice	Influenza vaccine versus placebo	Prevention of exacerbations of asthma	RCT	Prevention

RCT, randomized controlled trial; ED, emergency department.

vation, relapse, etc.), physiological parameters [peak expiratory flow (PEF), vital signs, oxygen saturation, etc.], adverse effects (e.g. tremor, nausea, tachycardia, etc.), medication use (e.g. β-agonist use, corticosteroid rescue, etc.), complications (e.g. intubation, pneumonia, etc.) and symptoms (e.g. quality of life, symptoms, etc.) may all be reported. The clinician must select appropriate primary and secondary outcomes before beginning the search. The primary outcome should reflect the outcome that is most important to the clinicians, patients, policy makers and/or consumers.

Often the clinician may also be interested in secondary outcomes, side-effects and patient preference. While patient preference is not often reported in clinical trials and therefore SRs, side-effects and secondary outcomes are commonly encountered. The importance of secondary outcomes is that, if their pooled results are concordant with that of the primary outcome, this adds corroborating evidence to the conclusion. In addition, side-effect profiles provide the patients, clinician and others with the opportunity to evaluate the risks associated with the treatment. Inclusion of other outcomes, which are either infrequently reported or clinically unhelpful, should be considered with caution.

Other question considerations

Two additional components to be considered in the development of an answerable question for a clinical case are the topic area and the study methodology or design.

Topic areas
While selecting between topic areas may initially appear straightforward, there can be confusion. For example, is pulmonary function a diagnostic or a prognostic topic? Clearly, the use of pulmonary function tests has been examined as a di-

agnostic tool compared with clinical examination, and a review in this area would encompass a diagnostic domain. However, whether spirometry testing is effective in predicting relapse after discharge would be a prognostic question. As there are other domains of SRs (including therapy, prevention and aetiology), by selecting the topic of the clinical question, this further clarifies the approach for the clinician.

Design
The design of the studies to be located should also be considered carefully in the initial question formulation. For example, if one is interested in a therapeutic topic, the best level of evidence (Level I) includes results from large RCTs or SRs.[7,21] The next level of evidence (Level II) would be small RCTs, which are insufficiently powered. Finally, cohort, case–control and case series would be considered lower levels of evidence for treatment. It is therefore appropriate and efficient for initial searches for therapy answers to be limited to SRs and RCTs.

Locating the evidence: literature searching

Searching for evidence is a complex and time-consuming task. For example, to ensure that one has identified all relevant possible citations pertaining to a clinical problem, simple searching is often ineffective.[22] Search of MEDLINE, the bibliographic database of the National Library of Medicine, for RCTs using a non-comprehensive search strategy will miss nearly half the relevant publications.[23] In addition, by not adding EMBASE (a European electronic database maintained by Elsevier) searching, clinicians may be missing an additional 40% of the available evidence.[24] Hand searching has been shown to increase the yield of RCT searches.[24] Finally, unpublished and foreign language literature may contain important information relevant to your patient's problem and should not be excluded. Given the volume of literature, the search strategies required and the need for multilingual detective work, it is hardly surprising that clinicians find it difficult to obtain all the relevant articles in a particular topic area. Several strategies can be used to address this issue. One strategy is to target searches, using designated filters (see Table 2).[6] Another strategy, and the choice of this text, is to search for high-quality SRs, especially in therapy, to answer the question.[25]

Interpreting the evidence for clinical practice

Evidence-based medicine relies on the reporting of evidence using terms that are at times unfamiliar to clinicians. For example, in diagnostic articles, terms such as sensitivity, specificity and likelihood ratios (LR) are often reported. In therapy articles, terms such as odds ratio (OR), relative risk (RR) or number needed to treat (NNT) are commonly reported. In this book, these terms will be applied regularly in an attempt to distil the evidence for the clinician. There are many internet-based resources freely available to the reader that can provide additional information, calculations and interpretations of these terms. A limited internet resource list is provided in Table 3.

Evidence-based medicine in respiratory care

We are excited about highlighting the approaches to the diagnosis and treatment of respiratory conditions that will be detailed in this book. The editors have selected experts in both respiratory conditions (content) as well as evidence-based medicine (methodology). Following this introductory chapter, the remainder of the chapters will focus on individual topic areas. Many of the chapters in this book have been organized in a similar fashion using the following format.

Case scenario

The chapter author has been asked to develop a patient scenario upon which the remainder of the chapter will be based. Authors have been instructed to provide a real-world clinical problem.

Questions

Using the PICO methodology described above, questions will be developed from each case. These clinical scenarios will be used to identify important questions relevant to the diagnosis, prognosis, therapy, adverse effects, cost-effectiveness, etc. of respiratory conditions.

Literature search

A brief description of the search strategies employed to identify the relevant research used to answer the clinical question will be provided. In general, the evidence from SRs, especially those available in the Cochrane Library, will be highlighted.

Table 2. Common search strategies for identifying evidence from electronic databases using search filters.

Topic	Highest level design	Search terms
Therapy	RCT	Publication type: RANDOMIZED CONTROLLED TRIAL; CONTROLLED CLINICAL TRIAL; CLINICAL TRIAL MeSH headings: RANDOMIZED CONTROLLED TRIALS; RANDOM ALLOCATION; DOUBLE BLIND; SINGLE BLIND; PLACEBO(S)
Therapy	SR	Publication type: REVIEW; SYSTEMATIC REVIEW; META-ANALYSIS MeSH headings: MEDLINE
Diagnosis	Prospective cohort	Publication type: DIAGNOSIS MeSH headings: SENSITIVITY AND SPECIFICITY Text word: sensitivity
Prevention	RCT, SR	See above for RCT and SR
Aetiology	Prospective cohort	Text word: risk

MeSH, Medical Subject Heading; RCT, randomized controlled trial; SR, systematic review.

Table 3. Selected EBM websites.

EBM	Website address
Cochrane Airway Group (airways progress and releases)	www.cochrane-airways.ac.uk
Bandolier (various EBM topics)	http://www.jr2.ox.ac.uk/bandolier/
VirtualRx (NNT calculations)	http://www.nntonline.com/ebm/visualrx/nnt.asp
Cochrane Collaboration	www.cochrane.org
ACP Journal/EBM Journal	http://ebm.bmjjournals.com/
Agency for Health Care Policy and Research (AHRQ)	http://www.ahrq.gov
Centre for Evidence-Based Medicine (Oxford, UK)	http://www.cebm.net
Centre for Health Evidence (CHE)	http://www.cche.net/che/home.asp
Centre for Reviews and Dissemination (CRD)	http://www.york.ac.uk/inst/crd/

This list is neither comprehensive nor complete; it represents some of the EBM resources of use to the authors.

Summary critical appraisal

A summary of the available evidence will be provided by the authors, focusing on the key results and their implications.

Answers/conclusions

A summary approach to the patient will be presented at the end of each chapter.

Summary

Much progress has been made in respiratory medicine over the past half century in the areas of aetiology, diagnosis, prevention, therapy and prognosis. The synthesis of this evidence has been undertaken by many researchers, and there is now good evidence for the management of many common respiratory conditions. This book attempts to summarize this evidence in a best evidence fashion using relevant examples from clinical practice.

Acknowledgements

The authors would like to thank Mrs Diane Milette for her secretarial support. In addition, the authors would like to acknowledge the work of the Airway Review Group staff (Stephen Milan, Toby Lasserson and Mrs Karen Blackhall) and the Review Group editors (Professor Paul Jones and Dr Christopher Cates) at the St George's Hospital Medical School for their support with the development of reviews.

Conflicts of interest

Dr Rowe is supported by the Canadian Institute of Health Research (CIHR; Ottawa, Canada) as a Canada Research Chair in Emergency Airway Diseases.

References

1 Sackett DL, Rosenberg WMC, Gray JAM, Haynes RB. Evidence based medicine: what it is and what it isn't. *BMJ* 1996; **312**:71–2.

2 Haynes RB, Devereaux PJ, Guyatt GH. Physicians' and patients' choices in evidence based practice: evidence does not make decisions, people do. *BMJ* 2002; **324**:1350.

3 Rowe BH, Spooner CH, Ducharme FM, Bretzlaff JA, Bota GW. Corticosteroids for preventing relapses following acute exacerbations of asthma (Cochrane Review). In: *The Cochrane Library*, Issue 4. Oxford, Update Software, 2003.

4 Edmonds ML, Camargo CA Jr, Brenner B, Rowe BH. Inhaled steroids in acute asthma following emergency department discharge (Cochrane Review). In: *The Cochrane Library*, Issue 4. Oxford, Update Software, 2003.

5 Gibson PG, Coughlan J, Wilson AJ *et al.* Self-management education and regular practitioner review for adults with asthma (Cochrane Review). In: *The Cochrane Library*, Issue 4. Oxford, Update Software, 2003.

6 Haynes RB, Haines A. Barriers and bridges to evidence based clinical practice. *BMJ* 1998; **317**:273–6.

7 Guyatt GH, Sackett DL, Sinclair JC *et al.* User's guide to the medical literature IX: a method of grading health care recommendations. *JAMA* 1995; **274**:1800–4.

8 LeLorier J, Gregoire G, Benhaddad A *et al.* Discrepancies between meta-analyses and subsequent large randomized, controlled trials. *N Engl J Med* 1997; **337**:536–42.

9 Rowe BH, Alderson P. The Cochrane Library: a resource for clinical problem solving in emergency medicine. *Ann Emerg Med* 1999; **34**:86–90.

10 Moher D, Schulz KF, Altman DG for the CONSORT Group. The CONSORT statement: revised recommendations for improving the quality of reports of parallel-group randomized trials. *JAMA* 2001; **285**:1987–91.

11 Moher D, Cook DJ, Eastwood S *et al*. Improving the quality of reports of meta-analyses of randomised controlled trials: the QUOROM statement. *Lancet* 1999; **354**:1896–900.

12 Chalmers I, Haynes RB. Reporting, updating, and correcting systematic reviews of the effects of health care. *BMJ* 1994; **309**: 862–5.

13 Jadad AR, Cook DJ, Jones A *et al*. Methodology and reports of systematic reviews and meta-analyses. *JAMA* 1998; **280**:278–80.

14 Olsen O, Middleton P, Ezzo J *et al*. Quality of Cochrane reviews: assessment of sample from 1998. *BMJ* 2001; **323**:829–32.

15 Jadad AR, Moher M, Browman GP *et al*. Systematic reviews and meta-analyses on treatment of asthma: critical evaluation. *BMJ* 2000; **320**:537–40.

16 Oxman AD, Cook DJ, Guyatt GH for the Evidence-Based Medicine Working Group. Users' guides to the medical literature VI. How to use an overview. *JAMA* 1994; **272**:1367–71.

17 Olkin L. Statistical and theoretical considerations in meta-analysis. *J Clin Epidemiol* 1995; **38**:133–46.

18 Laupacis A, Sackett DL, Roberts RS. An assessment of a clinically useful measure of the consequences of treatment. *N Engl J Med* 1988; **318**:1728–33.

19 Rowe BH, Spooner CH, Ducharme FM, Bretzlaff JA, Bota GW. The effectiveness of corticosteroids in the treatment of asthma: a meta-analysis of their effect on preventing admission (Cochrane Review). In: *The Cochrane Library*, Issue 4. Oxford, Update Software, 2003.

20 DerSimonian R, Laird N. Meta-analysis in clinical trials. *Control Clin Trials* 1986; **7**:177–88.

21 Sackett DL, Richardson WS, Rosenberg W, Haynes RB. *Evidence-based Medicine. How to Practice and Teach EBM*. New York, Churchill Livingstone, 1992.

22 Dickersin K, Chan S, Chalmers TC *et al*. Publication bias and clinical trials. *Control Clin Trials* 1987; **8**:343–53.

23 Dickersin K, Scherer R, Lefebvre C. Identifying relevant studies for systematic reviews. *BMJ* 1994; **309**:1286–91.

24 Suarez-Almazor ME, Belseck E, Homik J *et al*. Identifying clinical trials in the medical literature with electronic databases: MEDLINE alone is not enough. *Control Clin Trials* 2000; **21**:476–87.

25 Hunt DL, McKibbon KA. Locating and appraising systemic reviews. *Ann Intern Med* 1997; **126**:532–8.

CHAPTER 1.2
Diagnostic strategies

CHAPTER 1.2.1

Presenting symptoms

Michael Abramson

Many, perhaps most, patients do not present to a physician with clear-cut syndromes. The clinician frequently faces the challenge of first making a specific diagnosis in order to institute the most effective management. Traditional textbooks are replete with lengthy lists of differential diagnoses and specialized laboratory investigations that are not always widely available. This chapter will focus on a few of the more common respiratory symptoms (cough, haemoptysis, dyspnoea and wheeze) and outline diagnostic strategies that can be applied across a range of clinical settings.

There is good evidence that non-specific respiratory symptoms are indeed common in many western populations. For example, a survey of randomly selected 20- to 44-year-old adults in Melbourne, Australia, found that 28.6% reported nocturnal cough, 28% wheeze, 15.6% wheeze with breathlessness and 11.3% nocturnal dyspnoea within the last 12 months.[1] A subsequent survey of randomly selected 45- to 69-year-old adults also found high symptom prevalences: wheeze 20.5%, wheeze with breathlessness 11%, shortness of breath hurrying or walking uphill 27.2%, cough and sputum 12.5% and nocturnal dyspnoea 9%.[2]

Literature search

In order to identify relevant original diagnostic studies, MEDLINE searches were conducted from 1966 to 2002 using the keywords 'sensitivity' and 'specificity' and each of cough, haemoptysis, dyspnoea (or breathlessness) and wheeze in turn. A number of narrative reviews and consensus statements were also identified, but no systematic reviews or randomized controlled trials (RCTs) of diagnostic tests for any of these respiratory symptoms were found. No citations were found before the late 1980s. The Cochrane Library was searched for systematic reviews of specific therapies for underlying conditions such as gastro-oesophageal reflux, allergic rhinitis and sinusitis. Studies were selected if they reported diagnostic test properties. For practical reasons, the literature review was restricted to studies published in English.

Diagnostic strategies for cough

Conventionally, cough has been subdivided into acute and transient, acute and life-threatening, and chronic lasting more than 3 weeks.[3] Acute cough lasting less than 3 weeks is considered most frequently due to viral upper respiratory tract infections (URTIs), such as the common cold. However, the distinction is somewhat arbitrary as shown by a recent cohort study conducted in two general practices.[4] Jones and Stewart followed 131 patients without chronic chest problems who presented with an URTI until their cough resolved. Of these, 78% coughed for at least 1 week, 58% for 2 weeks, 35% for 3 weeks, 17% for 4 weeks and one patient coughed into the 10th week.

An 'anatomic diagnostic protocol' for chronic cough has been promoted by Irwin and colleagues at the University of Massachusetts in Worcester, MA, USA. This protocol is based upon current understanding of the anatomy of the afferent limb of the cough reflex (Fig. 1), rather than high-level evidence. It has now been applied successfully to selected series of patients in a number of countries. These case series constitute relatively weak evidence and are subject to referral bias, but are probably not unrepresentative of patients seen in specialist or hospital practice. The most common causes of chronic cough have proved to be:

- Postnasal drip syndrome (from allergic rhinitis ± chronic sinusitis);
- Gastro-oesophageal reflux disease;
- Asthma.

These three conditions, which often co-exist, account for 85% of all causes of chronic cough in older adults.[3] However, many of these case series exclude smokers, in whom cough may be the presenting symptom of chronic obstructive pulmonary disease (COPD), and patients on angiotensin-converting enzyme (ACE) inhibitors. The frequency of coughing in the general community is significantly related to cigarette smoking.[5] In this Norwegian case–control study, cough frequency was also associated with declines in peak expiratory flow (PEF), but not as strongly as was dyspnoea.

Less common causes of chronic cough include aspiration, bronchiectasis, occult pulmonary infection, industrial bronchitis, intraluminal or extraluminal mass affecting the trachea and bronchi, interstitial lung disease, occult congestive heart failure, disorders of the external auditory canal, diaphragm, pleura, oesophagus or stomach, nasal polyps, rhinoliths, uvular or tonsillar enlargement, and thyroid disorders.[6] However, many of these rarer conditions have only been reported in small case series. Psychogenic (or habit) cough is generally considered to be a diagnosis of exclusion.

The anatomic diagnostic protocol for immunocompetent patients with chronic cough[7,8] comprises the following steps:
• review the patient's history and perform a physical examination focusing on the upper and lower respiratory tracts;
• chest X-ray—carcinoma, sarcoidosis and bronchiectasis are unlikely to occur in the presence of a normal chest X-ray;
• withhold further investigation until smoking has been ceased and/or ACE inhibitors discontinued for 4 weeks;

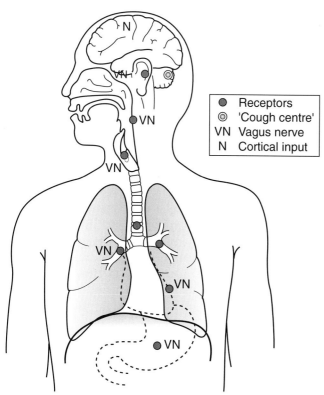

Figure 1. Current view of the anatomy of the afferent limb of the cough reflex. Solid dots, receptors; circled dot, cough centre; N, cortical input; VN, vagus nerve (reprinted from Irwin and Maddison,[8] Copyright ©2000, with permission from Excerpta Medica, Inc.).

• perform the following investigations as indicated by the initial evaluation: computerized tomography (CT) scan of the sinuses and skin tests for allergies; spirometry before and after bronchodilator, histamine or methacholine inhalation challenge; barium swallow or 24-hour ambulatory oesophageal pH monitoring;
• selected patients with abnormal chest X-rays may require sputum culture and cytology, flexible fibre-optic bronchoscopy, high-resolution CT scan of the chest or noninvasive cardiac studies. The investigation of recognized patterns of radiological abnormality is discussed further in Chapter 1.2.3;
• determine the cause(s) of cough by observing which specific therapy or therapies eliminate(s) the symptom.

This anatomic diagnostic protocol has been validated against the response to specific therapy. Given the lack of readily applicable 'gold standard' diagnostic tests for many of the conditions commonly responsible for chronic cough, this is probably a reasonable approach. The characteristics of some of the available diagnostic tests have been summarized in Table 1. However, it is doubtful whether the sensitivity, specificity or predictive values of any of the tests is really 100%. The protocol has evolved over time as newer, more sensitive tests have been introduced, such as CT scans of the sinuses and oesophageal pH monitoring. However, these more expensive technology-dependent investigations are not available in all clinical settings.

The treatment of all the specific conditions underlying chronic cough is beyond the scope of this chapter but, because a trial of treatment is often prescribed before diagnostic tests are performed, a few relevant systematic reviews will be mentioned briefly. The management of asthma is reviewed in detail in Part 2. More effective specific therapies have become available for gastro-oesophageal reflux disease. Proton pump inhibitors such as omeprazole provide significantly better relief of reflux symptoms than histamine 2 receptor antagonists, prokinetic agents,[9] antacids or conservative measures. However, the trials included in this systematic review focused on heartburn or dyspepsia rather than cough.

The best specific therapy for postnasal drip syndrome is unclear. A systematic review of RCTs of house dust mite avoid-

Table 1. Test characteristics of diagnostic protocol for cough (reprinted from Irwin and Maddison,[8] Copyright ©2000, with permission from Excerpta Medica, Inc.).

Test	Sensitivity (%)	Specificity (%)	PPV (%)	NPV (%)	PLR	NLR
Chest X-ray	100	54–76	36–38	100	2.2–4.2	0
Sinus X-ray	97–100	75–79	57–81	95–100	3.9–4.8	0–0.1
Inhalation challenge	60–100	67–71	60–82	100	3.0–3.4	0–0.6
Barium swallow	48–92	42–76	30–63	63–93	0.8–3.8	0.1–1.2
Oesophageal pH	<100	66–100	89–100	<100	>2.9	0
Bronchoscopy	100	50–92	50–89	100	2–12.5	0

PPV, positive predictive value; NPV, negative predictive value; PLR, positive likelihood ratio; NLR, negative likelihood ratio.

ance measures for perennial allergic rhinitis identified only four trials that satisfied the inclusion criteria, all of which were small and of poor quality.[10] The results suggested that the interventions may be effective in reducing some rhinitis symptoms, but it was not possible to provide a reliable summary estimate about the magnitude of such symptom reduction. A systematic review of allergen immunotherapy for seasonal allergic rhinitis is awaited.[11] Weiner *et al.*[12] found that intranasal corticosteroids provided more effective relief of nasal symptoms from allergic rhinitis, including postnasal drip, than did histamine 1 receptor antagonists (antihistamines). Antibiotics reduce persistent nasal discharge in children with rhinosinusitis, although around eight children must be treated in order to achieve one additional cure [number needed to treat (NNT) 8, 95% confidence interval (CI) 5–29].[13] A systematic review of decongestants and antihistamines will be published shortly.[13]

Case scenario

The patient was a 66-year-old retired engineer with a 15-year history of chronic cough. She presented following an upper respiratory tract infection complicated by 2 months of nocturnal bouts of non-productive cough and wheezing. She had been treated with inhaled salbutamol and inhaled corticosteroids, but did not find these medications to be of benefit. There was no history of early respiratory illness, allergies or postnasal drip. She was a non-smoker. There was no relevant family or occupational history.

The provisional diagnosis was late-onset asthma. Spirometry was normal with a vital capacity of 2.42 L (predicted 2.79 L) and forced expiratory volume in 1 s (FEV_1) of 1.84 L (76% of vital capacity). However, bronchial provocation testing was reported as negative—there was a 17% decline in FEV_1 after the inhalation of 2 mg (10 μmol) of methacholine.

At the next consultation, she was seen by another physician who noted occasional symptoms of gastro-oesophageal reflux. She was commenced on ranitidine (an H_2 antagonist) with some improvement in the nocturnal cough, but ceased this medication after a few months. She returned complaining of further coughing bouts resulting in urinary incontinence.

Ambulatory oesophageal pH monitoring revealed that pH was <4 12.4% of the time, and the De Meester score was 41.3 (normal <14.72). These findings were consistent with mild to moderate acid reflux. The patient was referred for upper gastrointestinal endoscopy, which showed moderate reflux oesophagitis (erosions less than 10% of the distal mucosa) and a small sliding hiatal hernia. She was then commenced on omeprazole (a proton pump inhibitor), but the cough persisted, and cisapride (a prokinetic agent) was added. Later that year, the manufacturer issued an alert warning that cisapride was associated with prolonged QT interval and ventricular tachycardia.

Questions

1 What is the probability of asthma following a negative methacholine challenge in adults with respiratory symptoms?
2 How does upper gastrointestinal endoscopy compare with 24-h pH monitoring in the diagnosis of gastro-oesophageal reflux?
3 What is the risk of cardiac arrhythmias from prokinetic agents such as cisapride?

Q1. Asthma following a negative methacholine challenge

The MEDLINE database was searched from 1996 to 2003 with the following strategy:

1 exp 'methacholine chloride'/ and exp 'bronchial provocation tests'/	547
2 exp 'sensitivity and specificity'/ or exp 'predictive value of tests'/	88 544
3 1 and 2	54
4 limit 3 to (human and English language and review articles)	2

One of these narrative reviews[14] was relevant to investigation of the patient described above. The abstract is reproduced in part below:

Using a cut-off value of 8 mg/mL or 8 μmol for PD_{20}, the tests will discriminate asthmatic from non-asthmatic subjects (based on questionnaire definitions of asthma) with a sensitivity of around 60% and a specificity of around 90%. These properties of the test result in positive and negative predictive values of 86% and 69% when the prevalence of asthma is high (50%, as in the clinical setting) and 40% and 95% when the prevalence of asthma is low (10%, as in general population studies). In the usual clinical setting, assessing the significance of atypical or non-specific symptoms, the tests are of intermediate value in predicting the presence of asthma and less useful in excluding asthma.

Thus, the sensitivity of methacholine challenge is not as high as often assumed. About 40% of patients with diagnosed asthma will have a negative challenge test. This can arise because of misdiagnosis, their asthma was well treated with inhaled corticosteroids or has remitted spontaneously. The pretest probability of asthma in our patient was around 80%. The negative likelihood ratio (NLR) = (1–sensitivity)/specificity = 0.44.

Using the nomogram (Fig. 2), following a negative challenge, the post-test probability was only reduced to 64%, not sufficient to exclude asthma in this case. Only a highly sensitive test that returned a negative result can be used to rule out a diagnosis, a property of diagnostic tests captured by the abbreviation SnOut.

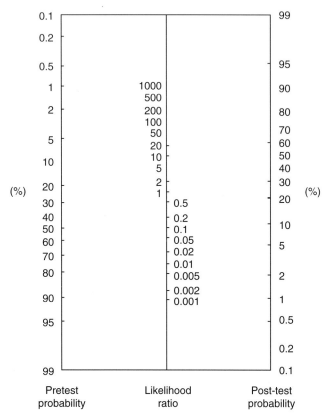

Figure 2. Nomogram for converting the pretest probability of disease to the post-test probability, given the likelihood ratio associated with a positive or negative result.

Q2. Diagnosis of gastro-oesophageal reflux

The MEDLINE database was searched from 1996 to 2003 for studies on the sensitivity and specificity of upper gastrointestinal endoscopy in gastro-oesophageal reflux. This yielded 10 citations, including four RCTs of omeprazole, that did not address the question. However, the gold standard test for gastro-oesophageal reflux has now become ambulatory oesophageal pH monitoring. As this was not a MESH term, the MEDLINE database was searched again from 1996 to 2003 for studies of 'sensitivity and specificity'/ and 'monitoring, ambulatory'/ and 'esophagus'/ and 'hydrogen-ion concentration'/, which yielded 12 citations. One of these studies[15] appeared to be directly relevant, and the abstract is reproduced below:

The aim of this study was to evaluate the accuracy of symptomatology and esophago-gastroduodenoscopy (EGD) in the diagnosis of proven gastroesophageal reflux disease (GERD). We evaluated the symptoms and EGD findings of 100 consecutive patients presenting with symptoms suggestive of GERD. Patients' symptoms were scored at their first visit with a standardized symptom scoring system (grades 0–3). Grade 3 symptoms were the most severe. EGD findings were classified according to

the modified Savary–Miller scale. Esophageal acid exposure was quantified using 24-hour esophageal pH monitoring; a positive composite score was considered evidence of GERD. Fifty-seven patients had positive pH scores, and 43 were negative. The combination of grade 2 or 3 heartburn and/or regurgitation with erosive esophagitis or Barrett's esophagus on EGD had a 97 per cent specificity and 64 per cent sensitivity for accurately diagnosing GERD. It is concluded that, in the presence of moderate to severe symptoms and endoscopic injury, the diagnosis of GERD can be made without further studies. However, 24-hour esophageal pH monitoring is still indicated in patients with mild typical symptoms, atypical symptoms, or when the combination of heartburn and regurgitation, regardless of their severity, occurs in the absence of severe mucosal damage.

This study would suggest that 36% of patients with reflux on oesophageal pH monitoring would not be diagnosed from the combination of heartburn and endoscopic abnormalities. As our patient had atypical symptoms (cough), oesophageal pH monitoring was the appropriate initial investigation. Upper gastrointestinal endoscopy did not add much diagnostic information. The approved indications for prescribing proton pump inhibitors in Australia have now been broadened, and endoscopy is no longer routinely required. Situations in which endoscopy is recommended include suspicion of oesophageal complications such as malignancy, Barrett's oesophagus and stricture.

Q3. Risk of cardiac arrhythmias from cisapride

The Cochrane Library was searched for systematic reviews of prokinetic agents. Augood et al. identified nine RCTs of cisapride for gastro-oesophageal reflux.[16] One trial found no difference in the QTc interval after 3–8 weeks of treatment.[17] As the library did not subscribe to the journal, an interlibrary loan request had to be made. Furthermore, this study related only to children, so a MEDLINE search (1996–2002) was conducted using the terms 'explode cisapride'/ae (adverse effects). This yielded 120 citations, which were then restricted to human English language review articles. Three of the 14 remaining narrative reviews appeared to be relevant.

The narrative review by Tonini et al.[18] could be consulted online as the library had an electronic subscription to the journal. This review stated:

The cardiotoxic potential of cisapride should be considered, particularly in newborns or children in patients with an idiopathic, congenital or acquired long QT interval, patients receiving Class III antiarrhythmic agents, phenothiazines, tricyclic antidepressants, H1-histamine receptor antagonists (e.g. terfenadine), those with renal or hepatic insufficiency, or finally, patients concomitantly treated with drugs known to inhibit the CYP3A4 isoenzyme.

The case described above had a normal electrocardiogram (ECG) and was not receiving any of the medications known to interact with cisapride or inhibit the cytochrome P450 isoenzyme. It was decided that it was safe to leave the patient on cisapride.

Diagnostic strategies for haemoptysis

Haemoptysis is the expectoration of blood from the tracheobronchial tree or pulmonary parenchyma. The history and examination need to distinguish haemoptysis from oral or dental bleeding, epistaxis with postnasal drip or even haematemesis, as the investigation of these conditions is very different. Globally, the commonest cause of haemoptysis is infection, particularly acute bronchitis, pneumococcal pneumonia, tuberculosis and mycetoma or sequelae such as bronchiectasis. However, in western countries, haemoptysis may be the presenting symptom of lung cancer. Less common causes include bronchial adenomas, pulmonary embolism (with infarction) and arteriovenous malformations. However, often no cause is found, particularly in patients with normal chest X-rays.

In the absence of systematic reviews or RCTs, clinical guidelines have been developed by consensus. The American College of Radiology (ACR)[19] recommended that the initial evaluation of patients with haemoptysis should include a chest X-ray. Patients with less than two risk factors for malignancy (male, > 40 years old, > 40 pack–year smoking history) and negative chest X-ray can be followed with observation. Chest CT scan and fibre-optic bronchoscopy (FOB) are complementary examinations in patients presenting with either two or more risk factors for malignancy or persistent or recurrent haemoptysis and a negative chest X-ray. The ACR also suggested that patients with two or more risk factors and positive X-ray findings should proceed to CT scan. The management of patients with abnormal chest X-rays is beyond the scope of this chapter (see Chapter 1.2.3).

A number of studies have compared bronchoscopy with CT scanning in the investigation of patients with haemoptysis. McGuinness *et al.*[20] reported a prospective series of 57 consecutive patients presenting with haemoptysis to an inner city hospital in the USA. FOB and high-resolution chest CT were performed within 48 hours of each other with the bronchoscopist and radiologist blinded to clinical and other data. The patients were older (mean age 59 years), with high prevalences of smoking, Mantoux positivity (65%), intravenous drug use and HIV seropositivity. Haemoptysis was attributed to bronchiectasis in 14 cases (25%), tuberculosis in nine (16%), lung cancer in seven (12%), fungal infection in seven (12%), bronchitis in four (7%), miscellaneous causes in three (5%) and multiple causes in two (4%). The cause of haemoptysis could not be identified in 11 cases (19%). CT was particularly helpful in identifying bronchiectasis, parenchymal masses, intracavitary filling defects due to aspergilloma

and active tuberculosis. FOB was required for diagnosis of endobronchial lesions (including Kaposi's sarcoma) and bronchitis. CT suggested the correct diagnosis in 63% and FOB in 43% of cases. However, the combined diagnostic yield was 81% suggesting that the two investigations were complementary.

Somewhat different results were reported by Tak *et al.*[21] from an Indian series of 50 patients with haemoptysis and a normal or non-localizing chest X-ray. Only one radiologist examined the CT scans, and it was not clear whether FOB was performed without knowledge of the CT results. The patients were younger than in other series (mean age 37.2 years), few smoked and there was a high prevalence (40%) of Mantoux positivity. Three (6%) patients demonstrated central airway lesions on CT, which proved to be bronchial adenomas after bronchoscopy. Bronchiectasis was found on CT in 12 cases (24%) without bronchoscopy contributing further information. One patient each was diagnosed with acute bronchitis and active tuberculosis following bronchoscopy and examination of bronchial washings. The authors again concluded that the two investigations were complementary. However, an unusual feature of this series was the complete absence of lung cancer.

In the absence of RCTs, Colice[22] performed a decision analysis in a hypothetical cohort of 100 patients with haemoptysis and a normal chest X-ray. Rather than assigning costs or utilities, the primary outcome was the number of tests needed to diagnose (NTND) lung cancer. Bronchoscopy was used to diagnose endobronchial abnormalities and transthoracic needle aspirate to diagnose parenchymal abnormalities. The most efficient strategy was to perform bronchoscopy first (Fig. 3). This conclusion was not affected by varying the prevalence or distribution of endobronchial or parenchymal cancers. However, reducing the false-positive rate of CT for airway lesions reduced the NTND of performing CT first. Adding sputum cytology as a guide for performing bronchoscopy substantially reduced the NTND for the bronchoscopy approach. Undiagnosed patients underwent serial chest X-ray follow-up, which should really be regarded as a diagnostic test in its own right.

'Massive' haemoptysis has been defined as bleeding more than 300 mL in 24 hours[19] and is potentially life-threatening. FOB was compared with bronchial angiography in a series of 36 patients, 12 of whom had bled more than 300 mL/24 hours, by Saumench and colleagues in Spain.[23] Causes included bronchiectasis (14), sequelae to tuberculosis (12), active tuberculosis (4), arteriovenous fistula and silicosis. Unfortunately, FOB was only performed in 25 patients, but identified the site of bleeding in 17 (68%). Angiography was abnormal in 31 (86%) patients, but identified the site of bleeding in 20 (65%). Angiographic and bronchoscopic findings coincided in 11 of the 17 patients in whom the bleeding site was identified by FOB. Angiography was only positive in two of the eight patients in whom FOB did not localize the site. Thus, consid-

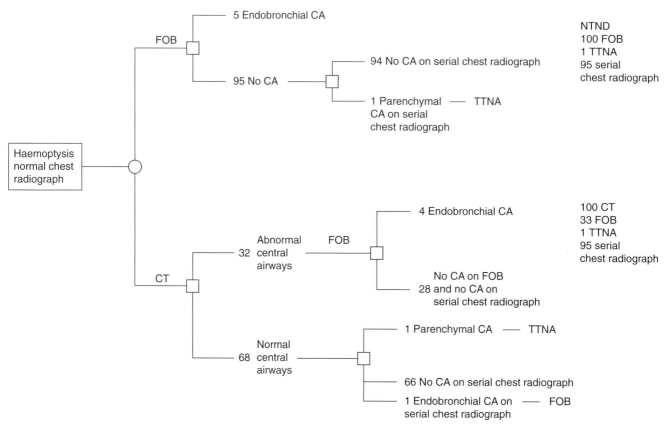

Figure 3. This schematic outlines the results of choosing either FOB or CT as the first diagnostic test for a patient presenting with haemoptysis and a normal chest X-ray. The NTND is larger for the CT first strategy because false-positive interpretations of abnormal central airways must be evaluated by FOB. The number of serial follow-up chest X-rays is the same for each approach (reprinted from Colice,[22] Copyright ©1997, with the permission of the American College of Chest Phycisians).

ering angiography to be the gold standard, the sensitivity of FOB was 85%, but the specificity only 50%.

Diagnostic strategies for dyspnoea

Dyspnoea or breathlessness is another common symptom in the community that often leads to referral to specialist physicians. Conventionally, it has been divided into acute and chronic dyspnoea, with chronic being considered as lasting more than 3 weeks. Acute causes of dyspnoea include acute exacerbations of asthma (see Part 2) or chronic obstructive pulmonary disease (COPD, Part 3), pneumonia (Part 4), pulmonary embolism (Chapter 1.2.4) and left ventricular failure, which is beyond the scope of this book.

Pulmonary function testing can be helpful in distinguishing respiratory from cardiac causes of acute dyspnoea. McNamara and Cionni conducted a prospective observational study of adult patients presenting with moderate or severe dyspnoea to an emergency department (ED) in Philadelphia, USA.[24] Peak expiratory flow (PEF) was measured with a mini-Wright meter, but five patients were unable to co-operate with the forced manoeuvre. The authors analysed 41 dyspnoeic epi-

sodes in 40 patients, with 18 episodes principally attributed to congestive heart failure (CHF) and 23 principally to chronic lung disease. An absolute PEF > 150 L/min had a sensitivity of 78%, specificity of 87% and positive predictive value (PPV) of 82% for a diagnosis of CHF. These test characteristics correspond to a positive likelihood ratio (PLR) of 6.0. A PEF ″ 150 L/min had a sensitivity of 87%, specificity of 78% and PPV of 83% for a diagnosis of chronic lung disease, corresponding to a PLR of 4.0. Limitations of this study included the lack of an independent diagnostic gold standard and the treating physician was not blinded to the PEF. The PEF was not adjusted for age, gender or height. The results should not be generalized to patients < 40 years old or those with mild dyspnoea.

A more elaborate dyspnoea differentiation index (DDI) was developed by Ailani et al.[25] This group reported a prospective series of 71 patients presenting with moderate or severe dyspnoea to an emergency department in Cleveland, OH, USA. Arterial blood gases were measured in room air as well as PEF. The DDI was defined as $PEF \times Pao_2 / 1000$. After excluding seven patients with multiple causes of dyspnoea and one with diabetic ketoacidosis, there were 24 with CHF and 39 with pulmonary causes including exacerbations of COPD or asthma and pneumonia. Receiver operator characteristic (ROC) curves were constructed for PEF, PEF %predicted, DDI and %DDI (Fig. 4). Using optimal cut points identified by ROC analysis, DDI had a higher sensitivity and negative predicted value (NPV) for pulmonary dyspnoea than did PEF (Table 2). Likelihood ratios were calculated using standard formulae from information provided in the paper. DDI more accurately predicted the cause of acute dyspnoea than PEF alone or the ED physician. One limitation was the need to withdraw oxygen for 15 minutes from dyspnoeic patients who had already been commenced on it. The DDI needs to be more widely applied in different clinical settings before it can be recommended.

Again, there are no systematic reviews or RCTs, so only consensus guidelines are available on the investigation of chronic dyspnoea. The ACR recommend that chest X-rays be performed when dyspnoea is chronic or severe or when there are associated risk factors such as age greater than 40 years, features of cardiovascular, pulmonary or neoplastic disease, other symptoms or positive findings on physical examination.[26] The ACR also suggested that CT scan should be considered when the initial evaluation was non-revealing or when it revealed an abnormality, but no definite diagnosis.

Limited evidence is available to support the ACR recommendations, which were based upon a few case series. Pratter et al.[27] prospectively studied 85 patients presenting with

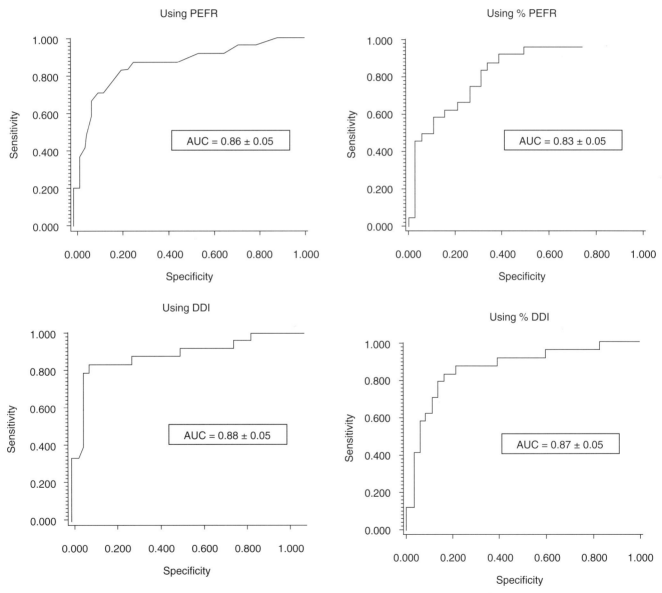

Figure 4. ROC curves of PEF, PEF %predicted, DDI and %DDI along with the area under the curve (AUC) for each graph. AUC for each parameter is shown along with the standard error (reprinted from Ailani et al.,[25] Copyright ©1999, with the permission of the American College of Chest Phycisians).

Table 2. ROC curve analysis of peak expiratory flow (PEF), PEF %predicted, dyspnoea discrimination index (DDI) and %DDI for patients presenting with acute dyspnoea (modified from Ailani et al.[25] — reprinted with permission from the American College of Chest Physicians).

Variable	Cut point	Sensitivity (%)	Specificity (%)	PPV (%)	NPV (%)	PLR	NLR
PEF	200	72	71	80	63	2.5	0.4
PEF%	42	59	78	81	54	2.7	0.5
DDI	13	82	74	84	71	3.2	0.4
%DDI	3	77	70	81	66	2.6	0.3

PPV, positive predictive value; NPV, negative predictive value; PLR, positive likelihood ratio; NLR, negative likelihood ratio.

Table 3. Predictive value and likelihood ratios for selected specific items in the diagnostic evaluation of chronic dyspnoea (reprinted from Pratter et al.,[27] Copyright ©1989, American Medical Association, All rights reserved).

Item	Diagnosis	PPV (%)	NPV (%)	PLR	NLR
Smoking	COPD	20	100	2.1	0
Wheezing	Asthma	42	83	1.7	0.5
Wheezing	Upper airway	5	88	0.5	4.7
Throat clearing	Upper airway	12	97	1.5	0.3
Postnasal drip	Upper airway	12	94	1.4	0.7
Spirometry	COPD	32	100	2.9	0
Spirometry	Asthma	18	72	1.3	0.9
Bronchoprovocation	Asthma	95	100	44	0
Diffusing capacity	Interstitial lung disease	79	95	18.3	0.09
Chest X-ray	Any diagnosis	75	91	9.0	0.3
Spirometry	Any diagnosis	80	56	3.1	0.6

chronic dyspnoea to the pulmonary clinic at the University of Massachusetts Medical Center in Worcester, MA, USA. The examining physician completed a questionnaire including the British Medical Research Council (MRC) and Mahler dyspnoea indices. Chest X-rays and spirometry were performed in all but one case. Other lung function tests included bronchoprovocation challenge, flow volume loops, lung volumes, single breath diffusing capacity and assessment of reversibility to bronchodilator. Less frequently performed investigations included exercise testing, barium swallow, bronchoscopy and cardiac investigations such as echocardiography or radionuclide ventriculography. A final diagnosis was reached in all 85 cases after two investigators independently reviewed the patients' files. However, a successful response to therapy was not necessarily required to confirm the diagnosis (unlike similar studies of chronic cough from the same group of investigators).

The 85 patients (48 men and 37 women) had dyspnoea for a mean of 2.9 years. The mean MRC dyspnoea index was 2.9 (out of 4) and the mean Mahler index 5.7 (out of 10). Dyspnoea was attributed to a respiratory cause in 64 (75%) and a non-respiratory cause in 21 (25%) patients. It is likely that the balance would have been different in another setting. The commonest causes of dyspnoea were asthma (29%), COPD (14%), interstitial lung disease (14%) and cardiomyopathy (10%). However, almost a third of cases were due to a wide range of other conditions including upper airway disorders, deconditioning, gastro-oesophageal reflux, psychogenic factors, chest wall disorders and miscellaneous conditions (bronchiectasis, lung cancer, bronchiolitis obliterans and unilateral hypolucent lung).

The physician's initial clinical impression was correct in only 56 (66%) of the 85 cases, confirming the importance of further investigation of dyspnoea. The predictive values of specific symptoms and investigations are summarized in Table 3. Likelihood ratios have again been calculated from information provided in the paper,[27] although this was not possible for all symptoms or investigations. A negative smoking history virtually ruled out a diagnosis of COPD in this case series. An absence of throat clearing or postnasal drip made an upper airway disorder extremely unlikely. Spirometry, particularly with assessment of reversibility, was a useful test for COPD. Bronchoprovocation was highly predictive of asthma in this series. However, as noted above, this has not been the experience in other settings.[14] Chest X-rays and diffusing capacity were predictive of interstitial lung disease. Exercise testing was particularly helpful in diagnosing psychogenic dyspnoea and deconditioning.

Diagnostic strategies for wheeze

Wheeze or whistling noises from the chest is asked about by most respiratory questionnaires. Wheeze particularly in the last 12 months has often been used as a surrogate for asthma in epidemiological studies, such as the International Study of Asthma and Allergies in Childhood (ISAAC).[28] However, in adult patients, there are many other causes including COPD, bronchiectasis and even acute pulmonary oedema ('cardiac asthma'). A case–control study in Norway[5] found that wheezing was significantly more frequent among patients with obstructive lung diseases than among healthy subjects. PEF was also significantly related to the frequency of wheezing, and more so in men than women.

The predictive value of wheezing and various combinations of respiratory symptoms for asthma was examined by Sistek *et al.*[29] The subjects were participants in a large cross-sectional study of Swiss adults aged 18–60 years who completed the validated European Community Respiratory Health Survey questionnaire. Current asthma was defined as the combination of doctor-diagnosed asthma and an attack within the last 12 months. The diagnostic values of individual symptoms are presented in Table 4, with likelihood ratios calculated as previously. Wheezing was the most prevalent symptom in asthmatics, but wheezing with dyspnoea and nocturnal dyspnoea had the highest PPV. Although the authors concluded that any type of wheezing predicted asthma, wheezing with dyspnoea or without a cold had the highest PLR.

The most sensitive combination of symptoms (80%) was wheezing and/or two nocturnal symptoms, which also had the best test properties. Combining wheezing with dyspnoea at rest produced the highest PPV (42%). Although almost all subjects underwent methacholine challenge, no data were presented in this paper, which relied solely on self-report for the 'gold standard'. However, a reasonable conclusion is that clinicians should ask patients presenting with wheeze about nocturnal dyspnoea, chest tightness and cough to diagnose asthma.

The combination of wheezing in the last 12 months and bronchial hyper-reactivity (BHR) has been proposed as a definition of current asthma for epidemiological studies.[30] However, it is now recognized that just as 'not all that wheezes is asthma', not all asthma patients demonstrate BHR all the time. The associations between BHR, wheezing and asthma have been examined recently in a large family-based cross-sectional study in rural China by Xu *et al.*[31] As has been found previously, there were significant reverse dose–response relationships between PD_{20} methacholine and either doctor-diagnosed asthma or persistent wheezing without a cold. A positive methacholine challenge ($PD_{20} < 150$ mg/mL) was associated with a 3.3- to 3.5-fold increase in the risk of asthma in adults, after adjusting for age, gender and smoking. Similarly, a positive challenge was associated with a 2.4- to 3.2-fold adjusted increase in the risk of wheezing in adults.

Examination of ROC curves showed that sensitivity in the highest cumulative dose ranged from 56.2% to 73.2% and declined with a reduction in cumulative dose. Conversely, specificity at the lowest cumulative dose ranged from 87.3% to 95.9% and declined with increasing dose. The lowest sensitivity (60.7%) for asthma was observed in young adults, as was the highest specificity. These data indicated that methacholine challenge was less sensitive for asthma than was suggested by previous clinical studies (see Table 1 in Chapter 1.2.1). Although the data were subject to misclassification of self-reported doctor-diagnosed asthma, there was virtually no use of inhaled steroids in rural China at the time. Thus, although bronchial challenge remains a useful investigation for patients presenting with wheeze, just as in cough, a negative result does not necessarily exclude asthma (see answer 1 to the Case scenario).

The predictive value of lower respiratory symptoms such as wheeze has been examined in a number of occupational populations. Meijer *et al.*[32] developed a model to predict COPD in dust-exposed workers in the rubber, concrete and paper industries. Spirometry was performed to European Respiratory Society (ERS) standards, but no bronchodilator was adminis-

Table 4. Diagnostic value of isolated symptoms for current asthma (reprinted from Sistek *et al.*,[29] Copyright ©2001, with permission from European Respiratory Society Journals).

Symptom	Sensitivity (%)	Specificity (%)	PPV (%)	NPV (%)	PLR	NLR
Wheezing	74.7	87.3	12.4	99.3	5.9	0.3
Wheezing with dyspnoea	65.2	95.1	23.9	99.1	13.3	0.4
Wheezing without a cold	59.8	93.6	18.2	99.0	9.3	0.4
Nocturnal chest tightness	49.3	86.4	8.0	98.6	3.6	0.6
Resting dyspnoea	47.1	94.9	18.0	98.7	9.2	0.6
Exercise dyspnoea	69.3	75.7	6.4	99.0	2.9	0.4
Nocturnal dyspnoea	46.2	96.0	21.5	98.7	11.6	0.6
Nocturnal cough	49.3	72.3	4.1	98.4	1.8	0.7
Chronic cough	21.5	95.2	9.6	98.1	4.5	0.8
Chronic sputum	22.7	93.3	7.5	98.1	3.4	0.8

tered to assess reversibility. COPD was stringently defined as FEV_1/forced vital capacity (FVC) < 5%le for age and height. Wheezing, shortness of breath, work-related lower respiratory symptoms and heavy smoking (≥ 17.5 pack–years) were independent predictors of COPD. The model was validated in another data set. The area under the ROC curve was 0.74 in the derivation set and 0.81 in the validation set, indicating acceptable discriminatory power. The authors suggested that this model could be used in occupational health surveillance to identify workers at risk of COPD who could be referred for spirometry.

Conclusions

Cough

Although patients commonly present with respiratory symptoms, only limited evidence is available on the best diagnostic strategies. No systematic reviews and very few relevant RCTs have been identified. An anatomic diagnostic protocol for chronic cough based on understanding of the cough reflex has been applied in several case series. The most common causes appear to be postnasal drip syndrome, gastro-oesophageal reflux and asthma. The protocol includes reviewing the history and performing a physical examination focusing on the upper and lower respiratory tracts and a chest X-ray. Further investigations are withheld until smoking has been ceased and/or ACE inhibitors discontinued. The following investigations are then performed as indicated by the initial evaluation: CT scan of the sinuses and skin tests for allergies; spirometry before and after bronchodilator, inhalation challenge; barium swallow or 24-hour ambulatory oesophageal pH monitoring. Selected patients with abnormal chest X-rays may require further investigation. The cause(s) of cough are finally determined by observing which specific therapy or therapies eliminate(s) the symptom.

Haemoptysis

Consensus guidelines for the investigation of haemoptysis recommend a chest X-ray as initial investigation. Patients with two or more risk factors for malignancy (male, > 40 years old, heavy smoking history) or persistent or recurrent haemoptysis should proceed to chest CT or fibre-optic bronchoscopy. Several case series have demonstrated that these two investigations are complementary. However, one decision analysis suggested that the most efficient approach in patients with normal chest X-rays was first to perform sputum cytology followed by bronchoscopy.

Dyspnoea

Consensus guidelines also recommend chest X-ray for patients with chronic dyspnoea. A CT scan can be considered if the initial evaluation is non-revealing or reveals a non-diagnostic abnormality. One case series found that the commonest causes of dyspnoea were asthma, COPD, interstitial lung disease and cardiomyopathy; however, almost a third of cases were due to a wide range of other conditions. A negative smoking history virtually ruled out a diagnosis of COPD. An absence of throat clearing or postnasal drip made an upper airway disorder extremely unlikely. Spirometry, particularly with assessment of reversibility, was a useful test for COPD.

Asthma and wheeze

Bronchoprovocation was highly predictive of asthma, but this has not been the experience in other settings. Chest X-rays and diffusing capacity predicted interstitial lung disease. Exercise testing was particularly helpful in diagnosing psychogenic dyspnoea and deconditioning.

There are many causes of wheezing in adults. Clinicians should ask patients presenting with wheeze about nocturnal dyspnoea, chest tightness and cough in order to diagnose asthma. Although a positive methacholine or histamine challenge significantly increases the likelihood of asthma, one negative challenge does not necessarily exclude the diagnosis. The combination of wheezing, shortness of breath, work-related lower respiratory symptoms and heavy smoking are predictive of COPD. This diagnosis can be confirmed by spirometry with assessment of reversibility to bronchodilator.

References

1 Abramson M, Kutin J, Czarny D *et al*. The prevalence of asthma and respiratory symptoms among young adults: is it increasing in Australia? *J Asthma* 1996; **33**:189–96.

2 Abramson M, Matheson M, Wharton C *et al*. Prevalence of respiratory symptoms related to chronic obstructive pulmonary disease and asthma amongst middle aged and older adults. *Respirology* 2002; **7**:325–31.

3 Smyrnios NA, Irwin RS, Curley FJ *et al*. From a prospective study of chronic cough: diagnostic and therapeutic aspects in older adults. *Arch Intern Med* 1998; **158**:1222–8.

4 Jones B, Stewart M. Duration of cough in acute upper respiratory tract infections. *Aust Fam Phys* 2002; **31**:971–3.

5 Gulsvik A, Refvem OK. A scoring system on respiratory symptoms. *Eur Respir J* 1988; **1**:428–32.

6 Pratter MR, Bartter T, Akers S *et al*. An algorithmic approach to chronic cough. *Ann Intern Med* 1993; **119**:977–83.

7 Irwin RS, Boulet LP, Cloutier MM *et al*. Managing cough as a defense mechanism and as a symptom. A consensus panel report of the American College of Chest Physicians. *Chest* 1998; **114**(2 Suppl Managing):133S–81S.

8 Irwin RS, Madison JM. Anatomical diagnostic protocol in evaluating chronic cough with specific reference to gastroesophageal reflux disease. *Am J Med* 2000; **108**(Suppl 4a):126S–30S.

9 van Pinxteren B, Numans ME, Bonis PA *et al*. Short-term treatment with proton pump inhibitors, H2-receptor antagonists and prokinetics for gastro-oesophageal reflux disease-like symptoms and endoscopy negative reflux disease (Cochrane Review). In: *The Cochrane Library*, Issue 4. Chichester, John Wiley & Sons, 2003.

10 Sheikh A, Hurwitz B. House dust mite avoidance measures for perennial allergic rhinitis (Cochrane Review). In: *The Cochrane Library*, Issue 4. Chichester, John Wiley & Sons, 2003.

11 Alves B, Sheikh A, Hurwitz B et al. Allergen injection immunotherapy for seasonal allergic rhinitis (Protocol for a Cochrane Review). In: *The Cochrane Library*, Issue 4. Chichester, John Wiley & Sons, 2003.

12 Weiner JM, Abramson MJ, Puy RM. Intranasal corticosteroids versus oral H1-receptor antagonists in allergic rhinitis: a systematic review of randomised controlled trials. *BMJ* 1998; **317**:1624–9.

13 Morris P, Leach A. Decongestants and antihistamines for persistent nasal discharge (rhinosinusitis) in children (Protocol for a Cochrane Review). In: *The Cochrane Library*, Issue 4. Chichester, John Wiley & Sons, 2003.

14 James A, Ryan G. Testing airway responsiveness using inhaled methacholine or histamine. *Respirology* 1997; **2**:97–105.

15 Tefera L, Fein M, Ritter MP et al. Can the combination of symptoms and endoscopy confirm the presence of gastroesophageal reflux disease? *Am Surg* 1997; **63**:933–6.

16 Augood C, MacLennan S, Gilbert R et al. Cisapride treatment for gastro-oesophageal reflux in children (Cochrane Review). In: *The Cochrane Library*, Issue 4. Chichester, John Wiley & Sons, 2003.

17 Levy J, Hayes C, Kern J et al. Does cisapride influence cardiac rhythm? Results of a United States multicenter, double-blind, placebo-controlled pediatric study. *J Pediatr Gastroenterol Nutr* 2001; **32**: 458–63.

18 Tonini M, De Ponti F, Di Nucci A et al. Review article: cardiac adverse effects of gastrointestinal prokinetics. *Aliment Pharmacol Therapeut* 1999; **13**:1585–91.

19 Fleishon H, Westcott J, Davis SD et al. Hemoptysis. American College of Radiology. ACR Appropriateness Criteria. *Radiology* 2000; **215**(Suppl):631–5.

20 McGuinness G, Beacher JR, Harkin TJ et al. Hemoptysis: prospective high-resolution CT/bronchoscopic correlation. *Chest* 1994; **105**:1155–62.

21 Tak S, Ahluwalia G, Sharma SK et al. Haemoptysis in patients with a normal chest radiograph: bronchoscopy-CT correlation. *Australas Radiol* 1999; **43**:451–5.

22 Colice GL. Detecting lung cancer as a cause of hemoptysis in patients with a normal chest radiograph: bronchoscopy vs CT. *Chest* 1997; **111**:877–84.

23 Saumench J, Escarrabill J, Padro L et al. Value of fiberoptic bronchoscopy and angiography for diagnosis of the bleeding site in hemoptysis. *Ann Thorac Surg* 1989; **48**:272–4.

24 McNamara RM, Cionni DJ. Utility of the peak expiratory flow rate in the differentiation of acute dyspnea. Cardiac vs pulmonary origin. *Chest* 1992; **101**:129–32.

25 Ailani RK, Ravakhah K, DiGiovine B et al. Dyspnea differentiation index: a new method for the rapid separation of cardiac vs pulmonary dyspnea. *Chest* 1999; **116**:1100–4.

26 Westcott J, Davis SD, Fleishon H et al. Dyspnea. American College of Radiology. ACR Appropriateness Criteria. *Radiology* 2000; **215**(Suppl):641–3.

27 Pratter MR, Curley FJ, Dubois J et al. Cause and evaluation of chronic dyspnea in a pulmonary disease clinic. *Arch Intern Med* 1989; **149**:2277–82.

28 The International Study of Asthma and Allergies in Childhood (ISAAC) Steering Committee. Worldwide variation in prevalence of symptoms of asthma, allergic rhinoconjunctivitis, and atopic eczema: ISAAC. *Lancet* 1998; **351**:1225–32.

29 Sistek D, Tschopp JM, Schindler C et al. Clinical diagnosis of current asthma: predictive value of respiratory symptoms in the SAPALDIA study. Swiss Study on Air Pollution and Lung Diseases in Adults. *Eur Respir J* 2001; **17**:214–19.

30 Toelle BG, Peat JK, Salome CM et al. Toward a definition of asthma for epidemiology. *Am Rev Respir Dis* 1992; **146**:633–7.

31 Xu X, Niu T, Chen C et al. Association of airway responsiveness with asthma and persistent wheeze in a Chinese population. *Chest* 2001; **119**:691–700.

32 Meijer E, Grobbee DE, Heederik DJ. Health surveillance for occupational chronic obstructive pulmonary disease. *J Occup Environ Med* 2001; **43**:444–50.

CHAPTER 1.2.2

Lung function testing

David P Johns and Alan J Crockett

Introduction

The cardinal function of the lungs is to arterialize mixed venous blood to meet the body's varying metabolic demands. Normal lungs have a large functional reserve and are able to arterialize venous blood even during vigorous exercise and often also in the presence of significant respiratory disease.

Clinical pulmonary function testing has an essential role in the management of patients with, or at risk of developing, respiratory dysfunction. Pulmonary function tests are not useful in making a 'diagnosis' in terms of a specific disease. Their value lies in the ability to quantify the degree of impairment imposed by the disease process. In evidence-based medicine, a highly sensitive test's negative result rules out the diagnosis (SnOut). A highly specific test's positive result rules in the diagnosis (SpIn). One of the dilemmas relating to determining sensitivity and specificity is the choice of the 'gold standard' for the comparison.

The 'diagnosis' related to the most common test, spirometry, is the physiological abnormality of airways obstruction rather than emphysema, chronic obstructive pulmonary disease (COPD) or asthma.

In this chapter, we will review both the usual approach taken in the interpretation of routinely performed lung function tests and the supporting evidence.

Literature search

A detailed search of PubMed, DARE, TRIP and CINAHL using the following search terms (lung function tests) AND systematic[sb] or individually (spirometry, lung volumes, diffusing capacity, oximetry) AND systematic[sb] field: MESH major topic, Limits: English, randomized controlled trial, human yielded no papers. When the term (spirometry) AND (sensitivity and specificity [MESH] OR sensitivity [WORD] OR (diagnosis [SH] OR diagnostic use [SH] OR specificity [WORD]) was used, 4598 papers were retrieved. The majority of these papers evaluated interventions using spirometry as one of several outcome variables. Further searching of lung function testing guidelines published by the major professional societies was also undertaken.

Routine lung function tests

There are several component processes that interact to determine the effectiveness of the lungs in arterializing venous blood; consequently, there is no single test of lung function that evaluates all aspects of function. Several tests are usually performed to assess the different, albeit overlapping, aspects of lung physiology:

• Spirometry: spirometry assesses the ventilatory capacity and displacement volume of the lungs. The most common indices are the forced expiratory volume in one second (FEV_1), vital capacity (VC or FVC), peak expiratory flow (PEF) and the FEV_1/FVC (or FEV_1/VC) ratio.

• Lung volumes: lung volumes assess lung size and represent the structural and physiological limits of the respiratory system. The most common indices are total lung capacity (TLC), functional residual capacity (FRC), residual volume (RV), vital capacity (VC), inspiratory capacity (IC), expiratory reserve volume (ERV) and the RV/TLC ratio.

• Diffusing capacity: the diffusing capacity for carbon monoxide (D_LCO) assesses the perfused surface area, thickness and integrity of the alveolar–capillary membrane. The common indices are D_LCO (also known as T_LCO or transfer factor, TF), which is a measure of the diffusing capacity for the whole lung, and D_LCO/VA, the diffusing capacity expressed per litre of accessible alveolar lung volume (VA). The results are usually reported after correction to a normal haemoglobin value.

Other commonly performed tests include assessment of respiratory muscle strength to determine the maximal inspiratory and expiratory pressures, and exercise testing to assess aerobic fitness.

Thus, only a relatively small number of lung function tests are used to assess the effect of many diseases on lung physiology. The tests are usually performed at rest but can be applied (some with difficulty) during exercise. Although lung function tests are rarely diagnostic by themselves, they can provide valuable clues about the mechanisms underlying the pathophysiological disease process. The clues to be gained from lung function testing depend on a sound understanding of the physiological basis of the measurement, test variability, comparison with normal reference values and knowledge of how lung disease alters the structure and function of the lungs.

The different lung function tests are often interpreted together. Of particular value is that recognizable patterns of abnormal lung function are often associated with specific lung diseases. For example, airflow limitation in people with emphysema and a significant smoking history is often associated with functional hyperinflation, raised RV and reduced D_LCO. However, for the same degree of airflow limitation, functional hyperinflation and RV, the D_LCO is often normal in never smokers when the cause is asthma.

The value of lung function testing is to detect, grade and manage patients with known or suspected lung disease (e.g. presence of abnormal chest X-ray, cough, dyspnoea, wheeze). They are also regarded as a significant aid to diagnosis, efficacy of therapeutic interventions and, in particular, assessment of disease progression and prognosis. However, it is often difficult to decide what constitutes a significant change as this varies depending on the index (FEV_1, FVC, TLC, D_LCO, etc.), time interval between repeat measurements and may differ in diseased and healthy subjects. They also play a very useful role in preoperative assessment, particularly for respiratory patients requiring thoracic or abdominal surgery and in patients undergoing lung resection.

Spirometry

Spirometry is the most commonly performed lung function test because impaired ventilatory capacity, particularly airflow limitation, is the hallmark of many common diseases affecting the lungs such as asthma and COPD. The most common cause of impaired ventilatory function is airway narrowing. This may be due to loss of traction from the surrounding lung tissue as in emphysema, inflammation of the walls of the airways, mucus plugging and bronchospasm as in asthma, or obstruction of the airway lumen. Other causes of impaired ventilatory function include respiratory muscle weakness or paralysis, cardiac enlargement, alterations to the lung, chest wall or pleura that limit full expansion or the rate of emptying of the lung. In these diseases, the FEV_1, VC, FVC, PEF and FEV_1/FVC (or FEV_1/VC) ratio are commonly reduced. It is recommended that the FEV_1 be used to determine the severity of airflow obstruction, the FEV_1/FVC ratio to confirm an obstructive defect and the FEV_1 (and FVC) to assess bronchodilator response.[1] The most commonly used indices of spirometry (FEV_1, FVC) are reproducible with a coefficient of variation of ″ 5%.[1] Evidence of airflow limitation is also a common finding in sarcoidosis, rheumatoid arthritis and eosinophilic granuloma, resulting in mixed ventilatory defects.[2]

Spirometry is used, often in conjunction with lung volumes, to classify abnormal ventilatory defects into one of three categories (see Table 1):

1 Obstructive ventilatory defect: characterized by a reduced capacity to ventilate the lungs due to airflow limitation. Typically, the FEV_1, FEV_1/FVC ratio and PEF are reduced, and there is a concavity towards the volume axis of the expiratory flow volume curve.

2 Restrictive ventilatory defect: characterized by loss of lung volume in the absence of airflow limitation. It is suggested by a low VC (or FVC) and normal or high FEV_1/FVC ratio and is confirmed if the TLC is reduced. Gilbert and Auchincloss[3] found that spirometry had specificity of 82% and sensitivity of 93% for detecting or excluding a restrictive defect when FVC was low and FEV_1/FVC was normal.

3 Mixed ventilatory defect: characterized by both airflow limitation and loss of lung volume. It is suggested when the VC and FEV_1/FVC ratio are reduced. Total lung capacity needs to be measured to confirm and quantify the restrictive component.

The shape of the flow–volume curve (see Fig. 1) can vary considerably between different lung diseases and often provides very useful additional and complementary information.

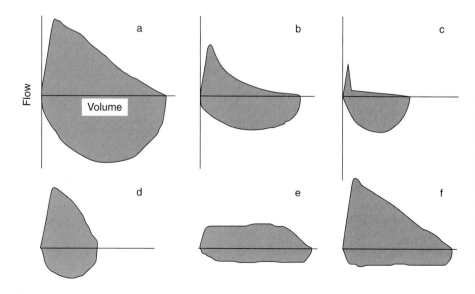

Figure 1. Normal flow volume loop is shown together with examples of how respiratory disease can alter its shape. (a) Normal subject. (b) Obstructive airway disease (e.g. asthma). (c) Severe obstructive disease (e.g. emphysema). (d) Restrictive lung disease (e.g. pulmonary fibrosis). (e) Fixed major airway obstruction (e.g. carcinoma of the trachea). (f) Floppy extrathoracic airway obstruction (e.g. tracheomalacia) (reprinted with permission from Johns and Pierce[90]).

Table 1. Classification and characteristics of abnormal ventilatory defects.

Ventilatory	Characterized by	Lung function	Clinical examples
Obstructive	Reduced capacity to ventilate the lungs due to airflow limitation	Spirometry: reduced FEV_1, FEV_1/FVC, PEF, $FEF_{25-75\%}$, scooped expiratory flow volume curve. Inspiratory flows are also reduced if the obstruction is intrinsic to the airways (e.g. asthma), but are often normal if the primary cause is lack of parenchymal support (e.g. emphysema). Lung volumes: TLC, FRC, RV and RV/TLC are often increased. In less severe disease, TLC may be within the normal range, but FRC is often elevated. In cystic fibrosis, TLC may be within normal limits even in the presence of severe airflow limitation. Diffusing capacity: in asthma, the D_LCO is often normal or it can be elevated. In emphysema, D_LCO and D_LCO/VA are usually reduced	Current asthma COPD (emphysema and chronic bronchitis) Cystic fibrosis
Restrictive	Loss of lung volume in the absence of airflow limitation	Spirometry: normal or high FEV_1/FVC ratio, reduced VC and FVC, well-maintained expiratory flows unless there is impaired respiratory muscle strength. Inspiratory flows are usually reduced if the restrictive pattern is due to lung disease but may be normal if due to external constraint to inspiration. Lung volumes: TLC, FRC, VC and RV are usually reduced, although FRC may be normal if the restrictive defect is due to respiratory muscle weakness. Diffusing capacity: D_LCO and D_LCO/VA are often reduced in restrictive lung diseases, although they are often within the normal range in mild cases. If the cause is non-pulmonary such as stiff chest wall or respiratory muscle weakness, then D_LCO/VA is often increased.	Fibrosis alveolitis Sarcoidosis Deformed chest Stiff chest wall Respiratory muscle disease Lung resection Lung transplant
Mixed	Both airflow limitation and loss of lung volume	Spirometry: reduced FEV_1, FEV_1/FVC, PEF, $FEF_{25-75\%}$, FVC and scooped expiratory flow volume curve. Lung volumes: reduced TLC. Diffusing capacity: D_LCO is usually reduced	

The shape varies between obstructive ventilatory defects, in which maximal expiratory flows are reduced and the curve is usually scooped out or concave to the volume axis, and restrictive diseases, in which expiratory flows may be increased in relation to lung volume and the shape is often convex away from the axes. Diminished expiratory flows as RV is approached are suggestive of obstruction in the small peripheral airways. There is evidence (from a case–control study) for truncation of both expiratory and inspiratory curves to detect fixed upper airway obstruction.[4] Examination of the shape of the flow–volume loop can also help to distinguish different disease states. Severe emphysema often causes a very rapid decrease in expiratory flow that is dependent on expiratory effort, whereas inspiratory flows are well preserved. In emphysema, the airways are prone to rapid collapse and/or narrowing during forced expiration due to loss of elastic tissue airway support with the obliteration of the alveolar walls. During inspiration, the airways are easily dilated preserving inspiratory flows. If the airflow limitation results from airways disease (e.g. asthma), the scalloping of the expiratory curve is usually more gradual (volume dependent) and less effort dependent. The inspiratory flows are also reduced, suggesting that the cause of the airflow limitation is relatively 'fixed'.

Gilbert and Auchincloss[5] demonstrated the accuracy of the spirogram in detecting or excluding airway obstruction prospectively in 200 subjects, 74 with obstruction and 126 without it. The 'gold standard' diagnosis of airway obstruction was based on a combination of clinical and body plethysmographic data. The ratio of forced expiratory volume in one second to forced vital capacity (FEV_1/FVC) had a sensitivity of 82% and a specificity of 98%. The use of a fixed lower limit of normal seemed better than a lower limit of normal based on prediction formulae. Because specificity was found to be higher than sensitivity, less precise clinical information may be required to confirm the presence of obstruction, if the FEV_1/FVC ratio is abnormal, than is needed to exclude obstruction if the FEV_1/FVC ratio is normal. They also found that the use of a combination of FEV_1/FVC and the ratio of forced expiratory flow (FEF) at 50% of FVC gave a higher sensitivity with a comparable specificity when compared with the use of the FEV_1/FVC ratio alone. A normal value for FEF between 25% and 75% of FVC virtually ruled out obstruction, but low values had poor specificity.

Spirometry also has a useful screening role in the early detection of airflow limitation in asymptomatic smokers[6] and subsequent management of people with COPD.[7] In smokers, the severity of airflow limitation correlates with the pathological changes in the lungs,[8] and high-resolution computerized tomography (CT) scans are moderately related to impaired spirometry and D_LCO.[9] Despite this, the use of spirometry in primary care continues to be very low.[10,11] It has now been established that spirometry can detect mild airflow limitation in asymptomatic smokers at risk of COPD and that, in such people, early smoking cessation had a positive effect in preserving ventilatory function.[12,13] Those people who managed to quit smoking over a 4-year period had an initial small increase in FEV_1 and then a normal rate of decline in FEV_1 of 34 mL/year compared with 63 mL/year for those who continued to smoke.[13]

Lung function tests are particularly useful for assessing disease severity and therefore play an important role in management and assessment of prognosis. In a 15-year follow-up study of adult asthmatics, the fall in FEV_1 was greater in asthmatic than in non-asthmatic subjects.[14] FEV_1 has also been reported to be a strong predictor of mortality from COPD[15,16] and is used to assess prognosis in COPD, with values < 0.75 L being associated with a mortality rate of 30% at 1 year and 95% at 15 years.[17] The prognosis in patients with COPD has been found to be less favourable when the airflow limitation is accompanied by a reduced D_LCO. Other tests such as the 6-minute walk test have been recommended as predictors of mortality and morbidity in COPD.[18] The FEV_1 has become the 'gold standard' in the measurement of airway narrowing and is a component of the severity scores in guidelines from the National Asthma Education and Prevention Program.[19] Interestingly, the guidelines from the Global Initiative for Asthma (GINA) and the British Thoracic Society use only PEF. In COPD, FEV_1 expressed as %predicted correlates with quality of life and exercise capacity.[20] The severity of airflow limitation based on FEV_1 when the FEV_1/VC ratio is below the normal range is: <34% of predicted is considered very severe; between 34% and 50% of predicted is severe; 60–70% of predicted is moderate; and ≥70% is mild.[1]

In a study of 24 patients with neuromuscular disease, Fromageot et al.[21] found that a >25% fall in VC when supine had a specificity and sensitivity for the diagnosis of diaphragmatic weakness of 90% and 79%, respectively, and therefore was helpful in detecting predominantly diaphragmatic weakness. Similarly, Lechtzin et al.[22] found that a supine FVC of <75% predicted was 100% specific and sensitive for predicting ab-

normally low transdiaphragmatic pressure in patients with amyotrophic lateral sclerosis.

Assessment of bronchodilator (BD) response in patients with airflow limitation is an important test that aids in the differentiation of asthma from COPD. A significant response indicates reversible airflow limitation and is characteristic of asthma, whereas in patients with COPD, the degree of reversibility is generally smaller and may be absent. However, the absence of reversibility does not necessarily exclude asthma because an asthmatic's response can vary from time to time and, at times, airway calibre is clearly normal and incapable of significant improvement. There are several guidelines available,[1,23–27] but none definitively describes the methodology to be used to assess BD response, and there is no agreement on what constitutes a significant response (Table 2) or how the response should be expressed.

The FEV_1 is the most common index used to assess reversibility and is usually expressed as percentage and absolute change from the prebronchodilator value[1,24,26] or as the percentage change in %predicted.[25] The use of the FEV_1/FVC ratio is not recommended, and the use of $FEF_{25-75\%}$ can be misleading if FVC changes.[1] In a retrospective study of asthmatics and patients with COPD, Quadrelli et al.[28] found that the absolute change in FEV_1 provided the best combination of sensitivity and specificity to separate asthma from COPD (Table 3). Also, although FEV_1 may not improve (e.g. in COPD), the degree of hyperinflation may decrease resulting in improved mechanics and greater capacity to ventilate during exercise.[29,30] Newton et al.[30] found that bronchodilators reduced hyperinflation and that the addition of lung volume measurements added sensitivity when assessing BD response. Not surprisingly, in COPD, the probability of a positive BD response is reduced in patients with a low D_LCO.[31]

Spirometry can be measured before and after exposure to direct stimuli such as methacholine or histamine to detect and quantify airway hyper-responsiveness, an important feature of clinical asthma, which is thought to reflect asthma severity quantitatively. However, some asthmatics may have a negative challenge, particularly if treated with corticosteroids, and normal subjects with no history of asthma or variability in spirometry may return positive challenge results particularly following recent upper respiratory tract infection.[32,33]

Indirect challenge tests, such as the inhalation of an aerosol of hypertonic saline, mannitol dry powder, exercise and eucapnic voluntary hyperventilation, are useful for detecting current asthma and have the advantage that they act on a wide range of mediators that contribute to airway narrowing.[34] A negative response to these challenges in asthmatic patients suggests that their asthma is well controlled.[34] Specific challenges can also be performed using allergen extracts (e.g. rye grass) or direct exposure to occupational allergens (e.g. bakers' flour) to determine the cause of asthma.

As people age, both FEV_1 and FVC progressively decrease. However, the rate of decrease in FEV_1 is greater than the de-

Table 2. National guidelines for a significant bronchodilator response.

Organization	VC	FVC	FEV$_1$	FEF$_{25-75\%}$	Comments
American Thoracic Society[1]	–	≥12% of baseline and ≥200 mL	≥12% of baseline and ≥200 mL	–	% of baseline and an absolute change in FEV$_1$ or FVC
European Respiratory Society[25]	–	>12% of % predicted and >200 ml	>12% of % predicted and >200 mL	–	% of %predicted and an absolute change in FVC or FEV$_1$
British Thoracic Society[26]	>330 mL	–	>160 mL	–	Absolute change in baseline VC or FEV$_1$
American College of Chest Physicians[23]	15–25% increase = slight reversibility 26–50% increase = moderate reversibility >50% increase = marked reversibility				% of baseline. Lung function index not specified
Intermountain Thoracic Society[24]	–	15–24% = improved ≥25% = markedly improved	12–24% = improved ≥25% = markedly improved	45–99% = improved ≥200% = markedly improved	% of baseline
Thoracic Society of Australia and New Zealand[27]	–	–	>12% of baseline and 200 mL	–	FEV$_1$ only

Table 3. Diagnostic properties of lung function measures.

Test	Condition	Sensitivity (%)	Specificity (%)	Reference
Spirometry				
FEV$_1$/FVC %	Airflow obstruction	82	98	5
FEV$_1$/FVC ratio combined with FEF$_{50}$	Airflow obstruction			5
FEV$_1$/FVC < 70% or FEF$_{50}$/FVC< 70%		92	91	
FEV$_1$/FVC < 70% or FEF$_{50}$/FVC< 60%		89	97	
VC > 25% fall when supine	Diaphragmatic weakness in neuromuscular disease	75	90	21
FVC < 75% predicted	Diaphragmatic weakness in neuromuscular disease	100	100	22
Absolute change in FEV$_1$	Bronchodilator responsiveness to distinguish asthma from COPD	70	71	28
Algorithm using FVC, FEV$_1$/VC ratio	Lung rejection after lung transplant	96	61	40
Bronchial hyper-responsiveness	Asthma in patients with dyspnoea	97		41
Bronchial hyper-responsiveness		91	90	50
PEF variability (daily)	Suspected asthma	10	100	48
Spirometry	Predicting postsurgical complications	15	47–92	79

crease in FVC; thus, the FEV$_1$/FVC ratio decreases with age. The rate of fall of FEV$_1$ over time is an important indicator of disease progression in people with COPD. In healthy non-smoking adults, the decrease is about 30 mL/year with an upper limit of about 50 mL/year.[35–37] A decrease greater than this suggests an abnormally rapid rate of deterioration, presumably due to the progression of underlying disease. Also,

changes over time have been shown to predict the risk of lung cancer.[38]

The early diagnosis of chronic rejection after lung transplantation is limited by the lack of a reliable test to detect early small airways disease (bronchiolitis obliterans).[39] However, a spirometry-based algorithm using FVC and the FEV$_1$/FVC ratio has been shown to have a high sensitivity (96%) for predicting restriction and a high negative predictive value (98%) for excluding restriction.[40] In a study of 22 stable lung transplant recipients, Cook et al.[39] concluded that high-resolution CT, V/Q scanning and $FEF_{25-75\%}$ were no more useful than FEV_1 for the early detection of rejection.

In a recent case–control study that determined the most useful tests for decision making in the diagnosis of asthma in patients with dyspnoea, bronchial hyper-responsiveness showed the highest values for sensitivity (97%), positive predictive value (PPV) (94%), negative predictive value (NPV) (92%) and diagnostic accuracy (93%).[41] However, other studies have not found such high predictive values (see previous chapter). The second most efficient test was skin prick testing, with PPV of 81% and diagnostic accuracy of 62%.[41]

There appear to be no published studies that have specifically examined the effects of measuring spirometry on outcomes in asthma. This would require a randomized control study in which patients were assigned to have spirometry measured (or not) as part of their usual care. Given the relatively poor uptake of spirometry in the management of asthma, a case–control study would be feasible. However, in a study of acute asthmatics, physicians in an emergency department were found to underestimate the degree of airflow limitation based purely on clinical examination and that subsequent knowledge of spirometry directly altered management in 20.4% of patients.[42]

Spirometry is often abnormal even in mildly asthmatic patients.[43] In a study of general practice in the UK, the measurement of spirometry was found to be feasible and was undertaken in 328 asthmatics on a national asthma register. Approximately one-third had normal spirometry, one-third had fixed airflow limitation and a quarter had reversible airflow limitation. Similarly, in children, one-fifth had airflow limitation as determined by a low FEV_1/FVC ratio, whereas approximately half had mild disease on the basis of a reduced $FEF_{25-75\%}$. In asthma, there are often large disparities between symptoms, measurements of spirometry and PEF variability; therefore, it is important to measure spirometric function in these patients.[42,44] Thus, given the disparity between subjective symptoms and objective lung function, it is likely that, by including spirometry as part of the treatment process, there may be real differences in subsequent outcomes such as symptoms and emergency department presentations.

There is evidence that early treatment with inhaled corticosteroids leads to be better spirometric function in subsequent years.[45] Furthermore, knowledge of parameters that reflect asthma severity, over and above simple clinical parameters such as symptom frequency and bronchodilator use, is beneficial for managing asthma. Measurement of airway hyper-responsiveness as an adjunct test for gauging asthma control as part of steroid dose adjustment was associated with better asthma outcomes compared with the use of GINA alone in one study.[46]

National guidelines on the diagnosis and management of asthma recommend that an excessive diurnal variation in PEF is an important indicator of asthma and that a progressive fall in PEF suggests treatment with corticosteroids.[19,47] One study of patients with normal spirometry who were suspected to have asthma found that variability in PEF and the improvement in FEV_1 after bronchodilator had a low sensitivity and high false-negative rates.[48] Also, PEF variability was poorly correlated with methacholine challenge, which questioned the validity of PEF variability as a diagnostic tool in asthma.

In contrast, Enright et al.[49] found that, in the elderly (≥65 years), mean PEF variability was significantly greater in current asthmatics (18%) compared with healthy people (12%). They concluded that a PEF variability of ≥30% was abnormal in the elderly and that it was associated with asthma. In a recent study to determine the level of evidence supporting commonly performed lung function tests, Borrill et al.[4] found that there was no high-quality evidence for the use of monitoring PEF to step-down treatment in asthma if there was low variability, but there was level 1b evidence (from a prospective cohort study) to support peak flow charting to diagnose asthma. Hunter et al.[50] compared different tests and reported that a methacholine challenge was the most sensitive (91%) and specific (90%) and therefore the most objective test in patients with mild asthma.

Methacholine and exercise challenges are widely used to determine airway hyper-responsiveness and exercise-induced bronchoconstriction.[18] Although methacholine has good sensitivity for asthma, it only has moderate PPV as a positive challenge is commonly seen in other diseases such as COPD.[51,52] However, it may be useful as an index of management outcome,[53] as is exercise challenge in assessing the efficacy of anti-inflammatory agents and other medications used to prevent exercise-induced bronchoconstriction.[18]

Lung volumes

Lung volumes are useful in detecting and grading the degree of hyperinflation (increased TLC) and lung restriction (reduced TLC) and for following disease progression and quantifying the response to therapy. The within-subject coefficients of variation of repeat measurements of TLC and FRC by plethysmography in healthy subjects are in the order of 4% and 7% respectively.[54]

TLC provides an absolute measure of the degree of hyperinflation. An increased FRC in the presence of normal TLC provides a measure of the degree of functional hyperinflation. In the absence of neuromuscular disease or a stiff chest wall and in the presence of airflow limitation, an increased RV and RV/TLC ratio can provide information about effective gas trapping due to poorly ventilated lung regions or premature and excessive airway narrowing during the expiratory manoeuvre. The difference between VC and FVC and between

TLC and VA can provide information about airway closure and the degree of effective gas trapping and non-uniformity of ventilation.

The combination of increased TLC, FRC, RV and decreased VC is a common pattern of more severe lung diseases causing airflow limitation. Total lung capacity is elevated in emphysema and has been shown to be associated with the severity of the disease.[55] In contrast, TLC is often normal in asthma although it can be elevated.[56]

Characteristically, all lung volume compartments (TLC, FRC, RV, VC) are proportionately reduced in restrictive lung disease due to loss of alveolar units and increased lung stiffness (e.g. fibrosing alveolitis), but can also occur from loss of lung tissue (e.g. lung resection), increased heart size and when space-occupying lesions are present. Lung volumes are also reduced in 50% of patients with precapillary pulmonary hypertension.[57]

Lung volumes can be abnormal in the presence of external constraints to inspiration (low TLC) or expiration (raised RV) such as increased chest wall stiffness, chest wall deformities, obesity and respiratory muscle weakness. In pure neuromuscular disease, FRC is often normal, but RV is usually increased in expiratory muscle weakness.[58] An elevated RV alone in the presence of normal spirometry has been proposed as an early indicator of peripheral airway disease.[59]

Lung volumes reach adult size at about 25 years old; thereafter, VC drops by an average of about 20 mL/year, but TLC remains fairly constant throughout adult life.[60] Thus, RV and the RV/TLC ratio increase with age.

Diffusing capacity

D_LCO is a useful test to detect, grade, monitor and manage diseases affecting the surface area and integrity of the alveolar capillary membrane. The measurement is useful for identifying and assessing obstructive diseases affecting the lung parenchyma such as emphysema. In obstructive lung disease, a reduced D_LCO has been shown to be useful in differentiating early emphysema from asthma and bronchitis.[61,62] It is also useful for assessing lung restriction (e.g. interstitial lung disease and pulmonary vascular disease) where there may be lung scarring and other causes that result in destruction or reduction in the size or number of pulmonary capillaries and thickening of the alveolar–capillary membrane. In interstitial disease, the reduced D_LCO is believed to be the earliest abnormal finding,[63] mainly due to loss of alveolar units rather than an increase in thickness of the alveolar–capillary membrane. A reduced D_LCO has also been shown to precede abnormal chest X-ray findings in idiopathic pulmonary fibrosis.[64] However, lung function tests cannot differentiate between the different types of interstitial lung disease.

Mismatching of perfusion and ventilation and alveolar filling (e.g. alveolar proteinosis, pneumonia) and anaemia are other causes of a reduced D_LCO. D_LCO is also commonly reduced in primary pulmonary hypertension, often with lung restriction.[65] It is also commonly reduced in pulmonary vascular occlusive disease and may be the only abnormal lung function test in recurrent multiple pulmonary emboli.[66,67]

Assessment of diffusing capacity is therefore useful in differentiating asthma from emphysema in patients with airflow limitation and between extrapulmonary (e.g. stiff or deformed chest wall) and intrapulmonary (e.g. fibrosing alveolitis) disease as the cause of lung restriction. However, an abnormal diffusing capacity is a common but non-specific finding.

D_LCO/VA is a more specific indicator of the integrity of those alveoli accessed during the test. A reduced D_LCO in the presence of a normal D_LCO/VA usually suggests that those alveoli participating in gas transfer are 'intact' and functionally normal in terms of CO transfer. The underlying mechanism may be that not all the available alveolar surface area was accessible to the inspired CO gas mixture (e.g. poorly ventilated lung regions) and/or there were a reduced number of alveoli. D_LCO and D_LCO/VA suggest interstitial lung disease and are usually low in emphysema and fibrosing alveolitis. In asthma, D_LCO is usually normal or even elevated. D_LCO and D_LCO/VA can be significantly elevated if the pulmonary capillary blood volume is increased through vascular recruitment or distension (e.g. during exercise, going from the sitting to the lying position and left to right shunt) and in the presence of fresh blood in the alveolar space (e.g. Goodpasture's syndrome). In any individual, there is an inverse relationship between D_LCO/VA and the degree of lung inflation. That is, D_LCO/VA will be 'overestimated' in the presence of an external (e.g. chest wall) constraint to inspiration or poor inspiratory effort. Therefore, when interpreting D_LCO/VA, it is important to check that the D_LCO test was performed at full lung inflation.

The determination of prognosis in the wide range of interstitial lung diseases (ILD) is less certain as lung function tests are less specific to an individual ILD and may be normal during the early stages of the disease.[68] However, one study found that a 20% decrease in D_LCO and a 10% decrease in VC in 1 year were associated with mortality.[69]

During the single breath D_LCO test, alveolar volume (VA) is also measured and represents the volume distribution within the lung of the inspired gas mixture. It provides information about the 'accessible' lung volume from which the uptake of CO occurs. Alveolar volume is nearly always lower than TLC (measured by body plethysmography or by multiple breath inert gas dilution). This is because VA does not include anatomical dead space V_D (about 150 mL) and not all lung regions are accessible during the 10-second breath-hold, particularly if airflow limitation is present. In the absence of airflow limitation and provided the patient inspires to full lung inflation, VA is typically 200–500 mL lower than TLC. A larger difference reflects non-uniform distribution and mixing of the inspired gas with the residual volume and is often referred to as 'effective gas trapping'.

The repeatability of D_LCO and D_LCO/VA measurements performed 7.2 ± 1.3 days apart in healthy subjects and people with emphysema by Robson and Innes[70] found that, like FEV_1 and VC,[71] between-session variability was independent of the magnitude of the measurement and was therefore preferred over %predicted. In the healthy group, the coefficients of repeatability for D_LCO and D_LCO/VA were ± 1.84 mmol/min/kPa (5.5 mL/min/mmHg) and 0.24 mmol/min/kPa/L (0.72 mL/min/mmHg/L) respectively. In people with emphysema, the variability was 1.30 mmol/min/kPa (3.9 mL/min/mmHg) and 0.20 mmol/min/kPa/L (0.6 mL/min/ mmHg/L) for D_LCO and D_LCO/VA respectively.

D_LCO reaches adult values at 20–25 years and decreases with age at the rate of about 0.5 mmol/min/kPa (1.5 mL/min/mmHg) per decade.

Preoperative risk assessment

A detailed review has been published by Smetana.[72] There is a relationship between the incidence of postoperative pulmonary complications and the distance of the surgical procedure from the diaphragm. The highest risks are associated with thoracic and upper abdominal surgery, which can result in large reductions in VC, RV, FRC and FEV_1.[73]

Although lung function testing has a role in preoperative assessment in resection (see below), the literature is unclear as to its role in predicting postoperative complications in thoracic and abdominal surgery.[74–76] This is also true for patients with COPD, even though this disease is a known risk factor for postoperative complications. A systematic review by Lawrence et al.[74] concluded that the literature failed to show that preoperative spirometry helped significantly in predicting and preventing complications. A case–control study found that patients with abnormal results of lung examination undergoing abdominal surgery were 5.8 times more likely to develop pulmonary complications, but no component of spirometry independently predicted risk.[76] A large study of well-managed asthmatics with a PEF > 80% predicted found no link between increased postoperative risk and lung function, although the frequency of complications increased in older patients with active asthma.[77] Despite suggestions of increased risk, there is no good-quality evidence to indicate that a lower level of lung function absolutely contraindicates surgery. However, the benefit has to be weighed against the risks, and spirometry is of value in identifying patients who would benefit from more rigorous preoperative and perioperative management.[72]

Although there is little consensus on the role of spirometry, lower limits for increased risk have been proposed (e.g. FEV_1 < 70%, FVC < 70%, FEV_1/FVC < 65%).[78] A review of patients undergoing abdominal surgery reported that the sensitivities and specificities of lung function tests in predicting complica-

tions ranged from 14 to 95% and 47 to 92%, respectively, and were of no greater benefit than clinical assessment alone.[79] Several retrospective studies of preoperative lung function tests used in the assessment of postoperative risk have found a modest benefit in risk assessment.[78] In a retrospective study of 480 patients after abdominal surgery, the incidence of postoperative pulmonary complications was 18%, and a combination of FEV_1 and Pa_{O_2} was found to be useful in identifying increased risk.[80] However, there have been no prospective randomized trials.[72]

A recent prospective study of 272 consecutive patients referred for non-thoracic surgery found that lung function tests were useful for identifying postoperative risk when they were performed at the discretion of the physician.[81] They found that complications occurred in 22 patients (8.1%) and significant lung function predictors (odds ratio) of postoperative complications were FVC < 1.5 L (OR 11.1), FEV_1 < 1.0 L (OR 7.9), forced expiratory time $\geq$ 9 seconds (OR 5.7). They also found that a $Pa_{CO_2} \geq 45$ mmHg was a strong predictor (OR 61.0), but this finding was based on only three hypercapnic patients.

Thus, the available evidence suggests that lung function tests should not be used to deny surgery, but may be a useful guide to preoperative workup and perioperative management. Further studies are clearly needed on the role of spirometry in predicting postoperative complications.

Lung resection

FEV_1 is the main index used for the assessment of patients requiring lung resection as it correlates with the degree of impairment due to COPD and provides an index of pulmonary reserve.[82] Patients undergoing pneumonectomy who have an FEV_1 > 2 L tolerate the procedure well, whereas an FEV_1 of 1.0–1.5 L is taken as the lower limit for patients undergoing lobectomy.[83,84] Postoperative lung function can be predicted based on either absolute or percentage preoperative FEV_1 and the estimated functional contribution of the resected lung tissue.[82]

D_LCO has been evaluated for predicting postoperative complications following pulmonary resection and has been reported as the most important predictor of mortality and postoperative complications.[82,85,86] By combining regional perfusion scanning to quantify the D_LCO of any resected lung tissue with the preoperative D_LCO, some studies have predicted the postoperative D_LCO.[86] High mortality and morbidity were associated with a predicted postoperative D_LCO below 40% predicted.

Exercise testing, including stair climbing and formal progressive exercise on a cycle ergometer, has been used to predict surgical risk.[82] A lower mortality has been reported in patients able to climb two flights of stairs compared with patients only able to climb one flight (11% versus 50%). In a progressive exercise test, the index that correlates best with postoperative complications is the level of work achieved as measured by

$V_{O_{2max}}$.[82,87] $V_{O_{2max}}$ is usually expressed per unit body weight (i.e. mL/kg/min), although it may also be reported as a percentage of predicted $V_{O_{2max}}$.[88] Bolliger *et al.*[88] found that eight out of nine patients undergoing lung resection had complications, whereas the probability of no complications was 0.9 for a $V_{O_{2max}}$ of >75%. Postoperative complications were found to be more common in patients with a $V_{O_{2max}}$ below 15 mL/kg/min.[89]

Conclusions

Like many tests used in clinical practice, pulmonary function tests provide little help in making a definitive diagnosis. However, these tests provide an objective assessment of the degree of impairment that may be associated with abnormal symptoms or signs and are helpful in confirming a diagnosis.

In terms of evidence-based medicine, the overall level of evidence is relatively low. One of the problems is the identification of the definitive 'gold standard' with which to compare the pulmonary function test result. The underlying feature of the 'obstructive' diseases is reduction in airflow related to reduced airway diameter. However, the mechanisms may be different in asthma and COPD.

The key to understanding pulmonary function testing is to have a systematic approach to interpreting the results. This approach should facilitate the recognition and significance of any parameter that falls outside the normal range. Pattern recognition is valuable in the interpretation of flow–volume curves, which are becoming the most common form of spirometry.

In selected circumstances, spirometry has been shown to have a high sensitivity and specificity. More studies are required to describe the specificity, sensitivity and repeatability of lung function tests in disease.

References

1 American Thoracic Society. Lung function testing: selection of reference values and interpretive strategies. *Am Rev Respir Dis* 1991; **144**:1202–18.

2 Alhamad EH, Lynch JP, Martinez FJ. Pulmonary function tests in interstitial lung disease: what role do the play? *Clin Chest Med* 2001; **22**:715–50.

3 Gilbert R, Auchincloss JH Jr. What is a 'restrictive' defect? *Arch Intern Med* 1986; **146**:1779–81.

4 Borrill Z, Houghton C, Sullivan PJ, Sestini P. Retrospective analysis of evidence base for tests used in the diagnosis and monitoring of disease in respiratory medicine. *BMJ* 2003; **327**:1136–38 .

5 Gilbert R, Auchincloss JH Jr. The interpretation of the spirogram. How accurate is it for 'obstruction'? *Arch Intern Med* 1985; **45**:1635–9.

6 Zielinski J. Early diagnosis of COPD. *Pol Arch Med Wewn* 2001; **105**(Suppl):225–6.

7 Ferguson GT, Enright PL, Buist AS, Higgins MW. Office spirometry for lung health assessment in adults: a consensus statement from the National Lung Health Education Program. *Chest* 2000; **117**:1146–61.

8 Thurlbeck WM. Pathophysiology of chronic obstructive pulmonary disease. *Clin Chest Med* 1990; **11**:389–403.

9 Gould GA, Redpath AT, Ryan M *et al.* Lung CT density correlates with measurements of airflow limitation and the diffusing capacity. *Eur Respir J* 1991; **4**:141–6.

10 Kesteb S, Chapman KR. Physician perceptions and management of COPD. *Chest* 1993; **104**:254–8.

11 Tirimanna PR, van Schayck CP, den Otter JJ *et al.* Prevalence of asthma and COPD in general practice in 1992: has it changed since 1977. *Br J Gen Pract* 1996; **46**:277–81.

12 Hankinson JL, Odencrantz JR, Fedan KB. Spirometric reference values from a sample of the general US population. *Am J Respir Crit Care Med* 1999; **159**:179–87.

13 Anthonisen NR, Connett JE, Kiley JP *et al.* Effects of smoking intervention and the use of an inhaled anticholinergic bronchodilator on the rate of decline of FEV_1. The lung health study. *JAMA* 1994; **272**:1497–505.

14 Lange P, Parner J, Vestbo J, Schnohr P, Jenson G. A 15-year follow-up study of ventilatory function in adults with asthma. *N Engl J Med* 1998; **339**:1194–200.

15 Traver GA, Cline MG, Burrows B. Predictors of mortality in chronic obstructive pulmonary disease. A 15-year follow-up study. *Am Rev Respir Dis* 1979; **119**:895–902.

16 Thomason MJ, Strachan DP. Which spirometric indices best predict subsequent death from chronic obstructive pulmonary disease? *Thorax* 2000; **55**:785-8.

17 Hodgkin JE. Prognosis in chronic obstructive pulmonary disease. *Clin Chest Med* 1990; **11**:555–69.

18 American Thoracic Society. Guidelines for methacholine and exercise challenge testing—1999. *Am J Respir Crit Care Med* 2000; **161**:309–29.

19 National Asthma Education and Prevention Program. *Expert Panel Report 2: Guidelines for the Diagnosis and Management of Asthma.* Publication No. 97-4051. Bethesda, MD, National Institutes of Health, 1997.

20 Wijkstra PJ, TenVergert EM, van der Mark ThW *et al.* Relation of lung function, maximal inspiratory pressure, dyspnoea, and quality of life with exercise capacity in patients with chronic obstructive pulmonary disease. *Thorax* 1994; **49**:468–72.

21 Fromageot C, Lofaso F, Annane D *et al.* Supine fall in lung volumes in the assessment of diaphragmatic weakness in neuromuscular disorders. *Arch Phys Med Rehabil* 2001; **82**:123–11.

22 Lechtzin N, Wiener CM, Shade DM, Clawson L, Diette GB. Spirometry in the supine position improves the detection of diaphragmatic weakness in patients with amyotrophic lateral sclerosis. *Chest* 2002; **121**:436–42.

23 American College of Chest Physicians. Committee report. Criteria for the assessment of reversibility in airways obstruction: report of the committee on emphysema. *Chest* 1974; **65**:552–3.

24 Morris AH, Kanner RE, Crapo RO, Gardner RM. *Clinical Pulmonary Function Testing: a Manual of Uniform Laboratory Procedures*, 2nd edn. Salt Lake City, UT, Intermountain Thoracic Society, 1984.

25 European Respiratory Society. Standardized Lung Function Testing. *Eur Respir J* 1993; **6**(Suppl 16).

26 British Thoracic Society, Society of Cardiothoracic Surgeons of Great Britain and Ireland Working Party. Guidelines on the selection of patients with lung cancer for surgery. *Thorax* 2001; **56**:89–108.

27 Thoracic Society of Australia and New Zealand and The Australian Lung Foundation. The COPDX Plan: Australian and New Zealand guidelines for the management of chronic obstructive pulmonary disease. *Med J Aust* 2003; **178**(Suppl):S1–S39.

28 Quadrelli SA, Roncoroni AJ, Montiel GC. Evaluation of bronchodilator response in patients with airflow obstruction. *Respir Med* 1999; **93**:630–6.

29 Chrystyn H, Mulley BA, Peake MD. Dose response relation to oral

theophylline in severe chronic obstructive disease. *BMJ* 1988; **297**:1506–10.

30 Newton MF, O'Donnell DE, Forkert L. Response of lung volumes to inhaled salbutamol in a large population of patients with severe hyperinflation. *Chest* 2002; **121**:1042–50.

31 Izquierdo-Alonso JL, Sanchez-Hernandez I, Fernandez Frances J, Castelao Naval J, Carrillo Arias F, Gallardo Carrasco J. Utility of transfer factor to detect different bronchodilator responses in patients with chronic obstructive pulmonary disease. *Respiration* 1998; **65**:282–8.

32 Juniper EF, Kline PA, Vanzieleghem MA, Ramsdale EH, O'Byrne PM, Hargreave F. Effect of long-term treatment with inhaled corticosteroids on airway hyperresponsiveness and clinical asthma in non-steroid dependent asthmatics. *Am Rev Respir Dis* 1990; **142**:832–6.

33 du Toit JI, Anderson SD, Jenkins CR, Woolcock AJ, Rodwell LT. Airway responsiveness in asthma: bronchial challenge with histamine and 4.5% sodium chloride before and after budesonide. *Allergy Asthma Proc* 1997; **18**:7–14.

34 Anderson SD, Brannan JD. Methods for 'indirect' challenge tests including exercise, eucapnic voluntary hyperapnea, and hypertonic saline. *Clin Rev Allergy Immunol* 2003; **24**:27–54.

35 Tager IB, Segal MR, Speizer FE, Weiss ST. The natural history of forced expiratory volumes. Effect of cigarette smoking and respiratory symptoms. *Am Rev Respir Dis* 1988; **138**:837–49.

36 Sherman CB, Xu X, Speizer FE, Ferris BG Jr, Weiss ST, Dockery DW. Longitudinal lung function decline in subjects with respiratory symptoms. *Am Rev Respir Dis* 1992; **146**:855–9.

37 Kerstjens HA, Rijcken B, Schouten JP, Postma DS. Decline of FEV_1 by age and smoking status: facts, figures, and fallacies. *Thorax* 1997; **52**:820–7.

38 Kuller LH, Ockene J, Meilahn E, Svendsen KH. Relation of forced expiratory volume in one second (FEV1) to lung cancer mortality in the Multiple Risk Factor Intervention Trial (MRFIT). *Am J Epidemiol* 1990; **132**:265–74.

39 Cook RC, Fradet G, Muller NL, Worsely DF, Ostrow D, Levy RD. Non-invasive investigations for the early detection of chronic airways dysfunction following lung transplantation. *Can Respir J* 2003; **10**:76–83.

40 Glady CA, Aaron SD, Lunau M, Clinch J, Dales RE. A spirometry-based algorithm to direct lung function testing in the pulmonary function laboratory. *Chest* 2003; **123**:1939–46.

41 Popovic-Grle S, Mehulic M, Pavicic F, Babic I, Beg-Zec Z. Clinical validation of bronchial hyperresponsiveness, allergy tests and lung function in the diagnosis of asthma in persons with dyspnea. *Coll Anthropol* 2002; **26**(Suppl):119–27.

42 Emerman CL, Cydulka RK. Effect of pulmonary function testing on the management of acute asthma. *Arch Intern Med* 1995; **155**:2225–8.

43 Griffiths C, Feder G, Wedzicha J, Foster G, Livingstone A, Marlowe GS. Feasibility of spirometry and reversibility testing for the identification of patients with chronic obstructive pulmonary disease on asthma registers in general practice. *Respir Med* 1999; **93**:903–8.

44 Rubinfeld AR, Pain MC. Perception of asthma. *Lancet* 1976; **1**(7965):882–4.

45 Haahtela, T, Jarvinen M, Kava T et al. Comparison of a β_2-agonist, terbutaline, with an inhaled corticosteroid, budesonide, in newly detected asthma. *N Engl J Med* 1991; **325**:388–92.

46 Sont JK, Willems LN, Bel EH et al. Clinical control and histopathological outcome of asthma when using airway hyperresponsiveness as an additional guide to long term treatment. *Am J Respir Crit Care Med* 1999; **159**:1043–51.

47 Guidelines on the management of asthma. *Thorax* 1993; **48**(Suppl): S1–S24.

48 Goldstein MF, Veza BA, Dunsky EH, Dvorin DJ, Belecanech GA, Haralabatos IC. Comparisons of peak diurnal expiratory flow variation, postbronchodilator FEV_1 responses, and methacholine inhalation challenges in the evaluation of suspected asthma. *Chest* 2001; **119**:1001–10.

49 Enright PL, McClelland RL, Buist AS, Lebowitz MD. Correlates of peak expiratory flow lability in elderly persons. *Chest* 2001; **120**:1861–8.

50 Hunter CJ, Brightling CE, Woltmann G, Wardlaw AJ, Pavord ID. A comparison of the validity of different diagnostic tests in adults with asthma. *Chest* 2002; **121**:1051–7.

51 Fish JE. Bronchial challenge testing. In: Middleton E. ed. *Allergy: Principles and Practice*, 4th edn. St Louis, MO, Mosby Year Book, 1993.

52 Ramsdell JW, Nachtwey FJ, Moser KM. Bronchial hyperreactivity in chronic obstructive bronchitis. *Am Rev Respir Dis* 1982; **126**:829–32.

53 Juniper EF, Frith PA, Hargreave FE. Airways responsiveness to histamine and methacholine: relationship to minimize treatment to control symptoms of asthma. *Thorax* 1981; **36**:575–9.

54 Viljanen AA, Viljanen BC, Halttunen PK, Kreus KE. Body plethysmographic studies in non-smoking, healthy adults. *Scan J Clin Lab Invest Suppl* 1982; **159**:35–50.

55 Boushy SF, Aboumrad MH, North LB, Helgason AH. Lung recoil pressure, airway resistance, and forced flows related to morphologic emphysema. *Am Rev Respir Dis* 1971; **104**:551–61.

56 Schlueter DP, Immekus J, Stead WW. Relationship between maximal inspiratory pressure and total lung capacity (coefficient of retraction) in normal subjects and in patients with emphysema, asthma, and diffuse pulmonary infiltration. *Am Rev Respir Dis* 1967; **96**:656–65.

57 Horn M, Ries A, Neveu C, Moser K. Restrictive ventilatory pattern in precapillary pulmonary hypertension. *Am Rev Respir Dis* 1983; **128**:163–5.

58 Bergofsky EH. Respiratory failure in disorders of the thoracic cage. *Am Rev Respir Dis* 1979; **119**:643–69.

59 Vulterini S, Bianco MR, Pellicciotti L, Sidoti AM. Lung mechanics in subjects showing increased residual volume without bronchial obstruction. *Thorax* 1980; **35**:461–6.

60 Stocks J, Quanjer PH. Reference values for residual volume, functional residual capacity and total lung capacity. ATS Workshop on Lung Volume Measurements. Official Statement of the European Respiratory Society. *Eur Respir J* 1995; **8**:492–506.

61 Gelb AF, Gold WM, Wright RR, Bruch HR, Nadel JA. Physiologic diagnosis of subclinical emphysema. *Am Rev Respir Dis* 1973; **107**:50–63.

62 Gonzalez E, Weill H, Ziskind MM, George RB. The value of the single breath diffusing capacity in separating chronic bronchitis from pulmonary emphysema. *Dis Chest* 1968; **53**:229–36.

63 Epler GR, McLoud TC, Gaensler EA, Mikus JP, Carrington CB. Normal chest roentgenograms in chronic diffuse infiltrative lung disease. *N Engl J Med* 1978; **298**:934–9.

64 Crystal RG, Fulmer JD, Roberts WC, Moss ML, Line BR, Reynolds HY. Idiopathic pulmonary fibrosis. Clinical, histologic, radiologic, physiologic, scintigraphic, cytologic, and biochemical aspects. *Ann Intern Med* 1976; **85**:769–88.

65 Rich S, Dantzker DR, Ayres SM et al. Primary pulmonary hypertension. A national prospective study. *Ann Intern Med* 1987; **107**:216–23.

66 Jones NL, Goodwin JF. Respiratory function in pulmonary thromboembolic disorders. *BMJ* 1965; **5442**:1089–93.

67 Nadel JA, Gold WM, Burgess JH. Early diagnosis of chronic pulmonary vascular obstruction. Value of pulmonary function tests. *Am J Med* 1968; **44**:16–25.

68 Doherty MJ, Pearson MG, O'Grady EA, Pellegrini V, Calverley PM. Cryptogenic fibrosing alveolitis with preserved lung volumes. *Thorax* 1997; **52**:998–1002.

69 Hanson D, Winterbauer RH, Kirtland SH, Wu R. Changes in pulmonary function test results after 1 year of therapy as predictors of

survival in patients with idiopathic pulmonary fibrosis. *Chest* 1995; **108**:305–10.

70 Robson AG, Innes JA. Short term variability of single breath carbon monoxide transfer factor. *Thorax* 2001; **56**:358–61.

71 Tweeddale PM, Alexander F, McHardy GJ. Short term variability of FEV1 and bronchodilator responsiveness in patients with obstructive ventilatory defects. *Thorax* 1987; **42**:487–90.

72 Smetana GW. Evaluation of preoperative pulmonary risk. UpToDate. http://uptodate.com, 2003.

73 Meyers JR, Lembeck L, O'Kane H, Baue AE. Changes in functional residual capacity of the lung after operation. *Arch Surg* 1975; **110**:576–83.

74 Lawrence VA, Page CP, Harris GD. Preoperative spirometry before abdominal operations. A critical appraisal of its predictive value. *Arch Intern Med* 1989; **149**:280–5.

75 Kroenke K, Lawrence VA, Theroux JF, Tuley MR, Hilsenbeck S. Postoperative complications after thoracic and major abdominal surgery in patients with and without obstructive lung disease. *Chest* 1993; **104**:1445–51.

76 Lawrence VA, Dhanda R, Hilsenbeck SG, Page CP. Risk of pulmonary complications after elective abdominal surgery. *Chest* 1996; **110**:744–50.

77 Warner DO, Warner MA, Barnes RD *et al.* Perioperative respiratory complications in patients with asthma. *Anesthesiology* 1996; **85**:460–7.

78 Gass GD, Olsen GN. Preoperative pulmonary function testing to predict postoperative morbidity and mortality. *Chest* 1986; **89**:127–35.

79 Zibrak JD, O'Donnell CR, Marton K. Indications for pulmonary function testing. *Ann Intern Med* 1990; **112**:763–71.

80 Fuso L, Cisternino L, Di Napoli A *et al.* Role of spirometric and arterial gas data in predicting pulmonary complications after abdominal surgery. *Respir Med* 2000; **94**:1171–6.

81 McAlister FA, Khan NA, Straus SE *et al.* Accuracy of the preoperative assessment in predicting pulmonary risk after nonthoracic surgery. *Am J Respir Crit Care Med* 2003; **167**:741–4.

82 Smetana GW. Preoperative evaluation for lung resection. UpToDate. http://uptodate.com. 2003.

83 British Thoracic Society and Association of Respiratory Technicians and Physiologists. Guidelines for the measurement of respiratory function. *Respir Med* 1994; **88**:165–94.

84 Miller JI, Grossman GD, Hatcher CR. Pulmonary function test criteria for operability and pulmonary resection. *Surg Gynecol Obstet* 1981; **153**:893–5.

85 Ferguson MK, Little L, Rizzo L. Diffusing capacity predicts morbidity and mortality after pulmonary resection. *J Thorac Cardiovasc Surg* 1988; **96**:894–900.

86 Pierce RJ, Copland JM, Sharpe K, Barter CE. Preoperative risk evaluation for lung cancer resection: predicted post-operative product as a predictor of surgical mortality. *Am J Respir Crit Care Med* 1994; **150**:947–55.

87 Ribas J, Diaz O, Barbera JA *et al.* Invasive exercise testing in the evaluation of patients at high risk for lung resection. *Eur Respir J* 1998; **12**:1429–35.

88 Bolliger CT, Jordan P, Soler M *et al.* Exercise capacity as a predictor of postoperative complications in lung resection candidates. *Am J Respir Crit Care Med* 1995; **151**:1472–80.

89 Walsh GL, Morice RC, Putnam JB Jr *et al.* Resection of lung cancer is justified in high-risk patients selected by exercise oxygen consumption. *Ann Thorac Surg* 1994; **58**:704–10.

90 Johns DP, Pierce R. *Pocket Guide to Spirometry*. Sydney, McGraw-Hill, 2003.

Chest radiographic and computerized tomography patterns

Johny A Verschakelen

Introduction

Chest radiographic patterns

The chest radiograph remains, despite the development of new and very sophisticated imaging techniques such as computerized tomography (CT) and magnetic resonance imaging (MRI), the basic imaging modality of the chest. The success of this technique is related to the fact that it is easy to perform, requires little co-operation from the patient, is not invasive and induces only a small amount of radiation. But, above all, it offers a lot of information on the cardiopulmonary status of the patient. The high X-ray attenuation differences between the bony structures, the soft tissues of chest wall and mediastinum and the lungs allow early detection of abnormalities and, especially within the lung, early changes in density can be appreciated very well. However, despite this and despite the fact that chest roentgenograms were one of the first radiological procedures available to the physician, the interpretation of a chest radiograph continues to be complex and challenging. As basically shadows of gross pathology are seen, it is not surprising that images are frequently non-specific and that there is usually no one-to-one histological correlation of the roentgenograms with the microscopic diagnosis. The concept of radiological differential diagnosis based on the recognition of various patterns was popularized by Reeder and Felson in their book *Gamuts in Radiology*.[1] This book provides a long list of the most common patterns of chest disease and their differential diagnosis.

Pattern recognition is indeed the first and a very important step in the interpretation of a chest radiograph.

Generally, the diagnosis of chest disease on a chest radiograph is based on five elements (Table 1).

Recognition of the disease pattern should allow the development of an appropriate differential diagnosis list that should include all the major categories of disease that might lead to the identified pattern.[2] Trying to determine whether the disease is located in the chest wall, pleura, diaphragm, mediastinum or lungs is the second step. However, this step is not always easy because chest radiographs provide us with projection images in which, for example, chest wall abnormalities that project on the lung can mimic lung disease. The localization of abnormalities should be made as precisely as possible, and one should try to decide whether the disease is focal or diffuse, peripheral or central, in the upper, middle or lower parts of the lung, affecting the airspaces or the interstitium, distributed along the blood vessels, the bronchi or the lymphatics. Careful analysis of the film for additional radiological findings can be very helpful in narrowing the differential diagnosis further. For example, the simultaneous detection of osteolytic lesions in the ribs and lung nodules could suggest metastatic disease. The examination of serial roentgenograms is of course very helpful when examining growth of lesions in comparison with older films. It can, however, also be interesting to wait for follow-up images before deciding on the diagnosis. When, in an intensive care patient, airspace opacities disappear rapidly after the administration of diuretics, a different diagnosis is suggested than when these opacities remained unchanged or increased in size. Finally, correlation with clinical and laboratory data, when available, is mandatory. The knowledge that a patient is immunocompromised will often change the differential diagnosis list. Although careful analysis of these five points can result in a diagnosis or a narrow differential diagnosis list, it is often not possible to make a definitive diagnosis because one or more of the discussed elements is unclear or missing: patterns can overlap and can change over time; disease can show an aberrant localization and distribution; additional findings can be misleading; previous examinations are not available or clinical history is aspecific. Nevertheless, even if a diagnosis cannot be made, it should be possible to suggest (imaging or other) procedures that may lead to the precise diagnosis.

Finally, it should be emphasized that checking the quality of the image is very important. Incorrect positioning of the patient, insufficient image collimation, the presence of life-supporting devices and especially incorrect exposure parameters are often responsible for a reduction in image quality and for a possible misinterpretation of the findings. Fortunately, the introduction of digital detectors has reduced the number of bad exposures and has made image quality more constant over time, which is of major importance in areas such as the emergency room and the intensive care unit. Of course, digitalization will not cope with the other mentioned causes of quality loss.

Computerized tomography patterns

Computerized tomography is the second most important im-

Table 1. Interpretation of abnormalities on a chest radiograph is based on:

1. Recognition of the pattern
2. Localization of the disease
3. Analysis of additional findings
4. Evaluation of serial roentgenograms
5. Correlation of radiological findings with clinical and laboratory data

Table 2. Indications for CT of the chest.

Abnormal chest X-ray
  Further evaluation of a chest wall, pleural, mediastinal or lung
    abnormality seen on a chest X-ray
  Rule out or confirm a lesion seen on a chest X-ray
  Lung cancer staging
  Assessment of thoracic vascular lesion

Normal chest X-ray
  Detection of diffuse lung disease
  Detection of pulmonary metastases from a known extrathoracic
    tumour
  Demonstration of pulmonary embolism
  Investigation of a patient with haemoptysis
  Investigation of patients with clinical evidence of a disease that
    might be related to the presence of chest abnormalities (e.g.
    thymoma in patients with biochemical evidence for the disease;
    pulmonary infection in an immunocompromised patient with
    fever)

aging modality of the chest. It is usually performed when a lesion is seen or suspected on a chest X-ray. However, there are indications when a CT scan of the chest is performed even when the chest X-ray could not reveal any abnormalities (Table 2). The advantage of CT in this situation relates to its cross-sectional format and its higher density resolution compared with the conventional chest radiograph. Also, other advantages are important: the intravenous administration of a relatively small amount of contrast helps to visualize the vascular structures in order to differentiate them from mediastinal structures and allows the study of the vascularization of normal and abnormal structures; X-ray attenuation can be measured, which can be helpful in determining the physical composition of the structure.

Since its introduction, CT has undergone several technical changes and improvements. The first scanners were 'incremental' CT scanners (also called conventional scanners). The patient suspends respiration for the few seconds needed to complete one scan. After that, the table moves and the next scan is performed. In this way, approximately 25 contiguous 5- to 10-mm-thick sections are usually required to image the en-

tire thorax.[3,4] Spiral scanning (also known as helical or continuous volume scanning) has radically altered the CT scanning protocols. This technique entails rapid acquisition of volumetric data through the chest. There is continuous patient movement with simultaneous scanning by a constantly rotating X-ray tube and detector system. This allows acquisition of a helix of raw projecting data; standard axial reconstructions are then possible.[5]

Spiral CT scanning has several advantages over incremental CT scanning:
1 rapid scan acquisition during one or two breath-holds;
2 reduced volume of contrast needed for optimal opacification of vessels;
3 no respiratory misregistration between scans, thus improving nodule detection;
4 potential for multiplanar and three-dimensional reconstructions.[6]

Recently, the multidetector CT (also known as multislice, multirow or multidetector row CT) was introduced. The most striking difference between the (single detector row) spiral CT technology and the multidetector CT is the configuration of the radiation detectors. In the (single detector row) spiral CT scanners, these detectors were long and narrow, with the length of a single detector element aligned in the longitudinal axis. Multidetector CT technology has incorporated a detector array that is segmented in the longitudinal axis. This allows for simultaneous acquisition of multiple images in the scan plane with one rotation of the X-ray tube around the patient.[7] Multidetector CT also offers flexible image reconstruction options. In contrast to the single row spiral CT scanners that only have the ability to reconstruct images of the same slice thickness, which has to be chosen before the acquisition of the data, with multidetector CT, it becomes possible to reconstruct images at various image thicknesses.

Major advantages of this technique over single row spiral CT are:
1 further decrease in examination time;
2 further improvement of blood vessel opacification in vascular studies;
3 faster and better multiplanar and three-dimensional reconstructions.[8]

High-resolution CT (HRCT), on the other hand, is not a different CT technique but is an acquisition technique that can be performed with all the above-mentioned scanners. Basically, HRCT uses 0.75–1 mm slice thickness and high-frequency reconstruction algorithms producing highly detailed images. In the chest, it is predominantly performed to evaluate diffuse pulmonary disease but is also used to produce high-detail images of specific regions of interest.

The interpretation of a CT scan is also based on the five elements that are used to interpret a chest X-ray:
1 recognition of the pattern;
2 study of localization and distribution of the disease;

3 careful analysis of CT examination for additional radiological findings;

4 examination of serial CTs;

5 correlation of findings with clinical and radiological data.

A major difference from the chest X-ray is that, because of the earlier mentioned advantages of the technique, CT can recognize the pattern better and is also a better technique for localizing the disease. It is not only easier to determine whether a lesion is located in the lung or in the pleura or chest wall but also, because of the higher detail, it is often possible to recognize vascular, airway or lymphatic distribution of the disease. In this way, HRCT is a significantly better imaging modality than the chest radiograph in the diagnosis of chest abnormalities.

Chest radiographic and computerized tomographic patterns and differential diagnosis

In this section, a review will be given of the most frequently occurring patterns seen in the chest. The description is organized according to the different chest radiographic patterns that can be recognized. For each pattern, the potential role of HRCT in the diagnosis and differential diagnosis of the diseases that can cause the pattern and, when applicable, the specific CT approach to the pattern are discussed. When necessary, the advantages of other imaging modalities will also be described briefly.

Chest wall

Abnormal increase in density

Chest wall opacities can be the result of both intrathoracic and extrathoracic normal and abnormal structures. Both the intrathoracic and the extrathoracic lesions become radiographically visible as soft-tissue opacities with an incomplete sharp border.[9,10] In the extrathoracic lesions, the border is produced by the interface of the mass with air and is lost where the mass is continuous with the soft tissues of the chest wall. Intrathoracic lesions are visible because of their interface with the aerated lung (Fig. 1a). This incomplete border is helpful in distinguishing chest wall lesions from pulmonary lesions. Intrathoracic extrapulmonary chest wall lesions can be distinguished from extrathoracic chest wall lesions by the presence of tapered superior and inferior borders. However, this tapered border may not be visible when the lesion is seen *en face*.[11] Also, pleural lesions can present as opacities with tapered superior and inferior borders. A key factor in the observation of chest wall lesions is the presence of rib destruction.[12,13] This excludes lipoma or other benign tumours such as neurofibroma from the diagnosis (Table 3).

Table 3. Chest wall opacities.

Nipples
Skin lesions (moles, neurofibroma)
Chest wall tumours
    Mesenchymal: lipomas, fibromas
    Neural: schwannoma, neurofibroma, neuroblastoma
    Lymphoma
    Haemangioma
    Bone: metastasis, plasmocytoma, chondrosarcoma, fibrous dysplasia, fibrosarcoma
    Askin tumour
Invasion by a contiguous mass (lung cancer, breast cancer)
Haematoma (rib fracture)
Infection

Because of its better density resolution and axial format, CT can better demonstrate the different tissues of the chest wall. CT has the advantage over magnetic resonance imaging (MRI) of higher spatial resolution and the ability to identify bony structures better[14,15] (CDROMFig. 1b and c). MRI, however, yields greater soft-tissue contrast, which can be important when soft-tissue abnormalities are examined.[16] Multiplanar imaging and three-dimensional reformation can be performed with both techniques and can be valuable in some selected cases.[15]

Ultrasound may also be used to examine the chest wall. In general, it provides less detailed and comprehensive information than the previous modalities, but it usually enables the lesion to be localized, allows a distinction to be made between cystic and solid lesions and enables guided aspiration/biopsy to be performed under imaging control. Ultrasound can also be helpful in clarifying suspicious or unclear findings during palpation of the chest.[17]

Abnormal decrease in density

Abnormal decrease in density of the chest wall is usually caused by a unilateral hypoplasia or absence of a breast or of muscles and can be seen after a mastectomy (CDROMFig. 2) when the pectoralis muscle is hypoplastic or absent.[18] Often an abnormal axillary fold can be recognized, which should also help to differentiate this entity from abnormal decrease in density caused by pleural or lung disease.

Subcutaneous emphysema of the chest wall is another cause of density decrease of the chest wall and is not uncommon following surgery, pleural drain placement and trauma or in cases of spontaneous or acquired pneumomediastinum.[19] Air dissects along tissue planes and between muscle bundles, giving an overall pattern of linear transradiancies, which can interfere significantly with the interpretation of the underlying structures (see Fig. 5). In this way, diagnosis of pneumothorax can become very difficult. In case of doubt, a CT scan can be performed.

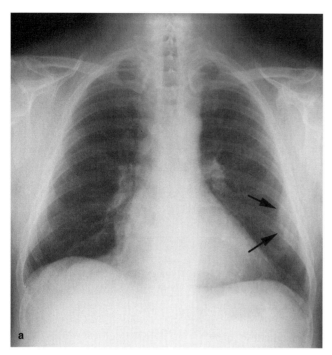

Figure 1. Abnormal increase in density of the chest wall. On a chest radiograph (a), a peripheral opacity with smooth incomplete tapered borders and obtuse angles (arrows) can be located either in the chest wall or in the pleura.

Pleura [20,21]

Abnormal increase in density

Pleural opacities

A pleural opacity should have a peripheral localization.[22] This localization is easily recognized when the mass is against the lateral chest wall, but the correct localization may be difficult to identify when the mass is located anterior, posterior or antero- or posterolateral.[23] Lateral and oblique views may be helpful, but sometimes a CT scan is required to confirm the peripheral location. A peripheral opacity can correspond to three locations: (a) the chest wall; (b) the pleura; and (c) the subpleural area of the lung. Smooth, incomplete tapered borders with obtuse pleural angles localize a mass to either the chest wall or the pleura (Fig. 1a). Irregular borders and acute pleural angles suggest a subpleural peripheral lung mass.[23,24] However, CT is often required for the precise localization of the abnormalities that are seen on the chest radiograph (CDROMFig. 1b and c). This is especially true for pleural lesions with a medial location that may mimic a mediastinal mass. CT is also valuable in distinguishing soft-tissue pleural opacities from fluid-containing opacities such as encapsulated pleural fluid collections, while density measurements can be helpful in making the diagnosis.[25,26] MRI can be indicated to study tumour extension into the chest wall.[27]

Table 4. Pleural opacities.

Solitary pleural opacity
  Loculated pleural effusion
  Metastasis
  Mesothelioma (benign or malignant)
  Lipoma
  Organized empyema
  Pleural haematoma
  Mesothelial cyst
  Localized fibrous tumour of the pleura

Multiple pleural opacities
  Loculated pleural effusions
  Metastases
  Malignant mesothelioma (pleural mass)
  Pleural plaques

Pleural lesions can also present as multiple, separate, smooth tapered opacities or as diffuse pleural thickening with lobulated inner borders (Table 4) (Fig. 3).

Pleural effusion

Although a loculated pleural effusion can present as a solitary pleural opacity or as multiple pleural opacities and in this way mimic other pleural disease (Table 4), a free pleural effusion often has typical signs, especially on an erect chest film.[28,29] Blunting of a lateral or posterior costophrenic angle typically suggests a free pleural effusion (CDROMFig. 4). However, other findings can be a complete opacification of the chest, an apparent elevation of the diaphragm or an opacity in the interlobar fissures. In case of doubt, a decubitus film can be performed, which should show a change in contour. Ultrasound is an easier and less invasive alternative, while CT and even MRI can be performed when the image remains difficult to interpret or when a tumour is suspected as being the cause of the pleural effusion.[27,30–32] Also, in case of empyema, ultrasound or CT can be performed. In addition, ultrasound is a good technique for guiding a transthoracic puncture and evacuation of the fluid and can demonstrate better than CT septations in the pleural fluid.

The differential diagnosis list of pleural effusions is long, and all types of pleural effusion are radiographically identical, although historical, clinical and other radiological features (Tables 5 and 6) may help to limit the diagnostic possibilities.[21] Sometimes, CT and MRI can also help to specify the diagnosis.[33]

Abnormal decrease in density

Pneumothorax

Typical signs of a pneumothorax are best seen on erect radiographs in which the pleural air rises to the lung apex and the

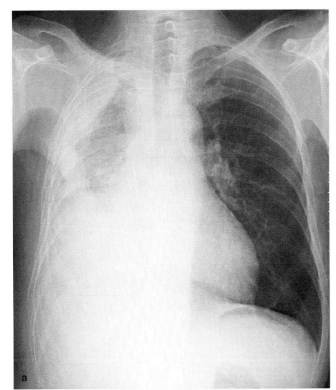

Table 5. Pleural effusion with a large cardiac silhouette.

Congestive heart failure
Pulmonary embolism
Myocarditis
Pericarditis
Systemic lupus
Rheumatoid arthritis
Metastatic tumour

Table 6. Pleural effusion with hilar enlargement.

Pulmonary embolism
Tumour
Tuberculosis
Sarcoidosis

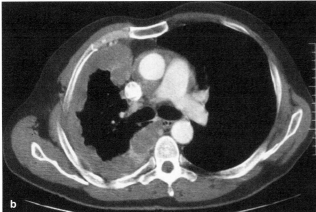

Figure 3. Abnormal increase in density caused by pleural opacity (a, chest radiograph; b, CT). Pleural malignant mesothelioma presenting as a diffuse pleural thickening with lobulated inner border.

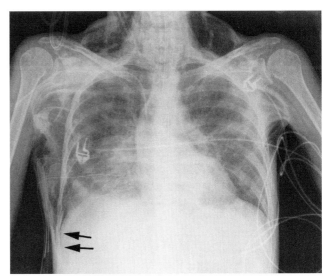

Figure 5. Patient with subcutaneous emphysema and a deep, finger-like right lateral costophrenic sulcus (arrows) suggesting a pneumothorax.

visceral pleural line at the apex becomes separated from the chest wall by a zone of abnormal decrease in density devoid of vessels.[34] Although this sounds a straightforward sign to assess, difficulties of interpretation can arise with avascular lung apices, as in bullous disease and when clothing or dressing artefacts, tubes and skin folds create linear shadows. Features that help to identify artefacts and skin folds include extension of the 'pneumothorax' line beyond the margin of the chest cavity, laterally located vessels and an orientation of a line that is inconsistent with the edge of a slightly collapsed lung. In indeterminate circumstances, a repeat chest radiograph, an ex-

piratory radiograph or one taken with the patient decubitus may clarify the situation.[34] Should doubt still remain, then CT is particularly helpful in distinguishing between bullae and a pneumothorax. CT can also be helpful in detecting the cause of the pneumothorax.[35] In particular, HRCT should be performed when small apical blebs are suspected as being the cause of the pneumothorax.[36]

Atypical signs arise when the patient is supine or when the pleural space is partly obliterated. In the supine position, pleural air rises and collects anteriorly, particularly medially and basally, and may not extend far enough posteriorly to separate lung from the chest wall at the apex or laterally. Signs that suggest a pneumothorax under these conditions are listed in Table 7[37,38] (Fig. 5).

Table 7. Atypical signs of pneumothorax.

Ipsilateral increased lucency
A deep, finger-like costophrenic sulcus laterally
A visible anterior costophrenic recess seen as an oblique line or
interface in the hypochondrium
A transradiant band parallel to the diaphragm and/or mediastinum
Visualization of the undersurface of the heart and of the cardiac fat
pads as rounded opacities suggesting masses
Diaphragm depression

Table 8. Bilateral symmetrical elevation of the diaphragm.

Supine position
Poor inspiration
Painful conditions
Bilateral diaphragmatic paralysis
Increased abdominal pressure or abdominal distension
Diffuse and basal pulmonary fibrosis
Bilateral pulmonary emboli

Table 9. Unilateral elevation of the diaphragm.

Posture (lateral decubitus position-dependent side)
Dorsal scoliosis
Distension of stomach or colon
Subphrenic mass or infection
Pulmonary embolism
Pulmonary hypoplasia
Pulmonary collapse
Pneumonia
Diaphragmatic paralysis
Eventration
Painful conditions (rib fracture)
Mimic: infrapulmonary pleural effusion

Hydropneumothorax

When air and liquid are present, the nomenclature depends on their relative volumes and the type of liquid. Small amounts of liquid are disregarded, and the condition is still called a pneumothorax; otherwise, the prefixes hydro-, haemo-, pyo- or chylo- are added, depending on the nature of the liquid. Typically, on the erect chest radiograph, one or more air–fluid levels are seen. Air may enter the pleural space by crossing any of its four major boundaries: the chest wall, mediastinum, lung or diaphragm.

Tension pneumothorax

The diagnosis of tension pneumothorax is usually made clinically, and treatment is instituted without a radiograph. Should a chest radiograph be taken, it will show contralateral mediastinal shift and ipsilateral diaphragm depression. Mild degrees of contralateral mediastinal shift are not unusual with a non-tension pneumothorax because of the negative pressure in the normal pleural space. However, moderate or gross mediastinal shift should be taken as indicating tension, particularly if the ipsilateral hemidiaphragm is depressed.

Table 10. Focal elevation (bulge).

Focal diaphragmatic dysfunction (paralysis, eventration)
Focal diaphragmatic adhesions
Herniation (congenital, acquired)
Diaphragmatic tumour
(Pleura tumour)
(Peripheral lung tumour)
(Mass in the liver, spleen)

Diaphragm

The diaphragm as such is not normally visualized on a postero-anterior (PA) or lateral chest radiograph. Only when air is present below and above it is the diaphragm visible as a distinct entity.[39] Ultrasonography, CT and MRI are the only imaging modalities that can visualize the diaphragm itself, although visualization is usually partial and dependent on the presence of pleural disease when using ultrasonography and on the presence of subdiaphragmatic fat when using CT and MRI.[40–42] Abnormalities of diaphragmatic height and configuration and loss of the normal clear outline provide important clues for the recognition of a variety of pathological changes not only in the diaphragm itself but also in the underlying lung, pleura and upper abdomen.[43,44]

1 Position of one or both leaves of the diaphragm can be abnormally high or abnormally low (CDROMFig. 6a and b, see also Fig. 6c). Severe pulmonary emphysema is a typical cause of an abnormally low position of the entire diaphragm. A unilateral depression of the diaphragm can be seen in ten-

sion pneumothorax. Causes of bilateral symmetrical and unilateral elevation of the diaphragm are listed in Tables 8 and 9.

2 A focal abnormality in diaphragmatic configuration often presents as a bulge on the contour (CDROMFig. 7). The cause of this focal bulge can be related to the pathology of the diaphragm itself but can also be related to lung or pleura pathology and even pathology of structures located below the diaphragm. A peripheral malignant lung tumour invading the diaphragm can present as a focal elevation of the diaphragm. Additional radiological signs such as pleural effusion or clinical signs such as pleural pain should alert the observer that the focal bulge is very likely not caused by a benign disease. Causes of a focal elevation are shown in Table 10.

3 Localized loss of clarity occurs when the diaphragm is not tangential to the X-ray beam, but usually indicates adjacent pulmonary or pleural disease, e.g. the costophrenic or

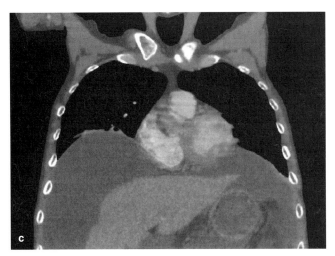

Figure 6. c) CT showing abnormal high position of both diaphragmatic leaves. The bilateral symmetrical elevation of the diaphragm is caused by abdominal distension resulting from an enormous amount of ascites, which is very well visulized on the CT scan.

costovertebral angles are obliterated by pleural fluid or the diaphragmatic outline may be obliterated by basal pneumonia.

Ultrasound and especially CT often allow a more specific diagnosis and should be performed when the chest radiograph is unable to make or suggest a definitive diagnosis. In particular, spiral CT and multidetector CT can be helpful because of their ability to produce high-quality reformations, which often allow a better study of the exact localization of the disease and its relationship to the diaphragm (Fig. 8).

Mediastinum

In most cases, imaging of the mediastinum is based on the combination of a chest radiograph and a CT scan in which the CT examination is used to confirm or deny the suspected abnormality seen on the chest radiograph. Moreover, CT, in addition to determining the exact localization of the abnormality, is often able to make a more specific diagnosis because this technique can also study tissue density and tissue enhancement after administration of intravenous contrast.[45] When problems are not resolved with CT, an additional magnetic resonance examination can be performed.[46]

Chest radiograph

On a chest radiograph, the mediastinum presents as a dense shadow located between the two lungs on a PA view and projecting on these lungs on the lateral view. This shadow is not a homogeneous density but, medial to its most lateral contours, several borders of mediastinal structures, which are referred to as 'mediastinal lines', in contact with the air-containing lung can be seen.[47] Table 11 shows how pathology can change the mediastinum on a chest radiograph.

Table 11. Signs of mediastinal pathology on a chest radiograph.

Shift of the mediastinum
Diffuse widening
Focal change in configuration of the mediastinal contour or of a mediastinal line
Focal change in integrity of the mediastinal contour or of a mediastinal line
Increased or decreased density

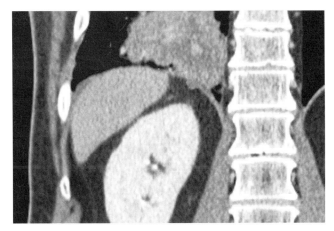

Figure 8. Multidetector CT-generated coronal reformatted images allow a very detailed study of the relationship between a lung tumour and the diaphragm.

Shift of the mediastinum

Shift of the mediastinum is identified by displacement of the entire mediastinal shadow and indicates an imbalance of pressure between the left and right sides of the thorax. The first step in the interpretation of a shifted mediastinum is to determine which side is abnormal. Associated findings such as atelectasis or hyperexpansion of the lung and elevation or depression of a hemidiaphragm are frequently helpful in making this determination. In case of doubt, an expiratory chest radiograph can be helpful. Table 12 shows the most frequent causes of mediastinal shift.

Widening of the mediastinum

Before deciding on the presence of a pathological diffuse widening of the mediastinum, it is important to rule out technical artefacts. Diffuse widening of the mediastinum is very often seen in chest radiographs obtained in the supine body position and when inspiration was insufficient. Also, a lordotic position of the patient can cause widening of the mediastinal shadow. Table 13 shows the most frequent causes of diffuse mediastinal widening (CDROMFigs 9a and b, 10a,b and 11a,c; see also Figs 10c and 11b).

Table 12. Causes of mediastinal shift.

Away from the pathological side
  Pleura:
    large pleural effusion
    tension pneumothorax
    large pleural mass
    large transdiaphragmatic herniation
  Lung:
    airway obstruction:
      large airway: foreign body (children)
      small airway: bronchiolitis obliterans (Swyer James syndrome:
        expiratory chest film)
    bullous emphysema
    large lung mass

Towards the pathological side
  Pleura:
    pneumothorax
  Lung:
    hypoplastic lung
    pneumonectomy (lobectomy)
    atelectasis

Table 13. Diffuse widening of the mediastinum.

Lipomatosis
Abnormal vascular structures including the heart
Haematoma
Neoplasm including enlarged lymph nodes, lymphoma
Inflammation

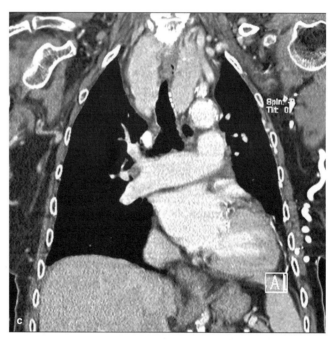

Figure 10. Widening of the upper part of the mediastinum caused by a goitre extending into the mediastinum. CT (c) confirms the presence of a strongly enhancing mass in the upper mediastinum surrounding the trachea and displacing the blood vessels laterally.

Changes in configuration and/or integrity of the mediastinal contour or of a mediastinal line

Focal changes in configuration and integrity of a mediastinal contour or of a mediastinal line can indicate the presence of a mediastinal mass that grows adjacent to and extends beyond this contour or line or pushes this contour or line laterally (Fig. 12a, CDROMFigs 12b and 13). They can also be caused by changes in the vascular structure that is responsible for this contour or line. The latter is seen for example when there is an aneurysm or a tortuous dilatation of the aorta. Changes in configuration and integrity can be very subtle and can often only be seen when comparison with a previous chest radiograph is possible. Localized loss of clarity can also occur when there is adjacent pulmonary or pleural disease.

Increased or decreased density

Diffuse increase in density of the mediastinum is often a technical artefact caused by underexposure of the chest film. Focal increase in density, however, especially when associated with a change in configuration or a loss of integrity of a mediastinal contour or line, usually indicates the presence of a mass or an

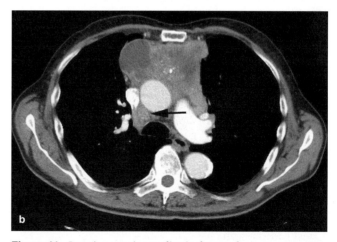

Figure 11. Invasive anterior mediastinal mass: thymosarcoma. CT (b) confirms the presence of the mass, which is irregularly enhancing and contains calcifications, and also low-attenuation areas corresponding with tumour necrosis. The malignant character of the mass is suggested by the fact that it is extending between the vessels and by the presence of an enlarged lymph node (arrow).

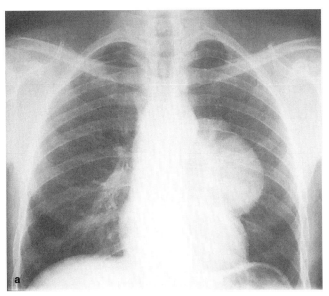

Figure 12. Congenital cyst. The chest radiograph (a) shows a change in configuration of the left mediastinal contour.

Table 14. Causes of an anterior, middle and posterior mediastinal mass.

Anterior mediastinal mass
    Thymic lesion
    Teratoid lesion
    Thyroid
    Lymph nodes
    Cardiovascular lesions

Middle mediastinal mass
    Enlarged lymph nodes
    Primary tumours (trachea, oesophagus)
    Vascular lesions
    Congenital cysts (bronchogenic)
    Other (hiatal hernia)

Posterior mediastinal mass
    Neoplasm (especially neural tumours)
    Lymph nodes
    Paraspinous abscess
    Congenital cysts (duplication)
    Aneurysm
    Abdominal diseases (Bochdalek hernia, pancreatic pseudocyst)
    Meningocoele

abnormal vascular structure (Fig. 12a). Sometimes, these masses can contain calcifications. Other causes of calcifications in the mediastinum are calcified cardiac valves, wall calcifications in the coronary arteries and constrictive pericarditis.

Focal decrease in density usually indicates the presence of free air in the mediastinum or the pericardium and can be caused by trauma and mediastinitis. Abnormal air collections can also be seen in the oesophagus in the case of a large hiatal herniation or achalasia.

Anterior, middle and posterior mediastinum
The diagnosis of mediastinal abnormalities on a chest radiograph is mainly based on their localization: anterior, middle or posterior mediastinum. The anterior mediastinum contains the thymus, lymph nodes, vessels and fat. The middle mediastinum is the area between the anterior border of the trachea and the posterior border of the heart and a line drawn 1 cm posterior to the anterior border of the vertebral bodies. This area includes the trachea, arch of the aorta, great vessels, pulmonary arteries, oesophagus and paratracheal and peribronchial nodes. The most common cause of a posterior mediastinal mass is a neural tumour (CDROMFig. 13a). Table 14 lists the most frequent causes of anterior, middle and posterior mediastinal masses.[48–52]

Computerized tomography
Computerized tomography (CT) is usually performed when a mediastinal mass is visible or suspected on the chest radiograph. CT can rule out other causes of mediastinal change but, when a mass is seen, the technique provides the most accurate assessment of the position of this mass together with a

description of its size, shape and characteristics such as CT density and contrast enhancement. In particular, the determination of this relative attenuation improves the ability to characterize masses (CDROMFigs 9b, 10b, see also Fig. 10c). In some cases, CT even permits a definitive diagnosis.

Based on the CT density characteristics, mediastinal masses can be divided into four major patterns:
1 fatty masses showing a fat density (CDROMFig. 9b);
2 'low' attenuation masses have a spontaneous low (water) density (CDROMFig. 12b);
3 'high' attenuation masses have a spontaneous (precontrast) high density (CDROMFig. 10b, see also Fig. 10c);
4 enhancing masses show important increase in density after administration of intravenous contrast[50–53] (Table 15) (CDROMFig. 10b, see also Fig. 10c).

Lung parenchyma and hilar structures

Chest radiograph

Abnormal increase in lung density

Opacities conforming to anatomic boundaries Some pathological processes are not transgressing anatomic boundaries and are limited to a segment, a lobe or one lung. When bounded by a fissure, often very typical radiological images occur. This is especially true when a segment or lobe becomes atelectatic. Each time an abnormal increase in lung density is seen that is

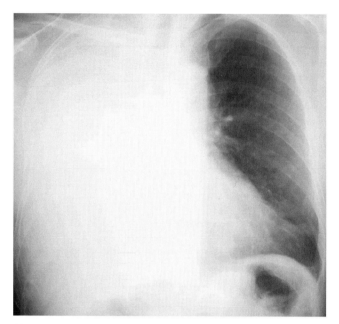

Figure 14. Complete opacification of a hemithorax can be caused by both pulmonary and pleural processes and is often the result of a combination of inflammatory or neoplastic infiltration of the entire lung in combination with pleural effusion. When the volume of the affected hemithorax is normal relative to the unaffected side, as in this patient, an inflammatory process of the lung or a combination of lung atelectasis and pleural effusion is suggested.

bound by anatomic structures, one should look carefully for signs that suggest volume loss because this volume loss could be the result of a process obstructing the feeding bronchus.[54]

Complete opacification of a hemithorax can be caused by an inflammatory or neoplastic infiltration of an entire lung or can be the result of atelectasis of an entire lung. The major differential diagnosis is a pleural process such as a pleural effusion, a fibrothorax or a large pleural tumour. When considering the differential diagnosis, it is important to note whether the volume of the hemithorax is increased (as in a massive pleural effusion, a large lung or pleural tumour), decreased (as in atelectasis of the entire lung) or normal relative to the unaffected side (as in inflammatory process of the lung or a combination of lung atelectasis and pleural effusion) (Fig. 14). It may be difficult to determine the cause in a given case, and further evaluation with CT is often necessary.

The most common cause of a segmental or lobar opacity is acute pneumonia[55,56] (CDROMFig. 15). The consolidated lobe or segment is a homogeneous, confluent opacity that obliterates the normal vascular markings and is bounded by the fissures that can be stretched. As the airways are frequently air filled and surrounded by airless lung, an air bronchogram is often seen.[57] Acute pneumonia can usually be diagnosed from the clinical history and the radiographic changes. When the infiltration does not resolve within 10 days after appropriate therapy, diagnosis becomes more difficult and further in-

Table 15. CT pattern of mediastinal masses.

Fatty masses
  Mediastinal lipomatosis
  Herniation of abdominal fat
  Neoplasms
    lipoma
    liposarcoma
    germ cell tumour
    thymolipoma

Low-attenuation masses
  Congenital cysts (bronchogenic, duplication, neurenteric, pericardial, thymic)
  Neoplasms (necrosis, cystic degeneration, old haemorrhage, intrinsic properties of neoplasm)
    primary tumour (peripheral nerve sheet tumour, lymphangioma)
    metastasis (testicular carcinoma)
    post treatment
  Intrathoracic meningocoele
  Inflammatory process (tuberculous lymphadenitis)
  Goitre (low-density areas)
  Mimics (thrombosed vein, fluid-filled oesophagus, localized pleural fluid, fluid within distended pericardial recess)

High-attenuation masses
  Calcification in lymph nodes, tumour and cyst wall
  Goitre
  Recent haematoma

Enhancing masses
  Vascular structures (normal and aneurysmatic)
  Neoplasms
    thymoma
    lymphoma
    germ cell tumour
    neural tumour
    goitre (strong enhancement)
    parathyroid mass (strong enhancement)
    haemangioma (strong enhancement)
    Castelmann tumour (strong enhancement)
    metastasis of sarcomas and melanomas (strong enhancement)

vestigation is necessary. Table 16 shows the most frequent causes of segmental and lobar opacities.

The radiographic signs of atelectasis include (Fig. 16a, CDROMFig. 16b):
1 increased opacity;
2 crowding and reorientation of pulmonary vessels;
3 displacement of fissures;
4 elevation of the diaphragm;
5 displacement of the hilum;
6 crowding of ribs;
7 compensatory overinflation of the normal lung;
8 shift of the mediastinum;
9 shift of the trachea.

Table 16. Causes of segmental and lobar opacities.

Bacterial pneumonia
Tuberculous pneumonia
Fungal pneumonia
Aspiration pneumonia
Pulmonary embolism (haemorrhage, oedema, infarction)
Neoplasm (obstructive pneumonia, bronchoalveolar cell carcinoma, lymphoma)
Pseudosegmental opacities (intralobar effusion, loculated pleural effusion, chest wall disease, lung tumours)

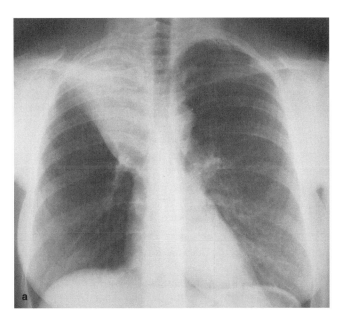

Figure 16. Atelectasis of the right upper lobe. Opacification and volume loss of the right upper lobe with displacement of the fissures and the hilum, elevation of the right hemidiaphragm and compensatory overinflation of the right middle and lower lobe. There is also some shift of the mediastinum and trachea to the right.

These signs are not always present but, when present and when the opacity is lobar and conforming to anatomic boundaries, typical patterns of upper, middle and lower lobe obstructive atelectasis on the right and of upper and lower lobe obstructive atelectasis on the left side will occur.[58,59]

Although airway obstruction is by far the most common cause of atelectasis, other causes are responsible for other types of atelectasis that are, however, not usually present as opacities conforming to anatomic boundaries.[60,61] Compressive atelectasis is caused by intrapulmonary abnormalities (e.g. a large lung mass) that compress surrounding lung. Changes in intrapleural pressure (e.g. pneumothorax) can cause passive atelectasis. Adhesive atelectasis means that the alveolar walls stick together and occurs when surfactant becomes deficient. Cicatrizing atelectasis is the result of scarring by fibrosis with the loss of volume as a secondary effect.

Table 17. Regional and multifocal, patchy consolidations.

Inflammation
  Bronchopneumonia
  Fungal pneumonia
  Tuberculosis
  Sarcoidosis
  Organizing pneumonia
  Eosinophilic lung disease
  Langerhans cell histiocytosis
  Mucoid impaction

Neoplasm
  Bronchoalveolar cell carcinoma
  Lymphoma
  Metastasis

Vascular
  Emboli (thromboemboli, septic emboli)
  Vasculitis (Wegener)
  Goodpasture syndrome
  Contusional haemorrhage

Inhalational
  Hypersensitivity pneumonitis
  Silicosis

Idiopathic
  UIP

Radiation reactions

UIP, usual interstitial pneumonia.

Opacities not conforming to anatomic boundaries

Regional, patchy multifocal and diffuse airspace consolidations
These opacities are usually homogeneous with ill-defined margins and may contain an air bronchogram. They may represent intra-alveolar oedema, inflammatory exudates, blood or tumour cells.[62,63]

Many pulmonary diseases can be responsible for the development of a regional consolidation (CDROMFig. 17) or patchy multifocal consolidations (CDROMFig. 18). These entities cause airspace filling but may also involve the peribronchovascular and septal interstitium. That is why an underlying fine nodular or reticular pattern can sometimes be seen. Table 17 lists the most frequent causes of this pattern.

The classic radiological appearance of diffuse airspace consolidation (Fig. 19) consists of diffuse coalescent or confluent opacities with ill-defined borders and often a perihilar distribution. Air-filled bronchi surrounded by the confluent opacities are seen as dark branching shadows (air bronchogram). Often, these airspace consolidations have a tendency to change in severity over a short period. Table 18 lists the most frequent causes of diffuse airspace consolidations.

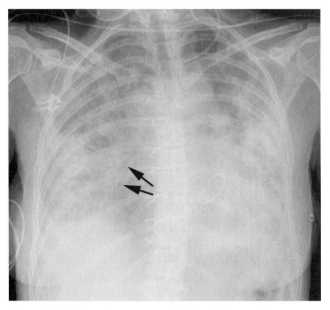

Figure 19. Diffuse airspace consolidation. Diffuse coalescent opacities with ill-defined borders located in a perihilar distribution are caused by pulmonary oedema. Notice the air bronchogram in the right lung (arrows).

Table 18. Diffuse airspace consolidation.

Oedema (cardiac failure, chronic renal failure, fluid overload, fat embolism, ARDS . . .)

Pneumonia (bacterial, viral, mycoplasma . . .)

Tumour (bronchoalveolar cell carcinoma, lymphoma)

Haemorrhage

Pulmonary alveolar proteinosis

Eosinophilic lung disease

ARDS, acute respiratory distress syndrome.

Nodular opacities Nodular opacities are more sharply circumscribed and homogeneous than patchy consolidations. They present as rounded, homogeneous densities that have relatively well-defined margins.

When a pulmonary nodule is seen, two questions should be raised:

1 Is this a solitary nodule or are there multiple pulmonary nodules?

2 Can it be lung cancer?

Solitary pulmonary nodules correspond with lung cancer in up to 30% of cases, and surgical resection may be appropriate. In contrast, the primary workup of multiple pulmonary nodules is non-surgical as these lesions often represent granulomas or metastases. CT plays an important role both in the search for additional nodules and in the differential diagnosis between benign and malignant nodular opacities.

Solitary pulmonary nodule The radiographic differential diagnosis between a benign and a malignant nodule is often impossible. However, there are some nodules that have a typical benign presentation while others have typical signs of a malignant tumour. In between are a lot of nodules in which differential diagnosis is difficult or impossible.[64–66]

Patient's age can be an indication because nodules in the adolescent population are rare whereas the proportion of malignant lesions increases rapidly over the age of 40 years.

Before looking at the specific radiological features of the nodule, it is important to compare serial films.[67,68] Nodules that enlarge very slowly are more likely to be benign. Also, a nodule that decreases in size is very probably a benign process even in the absence of calcifications, especially if this nodule also becomes more sharply defined. However, deciding that a growth rate is suspicious for tumour is often not so straightforward, especially as it is well known that a nodule must go through approximately 30 doublings to reach 1 cm of diameter and become radiographically visible.[69,70] Rate of growth is probably most useful in those cases in which an extremely rapid growth is observed. Very rapid growth is atypical for bronchogenic carcinoma and also unlikely in metastatic disease except in aggressive primary tumours such as osteosarcomas and choriocarcinomas. Very rapidly growing nodules suggest an infectious process and infarct.[71] Nevertheless, a growing nodule is a generally accepted indication for biopsy, while a solitary nodule that has not grown for 2 years may be considered benign.

Calcification is the most diagnostic feature of a pulmonary nodule. Central, laminated or complete calcification is virtually diagnostic of a granuloma. Popcorn-like calcifications may suggest a hamartoma (CDROMFig. 20). However, faint calcifications do not exclude malignancy.[72]

Border characteristics are valuable but rarely reliable in making a definitive diagnosis. The presence of irregular, speculated borders ('corona radiata'), although not pathognomonic, is strongly suggestive of malignancy especially when irregularity increases on follow-up films.[73] A very smooth border is not typical of primary lung carcinoma, but this appearance should not be used to exclude the diagnosis because it can be seen in well-differentiated adenocarcinomas and squamous cell tumour.[74] In addition, a sharply defined margin is the expected appearance for solitary metastasis (Fig. 21). Bronchial carcinoids, which most frequently occur in the proximal bronchi, may also arise from more peripheral bronchi and present as solitary nodules. Benign tumours such as hamartomas also have sharply defined borders, and granulomas become more sharply defined as the surrounding inflammatory reactions are replaced by fibrosis.[75]

The texture of a nodule is most frequently described as homogeneous, although intervening lucencies do occur. They can suggest that the process is spreading through the lung in an infiltrative way leaving some alveoli aerated or that central

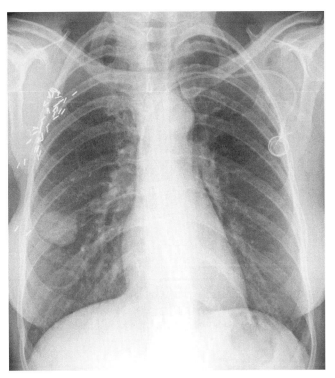

Figure 21. Solitary pulmonary nodule. A solitary pulmonary nodule with sharply defined margins in a patient who underwent surgery for cancer of the breast is very suspicious of metastatic disease.

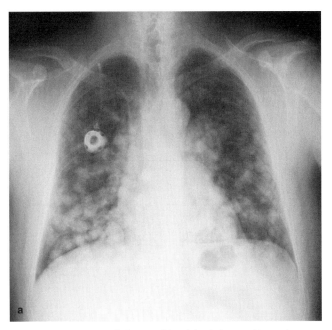

Figure 22. Coarse nodular opacities. (a) PA chest radiograph. Multiple pulmonary nodules caused by metastatic disease. Especially in both lower lobes, the nodules are superimposed and in this way mimic the patchy multifocal airspace consolidation pattern shown in CDROM Fig. 18.

Table 19. Coarse nodular opacities.

Neoplastic
  Malignant (metastasis, lymphoma, post-transplant
    lymphoproliferative disorders)
  Benign (hamartomas, amyloidosis, arteriovenous malformations)

Inflammatory
  Fungal infection
  Nocardiosis
  Tuberculosis
  Septic emboli
  Sarcoidosis

Vascular
  Rheumatoid nodules
  Wegener granulomatosis
  Organizing infarcts

Post-traumatic organizing haematomas

necrosis and cavitation has occurred.[76] This distinction usually requires CT for verification. An air bronchogram is usually considered in favour of an organizing process, although it should be emphasized that bronchoalveolar cell carcinoma and lymphoma can occasionally present as nodular opacities with an air bronchogram.

Sometimes, pulmonary nodules may assume a characteristic shape. The visualization of large vessels entering a nodule strongly suggests the diagnosis of an arteriovenous malformation, while a nodule in the medial portion of the lung just before the veins enter the left atrium should suggest a pulmonary vein varix.[77] A rounded mass in the lower third of the lung and broadly based on the chest wall together with pulmonary vessels extending as curvilinear densities towards this mass should suggest the diagnosis of rounded atelectasis.[78,79]

Multiple nodular opacities

Coarse nodular opacities Multiple pulmonary nodules are distinguished from multifocal patchy opacities in the same way as a solitary nodule is distinguished from a regional consolidation. They have a homogeneous appearance and sharply defined borders. Multiple coarse nodular opacities are most frequently the result of metastatic disease (Fig. 22a, CDROM-Fig. 22b). Other causes are listed in Table 19.[80] The presence of calcification may be diagnostic of a benign granuloma, but this does not prove that other nodules are also benign. Comparison with older films is necessary. Large, multifocal, ill-defined opacities evolving to smaller, sharply defined nodules indicate either healing granulomas or organizing infarcts to be the cause of the granulomas.

Table 20. Causes of fine and miliary interstitial opacities in the lung.

Infections
    Tuberculosis
    Fungus infections
    Viral pneumonia
    Bacterial (nocardia)
Metastatic tumour (thyroid, melanoma, adenocarcinoma)
Inhalational disease (silicosis, coal-worker's pneumoconiosis,
    allergic alveolitis)
Sarcoidosis
Bronchiolitis

Table 21. Diffuse fine reticular pattern.

Acute
    Oedema (interstitial oedema, ARDS)
    Infection (viral, mycoplasma, *Pneumocystis carinii*)

Chronic
    Chronic oedema
    Lymphangitic spread of tumour
    Lymphatic obstruction (mediastinal mass, hilar lymph nodes)
    Collagen vascular diseases (rheumatoid arthritis, scleroderma)
    Idiopathic interstitial lung disease (IPF, LIP, DIP)
    Granulomatous disease (sarcoidosis, eosinophilic granuloma)
    Lymphoma, leukaemia
    Inhalational disease (asbestosis, talcosis, silicosis, allergic
        alveolitis)
    Other (amyloidosis, alveolar proteinosis, lymphangiomyomatosis,
        increased markings emphysema)

ARDS, acute respiratory distress syndrome; IPF, idiopathic pulmonary fibrosis; LIP, lymphoid interstitial pneumonia; DIP, desquamative interstitial pneumonia.

Fine nodular opacities Fine nodular opacities can be defined as opacities with a diameter up to 3–4 mm (CDROMFig. 23). A nodular pattern with nodules smaller than 3 mm is usually called a miliary pattern. These miliary nodules are marginally detectable radiographically and may require CT. The nodules in this pattern may be caused by either small, sharply defined interstitial nodules or minimal involvement of the distal airspaces.[80,81]

In the case of ill-defined small nodules, one should think about pulmonary oedema, exudates and haemorrhage. Seeing ill-defined nodules should prompt examination of the radiograph for other signs of airspace-filling disease.

Sharply defined or discrete opacities suggest that the nodules are more likely to be interstitial (Table 20).

Linear opacities Linear opacities in the lung can be caused by vascular shadows, bronchial shadows, focal line shadows and interstitial line shadows (reticular pattern).[82–85]

Vascular shadows appear when vessels that are normally below the radiographic threshold of resolution become visible when dilated. This is seen in cardiac failure, cardiogenic pulmonary oedema and pulmonary hyperperfusion secondary to a left-to-right shunt (CDROMFig. 24).

Bronchial shadows occur when the bronchial wall is thickened and are seen in acute and chronic bronchitis. Ring shadows and tramline opacities are seen (CDROMFig. 25a) that respectively enlarge and become more widely separated when bronchiectasis develops (CDROMFig. 25b).

Focal line shadows are homogeneous linear or band-like densities. They have sharper edges than vascular markings and are frequently solitary. Causes are (thickened) interlobar fissures viewed tangentially, pulmonary scars and discoid atelectasis.

Interstitial line shadows: the diffuse fine reticular pattern. This pattern is one of the most reliable patterns for identifying diffuse interstitial lung disease (Table 21). In the early stage of disease, it can be difficult to distinguish this pattern from the normal pattern of blood vessels or from the vascular shadow pattern.[86] The reticular pattern refers to a fine network of markings that may be diffusely distributed through both lungs. It is due to the superposition of thickened interlobular septa (CDROMFig. 26). A very reliable sign to identify this linear interstitial pattern is the identification of Kerley-B lines.[54,87,88] These are short lines that are perpendicular to the pleura and contiguous with it and are best seen in the costophrenic angles on a PA chest radiograph. They are caused by thickening of the interlobular septa. These septa contain lymph vessels, pulmonary veins and interstitial tissue. Pathological thickening of these septa reflects pathology in one or more of these structures. Kerley-A and Kerley-C lines have also been described. While Kerley-A lines also correspond to thickened interlobular septa in the deep and apical part of the lungs, the anatomical definition of Kerley-C lines is not well defined.[54]

Besides a reticular pattern, other radiographic features characterizing interstitial lung disease can also be present. These include ill-defined hilar and vascular structures, accentuation of the interlobar fissures, a reticulonodular pattern and the honeycomb pattern. Ill-defined hilar and vascular structures are caused by the infiltration or thickening of the perivascular connective tissue, which also involves the adjacent alveoli, obscuring the normally sharp boundary between the vascular shadows and the aerated lung. Accentuation of the interlobar fissures is caused by infiltration or fibrosis of the subpleural connective tissues. The reticulonodular pattern is a reticular pattern combined with reticular nodulation. These small nodules are usually formed by small nodules in the interstitium but may also represent a summation effect caused by intersecting shadows. The honeycomb pattern is a coarse reticular pattern that characterizes the end stage of fibrosis.

Table 22. Causes of pulmonary hyperlucency.

Bilateral
  Overexposure
  Bilateral mastectomy
  Thin body status
  Emphysema
  Acute asthmatic attack
  Pulmonary embolism

Unilateral
  Rotation of the patient
  Mastectomy
  Muscular atrophy or absence
  Pneumothorax, subcutaneous emphysema
  Pulmonary embolism
  Emphysema
  Bronchial obstruction (neoplastic, granulomatous, mucocoele, foreign body)
  Bronchiolitis obliterans
  Compensatory overaeration

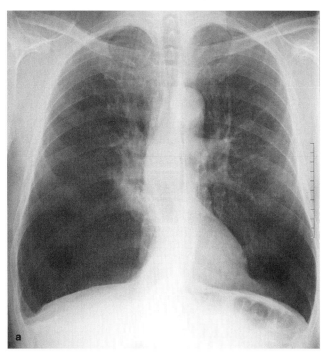

Figure 27. Bilateral lucent lungs. (a) PA chest radiograph. Reduction in calibre and number and abnormal spreading of the pulmonary vessels caused by overinflation in a patient with severe emphysema.

Table 23. Solitary and multiple lucent defects.

Infection (pyogenic, aspiration, fungal, tuberculosis)
Neoplasm (primary lung tumour, metastasis)
Vascular (rheumatoid, Wegener's granulomatosis, infarct, septic emboli)
Inhalation (excavating pseudotumour in silicosis and coal-miner's pneumoconiosis)
Pneumatocoele
Congenital cysts
Bullous emphysema
Cystic bronchiectasis
Honeycomb lung

Abnormal decrease in lung density

Unilateral or bilateral lucent lungs The first step in the evaluation of the apparently hyperlucent lung is to check whether this hyperlucency is really caused by lung disease and is not the result of a bad radiological technique or an extrapulmonary abnormality. An overexposed chest radiograph, a rotated patient or the absence of normal soft tissues of the chest wall can cause an apparent increase in lucency of one or both lungs. Real hyperlucency of the lung, whether generalized or regional, reflects a change in the pulmonary vascularity and is caused by a reduction in the calibre and number of the intrapulmonary vessels or by hyperinflation of the lung, which causes spreading (and reduced overall density) of the vascular shadows[89] (Fig. 27a, CDROMFig. 27b). The pulmonary and extrapulmonary causes of unilateral and bilateral pulmonary hyperlucency are listed in Table 22.

Solitary and multiple lucent defects Many diseases may give rise to the presence of one localized or multiple lucent lung defects surrounded by a band of opacity.[90,91] These may range from a few millimetres to several centimetres. Cavities, cysts, pneumatocoeles and bullae are terms that are often used to describe these 'holes' in the lung and reflect different pathogeneses. A cavity is formed when pus from an inflammatory process or liquefied necrotic material from a tumour erodes into a bronchus and is expectorated (CDROMFig. 28). A cyst usually presents as a ring shadow and is considered to be congenital or developmental. A pneumatocoele, especially in the early stage of the disease, cannot always be differentiated from a cavity. A pneumatocoele characteristically occurs in the healing phase of the disease, and the hole appears radiographically to enlarge while the patient appears to improve clinically.[92] The pathological mechanism has not yet been clearly defined. One postulate is that they are secondary to small airway obstruction with a sleeve valve mechanism that results in localized air trapping. Others believe that pneumatocoeles result from an alteration of the normal pulmonary elasticity. Bullae usually present as localized small or large areas of decreased density with a thin or a hardly perceptible wall. Finally, it should be emphasized that pseudocavities can also occur when extrapulmonary structures such as diaphragmatic hernias mimic a bulla or a cavity. Dilated bronchi may also be mistaken for cystic lesions (CDROMFig. 25) (Table 23).

Table 24. Hilar enlargement.

Large pulmonary vessels
    Pulmonary arterial hypertension
    Left-sided heart failure
    Pulmonary embolism
    Cardiac shunts

Hilar masses
    Unilateral
        neoplasm (primary, metastases, lymphoma)
        inflammatory lymph node enlargement (infection, sarcoidosis)
        congenital cysts
    Bilateral
        neoplasm (lymphoma, metastases, primary)
        inflammatory lymph node enlargement (sarcoidosis, silicosis)

Pathology of the hilum

Hilar enlargement, hilar mass The decision on the presence of an abnormal hilum is not always easy and is based on an abnormal increase in density and on recognizing an alteration in the configuration. Comparison with previous chest radiographs is very helpful in depicting an abnormal hilum. However, if not available, comparison with the opposite hilum is also a reliable method for detecting a subtle hilar abnormality. The next step is to determine whether the abnormal hilum is caused by an enlarged vascular structure or by one or more solid masses (CDROMFig. 29). This requires good understanding of the anatomy of the hilum on a PA and lateral chest radiograph. The most common causes of hilar enlargement caused by either abnormal vascular structures or a mass are shown in Table 24.[93]

The association of hilar adenopathy and the presence of a fine reticular pattern can be helpful in making a more specific differential diagnosis. This combination is seen in sarcoidosis, lymphoma and leukaemia, silicosis, metastases and some primary lung tumours.

Small hilar shadow Reduction in size of one or both hila is the result of a reduction in size of the vascular structures. Potential causes are surgery (lobectomy) (CDROMFig. 30), congenital aplasia of the pulmonary artery, oligaemia of a lobe or an entire lung (McLeod syndrome, emphysema), lobar collapse with hilum displacement behind the heart, normal variant, rotation (scoliosis, poor positioning) and, more rarely, a tumour or inflammatory process blocking a pulmonary artery.

Ill-defined hilar structures A hilar haze occurs when the hilar contours are partially obscured. Potential causes are pulmonary congestion and oedema, bronchial infection (CDROMFig. 31), thickening of the peribronchovascular interstitium, as seen, for example, in interstitial lung disease, and abutment of an ill-defined lung opacity on the hilum.

Table 25. Pulmonary calcifications.

Inflammation
    Tuberculosis
    Parenchymal scarring
    Sarcoidosis
    Varicella pneumonia
    Parasitism, histoplasmosis, coccidioidomycosis

Neoplasm
    Hamartoma
    Bronchial carcinoma
    Metastases (osteogenic sarcoma, chondrosarcoma, ovarian and thyroid carcinoma)

Vascular
    Thrombus
    Haemosiderosis
    Pulmonary arteriosclerosis

Miscellaneous
    Calcified bronchial cartilage
    Pneumoconiosis
    Bronchogenic cyst
    Alveolar microlithiasis
    Metabolic calcification

Pulmonary calcifications

Pulmonary calcifications are a very common finding on chest radiographs and can be either dystrophic, signifying an inactive or degenerative process, or metastatic (metabolic), which are less common and occur in patients with abnormalities of calcium metabolism. The most frequently occurring causes of pulmonary calcifications are listed in Table 25.[94,95]

Computerized tomography

Computerized tomography is, as already mentioned in the introduction, the second most important imaging modality for imaging of the lungs. Lung cancer detection and staging is probably the most frequent indication for performing a CT examination of the lungs. CT is indeed currently the procedure of choice for confirmation and evaluation of suspected pulmonary nodules.[96–98] It provides exact localization of the nodule and is reliable for the detection of other radiological features including calcification, cavitation and speculated borders.[99] The technique has been used to differentiate between benign and malignant solitary nodules but, although differences in enhancement after administration of intravenous contrast are seen that can allow differentiation between tumours and granulomas, measurement of nodule density is not performed routinely in every radiology department.[100,101]

When the diagnosis of a malignant mass is made, CT adds important information about the extent of the tumour (e.g.

extension into the mediastinum, the chest wall) and is also useful for detecting additional abnormalities (e.g. retro-obstructive atelectasis, hilar and mediastinal adenopathy, other nodules).[102]

As mentioned earlier, the higher diagnostic accuracy of HRCT is related to a better recognition of the pattern and of the distribution of disease.[103–107] Together with the clinical findings and the possible presence of associated radiological findings such as pleural effusion and enlarged lymph nodes, these are the major components used to make the diagnosis. Lung disease can be characterized by, either or in combination, by the presence of high- and low-attenuation lung changes. In the group of high-attenuation lung diseases, four patterns can be recognized: ground-glass opacity, consolidation, nodular pattern and reticular pattern. Lung destruction and emphysema, cystic airspaces, decreased lung attenuation, mosaic perfusion and air trapping belong to the group of low-attenuation lung changes. Because of its high detail, HRCT is often able to determine the exact localization and distribution pattern of the disease. It is possible to decide more accurately on the axial, central or peripheral localization of disease, on the preference for the apical or basal lung parts or on the predominant involvement of the dependent versus the non-dependent lung areas. Often, it also becomes possible to decide whether the disease shows a predominant (peri)lymphatic, an airway or a vascular distribution.[108] Knowledge of the secondary pulmonary lobule and its components is very important for this purpose. The secondary pulmonary lobule is defined as the smallest portion of the lung that is surrounded by connective tissue septa.[109] It is irregularly polyhedral and has a diameter between 0.5 and 3 cm. An important feature of this secondary pulmonary lobule is the 'core structure' comprising the supplying terminal bronchiole and the accompanying pulmonary artery branch, surrounded by lymph vessels. The secondary pulmonary lobules are demarcated by the 'interlobular septa' containing pulmonary veins, lymphatics and connective tissue stroma. Between the 'core' structures and the interlobular septa, numerous alveolar sacs, respiratory bronchioles and capillaries are found.

Ground-glass opacity

Ground-glass opacity is defined as a hazy increase in density of the lung with preservation of bronchial and vascular margins[110–112] (Fig. 32). Ground-glass opacities can be regional, multifocal patchy and diffuse, can be homogeneous or heterogeneous and can have sharp or blurred margins. The diseases that are characterized by the presence of ground-glass opacity are listed in Table 26.

Lung consolidation

Lung consolidation is characterized by an increase in pulmonary parenchymal attenuation that obscures the margins of the vessels and airway walls. The higher density and especially the obscuration of vessels and airway walls distinguish

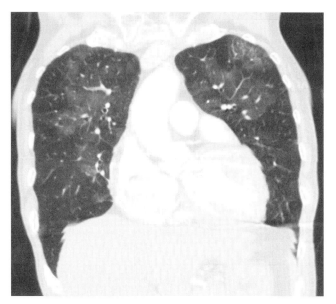

Figure 32. Multifocal patchy ground-glass opacity caused by pulmonary infection.

Table 26. Ground-glass opacity.

Acute
  Acute interstitial pneumonia
  ARDS
  Pulmonary oedema
  Pulmonary haemorrhage
  Pneumonia (viral, mycoplasma pneumonia, *Pneumocystis carinii*)
  Acute eosinophilic pneumonia
  Radiation pneumonitis

Subacute or chronic
  Hypersensitivity pneumonitis
  Organizing pneumonia (BOOP, COP)
  Idiopathic interstitial lung disease
    UIP
    NSIP
    DIP
    RBILD
  Chronic eosinophilic pneumonia
  Alveolar proteinosis
  Bronchoalveolar carcinoma
  Mosaic perfusion
  Lung fibrosis

Mimics
  Gravity- and expiration-induced increase in lung density

ARDS, acute respiratory distress syndrome; BOOP, bronchiolitis obliterans organizing pneumonia; COP, cryptogenic organizing pueumonia; UIP, usual interstitial pneumonia; NSIP, non-specific interstitial pneumonia; DIP, desquamative interstitial pneumonia; RBILD, respiratory bronchiolitis-associated interstitial lung disease.

Table 27. Lung consolidation.

Acute
  Acute interstitial pneumonia
  ARDS
  Pulmonary oedema
  Pulmonary haemorrhage
  Pneumonia (bacterial, mycoplasma pneumonia, *Pneumocystis carinii*)
  Acute eosinophilic pneumonia
  Radiation pneumonitis

Subacute/chronic
  Organizing pneumonia (BOOP, COP)
  Bronchoalveolar carcinoma
  Lymphoma
  Sarcoidosis
  Chronic eosinophilic pneumonia
  Idiopathic interstitial lung disease
    IPF
    NSIP
  Lipid pneumonia

ARDS, acute respiratory distress syndrome; BOOP, bronchiolitis obliterans organizing pneumonia; COP, cryptogenic organizing pneumonia; IPF, idiopathic pulmonary fibrosis; NSIP, non-specific interstitial pneumonia.

this pattern from the ground-glass pattern. Consolidation can be regional, multifocal, patchy or diffuse, may have sharp or blurred edges, is usually homogeneous but can show an air bronchogram[113–117] (Fig. 33). Table 27 lists diseases that are frequently associated with the presence of lung consolidation.

Linear opacities
There are many diseases that cause the appearance of linear opacities in the lung. According to their localization, they can be divided into (peri)bronchovascular thickening, interlobular septal lines, intralobular lines, subpleural thickening and 'other' linear opacities.

Honeycombing or honeycomb lung is a reticular pattern typically consisting of linear opacities and cystic airspaces that allows a confident diagnosis of lung fibrosis.[118,119]

(Peri)bronchovascular thickening The linear opacities belonging to this pattern are in close relationship to the bronchovascular structures that extend from the level of the pulmonary hila into the peripheral lung, where they correspond with centrilobular arterioles and bronchioles (Table 28). They are usually perceived on CT as an increase in bronchial or bronchiolar wall thickness, but are caused not only by thickening of the bronchial or bronchiolar wall but also by thickening of the peribronchovascular or 'axial' interstitium[120–122] (Fig. 34) and sometimes by an increase in diameter of the pulmonary artery branches. Enlarged bronchovascular structures present as tramlines or ring shadows when perpendicular to the scan-

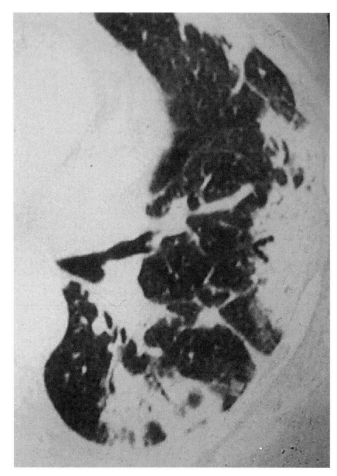

Figure 33. Multifocal peripheral areas of lung consolidation caused by cryptogenic organizing pneumonia. Notice the presence of an air bronchogram in the lesions.

Table 28. (Peri)bronchovascular thickening.

Bronchial and bronchiolar wall
  Bronchitis/bronchiolitis
  Bronchiectasis/broncholectasis

Artery/arterioles
  Increased perfusion (part of mosaic perfusion)
  Pulmonary hypertension
  Venous congestion

Peribronchovascular interstitium
  Lymphangitic spread of tumour
  Lymphoma
  Leukaemia
  Pulmonary oedema
  Sarcoidosis
  Silicosis
  Chronic hypersensitivity pneumonitis
  IPF, NSIP, LIP

IPF, idiopathic pulmonary fibrosis; NSIP, non-specific interstitial pneumonia; LIP, lymphoid interstitial pneumonia.

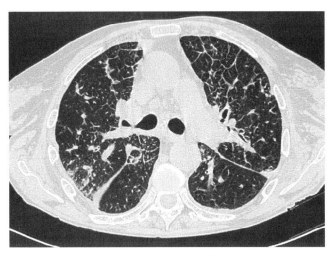

Figure 34. Peribronchovascular and septal lines in a patient with venous congestion and hydrostatic pulmonary oedema.

Table 29. Septal lines.

Lymphangitic spread of tumour
Lymphoma
Leukaemia
Hydrostatic pulmonary oedema
Central venous pulmonary obstruction
Increased lymphatic flow
(Sarcoidosis: usually nodular)
Pulmonary haemorrhage
Interstitial fibrosis (IPF)
Amyloidosis
Pneumonia (viral, PCP)

IPF, idiopathic pulmonary fibrosis; PCP, *Pneumocystis carinii* pneumonia.

ning plane; the smaller bronchovascular structures usually present as lines or dots when perpendicular to the scanning plane. It should be emphasized that these small lines or dots, when corresponding with the terminal arterioles and bronchioles, are located in the centre of the secondary pulmonary lobule and can be responsible for the development of intralobular lines (Table 31).

Septal lines Septal lines are caused by a thickening of the interlobular septa and can be seen in the presence of interstitial fluid (Fig. 34), cellular infiltration or fibrosis. Visibility of more than a few septal lines almost always indicates abnormality (Table 29).[123,124]

The combination of septal lines and ground-glass opacity results in an appearance termed crazy paving.[125,126] Although first described in patients with alveolar proteinosis, it is also seen in a variety of patients with other diseases (Table 30) (CDROMFig. 35).

Table 30. Crazy paving.

Alveolar proteinosis
Diffuse alveolar damage (superposed on UIP)
ARDS
(Cardiogenic) pulmonary oedema
Lymphatic obstruction
Drug-induced pneumonia
Pulmonary haemorrhage
Acute and chronic eosinophilic pneumonia
Organizing pneumonia (COP, BOOP)
Pneumonia (*P. carinii*, mycoplasma, bacterial)
Radiation pneumonitis
NSIP
Churg–Strauss syndrome

UIP, usual interstitial pneumonia; ARDS, acute respiratory distress syndrome; COP, cryptogenic organizing pneumonia; BOOP, bronchiolitis obliterans organizing pneumonia; NSIP, non-specific interstitial pneumonia.

Intralobular lines Intralobular lines are linear opacities located within the borders of the secondary pulmonary lobule. They can be the result of thickening of the intralobular interstitium (Fig. 36) and of the distal peribronchovascular interstitium (and are then part of the peribronchovascular pattern), but can also be the result of involvement of the small airways and arterioles[105,106,118,127]. When caused by thickening of the intralobular interstitium, a fine reticular pattern is seen with the lines separated by a few millimetres. Small airway involvement and involvement of the arterioles usually present as small branching lines spreading out from the centre to the periphery of the secondary pulmonary lobule (Table 31).[128]

Subpleural thickening Thickening of the subpleural interstitium occurs in the same diseases as interlobular septal thickening and is often associated with it (Table 29). It is best appreciated when the subpleural interstitium of the lung fissures is involved, when it presents as a thickening of this fissure. It is a frequent finding in idiopathic pulmonary fibrosis (IPF)[129] (CDROMFig. 37).

Other linear opacities The term parenchymal band has been used to describe a tapering, reticular opacity, usually several millimetres in thickness and from 2 to 5 cm in length in patients with atelectasis, pulmonary fibrosis or other causes of interstitial thickening. In some patients, these bands are continuous with septal thickening. They are frequently seen in patients with sarcoidosis, silicosis, scarring from previous tuberculosis and asbestosis.[106,130,131]

Subpleural curvilinear opacities were first described in patients with asbestosis but are also seen in patients with IPF and other causes of usual interstitial pneumonia (UIP). Transient subpleural lines are seen as a result of atelectasis in the dependent lung.[130,131]

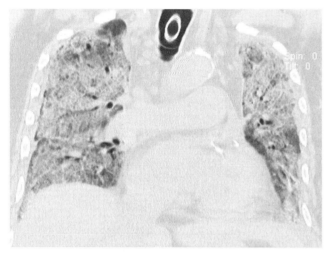

Figure 36. Ground-glass opacity and intralobular lines in a patient with acute respiratory distress syndrome (ARDS).

All other lines that cannot be characterized in one of the groups mentioned above are usually called irregular linear opacities and usually represent irregular areas of fibrosis.[132,133]

Honeycombing Honeycombing indicates the presence of end-stage lung fibrosis.[119,134,135] On HRCT, air-filled cystic structures averaging 1 cm in diameter are seen with clearly definable walls (CDROMFig. 37). The walls of these honeycomb cysts can be differentiated from intralobular lines because, in the latter, the reticulations are thinner and the spaces between the lines have lung density instead of air density. In the same way, the differential diagnosis between a reticular pattern caused by septal lines is based on the fact that this pattern is larger than the honeycombing pattern (Table 32).

Nodular opacities

A nodular opacity is defined as a rounded opacity, at least moderately well defined, with a maximum diameter of 3 cm. The (HR)CT assessment of multiple nodular opacities is predominantly based on their appearance (ill-defined or well-defined) and distribution (Tables 33 and 34).[136,137,138]

Recognizing the distribution pattern of the nodular opacities is extremely helpful in the differential diagnosis:

1 The (peri)lymphatic distribution means that the nodules can be found predominantly in relation to the pulmonary lymphatics, i.e. the perihilar peribronchovascular interstitium, the interlobular septa, the subpleural regions and the centrilobular interstitium (CDROMFig. 38).

2 Centrilobular opacities can be located either in the interstitium or in the airspaces, vary in size from a few millimetres to 1 cm and may be dense and homogeneous or of ground-glass density. When located in the airspace, the nodules are usually poorly defined and are often associated with an increased prominence and size of the centrilobular branching structures

Table 31. Intralobular lines.

Small airway involvement
    Infectious bronchiolitis (viral, mycoplasma, aspergillus, bacterial, tuberculosis)
    Asthma
    Chronic bronchitis
    Aspiration
    Acute fume and toxic exposure
    Cystic fibrosis
    Bronchoalveolar carcinoma
    Diffuse and interstitial lung diseases with a component of small airway involvement (RA, Sjögren, panbronchiolitis, smoking-associated bronchiolar disease, hypersensitivity pneumonitis)
    Organizing pneumonia

Involvement of the arterioles
    Vasculitis
    Haemorrhage
    Fat embolism
    Tumour thrombotic microangiopathy

Thickening of the intralobular interstitium
    Idiopathic interstitial lung disease
        IPF
        NSIP
        DIP
        Acute interstitial pneumonia
    Hypersensitivity pneumonitis
    Asbestosis
    Lymphangitic spread of tumour
    Leukaemia
    Lymphoma
    Oedema

RA, rheumatoid arthritis; IPF, idiopathic pulmonary fibrosis; NSIP, non-specific interstitial pneumonia; DIP, desquamative interstitial pneumonia.

Table 32. Honeycombing.

Idiopathic interstitial pneumonia
    IPF
    NSIP
    DIP
Organizing pneumonia
Collagen vascular diseases
Asbestosis
Chronic hypersensitivity pneumonitis
Sarcoidosis

IPF, idiopathic pulmonary fibrosis; NSIP, non-specific interstitial pneumonia; DIP, desquamative interstitial pneumonia.

Table 33. Appearance of nodular opacities.

> Sharply defined
>> Metastases
>> Sarcoidosis
>> Silicosis, coal-miner's pneumoconiosis
>> Langerhans cell histiocytosis
>> Amyloidosis
>> Bronchoalveolar carcinoma
>
> Ill-defined
>> Miliary tuberculosis
>> Bronchiolitis
>> Hypersensitivity pneumonitis
>> Alveolar bleeding
>> Bronchoalveolar carcinoma

Table 34. Nodular opacities.

Septal distribution
 Sarcoidosis
 Silicosis, coal-miner's pneumoconiosis
 Lymphangitic spread of tumour (usually associated with septal lines)

Centrilobular distribution
 Sarcoidosis
 Silicosis, coal-miner's pneumoconiosis
 Lymphangitic spread of tumour (usually associated with septal lines)
 Hypersensitivity pneumonitis (ill-defined, ground-glass)
 Bronchiolitis
  infectious: tuberculosis (endobronchial spread) (well- or ill-defined, dens)
  respiratory bronchiolitis (ill-defined, ground-glass)
  follicular bronchiolitis (well-defined, dens)
  allergic bronchopulmonary aspergillosis (ill-defined, ground-glass)
 Viral pneumonia (ill-defined, ground-glass)
 Cystic fibrosis (well- or ill-defined, dens)
 Langerhans cell histiocytosis (well-defined, dens)
 Organizing pneumonia (well- or ill-defined, dens or ground-glass)
 Endobronchial spread of tumour (well-defined, dens)
 Oedema (ill-defined, ground-glass)
 Haemorrhage (ill-defined, ground-glass)
 Vasculitis (ill-defined, ground-glass)

Random distribution
 Miliary infection (tuberculosis, fungus) (well-defined, dens)
 Haematogenous metastases (well-defined, dens)

and with an increased visibility and dilatation of the bronchioles and bronchi. In combination, these signs can produce a pattern that is described as 'tree in bud' (Fig. 39).

3 Sometimes, the nodules seem to be randomly distributed

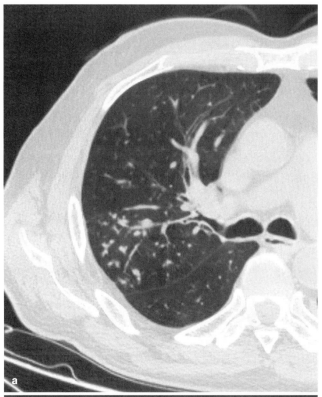
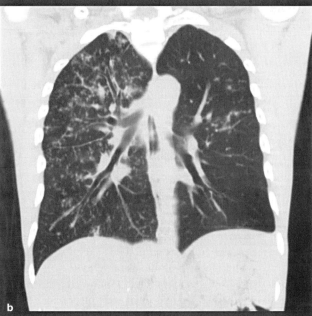

Figure 39. Centrilobular nodules and branching lines in two patients (a and b) with infectious bronchiolitis. In combination with the increased visibility and slight dilatation of the bronchioles and bronchi, these signs produce the 'tree in bud' sign (b).

in relation to the structures of the secondary pulmonary lobule and, although the causes of this pattern are limited, it is sometimes difficult to differentiate from the perilymphatic or centrilobular pattern especially when numerous nodules are present (CDROMFig. 40).

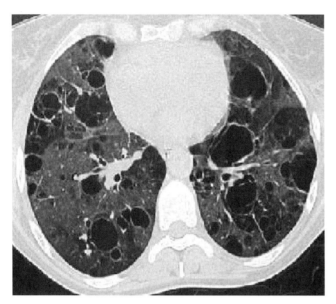

Figure 41. Cystic airspace pattern in a patient with lymphangioleiomyomatosis.

Table 35. Diseases with development of cystic airspaces.

Honeycombing
Cystic bronchiectasis
Lymphangioleiomyomatosis
Langerhans cell histiocytosis
Lymphocytic interstitial pneumonia
Pneumatocoeles

Other often helpful signs in the differential diagnosis are the density of the nodules, which can be a soft-tissue or a ground-glass density, and the nodule size.[139]

Cystic airspaces

The term cystic airspace is used to describe an air-containing lesion surrounded by a wall of variable thickness (Fig. 41). The wall may be thin or thick and, although the lumen usually contains air, it may also contain liquid, solid or semi-solid material.[106,140,141] This term is not usually used to describe emphysematous lung changes. Table 35 shows the differential diagnosis of lung diseases associated with the presence of cystic airspaces.[142]

Emphysema

The diagnosis of emphysema on CT is based on the presence of areas of abnormally low attenuation, typically without a visible wall, which reflect the presence of enlarged airspaces as a result of parenchymal destruction.[143–146]

Centrilobular emphysema is characterized by the presence of localized areas of very low attenuation measuring a few millimetres in diameter and located in the central portion of the secondary pulmonary lobule.[128,147,148] As the emphysema becomes more severe, these areas become confluent, and the centrilobular distribution is less apparent (CDROMFig. 42). At this stage, it may be difficult to differentiate centrilobular from panlobular emphysema. However, centrilobular emphysema typically affects the lungs unevenly, so that the typical and diagnostic early changes can usually also be found. In addition, there is usually an upper zonal predominance.[149]

The HRCT findings of panlobular emphysema typically consist of widespread areas of abnormally low attenuation and decreased vascularity most severe in the lower lobes.[150,151] In severe panlobular emphysema, the lung destruction and the reduction in vascular markings become extensive and can easily be differentiated from normal lung parenchyma. However, mild and even moderately severe disease can be very subtle and difficult to detect. Sometimes, the differential diagnosis with areas of hypoperfusion caused by small airways or vascular obstruction can be difficult.

In paraseptal emphysema, (HR)CT shows localized areas of low attenuation adjacent to interlobular septa, large bronchi and vessels, and pleura. Even mild paraseptal emphysema is easily detected in most cases because it is adjacent to high-density structures.

Cicatricial emphysema shows no consistent relationship to any portion of the secondary pulmonary lobule and is always associated with fibrosis.

Finally, bullae are manifested on HRCT as thin-walled, sharply defined areas of avascularity and, in the vast majority of patients, are associated with concomitant centrilobular and less frequently panlobular emphysema.[152]

Decreased lung attenuation, mosaic attenuation and air trapping

Areas of decreased density of the lung parenchyma and mosaic attenuation The reduction in the lung attenuation is an indirect sign of decrease of perfusion in the small vessels and capillaries that are beyond the resolution of HRCT (CDROM-Fig. 43).

These areas can be patchy or can be widespread and are usually poorly defined but can have a well-demarcated geographical outline as well. Redistribution of blood flow to the normal surrounding area causes increased density of these areas. In this way, a patchwork of regions of varied attenuation develops. These density differences between different adjacent lung areas give rise to the term 'mosaic attenuation'.[153]

Major features of the mosaic attenuation pattern are the difference in lung attenuation between the affected and non-affected lung areas and also the difference in vessel size in these areas: that is why the term 'mosaic perfusion' is also used to describe this entity (CDROMFig. 44). The reduction of the calibre of the larger vessels in the low-attenuation areas is often directly visible. Because of redistribution of flow to the normal areas, vessel calibre in these areas is typically increased. A very important differential diagnostic feature with emphysema is the fact that the vessels are not distorted. Although correct here, the term mosaic perfusion is not always correct. It should not be used in those cases where the inhomogeneous attenuation of the lung parenchyma is caused by a patchy distribution of the lung disease, for example when multiple areas of ground-glass opacity can be recognized in the lung. Mosaic attenuation is often the result of bronchiolar obstruction causing hypoxic vasoconstriction but can also be caused by direct vascular obstruction. The obstructed small vessels are then responsible for the low-attenuation areas while redistribution of blood to surrounding normal lung causes increased attenuation. In most cases of vascular disease leading to mosaic perfusion on HRCT, the cause is chronic thromboembolic disease or pulmonary artery hypertension. The differential diagnosis between a bronchiolar and a vascular cause is sometimes possible and based on the presence or absence of air trapping on expiratory CT respectively (CDROMFig. 44). However, the pattern has also been described in patients with primary pulmonary artery hypertension, pulmonary capillary haemangiomatosis, pulmonary venoocclusive disease, polyarteritis nodosa, scleroderma and intimal sarcoma of the pulmonary arteries.[153–157]

Air trapping at expiratory CT Air trapping at expiratory CT is defined as 'retention of excess gas (air) in all or part of the lung, especially during expiration, either as a result of complete or partial airway obstruction or as a result of local abnormalities in pulmonary compliance'.[106] The air is trapped and the cross-sectional areas of the affected parts of the lung do not decrease in size on expiratory CT. Usually, the regional inhomogenicity of the lung density (mosaic attenuation) seen at end-inspiration HRCT scans is accentuated on sections obtained at end, or during, expiration because the high-attenuation areas increase in density while the low-attenuation areas remain unchanged (CDROMFig. 44). Sometimes, however, the areas of decreased attenuation are not visible on inspiratory CT but are only detectable on expiratory CT when normal areas decrease in size and increase in density and the affected areas remain more or less unchanged.[158–162] As mentioned earlier, looking for air trapping on expiratory CT may be helpful in differentiating between occlusive vascular diseases and bronchiolar disease as a cause of mosaic attenuation. When caused by bronchiolar obstruction, mosaic perfusion is accentuated on expiratory CT because the low-attenuation areas show air trapping. In the case of occlusive vascular disease, air trapping does not usually occur.[163,164]

It should be emphasized that, in about 50–80% of individuals with normal pulmonary function tests, one or more areas of air trapping often limited to one or a few adjacent secondary pulmonary lobules can be seen.[162,165] These areas of air trapping are predominantly seen in the dependent parts of the lower lobes.[166] The frequency increases with age while severity increases with age and smoking.[162,166] Air trapping is usually

Table 36. Diseases associated with areas of low attenuation, mosaic perfusion and air trapping on expiratory HRCT.

Constrictive bronchiolitis (bronchiolitis obliterans)
  Idiopathic (rare)
  Healed infections (especially viral and mycoplasma)
  Component of chronic bronchitis, cystic fibrosis, bronchiectasis
  Inhalation of toxin or fume (including cigarette smoke)
  Connective tissue diseases (rheumatoid arthritis, Sjögren)
  Transplant-associated airway injury (bone marrow, heart–lung, lung)
  Drug reaction (penicillamine)
  Other conditions (inflammatory bowl disease)
Hypersensitivity pneumonitis
Sarcoidosis
Asthma
Acute pulmonary embolism
Vasculitis

considered to be abnormal when it affects a volume of lung equal to or greater than a pulmonary segment[167] (Table 36). It should be further emphasized that air trapping can also be a component of diffuse lung disease in which bronchiolar narrowing is caused by bronchiolar spasm or by granulomatous involvement of the bronchiolar wall.

References

1 Reeder MM (ed.). *Reeder and Felson's Gamuts in Radiology*, 4th edn. New York, Springer Verlag, 2003.
2 Reed JC (ed.). *Chest Radiology*, 5th edn. Mosby, 2003.
3 Kreel L. Computed tomography of the thorax. *Radiol Clin North Am* 1978; **16**:575–84.
4 Rosenblum LJ, Mauceri RA, Wellenstein DE *et al.* Computed tomography of the lung. A preliminary report. *Radiology* 1978; **129**:521–4.
5 Kalender WA, Polacin A, Süss C. A comparison of conventional and spiral CT: an experimental study on detection of spherical lesions. *J Comput Assist Tomogr* 1994; **18**:167–76.
6 Kalender WA, Seissler W, Vock P. Single-breath-hold spiral volumetric CT by continuous patient translation and scanner rotation. *Radiology* 1989; **173**(P):414.
7 Klingenbeck-Regn K, Schaller S, Flohr T *et al.* Subsecond multislice computed tomography: basics and applications. *Eur J Radiol* 1999; **31**:110–24.
8 Silverman PM, Kalender WA, Hazle JD. Common terminology for single and multislice helical CT. *Am J Radiol* 2001; **176**:1135–6.
9 Ellis R. Incomplete border sign of extrapleural masses. *JAMA* 1977; **237**:2748.
10 Jeung MY, Gangi A, Gasser B *et al.* Imaging of chest wall disorders. *Radiographics* 1999; **19**:617–37.
11 Felson B, Jacobson HG. Chest wall lesions mimicking intrapulmonary pathological conditions. *JAMA* 1978; **239**:535–6.
12 Sargent EN, Turner AF, Jacobson G. Superior marginal rib defects: an etiologic classification. *Am J Roentgenol* 1969; **106**:491–505.
13 Pearlberg JL, Sandler MA, Beute GH *et al.* Limitations of CT in evaluation of neoplasms involving chest wall. *J Comput Assist Tomogr* 1987; **11**:290–3.
14 Wechsler RJ. Cross-sectional imaging of the chest wall. *J Thorac Imaging* 1989; **4**:29–40.

15 Kuhlman JE, Bouchardy L, Fishman EK, Zerhouni EA. CT and MR imaging evaluation of chest wall disorders. *Radiographics* 1994; **14**:571–95.

16 Fortier M, Mayo JR, Swensen SJ et al. MR imaging of chest wall lesions. *Radiographics* 1994; **14**:597–606.

17 Mathis G. Thorax sonography. Part I: Chest wall and pleura. *Ultrasound Med Biol* 1997; **23**:1131–9.

18 Fokin AA, Robicsek F. Poland's syndrome revisited. *Ann Thorac Surg* 2002; **74**:2218–25.

19 Samlaska CP, Maggio KL. Subcutaneous emphysema. *Adv Dermatol* 1996; **11**:117–52.

20 McLoud TC, Flower CDR. Imaging the pleura: sonography, CT, and MR imaging. *Am J Roentgenol* 1991; **156**:1145–53.

21 Muller NL. Imaging of the pleura. *Radiology* 1993; **186**:297–309.

22 Vix VA. Roentgenographic manifestations of pleural disease. *Semin Roentgenol* 1977; **12**:277–86.

23 Theros EG, Feigin DS. Pleural tumors and pulmonary tumors: differential diagnosis. *Semin Roentgenol* 1977; **12**:239–47.

24 Dynes MC, White EM, Fry WA et al. Imaging manifestations of pleural tumors. *Radiographics* 1992; **12**:1191–1201.

25 England DM, Hochholzer L, McCarthy MJ. Localized benign and malignant fibrous tumors of the pleura. A clinicopathological review of 223 cases. *Am J Surg Pathol* 1989; **13**:640–58.

26 Epler GR, McLoud TC, Munn CS et al. Pleural lipoma: a diagnosis by computed tomography. *Chest* 1986; **90**:265.

27 Bittner RC, Schorner W, Loddenkemper C et al. Pleural diseases in magnetic resonance tomography. *Pneumologie* 1992; **46**:612–20.

28 Ruskin JA, Gurney JW, Thorsen MK, Goodman LR. Detection of pleural effusions on supine chest radiographs. *Am J Roentgenol* 1987; **148**: 681–83.

29 Raasch BN, Carsky EW, Lane EJ et al. Pleural effusion: explanation of some typical appearances. *Am J Roentgenol* 1982; **139**:899–904.

30 Yang P-C, Luh K-T, Chang D-B et al. Value of sonography in determining the nature of pleural effusion: analysis of 320 cases. *Am J Roentgenol* 1992; **159**:29–33.

31 Lomas DJ, Padley SG, Flower CDR. The sonographic appearances of pleural fluid. *Br J Radiol* 1993; **66**:619–24.

32 Bittner RC, Schnoy N, Schonfeld N et al. High-resolution magnetic resonance tomography (HR-MRT) of the pleura and thoracic wall: normal findings and pathological changes. *Rofo Fortschr Geb Rontgenstr Neuen Bildgeb Verfahr* 1995; **162**:296–303.

33 McLoud TC. CT and MR in pleural disease. *Clin Chest Med* 1998; **19**:261–76.

34 Greene R, McLoud TC, Stark P. Pneumothorax. *Semin Roentgenol* 1977; **12**:313–25.

35 Knisely BL, Kuhlman JE. Radiographic and computed tomography (CT) imaging of complex pleural disease. *Crit Rev Diagn Imaging* 1997; **38**:1–58.

36 Lesur O, Delorme N, Fromaget JM, Bernadac P, Polu JM. Computed tomography in the etiologic assessment of idiopathic spontaneous pneumothorax. *Chest* 1990; **98**:341–7.

37 Gordon R. The deep sulcus sign. *Radiology* 1980; **136**:25–7.

38 Rhea JT, van Sonnenberg E, McLoud TC. Basilar pneumothorax in the supine adult. *Radiology* 1979; **133**:593–5.

39 Tarver RD, Cones DJ, Cory DA, Vix VA. Imaging the diaphragm and its disorders. *J Thorac Imaging* 1989; **4**:1–18.

40 Verschakelen JA, Marchal G, Verbeken E, Baert AL, Lauweryns J. Sonographic appearance of the diaphragm in the presence of pleural disease: a cadaver study. *J Clin Ultrasound* 1989; **17**:222–7.

41 Brink JA, Heiken JP, Semenkovich J et al. Abnormalities of the diaphragm and adjacent structures: findings on multiplanar spiral CT scans. *Am J Roentgenol* 1994; **163**:307–10.

42 Bogaert J, Verschakelen J. Spiraal CT van het diafragma. *JBR-BTR* 1995; **78**:86–7.

43 Lennon FA, Simon G. The height of the diaphragm in the chest radiograph of normal subjects. *Br J Radiol* 1965; **38**:937–43.

44 Simon G, Bonnell J, Kazantzis G, Waller RE. Some radiological observations on the range of movement of the diaphragm. *Clin Radiol* 1969; **20**:231–3.

45 Oldham HN Jr. Mediastinal tumors and cysts (collective review). *Ann Thorac Surg* 1971; **11**:246–75.

46 Murayama S, Murakami J, Watanabe H et al. Signal intensity characteristics of mediastinal cystic masses on T1-weighted MRI. *J Comput Assist Tomogr* 1995; **19**:188–91.

47 Woodring JH, Daniel TL. Mediastinal analysis emphasizing plain radiographs and computed tomograms. *Med Radiogr Photogr* 1986; **62**:1–49.

48 Brown LR, Aughenbaugh GL. Masses of the anterior mediastinum: CT and MRI findings. *Am J Roentgenol* 1991; **157**:1171–80.

49 Strollo DC, Rosado-de-Christenson ML, Jett JR. Primary mediastinal tumors. Part 1. Tumors of the anterior mediastinum. *Chest* 1997; **112**:511–22.

50 Tecce PM, Fishman EK, Kuhlman JE. CT evaluation of the anterior mediastinum: spectrum of disease. *Radiographics* 1994; **14**:973–90.

51 Kawashima A, Fishman EK, Kuhlman JE, Nixon MS. CT of the posterior mediastinal masses. *Radiographics* 1991; **11**:1045–67.

52 Jeung M-Y, Gasser B, Gangi A et al. Imaging of cystic masses of the mediastinum. *Radiographics* 2002; **22**:S79–S93.

53 Cohen LM, Schwartz AM, Rockoff SD. Benign schwannomas: pathologic basis for CT inhomogeneities. *Am J Roentgenol* 1986; **147**:141–3.

54 Heitzman ER. *The Lung. Radiologic–pathologic Correlations*, 2nd edn. St Louis, The CV Mosby Co., 1984.

55 Tsirgiotis E, Ruffin R. Community acquired pneumonia. A perspective for general practice. *Aust Fam Phys* 2000; **29**:639–45.

56 Markowitz RI, Ruchelli E. Pneumonia in infants and children: radiological–pathological correlation. *Semin Roentgenol* 1998; **33**:151–62.

57 Reed JC. Pathologic correlations of the air-bronchogram: a reliable sign in chest radiology. *CRC Crit Rev Diagn Imag* 1977; **10**:235–55.

58 Proto AV, Tocino I. Radiographic manifestations of lobar collapse. *Semin Roentgenol* 1980; **15**:117–73.

59 Woodring JH, Reed JC. Radiographic manifestations of lobar atelectasis. *J Thorac Imag* 1996; **11**:109–44.

60 Woodring JH, Reed JC. Types and mechanisms of pulmonary atelectasis. *J Thorac Imag* 1996; **11**:92–108.

61 Westcott JL, Cole S. Plate atelectasis. *Radiology* 1985; **155**:1–9.

62 Felson B. The roentgen diagnosis of disseminated pulmonary alveolar diseases. *Semin Roentgenol* 1967; **2**:3–21.

63 Ziskind MM, George RB, Weill H. Acute localized and diffuse alveolar pneumonias. *Semin Roentgenol* 1967; **2**:49–60.

64 Bateson EM. An analysis of 155 solitary lung lesions illustrating the differential diagnosis of mixed tumors of the lung. *Clin Radiol* 1965; **16**:51–65.

65 Toomes H, Delphendahl A, Marike HG et al. The coin lesion of the lung: a review of 955 resected coin lesions. *Cancer* 1983; **51**:534–7.

66 Munden RF, Pugatch RD, Liptay MJ et al. Small pulmonary lesions detected at CT: clinical importance. *Radiology* 1997; **202**:105–10.

67 Nathan MH, Collins VP, Adams RA. Differentiation of benign and malignant pulmonary nodules by growth rate. *Radiology* 1962; **79**:221–32.

68 Meyer JA. Growth rate versus prognosis in resected primary bronchogenic carcinomas. *Cancer* 1973; **31**:1468–72.

69 Collins VP, Loeffler RK, Tivey H. Observations on growth rates of human tumors. *Am J Roentgenol* 1956; **76**:988–1000.

70 Weiss W. Tumor doubling time and survival of men with bronchogenic carcinoma. *Chest* 1974; **65**:3–8.

71 Ellis AR, Mayers DL, Martone WJ *et al.* Rapidly expanding pulmonary nodule caused by Pittsburgh pneumonia agent. *JAMA* 1981; **245**:1558–9.

72 Stewart JG, McMahon H, Vyborny CJ *et al.* Dystrophic calcification in carcinoma of the lung: demonstration by CT. *Am J Roentgenol* 1987; **148**:29–30.

73 Heitzman ER. Bronchogenic carcinoma: radiologic–pathologic correlations. *Semin Roentgenol* 1977; **12**:165–74.

74 Madewell JE, Feigin DS. Benign tumors of the lung. *Semin Roentgenol* 1977; **12**:175–85.

75 Rigler LG. The natural history of untreated lung cancer. *Ann NY Acad Sci* 1964; **114**:755–66.

76 Woodring JH, Fried AM. Significance of wall thickness in solitary cavities of the lung: a follow-up study. *Am J Roentgenol* 1983; **140**:473–4.

77 Ben-Menachem Y, Kuroda K, Kyger ER 3rd *et al.* The various forms of pulmonary varices. *Am J Roentgenol* 1975; **125**:881–9.

78 Hanke R, Kretzschmar R. Round atelectasis. *Semin Roentgenol* 1980; **15**:174–82.

79 Hillerdal G. Rounded atelectasis: clinical experience with 74 patients. *Chest* 1989; **95**:836–41.

80 Toh H, Tokunaga S, Asamoto H *et al.* Radiologic–pathologic correlations of small lung nodules with special reference to peribronchiolar nodules. *Am J Roentgenol* 1978; **130**:223–31.

81 Felson B. A new look at pattern recognition of diffuse pulmonary disease. *Am J Roentgenol* 1979; **133**:183–9.

82 Heitzman ER, Ziter FM, Markarian B *et al.* Kerley's interlobular septal lines: roentgen–pathologic correlation. *Am J Roentgenol* 1967; **100**:578–82.

83 Trapnell DH. The peripheral lymphatics of the lung. *Br J Radiol* 1963; **36**:660–72.

84 Trapnell DH. The differential diagnosis of linear shadows in chest radiographs. *Radiol Clin North Am* 1973; **11**:77–92.

85 Ried L. The connective tissue septa in the adult human lung. *Thorax* 1959; **14**:138–45.

86 Epler GR, McLoud TC, Gaensler EA *et al.* Normal chest roentgenograms in chronic diffuse infiltrative lung disease. *N Engl J Med* 1978; **298**:934–9.

87 Felson B. Lung torsion: radiographic findings in nine cases. *Radiology* 1987; **162**:631–8.

88 Fraser RG, Paré JAP, Paré PD *et al. Diagnosis of Diseases of the Chest*, 3rd edn. Philadelphia, WB Saunders, 1989.

89 Thurlbeck WM, Simon G. Radiographic appearance of the chest in emphysema. *Am J Roentgenol* 1978; **130**:429–40.

90 Putman CE, Godwin JD, Silverman PM *et al.* CT of localized lucent lung lesions. *Semin Roentgenol* 1984; **19**:173–88.

91 Godwin JD, Webb WR, Savoca CJ *et al.* Multiple, thin walled cystic lesions of the lung. *Am J Roentgenol* 1980; **135**:593–604.

92 Dines DE. Diagnostic significance of pneumatocele of the lung. *JAMA* 1968; **204**:79–82.

93 Murray JG, Breatnach E. Imaging of the mediastinum and hila. *Curr Opin Radiol* 1992; **4**:44–52.

94 Brown K, Mund DF, Aberle DR *et al.* Intrathoracic calcifications: radiographic features and differential diagnoses. *Radiographics* 1994; **14**:1247–61.

95 Chai JL, Patz EF Jr. CT of the lung: patterns of calcification and other high-attenuation abnormalities: pictorial essay. *Am J Roentgenol* 1994; **162**:1063–6.

96 Trotman-Dickenson B, Baumert B. Multidetector-row CT of the solitary pulmonary nodule. *Semin Roentgenol* 2003; **38**:158–67.

97 Tang AW, Moss HA, Robertson RJ. The solitary pulmonary nodule. *Eur J Radiol* 2003; **45**:69–77.

98 Leef JL 3rd, Klein JS. The solitary pulmonary nodule. *Radiol Clin North Am* 2002; **40**:123–43.

99 Zwirewich CV, Vedal S, Miller RR *et al.* Solitary pulmonary nodule: high-resolution CT and radiologic–pathologic correlation. *Radiology* 1991; **179**:469–76.

100 Swensen SJ. Functional CT: lung nodule evaluation. *Radiographics* 2000; **20**:1178–81.

101 Swensen SJ, Viggiano RW, Midthun DE *et al.* Lung nodule enhancement at CT: multicenter study. *Radiology* 2000; **241**:73–80.

102 Verschakelen JA, Bogaert J, De Wever W. Computed tomography in staging for lung cancer. *Eur Respir J Suppl* 2002; **35**:40s–48s.

103 Webb WR. High-resolution CT of the lung parenchyma. *Radiol Clin North Am* 1989; **27**:1085–97.

104 Zerhouni E. Computed tomography of the pulmonary parenchyma: an overview. *Chest* 1989; **95**:901–7.

105 Zerhouni EA, Naidich DP, Stitik FP *et al.* Computed tomography of the pulmonary parenchyma: part 2. Interstitial disease. *J Thorac Imag* 1985; **1**:54–64.

106 Austin JH, Müller NL, Friedman PJ *et al.* Glossary of terms for CT of the lungs: recommendations of the Nomenclature Committee of the Fleischner Society. *Radiology* 1996; **200**:327–31.

107 Bergin CJ, Müller NL. CT of insterstitial lung disease: a diagnostic approach. *Am J Roentgenol* 1987; **148**:9–15.

108 Collins J. CT signs and pattern of lung disease. *Radiol Clin North Am* 2001; **39**:1115–35.

109 Miller WS. *The Lung*, 2nd edn. Springfield, CC Thomas, 1947, pp 203–5.

110 Collins J, Stern EJ. Ground-glass opacity at CT: the ABCs. *Am J Roentgenol* 1997; **169**:355–67.

111 Engeler CE, Tashjian JH, Trenkner SW, Walsh JW. Ground-glass opacity of the lung parenchyma: a guide to analysis with high-resolution CT. *Am J Roentgenol* 1993; **160**:249–51.

112 Remy-Jardin M, Remy J, Giraud F, Wattinne L, Gosselin B. Computed tomography assessment of ground-glass opacity: semiology and significance. *J Thorac Imag* 1993; **8**:249–64.

113 Kjeldsberg KM, Oh K, Murray KA, Cannon G. Radiographic approach to multifocal consolidation. *Semin Ultrasound CT MR* 2002; **23**;288–301.

114 Genereux JP. CT of acute and chronic distal air space (alveolar) disease. *Semin Roentgenol* 1984; **19**:211–21.

115 Tomiyama N, Muller NL, Johkoh T, *et al.* Acute parenchymal lung disease in immunocompetent patients: diagnostic accuracy of high-resolution CT. *Am J Roentgenol* 2000; **174**:1745–50.

116 Ketai L, Washington L. Radiology of acute diffuse lung disease in the immunocompetent host. *Semin Roentgenol* 2002; **37**:25–36.

117 Hommeyer SH, Godwin JD, Takasugi JE. Computed tomography of air-space disease. *Radiol Clin North Am* 1991; **29**:1065–84.

118 Webb WR, Stein MG, Finkbeiner WE *et al.* Normal and diseased isolated lungs: high-resolution CT. *Radiology* 1988; **166**:81–7.

119 Müller NL, Miller RR, Webb WR *et al.* Fibrosing alveolitis: CT–pathologic correlation. *Radiology* 1986; **160**:585–8.

120 Murata K, Takahashi M, Mori M *et al.* Peribronchovascular interstitium of the pulmonary hilum: normal and abnormal findings on thin-section electron-beam CT. *Am J Roentgenol* 1996; **166**:309–12.

121 Bergin CJ, Müller NL. CT in the diagnosis of interstitial lung disease. *Am J Roentgenol* 1985; **145**:505–10.

122 Johkoh T, Ikezoe J, Tomiyama N *et al.* CT findings in lymphangitic carcinomatosis of the lung: correlation with histologic findings and pulmonary function tests. *Am J Roentgenol* 1992; **158**:1217–22.

123 Kang EY, Grenier P, Laurent F *et al.* Interlobular septal thickening: patterns at high-resolution computed tomography. *J Thorac Imag* 1996; **11**:260–4.

124 Bergin C, Roggli V, Coblentz C, Chiles C. The secondary pulmonary

lobule: normal and abnormal CT appearances. *Am J Roentgenol* 1988; **151**:21–5.

125 Murayama S, Murakami J, Yabuuchi H, Soeda H, Masuda K. 'Crazy paving appearance' on high resolution CT in various diseases. *J Comput Assist Tomogr* 1999; **23**:749–52.

126 Johkoh T, Itoh H, Muller NL *et al.* Crazy-paving appearance at thin-section CT: spectrum of disease and pathologic findings. *Radiology* 1999; **211**:155–60.

127 Kim TS, Lee KS, Chung MP *et al.* Nonspecific interstitial pneumonia with fibrosis: high-resolution CT and pathologic findings. *Am J Roentgenol* 1998; **171**:1645–50.

128 Murata K, Itoh H, Todo G *et al.* Centrilobular lesions of the lung: demonstration by high-resolution CT and pathologic correlation. *Radiology* 1986; **161**: 641–5.

129 Swensen SJ, Aughenbaugh GL, Douglas WW *et al.* High-resolution CT of the lungs: findings in various pulmonary diseases. *Am J Roentgenol* 1992; **158**:971–9.

130 Aberle DR, Gamsu G, Ray CS *et al.* Asbestos-related pleural and parenchymal fibrosis: detection with high-resolution CT. *Radiology* 1988; **166**:729–34.

131 Aberle DR, Gamsu G, Ray CS. High-resolution CT of benign asbestos-related diseases: clinical and radiographic correlation. *Am J Roentgenol* 1988; **151**:883–91.

132 Morimoto S, Takeuchi N, Imanaka H *et al.* Gravity dependent atelectasis: radiologic, physiologic and pathologic correlation in rabbits on high-frequency ventilation. *Invest Radiol* 1989; **24**:522–30.

133 Kubota H, Hosoya T, Kato M *et al.* Plate-like atelectasis at the corticomedullary junction of the lung: CT observation and hypothesis. *Radiat Med* 1983; **1**:305–10.

134 Primack SL, Hartman TE, Hansell DM *et al.* End-stage lung disease: CT findings in 61 patients. *Radiology* 1993; **189**:681–6.

135 Genereux GP. The end-stage lung: pathogenesis, pathology, and radiology. *Radiology* 1975; **116**:279–89.

136 Gruden JF, Webb WR, Naidich DP *et al.* Multinodular disease: anatomic localization at thin-section CT: multireader evaluation of a simple algorithm. *Radiology* 1999; **210**:711–20.

137 Lee KS, Kim TS, Han J *et al.* Diffuse micronodular lung disease: HRCT and pathologic findings. *J Comput Assist Tomogr* 1999; **23**:99–106.

138 Gruden JF, Webb WR, Warnock M. Centrilobular opacities in the lung on high-resolution CT: diagnostic considerations and pathologic correlation. *Am J Roentgenol* 1994; **162**:569–74.

139 Franquet T, Muller NL, Gimenez A, Martinez S, Madrid M, Domingo P. Infectious pulmonary nodules in immunocompromised patients: usefulness of computed tomography in predicting their etiology. *J Comput Assist Tomogr* 2003; **27**:461–8.

140 Naidich DP. High-resolution computed tomography of cystic lung disease. *Semin Roentgenol* 1991; **26**:151–74.

141 Worthy SA, Brown MJ, Müller NL. Technical report: cystic airspaces in the lung: change in size on expiratory high-resolution CT in 23 patients. *Clin Radiol* 1998; **53**:515–19.

142 Ryu JH, Swensen SJ. Cystic and cavitary lung diseases: focal and diffuse. *Mayo Clin Proc* 2003; **78**:744–52.

143 Robertson RJ. Imaging in the evaluation of emphysema. *Thorax* 1999; **54**:379.

144 Stern EJ, Frank MS. CT of the lung in patients with pulmonary emphysema: diagnosis, quantification, and correlation with pathologic and physiologic findings. *Am J Roentgenol* 1994; **162**:791–8.

145 Stern EJ, Song JK, Frank MS. CT of the lungs in patients with pulmonary emphysema. *Semin Ultrasound CT MR* 1995; **16**:345–52.

146 Foster WL Jr, Gimenez EI, Roubidoux MA *et al.* The emphysemas: radiologic–pathologic correlations. *Radiographics* 1993; **13**:311–28.

147 Hruban RH, Meziane MA, Zerhouni EA *et al.* High resolution computed tomography of inflation-fixed lungs. Pathologic–radiologic correlation of centrilobular emphysema. *Am Rev Respir Dis* 1987; **136**:935–40.

148 Foster WL Jr, Pratt PC, Roggli VL *et al.* Centrilobular emphysema: CT–pathologic correlation. *Radiology* 1986; **159**:27–32.

149 Gurney JW, Jones KK, Robbins RA *et al.* Regional distribution of emphysema: correlation of high-resolution CT with pulmonary function tests in unselected smokers. *Radiology* 1992; **183**:457–63.

150 Spouge D, Mayo JR, Cardoso W, Muller NL. Panacinar emphysema: CT and pathologic findings. *J Comput Assist Tomogr* 1993; **17**:710–13.

151 Guest PJ, Hansell DM. High resolution computed tomography (HRCT) in emphysema associated with α_1-antitrypsin deficiency. *Clin Radiol* 1992; **45**:260–6.

152 Morgan MD, Strickland B. Computed tomography in the assessment of bullous lung disease. *Br J Dis Chest* 1984; **78**:10–25.

153 Worthy SA, Muller NL, Hartman TE *et al.* Mosaic attenuation pattern on thin-section CT scans of the lung: differentiation among infiltrative lung, airway, and vascular diseases as a cause. *Radiology* 1997; **205**:465–70.

154 Primack SL, Muller NL, Mayo JR *et al.* Pulmonary parenchymal abnormalities of vascular origin: high-resolution CT findings. *Radiographics* 1994; **14**:739–46.

155 Mandel J, Mark EJ, Hales CA. Pulmonary veno-occlusive disease. *Am J Respir Crit Care Med* 2000; **162**:1964–73.

156 Sherrick AD, Swensen SJ, Hartman TE. Mosaic pattern of lung attenuation on CT scans: frequency among patients with pulmonary artery hypertension of different causes. *Am J Roentgenol* 1997; **169**:79–82.

157 Dennie CJ, Veinot JP, McCormack DG *et al.* Intimal sarcoma of the pulmonary arteries seen as a mosaic pattern of lung attenuation on high-resolution CT. *Am J Roentgenol* 2002; **178**:1208–10.

158 Stern EJ, Frank MS. Small-airways disease of the lungs: findings at expiratory CT. *Am J Roentgenol* 1994; **163**:37–41.

159 Arakawa H, Webb WR. Air trapping on expiratory high-resolution CT scans in the absence of inspiratory scan abnormalities: correlation with pulmonary function tests and differential diagnosis. *Am J Roentgenol* 1998; **170**:1349–53.

160 Desai SR, Hansell DM. Small airways disease: expiratory computed tomography comes of age. *Clin Radiol* 1997; **52**:332–7.

161 Lucidarme O, Coche E, Cluzel P *et al.* Expiratory CT scans for chronic airway disease: correlation with pulmonary function test results. *Am J Roentgenol* 1998; **170**:301–7.

162 Verschakelen JA, Scheinbaum K, Bogaert J *et al.* Expiratory CT in cigarette smokers: correlation between areas of decreased lung attenuation, pulmonary function tests and smoking history. *Eur Radiol* 1998; **8**:1391–9.

163 Arakawa H, Webb WR, McCowin M *et al.* Inhomogeneous lung attenuation at thin-section CT: diagnostic value of expiratory scans. *Radiology* 1998; **206**:89–94.

164 Stern EJ, Swensen SJ, Hartman TE *et al.* CT mosaic pattern of lung attenuation: distinguishing different causes. *Am J Roentgenol* 1995; **165**:813–16.

165 Webb WR, Stern EJ, Kanth N *et al.* Dynamic pulmonary CT: findings in healthy adult men. *Radiology* 1993; **186**:117–24.

166 Lee KW, Chung SY, Yang I *et al.* Correlation of aging and smoking with air trapping at thin-section CT of the lung in asymptomatic subjects. *Radiology* 2000; **214**:831–6.

167 Grenier PA, Beigelman-Aubry C, Fetita C *et al.* New frontiers in CT imaging of airway disease. *Eur Radiol* 2002; **12**:1022–44.

Diagnostic strategies in pulmonary embolism: an evidence-based approach

Martin Riedel

Abstract

The diagnosis of pulmonary embolism (PE) is formidably difficult, particularly when there is co-existing heart or lung disease, and it is notoriously inaccurate when based on clinical signs alone. About two out of three patients who present with suspected PE do not have this condition. Objective testing is necessary, but no single investigation has ideal properties and several tests must often be performed. Pulmonary angiography is still regarded as the final arbiter but, owing to its limited availability, costs and invasiveness, it is ill-suited for diagnosing a disease present in only a third of patients in whom it is suspected. Non-invasive diagnostic strategies have therefore been developed to forgo angiography in patients suspected of having PE. For optimal efficiency, choice of the initial diagnostic test should be guided by clinical assessment of the likelihood of PE and by patient characteristics that may influence test accuracy. Standardized clinical estimates can be used effectively to give a pretest probability to calculate, after appropriate objective testing, the post-test probability of PE.

A negative result of a highly sensitive D-dimer assay excludes PE in outpatients with low clinical likelihood of PE; such patients do not require imaging for thromboembolism. Normal lung perfusion scintigraphy excludes PE. A high-probability scan warrants the institution of anticoagulant therapy especially when paired with high clinical likelihood of PE. Yet, only a minority of patients with confirmed PE have high-probability scans. Scintigraphic abnormalities other than those of the high-probability scan must be regarded as non-diagnostic. Under these circumstances, documentation of deep vein thrombosis by leg testing warrants anticoagulation without the need for further lung imaging. However, a single negative venous study result does not permit one to rule out PE in patients with non-diagnostic scintigraphy. Spiral computerized tomography (CT) detects all clinically relevant emboli and also, very importantly, the angiographically and scintigraphically undetectable alternative diagnoses. Multislice spiral CT can replace both scintigraphy and pulmonary angiography for the exclusion and diagnosis of this disease and should now be considered the central imaging investigation in suspected PE. Suspected massive PE with haemodynamic instability is a distinct clinical situation requiring a specific diagnostic approach, in which echocardiography plays a major role.

Introduction

Pulmonary embolism (PE) can produce widely differing clinical pictures, often mimicking other cardiopulmonary disorders. Objective testing for PE is necessary because clinical assessment alone is unreliable and the consequences of misdiagnosis are serious. Failure to diagnose PE is associated with high mortality, and incorrect diagnosis of the condition unnecessarily exposes patients to the risks of anticoagulant therapy.[1] No single investigation for the diagnosis of PE has ideal properties (100% sensitivity and specificity, no risk, low cost, ready availability), and several tests are often performed, either sequentially or in combination.

The world of diagnostic tests for PE is highly dynamic. New tests are developed at a fast rate, and the technology of existing tests is continuously being improved. Exaggerated and biased results from poorly designed and reported diagnostic studies can trigger premature dissemination of a test and lead physicians into making incorrect treatment decisions. In studies of diagnostic accuracy, the results from one or more tests under evaluation (index test) are compared with results from a reference ('gold') standard, both measured in subjects who are suspected of having PE. The reference standard is considered to be the best available method for establishing the presence or absence of PE; it can be a single method or a combination of methods, and it can include imaging tests, laboratory tests and pathology, but also dedicated follow-up of subjects. The term accuracy refers to the amount of agreement between the index test and the reference standard. Diagnostic accuracy can be expressed in many ways, including specificity and sensitivity, predictive values, likelihood ratios, diagnostic odds ratio and the area under a receiver–operator characteristic (ROC) curve.[2] In this chapter, the methodological aspects and technical details of index tests and reference standards are not described in detail; it should be remembered that, in most studies of diagnostic accuracy, the newest equipment and methodology are usually used and meticulous attention to detail applied, which might not be the case in the imperfect real world.

Also, although the information in this chapter was extracted predominantly from prospective cohort studies using a criterion standard and satisfying basic methodological quality, not all studies are methodically flawless and report satisfactorily on all key elements of design, selection bias, conduct and analysis.[2,3] Finally, publication of articles is often related to a more positive outcome; this problem is impossible to overcome, and therefore one should remain cautious of the findings of a critical literature review.

Specific problems in diagnosing pulmonary embolism

A general consensus regarding the diagnostic procedures for PE has not yet been developed. Different authors emphasize different approaches to this frequent and potentially life-threatening disease and, therefore, different and often contrasting opinions are continuously reported in the literature. This is a peculiarity of PE, which, after acute myocardial infarction and stroke, is the third commonest acute cardiovascular emergency. Whereas myocardial infarction and stroke are diagnosed according to widely accepted and simple guidelines, no simple guidelines exist for PE.

There are several reasons for the difficulties in diagnosing PE and for the problems in the evaluation of specific diagnostic tests. First, the clinical presentation of PE is highly variable and non-specific. Whereas acute myocardial infarction usually presents with a single relatively specific symptom (typical chest pain), none of the individual symptoms (Fig. 1) and signs (Fig. 2) of PE are either sufficiently sensitive or specific or frequent to raise a well-grounded suspicion of the disease.[4] As a consequence, depending on the clinical experience and acumen of the physicians, the real frequency of PE varies between 5% and 60% of those in whom it is suspected. This is an important issue, because the frequency of the disease in the examined population influences the predictive value of a given test (Table 1). For instance, a recent study confirmed that the D-dimer test has a high sensitivity in outpatients suspected of having acute PE.[5] However, in this study, PE was eventually confirmed in only 50 of the 1106 consecutive patients (i.e. 4.5 %) originally suspected of having PE. The final diagnoses in those 1056 patients suspicious of PE in whom the diagnosis

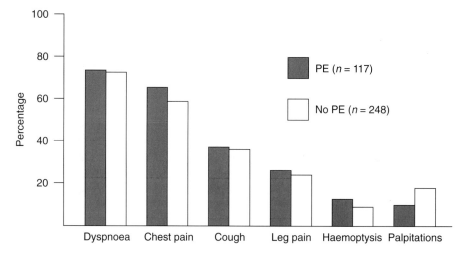

Figure 1. Frequency of symptoms in patients with suspected PE and without previous cardiopulmonary disease. The diagnosis of PE was subsequently confirmed or excluded by objective testing (after Stein *et al.*[4]).

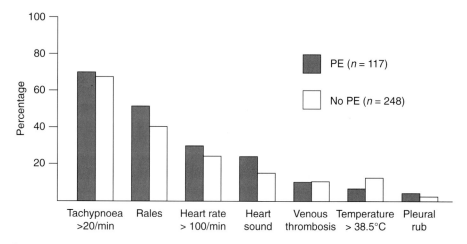

Figure 2. Frequency of clinical signs in patients with suspected PE and without previous cardiopulmonary disease. The diagnosis of PE was subsequently confirmed or excluded by objective testing (after Stein *et al.*[4]).

Table 1. Effect of prevalence of the disease on positive predictive value (PPV) of a test*.

Prevalence of disease (%)	PPV of a test (%)			
20	50.0	69.2	82.6	96.1
10	30.8	50.0	67.9	91.7
5	17.4	32.1	50.0	83.9
1	3.9	8.3	16.1	50.0
Specificity (%)	80	90	95	99
Sensitivity (%)	80	90	95	99

*Positive predictive value is the percentage of patients with a positive test result who actually have the disease. Prevalence does not affect the sensitivity or specificity.

was eventually excluded were not stated. The fact that the authors erred in 96 out of 100 cases of suspected PE points to a low level of diagnostic skills (history taking and clinical examination) of the physicians involved in this study,[5] with the consequence of wasting resources through ordering many unnecessary studies, most of them involving radiation burden. The same diagnostic accuracy in differentiating chest pain would lead to 96 out of 100 unnecessary coronary angiographies. One wonders if the opposite and, for the patient more dangerous, type of diagnostic inaccuracy, namely not suspecting PE in patients who actually have it, was equally frequent. In studies from emergency departments in Europe, the frequency of objectively confirmed PE is in the range of 27–48% of the outpatients originally suspected of having the disease.[6–12] It ranges from 9.5%[13] to 16.8%[14] in North American emergency departments. In valuable studies, the frequency of confirmed PE should be between 30% and 50% of all patients suspected of having the disease.

The second problem lies in the widely variable haemodynamic consequences of acute PE. In patients with massive PE, there is usually right ventricular strain and, therefore, methods capable of proving this strain (e.g. echocardiography or ECG) might be indirectly valuable in the diagnosis of PE. In contrast, in minor PE, there is no real haemodynamic stress and, thus, these investigations are useless for diagnosing PE (although they retain their value for the differential diagnosis).

The third problem refers to the diagnostic reference standard. Pulmonary angiography is regarded as the final arbiter but, because of its limited availability, costs and invasiveness, it is ill-suited for diagnosing a disease present in only a third of patients in whom it is suspected. Other standards (e.g. autopsy or clinical follow-up, see below) are applicable only in a minority of patients with suspected PE, and therefore of limited help in evaluating other diagnostic tests.

Fourth, because pulmonary angiography for definitive confirmation or exclusion of PE cannot be used in all subjects suspected of having PE, other tests with lower accuracy are being used instead, with some doubt left after these tests. This doubt can be lessened by taking into account the clinical likelihood (pretest probability) of venous thromboembolism (VTE). By adopting a thorough stratification system, the clinician can more appropriately select further investigations to prove or exclude PE, and predict the probability of PE after further objective testing (post-test probability). The benefit of clinical likelihood estimate can be illustrated by the effect of prevalence of disease on the positive predictive value (PPV) of a diagnostic test (Table 1). Prevalence does not affect the sensitivity or specificity of a test, but it does affect the positive and negative predictive values. When the prevalence of a disease falls well below 20%, the PPV of the diagnostic test falls dramatically. Consequently, when the test is used in a low-prevalence population, its usefulness declines because of a loss of PPV. Assessment of clinical likelihood of VTE helps to triage patients into clinically useful groups to avoid unnecessary testing and costs, while minimizing risk.[15]

Finally, another peculiarity in PE diagnosis lies in the fact that thrombotic PE is not an isolated disease of the chest but a complication of venous thrombosis. Deep venous thrombosis (DVT) and PE are therefore parts of the same process, VTE. Evidence of leg DVT (by contrast venography) is found in about 70% of patients who have sustained a PE.[16,17] Conversely, PE occurs in up to 50% of patients with proximal DVT of the legs (involving the popliteal and/or more proximal veins),[18–21] and is less likely when the thrombus is confined to the calf veins. Rarely, the source of emboli is the iliac veins, renal veins, right heart or upper extremity veins; the clinical circumstances usually point to these unusual sites.[1] The sequential course of most cases of VTE, with progression from DVT in the calf to proximal DVT and subsequently to PE, has some important diagnostic and management implications. First, identifying asymptomatic DVT can, indirectly, establish the diagnosis of PE; this is helpful when initial tests for PE are non-diagnostic.[22,23] Second, if proximal DVT can be excluded, there is a low short-term risk of PE with non-diagnostic test for PE at presentation.[13,24,25] Third, if proximal DVT is excluded at presentation and does not develop within 2 weeks, patients with non-diagnostic tests for PE have a low long-term risk of subsequent VTE.[13,24,25] Fourth, without treatment, about one-half of patients with symptomatic proximal DVT or PE are expected to have recurrent VTE within 3 months.[1]

The approaches to the diagnosis of PE that minimize the use of pulmonary angiography are based on two guiding principles. In order for a test, or a combination of tests, to be considered accurate enough to diagnose the presence of PE, it should have a PPV of more than 95%, compared with pulmonary angiography. To exclude the presence of PE, such a test should have a negative predictive value (NPV) of more than 99%, compared with pulmonary angiography, or be associated with less than 2% incidence of VTE during follow-up if it is the base for withholding treatment. Near-perfect sensitivity is important because, for every 2% decrease in sensitivity, 1 per

Table 2. Test results that effectively exclude or confirm pulmonary embolism.

Pulmonary embolism is excluded by
  Normal pulmonary angiogram
  Normal perfusion scan
  Normal thin-collimation (multislice) CTPA
  Normal single-detector spiral CTPA and compression
    ultrasonography (or CT venography)
  Normal D-dimer level (assay with high sensitivity) and low clinical
    likelihood
  Low-probability scan and low clinical likelihood
  Non-diagnostic lung scan and normal results on serial leg testing
  Non-diagnostic lung scan and normal single-leg testing and low
    clinical likelihood

Pulmonary embolism is confirmed by
  Intraluminal filling defect on pulmonary angiogram
  Intraluminal filling defect on spiral CTPA
  High-probability scan and high clinical likelihood
  Apparative evidence of acute DVT with non-diagnostic scan or
    spiral CTPA

CTPA, computerized tomography pulmonary angiogram; DVT, deep vein thrombosis.

1000 patients studied will die of recurrent PE as a result of inappropriately withholding anticoagulation. The test results that effectively exclude or confirm PE are summarized in Table 2.

Reference standards

It is difficult to assess the value of a diagnostic test if it is commonly regarded as a reference standard.

Pulmonary angiography

Conventional pulmonary angiography (either film screen or digital subtraction) has been seen as the standard against which other imaging modalities have historically been evaluated.[26] Of patients with normal pulmonary angiograms, about 1% have an episode of symptomatic VTE during the following 6 months;[27–29] this is the standard against which the safety of withholding anticoagulants following negative tests for PE is assessed. However, animal models that mimic subsegmental emboli have found sensitivity and PPV of only 87–88% compared with necropsy.[30] Also, interobserver agreement of an angiographically documented subsegmental embolus is only about 70%.[31] Consequently, pulmonary angiography remains the gold standard for central and segmental PE, but not for subsegmental PE (which occurs isolated in 17–20% of patients with PE[31,32]). Comparable to asymptomatic calf vein thrombosis, an isolated subsegmental embolus may remain clinically asymptomatic without the need for anticoagulation. Prospective clinical outcome studies as to whether it will be safe to withhold anticoagulation in cases of isolated subsegmental embolism are lacking.

In routine practice, catheter pulmonary angiography should now be considered only when other investigations are inconclusive.[28] Angiography has the disadvantages of limited availability, invasiveness and a small (<0.3%) but definite risk of mortality.[26,33–35] The use of intravenous digital subtraction angiography (DSA) avoids the need for pulmonary artery catheterization but has been disappointing because opacification of the pulmonary vessels is poor. Although intravenous DSA may be adequate for showing large proximal arterial occlusions, resolution is inadequate to identify an embolus in the segmental vessels and beyond. Thus, minor PE cannot be excluded on the basis of a normal DSA with peripheral contrast application.[26]

Autopsy

More than two-thirds of the major (either fatal or contributing to death) embolic events diagnosed at autopsy are overlooked *in vivo* by the attending physicians.[1,36] Autopsy can obviously be used to detect PE only in deceased patients and, therefore, when used in diagnostic studies as a reference standard for the presence of PE, it must be combined with some other standard in survivors. Even if autopsy may represent the true gold standard for the presence of PE, it is not without a degree of tarnish. Emboli may easily be missed if the pulmonary arteries are not opened with care far into the periphery; sometimes, it may be difficult to distinguish premortem from postmortem thrombus or even thromboemboli from thrombi formed primarily *in situ* in small pulmonary arteries. Especially for the exclusion of PE, the time interval between the clinical event leading to suspicion of PE and the time of death must be short.

Composite reference standard

When it is not possible to subject all patients to pulmonary angiography for practical or ethical reasons, authors often use a composite reference standard. The components reflect different strategies for diagnosing PE. For instance, all patients are subjected to pulmonary scintigraphy and venous ultrasonography, with pulmonary angiography applied only in patients with inconclusive results from the first two tests.

Clinical follow-up (management or outcome studies)

The goal of the first diagnostic strategies introduced was to confirm rather than exclude the presence of PE. Because usually less than a third of patients with suspected PE have the disease confirmed by objective testing[13,14,17,37–43] and because wide use of pulmonary angiography is unfeasible, not only in routine practice but also in clinical studies, the more recently evaluated diagnostic approaches have focused on identifying patients who probably do not have PE and therefore do not require anticoagulant therapy.[38,44] Indeed, not all venous thromboembolic events carry the same risk of an unfavourable outcome when left untreated,[24,45–47] whereas the risk of major bleeding due to anticoagulant treatment is always present. Hence, management studies on PE diagnosis have focused on the identification of those patients in whom anticoagulation could safely be withheld, rather than on the pursuit of all thromboemboli, whatever their size and localization. To exclude the presence of PE, an index test should be associated with no more than a 1–2% frequency of VTE during rigorous follow-up (usually 3–6 months) if it is the basis for withholding treatment.

Estimating pretest clinical likelihood of thromboembolism

Until the 1970s, the diagnosis or exclusion of PE was made on clinical grounds alone. In the urokinase pulmonary embolism trial (UPET), several clinical findings, previously considered valuable in the diagnosis of PE, were not present in many patients with the disease.[39] These results led clinicians to virtually abandon clinical examination and diagnose PE solely based on the results of objective tests. A number of recent studies, however, have suggested that combining the individual components of clinical assessment, risk factors for VTE, possible alternative diagnoses and simple investigations reliably categorizes the likelihood of PE in an individual patient as low, moderate or high.[7,25,37,48–50]

Clinical likelihood of PE is determined after consideration of major risk factors[1,51] (the commonest being immobilization, hip or leg fractures and recent major trauma or surgery; Table 3), presentation (including presence or absence of another reasonable clinical explanation) and basic investigations (ECG and plain chest radiograph). The generally accepted characteristics of these clinical estimates are given in Table 4.

Nearly all patients with PE will have one or more of dyspnoea of sudden onset, tachypnoea (>20 breaths/min) or chest pain (pleuritic or substernal);[4] if the clinician remembers these three features, the possibility of PE will rarely be overlooked. When these clinical features are associated with ECG signs of right ventricular strain and/or radiological signs of plump hilum, pulmonary infarction or oligaemia, the likelihood of PE is high (>70%), and it is further strengthened in the presence of risk factors for VTE as well as in the presence of arterial hypoxaemia with hypocapnia. In contrast, the absence of

Table 3. Risk factors for venous thromboembolic disease.[1,51]

Strong risk factors (odds ratio >10):
  Hip or leg fracture
  Hip or knee replacement
  Major trauma or general surgery within 4 weeks

Moderate risk factors (odds ratio 2–9):
  Immobilization (>2 days) or other cause of venous stasis (e.g. paralytic stroke)
  Active malignancy (treatment within previous 6 months or palliative therapy)
  Indwelling catheters and electrodes in great veins and right heart
  Reduced cardiac output (congestive heart failure)
  Puerperium
  Oral contraception, hormone replacement therapy
  Previous proven venous thromboembolism
  Hereditary thrombophilia
  Acquired thrombotic disorders (e.g. antiphospholipid antibodies, heparin-induced thrombocytopenia, thrombocytosis, post-splenectomy)
  Arthroscopic knee surgery

Weak risk factors (odds ratio <2):
  Obesity
  Advanced age
  Pregnancy
  Immobility due to long sitting (e.g. prolonged travel)
  Laparoscopic surgery (e.g. cholecystectomy)

Table 4. Estimation of the (pretest) clinical likelihood of PE.

High (>70 % likely)	Otherwise unexplained sudden onset of dyspnoea, tachypnoea or chest pain and at least two of the following:
	  Significant risk factor present (immobility, leg fracture, major surgery)
	  Fainting with new signs of right ventricular overload in ECG
	  Signs of possible leg DVT (unilateral pain, tenderness, erythema, warmth or swelling)
	  Radiographic signs of infarction, plump hilum or oligaemia

Intermediate (15–70 % likely)	Neither high nor low clinical likelihood
Low (<15 % likely)	Absence of sudden onset of dyspnoea and tachypnoea and chest pain Dyspnoea, tachypnoea or chest pain present but explainable by another condition Risk factors absent Radiographic abnormality explainable by another condition Adequate anticoagulation (INR >2 or a PTT >1.5 times control) during the previous week

ECG, electrocardiogram; DVT, deep venous thrombosis; INR, international normalized ratio; PTT, partial thromboplastin time.

all these three clinical features virtually excludes the diagnosis of PE.[1,52,53] In the absence of major risk factors for VTE, paucity of typical signs for PE and/or DVT and positive indications for the presence of an alternative diagnosis (e.g. fever, radiographic evidence of pulmonary oedema or consolidation), the predicted likelihood of PE is low (<15%).

Several studies have shown that well-characterized clinical empirical estimates[7,37,48,50,54] or explicit prediction rules[9,25,55–57] of pretest likelihood of PE can be used for the safe management of patients suspected of having the disease (Tables 5 and 6).[53,58,59] However, these studies involved experienced clinicians using defined criteria under a research protocol; this is very different from the emergency room situation where decisions are often made by junior doctors whose ability to make an accurate estimate of the likelihood of PE is much less than that of their seniors. It is not clear whether explicit prediction rules offer enough of an advantage over empirical assessment.[59]

When the independent clinical estimate of likelihood is high or low, it seems to move the patient into a high- or low-prevalence category where the positive or negative predictive value of an appropriate test is more useful (Table 1). In this way, the high clinical likelihood seems to ensure a sufficiently high prevalence of PE to make PPV of the appropriate test use-

Table 5. Scoring prediction rules for the estimation of clinical likelihood of PE.

Wells et al.[13,25]		Wicki et al.[9]	
Variable	Points	Variable	Points
Signs and symptoms of DVT	3	Recent surgery	3
Previous DVT or PE	1.5	Previous DVT or PE	2
Immobilization or surgery	1.5	Heart rate >100 beats/min	1
Heart rate >100 beats/min	1.5	Age 60–79 years	1
Haemoptysis	1	Age ≥80 years	2
Malignancy	1	Plate atelectasis	1
PE more likely than alternative diagnosis	3	Elevation of diaphragm	1
		$Paco_2$ <36 mmHg	2
		$Paco_2$ 36–39 mmHg	1
		Pao_2 <50 mmHg	4
		Pao_2 50–59 mmHg	3
		Pao_2 60–70 mmHg	2
		Pao_2 71–82 mmHg	1
Pretest PE likelihood	Total points		Total points
Low	>2		<5
Moderate	2–6		5–8
High	>6		>8

Table 6. Accuracy of pretest clinical estimates of PE likelihood.

Study	PIOPED[37]	Miniati et al.[48]	Perrier et al.[7]	Wicki et al.[9]	Wells et al.[55]	Miniati et al.[56]
Patient spectrum	Outpatients and inpatients	Outpatients and inpatients	Only outpatients	Only outpatients	Outpatients and inpatients	Outpatients and inpatients
No. of patients	887	583	1034	986	972	1100
Method of assessment	Empirical	Empirical	Empirical	Score (Table 5)	Score (Table 5)	Score
Frequency of PE (%)						
Low probability	9	6	8	10	4	4
Moderate probability	30	46	36	38	21	34
High probability	68	97	67	81	67	98
Total	27	52	27	27	17	40

ful. Conversely, the low clinical likelihood probably ensures a sufficiently low prevalence of VTE to make the NPV of a test useful. These relationships have been validated for the lung scanning, D-dimer assay and venous ultrasonography in the diagnosis of VTE, but probably also hold for all other tests. For instance, when combined with a negative D-dimer test, the stratification excludes PE in outpatients with low pretest probability;[13] in those with intermediate or high clinical probability, further testing is required. Conversely, a high-probability scan actually represents PE in 87% of all patients suspected of having PE (i.e. there are 13% false-positive results), but in 96% of those with high clinical likelihood of the disease.[37] Of course, the estimation of the pretest clinical likelihood of PE is highly dependent on the acumen of the physician.

Lung scintigraphy

Lung scanning is still the most commonly used technique in the diagnostic workup of patients with clinical suspicion of PE. A normal perfusion scan essentially excludes the diagnosis of a recent PE because occlusive PE of all types produces a defect of perfusion. Normal results are almost never associated with recurrent PE, even if anticoagulants are withheld.[10,25,44,60–66] However, a normal perfusion scan is found only in a minority (about a quarter) of patients suspected of having PE.[25,37]

The perfusion scan is an indirect method of diagnosis as it does not detect the embolus itself but only its consequence, the perfusion abnormality. Many conditions other than PE, such as tumours, consolidation, left heart failure, bullous lesions, lung fibrosis and obstructive airways disease,[67] can also produce perfusion defects. Addition of a ventilation scan increases the specificity of scintigraphy. PE usually produces a defect of perfusion but not ventilation ('mismatch') whereas most of the other conditions produce a ventilation defect in the same area as the perfusion defect (matched defects). PE can also produce matched defects when infarction has occurred but, in this situation, the chest radiograph nearly always shows shadowing in the area of scan defect.

The probability that perfusion defects are due to PE can be assessed as high, intermediate or low depending on the type of scan abnormality.[33,37] If the scan is of a high-probability type (multiple segmental or larger perfusion defects with normal ventilation), there is a >85% chance that the patient has PE. This implies that about 15% of patients with a high-probability scan do not have PE and are therefore overtreated. The majority of patients with clinically suspected PE do not have a high-probability scan and instead have one that suggests either low or intermediate probability (= non-diagnostic scan) and, in these patients, the prevalence of PE is about 25%.[37,50] Taking the clinical assessment into account improves diagnostic accuracy (when the clinical likelihood of PE and scan interpretation is concordant, the ability to diagnose

Table 7. Probability (%) of underlying PE according to the criteria of the PIOPED study.

	Scan probability			
	Normal/ very low	'Non-diagnostic'		High
		Low	Intermediate	
Clinical likelihood:				
Low	2	4	16	56
Intermediate	6	16	28	88
High	0	40	66	96

Data from PIOPED.[37]

Table 8. Probability (%) of underlying PE according to the criteria of the PISA-PED study.

	Scan probability	
	PE–	PE+
Clinical likelihood:		
Low	3	55
Intermediate	12	92
High	39	99

Data from Miniati et al.[54]

or exclude PE is optimized; Table 7), but the diagnosis can still be made or excluded with accuracy in only about 40% of patients. A low-probability scan does not rule out PE but, in fact, there is up to a 40% probability of PE when clinical likelihood is high.[37,56,59]

A ventilation scan is not indicated in cases with a subsegmental defect on the perfusion scan because, by definition,[33] this cannot lead to a high-probability ventilation–perfusion scan. A ventilation scan is indicated in cases with segmental defects on the perfusion scan; otherwise, it cannot lead to a high-probability ventilation–perfusion scan. In theory, the addition of ventilation scanning should improve the usefulness of perfusion imaging, but the PIOPED study showed such benefit to be marginal (because perfusion defects in PE were often associated with ventilation abnormalities).[37] Perfusion defects due to PE are most often wedge-shaped. In the PISA-PED study, when only wedge-shaped defects were classified as indicative of PE, perfusion scintigraphy without the use of ventilation scans, combined with clinical assessment of PE likelihood (Table 8), enabled confirmation or exclusion of PE in 76% of patients with abnormal scans, with an accuracy of 97%.[48,54] This suggests that, where ventilation imaging is unavailable, perfusion scanning alone is acceptable. The simple PISA-PED criteria are an attractive alternative to the complex PIOPED criteria.[52]

Although the lung scan is often an imprecise guide, it is useful in clinical decision making: a normal scan or a low-probability scan with low clinical likelihood of PE means that treatment for suspected PE can be withheld, and a high-probability scan with a high clinical likelihood of PE means that treatment is mandatory (Table 2). Further objective tests for DVT and/or PE must be used to decide on the therapy in patients between these extremes and in whom the clinical likelihood of PE and scan interpretation are discordant. An important principle is that, in abnormal lung scans, the knowledge of clinical probability is essential in interpreting the report's meaning but must not influence its description.

Planar scintigraphy is the standard technology in most institutions. With SPECT (single photon emission CT) technology, pictures can be reconstructed in any plane, and the specificity of scintigraphy improves as a result of the reduction in the frequency of non-diagnostic scans.[68,69] Scanning should be performed within 24 hours of the onset of symptoms suspected of PE, as some scans revert to normal quickly. A follow-up scan at the time of discharge (or termination of anticoagulant therapy) is helpful in establishing a new baseline for subsequent episodes of suspected PE.[70] One clinically important cause of a false-positive study is prior PE that has not resolved, leaving a lung scan pattern that remains in the high-probability category.[1]

Spiral computerized tomography

Spiral CT with injection of contrast medium into an arm vein (CT pulmonary angiography, CTPA) has emerged as a valuable method for diagnosing PE and, because of its availability, it is becoming the first-choice method at many institutions. The technique is faster, less complex, less invasive and less operator dependent than conventional pulmonary angiography and has about the same frequency of technically insufficient examinations (about 5%).[71] The thorax can be scanned during a single breath-hold. There is better interobserver agreement in the interpretation of CTPA than for scintigraphy.[72] Another advantage of CTPA over scintigraphy is that, by imaging the lung parenchyma and great vessels, an alternative diagnosis (e.g. pulmonary mass, pneumonia, emphysema, pleural effusion, mediastinal adenopathy) can be made if PE is absent.[43,70] This advantage of CTPA also pertains to conventional pulmonary angiography, which images only the arteries. CT can also detect right ventricular dilatation, thus indicating severe, potentially fatal PE. Whereas the accuracy of lung scintigraphy, assessed by comparison with pulmonary angiography in large prospective trials,[37,54] will not change significantly in the future, both the accuracy and the clinical utilization of CTPA are likely to increase with technological advancements leading to improvement in data acquisition, particularly with the use of thinner section collimation and multidetector CT.[73–75]

Criteria for a positive CTPA result are similar to those of a conventional angiography and include a partial filling defect (defined as intraluminal area of low attenuation surrounded by contrast medium), a complete filling defect and the 'railway track sign' (masses seen floating in the lumen, allowing the flow of blood between the vessel wall and the embolus). CTPA also allows a quantitative assessment of PE severity, which correlates well with clinical severity.[76,77] The procedure has over 90% specificity and sensitivity in diagnosing PE in the main, lobar and segmental pulmonary arteries.[71,72] When CTPA is used to evaluate patients with a non-diagnostic lung scan, the sensitivity is lower.[74,78,79]

Although recent advances in CT technology (multidetector scanners) with 1- to 2-mm multiplanar image reconstruction enable better visualization of subsegmental arteries,[73–75] these small vessels remain difficult to evaluate. The clinical significance of isolated subsegmental emboli (which account for about 17–20% of symptomatic PE[31,32]) is unclear, but it is not current practice to ignore them. They may be of importance in patients with poor cardiopulmonary reserve, and their presence is an indicator of current VTE, which thus potentially heralds more severe emboli. Recent studies have shown, however, that patients with PE-negative CTPA do well without anticoagulation therapy.[80–87] This should be especially true when these patients also have a leg venous study that is negative for thrombus.[43,72,88]

After performing CTPA to diagnose PE, sufficient opacification of the venous system remains to evaluate the veins of the legs, pelvis and abdomen for DVT, without additional venepuncture or contrast medium. Such an examination is a continuous study, adding approximately 5 min to pulmonary scanning, with the added expense of only one sheet of film. The pelvic and abdominal images screen the iliac veins and vena cava for thrombosis, an important advantage over sonography, particularly when caval filter placement is considered.[89–91] If the accuracy of venous imaging after lung scanning is confirmed in large studies, its use should be considered whenever CTPA is indicated. A disadvantage is an increased radiation dose, particularly to the gonads.

D-dimer

Endogenous fibrinolysis is indicated by the sensitive assay of cross-linked fibrin degradation products (D-dimers). However, this test has low specificity and is positive not only when there is VTE but also in the presence of disseminated intravascular coagulation, many inflammatory diseases, malignancy and after trauma or surgery. Although a negative test may be strong enough evidence that clotting has not occurred and that anticoagulants can be withheld, a positive test cannot confirm VTE. The test can safely reduce the number of imaging investigations in patients with suspected PE and a low pretest likelihood of VTE.[12,13,38,40,41,44,49,92] However, if there is a high clinical suspicion of acute PE, diagnostic tests should proceed in spite of a normal D-dimer (in fact, D-dimer assay is useless in those with high clinical probability of PE). Not surprisingly, false-negative results are more common in patients with subsegmental than in those with larger emboli.[42] In elderly or inpatients, D-dimer retains a high NPV, but is normal in less than 20% of patients and, hence, not very useful.[60,93,94]

Many different assays are now commercially available, and clinicians should appreciate that these cannot necessarily be used interchangeably. Not all D-dimer testing methods have sufficient sensitivity, but the rapid assays with a NPV approaching 100% (e.g. VIDAS DD) are comparable to the reliable but labour- and time-consuming conventional enzyme-linked immunosorbent assay (ELISA) tests.[53,59,92,95] Clinicians should know the characteristics of the test used in their own institution.

Search for (residual) deep venous thrombosis

Venous thrombosis cannot be diagnosed reliably on the basis of the history and physical examination. Patients with lower extremity DVT often do not exhibit pain, tenderness, redness, warmth or swelling. When present, however, these findings merit further evaluation. Impedance plethysmography, compression ultrasonography, indirect CT venography and magnetic resonance imaging (MRI) are established non-invasive methods for diagnosing DVT.[96] While contrast venography remains the gold standard, it is rarely performed because it is invasive and difficult to carry out in the acutely ill patient.[17] Venography should only be performed whenever non-invasive testing is non-diagnostic or impossible to perform. While plethysmography and ultrasound are reliable for the diagnosis of symptomatic proximal DVT,[97] they are much less reliable for recognizing asymptomatic or distal DVT. They are also not able to detect floating thrombus in the vena cava. Plethysmography is inferior to the latest ultrasound techniques; it is now used in only a few institutions. The single well-validated criterion for DVT on ultrasonography is the absence of full compressibility of the vein when applying pressure through the ultrasound transducer. Doppler studies do not add significant diagnostic accuracy, as reduced flow is not specific for DVT and clots may be non-occlusive.[96]

Indirect CT venography is very accurate, providing good visualization of the proximal venous system and deep calf veins. As an added advantage, CT venography can be combined with CTPA for a simultaneous investigation of both DVT and PE.[89–91] MR venography, performed with time-of-flight and phase-contrast imaging, is highly accurate at showing blood flow in the proximal venous system. MR direct thrombus imaging uses high signal generated from the thrombi to calculate the volume of intravenous clots and assess the risk of subsequent PE.[98,99] Evaluation of pregnant women and patients with plaster casts is possible, as is differentiation between acute and chronic DVT and mimicking pathology.

On the down side, the costs of MRI are high, and the modality is not sufficiently available to be considered as a screening tool.

Although none of the above methods for detecting thrombus in the deep veins establishes the diagnosis of PE, the confirmation of DVT is of major importance in management decisions. The logic of leg vein imaging is that many patients with PE have residual proximal clot even in the absence of clinical evidence of DVT, itself an indication for treatment even if there is no direct proof of PE. If there is no thrombosis in the proximal leg or pelvic veins, the chance of a further significant PE is low[13,24,25] and, therefore, even if a small PE has occurred already, anticoagulation can be omitted. This approach may be inappropriate if the patient has inadequate cardiorespiratory reserve, is likely to remain immobile or if there could be an embolic source elsewhere (e.g. right atrium or vena cava).[24] Also, a negative single examination by ultrasound does not reliably exclude VTE,[100] except in the few patients with no major risk factors and no clinical suspicion of DVT. A normal repeat ultrasonography, while it does not rule out distal thrombosis, identifies subjects with a very low risk (<1%) of recurrent thromboembolism when left untreated. However, the diagnostic yield of serial ultrasound studies is very low, making this strategy unlikely to be cost-effective.

Failure to identify thrombosis of the calf veins rarely has serious sequelae, and the investigation can be repeated if there is persisting clinical concern. In patients with documented isolated calf vein thrombosis, repeated compression ultrasonography can be used to separate the 20% of patients who develop proximal extension (and require treatment) from the remaining 80% of patients who do not and in whom the risks of anticoagulant therapy may outweigh the benefits (e.g. in patients at high risk of bleeding).[24,25,96]

Non-diagnostic but useful techniques

Electrocardiography

In minor PE, there is no real haemodynamic stress and thus the only finding is sinus tachycardia. In massive PE, evidence of right heart strain may be seen (rightward shift of the QRS axis, transient right bundle branch block, Qr pattern in V1, T-wave inversion in leads V1–3, SIQIIITIII pattern, P pulmonale), but these signs are non-specific.[4,48,101,102] The main value of ECG is in excluding other potential diagnoses, such as myocardial infarction or pericarditis.

Chest radiography

Chest radiographic findings are also non-specific but may be helpful.[37,48] A normal film is compatible with all types of PE; in fact, a normal film in a patient with severe acute dyspnoea without wheezing is very suspicious of PE. The lung fields may show evidence of pulmonary infarction: peripheral opacities, sometimes wedge-shaped or semicircular, arranged along the pleural surface (so called Hampton's hump). Atelectasis, small pleural effusions and raised diaphragm have low specificity for PE. In massive PE, a plump pulmonary artery shadow may be seen when the pulmonary artery pressure is elevated. It may be possible to detect areas of oligaemia in the parts of the lung affected by emboli (Westermark sign), but this is difficult on the type of film usually available in the acute situation. The radiograph is especially valuable in excluding other conditions mimicking PE (pneumothorax, pneumonia, left heart failure, tumour, rib fracture, massive pleural effusion, lobar collapse), but PE may co-exist with other cardiopulmonary processes. The radiograph is also necessary for the proper interpretation of the lung scan.[1,52]

Echocardiography

Transthoracic echocardiography rarely enables direct visualization of the pulmonary embolus[63,103] but may reveal thrombus floating 'in transit' in the right atrium or ventricle.[104–106] With transoesophageal echocardiography, it is possible to visualize massive emboli in the central pulmonary arteries with high specificity,[107] but its sensitivity has not been evaluated in larger studies of unselected patients with suspected PE.[108]

In massive PE, the right ventricle is dilated and hypokinetic, with a corresponding decrease in left heart dimensions.[109] There will be interventricular septum flattening or bulging towards the left ventricle in diastole. The dilated inferior vena cava does not collapse during inspiration. In patients with normal blood pressure on presentation, this right ventricular dysfunction provides indirect evidence of severe pulmonary artery obstruction and impending haemodynamic failure.[106,110–113] Unfortunately, the finding of right ventricular dysfunction is non-specific,[63,103] and certain conditions commonly confused with PE [such as chronic obstructive pulmonary disease (COPD) exacerbations or cardiomyopathy] are also associated with abnormal right ventricular function. The Doppler technique allows the detection of pulmonary hypertension and, together with contrast echocardiography, it is useful in diagnosing patent foramen ovale, which may indicate impending paradoxical embolism.[1]

Although direct echocardiographic visualization of intraluminal thrombi in patients with suspected PE is an almost exceptional event and even when echocardiography provides only indirect signs compatible with haemodynamic consequences of massive PE, it is helpful in excluding or suggesting alternative causes for haemodynamic instability (aortic dissection, ventricular septal rupture, cardiac tamponade, etc).[114] In an unstable hypotensive patient requiring immediate treatment, such information is of great importance.[11] However, because the right ventricle may show no dysfunction even in patients with massive PE, echocardiography is an ancillary rather than a principal diagnostic test for PE.[1,63]

Alveolar dead-space measurements

An elevated alveolar dead-space value suggests the presence of pulmonary vascular obstruction.[1] Two studies in haemodynamically stable patients found that the combination of normal alveolar dead-space fraction and normal D-dimer assay safely excludes PE (sensitivity 98.4% and 97.8%). However, the sensitivity of the alveolar dead-space fraction measurement alone was very low (67.2% and 79.5%).[14,115] Owing to the fast redistribution of ventilation away from the embolized areas and the requirements of a fairly co-operative patient able to achieve a steady state, careful calibration of the equipment and staff experienced with this test available on all shifts, the technique will be unlikely to find application in clinical routine.

Useless diagnostic procedures

Arterial blood gases

The characteristic changes are a reduced Pa_{O_2} and a Pa_{CO_2} that is normal or reduced because of hyperventilation. The Pa_{O_2} is almost never normal in the patient with massive PE but can be normal in minor PE, mainly because of hyperventilation. In such cases, the widening of the alveolo-arterial P_{O_2} gradient (AaP_{O_2} >20 mmHg) may be more sensitive than Pa_{O_2} alone. Both hypoxaemia and a wide AaP_{O_2} may obviously be due to many other causes. Blood gases, therefore, may heighten the suspicion of PE and contribute to the clinical assessment, but they are of insufficient discriminant value to permit proof or exclusion of PE.[4,9,48,52,116,117]

Cardiac biomarkers

Patients with significant right ventricular overload due to massive PE may show increased concentrations of cardiac troponin in blood, even in the absence of right coronary artery atherosclerosis. Troponin is a sensitive indicator of myocardial damage, and its elevated concentration in PE reflects the right heart overload and has prognostic significance.[118–122] Similar to the examination of cardiac troponin, the assay of brain natriuretic peptide (BNP) does not contribute to the diagnosis of PE but enables the assessment of its haemodynamic significance. Whereas troponin is released due to myocardial damage, the initiating factor for the release of BNP is increased tension in the right ventricle, which antedates ventricular failure. Patients with stable haemodynamics but increased blood concentrations of BNP at admission have a higher mortality within 3 months after PE[123] and should perhaps be treated more aggressively during the acute stage.

Transthoracic sonography

Transthoracic sonography does not fulfil satisfactory performance criteria for application in patients with suspected PE.[124] It has not been compared with a recognized reference standard in unselected patients with suspected PE.

Possible developments

Magnetic resonance imaging (MRI)

MRI offers both morphological and functional information on lung perfusion and right heart function, but its image quality still needs improvement to be comparable with CT. An attractive advantage is the avoidance of nephrotoxic iodinated contrast and ionizing radiation. This technique may ultimately allow simultaneous and accurate detection of both DVT and PE. A disadvantage of MRI compared with CT is the long time needed to perform the examination, which is not suitable for clinically unstable patients. Improvements in MRI angiographic techniques will inevitably produce better results in the future,[99,125,126] but limited access is likely to continue for several years.

Thrombus Imaging
Scintigraphic thrombus imaging with tracers that target either platelets or fibrin may locate both PE and DVT in the future.[127,128]

The integrated diagnostic approach with management options

The diagnosis requires a high level of clinical suspicion, estimation of the pretest clinical likelihood of PE and the judicious use of objective investigations to confirm or refute the suspicion. Pulmonary angiography is regarded as the final arbiter but is not often performed on account of its limited availability, costs and invasiveness. Therefore, treatment is often based on clinical probability of PE rather than on a definite diagnosis or ruling out of the condition. Consequently, some patients receive anticoagulants without proof of PE, and other patients are not treated although they may have PE. For these reasons, much effort has been invested to determine how clinicians could reliably use non-invasive tests, alone or in combination, to replace pulmonary angiography as a diagnostic tool. The elusive quest for an ideal, single, non-invasive test has been replaced by more realistic endeavours to design and validate algorithms combining several tests in a rational manner.

Various combinations of tests have resulted in many elaborate diagnostic algorithms,[7,10,11,13–15,17,24,25,41,43,44,49,52,53,59,60,67,70,88,115,129] which, however, are seldom followed in clinical routine. Algorithms that inevitably result in large numbers of patients being referred for angiography are unhelpful.[10,60] Co-morbidity leads to less favourable cost-effectiveness of algorithms using D-dimer or scintigraphy as the first step. The availability of, and familiarity with, a certain technology may influence the diagnostic approach. The specific clinical scenario also impacts on the diagnostic procedure that is chosen. There is no single algorithm to be recommended for all situations; rather, the investigations should be chosen according to the haemodynamic state of the patient (suspicion of massive versus minor PE), the onset of symptoms (in versus out of hospital), the presence or absence of other cardiopulmonary diseases and the availability of specific tests.[15]

Basic tests
Basic tests include the ECG and plain chest radiograph. These must be performed in all patients both to support clinical suspicion of PE and, in particular, to exclude alternative diagnoses. As ECG and chest radiographic abnormalities in PE may be non-specific, absent, transient or delayed, they cannot confirm the diagnosis. However, they are important in estimating the prior probability of the disease.[56] Normal blood gases do not rule out PE; findings of hypoxaemia or hypocapnia may increase the physician's level of suspicion, but they are not specific for PE.[117] More specific investigations are always required, but choosing which road to follow from the many possibilities can be confusing.

Haemodynamic instability
Acute massive PE is an emergency requiring immediate treatment by thrombolytic therapy, perhaps combined with mechanical fragmentation of the clot through catheter techniques, or by embolectomy. All these measures have inherent risks and must therefore be applied only in patients with unequivocal evidence that the acute haemodynamic failure is caused by massive PE. In order to initiate aggressive treatment without delay, it is a great challenge to diagnose this disorder promptly. The problems are magnified by the fact that patients with massive PE are often too ill for transportation to diagnostic tests. Acute massive PE should be suspected in hypotensive, cyanotic and dyspnoeic patients when there is evidence of (or predisposing factors for) venous thrombosis, clinical evidence of acute right heart failure (high jugular venous pressure, an S3 gallop at lower sternum, tachycardia and tachypnoea) and electrocardiographic signs of right heart strain. The differential diagnosis includes all conditions that can lead to acute circulatory collapse, particularly if they are also likely to cause acute dyspnoea. The most important are left heart failure, cardiac tamponade, ventricular septal rupture, myocardial infarction, aortic dissection, tension pneumothorax and severe asthma. The absence of pulmonary rales is the warning that the haemodynamic problems do not result from left ventricular impairment, but a pattern similar to acute massive PE can result from right ventricular infarction.[1]

There are no trials and there never will be any of appropriate size or design comparing different investigations in emergency diagnosis of life-threatening PE. The diagnostic approach will be influenced by the ready availability of and experience with a certain technology. In critically ill patients suspected of having massive PE, particularly those with cardiovascular collapse, transthoracic echocardiography should be performed rapidly at the bedside to exclude other diseases or, occasionally, to establish the diagnosis by finding clots in the central pulmonary arteries or the right heart.[104–106] By visualization of thrombi, further investigations are not necessary. The finding of right ventricular dysfunction in a shocked patient with a normal left ventricular contractility would support (but not confirm) a diagnosis of PE, whereas its absence would make haemodynamically significant PE unlikely.[11] When evidence of significant and otherwise unexplainable right heart strain without clots is present on transthoracic echocardiography, transoesophageal echocardiography should follow rapidly at the bedside. The finding of unequivocal thrombus in the pulmonary arteries by transoesophageal echocardiography warrants treatment without further testing if the diagnosis fits clinically.[107] If transoesophageal echocardiography is unavailable, negative for PE or inconclusive, spiral CTPA or catheter pulmonary angiography should follow, depending on which is available with least delay. Should major PE be excluded, the correct diagnosis is usually evident with either procedure. Both procedures, however, may be constrained by logistical problems, including patient transportation. Catheterization enables immediate rapid fragmentation of central emboli.[1]

In patients with life-threatening instability where emergency treatment is necessary and CTPA or cardiac catheterization is unavailable, intravenous DSA may be adequate for showing large proximal arterial occlusions. Image quality can be improved by delivering the contrast to the pulmonary artery via a flow-directed, balloon-tipped catheter.[130] The floating catheter may also be useful in showing the characteristic haemodynamic changes with massive PE and suggesting an alternative diagnosis.[131,132]

Haemodynamically stable patients

The principal challenge in stable patients is to develop a logical sequence of investigations that allow early, cost-effective[15] diagnosis and are associated with the most favourable markers of outcome. Depending on timely availability of tests, expertise required for their use and on patient presentation, several approaches are possible:

Proof of DVT without definitive diagnosis of PE

This should be the preferred first procedure in patients with clinical suspicion of DVT in addition to the suspicion of PE.[133] If sonography, MRI or impedance plethysmography confirms thrombosis, therapy can be started without recourse to lung imaging.[53,96] Because the therapy of DVT and PE is the same in most patients with stable circulation, establishing the diagnosis of DVT is sufficient reason for full anticoagulation and avoids the need for additional studies. If the leg study is negative or inconclusive, however, further investigations are imperative.

Leg vein imaging can also be performed as the initial investigation for suspected PE in patients with previous PE or chronic cardiopulmonary disease, where the frequency of non-diagnostic scans is high. Adding ultrasonography to the diagnostic approach before lung scanning in patients without symptoms of DVT would avoid approximately 14% of lung scans and 9% of angiograms, but would lead to unnecessary treatment of 13% of patients who have an abnormal ultrasonographic result (3% of all those receiving anticoagulation).[23]

D-dimer

In outpatients with a low clinical likelihood of PE, a normal level of D-dimer rules out any significant thromboembolism; further investigations are not necessary.[13,38,40,41,44,92] The use of a D-dimer test in combination with clinical likelihood assessment is rapid, convenient for the patient and cost-effective. However, an elevated D-dimer level is a frequent non-specific finding in elderly[94] and hospitalized[60, 93] patients, in whom the clinical usefulness of this test is low.

Lung scintigraphy

In about 40% of cases, lung scan either rules out the diagnosis (normal perfusion or low-probability scan with low clinical likelihood of PE) or suggests a high enough probability of PE that, in case of concurrent high clinical likelihood of PE, therapy can be undertaken on the basis of its results without further investigations.[33,37,48,54,60,134] The frequency of such diagnostic scans is greater in outpatients with no prior cardiopulmonary disease who have a normal chest radiograph and, especially in these patients, scintigraphy is the preferred initial examination. By limiting the patients who undergo scintigraphy to those without demonstrable lung disease at chest radiography, one can reduce the number of indeterminate studies and select a group of patients whose scintigrams are likely to show normal or high-probability results. However, the presence of cardiopulmonary disease or indeed any critical illness should not deter clinicians from requesting a lung scan, if it is readily available.[67]

In patients with non-diagnostic scan, or whose clinical likelihood of PE does not correlate with the scan result, further investigation is necessary. Of these patients, about 25% will prove to have PE and require anticoagulants; the rest will have another disease as the cause of lung scan defects. Conventional pulmonary angiography as the next step is reliable[17,29,63] but difficult and expensive to implement in daily clinical practice. CTPA may be useful in these patients owing to its efficacy in imaging alternative pulmonary pathology; however, single-detector CTPA has limited value as a second diagnostic test in a routine clinical setting because of low sensitivity for subsegmental emboli.[79] In outpatients with non-diagnostic scan, low clinical likelihood of PE and no prior cardiopulmonary disease, the finding of a normal D-dimer level (measured by a test with nearly 100% sensitivity) can be used to reliably exclude VTE.[59,60]

When compression ultrasonography is done in patients with non-diagnostic scan, 9% of angiographies are prevented at the cost of unnecessarily treating 26% of patients who have an abnormal ultrasonographic result (2% of all patients receiving anticoagulation).[23] If the scan is non-diagnostic, anticoagulation can probably be withheld in patients with low clinical likelihood of PE if repeated examination of leg veins over a week is normal and the patient has adequate cardiopulmonary reserve.[7,17,24,25,44,62,135] If the leg veins are clear, it is reasonable to assume that the patient is not in imminent danger of a fatal recurrence. Those with underlying cardiopulmonary disease, where only a medium-sized embolus could be fatal, require a more aggressive diagnostic approach.[24]

Spiral CTPA

Because the results of scintigraphy are inconclusive in most cases, CTPA should be the initial imaging modality of choice, especially in patients known to have a high rate of indeterminate scintigrams (e.g. all inpatients, patients with radiographic abnormalities and patients with COPD).[86] If single-detector CTPA is positive for PE, no further examination is necessary. Also, if it is negative down to the subsegmental arteries, it is not necessary to perform another investigation.[43,83–86] However, if the CTPA findings are normal in the presence of a high clinical likelihood of PE, the patient may undergo leg imaging to detect the presence of a DVT. If this test is negative and the clinical likelihood of PE remains high, catheter angiography that focuses on the distal pulmonary vasculature should be performed. Multislice CTPA with thin collimation probably reliably confirms and excludes any clinically relevant subsegmental emboli.[73–75]

Pulmonary angiography

Depending on local capabilities, this may sometimes be the most readily available investigation (especially in centres specialized in catheter treatment of acute coronary syndromes). It pinpoints the diagnosis in cases of high clinical likelihood of PE despite non-diagnostic findings on lung and leg imaging. Occasionally, pulmonary angiography is used when the clinical likelihood is low despite the fact that other tests indicate PE. Angiography is also indicated if there are special reasons why the diagnosis must be confirmed beyond doubt (e.g. when the risk from anticoagulation is higher than normal or when suspected recurrent emboli have led to frequent admissions to hospital often in the absence of any firm evidence of VTE). Angiography may also be the preferred option where serial testing is not feasible (e.g. patient scheduled for surgery, geographical inaccessibility).

Summary

Pulmonary embolism remains a challenging diagnostic problem. The clinical diagnosis of PE is an insufficient basis for initiating long-term anticoagulant therapy; objective testing is required. The goal of cost-effective diagnosis is to restrict the need for angiography to a minority of patients with suspected PE. With scintigraphy, PE can only be diagnosed or excluded in a minority of patients, and continuing attempts to refine technology and to redefine interpretative criteria will not materially improve this. On the contrary, the diagnosis of PE by CT and MRI will continue to improve.

Clinicians are increasingly interested in working with a simple strategy that can be performed quickly in every setting. The first goal of this strategy will be to exclude PE safely in as many patients as possible. This can be done using either normal D-dimer levels in patients with low clinical likelihood or a normal perfusion scan. The next goal is to apply a reliable, simple method to confirm the presence of PE; most probably, this will be multislice CTPA in the near future. However, the choice of a diagnostic strategy should depend not only on the strategy's accuracy but also on the local facilities and expertise required for its use. Bearing in mind that an effective diagnostic strategy should be as flexible as possible in order to be applied in every clinical setting, a list of evidence-based criteria for the safe confirmation or exclusion of PE is given in Table 2. To prevent haphazard and cost-ineffective investigation of this commonly poorly managed condition, there should be at least one interested physician and radiologist who together review and refine both the hospital's policy and its application in practice.

References

1 Riedel M. Pulmonary embolic disease. In: Gibson GJ, Geddes DM, Costabel U et al. eds. Respiratory Medicine. London, Saunders, 2003:1711–58.

2 Bossuyt PM, Reitsma JB, Bruns DE et al. Towards complete and accurate reporting of studies of diagnostic accuracy: the STARD initiative. Ann Intern Med 2003; 138:40–44.

3 Hartmann IJ, Prins MH, Buller HR et al. Acute pulmonary embolism: impact of selection bias in prospective diagnostic studies. ANTELOPE study group. Advances in new technologies evaluating the localization of pulmonary embolism. Thromb Haemost 2001; 85:604–8.

4 Stein PD, Terrin ML, Hales CA et al. Clinical, laboratory, roentgenographic, and electrocardiographic findings in patients with acute pulmonary embolism and no pre-existing cardiac or pulmonary disease. Chest 1991; 100: 598–603.

5 Dunn KL, Wolf JP, Dorfman DM et al. Normal D-dimer levels in emergency department patients suspected of acute pulmonary embolism. J Am Coll Cardiol 2002; 40:1475–8.

6 Pacouret G, Marie O, Alison D et al. Association of D-dimer and helicoidal thoracic scanner for diagnosis of pulmonary embolism. Prospective study of 106 ambulatory patients. Presse Med 2002; 31:13–18.

7 Perrier A, Miron M-J, Desmarais S et al. Using clinical evaluation and lung scan to rule out suspected pulmonary embolism. Arch Intern Med 2000; 160:512–16.

8 Tardy B, Tardy Poncet B, Viallon A et al. Evaluation of D-dimer ELISA test in elderly patients with suspected pulmonary embolism. Thromb Haemost 1998; 79:38–41.

9 Wicki J, Perneger TV, Junod AF et al. Assessing clinical probability of pulmonary embolism in the emergency ward: a simple score. Arch Intern Med 2001; 161:92–7.

10 Perrier A, Bounameaux H, Morabia A et al. Diagnosis of pulmonary embolism by a decision analysis-based strategy including clinical probability, D-dimer levels, and ultrasonography: a management study. Arch Intern Med 1996; 156:531–6.

11 Kucher N, Luder CM, Dornhofer T et al. Novel management strategy for patients with suspected pulmonary embolism. Eur Heart J 2003; 24:366–76.

12 Perrier A, Desmarais S, Goehring C et al. D-dimer testing for suspected pulmonary embolism in outpatients. Am J Respir Crit Care Med 1997; 156:492–6.

13 Wells PS, Anderson DR, Rodger M et al. Excluding pulmonary embolism at the bedside without diagnostic imaging: management of

patients with suspected pulmonary embolism presenting to the emergency department by using a simple clinical model and d-dimer. *Ann Intern Med* 2001; **135**:98–107.

14 Kline JA, Israel EG, Michelson EA *et al*. Diagnostic accuracy of a bedside D-dimer assay and alveolar dead-space measurement for rapid exclusion of pulmonary embolism: a multicenter study. *JAMA* 2001; **285**:761–8.

15 Perrier A, Nendaz MR, Sarasin FP *et al*. Cost-effectiveness analysis of diagnostic strategies for suspected pulmonary embolism including helical computed tomography. *Am J Respir Crit Care Med* 2003; **167**:39–44.

16 Girard P, Musset D, Parent F *et al*. High prevalence of detectable deep venous thrombosis in patients with acute pulmonary embolism. *Chest* 1999; **116**:903–8.

17 Hull RD, Hirsh J, Carter CJ *et al*. Pulmonary angiography, ventilation lung scanning, and venography for clinically suspected pulmonary embolism with abnormal perfusion lung scan. *Ann Intern Med* 1983; **98**:891–9.

18 Girard P, Decousus M, Laporte S *et al*. Diagnosis of pulmonary embolism in patients with proximal deep vein thrombosis: specificity of symptoms and perfusion defects at baseline and during anticoagulant therapy. *Am J Respir Crit Care Med* 2001; **164**:1033–7.

19 Meignan M, Rosso J, Gauthier H *et al*. Systematic lung scans reveal a high frequency of silent pulmonary embolism in patients with proximal deep venous thrombosis. *Arch Intern Med* 2000; **160**: 159–64.

20 Moser KM, Fedullo PF, LitteJohn JK *et al*. Frequent asymptomatic pulmonary embolism in patients with deep venous thrombosis. *JAMA* 1994; **271**:223–5.

21 Monreal M, Ruiz J, Fraile M *et al*. Prospective study on the usefulness of lung scan in patients with deep vein thrombosis of the lower limbs. *Thromb Haemost* 2001; **85**:771–4.

22 Kearon C, Julian JA, Math M *et al*. Noninvasive diagnosis of deep venous thrombosis. *Ann Intern Med* 1998; **128**:663–77.

23 Turkstra F, Kuijer PMM, van Beek EJR *et al*. Diagnostic utility of ultrasonography of leg veins in patients suspected of having pulmonary embolism. *Ann Intern Med* 1997; **126**:775–81.

24 Hull RD, Raskob GE, Ginsberg JS *et al*. A noninvasive strategy for the treatment of patients with suspected pulmonary embolism. *Arch Intern Med* 1994; **154**:289–97.

25 Wells PS, Ginsberg JS, Anderson DR *et al*. Use of a clinical model for safe management of patients with suspected pulmonary embolism. *Ann Intern Med* 1998; **129**:997–1005.

26 Greenspan RH. Pulmonary angiography and the diagnosis of pulmonary embolism. *Prog Cardiovasc Dis* 1994; **37**:93–105.

27 Stein PD, Athanasoulis C, Alavi A *et al*. Complications and validity of pulmonary angiography in acute pulmonary embolism. *Circulation* 1992; **85**:462–8.

28 van Beek EJ, Brouwerst EM, Song B *et al*. Clinical validity of a normal pulmonary angiogram in patients with suspected pulmonary embolism — a critical review. *Clin Radiol* 2001; **56**:838–42.

29 van Beek EJ, Reekers JA, Batchelor DA *et al*. Feasibility, safety and clinical utility of angiography in patients with suspected pulmonary embolism. *Eur Radiol* 1996; **6**:415–19.

30 Baile EM, King GG, Müller NL *et al*. Spiral computed tomography is comparable to angiography for the diagnosis of pulmonary embolism. *Am J Respir Crit Care Med* 2000; **161**:1010–15.

31 Diffin DC, Leydendecker JR, Johnson SP *et al*. Effect of anatomic distribution of pulmonary emboli on inter-observer agreement in the interpretation of pulmonary angiography. *Am J Roentgenol* 1998; **171**:1085–9.

32 de Monyé W, van Strijen MJ, Huisman MV *et al*. Suspected pulmonary embolism: prevalence and anatomic distribution in 487 consecutive patients. Advances in New Technologies Evaluating the Localisation of Pulmonary Embolism (ANTELOPE) Group. *Radiology* 2000; **215**:184–8.

33 Worsley DF, Alavi A. Comprehensive analysis of the results of the PIOPED study. *J Nucl Med* 1995; **36**:2380–7.

34 Nilsson T, Carlsson A, Mare K. Pulmonary angiography: a safe procedure with modern contrast media and technique. *Eur Radiol* 1998; **8**:86–9.

35 Hudson ER, Smith TP, McDermott VG *et al*. Pulmonary angiography performed with iopamidol: complications in 1,434 patients. *Radiology* 1996; **198**:61–5.

36 Karwinski B, Svendsen E. Comparison of clinical and post-mortem diagnosis of pulmonary embolism. *J Clin Pathol* 1989; **42**:135–9.

37 The PIOPED Investigators. Value of the ventilation/perfusion scan in acute pulmonary embolism. Results of the prospective investigation of pulmonary embolism diagnosis (PIOPED). *JAMA* 1990; **263**:2753–9.

38 MacGillavry MR, Lijmer JG, Sanson BJ *et al*. Diagnostic accuracy of triage tests to exclude pulmonary embolism. ANTELOPE Study Group. *Thromb Haemost* 2001; **85**:995–8.

39 Urokinase Pulmonary Embolism Trial. A national cooperative study. *Circulation* 1973; **47** and **48**:1–108.

40 Kruip MJHA, Slob MJ, Schijen JHEM *et al*. Use of clinical decision rule in combination with d-dimer concentration in diagnostic workup of patients with suspected pulmonary embolism. *Arch Intern Med* 2002; **162**:1631–5.

41 Leclercq MG, Lutisan JG, Van Marwijk Kooy M *et al*. Ruling out clinically suspected pulmonary embolism by assessment of clinical probability and D-dimer levels: a management study. *Thromb Haemost* 2003; **89**:97–103.

42 De Monye W, Sanson BJ, MacGillavry MR *et al*. Embolus location affects the sensitivity of a rapid quantitative D-dimer assay in the diagnosis of pulmonary embolism. *Am J Respir Crit Care Med* 2002; **165**:345–8.

43 Van Strijen MJ, De Monye W, Schiereck J *et al*. Single-detector helical computed tomography as the primary diagnostic test in suspected pulmonary embolism: a multicenter clinical management study of 510 patients. *Ann Intern Med* 2003; **138**:307–14.

44 Kruip MJHA, Leclercq MG, van der Heul C *et al*. Diagnostic strategies for excluding pulmonary embolism in clinical outcome studies. A systematic review. *Ann Intern Med* 2003; **138**:941–51.

45 Nielsen HK, Husted SE, Krusell LR *et al*. Silent pulmonary embolism in patients with deep venous thrombosis. Incidence and fate in a randomized, controlled trial of anticoagulation versus no anticoagulation. *J Intern Med* 1994; **235**:457–61.

46 Stein PD, Henry JW, Relyea B. Untreated patients with pulmonary embolism. Outcome, clinical and laboratory assessment. *Chest* 1995; **107**:931–5.

47 Johnson R, Charnley J. Treatment of pulmonary embolism in total hip replacement. *Clin Orthop Rel Res* 1977; **124**:149–54.

48 Miniati M, Prediletto R, Formichi B *et al*. Accuracy of clinical assessment in the diagnosis of pulmonary embolism. *Am J Respir Crit Care Med* 1999; **159**:864–71.

49 Perrier A, Desmarais S, Miron MJ *et al*. Non-invasive diagnosis of venous thromboembolism in outpatients. *Lancet* 1999; **353**: 190–5.

50 Hull RD, Hirsh J, Carter CJ *et al*. Diagnostic value of ventilation–perfusion lung scanning in patients with suspected pulmonary embolism. *Chest* 1985; **88**:819–28.

51 Anderson FA, Spencer FA. Risk factors for venous thromboembolism. *Circulation* 2003; **107**:I9–I16.

52 Pistolesi M, Miniati M. Imaging techniques in treatment algorithms of pulmonary embolism. *Eur Respir J* 2002; **19**:28s–39s.

53 Perrier A, Bounameaux H. Cost-effective diagnosis of deep vein

thrombosis and pulmonary embolism. *Thromb Haemost* 2001; **86**:475–87.

54 Miniati M, Pistolesi M, Marini C *et al.* Value of perfusion lung scan in the diagnosis of pulmonary embolism: results of the prospective investigative study of acute pulmonary embolism diagnosis (PISA-PED). *Am J Respir Crit Care Med* 1996; **154**:1387–93.

55 Wells PS, Anderson DR, Rodger M *et al.* Derivation of a simple clinical model to categorize patients' probability of pulmonary embolism: increasing the model's utility with the SimpliRED D-dimer. *Thromb Haemost* 2000; **83**:416–20.

56 Miniati M, Monti S, Bottai M. A structured clinical model for predicting the probability of pulmonary embolism. *Am J Med* 2003; **114**:173–9.

57 Hoellerich VL, Wigton RS. Diagnosing pulmonary embolism using clinical findings. *Arch Intern Med* 1986; 146:1699–1704.

58 Chagnon I, Bounameaux H, Aujesky D *et al.* Comparison of two clinical prediction rules and implicit assessment among patients with suspected pulmonary embolism. *Am J Med* 2002; **113**:269–75.

59 Michiels JJ, Schroyens W, De Backer W *et al.* Non-invasive exclusion and diagnosis of pulmonary embolism by sequential use of the rapid ELISA D-dimer assay, clinical score and spiral CT. *Int Angiol* 2003; **22**:1–14.

60 Miron M-J, Perrier A, Bounameaux H *et al.* Contribution of noninvasive evaluation to the diagnosis of pulmonary embolism in hospitalized patients. *Eur Respir J* 1999; **13**:1365–70.

61 van Beek EJR, Kuyer PMM, Chenk BE *et al.* A normal perfusion lung scan in patients with clinically suspected pulmonary embolism. Frequency and clinical validity. *Chest* 1995; **108**:170–3.

62 Kruit WH, de Boer A, Sing AK *et al.* The significance of venography in the management of patients with clinically suspected pulmonary embolism. *J Intern Med* 1991; **230**:333–9.

63 Miniati M, Monti S, Pratali L *et al.* Value of transthoracic echocardiography in the diagnosis of pulmonary embolism: results of a prospective study in unselected patients. *Am J Med* 2001; **110**:528–35.

64 van Beek EJ, Kuijer PM, Buller HR *et al.* The clinical course of patients with suspected pulmonary embolism. *Arch Intern Med* 1997; **157**:2593–8.

65 Hull RD, Raskob GE, Coates G *et al.* Clinical validity of a normal perfusion lung scan in patients with suspected pulmonary embolism. *Chest* 1990; **97**:23–6.

66 Kipper MS, Moser KM, Kortman KE *et al.* Longterm follow-up of patients with suspected pulmonary embolism and a normal lung scan. Perfusion scans in embolic suspects. *Chest* 1982; **82**:411–15.

67 Hartmann IJ, Hagen PJ, Melissant CF *et al.* Diagnosing acute pulmonary embolism. Effect of chronic obstructive pulmonary disease on the performance of d-dimer testing, ventilation/perfusion scintigraphy, spiral computed tomographic angiography, and conventional angiography. *Am J Respir Crit Care Med* 2000; **162**:2232–7.

68 Corbus HF, Seitz JP, Larson RK *et al.* Diagnostic usefulness of lung SPET in pulmonary thromboembolism: an outcome study. *Nucl Med Commun* 1997; **18**:897–906.

69 Lemb M, Pohlabeln H. Pulmonary thromboembolism: a retrospective study on the examination of 991 patients by ventilation/perfusion SPECT using Technegas. *Nuklearmedizin* 2001; **40**:179–86.

70 Lorut C, Ghossains M, Horellou MH *et al.* A noninvasive diagnostic strategy including spiral computed tomography in patients with suspected pulmonary embolism. *Am J Respir Crit Care Med* 2000; **162**:1413–18.

71 Ruiz Y, Caballero P, Caniego JL *et al.* Prospective comparison of helical CT with angiography in pulmonary embolism: global and selective vascular territory analysis. Interobserver agreement. *Eur Radiol* 2003; **13**:823–9.

72 Blachere H, Latrabe V, Montaudon M *et al.* Pulmonary embolism revealed on helical CT angiography: comparison with ventilation–perfusion radionuclide lung scanning. *Am J Roentgenol* 2000; **174**:1041–7.

73 Patel S, Kazerooni EA, Cascade PN. Pulmonary embolism: optimization of small pulmonary artery visualization at multi-detector row CT. *Radiology* 2003; **227**:455–60.

74 Qanadli SD, El Hajjam M, Mesurolle B, *et al.* Pulmonary embolism detection: prospective evaluation of dual-section helical CT versus selective pulmonary arteriography in 157 patients. *Radiology* 2000; **217**: 447–55.

75 Schoepf UJ, Holzknecht N, Helmberger TK *et al.* Subsegmental pulmonary emboli: improved detection with thin-collimation multidetector row spiral CT. *Radiology* 2002; **222**:483–90.

76 Mastora I, Remy-Jardin M, Masson P *et al.* Severity of acute pulmonary embolism: evaluation of a new spiral CT angiographic score in correlation with echocardiographic data. *Eur Radiol* 2003; **13**:29–35.

77 Qanadli SD, El Hajjam M, Vieillard-Baron A *et al.* New CT index to quantify arterial obstruction in pulmonary embolism: comparison with angiographic index and echocardiography. *Am J Roentgenol* 2001; **176**:1415–20.

78 Mullins MD, Becker DM, Hagspiel KD *et al.* The role of spiral volumetric computed tomography in the diagnosis of pulmonary embolism. *Arch Intern Med* 2000; **160**:293–8.

79 Van Strijen MJ, De Monye W, Kieft GJ *et al.* Diagnosis of pulmonary embolism with spiral CT as a second procedure following scintigraphy. *Eur Radiol* 2003; **13**:1501–7.

80 Goodman LR, Lipchik RJ, Kuzo RS *et al.* Subsequent pulmonary embolism: risk after a negative helical CT pulmonary angiogram—prospective comparison with scintigraphy. *Radiology* 2000; **215**:535–42.

81 Gottsater A, Berg A, Centergard J *et al.* Clinically suspected pulmonary embolism: is it safe to withhold anticoagulation after a negative spiral CT? *Eur Radiol* 2001; **11**:65–72.

82 Ost D, Rozenshtein A, Saffran L *et al.* The negative predictive value of spiral computed tomography for the diagnosis of pulmonary embolism in patients with nondiagnostic ventilation–perfusion scans. *Am J Med* 2001; **110**:16–21.

83 Swensen SJ, Sheedy PF, Ryu JH *et al.* Outcomes after withholding anticoagulation from patients with suspected acute pulmonary embolism and negative computed tomographic findings: a cohort study. *Mayo Clin Proc* 2002; **77**:130–8.

84 Nilsson T, Olausson A, Johnsson H *et al.* Negative spiral CT in acute pulmonary embolism. *Acta Radiol* 2002; **43**:486–91.

85 Bourriot K, Couffinhal T, Bernard V *et al.* Clinical outcome after a negative spiral CT pulmonary angiographic finding in an inpatient population from cardiology and pneumology wards. *Chest* 2003; **123**:359–65.

86 Tillie-Leblond I, Mastora I, Radenne F *et al.* Risk of pulmonary embolism after a negative spiral CT angiogram in patients with pulmonary disease: 1-year clinical follow-up study. *Radiology* 2002; **223**:461–7.

87 Garg K, Sieler H, Welsh CH *et al.* Clinical validity of helical CT being interpreted as negative for pulmonary embolism: implications for patient treatment. *Am J Roentgenol* 1999; **172**:1627–31.

88 Musset D, Parent F, Meyer G *et al.* Diagnostic strategy for patients with suspected pulmonary embolism: a prospective multicentre outcome study. *Lancet* 2002; **360**:1914–20.

89 Coche EE, Hamoir XL, Hammer FD *et al.* Using dual-detector helical CT angiography to detect deep venous thrombosis in patients with suspicion of pulmonary embolism: diagnostic value and additional findings. *Am J Roentgenol* 2001; **176**:1035–9.

90 Loud PA, Katz DS, Bruce DA *et al.* Deep venous thrombosis with suspected pulmonary embolism: detection with combined CT

venography and pulmonary angiography. *Radiology* 2001; **219**: 498–502.

91 Begemann PG, Bonacker M, Kemper J *et al.* Evaluation of the deep venous system in patients with suspected pulmonary embolism with multi-detector CT: a prospective study in comparison to Doppler sonography. *J Comput Assist Tomogr* 2003; **27**:399–409.

92 Kelly J, Rudd A, Lewis RR *et al.* Plasma d-dimers in the diagnosis of venous thromboembolism. *Arch Intern Med* 2002; **162**:747–56.

93 Brotman DJ, Segal JB, Jani JT *et al.* Limitations of D-dimer testing in unselected inpatients with suspected venous thromboembolism. *Am J Med* 2003; **114**:276–82.

94 Righini M, Goehring C, Bounameaux H *et al.* Effects of age on the performance of common diagnostic tests for pulmonary embolism. *Am J Med* 2000; **109**:357–61.

95 van der Graaf F, van den Borne H, van der Kolk M *et al.* Exclusion of deep venous thrombosis with D-dimer testing. *Thromb Haemost* 2000; **83**:191–8.

96 Hirsh J, Lee AY. How we diagnose and treat deep vein thrombosis. *Blood* 2002; **99**:3102–10.

97 Heijboer H, Büller HR, Lensing WA *et al.* A comparison of real-time compression ultrasonography with impedance plethysmography for the diagnosis of deep-vein thrombosis in symptomatic outpatients. *N Engl J Med* 1993; **329**:1365–9.

98 Fraser DGW, Moody AR, Morgan PS *et al.* Diagnosis of lower limb deep venous thrombosis: a prospective blinded study of magnetic resonance direct thrombus imaging. *Ann Intern Med* 2002; **136**:89–98.

99 Kelly J, Hunt BJ, Moody A. Magnetic resonance direct thrombus imaging: a novel technique for imaging venous thromboemboli. *Thromb Haemost* 2003; **89**:773–82.

100 MacGillavry MR, Sanson BJ, Buller HR *et al.* Compression ultrasonography of the leg veins in patients with clinically suspected pulmonary embolism: is a more extensive assessment of compressibility useful? *Thromb Haemost* 2000; **84**:973–6.

101 Kucher N, Walpoth N, Wustmann K *et al.* QR in V1 — an ECG sign associated with right ventricular strain and adverse clinical outcome in pulmonary embolism. *Eur Heart J* 2003; **24**:1113–19.

102 Rodger M, Makropoulos D, Turek M *et al.* Diagnostic value of the electrocardiogram in suspected pulmonary embolism. *Am J Cardiol* 2000; **86**:807–9.

103 Perrier A, Tamm C, Unger P-F *et al.* Diagnostic accuracy of Doppler-echocardiography in unselected patients with suspected pulmonary embolism. *Int J Cardiol* 1998; **65**:101–9.

104 Casazza F, Bongarzoni A, Centonze F *et al.* Prevalence and prognostic significance of right-sided cardiac mobile thrombi in acute massive pulmonary embolism. *Am J Cardiol* 1997; **79**:1433–5.

105 Chartier L, Bera J, Delomez M *et al.* Free-floating thrombi in the right heart: diagnosis, management, and prognostic indexes in 38 consecutive patients. *Circulation* 1999; **99**:2779–83.

106 Cheriex EC, Sreeram N, Eussen YF *et al.* Cross sectional Doppler echocardiography as the initial technique for the diagnosis of acute pulmonary embolism. *Br Heart J* 1994; **72**:52–7.

107 Pruszczyk P, Torbicki A, Kuch-Wocial A *et al.* Diagnostic value of transoesophageal echocardiography in suspected haemodynamically significant pulmonary embolism. *Heart* 2001; **85**:628–34.

108 Steiner P, Lund GK, Debatin JF *et al.* Acute pulmonary embolism: value of transthoracic and transesophageal echocardiography in comparison with helical CT. *Am J Roentgenol* 1996; **167**:931–6.

109 Mansencal N, Joseph T, Vieillard-Baron A *et al.* Comparison of different echocardiographic indexes secondary to right ventricular obstruction in acute pulmonary embolism. *Am J Cardiol* 2003; **92**:116–19.

110 Grifoni S, Olivotto I, Cecchini P *et al.* Short-term clinical outcome of patients with acute pulmonary embolism, normal blood pressure, and echocardiographic right ventricular dysfunction. *Circulation* 2000; **101**:2817–22.

111 Kasper W, Konstantinides S, Geibel A *et al.* Prognostic significance of right ventricular afterload stress detected by echocardiography in patients with clinically suspected pulmonary embolism. *Heart* 1997; **77**:346–9.

112 Ribeiro A, Lindmarker P, Juhlin-Dannfeld A *et al.* Echocardiography Doppler in pulmonary embolism: right ventricular dysfunction as a predictor of mortality rate. *Am Heart J* 1997; **134**:479–87.

113 Rudoni RR, Jackson RE, Godfrey GW *et al.* Use of two-dimensional echocardiography for the diagnosis of pulmonary embolus. *J Emerg Med* 1998; **16**:5–8.

114 Nazeyrollas P, Metz D, Jolly D *et al.* Use of transthoracic Doppler echocardiography combined with clinical and electrocardiographic data to predict acute pulmonary embolism. *Eur Heart J* 1996; **17**:779–86.

115 Rodger MA, Jones G, Rasuli P *et al.* Steady-state end-tidal alveolar dead space fraction and D-dimer: bedside tests to exclude pulmonary embolism. *Chest* 2001; **120**:115–19.

116 Rodger MA, Carrier M, Jones GN *et al.* Diagnostic value of arterial blood gas measurement in suspected pulmonary embolism. *Am J Respir Crit Care Med* 2000; **162**:2105–8.

117 Stein PD, Goldhaber SZ, Henry JW *et al.* Arterial blood gas analysis in the assessment of suspected acute pulmonary embolism. *Chest* 1996; **109**:78–81.

118 Douketis JD, Crowther MA, Stanton EB *et al.* Elevated cardiac troponin levels in patients with submassive pulmonary embolism. *Arch Intern Med* 2002; **162**:79–81.

119 Konstantinides S, Geibel A, Olschewski M *et al.* Importance of cardiac troponins I and T in risk stratification of patients with acute pulmonary embolism. *Circulation* 2002; **106**:1263–8.

120 Giannitsis E, Müller-Bardorff M, Kurowski V *et al.* Independent prognostic value of cardiac troponin T in patients with confirmed pulmonary embolism. *Circulation* 2000; **102**:211–17.

121 Meyer T, Binder L, Hruska N *et al.* Cardiac troponin I elevation in acute pulmonary embolism is associated with right ventricular dysfunction. *J Am Coll Cardiol* 2000; **36**:1632–6.

122 Pruszczyk P, Bochowicz A, Torbicki A *et al.* Cardiac troponin T monitoring identifies high-risk group of normotensive patients with acute pulmonary embolism. *Chest* 2003; **123**:1947–52.

123 ten Wolde M, Tulevski II, Mulder JW *et al.* Brain natriuretic peptide as a predictor of adverse outcome in patients with pulmonary embolism. *Circulation* 2003; **107**:2082–4.

124 Mohn K, Quiot JJ, Nonent M *et al.* Transthoracic sonography of the lung and pleura in view of a suspected pulmonary embolism: a pilot study. *J Ultrasound Med* 2003; **22**:673–8.

125 Oudkerk M, van Beek EJ, Wielopolski P *et al.* Comparison of contrast-enhanced magnetic resonance angiography and conventional pulmonary angiography for the diagnosis of pulmonary embolism: a prospective study. *Lancet* 2002; **359**:1643–7.

126 Stern J-B, Abehsera M, Grenet D *et al.* Detection of pelvic vein thrombosis by magnetic resonance angiography in patients with acute pulmonary embolism and normal lower limb compression ultrasonography. *Chest* 2002; **122**:115–21.

127 Knight LC, Baidoo KE, Romano JE *et al.* Imaging pulmonary emboli and deep venous thrombi with 99mTc-bitistatin, a platelet-binding polypeptide from viper venom. *J Nucl Med* 2000; **41**:1056–64.

128 Ciavolella M, Tavolaro R, Di Loreto M *et al.* Immunoscintigraphy of venous thrombi: clinical effectiveness of a new antifibrin D-dimer monoclonal antibody. *Angiology* 1999; **50**:103–9.

129 Egermayer P, Town GI, Turner JG *et al.* Usefulness of D-dimer, blood gas, and respiratory rate measurements for excluding pulmonary embolism. *Thorax* 1998; **53**:830–4.

130 van Rooij WJ, den Heeten GJ, Sluzewski M. Pulmonary embolism: diagnosis in 211 patients with the use of selective pulmonary digital subtraction angiography with a flow-directed catheter. *Radiology* 1995; **195**:793–7.

131 Cozzi PJ, Hall JB, Schmidt GA. Pulmonary artery diastolic-occlusion pressure gradient is increased in acute pulmonary embolism. *Crit Care Med* 1995; **23**:1481–4.

132 Stanek V, Riedel M, Widimsky J. Hemodynamic monitoring in acute pulmonary embolism. *Bull Eur Physiopathol Respir* 1978; **14**:561–72.

133 Sheiman RG, McArdle CR. Clinically suspected pulmonary embolism: use of bilateral lower extremity US as the initial examination—a prospective study. *Radiology* 1999; **212**:75–8.

134 Barghouth G, Yersin B, Boubaker A *et al*. Combination of clinical and V/Q scan assessment for the diagnosis of pulmonary embolism: a 2-year outcome prospective study. *Eur J Nucl Med* 2000; **27**:1280–5.

135 Ginsberg JS, Brill EP, Demers C *et al*. D-dimer in patients with clinically suspected pulmonary embolism. *Chest* 1993; **104**:1679–84.

CHAPTER 1.2.5

Screening for lung cancer

John K Gohagan, Pamela M Marcus, Richard M Fagerstrom, William C Black,
Barnett S Kramer, Paul F Pinsky and Philip C Prorok

How important is lung cancer in public health terms?

Internationally, lung cancer statistics are bleak.[1] Annually, more than a million new cases of lung cancer are diagnosed worldwide, and more than 900 000 people die of the disease. Five-year survival following diagnosis is dismal −14% in the USA and even lower in Europe. Most lung cancers are diagnosed as locally advanced or metastatic disease, with only 22% of cases presenting at an early, and potentially curable, stage. Lung cancer is the leading cancer killer in the USA for both men and women. For males, the USA ranks fifth in World Health Organization age-adjusted standard population mortality statistics behind Hungary, Poland, the Netherlands and Italy. Canada, the UK and most of Europe rank closely below the USA. For females, the USA ranks first, with Denmark, Canada and the UK next in order.

Cigarette smoking is the principal cause of lung cancer. In the USA, where this point has been emphasized for nearly 40 years, cigarette packages by law warn of the risks of smoking, smoking cessation programmes are pervasive, former smokers nearly equal in number current smokers (roughly 46 million), and huge settlements have been awarded in litigation against tobacco companies. Despite these measures, lung cancer persists as the leading cause of cancer-related mortality in the USA, with an increasing fraction of new lung cancers diagnosed in former smokers.

In October 2000, the National Cancer Institute (NCI) of the USA convened its Lung Cancer Progress Review Group (PRG). The PRG was charged with identifying areas of high priority in lung cancer research. The PRG's members—clinicians, scientists, industry representatives and consumer advocates—reviewed the current lung cancer problem and identified research strategies in prevention, early detection and treatment that have the greatest potential to reduce disease burden. The PRG report began with this troubling picture of lung cancer in the US today:[2]

> Lung cancer is the leading cause of cancer death for both men and women in the USA, killing more people than breast, prostate, colon and pancreas cancers combined:

Fully 85 percent of patients who develop lung cancer die from it. We are still largely ignorant of the molecular events underlying the development of lung cancer and the mechanisms of resistance to drug and radiation therapy; no agent has been found useful in the prevention of lung cancer; and the benefits of lung cancer screening and early detection are mired in controversy. With half of all lung cancers in the USA now diagnosed in former smokers, it is a sobering reality that tobacco control will ameliorate but not, in the foreseeable future, eliminate the problem of lung cancer.

The PRG characterized the lung cancer problem as 'enormous' in scope and noted that:
- 'Chemotherapy, surgery, and radiation therapy have had a modest effect on patient outcomes'.
- 'Molecular events underlying the development of lung cancer are largely unknown'.
- 'Patients with the earliest surgical stage (T1N0) have disseminated disease between 15 and 30 percent of the time'.

How much is known about the natural history of the disease and the potential of early intervention?

In addition to emphasizing the need for smoking cessation initiatives and genetic and aetiological research, the PRG stressed the importance of research concerning early detection, stating that new imaging:

> approaches (and in particular the application of spiral CT) have the potential to identify small and early lesions that have not been readily accessible in clinical practice through more conventional detection methods . . . spiral CT screening offers a unique opportunity to study early carcinogenesis, and potentially to reduce lung cancer mortality. However, the clinical and biological significance of these small and early lesions is not well understood.

Although the search for an efficacious lung cancer screening modality dates back more than 50 years, no screening modality has been shown in randomized controlled trials (RCTs) to reduce lung cancer mortality. Three influential

RCTs, constituting the NCI's Early Lung Cancer Detection Project, were conducted in the 1970s and 1980s. Two of them, Johns Hopkins[3] and Memorial Sloan–Kettering,[4] showed no reduction in lung cancer mortality with a regimen of annual chest X-ray and sputum cytology every 4 months versus annual chest X-ray alone, indicating that sputum cytology in addition to chest X-ray was not useful. The third trial, the Mayo Lung Project (MLP), showed no reduction in lung cancer mortality with chest X-ray and sputum cytology every 4 months versus usual care (with participants in the usual care arm receiving only a recommendation at study entry to receive the two tests annually).[5] As no benefit of sputum cytology was observed in the Johns Hopkins and Memorial Sloan–Kettering trials, the results of the MLP were interpreted to indicate that screening chest X-ray does not reduce lung cancer mortality.

When the Early Lung Cancer Detection Project was conceived, opinions regarding the usefulness of lung cancer screening were varied. Some institutions, including the Mayo Clinic, recommended annual screening for lung cancer using chest X-ray and sputum cytology. However, Robert Fontana, a Mayo Clinic physician and Principal Investigator for the MLP, stated that '. . . when the three NCI-sponsored trials were in the formative stages, it was generally accepted that yearly chest radiography had no appreciable effect on lung cancer mortality'.[6] Nevertheless, the trials were carried out. In response to screening enthusiasts, the US National Institutes of Health (NIH) held a consensus development conference on screening for lung cancer while the three trials were still several years away from reporting results. This conference, chaired by Howard Anderson of the Mayo Clinic and John Bailar of the NCI, issued a cautionary report regarding lung cancer screening, in which it was stated that:[7]

> Until the value of screening for lung cancer by these methods has been demonstrated, mass screening programs should be limited to well-designed, controlled clinical trials, with provision for analysis of results and for further diagnostic workup and treatment when indicated. While some screening programs for lung cancer have been initiated among workers in certain industries, caution is strongly recommended in starting any new ones. Screened workers cannot be assured of an overall benefit on the basis of existing data.

A fourth RCT, conducted in Czechoslovakia, provided further evidence that screening with chest X-ray did not reduce lung cancer mortality (19 lung cancer deaths among 3172 in the screened arm and 13 among 3174 in the control arm).[8] As in the MLP, more lung cancers were diagnosed in the screened arm (108 versus 82), more screen-detected cancers were resectable (25% versus 16%), and survival after diagnosis was substantially longer in the screened arm. However, mortality was not reduced in the screened arm. As in the MLP, a larger

trial would have been necessary to detect a small reduction in mortality. This trial compared semi-annual screening by posteroanterior chest photofluorogram and sputum cytology with 3-year annual screening and no screening in a high-risk population of men aged 40–64 years.

Over the past 20 years, the findings of NCI's Early Lung Cancer Detection Project and the Czechoslovakian trial have played a central role in shaping policy decisions concerning lung cancer screening. The results of the three US trials convinced the majority of the medical community that screening with either chest X-ray or state-of-the-art sputum cytology was not effective in reducing lung cancer mortality, and the Czechoslovakian trial added international credence to this conclusion. In 1980, the American Cancer Society revised its previous lung cancer screening recommendations, stating that early detection of lung cancer was not recommended.[9] The national research focus shifted to smoking prevention, with the realization that cigarette smoking was the primary cause of lung cancer.

The principal investigators of the Memorial Sloan–Kettering trial disagreed with the conclusions of the Early Lung Cancer Detection Project. Maintaining that it was wrong to conclude from these trials that early detection by chest X-ray or sputum cytology did not lower the probability of death from lung cancer, Melamed and Flehinger wrote:[10]

> A realistic assessment of the current status of lung cancer in the USA, however, permits us only to reaffirm the present importance of identifying lung cancer while the patient is still asymptomatic, and to re-state our view that a decision to advise against efforts to detect lung cancer early is equivalent to a decision not to treat for cure. The weight of evidence continues to support the prudent medical practitioner who recommends regular screening of asymptomatic persons at high risk for lung cancer.

What are the possible treatment options following screening?

When a lung tumour is limited to the hemithorax and can be completely excised, surgery is the preferred treatment. Screening, as evidenced in the MLP, identifies more early stage (stage I and II) tumours that can be resected. Disseminated disease, as evidenced by involved lymph nodes, for which chemotherapy is standard treatment, offers much poorer survival prognosis.

How effective are screening/treatment options in terms of mortality and morbidity?

Post hoc mathematical modelling of the progression kinetics of lung cancer using the Memorial Sloan–Kettering trial data hypothesized that there could be a small mortality reduction attendant on X-ray screening of less than 20%.[11] Unfortunately, the MLP had inadequate statistical power to identify such a small but clinically important effect. The NCI is currently revisiting this question of effectiveness of lung cancer screening in the Prostate, Lung, Colorectal, and Ovarian (PLCO) Cancer Screening Trial.[12] In the PLCO Trial, the intervention arm is offered an initial and three subsequent annual chest X-rays (participants who have never smoked receive only two annual chest X-rays) while the control arm receives usual care. This trial has 90% statistical power to detect a 20% reduction in lung cancer mortality. PLCO randomization concluded at almost 155 000 participants on 2 July 2001; lung cancer screening ended in July 2004.

Although lacking the statistical power to identify a small but important reduction in lung cancer mortality, data from the MLP have provided important insights on other issues concerning lung cancer screening. More lung cancers were detected in the screened arm (206 versus 160 in the usual care group) and a greater percentage were completely resectable (46% versus 32% in the usual care arm). Nevertheless, the cumulative numbers of late-stage, unresectable lung cancers in the two groups were almost identical year by year, and at no point in the trial was lung cancer mortality significantly lower for the intervention arm.[6] In fact, mortality was a little higher (although not significantly different) in the screened arm (3.2/1000 person–years versus 3.0/1000 person–years) at the end of the trial. Strauss et al.[13] have interpreted this constellation of findings as an indication of a screening benefit and evidence of study flaws, including group incomparability. Others recognize a pattern that strongly suggests overdiagnosis, that is the diagnosis of cancers that would never have been diagnosed in the absence of screening.[14]

Extended follow-up and reanalysis of the Mayo Lung Project

Marcus and Prorok[15] investigated the possibility that the negative results of the MLP were due to an imbalance of lung cancer risk and prognostic factors across study arms. Using proportional hazards models, the authors examined whether age at entry, history of cigarette smoking, exposure to non-tobacco lung carcinogens and previous pulmonary illnesses confounded the relationship of screening and lung cancer mortality; they also examined whether this relationship was modified by those factors. Neither adjustment for, nor stratification by, these factors altered the original findings of the MLP. To address the possibility that longer follow-up of the MLP participants might reveal a mortality reduction, Marcus and colleagues, using a National Death Index Plus search, conducted an additional 14 years of lung cancer mortality follow-up for the MLP participants.[16] The result remained the same: lung cancer mortality was slightly higher for the intervention arm (4.4 deaths per 1000 person–years versus 3.9 per 1000 person–years in the usual care arm; P value = 0·08). These two

analyses addressed the major criticisms levelled at the MLP and reinforced the original finding of no reduction in lung cancer mortality with an intense regimen of screening.

All evidence argues against recommending screening for lung cancer by chest X-ray or sputum cytology.

Low-dose spiral computerized tomography as a lung cancer screening modality

Low-dose helical computerized tomography (helical CT or spiral CT), an advance in CT technology introduced during the 1990s, has been observed to be more sensitive than chest X-ray for identifying lesions in the lung. Low-dose spiral CT offers rapid image acquisition at radiation doses substantially below standard high-resolution CT, making it a candidate for lung cancer screening.[17] The potential for mass screening using spiral CT in Japan was investigated in 1996.[18] Of 5483 smokers and non-smokers between the ages of 40 and 74 years screened in a mobile unit, 279 received workups for suspicious findings, 29 underwent surgery, and 23 cancers were diagnosed on the first screen. Some patients received one repeat screen over a 2-year period and, of the 60 cancers detected throughout the period, 40 (two-thirds) were not seen on retrospective interpretation of chest radiographs.

The most publicized results regarding the use of low-dose spiral CT as a lung cancer screening modality were reported by the NCI-supported Early Lung Cancer Action Project (ELCAP).[19] ELCAP recruited 1000 volunteers at elevated risk of lung cancer (at least 10 pack–years of smoking) and screened them with both chest X-ray and low-dose spiral CT. In this group, the baseline (prevalence) spiral CT screen detected all non-calcified nodules visible on chest X-ray and also identified other lesions: spiral CT detected non-calcified nodules in 233 participants (malignant disease confirmed in 27), while chest X-ray detected non-calcified nodules in only 68 participants (malignant disease confirmed in seven). Additionally, four cancers not characterized as nodules were detected by spiral CT. The findings of ELCAP suggest that spiral CT is more sensitive than chest X-ray. ELCAP reported finding an additional seven cancers (six non-small cell and one small cell) in this population on repeat screens.[20] Thirty positive screens out of the 1184 annual repeat screens resulted in six non-small cell cancers (five of stage IA) and one small cell cancer. In two instances, the patient died of other causes before diagnostic workup, the nodules resolved spontaneously in 12, nodules were not enlarging in eight, and eight underwent biopsy for possible cancer. But, because the ELCAP incorporates no equivalent control group for comparison, it lacks the ability to determine the impact of spiral CT screening on mortality or directly to compare harms against possible benefits of screening.

The NCI is also funding a project at the Mayo Clinic in which men and women over 50 years of age with a smoking

Table 1. New randomized controlled trials initiatives.

Country (status)	Smoking history (pack–years)	Size (I/C)	Randomized by	Calculated effect (%)/ power (%)	Screens	Intervention
Denmark (P;m)	20	5000/5000	Individual	25/??	T0 and annual × 5	SCT versus UC
France (P;m)	30	10 000/10 000	Individual	44/90	T0 and annual × 5	SCT versus UC
Germany (P;m)	40 years	20 000/20 000	Individual	20/90	T0 and annual × 4	SCT versus CXR
Italy (P;m)	20	6000/6000	Individual	35/80	T0 and annual × 3	SCT versus UC
Israel (A;$;m)	20	2500/2500	Individual	NA	T0 and annual × 5	SCT versus UC
Netherlands (P;m)	20	8000/16 000	Individual	20/90	T0 and annual × 2	SCT versus UC
Norway (P;m)	20	12 000/24 000	Individual	?/80	T0 and annual × 5	SCT versus UC
UK (P;f)	Smokers	1000/1000	Individual	NA	T0 and annual × 1	SCT versus UC
UK (P;m)		25 000/25 000	Individual	NA	T0 and annual × 5	SCT versus UC
USA (A;$;f)	30	1600/1600	Individual	NA	T0 and annual × 2	SCT versus CXR
USA (P;m)		25 000/25 000	Individual	20/90	T0 and annual × 2	SCT versus CXR

Status: A, active; P, proposed; $, funded; f, feasibility project; m, mortality endpoint trial; T0, baseline prevalence screen; SCT, spiral CT; CXR, chest X-ray; UC, usual care; I/C, intervention/control.

history of at least 20 pack–years are being screened with spiral CT and sputum cytology.[21] This study enrolled 1520 individuals in 1 year, almost two-thirds of whom were current smokers and the rest former smokers. Indeterminate nodules were found in 775 subjects, and 13 lung cancers were diagnosed (12 identified on CT). As with ELCAP, no comparison arm exists in the study for the purpose of assessing the impact of screening on mortality.

There is widespread appreciation that an RCT is needed to determine the mortality-reducing efficacy and risks of spiral CT screening for lung cancer. Since early 2000, NCI has sponsored several workshops at which the need for an RCT with ample statistical power to detect a modest reduction in lung cancer mortality was debated and endorsed.[21] The need for an RCT has been argued in the peer-reviewed literature by independent radiologists as well.[14,22]

To assess the feasibility of conducting an RCT of spiral CT for lung cancer screening, the Lung Screening Study (LSS), a 12-month special study within the PLCO Trial, was undertaken in September 2000. The goals were to determine the ability to randomize high-risk candidates around the nation to spiral CT versus chest X-ray, determine background use of spiral CT, measure crossover contamination between screening arms and assess downstream follow-up burden. The accrual goal was to randomize 3000 non-PLCO participants aged 55–74 years over a 2-month period at six PLCO screening centres. Randomized individuals received either a single spiral CT or a chest X-ray screen. Screening was completed on 31 January 2001. Medical record abstracting of diagnostic follow-up to positive screens was completed by the end of May 2001. Interest was twice as great as projected, and recruitment mailings had to be discontinued ahead of schedule: 3373 eligible participants were randomized. Previous use of spiral CT by interest-

ed participants was very low at all centres (<3%). Compliance with screening examinations exceeded 95%. Crossover contamination from the chest X-ray to spiral CT was less than 2%. Positivity rates for the initial screen were 20.5% for spiral CT and 9.8% for chest X-ray, resulting in 30 cancers diagnosed in the CT arm and seven in the X-ray arm. At the first annual screen, the positivity rates were 25.8% for spiral CT and 8.7% for chest X-ray, resulting in eight additional cancers detected in the CT arm and nine in the X-ray arm. Compliance with screening declined from 93% at baseline to 86% at the first annual screen in the CT arm and from 93% to 80% in the X-ray arm.[23,24]

New initiatives to evaluate spiral CT

Publication of the ELCAP findings sparked intense international interest in spiral CT for lung cancer screening. Several European countries and the USA are developing RCT designs to assess the effect of spiral CT screening on mortality. The trial designs under consideration vary by country, as shown in Table 1 and the following text. Designs comparing spiral CT with chest X-ray reflect the possibility that chest X-ray may have a small, but as yet unknown, impact on lung cancer mortality. If chest X-ray in the PLCO Trial is found to have no effect, these designs will be equivalent to the spiral CT versus usual care design (apart from harm incurred by screening chest X-ray and medical management). As described above, the National Cancer Institute of the United States (NCI) conducted a 12-month feasibility project, beginning September 2000, in which 3373 consenting individuals were randomized to either spiral CT or chest X-ray screening. Results of this project are being prepared for publication in 2002. In the feasibility project, only an initial (T0) screen was offered, but the

NCI extended the project for a second 12 months to include a first annual incidence (T1) screen and follow-up.

Denmark. Randomize men and women (age 50–65 years) to spiral CT or no screening. Participants must be judged physically fit for surgery, as judged by their ability to climb two flights of stairs with no pausing within 30 seconds, have an a forced expiratory volume in 1 second of at least 1000 mL, be current smokers with a 20 pack–year smoking history and consent to be randomized. Subjects are excluded for a history of lung cancer or other malignancy, other than basal cell carcinoma, or for cardiac or other disease that would preclude surgery for lung cancer. Recruitment (10 000 subjects) will be completed in 24 months. Subjects will be invited by mail from Copenhagen, Frederiksberg and Copenhagen County. Screening will consist of an initial plus five repeat annual screens; control subjects will not receive a prevalence screen. Both screen and control groups will be invited annually for spirometry, smoking cessation counselling and quality of life assessment. First interim analysis for mortality planned following year 4.

France. Recruit 26 000 men and women (age 50–75 years) through 1000 general practices for a prevalence spiral CT screen. Participants must be judged physically fit, as judged by their ability to climb two flights of stairs without significant breathlessness, and have no current signs of cancer or prior history of cancer. Current and former heavy smokers with a 20 pack–year history are eligible. Informed consent is required. Subjects with negative findings on the prevalence screen will be eligible for randomization. Both screen and control groups will receive smoking cessation counselling. At T5, both arms will receive a final spiral CT screen.

Germany. Recruit 40 000 men and women (age 55–69 years) by media advertising or direct mail to 12 screening centres in Germany and two in Vienna, Austria. Participants must have no serious illnesses and have a life expectancy of at least 10 years, must be healthy enough to undergo chest surgery and have no history of lung cancer. Subjects must have at least a 40-year history of smoking and, if under 60 years of age, must be current smokers or have quit within the last 5 years. Informed consent is required for randomization. Subjects will be asked to donate blood for future research. The first interim analysis for mortality is planned when all subjects have been enrolled for 5 years.

Italy. Recruit 12 000 men and women (age 55–69 years) through general practices. Current and former smokers (quitting within last 10 years) who are healthy enough to undergo curative surgery for lung cancer. Post-randomization consent is proposed. All subjects will receive smoking cessation counselling. Randomization is to be accomplished within 12 months. The first interim analysis for mortality is proposed at year 6.

Israel. Recruit 5000 men and women (age 45–70 years) by media and advertising in general practitioners' offices. Current smokers with at least 20 pack–year history and former smokers (having quit smoking within 5 years after smoking at least 20 pack–years). Individuals with active cancer (except skin), a severe heart condition or life expectancy less than 7 years are excluded. Screened persons undergo spirometry, sputum cell examination and low-radiation spiral CT (after October 2001, spiral CT will be via multislice systems). About 1000 subjects have been screened. Five annual rescreens are planned.

Netherlands. Recruit 24 000 men and women (age 50–75 years) by mail questionnaire through population registries in Rotterdam, Utrecht and Groningen. Participants must be able to climb three flights of stairs, have no history of recent myocardial infarct and be judged able to undergo surgical treatment for lung cancer. Current and former smokers (<5 years since quitting) with a 20 pack–year history are eligible. Subjects with a previous history of cancer, excepting basal cell carcinoma of the skin, are excluded. Blood samples will be collected from the screened group for future research. Randomization will be stratified by asbestos exposure only. Informed consent is required for randomization.

Norway. Recruit 24 000 men and women (age 60–69 years) from previously identified high-risk (at least 20 pack–years) cohort of current smokers or smokers who have quit within 5 years of randomization. Subjects invited to screen will receive spirometry, receive counselling on diet if blood lipids are high and will donate blood for future research. Blood and sputum samples from the screened group will be archived. Smoking cessation counselling will be restricted to the screening arm.

United Kingdom. A pilot study is proposed to include 2000 subjects (age 60 years and older) from two large general practices randomized to spiral CT versus usual care for an initial and one annual screen. If feasibility is shown, the pilot will be expanded without interruption into a mortality endpoint RCT with 40 000 to 60 000 subjects randomized to usual care or spiral CT (initial and five annual screens). Recruitment through designated general practices identified through the MRC General Practice Research Framework. Smoking cessation programme will be offered to all subjects in the pilot and main trial. Eligibility restricted to current smokers. Individuals unlikely to benefit from screening or with current serious illness excluded. The pilot was not funded as of 2005. There remains interest in revisiting the issue.

United States. Twelve-month feasibility study completed 30 September 2001: 3373 individuals (age 55–74 years; at least 30 pack–year smoking history; current or former smokers who quit within last 10 years) randomized at six centres to an initial screen of either spiral CT or chest X-ray. Background use of spiral CT and crossover contamination between arms measured. Feasibility study extended to 31 October 2002 to include first annual screen and appropriate follow-up. A definitive mortality endpoint RCT with an initial and two annual screens with subjects in the feasibility study becoming the vanguard group, is under consideration for funding with a proposed start date of December 2001. Informed consent is required for randomization. Recruitment is by direct mail. Individuals are excluded if they have a history of lung cancer or are being treated for other cancer, except non-melanoma skin cancer. Subjects are referred to smoking cessation programmes. Annual interim analyses for mortality planned to begin March 2004. Randomization began in the autumn of 2002 and finished at the end of April 2004 with a total of 53 476 participants who have all received their initial screens. Sceening is expected to be completed (all three screens) by December 2006.

How acceptable are screening methods?

Chest X-ray is a standard clinical procedure and is widely considered to confer low radiation risk (7–12 mrem, compared with annual ambient exposures of about 500 mrem in the USA). The production of sputum for cytological analysis requires substantial uncomfortable effort from subjects. Spiral CT is a quick and painless screening procedure requiring a 25-second breath-hold, which most heavy smokers can achieve when coached effectively.

What are the costs of screening and subsequent workup?

Spiral CT screening can cost anywhere from $350 to two or three times that amount in private practice settings. Chest X-ray may cost about a third as much. Sputum cytology, not a typical procedure, may fall somewhere in the middle. The costs of screening are only the beginning. Follow-up procedures to differentially diagnose and treat screen-detected cancers can generate tens of thousands of dollars in charges.

What is the cost-effectiveness of screening?

Cato et al.[25] and Okamoto[26] have attempted to evaluate the potential cost-effectiveness of screening for lung cancer in the USA and Japan respectively. Each concluded that screening was potentially cost-effective; however, as the true effectiveness of spiral CT or chest X-ray screening in reducing lung cancer mortality is not known, these analyses relied on postulated benefits of screening. Currently, plans for cost-effectiveness analyses in both PLCO and NLST are being developed. Such analyses will try to estimate the costs associated with a screening programme and weigh these against the beneficial effects of screening, if any. Costs of a screening programme include the costs of the screen, as well as the costs of diagnostic follow-up and the costs of treating overdiagnosed cases.

Unresolved issues

Many issues are yet to be addressed regarding spiral CT screening. Will the high sensitivity of spiral CT result in substantial overdiagnosis, overtreatment and unacceptable harm, or will it be possible to refine the diagnostic process in order to achieve acceptable specificity? ELCAP is applying imaging-based algorithms to determine whether lesions detected on spiral CT are growing. Those that appear to be static are considered safe to follow by periodic rescreens. Those that appear to be growing are considered potentially malignant and in need of immediate treatment. It is unclear whether this approach will be adequate to minimize harm without diminishing potential efficacy. Uncertainty among experts regarding how to manage the assessment of lesions less than 3 mm in diameter and so-called ground-glass opacities was a topic of extensive discussion at the Fifth International Conference on Screening for Lung Cancer, 26–28 October 2001.[27] Investigators proposing RCTs to evaluate spiral CT are also planning to address screening risks, reliability of image interpretation, optimizing the sensitivity/specificity relationship and cost-effectiveness.

In the meantime, advocates of spiral CT screening for lung cancer are active. In the USA, newspapers and television advertisements impute benefits to screening. Laypersons and medical professionals are advocating screening, in the belief that screening, if not of proven benefit, is at least not harmful and should be available to all. Waiting to learn whether screening is more beneficial than harmful is often considered unacceptable, while doing trials to 'further characterise and quantify the risks involved' is acceptable, but should not impede the widespread application of spiral CT screening, some argue.[28]

Recently resurrected enthusiasm for lung cancer screening is based upon intuition and logic rather than carefully controlled trials assessing health outcomes — both good and bad. The history of medicine, for example national neuroblastoma screening in Japan,[29,30] tells us that enthusiastic embracement of medical technology — even when well intended — can lead to unintended harm. In the case of lung cancer screening, in particular, trials using chest X-ray and sputum cytology documented how early calls for widespread implementation were misplaced. The consequences of misplaced enthusiasm can cause harm as well as benefit. It is important to get the answer right. Meticulous application of the scientific method in rigorously designed and conducted trials will not fail us.

References

1 van Klaveren RJ, Habbema JDF, Pedersen JF, de Koning HJ, Oudkerk M, Hoogsteden HC. Lung cancer screening by low-dose spiral computed tomography. *Eur Respir J* 2001; **18**:857–66.

2 The Report of the Lung Cancer Progress Review Group, 2001. Available online at http://osp.nci.nih.gov/prg_assess/prg/lungprg/lung_rpt.htm.

3 Frost JK, Ball WCJ, Levin ML *et al.* Early lung cancer detection: results of the initial (prevalence) radiologic and cytologic screening in the Johns Hopkins study. *Am Rev Respir Dis* 1984; **130**:549–54.

4 Flehinger BJ, Melamed MR, Zaman MB, Heelan, RT, Perchick, WB,

Martini, N. Early lung cancer detection: results of the initial (prevalence) radiologic and cytologic screening in the Memorial Sloan-Kettering study. *Am Rev Respir Dis* 1984; **130**:555–60.

5 Fontana RS, Sanderson DR, Woolner LB, Taylor WF, Miller WE, Muhn JR. Lung cancer screening: the Mayo program. *J Occup Med* 1986; **28**:746–50.

6 Fontana RS, Sanderson DR, Woolner LB *et al.* Screening for lung cancer: a critique of the Mayo Lung Project. *Cancer* 1991; **67**:1155–64.

7 Gordon RS. Lung cancer mortality appears unaffected by roentgenographic and sputum screening in asymptomatic persons. *JAMA* 1979; **241**:1582.

8 Kubik A, Polak J. Lung cancer detection results of a randomized prospective study in Czechoslovakia. *Cancer* 1986; **57**:2427–37.

9 American Cancer Society Report on the cancer-related health check-up: cancer of the lung. *Cancer J Clin* 1980; **30**:199–207.

10 Melamed MR, Flehinger, BJ. Letter to the Editor. *Ann Intern Med* 1989; **111**:764–5.

11 Flehinger BJ, Kimmel M. The natural history of lung cancer in a periodically screened population. *Biometrics* 1987; **111**:127–44.

12 Gohagan JK, Levin DL, Prorok PC, Sullivan DA (eds) The Prostate, Lung, Colorectal and Ovarian (PLCO) cancer screening trial. *Control Clin Trials* 2000; **21**(Suppl):249S–406S.

13 Strauss GM, Gleason RE, Shugarbaker DJ. Screening for lung cancer: another look; a different view. *Chest* 1997; **111**:754–68.

14 Black WC. Overdiagnosis: an unrecognized cause of confusion and harm in cancer screening. *J Natl Cancer Inst* 2000; **92**:1280.

15 Marcus PM, Prorok PC. Reanalysis of the Mayo Project data: the impact of confounding and effect modification. *J Cancer Screen* 1999; **6**:47–9.

16 Marcus PM, Bergstralh EJ, Fagerstrom RM *et al.* Lung cancer mortality in the Mayo Lung Project: impact of extended follow-up. *J Natl Cancer Inst* 2000; **92**:1308–16.

17 Naidich DP, Marshall CH, Gribbin C, Arams RS, McCauley DI. Low-dose CT of the lungs: preliminary observations. *Radiology* 1990; **175**:729–31.

18 Sone S, Takashima S, Li F *et al.* Mass screening for lung cancer with mobile spiral computed tomography scanner. *Lancet* 1998; **351**:1242–5.

19 Henschke CI, McCauley DI, Yankelevitz DF *et al.* Early Lung Cancer Action Project: overall design and findings from baseline screening. *Lancet* 1999; **354**:99–105.

20 Henschke CI, Naidich DP, Yankelevitz DF *et al.* Early Lung Cancer Action Project: initial findings on repeat screening. *Cancer* 2001; **92**:153–9.

21 Division of Cancer Prevention, National Cancer Institute. Proceedings of the Spiral CT Screening for Lung Cancer Workshop, Internal Document, October 26 1999.

22 Patz EF Jr, Rossi S, Harpole DH, Herndon JE, Goodman PC. Correlation of tumor size and survival in patients with stage 1A non-small cell lung cancer. *Chest* 2000; **117**:1568–71.

23 Gohagan J, Marcus P, Fagerstrom R, Pinsky P, Kramer B, Prorok P, for the Lung Screening Study Research Group. Baseline findings of a randomized feasibility trial of lung cancer screening with spiral CT scan vs chest tradiograph. *Chest* 2004; **126**:114–21.

24 Gohagan JK, Marcus PM, Fagerstrom RM *et al.* Final results of the Lung Screening Study, a randomized feasibility study of spiral CT versus chest X-ray screening for lung cancer. *Lung Cancer* 2005; **47**:9–15.

25 Cato JJ, Klittich WS, Strauss G. Could chest x-ray screening for lung cancer be cost effective? *Cancer* 2000; **89**:2502–5.

26 Okamoto N. Cost-effectiveness of lung cancer screening in Japan. *Cancer* 2000; **89**:2489–93.

27 5th International Conference on Screening for Lung Cancer, October 26–28, 2001, Weill Medical College of Cornell University, New York.

28 Parles K. Low-dose spiral CT screening. Letter to the Editor. *Chest* 2001; **120**:1042–3.

29 Yamamoto K, Hanada R, Kikuchi A *et al.* Spontaneous regression of localized neuroblastoma detected by mass screening. *J Clin Oncol* 1998; **16**: 1265–9.

30 Bessho F. Effect of mass screening on age-specific incidence of neuroblastoma. *Int J Cancer* 1996; **67**:520–2.

CHAPTER 1.3
Therapeutics: general issues

CHAPTER 1.3.1
Adherence and self-management

Liesl M Osman and Michael E Hyland

Summary

Objective measures of adherence (such as electronic monitoring) suggest that common levels of adherence to prophylactic medication are between 60% and 80% of prescribed dose, taken on 50–60% of days prescribed. Studies introducing oral therapy have shown that it is more likely to be more adhered to than inhaled therapy, in those patients for whom it is suitable as therapy. Adherence to peak flow monitoring is at similar levels.

Sociodemographic characteristics such as age, income and education are related to higher levels of adherence. They are likely to reflect differences in quality of health care provided and factors such as continuity of relationship with a doctor and experience of prophylactic medication.

Non-adherence cannot be shown inevitably to lead to poor outcome. Many patients effectively control their asthma at adherence levels of 60–80% of use. However, very low levels of adherence (40% or less) are characteristic of symptomatic patients who have frequent hospitalizations and emergency attendances, and non-adherence has been identified as a factor in fatal asthma. Thus, non-adherence can be successful or unsuccessful, and this can only be gauged by looking at patient outcomes.

Low usage of prescribed preventive medication can be conceptualized as resulting from non-intentional non-adherence (forgetting), reasoned or intentional non-adherence (refusal) and unwillingness to accept an asthma identity by patients (denial). Actual non-adherence by a patient can have elements of all these factors.

The self-management approach addresses all these aspects of non-adherence. Unintentional non-adherence is reduced by the provision of simple written instruction on medication taking; reasoned non-adherence and denial are addressed by the requirement to reach concordance between doctor and patient in drawing up a self-management plan (action plan). This approach has been shown successfully to improve patient outcomes in studies with children and adults.

Introduction

Asthma is an illness that is usually well controlled by the use of regular preventive medication. However, we know that many people do not use regular asthma medication at the level at which it has been prescribed. This underusage may be 'unintentional', as some patients find it difficult to remember to take medication every day, or it may be 'intentional', with some patients being reluctant to use regular medication for a variety of reasons.

The underusage of prescribed regular medication by asthma patients is commonly referred to as 'non-adherence' or 'non-compliance'. The terms non-adherence and non-compliance are also used to describe two other aspects of self-management: first, where the use of peak flow meters is less frequent than that requested or recommended by clinicians; and second, where patients do not follow an action plan recommending increase in medication when symptoms increase. Non-adherence is also used in a wider and vaguer sense to refer to occasions when patients do not follow other health advice given to them by professionals. The main areas that this chapter will consider are medication underusage (including action plan non-adherence) and less than recommended use of peak flow monitoring. Non-adherence and non-compliance are used interchangeably in this paper to refer to underusage of preventive medication, undermonitoring of peak expiratory flow (PEF) and non-following of action plan recommendations to alter medication when symptoms alter.

A term sometimes used in discussing patient self-care behaviour is 'concordance'. This refers to the degree of agreement between patient and clinician on actions to be taken in self-management. The degree of concordance between health professional and patient may influence level of adherence, but concordance (agreement) is not equivalent to adherence (usage behaviour). It is logically and empirically possible that there is concordance between doctor and patient, but that patients are non-adherent, either intentionally or unintentionally.

To most health professionals working in the field of asthma, non-adherence is believed to lead to unnecessary morbidity for patients. Health professionals want information on effective strategies to use to encourage patients to follow preventive medication regimens that are consistent with guidelines. Health professionals want to help patients improve their self-management.

This chapter first examines evidence in relation to these questions:

- How is adherence with prescribed regular medication assessed, and what levels of non-adherence are found in asthmatics? What medication and patient characteristics are associated with adherence?
- What is the relationship between adherence and outcome? Is non-adherence inevitably associated with poor outcome?

Finally, we examine the evidence for different styles of non-adherence and address the question:

- What is the relationship between styles of non-adherence and outcome?

Literature search

We searched MEDLINE using a search strategy of ['compliance' or 'adherence' or 'concordance'] and [asthma]. This search identified 810 journal articles for the period from January 1993 to November 2003. From this database, articles referring to physician compliance or adherence to clinical guidelines, commentaries and review articles that were not systematic reviews were excluded (as were studies referring to lung compliance or genetic concordance). This left 477 articles. Further examination excluded articles that referred to compliance or adherence or concordance only as part of general comments on the interpretation of study results. This left 136 studies. Selecting studies with a defined measure of adherence/compliance, which were observational clinical, epidemiological or randomized controlled trials and excluding multiple reports of the same trial left 55 trials. Six additional trials before 1993 were included.[1-6] Most of the studies referred to the use of inhaled steroids, with only a small number describing adherence to other preventive medications such as antileukotrienes, theophyllines or sodium nedocromil.

The additional papers referred to in this chapter are systematic reviews or qualitative or attitude studies investigating patient attitudes to self-care, including medication use, PEF meter use and action plan use. These included Ley's seminal studies in the 1970s and 1980s of information given in medical encounters, and controlled trials of strategies to improve recall of medication instructions.[7-15]

How is adherence with prescribed regular medication and peak flow meter use assessed, and what levels of adherence are found in asthmatics?

Measurement issues

There are four common ways of measuring adherence: electronic monitoring; canister weighing; use of prescription records (all objective measures); or patient report (subjective assessment). Table 1 summarizes 35 studies that used one of the three objective measurement techniques. Results from 22 studies using self-report are shown in Table 2. Most of the

studies investigated medication usage, but there were also studies of peak flow meter use and action plan use.

Each of these four methods of assessing adherence has advantages and disadvantages. The advantage of patient report is that patients can provide information about their strategy for dealing with, for example, exacerbations; the disadvantage is that patients often forget or can purposely mislead in order to please the experimenter or clinician, and self-report correlates poorly with objective measures of use such as electronic monitoring.[16-18] The advantage of electronic monitoring is that an electronic record is made of the time of actuation; the disadvantage is that one cannot be sure the actuation was accompanied by inhalation. Canister weighing can be performed without the need for specialized inhalers, but suffers the same disadvantage as electronic inhalers. The advantage of prescription monitoring is that it allows large-scale surveys with existing data; the disadvantage is that prescriptions are not always used, and inhalers can be shared between family members.

For each of these methods of assessment, there is also a problem in summing up levels of adherence among patients. Different studies use different definitions of adherence. Self-report studies usually ask patients how often they take their regular medication, and then set a level at which patients are described as adherent. Thus, patients may be classified as adherent if they report taking medication twice a day every day, or as adherent if they report they usually take what can be calculated to be about 70% of the dosage that the researchers estimate to be required. However, some self-report studies ask patients if they take medication 'as prescribed', and some use 'adherence scales', which ask general questions about attitudes to medication taking.

Where adherence is calculated from objective measures such as electronic metering of inhaler use, canister weights or number of prescriptions taken, the most common definition is percentage of doses taken divided by 'ideal' number of doses that would have been taken if prescribing guidelines had been followed. Others define patients as 'adherent' if they have taken 100% of prescribed doses or 70% of prescribed doses. One study[19] defined adherence separately for morning and evening doses, but most studies calculate adherence from daily use.

Levels of adherence: findings from objective studies

Electronic monitors for inhaler use became available in the 1980s and allowed precise assessment of inhaler use. Early studies in this period include that of Mawhinney et al.[3] among patients who were using inhaled steroids for the first time, who found that patients took their medication fully as instructed on 37% of study days. In 1992, Rand et al.[6] reported a mean of 62% of required activations across the patient group, but also noted that dumping (repeated activation before clinic attendance) occurred in 14% of participants. Milgrom et al.[20]

Table 1. Studies using objective measures of medication adherence.

Author and date	Participants	Compliance measured by	Average compliance level	Compliance morbidity relationship?
Apter et al. (2003)[23]	85 adults	EM Dosage per person as %total prescribed per day	60%	Not reported
Ashkenazi et al. (1993)[85]	150 children	Therapeutic serum levels	22% Children attending ER 73% Comparison group at clinic attendance	ER attenders had lower adherence than clinic attenders
Bartlett et al. (2002)[105]	15 children	EM Using inhaler daily	54%	Not reported
Bender et al. (1998)[33]	24 children	EM Number of days on which inhaler used at least once	52%	Not reported
Bender et al. (2000)[17]	27 children	Canister weight as %total prescribed	69%	Not reported
Berg et al. (1998)[16]	55 adults	Activations as %prescribed/correct intervals as %activated	96%/37%	Not reported
Bosley et al. (1994)[76]	102 adults	EM %subjects taking at least 70% total prescribed	63%	Not reported
Braunstein et al. (1996)[77]	201 children	EM mean number double actuations per day (four prescribed)	2.1	Not reported
Celano et al. (1998)[34]	55 children	Canister weight as proportion of expected	44%	Not reported
Chung and Naya (2000)[106]	57 adults	EM % days with two dosing events	71%	Not reported
Dickinson et al. (1998)[26]	87 adults	DC Total dose issued as %total prescribed	69%	Not reported
Dompeling et al. (1992)[4]	26 adults	DC Discs used as %discs prescribed	46% 'non-compliant'	Adherence not related to morbidity
Gallefoss and Bakke (2000)[107]	78 adults	PC Total dose issued as %total prescribed: Mean > 75%	32% (control group) 57% (intervention group)	Not reported
Gibson et al. (1995)[21]	29 children	EM Dosage per person as %total prescribed	Mean 77%	No relation of symptom score to adherence
Jonasson et al. (1999)[108]	163 children	EM Dosage per person as %total prescribed	Median 77%	No relation of symptom score to adherence
Jonasson et al. (2000)[19]	122 children	EM Dosage per person as %total prescribed	Median 40% morning dose 47% evening dose	No relation of symptom score to adherence

Table 1. *Continued*

Author and date	Participants	Compliance measured by	Average compliance level	Compliance morbidity relationship?
Jones *et al.* (2003)[72]	48 751 children and adults	PC % Drug supply days after starting therapy	68%	Not reported
Kelloway *et al.* (2000)[109]	67 adults	PC Total dose issued as %total prescribed	58%	Not reported
Mann *et al.* (1992)[5]	16 adults	EM Days with prescribed dose as %total days	80% twice-daily regimen 43% four-daily regimen	Not reported
Mawhinney *et al.* (1991)[3]	34 adults	EM Days activated as %total days	37%	Not reported
McQuaid *et al.* (2003)[22]	106 teenagers	EM Dosage per person as %total prescribed	48%	Not reported
Milgrom *et al.* (1996)[20]	24 children	EM Dosage per person as %total prescribed	Mean 58%	No overall adherence–morbidity relationship. But those requiring oral steroids 14% compliance versus no steroids 68% compliance
Nides *et al.* (1993)[102]	251 adults	EM Daily activations as mean of three prescribed daily activations	1.95 (~66%)	Not reported
Onyirimba *et al.* (2003)[83]	19 adults	EM Dosage per person as %total prescribed	Mean intervention 70%+ Mean control <47%	No relation of symptom score or quality of life to adherence
Osman *et al.* (1999)[90]	754 adults	ICS prescription requests over 12 months among high bronchodilator users	50%	High bronchodilator/low ICS, usage group had more hospitalizations, more symptoms, more family practice contact
Rand *et al.* (1992)[6]	165 adults	EM Activations as %daily required activations	Adherent usage = 5 + ICS prescriptions per year	Not reported
Sherman *et al.* (2001)[38]	171 children	PC %doses of doses prescribed	15% used more than twice per day	Not reported
Van Der Palen *et al.* (1997)[110]	22 adults	EM Dosage per person as %total prescribed	57% oral median, 44% ICS median	Not reported
van der Woude and Aalbers (2001)[111]	15 760 adults	PC Actual time to refill prescription/expected time	83% in run in, 95% main trial	Not reported
Van Grunsven *et al.* (2000)[24]	29 adults	DC Discs used as %discs prescribed	100%	Not reported
Van Schayck *et al.* (2002)[25]	34 adults	EM Doses per person as %total prescribed	72% (2-year trial) 91% bd 79% qd	Not reported

EM, electronic monitor; DC, dose count Turbohaler/Rotadisk; CW, canister weight; PC, prescription counting; ICS, inhaled corticosteroids.

Table 2. Studies using self-report measures.

Author and date	Number of patients	Compliance defined as	Compliance level	Compliance morbidity relationship?
Alessandro et al. (1994)[112]	288 children	'Full compliance'	63%	Not reported
Bailey et al. (1990)[2]	267 adults	Agreement to at least 5/6 items on adherence scale	96%/83% (intervention/control)	Intervention group more adherent, less symptomatic
Bauman et al. (2002)[84]	1199 children	Risk for non-adherence scale	54% 'Takes more than one medicine per day'	Children of parents with high non-adherence scores significantly worse on morbidity measures
Cerveri et al. (1997)[113]	116 adults	'Taking ICS as prescribed'	65–74% 'took as prescribed'	Not reported
Cerveri et al. (1999)[40]	1771 adults	'Do you normally take all your medicines' yes = adherent	Median 67% across 14 countries, 40% USA–78% Iceland	Not reported
Chambers et al. (1999)[114]	394 adults	'ICS twice a day most days'	38% ICS 'twice a day most days'	Not reported
Chan and Debruyne (2000)[115]	170 children	'Have not missed > 25% of doses'	38% 'missed >25% of ICS doses'	Not reported
Cheng et al. (2002)[116]	73 children	'Spacer use as recommended'	69% used spacer as recommended	Not reported
Couturaud et al. (2002)[117]	72 adults	Followed action plan	5/54 complied	More symptom-free days in the five high compliers
Diette et al. (1999)[36]	6612 adults	At least four puffs per day every day	36%	Underuse was associated with fewer symptoms
Farber et al. (2003)[44]	571 children	'Misunderstand role of ICS'	23% of parents misunderstood role of ICS	Not reported
Finkelstein et al. (2002)[37]	1083 children	No use of ICS/less than daily use of ICS	41% no use, 24% less than daily use	Not reported
Leickly et al. (1998)[118]	344 children	'Followed action plan after ER attendance'	69% attended appointment after ER, 85% reported following ER recommendations	Not reported
Lozano et al. (2003)[119]	638 children	Using controllers 5+ days per week	66%	Among group with evidence of symptoms/poor control, 34% used controllers 5+ days per week
Smith et al. (1986)[1]	196 children	Doses taken as % prescribed dose	78% intervention, 54% control	Not reported
Soussan et al. (2003)[87]	167 children	'Taking prescribed dose'	OR 4.82 for symptom control among compliant compared with non-compliant	Clinician-assessed non-compliant had poorer control
Van Ganse et al. (1997)[88]	53 adults	'Suboptimal use of ICS' reported from questionnaire	OR 5.5 for suboptimal use among hospitalized compared with non-compliant	Hospitalized more likely to report suboptimal use of ICS than matched non-hospitalized
Wraight et al. (2002)[99]	163 adults	Increase or decrease dose in response to symptoms	78% adherence in severe episodes, 31% in mild episodes	Compliance followed symptoms

ICS, inhaled corticosteroids; OR, odds ratio.

Table 3. Studies of peak flow monitoring.

Author and date	Participants	Compliance measured by	Compliance level	Compliance morbidity relationship?
Electronic peak flow monitoring (EPFM)				
Burkhart et al. (2000)[28]	42 children	EPFM Days measured as % total days	79% (intervention) 64% (control)	Not reported
Cote et al. (1998)[27]	26 adults	EPFM Days measured as % total days	33%	Not reported
Kamps et al. (2001)[30]	40 adults	EPFM Days measured as % total days	77%	Not reported
Malo et al. (1995)[31]	21 adults	EPFM Times measured 2-hourly as % total 2-hourly times requested	80%	Not reported
Reddel et al. (2002)[32]	61 adults	EPFM % scheduled sessions recorded	89%	Not reported
Redline et al. (1996)[120]	65 children	EPFM Days with record as % total days	48%	Not reported
Verschelden et al. (1996)[121]	20 adults	EPFM % scheduled sessions recorded	44%	Not reported
Hyland et al. (1993)[29]	24 adults	EPFM % scheduled sessions recorded	80%	Not reported
Self-report				
Mcmullen et al. (2002)[122]	168 children	Reported 'useful in monitoring'	69% at 1 year	Not reported
Chmelik and Doughty (1994)[35]	20 adults	'complied with protocol for PEF monitor use'	50%	Not reported
Mendenhall and Tsien (2000)[123]	54 adults and children	Using PEF as recommended	79%	Not reported

reported in 1996 that, among 24 children aged 8–12 years, inhaled steroid use over 13 weeks was 58% of that prescribed. Gibson et al.[21] found that there was full compliance on a median of 50% of days among 29 children, with 77% of doses taken overall. Most of these studies compared electronic monitoring with usage as reported in diaries kept by patients in the studies, and found that self-report overestimated usage by 30% or more.

More recently, McQuaid et al.[22] found that, among teenagers using an electronic monitor, only 48% of prescribed doses were taken. Apter et al.[23] reported 64% usage among American adults in 2003. Van Grunsven et al.[24] found a usage rate of 71% of prescribed among 29 adults with asthma, and Van Schayk et al.[25] found 91% usage among 34 adults with asthma.

Prescription counting studies find similar results. In a study published in 1998, Dickinson et al.[26] monitored prescription take up of inhaled steroid over 1 year in a UK general practice, and found that it was 69% of the recommended dosage.

Summary: Electronic monitoring of inhaler use and prescription counting suggests that common usage is between 60% and 80% of dose prescribed, with inhaler used on 50% or more days.

Levels of adherence: findings from self-report studies

Table 2 shows that self-report is influenced by the way the adherence question is asked. Generally, about one-third of pa-

tients surveyed define themselves as 'taking medication every day', but 70% or more agree if the question is 'do you use medication as prescribed?'. Many of the studies using objective measures also ask patients to self-rate their adherence, and consistently find that patients overestimate frequency of usage by about 20–30%. Self-report is not reliable if a strictly accurate measure of adherence is sought. However, it is interesting to note that a large group of patients confirm that they do not use medication every day, but say that they use medication as prescribed. Rather than dismiss this as confabulation, we should consider whether these patients (and for some of them, their health professionals also) think that their pattern of use, although it may not be fully adherent by a strict definition, is appropriate and effective in producing the outcomes they want, and does not result in loss of control of their asthma.

Summary: Patient self-report is imprecise by comparison with objective measures, but patient self-classification of their own adherence is important in evaluating adherence behaviour. Seventy per cent of patients believe they take medication as directed.

Peak flow meter use: self-report and objective assessment

Table 3 shows that similar patterns of use are found in studies of peak flow meters (PFMs). Studies using electronic PFMs find days used vary from 33%[27] to over 75%[28–32] and that 30% or more peak flow diary entries are made retrospectively.

Hyland *et al.*[29] found that more sessions were missed in the evening than in the morning, and more retrospective entries were made in the evening. This study also found that anxiety score was significantly related to number of missing days.

Reddel *et al.*,[32] however, found that, in a 72-week trial, adherence to monitoring was 96% in the first 2 months of the trial, declining to 89% at 18 months. Fifteen per cent of participants were withdrawn because of non-adherence, indicating that overall adherence in a committed group was 70–80% over 18 months.

Summary: Peak flow meter adherence, as with medication adherence, varies from complete confabulation to high levels of continued adherence. Rates of 80% to almost 100% can be sustained among some groups of patients for several months.

Patient and medication characteristics associated with adherence

Cultural and national differences

In the studies reviewed for this chapter, adherence tended to be lower in American studies[22,33–38] than in the European and Australasian studies.[1,24,25,32,39] The international survey by Cerveri *et al.*[40] similarly found lower adherence in the US. These national differences may reflect differences among groups studied in their experience of prophylactic medication, and differences in the way medical care is delivered. Mougdil and Honeybourne[41] found in a study of 345 white European British (WEB) and 344 Indian Subcontinent British (ISCB) asthma patients that self-reported compliance, understanding of asthma medication and understanding of self-management were all lower among the ISCB patients, and ISCB patients were more likely than WEB patients to receive treatment from hospital settings such as emergency departments. If the service used by an asthma patient does not provide continuity, it cannot provide feedback to patients on how their usage patterns are related to their symptoms, or give good supportive information explaining the purpose of preventive medication.

Summary: Cultural differences are fluid, cannot be expected to be permanent and are intertwined with experience of different levels of care and types of care.

Education and income

Educational level is associated with levels of adherence.[42] Education is probably associated with good communication between health professionals and their patients influencing adherence. In an observational study of communication in clinical settings, Steele *et al.*[43] found that more educated patients were more likely to ask questions of their doctors, and doctors were more likely to give information to more educated patients.

Farber *et al.*[44] found that misunderstanding of the role of anti-inflammatory medication was associated with decreased adherence, and that misunderstanding in its turn was more common among patients who had not completed high school. Scherer and Bruce[45] found that attitudes to asthma management (rather than asthma knowledge per se) had the greatest influence on adherence to medication use, and that positive attitudes to asthma management were related to educational level.

Lower income and education are associated with undertreatment of asthma and failure to follow guidelines by health professionals.[46] Adams *et al.*[47] carried out a study of 2509 people with asthma in a community survey and found that a range of socioeconomic factors (income, education, unemployment and ethnicity) was associated with lower use of inhaled corticosteroids (ICS), where lower use included less prescribing of preventive medication and less adherence when ICS had been prescribed.

Summary: Education and income are related to adherence and probably reflect better experience of care, and delivery of care, to higher income/more educated patients, influencing adherence.

Age

Older patients are more likely than younger patients to adhere to regular medication use.[48] Lindberg *et al.*[49] found that age, gender and duration of asthma were significantly associated with attitudes to adherence, but equally significant was perception that 'the staff listened and took patient's views into account' and that 'the patient perceived they had received information about asthma'. Abdulwadud *et al.*[50] found that older patients were six times more likely than young adults with asthma to attend an educational programme. However, older patients are also more likely to be undertreated and underprescribed preventive medication.[51]

Parents are often uneasy about the use of regular medication, particularly steroids, with children. Donnelly *et al.*[52,53] found that, even when parents accepted the need for regular preventive medication, they were reluctant to give any medicine to their child on a daily basis. They judged that 47% of parents in their study had a basic understanding of when to use ICS.

Anecdotally, teenagers are reported to have difficulties with adherence. In part, this may reflect issues in handing over responsibility for self-care from parent to child, which may be done inappropriately.[54] But it may also be the case that most teenagers manage competently, and only a small group contribute to the belief that teenagers are difficult patients. Kyngas[55] found, in a Finnish study of 266 adolescents, that only 18% reported poor compliance with asthma medication. Support from parents, physicians and nurses had a significant positive relationship with self-perceived adherence.

Slack and Brooks[56] studied issues related to medication use by teenagers with asthma in a series of focus groups. The teenagers considered themselves to be compliant with medication therapy. Focus group responses indicated that teenagers wanted complete responsibility for taking their medication and experienced conflict with adults—parents, teachers, school nurses and physicians—about medication use. The teenagers reported that they did not disobey their parents or physicians by refusing to take their medication, and peers did not have a negative influence on the teenagers' asthma management. The primary medication issue for this group of adolescents was managing their medication to control their asthma in spite of inappropriate rules or behaviour by adults.

Summary: Middle-aged and older patients are more adherent than teenagers and young adults. There are special issues of handing over control of self-care to teenagers. If these are not addressed carefully, this may result in non-adherence for teenagers.

Psychological factors and adherence

Patients who are depressed or psychologically distressed are not likely to use medication effectively. Dimatteo et al.[57] carried out a meta-analysis of studies of medication taking (although not including any asthma-specific studies) and found that depression was significantly related to non-adherence to regular medication taking, but no evidence for an anxiety–non-adherence relationship. In asthma, Bosley et al.[58] found that depression scores on the Hospital Anxiety and Depression Scale[59] were significantly higher among non-adherent patients. Apter et al.[23] found that depression was associated with non-adherence among African- and non-African-Americans, but the relationship disappeared when adjusted for race and attitudes to medication. Depression is probably one of several intercorrelated factors that contribute to non-effective use of medication.

It is also known that non-adherence contributes to asthma deaths. Denial, delay in responding to worsening symptoms and underuse of preventive medication have been found among patients in two UK Confidential Enquiries into Asthma Deaths[60,61] and several studies from Australia of near-fatal asthma.[62]

Patient satisfaction with their communication with their clinician is related to adherence:[9,63,64] this is especially important for the use of preventive asthma medication.[65]

Studies have found that, among asthma patients, the most characteristic psychological response to self-care is a reluctance to use any preventive medication regularly;[66,67] this dislike is more prevalent than a specific steroid phobia. The question we need to address is why most patients overcome this reluctance and are able to commit to a more or less regular regimen of use, achieving adequate asthma control.

Summary: Regular medication taking is a difficult pattern of behaviour to adopt for most patients. Any psychological co-morbidity, but particularly depression, makes it more likely that a patient will not be able to achieve adherence.

Medication delivery and adherence

Patients express preference for oral therapy,[68–70] and higher adherence rates have been found than for inhaled therapy.[71] Sherman et al.[38] used prescription refill data histories and found that, over about 7 months, 59% of prescribed montelukast therapy was used and 44% of fluticasone. In a prescription study among 48 751 children and adults, Jones et al.[72] reported that the proportion of 'drug supply days' was 68% for new-start leukotriene monotherapy, 34% for continuing inhaled steroid therapy and 40% for inhaled long-acting β agonists (LABA).

There are methodological caveats in relying too much on the present data. Oral therapy was new to patients in these studies and, as pointed out above, usage may decline as length of time the patient has used the medication increases. Long-term studies are needed to test whether adherence to oral therapy continues to be higher than adherence to inhaled therapy in everyday use.

Although patients express preferences for taking fewer medications or combined treatments,[73] and combined treatments may offer therapeutic advantages,[74] combined treatments have not yet been shown to offer any adherence advantages.[75] Bosley[76] found that average compliance with combined terbutaline/budesonide was 60–70%, no different from rates among patients using individual inhalers. Braunstein et al.[77] found that 34% of patients used a combined nedocromil sodium/salbutamol inhaler as prescribed for more than 60% of days, no different from patients with individual inhalers. As of December 2003, no other studies have been reported that compare adherence levels with combined and non-combined medication.

Requiring patients to take medication more frequently in a day is associated with non-adherence. Once-daily medication regimes are better adhered to than twice or four times daily, but symptom outcomes have been found to be poorer for patients using once-daily prophylactic regimens,[78,79] and for patients using twice daily compared with four times daily.[80]

Summary: Oral medication may be preferred by patients, but long-term pragmatic studies have not yet been carried out to show whether the advantages found in studies introducing oral medication to selected groups persist for general asthma management. Studies have not yet shown that combined inhalers offer greater advantages in adherence.

Commentary

Tentatively, we might suggest that a 'usual' usage level of adherence is around 60–70% of prescribed medication, with actual days adherent lower than this, at about 50%. These rates can vary. The studies surveyed ranged from 20% of patients using medication just as prescribed to 90–100%. Cochrane et al.[81] in a systematic literature review also concluded that days on which patients took medication as prescribed varied between 20% and 73% across different studies. The variations across studies in adherence rates are not explained by differences in definition of adherence, or means of measuring adherence, as wide variation is found among studies that use the same methods (such as electronic monitors) and define adherence in the same way.

Patient characteristics such as nationality, culture, age, income and education are associated, at a group level, with differences in average level of adherence, but we suspect that these differences are not fixed and that they largely reflect differences in delivery of care and health experience of these groups.

Among patients with severe asthma, a small subgroup appears to be unable to manage their self-care effectively, and non-adherence is part of this ineffective self-care. In this group, psychopathology is associated with denial and non-adherence to a preventive regime.

What is the relationship between adherence and outcome? Is non-adherence inevitably associated with poor outcome?

Does good clinical management need 100% adherence? It was noted earlier that pragmatically 70% adherence, or even 60%,[82] is usually considered to be 'good enough'. What evidence is there for the belief that full adherence is necessary for effective asthma control?

Clinical observational studies: association of medication usage and morbidity levels

Of the studies shown in Table 1, five (Gibson et al.,[21] Milgrom et al.,[20] Onyrimba et al.,[83] Jonasson et al.[19] and Mawhinney et al.[3]) examined morbidity in relation to adherence assessed with an electronic monitor. None of them found that morbidity was related to electronically measured adherence rates.

A further four studies related patient self-report of adherence to patient morbidity. Diette et al.[36] found that patients who reported underusing inhaled steroids had fewer symptoms and used fewer bronchodilators. Dompeling et al.[4] found no relationship between symptoms and adherence.

On the other hand, Baumann et al.[84] found that parents who reported attitudes of non-adherence (measured by a validated scale) had children with more symptoms. Jones et al.[72] noted that the proportion of drug supply days increased with increasing using of short-acting β agonist, used as an indicator of severity among the population. That is, medication adherence was associated with the presence of symptoms.

Summary: Observational studies across patient cohorts do not show that low adherence is related to increased symptoms. If anything, they suggest the opposite relationship: that adherence increases as symptoms increase.

Case–control studies and comparative studies

More convincing evidence that for some patients underusage of preventive medication is associated with increased risk of morbidity is given by case–control and comparative studies. Comparative studies show that, if we identify patients as having poorly controlled asthma, they are more likely to be non-adherent than patients classified as having good control. Four comparative or case–control studies[85–88] and one prescription counting study[89] have examined self-rated adherence between different 'asthma control' groups, such as comparisons between emergency department (ED) attenders and clinic outpatients attending regular review, or between hospitalized and non-hospitalized patients. All of these found that patients with moderate to severe asthma identified as having poor control reported using inhaled steroid less regularly than patients of similarly severity with higher control. For instance, Segala et al.[86] and Soussan et al.[87] found, over 3 years in a cohort of French adults and children, that symptom severity was significantly correlated with annually assessed adherence in clinical interview, using a standardized questionnaire. Van Ganse et al.[88] found that hospitalized 'cases' differed significantly from non-hospitalized control subjects in lower reported adherence to inhaled steroid medication and greater preference for bronchodilators to control their asthma. Ashkenazi et al.[85] found that ED attenders reported less adherence to inhaled steroid than clinic outpatients. Put et al.[89] also identified a patient subgroup that catalogued itself as non-compliant who were at risk of hospitalization and were characterized by emotional distress associated with disease and treatment.

Osman et al.[90] found that, over a 12-month period among 754 clinic outpatients, the 25% who were high users of bronchodilators and used less than 50% of their prescribed inhaled steroid were significantly more likely to have a hospital admission and made more acute asthma contacts than patients who did not fit this pattern. However, patients who were low bronchodilator users and non-adherent to their prescribed inhaled steroid had no worse outcome than the adherent users. Non-adherence did not put all patients at risk of acute exacerbations.

Summary: Case–control and comparative studies show that subgroups of patients exist who have high symptoms and frequent exacerbation, but are irregular users of preventive medication. These poorly controlled patients do not follow the usual pattern of increasing adherence as symptoms increase. Usage among these patients on average is no greater than 30–40% of prescribed dose.

Commentary

The above studies show that patients who have unsatisfactory asthma control are likely to be non-adherent. They do not show that patients who are non-adherent are likely to have unsatisfactory control. Observational studies show that most non-adherent patients are achieving satisfactory outcomes. These findings are more complex than the assumption informing many health professionals, namely 'adherence is good and non-adherence bad'.

The studies do not support the hypothesis that the relationship between adherence and symptoms is a straightforward one in which higher levels of adherence are matched by decreasing symptoms. Most patients with low adherence are less symptomatic than patients with high adherence. Among the majority of patients, 'good enough' adherence, which gives effective control, may begin at about 60% of prescribed doses. The several action plan studies that have shown that action plans improve patients' outcomes have not demonstrated for most patients a high degree of increase in adherence. It rather appears that the key is knowing when to take appropriate action and when to respond to increasing symptoms by increasing preventive medication.

The minority group of low adherers who have markedly poor control have symptoms, but their preventive medication usage continues to be low and irregular. They contravene the usual patient behaviour of increasing medication as symptoms increase. For symptomatic patients, persistence in low adherence is associated with frequent acute events and high use of health care resources.

The data suggest that non-adherence often leads to satisfactory outcomes but sometimes it does not. The question that remains is: what makes some patients able to be 'safely' non-adherent, and not others?

Differences in style of self-management and outcome

The review above suggests that, for some patients, non-adherence leads to satisfactory self-management, but for others it does not. It seems likely that there are differences between non-adherent patients in the reasons for their non-adherence, the behaviour of non-adherence and outcome. Several authors have described ways in which patients differ. There is a good deal of overlap in the terms used in their descriptions and, in this section, we have combined the underlying concepts in these different descriptions. This combination produces three different ways in which non-adherence leads to unsatisfactory self-management. Any individual patient can be described in terms of these three different ways or dimensions of non-adherence: (a) low versus high non-intentional non-adherence; (b) non-adherence based on reasoning that is either successful or unsuccessful; (c) acceptance versus denial (Fig. 1).

Non-intentional non-adherence

Non-intentional non-adherence includes forgetting the use of inhalers (e.g. mixing up the brown and blue) and forgetting to take the inhaler. There is much evidence from Ley's group 20 years ago that forgetting of instructions for medicine use is common across disease management, and that simple strategies (such as specific instructions rather than general rules, and the use of understandable language as determined by a readability formula) can be used to reduce forgetting by patients.[1,7,8,10–15,91]

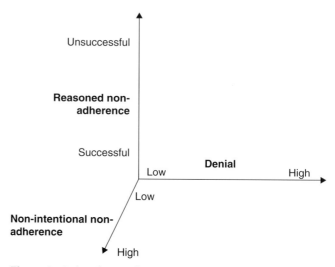

Figure 1. Styles of non-adherence.

Patients who live difficult or disregulated lives may forget to self-manage effectively[92] simply because asthma management is just one other burden in a burdensome life, and this is consistent with the association between non-adherence and psychological morbidity.[42,57,58]

Incorrect reasoning

Several authors have noted that some patients make a reasoned decision not to take their medication as instructed. Patients make a trade-off between the advantages and costs of adherence;[93,94] these patients are also referred to as 'pragmatists'[95] or problem-focused copers.[96] Making a reasoned decision may or may not lead to good self-management.[95] However, we have been unable to find research that shows why some reasoned decisions lead to good and others to poor outcomes. Severity is likely to be one factor that affects outcome. For example, milder patients within the step 2 category of treatment are likely to more tolerant of non-adherence compared with severer patients within the same step, and this is probably the reason for lack of a positive association between adherence and good outcome in clinical observational studies.[36] Similarly, mild patients with seasonal asthma may be able to avoid taking prophylactic medicine at certain times of the year without risk.

Another factor that may be important is the actual behaviour of non-adherence—there are several types of non-adherence behaviour that may lead to different outcomes, for example symptom-directed prophylactic use, using a constant but lower dose, taking occasional drug holidays, etc. Some types of behaviour may be more successful than others, but there is no evidence to suggest which are more or less effective. All we can say is that many non-adherent asthmatics manage their asthma successfully.

Denial

Many authors have noted the tendency of some patients to deny that they have asthma, labelling them 'deniers',[97] 'ignoring asthma'[98] or 'anonymous stream'.[95] Such patients employ an 'emotion-focused coping strategy'[96] of avoiding negative emotions generated from a diagnosis of asthma rather than dealing with the problem of asthma itself. Thus, denial is a way of maintaining positive self-esteem and avoiding the negative emotions generated by having asthma. Patients therefore undermedicate and fail to attend appointments. The association between denial and poor outcome has been found in two UK Confidential Enquiries into Asthma Deaths[60,61] and several studies from Australia of near-fatal asthma.[62]

Commentary and implications for education

The above analysis suggests that every patient can be located at a point in three-dimensional space: (a) the extent to which they forget; (b) the success or otherwise of the non-adherent style of self-management that the patient reasons is best; and (c) the level of denial. This model is shown in Figure 1. It suggests that the only successfully non-adherent patients are those who have made a reasoned decision to non-adhere as part of a self-management strategy which is, for one reason or another, suitable for that individual patient. The lack of relationship observed in some clinical observational studies[4,36,72,89,99] between non-adherence and poor outcome is likely to be due to this group being the largest group of non-adherent patients in that population. Studies showing that asthma education improves adherence but does not reduce symptoms[82] are also consistent with the suggestion that many patients adopt successful patterns of non-adherence. On the other hand, not all patients who reason not to adhere actually adopt a successful self-management strategy, and Gallefoss and Bakke's[39] study showing that education improves both adherence and outcome would indicate that larger numbers of unsuccessfully reasoned patients are in the population. Different results in different studies could be caused by population effects, depending on the proportion of successful and unsuccessful non-adherent patients.

Both non-intentional non-adherence and denial are likely to lead to poor outcome. In the case of non-intentional non-adherence, education may be of benefit if the educational package focuses on forgetting and reasons for forgetting, but is unlikely to compensate for dysfunctional lives. Conventional asthma education is unlikely to be of much benefit to deniers, because these patients manage their lives by avoiding the negative emotions that may be aroused by asthma education. More broadly based, psychological management strategies may help those high in denial and non-intentional non-adherence, but generally management strategies have not been well developed for these patients. The association between denial and near-fatal asthma suggests that these are a particularly problematic group of patients, for whom conventional asthma clinics do not provide a satisfactory solution.

Addressing non-adherence within a self-management approach

The self-management approach requires providing an individualized action plan to each patient. There is now good evidence that this approach improves patient outcomes[39,100] if patients are allowed to discuss and ask questions about the plan.[101] Action plans are effective because they address each of the contributing factors that lead to unsuccessful non-adherence.

1 Action plans help to reduce non-intentional non-adherence by giving clear written instructions for medication use both when asthma is controlled and when it begins to deteriorate. This helps to reduce non-intentional non-adherence. They follow the simple principle, first elucidated and shown 20 years ago in numerous studies by Ley and co-workers,[1,7,8,10–15,91] that communicating clearly and giving written information increases the likelihood that medication will be used as prescribed.

2 Action plans address intentional or reasoned non-adherence by requiring patients and health professionals to reach concordance on goals. They facilitate discussion between patients and health professionals on the efficacy of the regimen prescribed. Nides *et al*.[102] examined the benefit of giving feedback to patients on their pattern of inhaler usage and found 80% usage rates among patients given feedback, compared with 60% among patients not given feedback. Gavin *et al*.[103] showed that a positive treatment partnership between parents and physician was associated with better outcome. Clark *et al*.[104] have shown that training physicians in the skills to develop a management plan with patients is associated with improved outcomes. Cote *et al*.[101] showed that giving an action plan alone, without educational discussion, was not effective in improving outcome.

3 Action plans also have the potential for addressing non-adherence resulting from denial, although this is an area where evidence is lacking. The difficulty with denial is that such patients may fail to attend review clinics and maintain an action plan as part of denying: emotion-focused coping strategy. Conventional management plans may be less effective compared with action plans recognizing the increased likelihood of emergency care needed in these patients.

Conclusion

Non-adherence is common among asthma patients. For most patients, non-adherence produces no adverse effects; for a minority, non-adherence leads to life-threatening exacerbations or death. Health professionals need to be sensitive to the difference between these two types of patient. The simplistic belief that 'adherence is good and non-adherence bad' has led to insufficient research on (a) why non-adherence is sometimes successful or not and (b) how to manage those denying patients whose emotion-focused coping style makes them unsuited for conventional, problem-focused asthma education programmes which, for many other patients, produce successful results.

References

1 Smith NA, Seale JP, Ley P, Shaw J, Bracs PU. Effects of intervention on medication compliance in children with asthma. *Med J Aust* 1986; **144**:119–22.

2 Bailey WC, Richards JM Jr, Brooks CM, Soong SJ, Windsor RA, Manzella BA. A randomized trial to improve self-management practices of adults with asthma. *Arch Intern Med* 1990; **150**: 1664–8.

3 Mawhinney H, Spector SL, Kinsman RA *et al.* Compliance in clinical trials of two nonbronchodilator, antiasthma medications. *Ann Allergy* 1991; **66**:294–9.

4 Dompeling E, Van Grunsven PM, Van Schayck CP, Folgering H, Molema J, Van Weel C. Treatment with inhaled steroids in asthma and chronic bronchitis: long-term compliance and inhaler technique. *Fam Pract* 1992; **9**:161–6.

5 Mann M, Eliasson O, Patel K, ZuWallack RL. A comparison of the effects of bid and qid dosing on compliance with inhaled flunisolide. *Chest* 1992; **101**:496–9.

6 Rand CS, Wise RA, Nides M *et al.* Metered-dose inhaler adherence in a clinical trial. *Am Rev Respir Dis* 1992; **146**:1559–64.

7 Ley P, Bradshaw PW, Eaves D, Walker CM. A method for increasing patients' recall of information presented by doctors. *Psychol Med* 1973; **3**:217–20.

8 Bradshaw PW, Ley P, Kincey JA. Recall of medical advice: comprehensibility and specificity. *Br J Soc Clin Psychol* 1975; **14**:55–62.

9 Kincey J, Bradshaw P, Ley P. Patients' satisfaction and reported acceptance of advice in general practice. *J R Coll Gen Pract* 1975; **25**:558–66.

10 Ley P, Jain VK, Skilbeck CE. A method for decreasing patients' medication errors. *Psychol Med* 1976; **6**:599–601.

11 Ley P, Bradshaw PW, Kincey JA, Atherton ST. Increasing patients' satisfaction with communications. *Br J Soc Clin Psychol* 1976; **15**:403–13.

12 Ley P. Memory for medical information. *Br J Soc Clin Psychol* 1979; **18**:245–55.

13 Ley P. Satisfaction, compliance and communication. *Br J Clin Psychol* 1982; **21** (Pt 4):241–54.

14 Ley P. Doctor–patient communication: some quantitative estimates of the role of cognitive factors in non-compliance. *J Hypertens Suppl* 1985; **3**:S51–S55.

15 Smith NA, Ley P, Seale JP, Shaw J. Health benefits, satisfaction and compliance. *Patient Educ Couns* 1987; **10**:279–86.

16 Berg J, Dunbar JJ, Rohay JM. Compliance with inhaled medications: the relationship between diary and electronic monitor. *Ann Behav Med* 1998; **20**:36–8.

17 Bender B, Wamboldt FS, O'Connor SL *et al.* Measurement of children's asthma medication adherence by self report, mother report, canister weight, and Doser CT. *Ann Allergy Asthma Immunol* 2000; **85**:416–21.

18 Hamid S, Kumaradevan J, Cochrane GM. Single centre open study to compare patient recording of PRN salbutamol use on a daily diary card with actual use as recorded by the MDI compliance monitor. *Respir Med* 1998; **92**:1188–90.

19 Jonasson G, Carlsen KH, Mowinckel P. Asthma drug adherence in a long term clinical trial. *Arch Dis Child* 2000; **83**:330–3.

20 Milgrom H, Bender B, Ackerson L, Bowry P, Smith B, Rand C. Noncompliance and treatment failure in children with asthma. *J Allergy Clin Immunol* 1996; **98**:1051–7.

21 Gibson NA, Ferguson AE, Aitchison TC, Paton JY. Compliance with inhaled asthma medication in preschool children. *Thorax* 1995; **50**:1274–9.

22 McQuaid EL, Kopel SJ, Klein RB, Fritz GK. Medication adherence in pediatric asthma: reasoning, responsibility, and behavior. *J Pediatr Psychol* 2003; **28**:323–33.

23 Apter AJ, Boston RC, George M *et al.* Modifiable barriers to adherence to inhaled steroids among adults with asthma: it's not just black and white. *J Allergy Clin Immunol* 2003; **111**:1219–26.

24 Van Grunsven PM, Van Schayck CP, Van Deuveren M, van Herwaarden CL, Akkermans RP, Van Weel C. Compliance during long-term treatment with fluticasone propionate in subjects with early signs of asthma or chronic obstructive pulmonary disease (COPD): results of the Detection, Intervention, and Monitoring Program of COPD and Asthma (DIMCA) Study. *J Asthma* 2000; **37**:225–34.

25 Van Schayck CP, Bijl-Hofland ID, Folgering H *et al.* Influence of two different inhalation devices on therapy compliance in asthmatic patients. *Scand J Prim Health Care* 2002; **20**:126–8.

26 Dickinson J, Hutton S, Atkin A. Implementing the British Thoracic Society's guidelines: the effect of a nurse-run asthma clinic on prescribed treatment in an English general practice. *Respir Med* 1998; **92**:264–7.

27 Cote J, Cartier A, Malo Jl, Rouleau M, Boulet LP. Compliance with peak expiratory flow monitoring in home management of asthma. *Chest* 1998; **113**:968–72.

28 Burkhart PV, Dunbar-Jacob JM, Fireman P, Rohay J. Children's adherence to recommended asthma self-management. *Pediatr Nurs* 2002; **28**:409–14.

29 Hyland ME, Kenyon CA, Allen R, Howarth P. Diary keeping in asthma: comparison of written and electronic methods. *BMJ* 1993; **306**:487–9.

30 Kamps AW, Roorda RJ, Brand PL. Peak flow diaries in childhood asthma are unreliable. *Thorax* 2001; **56**:180–2.

31 Malo JL, Trudeau C, Ghezzo H, L'Archeveque J, Cartier A. Do subjects investigated for occupational asthma through serial peak expiratory flow measurements falsify their results? *J Allergy Clin Immunol* 1995; **96**:601–7.

32 Reddel HK, Toelle BG, Marks GB, Ware SI, Jenkins CR, Woolcock AJ. Analysis of adherence to peak flow monitoring when recording of data is electronic. *BMJ* 2002; **324**:146–7.

33 Bender B, Milgrom H, Rand C, Ackerson L. Psychological factors associated with medication nonadherence in asthmatic children. *J Asthma* 1998; **35**:347–53.

34 Celano M, Geller RJ, Phillips KM, Ziman R. Treatment adherence among low-income children with asthma. *J Pediatr Psychol* 1998; **23**:345–9.

35 Chmelik F, Doughty A. Objective measurements of compliance in asthma treatment. *Ann Allergy* 1994; **73**:527–32.

36 Diette GB, Wu AW, Skinner EA *et al.* Treatment patterns among adult patients with asthma: factors associated with overuse of inhaled β-agonists and underuse of inhaled corticosteroids. *Arch Intern Med* 1999; **159**:2697–704.

37 Finkelstein JA, Lozano P, Farber HJ, Miroshnik I, Lieu TA. Underuse of controller medications among Medicaid-insured children with asthma. *Arch Pediatr Adolesc Med* 2002; **156**:562–7.

38 Sherman J, Patel P, Hutson A, Chesrown S, Hendeles L. Adherence to oral montelukast and inhaled fluticasone in children with persistent asthma. *Pharmacotherapy* 2001; **21**:1464–7.

39 Gallefoss F, Bakke PS. How does patient education and self-management among asthmatics and patients with chronic obstruc-

tive pulmonary disease affect medication? *Am J Respir Crit Care Med* 1999; **160**:2000–5.

40 Cerveri I, Locatelli F, Zoia MC, Corsico A, Accordini S, De Marco R. International variations in asthma treatment compliance: the results of the European Community Respiratory Health Survey (ECRHS). *Eur Respir J* 1999; **14**:288–94.

41 Moudgil H, Honeybourne D. Differences in asthma management between white European and Indian subcontinent ethnic groups living in socioeconomically deprived areas in the Birmingham (UK) conurbation. *Thorax* 1998; **53**:490–4.

42 Apter AJ, Reisine ST, Affleck G, Barrows E, ZuWallack RL. Adherence with twice-daily dosing of inhaled steroids. Socioeconomic and health-belief differences. *Am J Respir Crit Care Med* 1998; **157**: 1810–17.

43 Steele DJ, Jackson TC, Gutmann MC. Have you been taking your pills? The adherence-monitoring sequence in the medical interview. *J Fam Pract* 1990; **30**:294–9.

44 Farber HJ, Capra AM, Finkelstein JA *et al.* Misunderstanding of asthma controller medications: association with nonadherence. *J Asthma* 2003; **40**:17–25.

45 Scherer YK, Bruce S. Knowledge, attitudes, and self-efficacy and compliance with medical regimen, number of emergency department visits, and hospitalizations in adults with asthma. *Heart Lung* 2001; **30**:250–7.

46 Hartert TV, Windom HH, Peebles RS Jr, Freidhoff LR, Togias A. Inadequate outpatient medical therapy for patients with asthma admitted to two urban hospitals. *Am J Med* 1996; **100**:386–94.

47 Adams RJ, Fuhlbrigge A, Guilbert T, Lozano P, Martinez F. Inadequate use of asthma medication in the United States: results of the asthma in America national population survey. *J Allergy Clin Immunol* 2002; **110**:58–64.

48 Arnsten JH, Gelfand JM, Singer DE. Determinants of compliance with anticoagulation: a case–control study. *Am J Med* 1997; **103**: 11–17.

49 Lindberg M, Ekstrom T, Moller M, Ahlner J. Asthma care and factors affecting medication compliance: the patient's point of view. *Int J Qual Health Care* 2001; **13**:375–83.

50 Abdulwadud O, Abramson M, Forbes A *et al.* Attendance at an asthma educational intervention: characteristics of participants and non-participants. *Respir Med* 1997; **91**:524–9.

51 Barr RG, Somers SC, Speizer FE, Camargo CA Jr. Patient factors and medication guideline adherence among older women with asthma. *Arch Intern Med* 2002; **162**:1761–8.

52 Donnelly JE, Donnelly WJ, Thong YH. Parental perceptions and attitudes toward asthma and its treatment: a controlled study. *Soc Sci Med* 1987; **24**:431–7.

53 Donnelly JE, Donnelly WJ, Thong YH. Inadequate parental understanding of asthma medications. *Ann Allergy* 1989; **62**:337–41.

54 Winkelstein ML, Huss K, Butz A, Eggleston P, Vargas P, Rand C. Factors associated with medication self-administration in children with asthma. *Clin Pediatr* 2000; **39**:337–45.

55 Kyngas HA. Compliance of adolescents with asthma. *Nurs Health Sci* 1999; **1**:195–202.

56 Slack MK, Brooks AJ. Medication management issues for adolescents with asthma. *Am J Health Syst Pharm* 1995; **52**:1417–21.

57 DiMatteo MR, Lepper HS, Croghan TW. Depression is a risk factor for noncompliance with medical treatment: meta-analysis of the effects of anxiety and depression on patient adherence. *Arch Intern Med* 2000; **160**:2101–7.

58 Bosley CM, Fosbury JA, Cochrane GM. The psychological factors associated with poor compliance with treatment in asthma. *Eur Respir J* 1995; **8**:899–904.

59 Lowe B, Grafe K, Zipfel S *et al.* Detecting panic disorder in medical and psychosomatic outpatients. Comparative validation of the Hos-

pital Anxiety and Depression Scale, the Patient Health Questionnaire, a screening question, and physicians' diagnosis. *J Psychosom Res* 2003; **55**:515–19.

60 Bucknall CE, Slack R, Godley CC, Mackay TW, Wright SC. Scottish Confidential Inquiry into Asthma Deaths (SCIAD), 1994–6 [comment]. *Thorax* 1999; **54**:978–84.

61 Sturdy PM, Victor CR, Anderson HR *et al.* Psychological, social and health behaviour risk factors for deaths certified as asthma: a national case–control study. *Thorax* 2002; **57**:1034–9.

62 Campbell DA, Yellowlees PM, McLennan G *et al.* Psychiatric and medical features of near fatal asthma. *Thorax* 1995; **50**:254–9.

63 Bultman DC, Svarstad BL. Effects of physician communication style on client medication beliefs and adherence with antidepressant treatment. *Patient Educ Couns* 2000; **40**:173–85.

64 Street RL. Communicative styles and adaptations in physician–parent consultations. *Soc Sci Med* 1992; **34**:1155–63.

65 Hand CH, Bradley C. Health beliefs of adults with asthma: toward an understanding of the difference between symptomatic and preventive use of inhaler treatment. *J Asthma* 1996; **33**:331–8.

66 Osman LM, Russell IT, Friend JA, Legge JS, Douglas JG. Predicting patient attitudes to asthma medication. *Thorax* 1993; **48**:827–30.

67 Van Grunsven PM, Van Schayck CP, van Kollenburg HJ *et al.* The role of 'fear of corticosteroids' in nonparticipation in early intervention with inhaled corticosteroids in asthma and COPD in general practice. *Eur Respir J* 1998; **11**:1178–81.

68 Bukstein DA, Bratton DL, Firriolo KM *et al.* Evaluation of parental preference for the treatment of asthmatic children aged 6 to 11 years with oral montelukast or inhaled cromolyn: a randomized, open-label, crossover study. *J Asthma* 2003; **40**:475–85.

69 Lim SH, Goh DY, Tan AY, Lee BW. Parents' perceptions towards their child's use of inhaled medications for asthma therapy. *J Paediatr Child Health* 1996; **32**:306–9.

70 Weinberg EG, Naya I. Treatment preferences of adolescent patients with asthma. *Pediatr Allergy Immunol* 2000; **11**:49–55.

71 Maspero JF, Duenas-Meza E, Volovitz B *et al.* Oral montelukast versus inhaled beclomethasone in 6- to 11-year-old children with asthma: results of an open-label extension study evaluating long-term safety, satisfaction, and adherence with therapy. *Curr Med Res Opin* 2001; **17**:96–104.

72 Jones C, Santanello NC, Boccuzzi SJ, Wogen J, Strub P, Nelsen LM. Adherence to prescribed treatment for asthma: evidence from pharmacy benefits data. *J Asthma* 2003; **40**:93–101.

73 Barnes PJ, O'Connor BJ. Use of a fixed combination β_2-agonist and steroid dry powder inhaler in asthma. *Am J Respir Crit Care Med* 1995; **151**:1053–7.

74 Kavuru M, Melamed J, Gross G *et al.* Salmeterol and fluticasone propionate combined in a new powder inhalation device for the treatment of asthma: a randomized, double-blind, placebo-controlled trial. *J Allergy Clin Immunol* 2000; **105**:1108–16.

75 Garcia-Marcos L, Schuster A, Cobos BN. Inhaled corticosteroids plus long-acting β_2-agonists as a combined therapy in asthma. *Expert Opin Pharmacother* 2003; **4**:23–39.

76 Bosley CM, Parry DT, Cochrane GM. Patient compliance with inhaled medication: does combining β-agonists with corticosteroids improve compliance? *Eur Respir J* 1994; **7**:504–9.

77 Braunstein GL, Trinquet G, Harper AE. Compliance with nedocromil sodium and a nedocromil sodium/salbutamol combination. Compliance Working Group. *Eur Respir J* 1996; **9**:893–8.

78 Dubus JC, Anhoj J. A review of once-daily delivery of anti-asthmatic drugs in children. *Pediatr Allergy Immunol* 2003; **14**:4–9.

79 Weiner P, Weiner M, Azgad Y. Long term clinical comparison of single versus twice daily administration of inhaled budesonide in moderate asthma. *Thorax* 1995; **50**:1270–3.

80 Malo JL, Cartier A, Ghezzo H, Trudeau C, Morris J, Jennings B. Com-

parison of four-times-a-day and twice-a-day dosing regimens in subjects requiring 1200 micrograms or less of budesonide to control mild to moderate asthma. *Respir Med* 1995; **89**:537–43.

81 Cochrane MG, Bala MV, Downs KE, Mauskopf J, Ben Joseph RH. Inhaled corticosteroids for asthma therapy: patient compliance, devices, and inhalation technique. *Chest* 2000; **117**:542–50.

82 Cote J, Cartier A, Robichaud P *et al*. Influence on asthma morbidity of asthma education programs based on self-management plans following treatment optimization. *Am J Respir Crit Care Med* 1997; **155**:1509–14.

83 Onyirimba F, Apter A, Reisine S *et al*. Direct clinician-to-patient feedback discussion of inhaled steroid use: its effect on adherence. *Ann Allergy Asthma Immunol* 2003; **90**:411–15.

84 Bauman LJ, Wright E, Leickly FE *et al*. Relationship of adherence to pediatric asthma morbidity among inner-city children. *Pediatrics* 2002; **110**:e6.

85 Ashkenazi S, Amir J, Volovitz B, Varsano I. Why do asthmatic children need referral to an emergency room? *Pediatr Allergy Immunol* 1993; **4**:93–6.

86 Segala C, Soussan D, Priol G *et al*. [Factors predicting the severity and the degree of symptom control of asthma in a recently diagnosed cohort of adult patients (ASMA study)]. *Rev Mal Respir* 2003; **20**:191–9.

87 Soussan D, Liard R, Zureik M, Touron D, Rogeaux Y, Neukirch F. Treatment compliance, passive smoking, and asthma control: a three year cohort study. *Arch Dis Child* 2003; **88**:229–33.

88 Van Ganse E, Hubloue I, Vincken W, Leufkens HG, Gregoire J, Ernst P. Actual use of inhaled corticosteroids and risk of hospitalisation: a case–control study. *Eur J Clin Pharmacol* 1997; **51**:449–54.

89 Put C, van den Bergh O, Demedts M, Verleden G. A study of the relationship among self-reported noncompliance, symptomatology, and psychological variables in patients with asthma. *J Asthma* 2000; **37**:503–10.

90 Osman LM, Friend JA, Legge JS, Douglas JG. Requests for repeat medication prescriptions and frequency of acute episodes in asthma patients. *J Asthma* 1999; **36**:449–57.

91 Smith NA, Seale JP, Ley P, Mellis CM, Shaw J. Better medication compliance is associated with improved control of childhood asthma. *Monaldi Arch Chest Dis* 1994; **49**:470–4.

92 Irvine L, Crombie IK, Alder EM, Neville RG, Clark RA. What predicts poor collection of medication among children with asthma? A case–control study. *Eur Respir J* 2002; **20**:1464–9.

93 Horne R, Weinman J. Patients' beliefs about prescribed medicines and their role in adherence to treatment in chronic physical illness. *J Psychosom Res* 1999; **47**:555–67.

94 Horne R, Hankins M, Jenkins R. The Satisfaction with Information about Medicines Scale (SIMS): a new measurement tool for audit and research. *Qual Health Care* 2001; **10**:135–40.

95 Harris GS, Shearer AG. Beliefs that support the behavior of people with asthma: a qualitative investigation. *J Asthma* 2001; **38**:427–34.

96 Hyland ME. Quality of life, compliance and patient satisfaction. In: Scadding G, O'Connor B, eds. *Key Advances in the Effective Management of Asthma*. London, Royal Society of Medicine Press, 1998, pp. 33–6.

97 Adams S, Pill R, Jones A. Medication, chronic illness and identity: the perspective of people with asthma. *Soc Sci Med* 1997; **45**:189–201.

98 Aalto AM, Harkapaa K, Aro AR, Rissanen P. Ways of coping with asthma in everyday life: validation of the Asthma Specific Coping Scale. *J Psychosom Res* 2002; **53**:1061–9.

99 Wraight JM, Cowan JO, Flannery EM, Town GI, Taylor DR. Adherence to asthma self-management plans with inhaled corticosteroid and oral prednisone: a descriptive analysis. *Respirology* 2002; **7**:133–9.

100 Osman LM, Calder C, Godden DJ *et al*. A randomised trial of self-management planning for adult patients admitted to hospital with acute asthma. *Thorax* 2002; **57**:869–74.

101 Cote J, Bowie DM, Robichaud P, Parent JG, Battisti L, Boulet LP. Evaluation of two different educational interventions for adult patients consulting with an acute asthma exacerbation. *Am J Respir Crit Care Med* 2001; **163**:1415–19.

102 Nides MA, Tashkin DP, Simmons MS, Wise RA, Li VC, Rand CS. Improving inhaler adherence in a clinical trial through the use of the Nebulizer Chronolog. *Chest* 1993; **104**:501–7.

103 Gavin LA, Wamboldt MZ, Sorokin N, Levy SY, Wamboldt FS. Treatment alliance and its association with family functioning, adherence, and medical outcome in adolescents with severe, chronic asthma. *J Pediatr Psychol* 1999; **24**:355–65.

104 Clark NM, Gong M, Schork MA *et al*. Long-term effects of asthma education for physicians on patient satisfaction and use of health services. *Eur Respir J* 2000; **16**:15–21.

105 Bartlett SJ, Lukk P, Butz A, Lampros-Klein F, Rand CS. Enhancing medication adherence among inner-city children with asthma: results from pilot studies. *J Asthma* 2002; **39**:47–54.

106 Chung KF, Naya I. Compliance with an oral asthma medication: a pilot study using an electronic monitoring device. *Respir Med* 2000; **94**:852–8.

107 Gallefoss F, Bakke PS. Impact of patient education and self-management on morbidity in asthmatics and patients with chronic obstructive pulmonary disease. *Respir Med* 2000; **94**:279–87.

108 Jonasson G, Carlsen KH, Sodal A, Jonasson C, Mowinckel P. Patient compliance in a clinical trial with inhaled budesonide in children with mild asthma. *Eur Respir J* 1999; **14**:150–4.

109 Kelloway JS, Wyatt R, DeMarco J, Adlis S. Effect of salmeterol on patients' adherence to their prescribed refills for inhaled corticosteroids. *Ann Allergy Asthma Immunol* 2000; **84**:324–8.

110 Van Der Palen J, Klein JJ, Rovers MM. Compliance with inhaled medication and self-treatment guidelines following a self-management programme in adult asthmatics. *Eur Respir J* 1997; **10**:652–7.

111 van der Woude HJ, Aalbers R. Compliance with inhaled glucocorticoids and concomitant use of long-acting β_2-agonists. *Respir Med* 2001; **95**:404–7.

112 Alessandro F, Vincenzo ZG, Marco S, Marcello G, Enrica R. Compliance with pharmacologic prophylaxis and therapy in bronchial asthma. *Ann Allergy* 1994; **73**:135–40.

113 Cerveri I, Zoia MC, Bugiani M *et al*. Inadequate antiasthma drug use in the north of Italy. *Eur Respir J* 1997; **10**:2761–5.

114 Chambers CV, Markson L, Diamond JJ, Lasch L, Berger M. Health beliefs and compliance with inhaled corticosteroids by asthmatic patients in primary care practices. *Respir Med* 1999; **93**:88–94.

115 Chan PW, Debruyne JA. Parental concern towards the use of inhaled therapy in children with chronic asthma. *Pediatr Int* 2000; **42**:547–51.

116 Cheng NG, Browne GJ, Lam LT, Yeoh R, Oomens M. Spacer compliance after discharge following a mild to moderate asthma attack. *Arch Dis Child* 2002; **87**:302–5.

117 Couturaud F, Proust A, Frachon I *et al*. Education and self-management: a one-year randomized trial in stable adult asthmatic patients. *J Asthma* 2002; **39**:493–500.

118 Leickly FE, Wade SL, Crain E, Kruszon-Moran D, Wright EC, Evans R III. Self-reported adherence, management behavior, and barriers to care after an emergency department visit by inner city children with asthma. *Pediatrics* 1998; **101**:E8.

119 Lozano P, Finkelstein JA, Hecht J, Shulruff R, Weiss KB. Asthma medication use and disease burden in children in a primary care population. *Arch Pediatr Adolesc Med* 2003; **157**:81–8.

120 Redline S, Wright EC, Kattan M, Kercsmar C, Weiss K. Short-term

compliance with peak flow monitoring: results from a study of inner city children with asthma. *Pediatr Pulmonol* 1996; **21**:203–10.

121 Verschelden P, Cartier A, L'Archeveque J, Trudeau C, Malo JL. Compliance with and accuracy of daily self-assessment of peak expiratory flows (PEF) in asthmatic subjects over a three month period. *Eur Respir J* 1996; **9**:880–5.

122 McMullen AH, Yoos HL, Kitzman H. Peak flow meters in childhood asthma: parent report of use and perceived usefulness. *J Pediatr Health Care* 2002; **16**:67–72.

123 Mendenhall AB, Tsien AY. Evaluation of physician and patient compliance with the use of peak flow meters in commercial insurance and Oregon health plan asthmatic populations. *Ann Allergy Asthma Immunol* 2000; **84**:523–7.

CHAPTER 1.3.2

Corticosteroid-induced osteoporosis

Michael L Burr and Michael Stone

Introduction

During the last 50 years, corticosteroids have become the most effective form of treatment for a wide range of chronic inflammatory diseases, including asthma and chronic obstructive pulmonary disease (COPD). Inhaled corticosteroids (ICS) are now the mainstay of treatment to prevent the symptoms of asthma, while oral preparations are mainly used for the more severe forms of the disease. Concerns have arisen about their adverse effects, particularly on bone metabolism. The evidence for these effects will be considered separately for oral and inhaled corticosteroids.

There are inevitable limitations in the types of evidence that are available to investigate the extent to which corticosteroids promote osteoporosis. It would obviously be unethical to conduct randomized controlled trials specifically to investigate serious adverse effects. Some evidence is available from trials that were conducted to investigate therapeutic actions of corticosteroids, with adverse effects also being monitored. But such trials tend to be fairly short term, whereas the more important adverse effects could be long term. The only trials conducted specifically to examine potentially adverse effects use biochemical markers of bone turnover as endpoints. The results of these trials are of only indirect relevance to issues of clinical importance such as bone fracture. Most of the evidence to be considered here is therefore derived from observational studies rather than controlled trials, except in relation to the prevention and treatment of osteoporosis.

Osteoporosis

Definition and prevalence

By international agreement, osteoporosis is defined as a progressive systemic skeletal disease characterized by low bone mass and micro-architectural deterioration of bone tissue, with a consequent increase in bone fragility and susceptibility to fracture.[1] For practical purposes, an arbitrary definition is used: a bone mineral density (BMD) of 2.5 or more standard deviations below the mean value in young adults (i.e. a T score of −2.5). According to this definition, the prevalence of osteoporosis at any site in white western women is 14.8% at ages 50–59 years, rising to 70.0% over the age of 80 years.[1] In men,

the condition is much less common; there is some uncertainty about the appropriate diagnostic cut-off values, so prevalence figures are not usually quoted.

The major determinants of osteoporosis are age and gender: men lose 14–45% of cancellous bone and 5–15% of cortical bone with advancing age, while women lose 35–50% and 25–30% respectively. There is a sharp increase in the rate of bone loss at the menopause. Other factors include thinness, physical inactivity, smoking, alcohol consumption, low calcium intake, low vitamin D status and poor calcium absorption.[2]

Risk of fracture

Osteoporosis is clinically important because it greatly increases the risk of fracture. There is an inverse and continuous relationship between bone mass and fracture risk. A meta-analysis of 11 cohort studies showed that the risk of a hip fracture increases by a factor of about 2.6 for each standard deviation (SD) decrease in hip BMD, with 95% confidence interval (CI) 2.0–3.5, and the risk of vertebral fracture by a factor of 2.3 (95% CI 1.9–2.8) for each SD decline in spine BMD.[3] The overall relative risk of fracture is about 1.5 (95% CI 1.4–1.6) for every SD decrease in BMD measured at a single site.

The risk factors for fracture reflect those for osteoporosis. For a British woman aged 50 years, the risk that she will suffer a fracture during the remainder of her life is 13% for the forearm, 11% for vertebrae and 14% for the femoral neck; the corresponding risk for a man is 2%, 2% and 3%.[4] Many vertebral fractures are undiagnosed even though they may cause symptoms, so the true risk is higher.

Osteoporotic fractures of the spine and forearm cause considerable pain and distress, but the most serious consequences arise from hip fractures, which carry 15–20% increase in mortality.[2] For women over the age of 45 years, they account for a higher proportion of bed occupancy than many other common conditions, including breast cancer and diabetes. It is obviously important to avoid any additional risk in people who already have a high probability of incurring this condition.

Biochemical markers

Osteoporosis occurs as a result of an imbalance between bone resorption and bone formation. In consequence, biochemical tests of these two processes can be used to indicate the risk of osteoporosis. They are particularly useful in showing the effects of interventions (including corticosteroid administration), in that a change in either process is likely to result in an increase or decrease in BMD. Commonly used markers of bone resorption include pyridinoline cross-links, deoxypyridinoline and telopeptides; markers of bone formation include the procollagen propeptides of type I collagen, osteocalcin and the bone isoenzyme of alkaline phosphatase.[2]

Oral corticosteroids

Scale of use

For many years, oral corticosteroids have played an important part in the treatment of respiratory disease. The evidence-based British Guideline on the Management of Asthma recommends their use in Step 5 of the management of asthma and in the treatment of the severe acute attack.[5] When given during an exacerbation of COPD in patients with moderate or severe disease, they shorten recovery time and hasten the recovery of lung function.[6] They are therefore taken intermittently by many people with respiratory disease, and continuously by a smaller number.

The extent to which various medications are used in the population can be estimated by means of medical records held on computer by general practitioners. Information from the General Practitioner Research Database suggested that, at any point in time, oral corticosteroids are being used by 0.9% of the adult population in England and Wales.[7] The most frequently recorded indication for their use was respiratory disease (40% of users), although continuous long-term treatment was more common among patients with arthropathies. Similar estimates were obtained in a study in Nottinghamshire, which found that oral corticosteroids were taken continuously (for at least 3 months) by 0.5% of the total population and by 1.4% of persons aged 55 years or more, with a higher proportion in women than in men.[8]

The highest usage (2.5%) is among persons aged 70–79 years,[7] an age group with a high prevalence of osteoporosis in any case, so the possibility of further reduction in bone density must be taken very seriously.

Mechanisms of action on bone

Corticosteroids act on the skeleton in a variety of ways.

The overall effect depends on several factors, including the dose, the duration, the type of corticosteroid and individual susceptibility.

The most important effect is the suppression of bone formation. This seems to involve several mechanisms:[9]
- the differentiation and activity of osteoblasts and other cells in bone;
- modulating the transcription of genes that govern the synthesis of type I collagen and osteocalcin by osteoblasts;
- influencing the synthesis and activity of locally acting factors, such as cytokines, that affect osteoblasts;
- shortening the lifespan of osteoblasts and osteocytes.

Corticosteroids also increase bone resorption, by promoting osteoclast survival. Other relevant actions include reduced calcium absorption, increased renal calcium excretion and osteonecrosis.[9]

Effect on bone

In 2002, the Royal College of Physicians, in collaboration with other interested parties, published evidence-based guidelines on the prevention and treatment of glucocorticoid-induced osteoporosis.[9] These guidelines included a review of the evidence linking corticosteroid use with osteoporosis.

Systematic reviews with meta-analyses have been conducted, and the results seem to convey a consistent message.[10,11] The relevant randomized controlled trials used BMD rather than fractures as endpoints and comprised only a small number of subjects; they suggest that 6 months of corticosteroid treatment produces an extra 3.9% of bone loss in the lumbar spine (95% CI 1.9–6.0%).[10]

More extensive evidence is derived from large observational studies. Two cohorts were retrospectively defined within the General Practice Research Database, one consisting of 244 235 oral corticosteroid users and the other of control subjects matched for age and sex. Patients taking oral corticosteroids were at significantly higher risk of fractures, the relative risks (with 95% CI) being 1.61 (1.47–1.76) for hip fracture and 2.60 (2.31–2.92) for vertebral fracture.[12] There was a clear dose–response relationship (see Table 1); for patients taking at least 7.5 mg of prednisolone (or the equivalent dose of another corticosteroid), the risk of hip fracture more than doubled and that for vertebral fracture increased fivefold in comparison with those not taking corticosteroids. The increased risk of vertebral fractures even for daily doses of under 2.5 mg indi-

Table 1. Relative risks for hip and vertebral fractures in users of oral corticosteroids.[12]

Daily dose of prednisolone or equivalent	Relative risk (95% CI)	
	Hip fracture	Vertebral fracture
<2.5 mg	0.99 (0.82–1.20)	1.55 (1.20–2.01)
2.5–7.5 mg	1.77 (1.55–2.02)	2.59 (2.16–3.10)
7.5 mg or more	2.27 (1.94–2.66)	5.18 (4.25–6.31)

cates that there is no 'safe dose'. All fracture risks declined rapidly towards baseline following cessation of treatment with oral corticosteroids.

Meta-analyses of mostly observational evidence broadly support these findings: thus, data from 66 papers on bone density and 23 papers on fractures showed strong correlations between cumulative dose and loss of BMD and between daily dose and incidence of fracture.[11] The risk of fracture increased rapidly after the onset of corticosteroid therapy (within 3–6 months) and decreased when treatment ceased. There is some evidence that bone loss occurs early in the course of corticosteroid therapy and stabilizes thereafter, and that it is partly or completely reversed when the treatment stops.[10]

There is some evidence to suggest that corticosteroids induce fractures at higher thresholds of BMD than those for age-related or postmenopausal osteoporosis. The Royal College of Physicians' guidelines reviewed data from a variety of studies and concluded that 'for a given BMD, the risk of fracture is higher in glucocorticoid-induced osteoporosis than in postmenopausal osteoporosis'.[9] Thus, a meta-analysis of data from seven large population-based studies showed that corticosteroid treatment significantly raised fracture risk independently of BMD; the relative risk for fracture was 1.62–2.09 at different ages after adjustment for BMD, in relation to the risks in the general population.[13]

Effects in patients with respiratory disease

Corticosteroid treatment is indicated for a variety of diseases, and its adverse effects may not be exactly the same in all of them. It is therefore important to examine its effects specifically in patients being treated for respiratory conditions. A systematic review of the literature assessed the evidence for the suggestion that asthma and COPD are associated with osteoporosis and fractures, with particular reference to treatment with oral corticosteroids.[14] One cohort study and nine cross-sectional studies provided data on the relationship between respiratory disease and bone density. They demonstrated clinically important reductions in BMD at various bone sites in patients with asthma or COPD who took oral corticosteroids daily. Three studies of asthmatic patients dependent on oral corticosteroids suggested an increased risk of vertebral fracture. There was less consistent evidence of a reduction in BMD in the absence of treatment with oral corticosteroids.

A subsequent study examined the relationship between use of oral corticosteroids and incidence of fracture in patients with chronic respiratory disease.[15] A questionnaire asking about fractures and relevant aspects of lifestyle was administered to 367 patients taking continuous or frequent oral corticosteroids for asthma, COPD or alveolitis, and to 734 subjects matched for age and sex who had never had oral corticosteroids or a diagnosis of lung disease. The cumulative incidence of fractures since the time of diagnosis was 23% in the treated group and 15% in the control subjects, with an odds ratio (OR) of 1.8 (95% CI 1.3–2.6). The respiratory patients were much more likely to have had a fracture of the vertebrae (OR 10, 95% CI 2.9–34), hip (OR 6, 95% CI 1.2–30) and ribs or sternum (OR 3.2, 95% CI 1.6–6.6) than the control subjects. Within the treated group, the effects of oral corticosteroids were dose related; the OR for the highest versus the lowest cumulative dose quartile was 2 for all fractures and 9 for vertebral fractures.

Another cross-sectional study examined the relationship between corticosteroid use and vertebral fractures in men aged 50 years and over who had COPD.[16] Men who took oral corticosteroids were twice as likely to have a vertebral fracture as those who never used corticosteroids, and the relationship was primarily due to continuous use of corticosteroids. Furthermore, the fractures in the oral corticosteroid group were more likely to be multiple and more severe.

Effects on biochemical markers

Three randomized controlled trials have investigated the effects of oral corticosteroids on biochemical markers of bone metabolism. All the studies showed a fall in serum osteocalcin, two after a week's treatment with 10 mg of prednisolone daily in healthy volunteers,[17,18] and one after a month's treatment with 15 mg of prednisone daily in patients with rheumatoid arthritis.[19] Other effects in these trials included rapid reductions in serum calcium[18] and serum alkaline phosphatase,[19] and increases in serum 1,25-dihydroxyvitamin D_3 and urinary hydroxyproline at a higher dose (40 mg daily), which produced a greater reduction in osteocalcin.[17] Thus, there is evidence of a reduction in bone formation and an increase in bone resorption.

Conclusions

There is strong evidence to suggest that oral corticosteroids induce osteoporosis and increase the risk of fractures, particularly of the spine and hip.

Inhaled corticosteroids

Scale of use

Inhaled corticosteroids are the most suitable drugs for preventing attacks of asthma and are recommended for use at stage 2 in the treatment of the disease.[5] In COPD, it is recommended that they be given to patients with a demonstrable response in forced expiratory volume at 1 second (FEV_1) or with moderate to severe disease and repeated acute exacerbations.[6] The apparent rise in the prevalence of asthma and the growing perception of the effectiveness of these preparations have produced a steady rise in the numbers being prescribed. It is estimated that they are used by 3% of the total population of the UK, and a fifth of these patients take 1000 µg or more every day.[20]

Patients for whom ICS are prescribed tend to take them long term, and not only when symptoms occur, as the intention is to prevent rather than to relieve symptoms by their use. In consequence, an increasing number of people have used these preparations for a substantial proportion of their lives, including many who are using them during the latter part of life when the incidence of osteoporosis is greatest. It follows that, even if ICS have only a small effect on bone density, it could be of major public health importance in terms of extra fractures, particularly of the hip and spine.

Systemic bioavailablility

Compared with oral administration, inhalation is a more efficient method of conveying corticosteroids to the lung where their actions are required. In this way, relatively small doses of the drug can be used to produce high local concentrations in the airways while minimizing systemic exposure. Nevertheless, some systemic absorption occurs, the extent depending on the preparation and mode of delivery.[21] Most of the dose is usually swallowed, but it is then largely metabolized in the liver (about 80% for beclomethasone, 89% for budesonide and 99% for fluticasone). Some direct absorption occurs via the buccal mucosa, although this can be reduced by mouth rinsing. Corticosteroid deposited in the lung is absorbed unmetabolized into the systemic circulation, so that any inhaler device that improves delivery to the lung will increase systemic bioavailability to a proportionately greater degree.

Effect on bone

A systematic Cochrane Review identified two randomized controlled trials that investigated the effects of ICS on fractures.[22] One was the EUROSCOP trial of budesonide for 3 years in 1277 smokers with mild COPD.[23] The other involved 374 patients with mild asthma who were randomized to receive inhaled budesonide, inhaled beclomethasone or non-corticosteroid treatment for 2 years; 239 completed the study.[24] No significant effect on vertebral fractures was detected in either study or in their combined results.

Together with another randomized trial (in 64 patients with asthma, followed up for 2 years),[25] these studies examined the effect on BMD as measured by dual-energy X-ray absorptiometry. A meta-analysis found no significant differences at the lumbar spine or femoral neck.[22] In one of these studies, within the groups treated with ICS, the mean daily dose was significantly related to the fall in BMD at the lumbar spine although not at the femoral neck.[24] The authors pointed out that, as the dose was inversely related to lung function, a direct effect of asthma severity on bone density was possible. If so, an effect of ICS might be masked by the better control of asthma that was achieved by this type of medication.

The results of two further trials were not included in this review. In one, 912 patients with mild COPD were randomly allocated to receive inhaled budesonide or placebo and followed up for 3 years.[26] No significant changes in BMD occurred at any site in budesonide-treated patients in comparison with the placebo group. But the other trial showed lower BMD of the lumbar spine and femur after 3 years' treatment with inhaled triamcinolone in 412 patients with COPD.[27]

Evidence from randomized trials is limited in respect of duration and dosage of treatment. In order to examine the possible effects of treatment over many years and at higher dosages, it is necessary to use data from observational studies. The largest study to investigate the possible effects of ICS on fracture incidence is probably that by van Staa and colleagues,[28] using the UK General Practice Research Database. This study examined the incidence of fractures in three retrospectively defined cohorts, comprising 170818 users of ICS, 170818 matched control subjects and 108786 users of bronchodilators who did not use corticosteroids. Patients who used oral corticosteroids were excluded. The patients taking ICS had a significantly higher incidence of fractures than the control group, with the relative risks being 1.22 (95% CI 1.04–1.43) for hip fractures and 1.51 (95% CI 1.22–1.85) for vertebral fractures. But there were no differences between the incidence rates of the ICS and bronchodilator groups. The excess risk associated with ICS might therefore be attributable to the underlying respiratory disease rather than to the treatment.

Another study used the same database to conduct a population-based case–control study.[29] Prior use of ICS was compared between 16341 cases of hip fracture and 29889 control subjects, individually matched for age, sex and general practice. Hip fracture was associated with exposure to ICS, with an odds ratio of 1.26 (95% CI 1.17–1.36). Various potential confounders were considered, including other drug use and comorbid illness; the only one that had an important effect was annual courses of oral corticosteroids and, after adjusting for that, the odds ratio was reduced to 1.19 (95% CI 1.10–1.28). There was a significant dose–response relationship between ICS and hip fracture that persisted after adjusting for annual number of courses of oral corticosteroids. In these elderly subjects (mean age 79 years), there was therefore evidence that ICS increased the risk of hip fracture.

A systematic review and meta-analysis by Lipworth[30] examined the findings of studies (mostly observational) relating ICS to various adverse effects, including reduction in bone density. Five out of seven cross-sectional or cohort studies in adults found an association between ICS and a reduction in BMD. Three further studies showed similar associations,[31–33] particularly in women, in whom the use of ICS alone was associated with bone densities that were intermediate between those of oral corticosteroid users and those of women who had never taken corticosteroids.[30]

Effects on biochemical markers

The Cochrane Review identified five randomized controlled trials from which data on biochemical markers could be used for the meta-analysis.[22] Three of these studies related to healthy subjects who were treated for 1–9 weeks,[17,34,35] whereas two dealt with patients with COPD or asthma who were followed up for 2–2.5 years.[24,36] Overall, with all data at all doses of ICS combined, there was no significant effect on serum osteocalcin. When the meta-analysis was conducted separately according to dose, a statistically significant adverse effect on osteocalcin was found when the dose exceeded that recommended in the British Thoracic Society Guidelines (as occurred in a subset of subjects in two studies), but not otherwise. One study reported an adverse effect on serum alkaline phosphatase, but this paradoxically occurred at the lower but not the higher dose and may have been an artefact of the study design. No significant effects were detected on other biochemical markers, including urinary hydroxyproline.

In one of these trials, two corticosteroid preparations were used, beclomethasone and budesonide. In comparison with the non-corticosteroid group, patients randomized to beclomethasone had lower osteocalcin levels and higher urinary markers over the 2 years of treatment, allowing for baseline values; no significant effects appeared in the budesonide group.[24] This concurs with some limited evidence that budesonide has bone-sparing properties.[9]

Lipworth's systematic review[30] included a number of observational studies that examined the effects of ICS on markers of bone metabolism. Short- and medium-term studies of healthy volunteers and asthmatic patients have detected dose-related effects on biochemical markers, occurring less frequently with inhaled than with oral corticosteroids. Cross-sectional studies of asthmatic patients receiving long-term beclomethasone or budesonide therapy have shown lower osteocalcin levels compared with control subjects.

Conclusions

There is no clear evidence that ICS induce osteoporosis or increase the risk of fractures. Some observational studies suggest that these preparations reduce BMD and increase the risk of hip fracture in elderly people and postmenopausal women. Randomized trials tend to be fairly short term in comparison with the usual duration of treatment, so their results could be misleading in two opposite ways. On the one hand, they will not reveal cumulative effects that take many years to occur; on the other hand, the short-term effects may not continue indefinitely when treatment is prolonged. Observational studies provide evidence on long-term effects but are potentially flawed by confounding factors: patients who frequently need medication are likely to have more severe disease, which may increase their risk of osteoporosis in other ways (e.g. by reducing their exercise level). Thus, there is some uncertainly about whether reduction in BMD occurs, particularly with certain preparations and in susceptible groups.

Management

Prevention and treatment

In this context, prevention usually refers to interventions designed to prevent bone loss in persons commencing corticosteroid therapy (primary prevention), and treatment

(or secondary prevention) relates to interventions given to persons who are already established on corticosteroids and in whom some loss of bone density or fracture has occurred.[9] The same interventions are appropriate for both situations, although the criteria for using them may differ. The evidence for their effectiveness will be reviewed briefly, and the recommendations for their use will then be considered.

General principles

In view of the known effects of oral corticosteroids, it is obviously prudent to restrict their use and dose to the minimum necessary. 'The aim of treatment is to control the asthma using the lowest possible dose, or if possible, to stop long term steroid tablets completely'.[5] Uncertainties about possible effects of ICS suggest a similar prudence regarding dose: 'Patients should be maintained at the lowest possible dose of inhaled steroid'.[5]

There are good reasons to believe that the risk of osteoporosis can be affected by lifestyle factors such as diet and exercise. The evidence is mostly observational and relates to postmenopausal rather than corticosteroid-induced osteoporosis, so the effects of these factors in the present context cannot be quantified. Nevertheless, in view of the weight of evidence combined with other known benefits of these measures, it is reasonable to advise physical exercise, adequate nutrition, cessation of smoking and moderation in alcohol intake for people using corticosteroids, especially postmenopausal women and the elderly.[9]

Bisphosphonates

The bisphosphonate drugs are adsorbed on to the surface of bone, primarily inhibiting osteoclastic function and thus reducing the rate of bone turnover. They comprise alendronate, clodronate, etidronate, pamidronate and risedronate, all of which have been used in the management of corticosteroid-induced osteoporosis.

The use of bisphosphonates in the prevention and treatment of corticosteroid-induced osteoporosis was examined in a Cochrane systematic review and meta-analysis (Table 2).[37] Thirteen controlled trials were identified, including 842 patients. The results were presented as weighted mean differences between the percentage changes in BMD in the treated and placebo groups. Statistically significant effects were reported for the lumbar spine and the femoral neck, the weighted mean differences being 4.3% (95% CI 2.7–5.9) and 2.1% (0.01–3.8) respectively. Some of the trials were not randomized, but their results were included as they tended to underestimate rather than overestimate the effect size. The incidence of spinal fractures was also lower in the treated group, but the difference was not statistically significant (odds ratio 0.76, 95% CI 0.37–1.53).

The authors concluded that bisphosphonates are effective in preventing and treating corticosteroid-induced bone loss at the lumbar spine and femoral neck. Long-term effects beyond

Table 2. Trial inclusion criteria for the Cochrane systematic reviews.[37–39]

Bisphosphonates for steroid-induced osteoporosis[37]	Calcitonin for preventing and treating corticosteroid-induced osteoporosis[38]	Calcium and vitamin D for corticosteroid-induced osteoporosis[39]
Types of trials: randomized and quasi-randomized controlled trials	Types of trials: randomized and quasi-randomized controlled trials	Types of trials: randomized and quasi-randomized controlled trials
Types of participants: adults over 18 years of age with underlying inflammatory disorders treated with systemic corticosteroids	Types of participants: adults over 18 years of age with an underlying disease requiring systemic corticosteroids	Types of participants: adults over 18 years of age with an underlying disease requiring systemic corticosteroids who had not used concomitant therapy in the past 6 months
Types of interventions: bisphosphonates (first or second generation) alone or in combination with calcium and/or vitamin D, compared with the control group taking placebo alone or in combination with calcium and/or vitamin D	Types of interventions: calcitonin therapy for treatment or prevention of osteoporosis, compared with usual care or placebo. Calcium and vitamin D were allowed if both groups received the same co-intervention in the same doses	Types of interventions: vitamin D (cholecalciferol), dihydroxy vitamin D (calcitriol), with calcium, compared with calcium alone or placebo in the treatment of corticosteroid-induced osteoporosis
Effeets: BMD improved by 4.3% Fractures: not reported	Effects: BMD improved by 3.2% Fractures: lower RR 0.71 (0.26–1.89)	Effects: BMD improved by 2.6% Fractures: no difference

BMD, bone mineral density.

1 year, and efficacy against spinal fractures, cannot be known except by extrapolation from the above findings and randomized trials in other types of osteoporosis.[2] The data suggest that primary prevention is more efficacious than secondary prevention. It cannot be assumed that all bisphosphonates have equal potency; there is some reason to think that pamidronate is more effective than etidronate (which was used in most of these studies), although not on the basis of this analysis.

Calcitonin

Calcitonin can be given by injection or nasal spray and has been shown to prevent bone loss and fractures in post-menopausal women.[2] A Cochrane systematic review examined its effectiveness in corticosteroid-induced osteoporosis (Table 2).[38] Nine randomized controlled trials were identified, including 441 patients. The meta-analysis showed that calcitonin was more effective than placebo in preserving bone mass at the lumbar spine after 6 and 12 months of therapy, the weighted mean differences being 2.8% (95% CI 1.4–4.3) and 3.2% (0.3–6.1) respectively. At 24 months, the weighted mean difference was still greater (4.5%), but the confidence interval was wider (–0.6 to 9.5), and the difference was not statistically significant. Bone density at the distal radius was also higher with calcitonin at 6 months, but no significant effect occurred at the femoral neck. The incidence of fractures was lower in the calcitonin group, but the differences were not statistically significant, the relative risks being 0.71 (95% CI 0.26–1.89) and 0.52 (0.14–1.96) for vertebral and non-vertebral fractures respectively. The effects appeared to be greater among patients who had been taking corticosteroids for more than 3 months,

although these trials were of poorer quality. There was no consistent relationship with dosage, but subcutaneous administration was associated with greater effects.

The reviewers concluded that calcitonin preserves bone mass at the lumbar spine by about 3% compared with placebo during the first year, but not at the femoral neck. The efficacy in preventing corticosteroid-induced fractures remains to be established.

Calcium and vitamin D

There is evidence that calcium salts can reduce bone loss in postmenopausal osteoporosis. The effects of vitamin D and its derivatives are uncertain, as the results of trials have been inconsistent. A combination of calcium and vitamin D has been shown to reduce the incidence of fractures in older people.[2]

A Cochrane systematic review examined the effectiveness of calcium and vitamin D, in comparison with calcium alone or placebo, in the prevention of corticosteroid-induced bone loss (Table 2).[39] Five randomized controlled trials were included, with 274 patients. There were significant weighted mean differences between treated and control groups in lumbar BMD (2.6, 95% CI 0.7–4.5) and in radial BMD (2.5, 95% CI 0.6–4.4). There were no significant differences in femoral neck bone mass, fracture incidence or biochemical markers of bone resorption. The authors concluded that a combination of calcium and vitamin D prevents bone loss in patients receiving corticosteroids. They recommended that all patients being started on systemic corticosteroids should receive prophylactic therapy with calcium and vitamin D because of its low toxicity and cost.

Fluoride

Administration of fluoride preparations causes a dramatic increase in cancellous bone density in the spine and femoral neck, but the effects on fracture incidence are less consistent.[2] A Cochrane Review of its effects in postmenopausal women concluded that it increases lumbar spine BMD without reducing the incidence of vertebral fractures, and it increases the risk of non-vertebral fractures, especially if given at high doses.[40] Randomized trials have been conducted in patients receiving oral corticosteroids; spine BMD increases after a year or two of treatment, but no significant effect has been found in the femoral neck or forearm BMD.[9] In view of the findings in postmenopausal women, its use in corticosteroid-induced osteoporosis does not seem justifiable.

Hormone replacement therapy

There is strong evidence that hormone replacement therapy, in the form of oestrogen preparations, maintains or improves bone density and reduces the incidence of non-vertebral fractures in postmenopausal women.[41] A few randomized controlled trials have been carried out in women receiving corticosteroids; BMD increased in the lumbar spine and the femoral neck.[9]

A few studies have shown an increase in vertebral BMD in men treated with testosterone. A crossover randomized controlled trial was conducted in 15 asthmatic men receiving long-term corticosteroids.[42] Mean BMD in the lumbar spine increased by 5.0% during 12 months of treatment but did not change during the control period; biochemical markers of bone turnover declined during treatment. No significant benefit occurred in the femoral neck.

Summary critical appraisal

The UK guidelines contained a number of recommendations, which were graded A–C according to the level of the supporting evidence:[9]
- People who are at high risk should be advised to commence bone-protective therapy at the time of starting oral corticosteroids: for example those aged 65 years and over and those who have already had a fragility fracture. This recommendation is grade A, being based on the results of randomized controlled trials, particularly in relation to the actions of bisphosphonate preparations.
- Bone densitometry (using dual-energy X-ray absorptiometry) should be considered for other people taking oral corticosteroids if the treatment is expected to continue for at least 3 months. This recommendation, like those below, is grade C, being based on expert opinion and clinical experience rather than on specific studies of experimental or observational design.
- Use of a bone-sparing agent should be considered if the BMD at the spine or hip has a T score of −1.5 or less. This cut-off level is arbitrary and represents the view of a British expert group; American guidelines recommend a T score of −1 for this pur-

pose. Age and sex need to be taken into account, as they greatly modify the predictive implications of a given T score. Tables are available (reproduced in the Guidelines) showing the 10-year probability of fracture according to age, sex and T score, but they are based on data in persons not receiving corticosteroids, which seem to increase the risk independently of the other factors. Thus, there is much uncertainty about the criteria that should be used.
- Good nutrition, an adequate dietary intake of calcium and appropriate physical activity should be encouraged, and tobacco smoking and alcohol abuse should be discouraged.

References

1 World Health Organization. *Assessment of Fracture Risk and its Application to Screening for Postmenopausal Osteoporosis.* WHO Technical Report Series 843. Geneva, WHO, 1994.

2 Royal College of Physicians. *Osteoporosis: Clinical Guidelines for Prevention and Treatment.* London, Royal College of Physicians of London, 1999.

3 Marshall D, Johnell O, Wedel H. Meta-analysis of how well measures of bone mineral density predict occurrence of osteoporotic fractures. *BMJ* 1996; **312**:1254–9.

4 Cooper C. Epidemiology and definition of osteoporosis. In: Compston JE, ed. *Osteoporosis: New Perspectives on Causes, Prevention and Treatment.* London, Royal College of Physicians, 1996

5 British Thoracic Society, Scottish Intercollegiate Guidelines Network. British guideline on the management of asthma. *Thorax* 2003; **58**(Suppl I):i1–i94.

6 MacNee W, Calverley PMA. Chronic obstructive pulmonary disease. 7: Management of COPD. *Thorax* 2003; **58**:261–5.

7 van Staa TP, Leufkens HG, Abenhaim L, Begaud B, Zhang B, Cooper C. Use of oral corticosteroids in the United Kingdom. *QJM* 2000; **93**: 105–11.

8 Walsh LJ, Wong CA, Pringle M, Tattersfield AE. Use of oral corticosteroids in the community and the prevention of secondary osteoporosis: a cross-sectional study. *BMJ* 1996; **313**:344–6.

9 Working Group in collaboration with The Royal College of Physicians, The Bone and Tooth Society of Great Britain, and The National Osteoporosis Society. *Glucocorticoid-induced Osteoporosis: Guidelines for Prevention and Treatment.* London, Royal College of Physicians, 2002.

10 Verhoeven AC, Boers M. Limited bone loss due to corticosteroids; a systematic review of prospective studies in rheumatoid arthritis and other diseases. *J Rheumatol* 1997; **24**:1495–503.

11 van Staa TP, Leufkens HGM, Cooper C. The epidemiology of corticosteroid-induced osteoporosis: a meta-analysis. *Osteoporos Int* 2002; **13**:777–87.

12 van Staa TP, Leufkens HGM, Abenhaim L, Zhang B, Cooper C. Use of oral corticosteroids and risk of fractures. *J Bone Miner Res* 2000; **15**: 993–1000.

13 Johnell O, De Laet C, Johansson H *et al.* Oral corticosteroids increase fracture risk independently of BMD. *Osteoporos Int* 2002; **13**(Suppl 1): S14.

14 Smith BJ, Phillips PJ, Heller RF. Asthma and chronic obstructive airway diseases are associated with osteoporosis and fractures: a literature review. *Respirology* 1999; **4**:101–9.

15 Walsh LJ, Wong CA, Oborne J *et al.* Adverse effects of oral corticosteroids in relation to dose in patients with lung disease. *Thorax* 2001; **56**:279–84.

16 McEvoy CE, Ensrud KE, Bender E *et al.* Association between cortico-

steroid use and vertebral fractures in older men with chronic obstructive pulmonary disease. *Am J Resp Crit Care Med* 1998; **157**:704–9.

17 Hodsman AB, Toogood JH, Jennings B, Fraher LJ, Baskerville JC. Differential effects of inhaled budesonide and oral prednisolone on serum osteocalcin. *J Clin Endocrinol Metab* 1991; **72**:530–40.

18 Lems WF, Jacobs JW, Van Rijn HJ, Bijlsma JW. Changes in calcium and bone metabolism during treatment with low dose prednisone in young, healthy, male volunteers. *Clin Rheumatol* 1995; **14**:420–4.

19 van Schaardenburg D, Valkema R, Dijkmans BAC *et al.* Prednisone treatment of elderly-onset rheumatoid arthritis: disease activity and bone mass in comparison with chloroquine treatment. *Arthritis Rheum* 1995; **38**:334–42.

20 Tattersfield AE. Limitations of current treatment. *Lancet* 1997; **350** (Suppl II):24–7.

21 Lipworth BJ. New perspectives on inhaled drug delivery and systemic bioactivity. *Thorax* 1995; **50**:105–10; corrections *Thorax* 1995; **50**:592.

22 Jones A, Fay JK, Burr M, Stone M, Hood K, Roberts G. Inhaled corticosteroid effects on bone metabolism in asthma and mild chronic obstructive pulmonary disease (Cochrane Review). In: *The Cochrane Library*, Issue 1. Oxford, Update Software, 2003.

23 Pauwels RA, Lofdahl C-G, Laitinen L *et al.* Long-term treatment with inhaled budesonide in persons with mild chronic obstructive pulmonary disease who continue to smoke. *N Engl Med J* 1999; **340**:1948–53.

24 Tattersfield AE, Town GI, Johnell O *et al.* Bone mineral density in subjects with mild asthma randomised to treatment with inhaled corticosteroids or non-corticosteroid treatment for two years. *Thorax* 2001; **56**:272–8.

25 Li JTC, Ford LB, Chervinsky P *et al.* Fluticasone proprionate powder and lack of clinically significant effects on hypothalamic–pituitary–adrenal axis and bone mineral density over 2 years in adults with mild asthma. *J Allergy Clin Immunol* 1999; **103**:1062–8.

26 Johnell O, Pauwels R, Lofdahl CG *et al.* Bone mineral density in patients with chronic obstructive pulmonary disease treated with budesonide Turbuhaler. *Eur Respir J* 2002; **19**:1058–63.

27 The Lung Health Study Research Group. Effect of inhaled triamcinolone on the decline in pulmonary function in chronic obstructive pulmonary disease. *N Engl J Med* 2000; **343**:1902–9.

28 van Staa TP, Leufkens HG, Cooper C. Use of inhaled corticosteroids and risk of fractures. *J Bone Miner Res* 2001; **16**:581–8.

29 Hubbard RB, Smith CJ, Smeeth L, Harrison TW, Tattersfield AE. Inhaled corticosteroids and hip fracture: a population-based case–control study. *Am J Resp Crit Care Med* 2002; **166**:1563–6.

30 Lipworth BJ. Systemic adverse effects of inhaled corticosteroid therapy: a systematic review and meta-analysis. *Arch Intern Med* 1999; **159**:941–55.

31 Marystone JF, Barrett-Connor EL, Morton DJ. Inhaled and oral corticosteroids: their effects on bone mineral density in older adults. *Am J Public Health* 1995; **85**:1693–5.

32 Wong CA, Walsh LJ, Smith CJP *et al.* Inhaled corticosteroid use and bone-mineral density in patients with asthma. *Lancet* 2000; **355**: 1399–403.

33 Israel E, Banerjee TR, Fitzmaurice GM, Kotlov TV, LaHive K, LeBoff MS. Effects of inhaled glucocorticoids on bone density in premenstrual women. *N Engl J Med* 2001; **345**:941–7.

34 Toogood JH, Jennings B, Hodsman AB, Baskerville J, Fraher LJ. Effects of dose and dosing schedule of inhaled budesonide on bone turnover. *J Allergy Clin Immunol* 1991; **88**:572–80.

35 Leech JA, Hodder RV, Ooi DS, Gay J. Effects of short-term inhaled budesonide and beclomethasone dipropionate on serum osteocalcin in premenopausal women. *Am Rev Respir Dis* 1993; **148**:113–15.

36 Kerstjens HAM, Postma DS, van Doormaal JJ *et al.* Effects of short term and long term treatment with inhaled corticosteroids on bone metabolism in patients with airways obstruction. *Thorax* 1994; **49**:652–6.

37 Homik J, Cranney A, Shea B *et al.* Bisphosphonates for steroid induced osteoporosis (Cochrane Review). In: *The Cochrane Library*, Issue 1. Oxford, Update Software, 2003.

38 Cranney A, Welch V, Adachi JD *et al.* Calcitonin for preventing and treating corticosteroid-induced osteoporosis (Cochrane Review). In: *The Cochrane Library*, Issue 1. Oxford, Update Software, 2003.

39 Homik J, Suarez-Almazor ME, Shea B, Cranney A, Wells G, Tugwell P. Calcium and vitamin D for corticosteroid-induced osteoporosis (Cochrane Review). In: *The Cochrane Library*, Issue 1. Oxford, Update Software, 2003.

40 Haguenauer D, Welch V, Shea B, Tugwell P, Wells G. Fluoride for treating postmenopausal osteoporosis (Cochrane Review). In: *The Cochrane Library*, Issue 1. Oxford, Update Software, 2003.

41 Torgerson DJ, Bell-Syer SE. Hormone replacement therapy and prevention of nonvertebral fractures: a meta-analysis of randomized trials. *JAMA* 2001; **285**:2891–7.

42 Reid IR, Wattie DJ, Evans MC, Stapleton JP. Testosterone therapy in glucocorticoid-treated men. *Arch Intern Med* 1996; **156**:1173–7.

CHAPTER 1.3.3

Helping people to stop smoking

Tim Lancaster

Questions

In smokers, (population), what is the effect of smoking cessation advice from doctors or nurses (intervention) on smoking quit rates (outcome)?

In smokers (population), what is the effect of behavioural intervention (intervention) on smoking quit rates (outcome)?

In smokers (population), what is the effect of self-help programmes (intervention) on smoking quit rates (outcome)?

In smokers (population), what is the effect of individually tailored intervention programmes (intervention) compared with standard smoking cessation materials (comparison) on smoking quit rates (outcome)?

In smokers (population), what is the effect of nicotine replacement therapy (intervention) compared with brief smoking cessation advice (comparison) on smoking quit rates (outcome)?

In smokers (population), what is the effect of antidepressants (intervention) compared with brief smoking cessation advice (comparison) on smoking quit rates (outcome)?

In smokers (population), what is the effect of complementary therapies (intervention) on smoking quit rates (outcome)?

In smokers (population), what is the effect of combined therapies/nicotine replacement therapy (intervention) compared with brief smoking cessation advice (comparison) on smoking quit rates (outcome)?

Background

Smoking is the most important preventable risk factor for respiratory diseases including chronic obstructive pulmonary disease (COPD) and lung cancer. Smoking cessation is the single most effective, and cost-effective, way to reduce the risk of developing COPD and stop its progression.[1,2] Stopping smoking improves pulmonary function, and the rate of age-related decline in function is slowed.[3,4] It has been estimated that 85–90% of COPD deaths in the USA can be attributed to smoking.[5] Smoking also contributes significantly to morbidity and mortality from other conditions, particularly vascular disease and other cancers. These illnesses are among the commonest causes of death in the developing world. Increasing tobacco consumption in developing countries means that smoking-related mortality is on the rise in many of these areas. Peto and Lopez[6] have estimated that current patterns of cigarette smoking will cause about 450 million deaths worldwide in the next 50 years. A reduction of 50% in the number of current smokers would avoid about 20–30 million premature deaths in the first quarter of the century and about 150 million in the second quarter.[6] Preventing young people from starting smoking will also reduce tobacco-related mortality, but the effects will not be seen until after 2050. Quitting by current smokers is therefore the only way in which tobacco-related mortality can be reduced in the medium term. Although many ex-smokers report that they quit without formal help, there is evidence that an increasing number of successful quit attempts have been achieved using some form of behavioural, psychological, pharmacological or complementary treatment.[7] The aim of this chapter is to summarize what is known about the effectiveness of the available interventions.

Literature search

The conclusions of this review are based on meta-analyses of randomized controlled trials. Where there are insufficient trials for meta-analysis, we report the findings of individual randomized trials. The meta-analyses are based on work conducted by the Cochrane Tobacco Addiction Review group (http://www.dphpc.ox.ac.uk/cochrane_tobacco/), which seeks to identify and summarize the evidence for interventions to reduce and prevent tobacco use. The group produces and maintains systematic reviews to inform policymakers, clinicians and individuals wishing to stop smoking. The Cochrane Database of Systematic Reviews was searched for systematic reviews that included smoking cessation in the title. Twenty-six systematic reviews of interventions for smoking cessation have been published in the Cochrane Database of Systematic Reviews. They have contributed to the evidence base for smoking cessation guidelines in the UK and elsewhere.[8,9]

Details of the methods and results of each review are available in the Cochrane Library (abstracts at http://www.update-software.com/abstracts/TOBACCOAbstractIndex.htm). The reviews summarize results from randomized controlled trials with at least 6 months of follow-up. Trials must report data on smoking status, and not just the effects of treatment on withdrawal symptoms. We summarize treatment effects as odds ratios (OR). An OR greater than 1 indicates more quitters in the intervention group. Where appropriate, we use meta-

Table 1. Efficacy of smoking cessation interventions.

Intervention	Results Increased quit rate	
	Odds ratio	95% CI
Advice from doctors		
Simple advice[12]	1.69	1.45–1.98
Counselling[16]	1.62	1.35–1.94
Aversive therapy		
Silver acetate[19]	1.05	0.63–1.73
Self-help materials		
Individually tailored[21]	1.36	1.13–1.64
Pharmacotherapy		
Nicotine replacement therapy[11]	1.74	1.64–1.86
Bupropion[18]	1.97	1.67–2.34
Nortryptyline	2.77	1.73–4.44
Clonidine[34]	1.89	1.30–2.74
Naltrexone[37]	1.34	0.49–3.63

analysis to report pooled estimates of treatment effect as ORs with 95% confidence intervals (CI) using either the Peto or the Mantel–Haenszel method.[10] Although the absolute risk difference and number needed to treat are easier measures to interpret, they cannot be calculated reliably from the available data because of variations in baseline quit rates in different populations. There is evidence that the relative effects of treatment are constant, but the actual number of quitters achieved depends on the population offered the treatment. Treatment usually produces more quitters in populations with a higher baseline stopping rate (for example motivated patients attending a specialist smoking clinic) and fewer when the baseline rate is lower (for example all smoking patients attending a general practitioner).[11]

Interventions (Table 1)

Interventions from doctors and nurses
The effect of simple advice from doctors during routine clinical care has been studied in 31 trials including over 26 000 smokers. The studies took place in a variety of settings including primary care, hospital wards, outpatient clinics and industrial clinics.[12] The Cochrane Review found that simple advice increased the quit rate (OR 1.69, 95% CI 1.45–1.98). More intensive advice produced a slightly higher quit rate. There is some evidence that the main effect of advice is to motivate a quit attempt, rather than to increase the chances of a success.[13] A recent Cochrane Review found that interventions from nurses also increased quit rates.[14] Most of the studies included in this review assessed the impact of nurses providing specialized counselling rather than giving advice as part of routine

clinical care. Studies of advice from nurses as part of general health promotion have not shown a similar effect.

Behavioural and psychological interventions
Motivated smokers may seek further help from specialist smoking cessation counsellors or clinics. Treatment may be delivered one-to-one or in a group. Both individual counselling and group therapy increase the chances of quitting.[15,16] Nine out of 11 studies of individual counselling included in the Cochrane Review compared counselling with brief advice or usual care.[16] The combined results favoured counselling (OR 1.62, 95% CI 1.35–1.94). In 22 trials, group therapy programmes were more effective than self-help materials, but not consistently better than other interventions involving personal contact.[15] There was no difference between group and individual therapy in the two trials that included both. Groups are theoretically more cost-effective, but their usefulness may be limited by difficulties in recruiting and retaining participants.[17]

In the trials, the therapists were usually clinical psychologists, but the interventions drew on a variety of psychological techniques rather than a distinctive theoretical model. There is therefore little evidence about the relative effectiveness of different psychological approaches. The exception is aversion therapy, which pairs the pleasurable stimulus of smoking with an unpleasant stimulus with the goal of extinguishing the urge to smoke. The Cochrane Review of 24, mainly small, trials of aversion therapy failed to detect an effect of non-specific aversive stimuli (for example focusing on negative aspects of cigarettes while smoking). However, there was some evidence that rapid smoking (inhaling rapidly to induce nausea) increased the likelihood of quitting.[18] Silver acetate is a pharmacological method of aversive stimulation. It produces an unpleasant, metallic taste when combined with cigarettes and is analogous to the use of disulfiram for alcoholism. Two studies with 6-month or greater follow-up failed to detect a benefit with silver acetate although confidence intervals were wide (OR 1.05, 95% CI 0.63–1.73).[19]

Self-help
The approaches used in one-to-one or group counselling can be delivered through written materials, audiotapes, videotapes or computer programs. Self-help materials have the potential to reach many more people than therapist-delivered interventions. Many forms of self-help materials are available, ranging from brief leaflets to complex manuals. They may be given as an adjunct to brief advice or without any personal contact.[20] The Cochrane Review did not find evidence that self-help materials had an additional benefit over brief personal advice. However, in 11 trials with no face-to-face contact, there was a small effect of self-help materials compared with no intervention (OR 1.24, 95% CI 1.07–1.45).

More recent approaches have concentrated on ways of making self-help materials appropriate for the needs of individual smokers who differ in their reasons for smoking, level of addiction and motivation to quit. After collection of baseline information, smokers receive materials matched to their readiness to change,[21] or to other factors such as self-efficacy and motivation. In 10 trials that compared individually tailored materials with standard or stage-based materials, there was a benefit of the personalized intervention (OR 1.36, 95% CI 1.13–1.64). There was no evidence that materials tailored solely to group characteristics (such as age, gender or race) were better than standard materials.

Telephone contact may be an economical way of adding some personal contact to self-help materials. In 13 trials that compared proactive telephone counselling with a minimal intervention control, five showed a significant benefit and eight had non-significant differences. Four trials provided telephone support following a face-to-face intervention, and did not show that this significantly improved long-term quit rates. In four trials that compared telephone support with use of nicotine replacement therapy (NRT) alone, no additional benefit of the counselling was detected. Providing access to a hotline showed a significant benefit in one trial and was associated with lower quit rates in another. Varying the type of counselling provided did not affect outcome.[22]

Increasingly, self-help materials are available on computer or through the internet, although there is as yet little evidence of whether the method of delivery affects the effectiveness of the materials.

Nicotine replacement therapy

The aim of NRT is to replace nicotine from cigarettes, thus reducing withdrawal symptoms associated with stopping smoking. NRT is available as chewing gum, transdermal patch, nasal spray, inhaler, sublingual tablet and lozenge. Over 90 trials of NRT have been reported. Although there is some evidence of publication bias (negative trials not published), the Cochrane Review found that NRT helps people to stop smoking.[11] Overall, NRT increased the chances of quitting about one and a half to two times (OR 1.74, 95% CI 1.64–1.86), whatever the level of additional support and encouragement. The quit rate was higher in both placebo and NRT arms of trials that included intensive support, so the effect of NRT seems to be to increase the rate from whatever baseline is set by other interventions. As all the trials of NRT reported so far have included at least some form of brief advice, this is the minimum that should be offered in order to ensure its effectiveness. Most studies of NRT have involved smokers with evidence of nicotine dependence. Its usefulness for less heavily dependent smokers is uncertain.

There is little direct evidence that any NRT product is more effective than another (Fig. 1). Thus, the decision about which to use should be guided by individual preferences. The nicotine patch delivers a steady level of nicotine throughout the day and can be worn unobtrusively. The main side-effect is skin irritation. Wearing the patch only during waking hours (16 hours/day) is as effective as wearing it for 24 hours/day. Eight weeks of patch therapy is as effective as longer courses, and there is no evidence that tapered therapy is better than abrupt withdrawal. The nicotine inhaler resembles a cigarette and may be useful for individuals who want a substitute for the act of smoking. The nasal spray delivers nicotine more rapidly and may be suitable for satisfying surges of craving. Gum, spray, inhaler and lozenges may all cause local irritation in the nose or mouth. There is evidence that, for highly dependent smokers, a 4-mg dose of nicotine gum is more effective than a 2-mg dose.

Some clinicians recommend combinations of nicotine products (for example providing a background nicotine level with patches and controlling cravings with faster acting preparations such as gum or spray). There have been too few trials to provide clear evidence about the effectiveness of patch and gum combinations,[23,24] but one trial has shown significantly greater efficacy for nasal spray and patch than patch alone.[25]

Antidepressants

There is both scientific and commercial interest in the neurochemical and genetic basis of tobacco dependence and its implications for therapy. The Cochrane Review failed to detect an

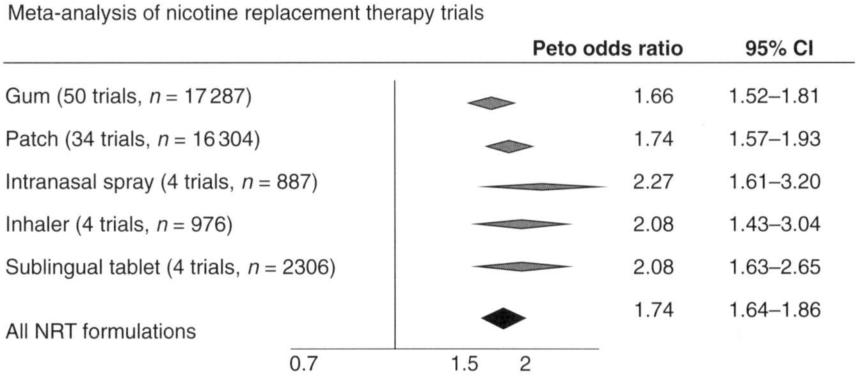

Meta-analysis of nicotine replacement therapy trials

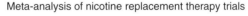

	Peto odds ratio	95% CI
Gum (50 trials, *n* = 17 287)	1.66	1.52–1.81
Patch (34 trials, *n* = 16 304)	1.74	1.57–1.93
Intranasal spray (4 trials, *n* = 887)	2.27	1.61–3.20
Inhaler (4 trials, *n* = 976)	2.08	1.43–3.04
Sublingual tablet (4 trials, *n* = 2306)	2.08	1.63–2.65
All NRT formulations	1.74	1.64–1.86

0.7   1.5   2

Figure 1. Meta-analysis of the effect of nicotine replacement therapy on smoking cessation.[11]

effect of anxiolytics,[26] but there is growing evidence that some antidepressants increase the likelihood of a quit attempt being successful.[18] Bupropion is an atypical antidepressant that is thought to inhibit neuronal uptake of noradrenaline and dopamine. A slow-release form is licensed for smoking cessation in many countries. There is evidence from 10 published trials and six unpublished studies that it increases the chances of quitting (Mantel–Haenszel OR 1.97, 95% CI 1.67–2.34). These trials recruited heavier smokers who were also offered behavioural support. One trial found that bupropion alone or combined with a nicotine patch was more effective than nicotine patch alone,[27] but a second unpublished trial did not detect a benefit.[28] One trial recruited patients with mild or moderate COPD. At 6-month follow-up from quit date, quit rates were 16% in the bupropion group and 9% for placebo.[29] Unpublished 12-month follow-up data showed that there had been more relapse in the bupropion group and differences were no longer significant (10% versus 9%; data from industry). Bupropion can cause dry mouth and insomnia, but serious side-effects were rare in the trials. The manufacturers report a 0.1% risk of seizures using sustained-release bupropion up to 300 mg/day, and this is approximately the level at which they have been observed in practice.[30] There may be a theoretical risk that bupropion might depress ventilatory responses in patients with severe COPD.[31] This effect was not detected in a study that included patients with mild to moderate COPD.[29] In the absence of evidence, clinical judgement is required when using it in patients with more severe disease.

Five trials have shown a benefit from the tricyclic antidepressant nortriptyline (OR 2.77, 95% CI 1.73–4.44). Selective serotonin reuptake inhibitors (SSRIs) do not appear to be effective.[32] Various other antidepressants have been tested for smoking cessation, but there is insufficient evidence to determine whether they are effective.

It is unclear how antidepressant drugs aid smoking cessation. Smoking and depression are known to be linked, but whether this reflects a common genetic predisposition or neurochemical effects of nicotine is uncertain.[33] In the trials, they were effective irrespective of whether depression was present. Whether efficacy for smoking cessation is drug specific, or shared by classes of antidepressant drugs, is unresolved.

Other pharmacological therapies

Although licensed primarily as an antihypertensive, clonidine shares some pharmacological effects with bupropion and tricyclic antidepressants. The Cochrane Review of six clinical trials has shown evidence of efficacy (OR 1.89, 95% CI 1.30–2.74), but its usefulness is limited by a significant incidence of sedation and postural hypotension.[34] The nicotine antagonist mecamylamine (used in the past for blood pressure reduction) has been investigated as a cessation aid in combination with nicotine replacement, but is not licensed for this

use. The evidence from two studies suggests that there is an effect of mecamylamine, started before cessation and continued after cessation, in aiding smoking cessation.[35] It is not clear whether this effect is significantly greater than that of nicotine replacement alone. The studies also suggest that the combination of mecamylamine with nicotine replacement, started before cessation, may increase the rates of cessation beyond those achieved with nicotine alone.

Lobeline is an alkaloid derived from the leaves of an Indian tobacco plant (*Lobelia inflata*). It was recognized in the early 1900s as a partial nicotinic agonist. The first reported use for smoking cessation was in the 1930s, and it has been used in proprietary smoking remedies. The Food and Drug Administration no longer permits it to be marketed in the United States, although Health Canada has recently licensed a quit aid containing lobeline. The Cochrane Review identified no trials that met the inclusion criteria of 6 months of follow-up. An unpublished multicentre study of a sublingual tablet found no evidence of efficacy at 6 weeks.[36]

The possibility that release of endogenous opioids may play some part in the rewarding effects of nicotine has led to interest in opioid antagonists for smoking cessation. Two trials of naltrexone reported long-term cessation data. Both trials failed to detect a significant difference in quit rates between naltrexone and placebo. Meta-analysis failed to detect a significant effect of naltrexone on long-term abstinence, although confidence intervals were wide (OR 1.34, 95% CI 0.49–3.63). No trials of naloxone reported long-term follow-up.[37]

Complementary therapies

The Cochrane Review of 20 trials failed to detect an effect of acupuncture compared with sham acupuncture. Acupuncture may be better than doing nothing, at least in the short term, but this may be a placebo effect.[38] The Cochrane Review of hypnotherapy failed to find an effect greater than other behavioural interventions.[39] The nine trials identified were small and of variable quality. Hypnotherapy is particularly difficult to evaluate in the absence of a sham procedure that can control for non-specific effects. A number of herbal preparations are advocated for smoking cessation, but none has been formally evaluated.

Combined approaches

Most trials have been designed to assess the impact of a single behavioural therapy or pharmacotherapy. Cochrane Reviews generally exclude trials that combine different approaches. The highest quit rates are, however, likely to be achieved by combining different approaches. In particular, there is a theoretical and practical rationale for combining behavioural interventions with pharmacotherapy. One trial has demonstrated the long-term benefit of this approach, on both cessation rates and pulmonary function. The Lung Health Study (LHS) recruited individuals aged 35–60 years who smoked and were thought to be at high risk of COPD as indicated by evidence of early airways obstruction. They were randomized to usual care (UC) or to 'special intervention' (SI), which consisted of physician advice to quit, a 12-session group programme and nicotine gum. Quitters entered a relapse prevention programme. Treatment was available throughout the 5-year study for those who failed to quit initially or who relapsed. After 5 years, sustained quit rates for those who quit at the time of the initial cessation programme were 22% in the SI condition compared with 5% in UC. Cross-sectional quit rates increased more in the UC group, but there was also a significant difference, 35% in SI versus 20% in UC, at 5 years. This rate of quitting was reflected in a significant effect on the primary outcome, decline in FEV_1, which was significantly smaller in the SI group.[3]

Longer term follow-up of participants in the LHS has shown that differences in lung function have persisted, even though the difference in smoking status between the groups was less pronounced with 52% of the SI group and 43% of the UC not smoking at the 11-year follow-up. There were large differences between sustained quitters and continuous smokers in percentage of predicted FEV_1. Whereas 38% of continuous smokers had a FEV_1 less than 60% of predicted normal, only 10% of sustained quitters fell into this category.[40] Thus, the LHS demonstrates benefits from early, intensive, multicomponent intervention, not only for achieving smoking cessation, but for preventing future morbidity, and is an important study for those caring for patients with COPD.

Interventions for smokers with respiratory disease may need to be intensive and to combine multiple approaches. Clinicians frequently believe that people with chronic lung disease find it harder to quit. However, the LHS shows that, at least in early disease, there is no reason for excessive pessimism when helping people with COPD to stop smoking.

Conclusions

Social attitudes, legislation and public health measures influence changes in tobacco use.[41] Against this background, many smokers give up without clinical intervention. Nevertheless, most health professionals believe they have an obligation to offer help to individuals seeking to stop.[42] Current evidence shows that there are an increasing number of effective strategies available to individuals seeking to stop smoking, and the health professionals who advise them. There are relatively few studies that have directly compared the available treatments, so it is difficult to recommend one approach over another. However, the Lung Health Study shows that, in patients with evidence of respiratory disease, intensive multimodal treatments increase quit rates and reduce morbidity.

Effective strategies for stopping smoking

Brief advice from a physician
Structured intervention from a nurse
Individual counselling
Group counselling
Self-help materials (effectiveness limited unless individually tailored)
Nicotine replacement therapy
Bupropion
Nortriptyline
Clonidine

Acknowledgements

The Cochrane Tobacco Addiction Review Group is supported by a grant from the National Health Service.

References

1 Pauwels R. Global initiative for chronic obstructive lung diseases (GOLD): time to act. *Eur Respir J* 2001; **18**:901–2.
2 Taylor DH Jr, Hasselblad V, Henley SJ, Thun MJ, Sloan FA. Benefits of smoking cessation for longevity. *Am J Public Health* 2002; **92**: 990–6.
3 Anthonisen NR, Connett JE, Kiley JP *et al.* Effects of smoking intervention and the use of an inhaled anticholinergic bronchodilator on the rate of decline of FEV_1. The Lung Health Study. *JAMA* 1994; **272**:1497–505.
4 Tashkin DP, Clark VA, Coulson AH *et al.* The UCLA population studies of chronic obstructive respiratory disease. VIII. Effects of smoking cessation on lung function: a prospective study of a free-living population. *Am Rev Respir Dis* 1984; **130**:707–15.
5 *The Health Consequences of Smoking: Chronic Obstructive Lung Disease.* A Report of the Surgeon General. US Department of Health and Human Services, 1984.
6 Peto R, Lopez AD. Future worldwide health effects of current smoking patterns. In: Koop CE, Pearson CE, Schwarz MR, eds. *Critical Issues in Global Health.* New York, Jossey-Bass, 2002, pp. 154–61.
7 Hughes JR. Four beliefs that may impede progress in the treatment of smoking. *Tob Control* 1999; **8**:323–6.
8 Raw M, McNeill A, West R. Smoking cessation guidelines for health professionals. A guide to effective smoking cessation interventions for the health care system. *Thorax* 1998; **53**:S1–S19.
9 Raw M, McNeill A, West R. Smoking cessation: evidence based recommendations for the healthcare system. *BMJ* 1999; **318**:182–5.
10 Yusuf S, Peto R, Lewis J, Collins R, Sleight P. β blockade during and after myocardial infarction: an overview of the randomized trials. *Prog Cardiovasc Dis* 1985; **27**:335–71.
11 Silagy C, Lancaster T, Stead LF, Mant D, Fowler G. Nicotine replacement therapy for smoking cessation (Cochrane Review). In: *The Cochrane Library*, Issue 4. Chichester, John Wiley & Sons, 2003.
12 Silagy C, Stead LF. Physician advice for smoking cessation (Cochrane Review). In: *The Cochrane Library*, Issue 4. Chichester, John Wiley & Sons, 2003.
13 Hughes JR, Goldstein MG, Hurt RD, Shiffman S. Recent advances in the pharmacotherapy of smoking. *JAMA* 1999; **281**:72–6.
14 Rice VH, Stead LF. Nursing interventions for smoking cessation (Cochrane Review). In: *The Cochrane Library*, Issue 4. Chichester, John Wiley & Sons, 2003.

15 Stead LF, Lancaster T. Group behaviour therapy programmes for smoking cessation (Cochrane Review). In: *The Cochrane Library*, Issue 4. Chichester, John Wiley & Sons, 2003.

16 Lancaster T, Stead LF. Individual behavioural counselling for smoking cessation (Cochrane Review). In: *The Cochrane Library*, Issue 4. Chichester, John Wiley & Sons, 2003.

17 Hollis JF, Lichtenstein E, Vogt TM, Stevens VJ, Biglan A. Nurse-assisted counseling for smokers in primary care. *Ann Intern Med* 1993; **118**:521–5.

18 Hughes JR, Stead LF, Lancaster T. Antidepressants for smoking cessation (Cochrane Review). In: *The Cochrane Library*, Issue 4. Chichester, John Wiley & Sons, 2003.

19 Lancaster T, Stead LF. Silver acetate for smoking cessation (Cochrane Review). In: *The Cochrane Library*, Issue 4. Chichester, John Wiley & Sons, 2003.

20 Lancaster T, Stead LF. Self-help interventions for smoking cessation (Cochrane Review). In: *The Cochrane Library*, Issue 4. Chichester, John Wiley & Sons, 2003.

21 Walsh RA, Redman S, Brinsmead MW, Byrne JM, Melmeth A. A smoking cessation program at a public antenatal clinic. *Am J Public Health* 1997; **87**:1201–4.

22 Stead LF, Lancaster T, Perera R. Telephone counselling for smoking cessation (Cochrane Review). In: *The Cochrane Library*, Issue 4. Chichester, John Wiley & Sons, 2003.

23 Kornitzer M, Boutsen M, Dramaix M, Thijs J, Gustavsson G. Combined use of nicotine patch and gum in smoking cessation: a placebo-controlled clinical-trial. *Prev Med* 1995; **24**:41–7.

24 Puska P, Korhonen HJ, Vartiainen E, Urjanheimo EL, Gustavsson G, Westin A. Combined use of nicotine patch and gum compared with gum alone in smoking cessation: a clinical trial in North Karelia. *Tob Control* 1995; **4**:231–5.

25 Blondal T, Gudmundsson LJ, Olafsdottir I, Gustavsson G, Westin A. Nicotine nasal spray with nicotine patch for smoking cessation: randomised trial with six year follow up. *BMJ* 1999; **318**:285–8.

26 Hughes JR, Stead LF, Lancaster T. Anxiolytics for smoking cessation. (Cochrane Review). In: *The Cochrane Library*, Issue 4. Chichester, John Wiley & Sons, 2003.

27 Jorenby DE, Leischow SJ, Nides MA *et al.* A controlled trial of sustained-release bupropion, a nicotine patch, or both for smoking cessation. *N Engl J Med* 1999; **340**:685–91.

28 Simon, JA, Duncan C, Carmody TP, Hudes ES. Bupropion for smoking cessation: a randomized trial. National Conference on Tobacco or Health, Nov 19–22 2002, San Francisco, CA.

29 Tashkin D, Kanner R, Bailey W *et al.* Smoking cessation in patients with chronic obstructive pulmonary disease: a double-blind, placebo-controlled, randomised trial. *Lancet* 2001; **357**:1571–5.

30 GlaxoSmithKline. Zyban (bupropion hydrochloride) Sustained-Release Tablets Product Information, 2001.

31 Garcia-Rio F, Serrano S, Mediano O, Alonso A, Villamor J. Safety profile of bupropion for chronic obstructive pulmonary disease. *Lancet* 2001; **358**:1009–10.

32 Niaura R, Spring B, Borrelli B *et al.* Multicenter trial of fluoxetine as an adjunct to behavioral smoking cessation treatment. *J Consult Clin Psychol* 2002; **70**:887–96.

33 Benowitz NL. Treating tobacco addiction — nicotine or no nicotine? *N Engl J Med* 1997; **337**:1230–1.

34 Gourlay, SG, Stead LF, Benowitz NL. Clonidine for smoking cessation (Cochrane Review). In: *The Cochrane Library*, Issue 4. Chichester, John Wiley & Sons, 2003.

35 Lancaster T, Stead LF. Mecamylamine for smoking cessation (Cochrane Review). In: *The Cochrane Library*, Issue 4. Chichester, John Wiley & Sons, 2003.

36 Stead LF, Hughes JR. Lobeline for smoking cessation (Cochrane Review). In: *The Cochrane Library*, Issue 4. Chichester, John Wiley & Sons, 2003.

37 David S, Lancaster T, Stead LF. Opioid antagonists for smoking cessation (Cochrane Review). In: *The Cochrane Library*, Issue 4. Chichester, John Wiley & Sons, 2003.

38 White AR, Rampes H, Ernst E. Acupuncture for smoking cessation (Cochrane Review). In: *The Cochrane Library*, Issue 4. Chichester, John Wiley & Sons, 2003.

39 Abbot NC, Stead LF, White AR, Barnes J, Ernst E. Hypnotherapy for smoking cessation (Cochrane Review). In: *The Cochrane Library*, Issue 4. Chichester, John Wiley & Sons, 2003.

40 Anthonisen NR, Connett JE, Murray RP. Smoking and lung function of Lung Health Study participants after 11 years. *Am J Respir Crit Care Med* 2002; **166**:675–9.

41 Chapman S. Unravelling gossamer with boxing gloves: problems in explaining the decline in smoking. *BMJ* 1993; **307**:429–32.

42 McAvoy BH, Kaner EF, Lock CA, Heather N, Gilvarry E. Our Healthier Nation: are general practitioners willing and able to deliver? A survey of attitudes to and involvement in health promotion and lifestyle counselling. *Br J Gen Pract* 1999; **49**:187–90.

PART 2

Asthma

CHAPTER 2.1

Acute exacerbations

Brian H Rowe

Case scenario

A 26-year-old women presents to the emergency department (ED) with a 3-day history of cough, shortness of breath and wheezing that began after symptoms of a common cold. She is alert and oriented but talking in short phrases only, with a respiratory rate of 32/min, heart rate of 110 and oxygen saturation of 91%. Examination of the chest reveals moderate intercostal and subcostal retractions. On auscultation, there is diffused expiratory wheezing throughout all lung fields with prolongation of the expiratory phase. The heart sounds are normal. The remainder of the physical examination is within normal limits. You diagnose her with an acute exacerbation of asthma and commence salbutamol therapy in addition to intravenous methylprednisolone. The medical student asks whether you would consider using magnesium sulphate or inhaled ipratropium bromide for this patient.

The patient improves rapidly with treatment using salbutamol and corticosteroids and asks what can be done to prevent her from relapsing back to the ED during this attack. Review of systems reveals that this young women has had several previous episodes of acute asthma in the past 12 months presenting to the ED as a result of upper respiratory tract infections. The patient describes her asthma as being worse with exertion, which has resulted in her being unable to lose what she considers to be excess weight. She describes using her salbutamol puffer several times a day before and after exertion and often in the middle of the night when she wakes with coughing episodes. She would also like to know how she could decrease her chances of having another exacerbation of this nature in the future and whether she regularly requires the inhaled corticosteroid she has recently restarted.

Background

Asthma is a common chronic condition and is characterized by intermittent exacerbations followed by variable degrees of 'stability'. The prevalence of asthma varies widely with demographics (more common in children and women), geography (regional variation is often noted) and socioeconomic status. The hallmark of exacerbation includes a history of asthma, increasing symptoms of dyspnoea, wheeze and/or cough and increasing need for short-acting β-agonists. Asthma

exacerbations are common presentations to the ED in many parts of the world,[1,2] and the costs associated with the care of asthma are enormous.[3-5] For example, in the United States, approximately six billion dollars per year is spent on asthma.[3] Twenty-five per cent of all asthma expenses are related to acute exacerbations (ED visits, hospitalizations).[5] As a result, it is clear that asthma and acute asthma are important health care problems.

Given the severe nature and importance of acute asthma as a respiratory condition, it is not surprising that there are a number of guidelines that have been developed to direct the management of this problem.[6-8] Despite the availability of these guidelines, there is a 'care gap' between what is known and what is practised, and the dissemination of evidence often does not reach the patient in the ED or other acute care setting. This is due in part to the rapidly changing understanding of the pathophysiology and treatment of asthma and the introduction of new management strategies in this field.

Formulating clinical questions

In order to address the issues of most relevance to your patient and to help in searching the literature for the evidence regarding these, you should structure your questions as recommended in Chapter 1.

Questions

1. In adults with acute asthma (population), does the measurement of pulmonary functions or oxygen saturation (tests) predict the need for hospital admission (outcome)? {prognosis}
2. In adults with acute asthma (population), does the delivery of β₂-agonists using inhalers with holding chambers (intervention) result in similar bronchodilation and admission to hospital (outcome) compared with treatment with nebulization of therapy? {therapy}
3. In adults with acute asthma (population), does the addition of nebulized anticholinergic agents (ipratropium bromide) (intervention) to nebulized β-agonist decrease the risk of admission to hospital (outcome) compared with treatment with β-agonist therapy alone? {therapy}

4. In adults with acute asthma (population), does the use of intravenous corticosteroids (intervention) in the ED reduce admissions to hospital? {therapy}

5. In adults with acute severe asthma (population), does intravenous magnesium sulphate (intervention) in addition to nebulized salbutamol and systemic corticosteroids improve the rate of recovery and reduce admissions to hospital (outcome)? {therapy}

6. In adult patients with acute asthma discharged from the ED (population), does treatment with systemic corticosteroids reduce relapse to additional care? {therapy}

7. In adult patients with acute asthma discharged from the ED (population), does the addition of inhaled corticosteroids (intervention) to routine therapy after discharge reduce relapse and improve quality of life (outcomes)?

8. In adult patients with acute asthma discharged from the ED (population), what is the role of patient education (intervention) in reducing further relapses and exacerbations of asthma (outcomes)? {therapy}

9. In adult patients with acute asthma seen in the ED (population), what is the role of newer agents such as long-acting β-agonists and leukotriene antagonists (intervention) in reducing admissions or relapses of asthma (outcomes)? {therapy}

General search strategy

You begin to address these questions by searching for evidence in the common electronic databases such as the Cochrane Library, MEDLINE and EMBASE looking specifically for systematic reviews and meta-analyses. The Cochrane Library is particularly rich in high-quality systematic review evidence on numerous aspects of acute and chronic asthma.[9] When a systematic review is identified, you also search for recent updates on the Cochrane Library and also search MEDLINE and EMBASE to identify randomized controlled trials that became available after the publication date of the systematic review. In addition, access to relevant, updated and evidence-based clinical practice guidelines (CPGs) on acute asthma are accessed to determine the consensus rating of areas lacking evidence.

Literature search

- Cochrane Library—asthma AND (Topic)
- MEDLINE—Asthma and AND MEDLINE AND (systematic review OR Meta-analysis OR metaanalysis) AND adult AND (Topic)
- EMBASE—Asthma and AND MEDLINE AND (systematic review OR Meta-analysis OR metaanalysis) AND adult AND (Topic)

Critical review of the literature

Your search strategy for the Cochrane Library identified no systematic reviews addressing Question 1 outlined above. Your MEDLINE search identified several articles relevant to this question; however, none was a systematic review.

Question

1. In adults with acute asthma (population), does the measurement of pulmonary functions or oxygen saturation (tests) predict the need for hospital admission (outcome)? {prognosis}

Literature search

- MEDLINE and EMBASE—asthma AND pulmonary functions OR spirometry and sensitivity or specificity

Physicians' estimates of severity of asthma, response to therapy and risk of relapse following discharge are often inaccurate in acute asthma. The assessment of asthma severity is recommended by all major acute asthma guidelines; however, the method of assessing severity is widely debated. For example, in some guidelines, pulmonary function testing is recommended. In others, severity determined objectively using spirometry, peak expiratory flow rates (PEFR) or both for patients over 5 years of age is recommended.[6]

This use of a pulmonary function measure has been encouraged, despite lack of evidence for the predictive value of individual measures.[10] Most EDs measure PEFR, rather than FEV_1, and follow this marker over the course of treatment during the acute visit. Not surprisingly, the cut points for severity vary among the different guidelines; however, all suggest that <50% predicted of either PEFR or FEV_1 indicates severe disease. Perhaps the more important issue relates to the change in pulmonary function over the acute treatment period. For example, blunted improvement in either FEV_1 or PEFR following initial bronchodilator therapy is predictive of a more prolonged attack course or the need for hospital admission.[11]

Pulse oximetry measurements (Sao_2) have previously been used extensively in children; however, recent research questions whether this measurement alone is a clinically useful predictor of hospital admission in children who present to the ED with acute asthma.[12] Low Sao_2 may indicate a need for admission to hospital, but normal levels do not exclude severe asthma or the possibility of relapse. Measurement of Sao_2 may help to guide treatment in adult patients; however, no studies were identified clearly demonstrating that Sao_2 predicted admission or relapse in adult asthmatic patients.

In summary, asthma severity is a multifactorial assessment in the emergency setting. Pulse oximetry, pulmonary function tests, vital signs, history, physical examination, response to

43

43

coarse

therapy and current medications are all required to determine the need for hospital admission and the risk of relapse after discharge.[13,14]

Question

2. In adults with acute asthma (population), does the delivery of β_2-agonists using inhalers with holding chambers (intervention) result in similar bronchodilation and admission to hospital (outcome) compared with treatment with nebulization of therapy? {therapy}

Literature search

• Cochrane Library—asthma AND holding chambers

Early treatment of acute asthma has generally focused on the use of inhaled (usually via nebulizer) short-acting β_2-agonists because of their undisputed and generally rapid effect on relieving bronchospasm. Whether the drug is most effec-tive when delivered via a nebulizer or a metered dose inhaler (MDI) with holding chamber or spacer device has been an area of intense research. A Cochrane Library systematic review of 22 trials involving 1520 subjects suggests that the use of either delivery method yields similar outcomes.[15] In adults, the relative risk (RR) of admission for holding chamber versus nebulizer was 0.88 [95% confidence interval (CI) 0.56–1.38; Fig. 1]. Length of stay in the ED for adults and FEV_1 or PEFR were also similar for the two delivery methods. Economic evaluations of these competing approaches demonstrate an advantage favouring the use of MDI with spacer over nebulized treatments.[16] Finally, the use of MDI was associated with fewer side-effects (e.g. tachycardia) than nebulizers, especially in children.

However, these data do not include patients with severe or near-fatal asthma. From a clinical perspective, these results suggest using MDI with a spacer device in patients with asthma who present with mild to moderate symptoms. For patients with severe asthma, the benefits and ease of continuous nebulization[17] and the need to focus on other issues may make

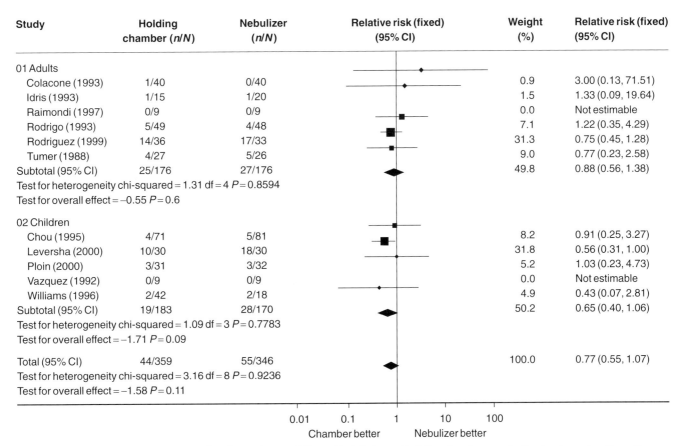

Figure 1. Similar hospital admissions when β-agonists are delivered by inhaler and holding chamber or nebulization in acute asthma. From Cates *et al*.[15]

nebulization an attractive alternative. Finally, employing MDI and spacer delivery in the acute setting affords a potential opportunity to assess inhaler technique and educate patients with regard to appropriate care.

Attempts to identify optimal doses or treatment intervals to achieve maximal bronchodilation or symptom relief have not been successful.[18] However, continuous treatment may have an advantage over intermittent treatment in the severe asthmatic.[17] In addition, lower doses appear to be equivalent to higher doses with regard to maximizing bronchodilation or clinical outcome.[19] A substantial number of patients achieve a bronchodilation 'plateau' and, in these people, additional β_2-agonist therapy only seems to cause more side-effects. Some guidelines now recommend that β-agonists be titrated to plateau using objective assessment of airway obstruction with pulmonary function measures.[6]

Despite this very strong evidence supporting the use of MDI and spacer devices, the convenience of and patient acceptance of nebulized salbutamol was entrenched in the past.[20,21] The recent worldwide severe acute respiratory syndrome (SARS) outbreak and its apparent spread following nebulization[22] has discouraged nebulization and should result in a rapid conversion to MDI.

Question

3. In adults with acute asthma (population), does the addition of nebulized anticholinergic agents (ipratropium bromide) (intervention) to nebulized β-agonist decrease the risk of admission to hospital (outcome) compared with treatment with β-agonist therapy alone? {therapy}

Literature search

• Cochrane Library and MEDLINE—asthma AND anticholinergics

There is increasing support, particularly in children, for *adding* anticholinergic agents (most commonly ipratropium bromide) to β_2-agonist therapy in moderate to severe acute asthma.[23,24] The best evidence for acute asthma arises from the Cochrane Review in children with acute asthma, in which ipratropium bromide plus β_2-agonists was compared with β_2-agonists alone.[23] Summary statistics indicate that multiple doses of ipratropium bromide effect a clinically significant improvement in FEV_1 of 16.1% (95% CI 6–27%) and 17.5% (95% CI 4–31%) at 60 min and 120 min respectively. Combined therapy reduced the risk of hospital admission by 25% (RR 0.75; 95% CI 0.62–0.89) in moderate and severe exacerbations. The number needed to treat (NNT) to prevent one admission was 12 (95% CI 8–32); the NNT decreased to 7 in

severe cases. These results were confirmed by the largest individual trial involved in an updated Cochrane Review.[25] There was no conclusive evidence for single or multiple doses of ipratropium bromide in children with mild exacerbations. Neither therapy group was associated with significant adverse effects.

A similar meta-analysis in adults also demonstrated a modest beneficial effect of adding ipratropium bromide to inhaled β_2-agonists.[24] The absolute increase in FEV_1 and PEFR was 7.3% (95% CI 4–11%) and 22.1% (95% CI 11–33%) over 45 to 90 min respectively. The risk of admission was decreased by 27% (RR 0.73; 95% CI 0.53–0.99). A large randomized controlled trial has since been completed that confirms the systematic review evidence.[26] The study observed a 21% (95% CI 3–38%) improvement in PEFR and a 48.1% (95% CI 20–76%) improvement in FEV_1 over the control group. High doses of ipratropium bromide reduced the risk of hospital admission by 49% (RR 0.51; 95% CI 0.31–0.83); the NNT to prevent a single admission was 5 (95% CI 3–17). Although questions still need to be resolved regarding ipratropium bromide therapy in the ED setting (such as the dose–response relationship), it seems prudent to use this agent with β_2-agonists for patients with moderate to severe acute asthma.

Question

4. In adults with acute asthma (population), does the use of intravenous corticosteroids (intervention) in the ED reduce admissions to hospital? {therapy}

Literature search

• Cochrane Library—acute asthma AND corticosteroids AND admission

The airway oedema and increased secretions associated with acute asthma are the result of inflammation and can be effectively treated with systemic corticosteroids. The early use (i.e. within 90 min of arrival) of corticosteroids delivered by either oral or intravenous (IV) routes is a principal treatment choice in published evidence-based asthma guidelines.[6,7] A Cochrane meta-analysis investigating this issue identified 12 studies involving 863 patients.[27] The authors determined that the early use of systemic corticosteroids for acute asthma in the ED significantly reduced admission rates (Fig. 2; OR 0.50; 95% CI 0.31–0.81), with the NNT being 8 (95% CI 5–20).[27] This benefit was more pronounced for those not already receiving corticosteroids (OR 0.37; 95% CI 0.19–0.70) and those experiencing a severe exacerbation (OR 0.35; 95% CI 0.21–0.59). The effects of corticosteroids on pulmonary functions were variable in the short term, mainly because of insuf-

Study	CS (n/N)	Placebo (n/N)	Odds ratio (random) (95% CI)	Weight (%)	Odds ratio (random) (95% CI)
Connett (1994a)	13/19	15/18		6.0	0.43 (0.09, 2.09)
Connett (1994b)	7/18	12/15		6.0	0.16 (0.03, 0.77)
Lin (1997)	7/23	5/22		7.4	1.49 (0.39, 5.65)
Lin (1999)	8/30	11/26		9.0	0.50 (0.16, 1.52)
Littenberg (1986)	9/48	23/49		10.8	0.26 (0.10, 0.65)
Rodrigo (1994)	4/49	5/49		7.1	0.78 (0.20, 3.11)
Scarfone (1993)	11/36	19/39		10.5	0.46 (0.18, 1.19)
Schneider (1988)	5/27	12/27		8.1	0.28 (0.08, 0.97)
Stein (1990)	21/44	23/47		11.7	0.95 (0.42, 2.17)
Storr (1987)	53/73	65/67		6.4	0.08 (0.02, 0.36)
Tal (1990)	4/17	4/13		5.8	0.69 (0.14, 3.52)
Wolfson (1994)	17/42	15/46		11.2	1.41 (0.59, 3.36)
Total (95% CI)	159/426	209/418		100.0	0.50 (0.31, 0.81)

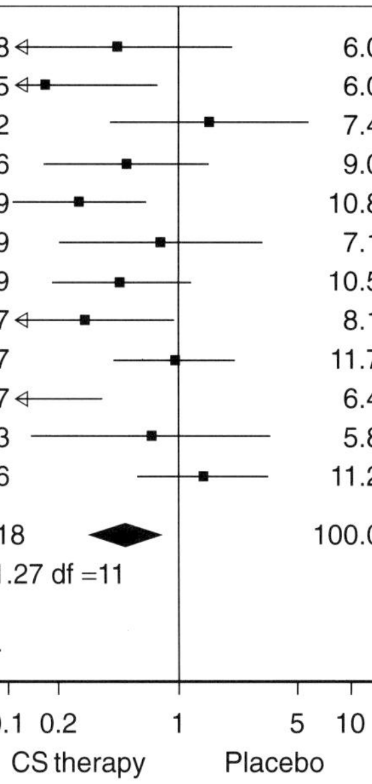

Test for heterogeneity chi-squared = 21.27 df = 11
  $P = 0.0307$
Test for overall effect = – 2.86 P=0.004

0.1 0.2   1   5 10
CS therapy   Placebo

Figure 2. Reduction in hospital admissions with early administration of systemic corticosteroids compared with placebo in acute asthma. From Rowe et al.[27]

ficient reporting of results in the individual trials. Side-effect profiles were similar between all corticosteroid treatment routes and placebo, suggesting that early treatment with corticosteroid is safe.

A debate regarding the use of IV versus oral corticosteroids in the ED persists; however, this now seems to be focused on identifying which patients require the IV route as opposed to the oral route. There is no evidence from controlled trials or meta-analyses to suggest that the advantage offered by corticosteroids in moderate to severe asthma is related to the route of administration.[27] Further systematic review evidence on dosing suggests that high-dose corticosteroids, at least in hospitalized patients, are no more effective than moderate and low doses.[28]

Applying this information in practice requires a clear understanding that not all levels of severity have been assessed with sufficient rigour to confirm equivalency of systemic routes. Until further evidence is available, it seems reasonable to select oral agents as the first-line choice while reserving IV corticosteroids for those who are too dyspnoeic to swallow, are obtunded or intubated or are unable to tolerate oral medications (e.g. vomiting). The agent and dose of corticosteroid administered does not appear to be as important, so the decision should be based on cost, availability and patient factors (Table 1). The main issue to remember is the need to start systemic corticosteroids early and consistently for patients with moderate to severe acute asthma.

Question

5. In adults with acute severe asthma (population), does intravenous magnesium sulphate (intervention) in addition to nebulized salbutamol and systemic corticosteroids improve the rate of recovery and reduce admissions to hospital (outcome)? {therapy}

Literature search

- Cochrane Library—acute asthma AND magnesium

Owing to their effect on smooth muscles and role in cellular calcium homeostasis, the use of IV and inhaled magnesium sulphate ($MgSO_4$) in unresponsive acute asthma has gained support over the past decade. There have been a number of systematic reviews, which all conclude that IV magnesium is not only safe but also effective in those patients with severe disease.[29,30] In the Cochrane Review, compared with β-agonist and IV systemic corticosteroids only, the *addition* of intravenous $MgSO_4$ reduced hospitalization (Fig. 3; OR 0.1; 95% CI 0.04–0.27) and improved pulmonary functions (mean increase in PEF 52 L/min; 95% CI 27–77) in severe asthma.[29] Overall, there were no adverse effects with respect to systolic blood pressure with this treatment, and side-effects were rare

Table 1. Acute asthma — drug dosing.

Drug	Admitted (severe)	Discharged (mild–moderate)
Methylprednisolone (Solumedrol)	80–125 mg IV	N/A
Hydrocortisone (Solucortef)	250–500 mg IV	N/A
Prednisone	40–60 mg/dose divided bid or once daily	40–60 mg/day (for outpatients: 5–7 days; tapering not required)
Methyl-xanthines	Not recommended	Not recommended
Salbutamol	Single treatment: 2.5–5.0 mg nebulized (0.5–1.0 mL of 0.5% solution) every 20 min. Inhaled: 4–6 activations via a holding chamber every 20 min	Inhaled: 1–2 activations using a holding chamber qid
Ipratropium bromide	Nebulizer: 250–500 µg qid. Inhaled: 4–6 activations via a holding chamber every 20 min	Inhaled: 1–2 activations using a holding chamber qid
Antibiotics	Not recommended	Not recommended
Inhaled corticosteroids	Recommended in addition to systemic corticosteroids; moderate doses. Budesonide: 400–1600 µg/day. Fluticasone: 500–100 µg/day. Flunisolide: 100–2000 µg/day	Recommended in addition to systemic corticosteroids; moderate doses. Budesonide: 400–1600 µg/day. Fluticasone: 500–100 µg/day. Flunisolide: 100–2000 µg/day
Magnesium sulphate	2-g IV bolus over 20 min; drip not required	N/A
NPPV	? Respiratory failure (see text)	N/A

NPPV, non-invasive positive pressure ventilation; IV, intravenous; N/A, not applicable; mg, milligrams; µg, micrograms; qid, four times daily; ED, emergency department.

Study	$MgSO_4$ (n/N)	Placebo (n/N)	Peto odds ratio (95% CI)	Weight (%)	Peto odds ratio (95% CI)
01 Severe					
Bloch (1995)	7/21	11/14		13.1	0.17 (0.05, 0.65)
Ciarallo (1997)	11/15	16/16		5.5	0.10 (0.01, 0.80)
Devi (1997)	9/15	15/16		8.5	0.15 (0.03, 0.81)
Skobeloff (1989)	7/19	15/17		13.3	0.12 (0.03, 0.46)
Subtotal (95% CI)	34/70	57/63		40.5	0.14 (0.07, 0.30)
Test for heterogeneity chi-squared = 0.24 df = 3 $P = 0.9701$					
Test for overall effect = −5.08 $P < 0.00001$					
02 Mild–moderate					
Bloch (1995)	14/46	13/54		30.1	1.38 (0.57, 3.32)
Green (1992)	13/58	11/62		29.4	1.34 (0.55, 3.26)
Subtotal (95% CI)	27/104	24/116		59.5	1.36 (0.72, 2.54)
Test for heterogeneity chi-squared = 0.00 df = 1 $P = 0.9627$					
Test for overall effect = 0.95 $P = 0.3$					
Total (95% CI)	61/174	81/179		100.0	0.54 (0.33, 0.88)
Test for heterogeneity chi-squared = 20.69 df = 5 $P = 0.0009$					
Test for overall effect = −2.49 $P = 0.01$					

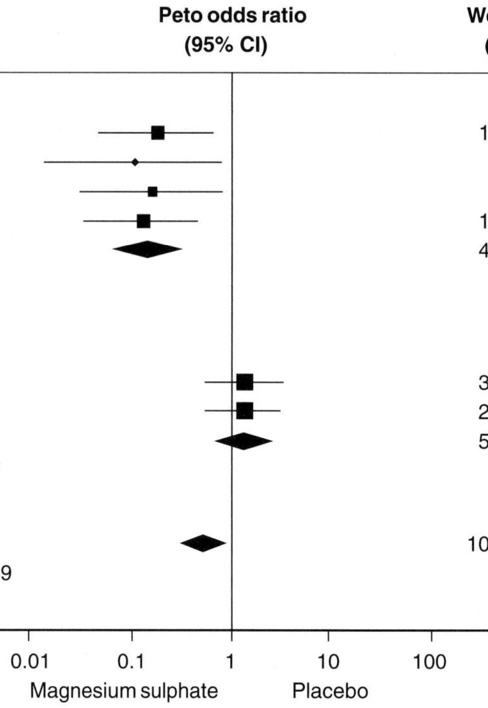

0.01 0.1 1 10 100
Magnesium sulphate   Placebo

Figure 3. Reduction in hospital admissions with early administration of intravenous magnesium sulphate compared with placebo in acute asthma. From Rowe et al.[29]

or minor. It is important to note that the *routine* use of $MgSO_4$ in all patients with asthma did produce clear beneficial effects (OR for admission 0.31; 95% CI 0.09–1.04). Adult patients with clinically severe asthma and/or pulmonary function testing < 30% predicted, who exhibit a poor response to initial bronchodilator therapy, appear to benefit most from IV $MgSO_4$ treatment. Since the publication of this study, there have been additional studies published; however, they do not alter the overall conclusion of the review.

As this agent has been shown to be easy to use, extremely safe and inexpensive, its early use in severe acute asthma should be considered. Currently, the recommended dose is 2 g IV over 20 min in adults (Table 1).[29]

Question

6. In adult patients discharged from the ED (population), does treatment with systemic corticosteroids (intervention) reduce relapse to additional care (outcome)? {therapy}

Literature search

• Cochrane Library—asthma AND corticosteroids AND discharge

Approximately 12–16% of patients treated for acute asthma will relapse within 2 weeks of ED discharge, many because of unresolved inflammation that leaves the airways sensitive to inhaled irritants.[31,32] Guidelines strongly encourage treatment with systemic corticosteroids following ED discharge for an acute exacerbation to reduce the risk of relapse.[6,7] Compelling evidence for this approach is found in a Cochrane systematic review of seven trials, involving 374 patients, comparing corticosteroid therapy with placebo following discharge.[32] Significantly fewer patients in the corticosteroid group relapsed in the first week (OR 0.35; 95% CI 0.17–0.73; Fig. 4). This reduced risk continued over the first 21 days (OR 0.33; 95% CI 0.13–0.82). The corticosteroid group also had less need for β_2-agonists (mean difference 3 activations/day; 95% CI −5.5 to −1.0). Changes in pulmonary function tests and side-effects, while rarely reported, showed no differences between the treatment groups. A subgroup analysis indicated that intramuscular (IM) corticosteroids and a 7- to 10-day tapering course of corticosteroids were similarly efficacious. IM therapy may be best reserved for those patients with questionable compliance, inability to afford the price of an oral prescription or those who are otherwise unreliable (cognitive impairment, intoxication, etc.). Thirteen (95% CI 7–91) patients would need to be treated to prevent one relapse after an exacerbation of asthma.[32,33]

Small sample sizes in the randomized control trials performed to date did not permit an examination of the relative

Study	CS (n/N)	Placebo (n/N)	Odds ratio (random) (95% CI)	Weight (%)	Odds ratio (random) (95% CI)
01 7- to 10-day follow-up					
Chapman (1991)	3/48	8/45		27.8	0.31 (0.08, 1.25)
Fiel (1983)	5/49	10/53		40.8	0.49 (0.15, 1.55)
Lee (1993a)	0/19	1/16		5.1	0.26 (0.01, 6.97)
Lee (1993b)	1/17	1/16		6.6	0.94 (0.05, 16.37)
McNamara (1993)	2/30	8/26		19.7	0.16 (0.03, 0.84)
Shapiro (1983)	0/11	0/15		0.0	Not estimable
Subtotal (95% CI)	11/174	28/171		100.0	0.35 (0.17, 0.73)
Test for heterogeneity chi-squared = 1.69 df = 4 P = 0.7933					
Test for overall effect = −2.80 P = 0.005					
02 21-day follow-up					
Chapman 1991	10/48	20/45		100.0	0.33 (0.13, 0.82)
Subtotal (95% CI)	10/48	20/45		100.0	0.33 (0.13, 0.82)
Test for heterogeneity chi-squared = 0.00 df = 0					
Test for overall effect = −2.39 P = 0.02					

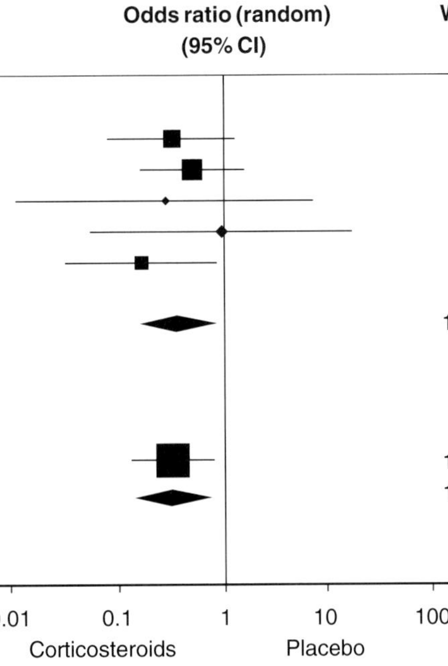

0.01   0.1   1   10   100
Corticosteroids   Placebo

Figure 4. Reduction in relapses with the addition of systemic corticosteroids after discharge from the emergency setting with acute asthma. From Rowe *et al.*[32]

effectiveness of various regimens, and definitive recommendation concerning dose or dosing protocol(s) cannot be provided. However, given the enhanced compliance associated with once-daily dosing and the availability of 40- or 50-mg tablets in many parts of the world, the use of oral corticosteroids for a short period (5–10 days) seems appropriate for most patients discharged with an acute asthma episode (Table 1). The need to 'taper' these oral corticosteroids over that period appears to be unwarranted,[34,35] especially when other anti-inflammatory agents are being used concurrently.[36]

Question

7. In adult patients with acute asthma discharged from the ED (population), does the addition of inhaled corticosteroids (intervention) to routine therapy after discharge reduce relapse and improve quality of life (outcomes)? {therapy}

Literature search

• Cochrane Library—acute asthma AND inhaled corticosteroids AND discharge

The majority of patients with acute asthma treated in an emergency setting are discharged and prescribed a short course (5–7 days) of oral corticosteroids.[2,31] Less information exists regarding the use of inhaled corticosteroids; however, the data that exist indicate impressive practice variation with respect to this treatment. For example, in US sites associated with a large North American ED airway research network, only 10% of discharged patients were prescribed an inhaled corticosteroid if they were not regularly taking one, whereas in Canadian sites, more than 50% of similar patients were treated with an inhaled corticosteroid at discharge.[37]

There is evidence to support using a combination of inhaled and oral corticosteroids after discharge from the ED.[36] There are three published randomized controlled trials,[36,38,39] which individually provide somewhat conflicting evidence for the addition of inhaled corticosteroids but, when combined in a systematic review, favour the combination.[40] The pooled effect demonstrates a trend in favour of the inhaled corticosteroid plus oral corticosteroid group having fewer relapses after discharge than the oral corticosteroid alone group (OR 0.68; 95% CI 0.46–1.02; Fig. 5).[40]

While the test for heterogeneity in the pooled result was not statistically significant ($P > 0.01$), it did appear that the results of the three trials were sufficiently different to warrant further scrutiny. The prospect of an OR as high as 46% favouring inhaled corticosteroid use cannot be ignored. Since the publication of the review, further non-randomized control trial evidence has been published supporting the role of inhaled corticosteroids at discharge. A recent administrative database study examining low-income patients who were discharged from the EDs suggested that a prescription for inhaled corticosteroids significantly reduced future relapses.[41]

Clinically, the results of this review indicate that patients already receiving inhaled corticosteroids should be counselled regarding compliance-enhancing interventions from the ED staff.[42–44] Keep in mind that many of the acute asthma patients who present to the ED exhibit features associated with poorly controlled chronic asthma.[44] They represent vulnerable patients who are ideal candidates for inhaled corticosteroids. Consequently, those patients not already on inhaled corticosteroid agents should be considered for short- or long-term inhaled corticosteroid therapy in conjunction with oral prednisone after discharge.[45] The dose and duration of inhaled corticosteroids should be based on recent history of symptom control, health care utilization and quality of life indicators (Table 1). For those patients with more severe illness, this would clearly be the optimal treatment strategy.

Study	ICS + oral CS (n/N)	Oral CS (n/N)	Odds ratio (fixed) (95% CI)	Weight (%)	Odds ratio (fixed) (95% CI)
Brenner (2000)	4/51	4/53		6.3	1.04 (0.25, 4.41)
Camargo (2000)	30/310	37/307		58.6	0.78 (0.47, 1.30)
Rowe (1999)	12/94	23/94		35.0	0.45 (0.21, 0.97)
Total (95% CI)	46/455	64/454		100.0	0.68 (0.46, 1.02)

Test for heterogeneity chi-squared = 1.72 df = 2
$P = 0.4239$
Test for overall effect = −1.85 $P = 0.06$

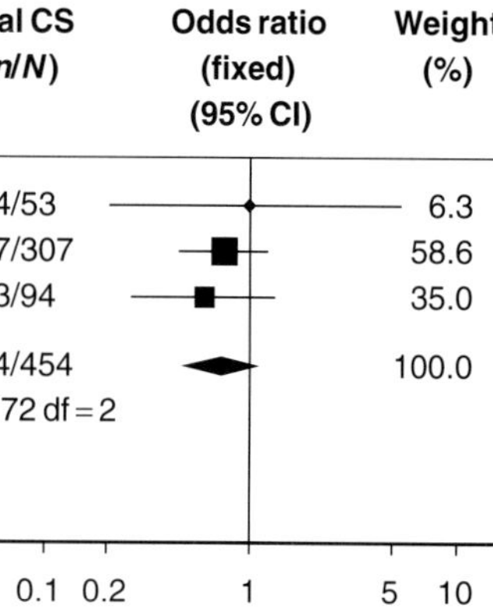

0.1 0.2   1   5   10

Figure 5. Comparison of relapses in patients with acute asthma discharged from the emergency department on systemic corticosteroids *in addition to* inhaled corticosteroids or systemic corticosteroids alone. From Edmonds *et al.*[40]

There are also several recent publications examining the effect of *replacing* oral corticosteroids with high-dose inhaled corticosteroid. These generally compare oral prednisone with very high doses of inhaled corticosteroids in acute mild asthma after discharge. While the systematic review failed to demonstrate a significant difference in asthma relapse between the two treatments (OR 1.0; 95% CI 0.48–1.42), these results need to be interpreted cautiously.[40] Although the evidence implies equivalence, these results are not conclusive because of the width of the confidence intervals and the inclusion of only patients with very mild asthma exacerbations. Given the limited data on this issue to date, use of inhaled corticosteroids alone should be reserved for those patients with very mild asthma and those who refuse or cannot take oral corticosteroids. Compared with the traditional short course of prednisone, inhaled corticosteroids are expensive and more difficult for patients and families to use. Given that there is potential for added benefit with combined therapy, future research should focus on this important comparison.

Question

8. In adult patients discharged from the ED (population), what is the role of patient education (intervention) in reducing further relapses and exacerbations of asthma (outcomes)? {therapy}

Literature search

• Cochrane Library and MEDLINE—acute asthma AND education

Providing asthma education is one of the key recommendations contained in many asthma guidelines.[6,7] In addition, when surveyed, acute care physicians felt that it was an important component of asthma care and rated many educational items as necessary.[43] In a narrative review of asthma education, authors have emphasized the need to educate asthma patients;[46] however, overall, the results of individual trials and systematic reviews regarding education have been disappointing. These disappointing results are especially true for the acute setting.

A Cochrane Review examined the impact of limited asthma education programmes (information only) for adults with asthma.[47] There was no effect on hospital admissions, doctor visits, lung function, medication use or normal activity days lost. Perceived asthma symptoms did improve in the education group (OR 0.40; 95% CI 0.18–0.86). One included study found that education was associated with reduced ED visits (mean decrease visits/person/year 2.8 visits; 95% CI –4.3 to 1.2). The reviewers concluded that the use of limited asthma education as it has been practised does not appear to improve health outcomes in adults. The usefulness of education in the

ED was encouraging; however, further research is required to confirm these findings.

A second review assessed the effects of adult asthma self-management programmes coupled with regular medical review.[48] Self-management education reduced hospitalizations (OR 0.57; 95% CI 0.38–0.88), ED visits (OR 0.71; 95% CI 0.57–0.90), unscheduled doctor visits (OR 0.57; 95% CI 0.40–0.82), missed work/school days (OR 0.55; 95% CI 0.38–0.79) and nocturnal asthma (OR 0.53; 95% CI 0.39–0.72). Pulmonary function measures, however, changed very little with these combined interventions. If a written action plan was added to this programme, there was an even greater reduction in hospitalization (OR 0.35; 95% CI 0.18–0.68). Patients who could self-adjust their medications using an individualized written plan had better lung function than those whose medications were adjusted by a doctor.

Overall, discussions regarding treatment compliance, follow-up visits with a regular physician and referral to asthma education services (including developing action plans) should be considered on every encounter; as further research in this area is urgently needed, the exact recommendations are necessarily vague.

Question

9. In adult patients with acute asthma seen in the ED (population), what is the role of newer agents such as long-acting β-agonists and leukotriene antagonists (intervention) in reducing admissions or relapses of asthma (outcomes)? {therapy}

Literature search

• Cochrane Library and MEDLINE—acute asthma AND long-acting β-agonists OR LABA
• Cochrane Library and MEDLINE—acute asthma AND leukotriene*

Despite the use of anti-inflammatory agents in acute asthma, admissions to hospital and relapses after discharge occur at an unacceptably high rate. Efforts to reduce these figures have recently focused on the newer agents that have been added to asthma management: long-acting β-agonists (LABA) and leukotriene receptor antagonists (LTRA). These new agents are currently enjoying increased use as *add-on* therapy in chronic asthma. To date, limited research has been conducted in the acute setting, and recommendations are based on those from either chronic management or consensus statements.

Overall, the acute asthma episode indicates that patients are unstable and out of control. Consequently, the use of these *add-on* agents may seem reasonable, especially in the case in which a patient is already receiving inhaled corticosteroids.

The best evidence for the use of LTRA in acute asthma was found in a randomized controlled trial of 201 patients treated with placebo, 7 or 14 mg of intravenous Montelukast.[49] The results suggested a small improvement in FEV_1 over the study period; however, ipratropium bromide and corticosteroids were not administered to all patients. While this research is encouraging, the jury is still out on whether intravenous Montelukast should be added to conventional current treatment. The effect of LTRA in chronic asthma has been summarized in a Cochrane Review, and the authors suggest that these agents have limited benefit compared with inhaled corticosteroids.[50]

The use of LABAs in the acute setting has been even less well examined. Only one randomized controlled trial reported as an abstract could be located in which improvements in quality of life were not observed by *adding* LABAs to systemic and inhaled corticosteroids in patients discharged from the ED.[51] Once again, while this treatment approach is encouraging in the chronic setting, its role in the treatment of acute asthma remains to be determined. As the evidence for and against the use of both LTRA and LABA accumulates, readers of this text are encouraged to search for updates in the Cochrane Library.

Conclusion

The patient mentioned above was treated with systemic corticosteroids, inhaled corticosteroids, education in the ED and close follow-up with her primary care provider. She recovered without incident and was motivated to continue to explore ways to reduce her asthma severity and the frequency of her ED visits. One year later, she was exercising regularly, had lost 12 kg and had avoided asthma exacerbations requiring ED visits.

Asthma is a common, chronic and often debilitating disease. The new treatment approaches to control bronchial inflammation summarized here provide hope for an early return to activities, reduced symptoms and improved quality of life in the subacute period following an exacerbation. Combining self-management skills and educational interventions with appropriate preventive medication provides patients with the best opportunity to maintain this health status and prevent an exacerbation or relapse in the future.

Acknowledgements

The author would like to thank Mrs Diane Milette for her secretarial support. In addition, the author would like to acknowledge the work of the Airway Review Group staff (Mr Stephen Milan and Toby Lasserson and Mrs Karen Blackhall) and the Review Group Editor (Professor Paul Jones: 1995–2003; Dr Christopher Cates: 2003–present) at the St George's Hospital Medical School for their support with the development of reviews.

Conflicts of interest

Dr Rowe is supported by the Canadian Institute of Health Research (CIHR; Ottawa, Canada) as a Canada Research Chair in Emergency Airway Diseases.

References

1 Mannino DM, Homa DM, Pertowski CA *et al.* Surveillance for asthma — United States, 1960–1995. CDC Surveillance Summaries, April 24, 1998. *MMWR* 1998; **47**:1–28.

2 Salmeron S, Liard R, Elkharrat D *et al.* Asthma severity and adequacy of management in accident and emergency departments in France: a prospective study. *Lancet* 2001; **358**:629–35.

3 Weiss KB, Sullivan SD, Lyttle CS. Trends in the cost of illness for asthma in the United States, 1985–1994. *J Allergy Clin Immunol* 2000; **106**:493–9.

4 Weiss KB, Sullivan SD. The health economics of asthma and rhinitis. I. Assessing the economic impact. *J Allergy Clin Immunol* 2001; **107**: 3–8.

5 Krahn MD, Berka C, Langlois P, Detsky AS. Direct and indirect costs of asthma in Canada. *Can Med Assoc J* 1996; **154**:821–31.

6 Boulet L-P, Becker A, Berube D *et al.* Canadian asthma consensus report, 1999. *Can Med Assoc J* 1999; **161**:S1–S61.

7 National Asthma Education Program. *Expert Panel Report II: Guidelines for the Diagnosis and Management of Asthma.* Bethesda, MD, National Institutes of Health, 1997.

8 British Thoracic Society, Scottish Intercollegiate Guidelines Network. British guideline on the management of asthma. *Thorax* 2003; **58**:1–94.

9 Jadad AR, Moher M, Browman GP *et al.* Systematic reviews and meta-analyses on treatment of asthma: critical evaluation. *BMJ* 2000; **320**:537–40.

10 Worthington JR, Ahuja J. The value of pulmonary function tests in the management of acute asthma. *Can Med Assoc J* 1989; **140**:153–6.

11 Rodrigo G, Rodrigo C. Early prediction of poor response in acute asthma patients in the emergency department. *Chest* 1998; **114**:1016–21.

12 Keahey L, Bulloch B, Becker AB *et al.* Initial oxygen saturation as a predictor of admission in children presenting to the emergency department with acute asthma. *Ann Emerg Med* 2002; **40**:300–7.

13 Beveridge B, Rowe BH. What is new since the last (1999) Canadian Asthma Consensus Guidelines? *Can Respir J* 2001; **8**:5A–27A.

14 Emerman CL, Woodruff PG, Cydulka RK *et al.* Prospective multicenter study of relapse following treatment for acute asthma among adults presenting to the emergency department. *Chest* 1999; **115**:919–27.

15 Cates CCJ, Bara A, Crilly JA, Rowe BH. Holding chambers versus nebulisers for β-agonist treatment of acute asthma (Cochrane Review). In: *The Cochrane Library,* Issue 4. Oxford, Update Software, 2003.

16 Turner MO, Gafni A, Swan D, Fitzgerald JM. A review and economic evaluation of bronchodilator delivery methods in hospitalized patients. *Arch Intern Med* 1996; **156**:2113–18.

17 Camargo CA Jr, Spooner CH, Rowe BH. Continuous versus intermittent β-agonists in the treatment of acute asthma (Cochrane Review). In: *The Cochrane Library,* Issue 4. Oxford, Update Software, 2003.

18 Emerman CL, Cydulka RK, McFadden ER. Comparison of 2.5 vs 7.5 mg of inhaled albuterol in the treatment of acute asthma. *Chest* 1999; **115**:92–6.

19 Stauss L, Hejal R, Galan G *et al.* Observations on the effects of aerosolized albuterol in acute asthma. *Am J Resp Crit Care* 1997; **155**:454–8.

20 Grunfeld A, Beveridge RC, Berkowitz J, Fitzgerald JM. Management of acute asthma in Canada: an assessment of emergency physician behavior. *J Emerg Med* 1997; 15:547–56.

21 Weber EJ, Silverman RA, Callaham ML *et al*. A prospective multi-center study of factors associated with hospital admission among adults with acute asthma. *Am J Med* 2002; **113**:371–8.

22 Varia M, Wilson S, Sarwal S *et al*. Investigation of a nosocomial outbreak of severe acute respiratory syndrome (SARS) in Toronto, Canada. *Can Med Assoc J* 2003; **169**:285–92.

23 Plotnick LH, Ducharme FM. Efficacy and safety of combined inhaled anticholinergics and β-2-agonists in the initial management of acute pediatric asthma (Cochrane Review). In: *The Cochrane Library*, Issue 4. Oxford, Update Software, 2003.

24 Stoodley RG, Aaron SD, Dales RE. The role of ipratropium bromide in the emergency management of acute asthma exacerbation: a meta-analysis of randomized clinical trials. *Ann Emerg Med* 1999; **34**:8–18.

25 Qureshi F, Pestian J, Davis P, Zaritsky A. Effect of nebulized ipratropium on the hospitalization rates of children with asthma. *N Engl J Med* 1998; **339**:1030–5.

26 Rodrigo GJ, Rodrigo C. First-line therapy for adult patients with acute asthma receiving a multiple-dose protocol of ipratropium bromide plus albuterol in the emergency department. *Am J Respir Crit Care Med* 2000; **161**:1862–8.

27 Rowe BH, Spooner C, Ducharme FM, Bretzlaff JA, Bota GW. Early emergency department treatment of acute asthma with systemic corticosteroids (Cochrane Review). In: *The Cochrane Library*, Issue 4. Oxford, Update Software, 2003.

28 Manser R, Reid D, Abramson M. Corticosteroids for acute severe asthma in hospitalised patients (Cochrane Review). In: *The Cochrane Library*, Issue 4. Oxford, Update Software, 2003.

29 Rowe BH, Bretzlaff JA, Bourdon C *et al*. Intravenous magnesium sulfate treatment for acute asthma in the emergency department (Cochrane Review). In: *The Cochrane Library*, Issue 4. Oxford, Update Software, 2003.

30 Alter HJ, Koepsell TD, Hilty WM. Intravenous magnesium as an adjunct in acute bronchospasm: a meta-analysis. *Ann Emerg Med* 2000; **36**:191–7.

31 Emerman CL, Woodruff PG, Cydulka RK *et al*. Prospective multicenter study of relapse following treatment for acute asthma among adults presenting to the emergency department. *Chest* 1999; **115**: 919–27.

32 Rowe BH, Spooner CH, Ducharme FM, Bretzlaff JA, Bota GW. Corticosteroids for preventing relapses following acute exacerbations of asthma (Cochrane Review). In: *The Cochrane Library*, Issue 4. Oxford, Update Software, 2003.

33 Laupacis A, Sackett DL, Roberts RS. An assessment of clinically useful measures of the consequences of treatment. *N Engl J Med* 1988; **318**:1728–33.

34 Verbeek PR, Gerts WH. Nontapering versus tapering prednisone in acute exacerbations of asthma: a pilot study. *J Emerg Med* 1995; **13**:715–19.

35 O'Driscoll BR, Karla S, Wilson M *et al*. Double-blind trial of steroid tapering in acute asthma. *Lancet* 1993; **341**:324–7.

36 Rowe BH, Bota GW, Fabris L *et al*. Inhaled budesonide in addition to oral corticosteroids to prevent relapse following discharge from the emergency department: a randomized controlled trial. *JAMA* 1999; **281**:2119–26.

37 Rowe BH, Bota GW, Pollack CV *et al*. Management of acute asthma among adults presenting to Canadian versus US emergency departments. *Ann Emerg Med* 1998; **32**:S2–S3.

38 Brenner BE, Chavda KK, Camargo CA Jr. Randomized trial of inhaled flunisolide versus placebo among asthmatics discharged from the emergency department. *Ann Emerg Med* 2000; **36**:417–26.

39 Camargo CA Jr for the MARC Investigators. Randomized trial of medium-dose fluticasone vs placebo after an emergency department visit for acute asthma. *J Allergy Clin Immunol* 2000; **105**:S262.

40 Edmonds ML, Camargo CA Jr, Brenner B, Rowe BH. Inhaled steroids in acute asthma following emergency department discharge (Cochrane Review). In: *The Cochrane Library*, Issue 4. Oxford, Update Software, 2003.

41 Sin DD, Man SFP. Low-dose inhaled corticosteroid therapy and risk of emergency department visits for asthma. *Arch Intern Med* 2002; **162**:1591–5.

42 Haynes RB, McDonald H, Garg AX, Montague P. Interventions for helping patients to follow prescriptions for medications (Cochrane Review). In: *The Cochrane Library*, Issue 4. Oxford, Update Software, 2003.

43 Emond SD, Reed CR, Graff LG *et al*. Asthma education in the emergency department. *Ann Emerg Med* 2000; **36**:204–11.

44 Emond SD, Camargo CA Jr, Nowak RM. 1997 national asthma education and prevention program guidelines: a practical summary for emergency physicians. *Ann Emerg Med* 1998; **31**:579–89.

45 Rowe BH, Edmonds ML. Inhaled corticosteroids for acute asthma after emergency department discharge. *Ann Emerg Med* 2000; **36**: 477–80.

46 Clark NM, Gotsch A, Rosenstock IR. Patient, professional and public education on behavioral aspects of asthma: a review of strategies for change and needed research. *J Asthma* 1993; **30**:241–55.

47 Gibson PM, Coughlan J, Wilson AJ *et al*. Limited (information only) patient education for adults with asthma (Cochrane Review). In: *The Cochrane Library*, Issue 4. Oxford, Update Software, 2003.

48 Gibson PM, Coughlan J, Wilson AJ *et al*. Self-management education and regular practitioner review for adults with asthma (Cochrane Review). In: *The Cochrane Library*, Issue 4. Oxford, Update Software, 2003.

49 Camargo CA Jr, Smithline HA, Malice MP, Green SA, Reiss TF. A randomized controlled trial of intravenous Montelukast in acute asthma. *Am J Respir Crit Care Med* 2003; **167**:528–33.

50 Ducharme FM, Hicks GC. Anti-leukotriene agents compared to inhaled corticosteroids in the management of recurrent and/or chronic asthma (Cochrane Review). In: *The Cochrane Library*, Issue 4. Oxford, Update Software, 2003.

51 Rowe BH, Travers A, Brown JB *et al*. Long-acting β-agonists following ED discharge: a randomized controlled trial. *Acad Emerg Med* 2001; **8**:531.

Chronic therapy: β-agonists, short-acting, long-acting β$_2$-agonists

Haydn Walters and Julia Walters

Introduction

β-Agonists are the most commonly used form of bronchodilator prescribed in the treatment of asthma. They have been available both orally and by inhalation but, because of the poor therapeutic ratio (good to bad effects) of the former, only the latter is recommended for conventional use.

β-Agonists used in asthma have their effects mainly through engagement of airway smooth muscle cell surface β-receptors. Through conformational changes in the receptor complex, an associated intracellular enzyme, adenylate cyclase, is activated to convert cytoplasmic adenosine triphosphate (ATP) to 3′ 5′ cyclic adenosine monophosphate (AMP). This acts as a second messenger to induce strategic cellular changes including inhibition of calcium mobilization and inhibition of actin–myosin molecular interactions, which are the basis of smooth muscle contraction. In allergic asthma, similar mechanisms are also operative at the level of mast cells, 'stabilizing' them to be less responsive to immunoglobulin E (IgE) cross-linking with environmental allergens.

The central mechanism of action and rationale for the use of β-agonists in asthma has been airway smooth muscle relaxation and secondary airway dilatation. More recently, however, there has been focus on potential anti-inflammatory and anti-airway remodelling effects of β-agonists in asthma,[1] especially when used regularly and chronically. The non-bronchodilator actions of β-agonists may result from direct effects upon non-muscle airway inflammatory or structural cells that have cell surface β-receptors, such as mast cells or epithelial cells. Alternatively, these may be secondary to a recognized potentiation of the anti-inflammatory effects of corticosteroids.[2] One suggestion for this enhanced steroid effect is increased rate of movement of steroid–steroid receptor complexes from the cytoplasmic compartment into the nucleus where they modify gene transcription.

Class definitions; clinical and historical issues

β-Agonists as therapeutic agents were derived from understanding of the sympathetic nervous system and especially the characteristic of adrenaline as having both α- and β-adrenoreceptor activity. Isoprenaline was designed to enhance the β-effects of adrenaline and was introduced in the 1960s as the first short-acting bronchodilator 'sympathomimetic' inhaler. However, isoprenaline had both β$_1$ effects, i.e. it caused cardiac inotropic and chronotropic stimulation, as well as β$_2$ effects, i.e. bronchodilatation. The epidemic of asthma deaths in Europe in the 1960s was blamed on the potential for isoprenaline to induce cardiac dysrhythmias. Whether this was actually the cause or not has never been definitely proved and is now mainly of historic interest only, because subsequently safer and relatively β$_2$-selective agents were introduced, such as salbutamol and terbutaline.

These drugs became established as the mainstay of β-agonist therapy for asthma during the 1970s and 1980s and have been highly successful. Because of their pharmacodynamic characteristics of rapid onset of action within a minute or so of inhalation, they were ideal as treatment for the acute relief of symptoms. However, their maximal effect would last only 30–60 min, with decline back to baseline in airway calibre over 2–4 hours. For sustained bronchodilator effects, repeated doses would be required every 2–4 hours, or even more frequently during acute attacks or exacerbations of asthma.

In the early 1990s, there were a number of epidemiological, clinical and laboratory-based studies to address worries that regular and frequent use of even β$_2$-selective agents, especially if used in high doses (e.g. via a nebulizer), might have detrimental effects in asthma. Indeed, epidemiological studies in both New Zealand and Canada did suggest that there was a potential for excess mortality related to short-acting β$_2$-agonist use.[3,4] Whether this phenomenon was due to death directly from poorly managed asthma, especially with inadequate use of anti-inflammatory medication with oral or inhaled corticosteroid, or whether there was a direct toxic effect from high blood concentrations of β-agonist drugs,[5] or a combination of these circumstances, is still controversial.

At much the same time, there was a highly publicized clinical study from New Zealand,[6] suggesting that regular use of fenoterol (a relatively non-β$_2$-selective short-acting agent) could lead to poorer control of asthma than if the same agent was used only as needed for relief of symptoms. This study had some unusual features in terms of a somewhat arbitrary set of criteria for evaluation of asthma control, but was backed up by a number of laboratory studies indicating that short-acting β_2-agonists if given regularly had potential for tachyphylaxis to their bronchodilator effects;[7] tachyphylaxis to their bronchoprotective effects against induced bronchoconstriction, both direct (muscle stimulation) and indirect (mast cell degranulation),[8] and could potentially enhance the underlying airway responsiveness to bronchoconstrictor agents.[9]

These studies gave rise to a major debate in the literature, with a host of narrative review and editorial articles, discussing the clinical relevance of these findings with short-acting β_2-bronchodilators. Although perhaps inevitably inconclusive, they did heavily influence the recommended use of β_2-agonists in subsequent clinical practice guidelines.

It was at the height of this 'β-agonist debate' that the newly designed long-acting β-agonists were introduced in the early to mid-1990s. The adverse environment and sentiment against the use of β_2-agonists at the time had some undoubted effect upon their reception by clinicians, and their subsequent clinical research development and placement in management guidelines. These agents are specifically designed for regular use, as they have a 12-hour duration of action and have been termed 'symptom controllers'. In contrast, inhaled corticosteroids (ICS) and other drugs designed to modify disease process have generally been designated as 'preventers', in the sense of changing the pattern of disease and decreasing the frequency of acute symptoms and both minor and major exacerbations of asthma.

Of the two long-acting β_2-agonists widely available, eformoterol is classified pharmacodynamically as a 'full agonist' with potential for a greater bronchodilator efficacy at high dose through full receptor occupancy, but with increased likelihood of tachyphylaxis development. Salmeterol, on the other hand, is a partial agonist, with a relatively slower onset of action, a less total bronchodilator capacity at high dose, due to less complete receptor engagement but, as a result, a lesser tendency to tachyphylaxis to its bronchodilator action. Although these differences have been emphasized to varying extents in competing commercial marketing strategies, it is unknown to what, if any, extent they matter clinically.

While these long-acting agents have been marketed predominantly for 'control' of symptoms, they have also been shown to have significant anti-inflammatory and anti-remodelling actions when used regularly in studies directly sampling the airways,[1,10,11] at least when used in combination with ICS, and to decrease the rate and severity of asthma exacerbations.[12] Good long-term studies are required on whether such effects of combinations have advantages in terms of the natural history of asthma and long-term airway damage to the airways in terms of development of fixed airflow obstruction.

Current guidelines: the nominated place of β_2-agonists

There are many national and supranational respiratory society guidelines for the management of asthma, but we have chosen to focus on just two as being especially prominent and established: the National Institutes of Health (NIH)-sponsored GINA guidelines and the British Thoracic Society (BTS) guidelines.

The GINA guidelines[13] classify asthma into four severity grades 'before treatment' on the basis of specific clinical features, lung function and, to some extent (in a rather circular way, i.e. treatment defining severity), by need for rapidly acting β_2-agonist relief medication, as follows:

Intermittent
Symptoms less than once a week
Brief exacerbations
Nocturnal symptoms not more than twice a month
- forced expiratory volume in 1 s (FEV_1) or peak expiratory flow (PEF) $\geq 80\%$ predicted
- FEV_1 or PEF variability $< 20\%$

Mild persistent
Symptoms more than once a week but less than once a day
Exacerbations may affect activity and sleep
Nocturnal symptoms more than twice a month
- FEV_1 or PEF $\geq 80\%$ predicted
- FEV_1 or PEF variability 20–30%

Moderate persistent
Symptoms daily
Exacerbations may affect activity and sleep
Nocturnal symptoms more than once a week
Daily use of inhaled short-acting β_2-agonist
- FEV_1 or PEF 60–80% predicted
- FEV_1 or PEF variability $> 30\%$

Severe persistent
Symptoms daily
Frequent exacerbations
Frequent nocturnal asthma symptoms
Limitation of physical activities
- FEV_1 or PEF $\leq 60\%$ predicted
- FEV_1 or PEF variability $> 30\%$

For intermittent asthma, a rapidly acting inhaled β_2-agonist 'may be' taken as needed to relieve asthma symptoms. Although not stated, this would presumably be in the form of short-acting agents usually, although eformoterol could potentially fall within the scope of this guideline.

For mild persistent asthma, some form of 'controller' medication is indicated, with an inhaled glucocorticosteroid preferred (sustained-release theophyllines, cromones and leukotriene modifiers are listed as alternatives). [Note, we consider the nomenclature for controller versus preventer in GINA to be rather confused.]

Long-acting β_2-agonists, given twice daily, are recommended to be introduced for the treatment of moderate persistent asthma in combination with inhaled glucocorticosteroid.

For severe persistent asthma, the therapy of choice is given as a higher dose of inhaled steroid together with long-acting inhaled β_2-agonist. Of note, oral β_2-agonists are given as an alternative or addition to the inhaled long-acting β_2-agonists, as are oral sustained-release theophylline and anti-leukotriene agents.

Thus, short-acting β_2-agonists, long-acting β_2-agonists and, to a lesser extent, oral β_2-agonists feature in GINA as asthma severity escalates.

The BTS Guidelines[14] are somewhat different and based upon five steps, each one related to a severity grade of asthma from Step 1: mild intermittent, in which short-acting β_2-agonists are used alone for symptom relief, to Step 5: (need for) continuous or frequent use of oral steroids. The clinical correlates for each step are considerably less precise than in the GINA Guidelines and are based upon treatment needs to a large extent. Inhaled steroids are recommended in Step 2 for patients with recent exacerbation, nocturnal asthma, 'impaired' lung function or using short-acting β_2-agonists more than once a day. Of note, long-acting inhaled β_2-agonists are offered at this point as a potential, though less effective, choice instead of inhaled corticosteroid, as are theophyllines, cromones, leukotriene modifiers, antihistamines and ketotifen.

Step 3: add-on therapy (in addition to ICS at 400 μg/day for adults and 200 μg/day for children). The first choice for add-on therapy is a long-acting β_2-agonist (in adults and children over 4 years). If symptoms are still inadequately controlled in spite of this combination, then the dose of ICS can be doubled and, if that does not work, oral slow-release β_2-agonist tablets (in adults only) should be considered, as might a sequential trial of other add-ons, namely leukotriene receptor antagonist and theophylline.

Step 4: poor control on moderate doses of inhaled steroid plus add-on therapy: addition of fourth drug. The options given are increasing the dose of ICS to 2000 μg/day for adults and 800 μg/day for children, oral leukotriene receptor antagonist, theophylline or slow-release β_2-agonist tablets (although it is emphasized that caution is needed in patients already on an inhaled long-acting β_2-agonist).

Thus, the BTS guidelines have some (marked) differences from GINA: long-acting β_2-agonist can be added as a 'regular preventer' at Step 2 as an alternative to ICS; oral β_2-agonist can be given at Step 2; and in Step 4, the oral β_2-agonist can be added as fourth drug even where an inhaled long-acting β_2-agonist is already being used.

Overall, however, with the two sets of guidelines, the sequence of drug use depending on disease severity is similar: as needed short-acting β_2-agonist inhaler; regular inhaled corticosteroids; addition of long-acting β_2-agonist in combination with ICS; and, if that is not sufficient even when the ICS component is increased to a high dose (up to 2000 μg/day), then various add-ons can be tried including an oral slow-release β_2-agonist.

Case scenarios

Question/problem

Although the available guidelines fairly unanimously recommend the use of short-acting β_2-agonist as relief medication only, are there circumstances in clinical practice where regular short-acting β_2-agonist would be a reasonable option? Would such an approach lead to general deterioration in asthma control?

Scenario 1

A 23-year-old student, who is fit but has had mild asthma for most of the last 15 years, which worsens with coryza. He usually only wheezes with exercise but does quite a lot of that, especially in the football season, e.g. he jogs each morning and trains with a team or plays several times per week. He frequently has to run between lectures. Should he be advised to use his metered dose inhaler [short-acting β_2-agonist (SABA), salbutamol] for relief in response to symptoms or regularly two or three times daily prophylactically to prevent his wheeze coming on? He is very reluctant to use ICS and, given his exercise-only symptoms, good pre-bronchodilator lung function with little bronchodilator reversibility on testing (because of good baseline spirometry), on GINA guidelines, he probably does not warrant ICS. On BTS guidelines, it would be worth considering ICS use on the basis of his daily use of SABA.

The evidence base for problem 1

We have published a systematic review[15] providing Level 1 evidence relevant to this question. It includes all available randomized control trials to define the relative merits of regular versus as-needed use of short-acting β_2-agonists. Studies compared regular use of inhaled short-acting β_2-agonist with matching placebo inhaled regularly while both groups also used an inhaled short-acting β_2-agonist as needed for relief of symptoms (rescue use). A subgroup of the review included studies in which both the experimental group and the placebo control group used an anticholinergic agent for rescue use.

Searches for relevant randomized control trials were carried out of the Cochrane Airways Group 'Asthma and Wheez* RCT' register in 1997, 1999 and 2002. Pharmaceutical companies and researchers with an interest in the area were asked for details of any studies that they knew of. Criteria for inclusion of a study were that participants, adults or children, had stable asthma for at least 6 months, diagnosed according to American Thoracic Society or another accepted standard, with documented evidence of reversibility to an inhaled short-acting β_2-agonist. Details of baseline severity of asthma and co-interventions being used by participants were recorded for subgroup analyses (see Table 1).

Table 1. Description of studies included in Cochrane Reviews of long-acting β-agonist treatment.

Features of studies in Cochrane Reviews of regular inhaled β_2-agonist use		Short-acting β_2-agonist versus placebo (as needed rescue)	Long-acting β_2-agonist versus short acting β-agonist	Long-acting β_2-agonist versus placebo	Long-acting β_2-agonist versus theophylline
No. of studies	Included	44	31	85	6
	Excluded	38	154	110	18
	Data used	28	28	74	6
Quality grading	Cochrane A	9	5	15	0
	Cochrane B	35	26	70	6
	Cochrane C	0	0	0	0
Study design	Parallel group	19	23	56	2
	Crossover	25	7	29	4
Age of participants (years)	12–80	41	28	71	6
	<12	3	3	14	0
Treatment period (weeks)	<6	24	8	32	5
	6–12	13	20	37	1
	>12–52	7	3	14	0
Baseline asthma severity	Mild	14	2	12	0
	Mild–moderate	19	23	51	6
	Moderate–severe	2	3	11	0
	Not classified	9	3	11	0
Co-interventions	No ICS	17	1	21	1
	All using ICS	11	6	34	0
	Mixed variety	21	24	35	5
Rescue agent	Inhaled short-acting β-agonist	28	29	71	6
	Inhaled anticholinergic	14	2	12	0

Cochrane grades: Grade A, adequate concealment; Grade B, unclear concealment; Grade C, obviously not adequate concealment. ICS, inhaled corticosteroids.

Forty-four studies meeting the inclusion criteria were included in the updated review in 2002, with 38 studies being excluded. Data were extracted, quality assessments were made, and parallel group and crossover trials were analysed separately.

No clinically or statistically significant differences were found in airway calibre measurements (Figs 1 and 2). The regular active treatment groups had fewer days with asthma symptoms, weighted mean difference (WMD) −6.7% (95% CI −2.7 to −10.7) (Fig. 3), but small advantages in asthma symptom scores were not statistically significant, either during the day or at night (Fig. 4). The regular active treatment group required less rescue medication, WMD −0.80 puffs/24 h (95% CI −0.07 to −1.30) and WMD −0.42 puffs/daytime (95% CI −0.12 to −0.72) (Fig. 5) but, not surprisingly, took more inhaled short-acting β-agonist overall.

There was no significant difference in the odds ratio for the occurrence of at least one major asthma exacerbation during treatment, in either parallel group or crossover studies (Fig. 6).

Airway reactivity was assessed as an indicator of potentially detrimental effects on the underlying disease process of regular treatment. There was a small increase in 'direct' airway reactivity found, of the order of 0.5 doubling doses (95% CI 0.1–0.8). There was some tachyphylaxis to the bronchopro-

tective effect of short-acting β2-agonist on direct airway reactivity, indicated by a significantly greater decrease in protection in the regular treatment group, of about one doubling dose magnitude. However, there remained clinically significant protection even after chronic regular use of short-acting agents. Bronchodilator responsiveness also appeared to show a small degree of tachyphylaxis with regular use. The regular group also showed a higher incidence of tremor, but the risk for other pharmacologically predictable effects was not greater.

Conclusion

If there are circumstances in which regular inhaled short-acting β2-agonist use would be convenient, reasonable and favoured by the patient, then there is no strong case against doing so and no consistent evidence for significant negative effects. There should be regular review and monitoring, however, to ensure that the circumstances of the patient do not change.

Two further clinical questions/problems are presented together, with an accompanying scenario for each, as the evidence base for each has a great deal of overlap.

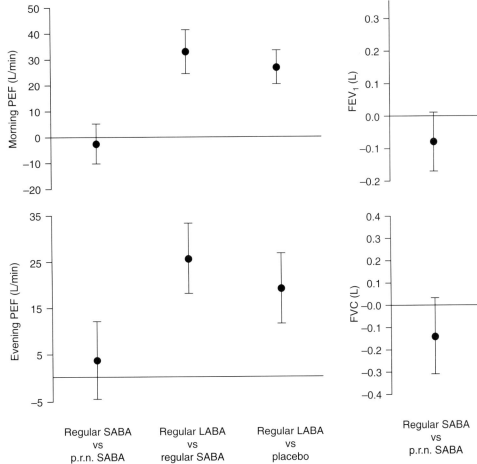

Figure 1. Mean difference in morning and evening PEF between treatments (WMD 95% CI).

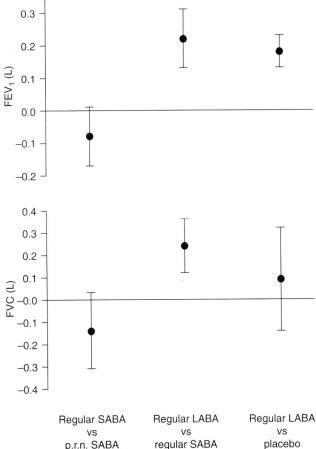

Figure 2. Mean difference in lung function between treatments (WMD, 95% CI).

Question/problem

The guidelines usually propose that, if symptoms require more than occasional use of inhaled short-acting β$_2$-agonist on an as-needed basis, patients should be prescribed ICS use before the introduction of a long-acting inhaled β$_2$-agonist. Are there circumstance in which it would be reasonable to use long-acting inhaled β$_2$-agonists before ICS for long-lasting prophylaxis against induced bronchospasm? Would such management have positive or negative effects in terms of overall asthma control?

Scenario 2

The same individual as in scenario 1, but he tends to forget to use his inhaler at midday and tends to wheeze with training in the afternoon. He has heard that there is now a long-acting form of the medication. Could he change to this long-acting inhaled β$_2$-agonist (LABA) safely and effectively, in spite of not being on ICS?

Question/problem

The guidelines generally agree that long-acting β$_2$-agonists should be introduced for symptom control when this is not adequate on moderate doses of ICS, rather than maximize the dose of ICS. However, what other add-on therapies should be considered?

Scenario 3

A 40-year-old female with asthma for 10 years. In spite of current ICS treatment (fluticasone proprionate 500 µg/day), she needs relief medication three or four times daily, mainly for exercise-induced symptoms on walking briskly and sometimes on exposure to cold air or irritants. She wakes at nights about once a week in cold weather. She is reluctant to increase the ICS dose due to previous experience with dysphonia. She wants advice on whether she should use β$_2$-agonist more regularly and, if so, what is available and what other alternative treatment there is in her case.

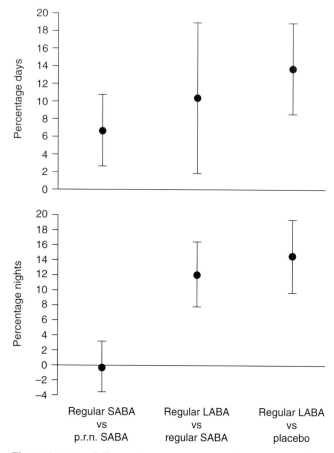

Figure 3. Mean difference between treatments in percentage of days and nights not affected by asthma (WMD, 95% CI).

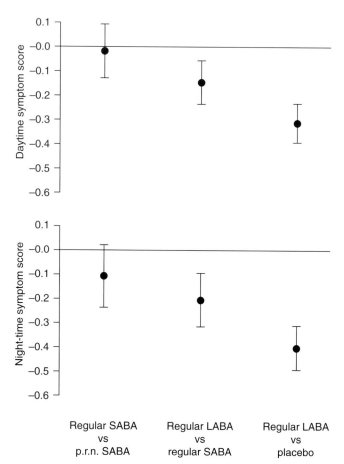

Figure 4. Mean difference in asthma symptom scores by day and night between treatments (SMD, 95% CI).

The evidence base for problems 2 and 3

Systematic reviews provide high-quality Level 1 evidence to assess the effects of inhaled long-acting β₂-agonists. Three relevant reviews are published in the Cochrane Library:

1 Inhaled long-acting β-agonists for stable chronic asthma.[16]

2 Regular treatment with long-acting β-agonists versus daily regular treatment with short-acting β-agonists in adults and children with stable asthma.[17]

3 Long-acting β-agonists versus theophylline for maintenance treatment of asthma.[18]

There are also three published structured abstracts of non-Cochrane Reviews, produced by Cochrane Reviewers on original publications that meet a set of quality criteria:

1 Long-acting β₂-agonists in the management of childhood asthma: a critical review of the literature.[19]

2 Meta-analysis of increased dose of inhaled steroid or addition of salmeterol in symptomatic asthma (MIASMA).[20]

3 The efficacy and safety of salmeterol compared with theophylline: meta-analysis of nine controlled studies.[21]

Further, a search of the database of the National Library of Medicine at PubMed for meta-analyses of long-acting β₂-agonists produced three more potentially relevant results:

1 Airway-stabilizing effect of long-acting β₂-agonists as add-on therapy to inhaled corticosteroids.[22]

2 Fluticasone versus salmeterol/low-dose fluticasone combination for long-term asthma control.[23]

3 Combined budesonide/formoterol turbuhaler treatment of asthma.[24]

Description of Cochrane Reviews

Inhaled long-acting β-agonists for stable chronic asthma

The objective of the review was to compare the effects of regular inhaled long-acting β₂-agonists versus placebo in chronic asthma.

Methods: searches of the Cochrane Airways Group trials register were carried out for all randomized studies of at least 2 weeks' duration, comparing a long-acting inhaled β-agonist given twice daily with a placebo, in chronic asthma, most recently in October 2002. Bibliographies of identified randomized controlled trials were searched and authors of identified trials contacted for other published and unpublished studies.

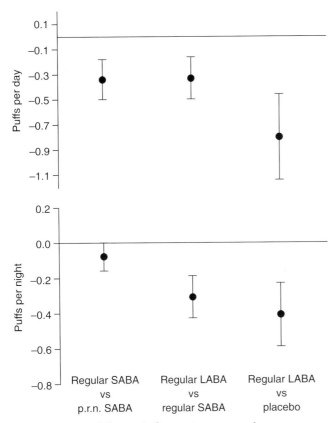

Figure 5. Mean difference in β_2-agonist rescue use between treatments (WMD, 95% CI).

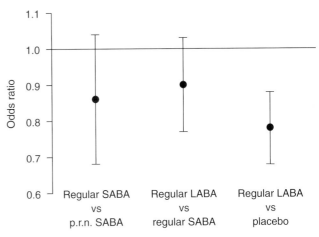

Figure 6. Odds ratio for risk of at least one major asthma exacerbation during treatment (OR, 95% CI).

Results: 85 studies recruiting 15 940 participants met the inclusion criteria, 56 parallel group and 29 crossover design, and 110 studies were excluded. Participants had a clinical diagnosis of asthma present for at least 3 months, and the nature of co-interventions for asthma was recorded. Seventy-one studies involved adult or adolescent participants, and 14 studies involved children aged less than 12 years. Salmeterol xinafoate was used as long-acting agent in 60 studies and formoterol fumarate in 25. The treatment period was 2–4 weeks in 32 studies and 12–52 weeks in 53 studies. Thirty-four studies used concurrent inhaled corticosteroid treatment, 21 studies did not permit their use, and 35 permitted either inhaled corticosteroid or cromones (see Table 1). Data were available and extracted from 74 studies and analysed separately for parallel group and crossover studies.

There were significant advantages to long-acting β_2-agonist treatment compared with placebo for a variety of measurements of airway calibre including morning PEF, WMD 26.8 L/min (95% CI 20.4–33.2), evening PEF WMD 19.2 L/min (95% CI 11.6–26.7) and FEV$_1$ WMD 0.18 L (95% CI 0.13–0.23) (Figs 1 and 2).

Long-acting β_2-agonists were associated with significantly fewer symptoms, in the daytime, standardized mean difference (SMD) –0.32 (95% CI –0.25 to –0.40), and at night, SMD –0.41 (95% CI –0.32 to –0.49) (Fig. 4), less use of rescue medication in the day, WMD –0.80 puffs/day (95% CI –0.46 to –1.14), and at night, WMD –0.41 puffs/night (95% CI –0.23 to –0.60) (Fig. 5). There were also significantly fewer days affected by asthma (Fig. 3) and higher quality of life scores as measured by an asthma-specific instrument. The WMD for the improvement in global score during treatment was 0.59 (95% CI 0.49–0.69). Results for improvements in the separate domains were: activity limitations WMD 0.41 (95% CI 0.31–0.50), symptoms WMD 0.68 (95% CI 0.56–0.80), emotional function WMD 0.62 (95% CI 0.47–0.77) and exposure to environmental stimuli WMD 0.52 (95% CI 0.39–0.65). The odds ratio for participants on LABA treatment assessing it as effective or very effective was OR 3.17 (95% CI 2.27–4.42).

In assessing possible detrimental effects, it was found that there was a lower risk of an exacerbation of asthma when on LABA, OR 0.78 (95% CI 0.69–0.88) when all studies were combined (Fig. 6), but subgroup analyses showed that this was significant only in adults using ICS, OR 0.76 (95% CI 0.62–0.93). Studies on children reported data on exacerbations, and the pooled analysis actually suggested an increased risk of exacerbations, OR 1.20 (95% CI 0.92–1.55), although the result was not statistically significant.

There was a significantly higher risk of headache occurring as an adverse event with active therapy, OR 1.35 (95% CI 1.01–1.81).

There was no evidence of an increase relative to baseline in airway reactivity in the long-acting β_2-agonist group. In fact, there was a greater increase in PD/PC 20, i.e. a larger fall in airway reactivity in the long-acting β_2-agonist group, relative to baseline during treatment, with a WMD of 0.48 doubling doses (DD) methacholine (95% CI 0.25–0.71). The high degree of protection against bronchoconstriction to directly acting agents after initial doses of long-acting β_2-agonist falls after regular use, but there remains a significant degree of bronchoprotection compared with placebo, WMD 1.83 DD methacholine (95% CI 0.99–2.67).

Regular treatment with long-acting β_2-agonists continued to give protection against exercise-induced bronchoconstriction. There was a significantly smaller fall in FEV_1 (measured in litres or as a percentage) with exercise in a standard exercise test, performed 6–12 hours after study drug dosing, SMD –0.61 (95% CI –1.15 to –0.07) in two studies in which most participants used ICS.

Results in those not using inhaled corticosteroids

In assessing the specific evidence pertinent to the question posed by scenario 2, examination of the subgroups analyses in the review does not provide evidence for the effectiveness of inhaled long-acting β_2-agonists in those not using ICS on airway calibre, symptoms or need for additional rescue short-acting β_2-agonist. However, the number of studies in which participants were not permitted to use ICS was small and consequently results were generally not significant or showed wide confidence intervals (Table 2).

While the reduction in exacerbations was confirmed in those using ICS in the active treatment group, OR 0.76 (95% CI 0.62–0.93), in four studies with 1020 participants not using ICS, the reduction was only of borderline significance, OR 0.72 (95% CI 0.52–1.00).

Regular treatment with long-acting β-agonists versus daily regular treatment with short-acting β-agonists in adults and children with stable asthma

The objective was to address the comparative benefit or detriment of treatment in chronic asthma with regular long-acting inhaled β_2-agonists versus regular short-acting inhaled β_2-agonists.

Methods: searches using the Cochrane Airways Group 'Asthma and Wheez' trial register were carried out (most recently in 2001) for randomized control trials (RCT) of at least 2 weeks' duration, comparing a long-acting inhaled β-agonist given twice daily with any short-acting inhaled β-agonist given regularly in chronic asthma. Inclusion criteria stated that participants needed a clinical diagnosis of asthma present for at least 6 months with documented reversibility to inhaled short-acting inhaled β-agonist. Bibliographies of identified RCTs were searched and authors contacted for other published and unpublished studies.

Results: 31 studies met the inclusion criteria, 24 of parallel group and seven of crossover design. One hundred and fifty-four studies were excluded (Table 1). The majority of studies were in mild to moderate asthmatics, and all participants were permitted to use co-interventions, usually inhaled corticosteroids (30/31). In only one study on children with mild asthma were all participants not on any inhaled corticosteroids. The majority of studies (28/31) were of 12 weeks' duration or less.

Long-acting β_2-agonists were significantly better than short-acting ones for a variety of lung function measurements including morning PEF, WMD 32.9 L/min (95% CI 24.8–41.5), or evening PEF, WMD 25.6 L/min (95% CI 18.0–33.3) (Fig. 1), FEV_1, WMD 0.22 L (95% CI 0.14–0.31), and forced vital capacity (FVC), WMD 0.24 L (95% CI 0.13–0.36) (Fig. 2). Long-acting β_2-agonist treatment gave significantly lower day and night-time asthma symptom

Table 2. Inhaled long-acting β-agonists for stable chronic asthma: results for subgroup analyses by inhaled corticosteroid (ICS) use.

Outcome (95% CI)	All on ICS WMD (95% CI)	None using ICS WMD
Morning PEF (L/min)	33.4 (21.3–45.4) $n=1151$	49.1 (6.2–91.95) $n=88$
Evening PEF (L/min)	29.1 (14.8–43.3) $n=942$	15.6 (–30.7 to 61.9) $n=66$
FEV_1 (L)	0.22 (0.13–0.3) $n=1392$	0.12 (–0.25 to 0.49) $n=70$
Day asthma symptom score	*–0.3 (–0.4 to –0.1) $n=998$	*–0.4 (–0.9 to 0.1) $n=79$
Night asthma symptom score	*–0.3 (–0.6 to –0.1) $n=992$	*–0.6 (–0.9 to –0.4) $n=66$
Increase in % days without asthma symptoms	18.1 (11.7–24.5) $n=1057$	12.7 (8.6–16.8) $n=789$
Increase in % nights without asthma symptoms	8.3 (1.2–15.3) $n=1047$	8.1 (4.5–11.3) $n=789$
Use of daytime rescue SABA (puffs/day)	–0.5 (–0.8 to –0.2) $n=1122$	–0.6 (–1.7 to 0.5) $n=23$
Use of night-time rescue SABA (puffs/day)	–0.3 (–0.4 to –0.1) $n=1122$	0.1 (–1.3 to 1.6) $n=23$
Risk of a major exacerbation of asthma	†0.76 (0.62–0.93) $n=1165$	†0.72 (0.52–1.00) $n=1020$

*SMD (95% CI).

†Odds ratio (95% CI).

PEF, peak expiratory flow; FEV_1, forced expiratory volume in 1 second; WMD, weighted mean difference; SABA, short-acting β-agonist.

scores and percentage of days and nights without symptoms (Figs 3 and 4). They were also associated with a significantly lower use of rescue medication during both day and night (Fig. 5).

The risk of an exacerbation was not different between the two types of agent, OR 0.9 (95% CI 0.78–1.03), but the short duration of most studies limited the power to test for such differences. The only pharmacologically predictable adverse event documented with a significant increase in odds ratio for long-acting compared with short-acting β-2 agonist treatment was found for headache, OR 1.28 (95% CI 1.02–1.62).

Long-acting β-agonists versus theophylline for maintenance treatment of asthma

The objective of this review was to assess the comparative efficacy and safety of long-acting β_2-agonists and theophylline in the maintenance treatment of asthma. The Cochrane Airways Group's register was searched, most recently in 2003, for all RCTs that compared the efficacy of theophylline (oral sustained-release and/or dose-adjusted) with long-acting β_2-agonists (salmeterol, eformoterol, bambuterol or bitolterol) in participants who were aged over 12 years with clinical evidence of asthma. Studies meeting inclusion criteria were assessed for validity (Table 1), and data were extracted and verified by the study authors.

Results showed that salmeterol improved FEV_1 significantly more than theophylline in five studies, but data from the different trials were not reported adequately for meta-analysis. Formoterol was used in two studies and was reported to be as effective as theophylline.

An increase in PEF from baseline was reported in eight studies on both theophylline and salmeterol but, in four studies, the increase was statistically significant with salmeterol compared with theophylline. One study demonstrated greater improvement in PEF with formoterol compared with theophylline. Meta-analysis was not possible to determine an overall result, but long-acting β_2-agonist and theophylline appeared to have comparable efficacy on lung function. The percentage of symptom-free nights was reported to be greater with long-acting β_2-agonist treatment than with theophylline in six studies, but incomplete data precluded meta-analysis. Nocturnal use of rescue medication fell by a greater amount with long-acting β_2-agonist use compared with theophylline in two studies, but the difference was not statistically significant.

Subjects taking salmeterol experienced fewer adverse events than those using theophylline, relative risk (RR) 0.44 (95% CI 0.30–0.63), NNT 9 (95% CI 6–14). Significant reductions were reported with salmeterol relative to theophylline for central nervous system adverse events, RR 0.50 (95% CI 0.29–0.86), NNT 14 (95% CI 8–50) and gastrointestinal adverse events, RR 0.30 (95% CI 0.17–0.55), NNT 9 (95% CI 6–16). The reviewers concluded that long-acting β_2-agonists are at least as effective as theophylline in reducing asthma

symptoms including night waking and improving lung function. There are fewer adverse events with long-acting β_2-agonists and, thus, for people with asthma who experience nocturnal symptoms and are able to use inhaled therapy, long-acting β_2-agonists are the preferred agents.

Published non-Cochrane Reviews — structured abstracts produced by Cochrane Reviewers on original publications

1. 'Long-acting β_2-agonists in the management of childhood asthma: a critical review of the literature' (original reference[19]). This is a narrative review of 30 RCTs in which an inhaled LABA, either salmeterol or formoterol, alone or in combination with inhaled corticosteroids, was compared with placebo, salbutamol, an inhaled corticosteroid, cromoglycate or nedocromil. The participants were children or adolescents with asthma, but inclusion criteria were not specified and no formal validity assessment was undertaken. The results from studies in which LABAs were used for regular treatment were not formally combined, which was appropriate given the heterogeneity in interventions between them. Individual study results were described, but no overall recommendation was made.

2. 'Meta-analysis of increased dose of inhaled steroid or addition of salmeterol in symptomatic asthma' (MIASMA) (original reference[20]). The objective was to examine the benefits of adding salmeterol compared with increasing the dose of inhaled corticosteroids in symptomatic asthma. The inclusion criteria were participants over 12 years of age with symptomatic asthma in primary or secondary care settings in randomized control trials comparing the addition of salmeterol and increased (at least doubling) dose of current inhaled steroid for a minimum of 12 weeks.

Data were extracted independently by two reviewers. Details of individual study designs were tabulated, but there were no details on whether or how quality was assessed. Heterogeneity was formally tested, P-values reported and causes explored in the analyses. Nine RCTs were included in the review with 3685 participants.

Compared with response to increasing steroids, in patients receiving salmeterol, morning PEF was greater at 3 months, with pooled WMD 22.4 L/min (95% CI 15.0–30.0). FEV_1 was also increased at 3 months, WMD 0.10 L (95% CI 0.04–0.16). The salmeterol treatment groups had fewer days and nights affected by asthma symptoms, WMD % days without asthma 12% (95% CI 9–15%); WMD % nights without asthma 5% (95% CI 3–7%). Fewer patients experienced any exacerbation with salmeterol, WMD 2.73% (95% CI 0.43–5.04%), and the proportion of patients with moderate or severe exacerbations was also lower with WMD 2.42% (95% CI 0.24–4.60%).

The conclusions of this review were that the addition of salmeterol in symptomatic patients, aged over 12 years, taking low to moderate doses of inhaled corticosteroids, improves lung function and control of asthma symptoms with no increase in exacerbations of any severity. It was noted that the review was funded by the company that manufactures salmeterol, and all included studies were sponsored by the company. They also employed or provided financial support for the authors.

3. 'The efficacy and safety of salmeterol compared with theophylline: meta-analysis of nine controlled studies' (original reference)[21]. The objective of the review was to compare the efficacy and safety of salmeterol versus theophylline in asthma management, and studies were selected for inclusion only if conducted by GlaxoSmithKline (Glaxo-Wellcome at the time), with no literature search for all relevant work. Nine studies in adult asthmatics were included, but no method was reported for assessing their validity. All patient data were available, and pooled results from the nine studies showed significantly greater increase in morning and evening PEF with salmeterol compared with theophylline and a greater percentage of symptom-free nights. There was a lower odds ratio for withdrawal due to an adverse event on salmeterol compared with theophylline, OR 0.56 (95% CI 0.38–0.83) and a lower incidence of gastrointestinal side-effects, OR 0.31 (95% CI 0.21–0.54). Despite the clear presentation of results in the review, the conclusion by the authors that salmeterol has a superior efficacy and safety profile than theophylline has to be somewhat compromised by the limited search for data and potential bias inherent in the selection of a single company's sponsored studies.

Other non-Cochrane reviews

1. 'Airway-stabilizing effect of long-acting β_2-agonists as add-on therapy to inhaled corticosteroids'.[22] This review aimed to determine the magnitude of residual bronchoprotection after chronic dosing with long-acting β_2-agonists. It combined results from 13 RCTs, the quality of which was formally assessed. The overall estimate of protection amounted to a 0.79 (95% CI 0.63–0.96) doubling dose/dilution shift from placebo, and the authors concluded that this stabilizing effect on airway smooth muscle may explain the beneficial effects on exacerbations.

2. 'Fluticasone versus salmeterol/low-dose fluticasone for long-term asthma control'.[23] This review compared fluticasone propionate monotherapy versus salmeterol in combination with low-dose fluticasone propionate for long-term asthma control in patients with moderate to severe persistent asthma. It identified four controlled clinical trials from a MEDLINE search from 1966 to 2002. The study design was summarized, but no formal quality assessment was made. The individual group results were presented but not pooled. Three studies showed greater improvements in FEV_1, PEF and symptom control for long-acting β_2-agonist combined with low-dose inhaled corticosteroid compared with monotherapy with increased inhaled corticosteroid dose. One study showed a lower risk of exacerbation of asthma, but the authors stated that the results are not conclusive because of study shortcom-

ings, although the nature of the review as presented does not allow the reader to make an assessment.

3. 'Combined budesonide/formoterol turbuhaler treatment of asthma'.[24] The objective of the review was to provide product information, review and analyse the clinical literature studying combination therapy with budesonide and formoterol in asthmatics. The inclusion criteria were all randomized, blinded, controlled studies of at least 3 months' duration exploring the efficacy of the combination of budesonide and formoterol (in one or separate formulations) compared with other treatments. The results of three included studies were presented in a narrative form, without details of quality assessments or any excluded studies. Only one study used a combination product in a single inhaler device, and no meta-analysis of outcome results was made. The results generally supported the view that the addition of formoterol to inhaled corticosteroids (ICS) in patients with moderate to severe asthma was more effective than monotherapy with a low or higher dose of ICS, but did not contain enough evidence to make any conclusion about their use in a single inhaler.

Other evidence

Data have recently emerged from the unpublished SMART study,[25,26] which suggest that salmeterol may lead to an increase in deaths or life-threatening asthma attacks in individuals with more severe asthma if they are not on inhaled corticosteroids. This seemed to be especially so in black rather than white Americans. This would also support the conclusions of the two relevant Cochrane Reviews.

Scenarios

Thus, in returning to the scenarios, what conclusions can we draw?

Scenario 2. Answer

The individual should be advised that regular treatment with long-acting β_2-agonists has been shown to be more effective than using regular short-acting β-agonist. This treatment is safe if ICS are being used regularly as prophylaxis, but there is not sufficient evidence that use of a long-acting agent regularly in the absence of ICS is safe, especially in more severe asthma and in ethnic groups who may be especially vulnerable.

Scenario 3. Answer

She should be advised that regular use of a long-acting inhaled β_2-agonist in addition to her current dose of ICS is more effective than increasing the dose of ICS and that there is evidence that a long-acting agent is more effective than regular use of a short-acting agent. There is evidence that both long-acting inhaled β$_2$-agonists and theophyllines are effective treatments for the control of nocturnal asthma, although long-acting inhaled β$_2$-agonists may more effectively reduce night waking and the need for rescue medication. The use of long-acting inhaled β$_2$-agonists is associated with fewer adverse events compared with the use of theophylline.

References

1 Li X, Ward C, Thien F *et al.* An antiinflammatory effect of salmeterol, a long-acting β$_2$-agonist, assessed in airway biopsies and bronchoalveolar lavage in asthma. *Am J Respir Crit Care Med* 1999; **160**:1493–9.

2 Eickelberg O, Roth M, Lorx R *et al.* Ligand-independent activation of the glucocorticoid receptor by β$_2$-adrenergic receptor agonists in primary human lung fibroblasts and vascular smooth muscle cells. *J Biol Chem* 1999; **274**:1005–10.

3 Crane J, Pearce N, Flatt A *et al.* Prescribed fenoterol and death from asthma in New Zealand, 1981–83: case–control study. *Lancet* 1989; **1**(8644):917–22.

4 Pearce N, Grainger J, Atkinson M *et al.* Case–control study of prescribed fenoterol and death from asthma in New Zealand, 1977–81. *Thorax* 1990; **45**:170–5.

5 Abramson M, Bailey M, Couper F *et al.* Are asthma medications and management related to deaths from asthma? *Am J Respir Crit Care Med* 2001; **163**:12–18.

6 Sears MR, Taylor DR, Print CG *et al.* Regular inhaled β-agonist treatment in bronchial asthma. *Lancet* 1990; **336**:1391–6.

7 Lipworth BJ, Struthers AD, McDevitt DG. Tachyphylaxis to systemic but not to airway responses during prolonged therapy with high dose inhaled salbutamol in asthmatics. *Am Rev Respir Dis* 1989; **140**: 586–92.

8 O'Connor BJ, Aikman SL, Barnes PJ. Tolerance to the nonbronchodilator effects of inhaled β$_2$-agonists in asthma. *N Engl J Med* 1992; **327**:1204–8.

9 Vathenen AS, Knox AJ, Higgins BG, Britton JR, Tattersfield AE. Rebound increase in bronchial responsiveness after treatment with inhaled terbutaline. *Lancet* 1988; **1**:554–8.

10 Wallin A, Sandstrom T, Soderberg M *et al.* The effects of regular inhaled formoterol, budesonide, and placebo on mucosal inflammation and clinical indices in mild asthma. *Am J Respir Crit Care Med* 1999; **159**:79–86.

11 Faurschou P, Dahl R, Jeffery P *et al.* Comparison of the anti-inflammatory effects of fluticasone and salmeterol in asthma: a placebo controlled, double blind crossover study with bronchoscopy, bronchial methacholine provocation and lavage. *Eur Respir J* 1997; **10**:243S.

12 Taylor DR, Town GI, Herbison GP *et al.* Asthma control during long term treatment with regular inhaled salbutamol and salmeterol. *Thorax* 1998; **53**:744–52.

13 NHLBI. *Global Strategy for Asthma Management and Prevention (Update); April 2002.* Report No. NIH 023659. NHLBI, 2002.

14 British Thoracic Society, National Asthma Campaign, Royal College of Physicians *et al.* The British guidelines on asthma management: 1995 review and position statement. *Thorax* 1997; **52**:S1.

15 Walters EH, Walters J, Gibson P, Jones PW. Inhaled short acting β-2 agonist use in asthma: regular versus as-needed treatment. *Cochrane Database of Systematic Reviews* 2003, Issue 1.

16 Walters EH, Walters JAE, Gibson MDP. Inhaled long acting β agonists for stable chronic asthma. *Cochrane Database of Systematic Reviews* 2003, Issue 3.

17 Walters EH, Walters JAE, Gibson PW. Regular treatment with long acting β agonists versus daily regular treatment with short acting β agonists in adults and children with stable asthma. *Cochrane Database of Systematic Reviews* 2003, Issue 3.

18 Shah L, Wilson A, Gibson P, Coughlan J. Long acting β-agonists versus theophylline for maintenance treatment of asthma. *Cochrane Database of Systematic Reviews* 2003, Issue 3.

19 Bisgaard H. Long-acting β$_2$-agonists in management of childhood asthma: a critical review of the literature. *Pediatr Pulmonol* 2000; **29**:221–34.

20 Shrewsbury S, Pyke S, Britton M. Meta-analysis of increased dose of inhaled steroid or addition of salmeterol in symptomatic asthma (MIASMA). *BMJ* 2000; **320**:1368–73.

21 Davies B, Brooks G, Devoy M. The efficacy and safety of salmeterol compared to theophylline: meta-analysis of nine controlled studies. *Respir Med* 1998; **92**:256–63.

22 Currie GP, Jackson CM, Ogston SA, Lipworth BJ. Airway-stabilizing effect of long-acting β$_2$-agonists as add-on therapy to inhaled corticosteroids. *QJM* 2003; **96**:435–40.

23 Heyneman CA, Crafts R, Holland J, Arnold AD. Fluticasone versus salmeterol/low-dose fluticasone for long-term asthma control. *Ann Pharmacother* 2002; **36**:1944–9.

24 Remington TL, Heaberlin AM, DiGiovine B. Combined budesonide/formoterol turbuhaler treatment of asthma. *Ann Pharmacother* 2002; **36**:1918–28.

25 GlaxoSmithKline. http://www.fda.gov/medwatch/SAFETY/2003/serevent.htm. In: FDA, 2003.

26 Wooltorton E. Salmeterol (Serevent) asthma trial halted early. *Can Med Assoc J* 2003; **168**:738.

CHAPTER 2.3

Inhaled corticosteroids in the treatment of asthma

Nick Adams

Introduction

A phenotype characterized by persistent inflammation of the airway mucosa and allied structures is common to all asthmatic individuals. Resulting airway hyper-responsiveness with variable airway calibre probably accounts for the majority of symptoms experienced by asthmatic patients. Avoidance of the specific exacerbating factors (where they can be identified) may help some patients but is often difficult to achieve; altering the genetic predisposition to asthma development is not currently a therapeutic option. Pharmacological treatment to reduce airway inflammation is therefore the cornerstone of therapy for most asthmatic patients. In the early 1930s, investigators experimented with adrenal cortical extracts for the treatment of asthma because it was reasoned that the fatigue and weakness experienced by asthma sufferers resembled that seen in adrenal insufficiency.[1] Further experiments with intramuscular adrenocorticotrophic hormone (ACTH) and cortisone, based on a recognition of their anti-inflammatory properties, suggested promise in asthma,[2] and small uncontrolled studies with hydrocortisone in the 1950s hinted at the potential benefits of corticosteroids delivered via the inhaled route. Different drug preparations and delivery methods (dry powder and aerosol) were used and, while some studies reported apparent beneficial effects with regard to symptom improvement,[3,4] others did not.[5–7] These conflicting findings may have resulted in lack of early enthusiasm for this class of agent. However, the last three decades have seen the development of a range of newer, potent, synthetic corticosteroids. Beclomethasone dipropionate (BDP) was introduced in 1969 for topical use in skin diseases, but was later adapted for aerosol administration for the treatment of asthma in 1972. Budesonide (BUD) was introduced in the early 1980s. Fluticasone propionate (FP) is a recently licensed synthetic inhaled corticosteroid (ICS) for the treatment of children and adults and is widely used in the UK, Europe, the United States and elsewhere. Experience with these drugs with a variety of oral inhaler delivery devices has led to a consensus that these are effective agents for the treatment of asthma.

Many controlled studies have been undertaken to assess the efficacy and safety of ICS using a wide range of outcome measures. In recent years, ICS have become the cornerstone of pharmacotherapy in the treatment of chronic asthma. Their importance is highlighted in all recent asthma management guidelines, and they are recommended as prophylactic therapy for all but the mildest disease with intermittent symptoms. However, despite the undoubted value of ICS, a number of questions remain. This chapter will examine eight Cochrane systematic reviews that have addressed these questions. These reviews share important (a priori defined) inclusion criteria. Only prospective, randomized controlled trials (RCTs) incorporating a treatment period of at least 1 week using a handheld delivery system (metered dose aerosol inhalers or dry powder devices) were included. Studies including children and adults were assessed, but trials recruiting infants under the age of 2 years were excluded.

Questions

1. Which outcome measures improve when treating asthmatic patients with ICS?

A wide variety of outcome measures has been used in trials to assess treatment response in chronic asthma. These include various symptom scales, measures of airway calibre, health status and exacerbation rates. No single study has examined all outcomes, yet it would be desirable to assess quantitatively the magnitude of response across the available outcome measures in order to gain a clearer idea of which aspects of disease control improve relative to others. Three reviews have been conducted to answer these questions in which the effects of BDP, BUD and FP have been compared with placebo.[8–10]

2. Do ICS exhibit a clinically meaningful dose response for useful outcome measures?

All the ICS are available in a range of formulations by metered dose inhaler (MDI) and various dry powder inhaler (DPI) devices. The nominal daily dose that a patient can be prescribed falls over a 40-fold difference in dose from 50 μg/day to 2000 μg/day. The term 'dose–response' refers to significant improvements in the size of a given outcome with increasing dose. When considering inhaled ICS, the issue of whether an important dose–response effect exists can be framed as two clinical questions: (a) do patients with poorly controlled asthma gain additional benefit by starting ICS treatment at higher as opposed to lower doses? and (b) for patients in whom asthma is not adequately controlled on a given dose of ICS, are additional benefits gained by increasing the dose? Current asthma guidelines[11-13] recommend higher starting doses in patients with more severe symptoms and increasing the daily dose if symptoms are uncontrolled. This advice is based on the assumption that beneficial effects increase with dose. Three reviews have been conducted to assess the evidence for this approach.[14-16]

3. What is the relative efficacy and safety of the different available ICS?

With an expanding range of drugs to choose from, it is important to establish their relative efficacy and safety. All ICS share close chemical and structural similarities. However, pharmacodynamic differences could lead to differences in their clinical effects. In vitro studies have shown differences between individual ICS. Receptor affinity is a measure of the strength with which an active molecule binds to the glucocorticoid receptor (GR). This is 1.5-fold higher for 17-beclomethasone monopropionate (17-BMP), the bronchially active metabolite of BDP, compared with BUD.[17] However, when assessing drugs in terms of their relative in vitro potency, i.e. the concentration of drug required to produce a standard effect, BUD appears to be more potent than BDP. This has been shown for the MacKenzie skin blanching test[18] and for several in vitro assays of anti-inflammatory action including eosinophil survival, basophil histamine release and expression of vascular cell adhesion molecule-1 (VCAM-1).[19] FP exhibits considerably greater GR binding affinity when compared with BDP and BUD[20] and has a greater potency than either BDP or BUD. When assessed in the in vitro skin blanching test, FP is twice as potent as BDP[21] and 25% more potent than BUD.[20] Similar rank order potencies have been shown for other assays of anti-inflammatory activity. Do these differences in in vitro pharmacodynamics translate into differences in clinical efficacy? This may depend on dose. At low inhaled dose, more likely to be on the 'steep' area of the dose–response curve for each drug, differences in potency might lead to differences in clinical efficacy. Conversely, at higher inhaled dose (approaching or on the 'plateau' of the dose–response curve for each drug), differences in clinical efficacy may not be apparent. Differences in potency may also have a bearing on the relative safety of ICS. The potential beneficial effects of high-potency ICS such as FP at active sites in the lung may be offset by systemic side-effects. Higher potency at the site of the pulmonary GRs will be mirrored by higher potency at the site of systemic GRs. This factor, associated with the longer elimination half-life[22] and higher lipophilicity[20] of FP compared with the older inhaled steroids, should lead to longer tissue retention times, and could lead to enhanced endogenous glucocorticoid suppression and increased exogenous steroid-related side-effects. Two Cochrane Reviews have been undertaken to compare the relative effects of BDP versus BUD, and FP versus BDP or BUD to determine whether these experimental differences lead to important differences with regard to clinical efficacy and safety.[23,24]

ICS efficacy

Fifty-two studies (3415 subjects)[25-79] were included in the review assessing BDP versus placebo; 43 studies (2833 subjects)[80-127] in the review assessing BUD versus placebo and 28 studies (5836 subjects)[81,128-167] in the review comparing FP versus placebo (Table 1).

Airway function

BDP resulted in a significant improvement in forced expiratory volume in 1 second (FEV_1) when compared with placebo of 0.34 L [95% confidence interval (CI) 0.19–0.5 L]. BUD resulted in significant improvement in FEV_1 compared with placebo when expressed as a % predicted value, weighted mean difference (WMD) 3.7% (95% CI 0.1–7.2%) or as change compared with baseline, WMD 0.20 L (95% CI 0.07–0.33 L) (Table 1).

FP also led to improvements in FEV_1. Trials reporting this outcome usually did so in the form of change compared with baseline. The relative improvement in FEV_1 ranged from 0.31 L (95% CI 0.27–0.36 L) for FP 100 µg/day or less to 0.53 L (95% CI 0.43–0.63 L) for FP 1000 µg/day. BDP and BUD led to significantly greater morning peak expiratory flow (PEF) compared with placebo of 50 L/min (95% CI 8–92 L/min) and 29 L/min (95% CI 22–36 L/min). FP led to improvements in morning PEF of between 29 L/min and 49 L/min over the dose range of 100–1000 µg/day (Fig. 1), with corresponding improvements in evening PEF of between 18 and 41 L/min for the same dose range. Rescue β_2-agonist use was consistently lower in BDP-, BUD- and FP-treated subjects compared with placebo. Significantly less rescue β_2-agonist was required in BDP- and BUD-treated patients: 1.8 puffs/day (95% CI 1.4–2.4 puffs/day) and 0.43 puffs/daytime (95% CI 0.06–0.80 puffs/daytime) respectively. For FP, reductions in rescue β_2-agonist use ranged between 1.1 puffs/day (95% CI 0.9–1.4 puffs/day) for FP 100 µg/day and 1.4 puffs/day (95% CI 1.0–1.8 puffs/day) for FP 1000 µg/day.

Symptoms and asthma exacerbations

For studies assessing BDP versus placebo, a wide variety of scales was used to assess symptoms, and the quality of reporting was poor with a substantial number of trials failing to provide standard deviation values for mean treatment effects. The data for daily asthma symptoms, where available, suggest that BDP results in significantly fewer symptoms (Table 2). For studies assessing BUD versus placebo, symptoms were reported using a diverse set of measures, and it was inappropriate to pool different measures used in individual studies. However, all the studies of good methodological quality (Jadad score[168] > 3) that reported any symptom measure showed a significant reduction in BUD-treated patients compared with placebo. FP led to reductions in the daily asthma symptom score compared with placebo ranging from 0.59 (95% CI 0.47–0.71) to 0.85 (95% CI 0.63–1.07) for a dose range from 100 to 1000

Table 1. Characteristics of ICS reviews.

Reference (no. of studies)	Population (no. of subjects)	Intervention	Control comparison	Outcomes	Design
8 (52)	Children >2 years and adults (3459)	Beclomethasone dipropionate	Placebo	FEV$_1$, PEF, symptoms, rescue bronchodilator use, quality of life, exacerbations (hospitalizations, unscheduled doctor visits, days off work), safety outcomes, oropharyngeal side-effects	Parallel and crossover RCTs
9 (43)	Children >2 years and adults (2801)	Budesonide	Placebo	FEV$_1$, PEF, symptoms, rescue bronchodilator use, bronchial hyper-responsiveness (BHR), quality of life, exacerbations (hospitalizations, unscheduled doctor visits, days off work), safety outcomes, oropharyngeal side-effects	Parallel and crossover RCTs
10 (28)	Children >2 years and adults (5788)	Fluticasone propionate	Placebo	FEV$_1$, PEF, symptoms, rescue bronchodilator use, BHR, quality of life, exacerbations (hospitalizations, ED visits, unscheduled doctor visits, days off work), safety outcomes, oropharyngeal side-effects, skin bruising	Parallel and crossover RCTs
14 (11)	Children >2 years and adults (1614)	Beclomethasone dipropionate	Beclomethasone dipropionate (<2-fold, 2-fold, 4-fold dose)	FEV$_1$, PEF, symptoms, rescue bronchodilator use, BHR, quality of life, exacerbations (hospitalizations, ED visits, unscheduled doctor visits, days off work), safety outcomes, oropharyngeal side-effects	Parallel and crossover RCTs
15 (24)	Children >2 years and adults (3907)	Budesonide	Budesonide (2-fold, 4-fold dose)	FEV$_1$, PEF, symptoms, rescue bronchodilator use, BHR, quality of life, exacerbations (hospitalizations, unscheduled doctor visits, days off work), safety outcomes, oropharyngeal side-effects	Parallel and crossover RCTs
16 (20)	Children >2 years and adults (>6000)	Fluticasone propionate	Fluticasone propionate (2-fold, 4-fold dose)	FEV$_1$, PEF, symptoms, rescue bronchodilator use, BHR, quality of life, exacerbations (hospitalizations, unscheduled doctor visits, days off work), safety outcomes, oropharyngeal side-effects, skin bruising	Parallel and crossover (one study) RCTs
23 (24)	Children >2 years and adults (1174)	Beclomethasone dipropionate	Budesonide (same daily dose)	FEV$_1$, PEF, symptoms, rescue β_2 agonist use, BHR, quality of life, exacerbations (hospitalizations, unscheduled doctor visits, days off work), safety outcomes, oropharyngeal side-effects	Parallel and crossover RCTs
24 (48)	Children >2 years and adults (11 479)	Fluticasone propionate	Beclomethasone dipropionate	FEV$_1$, PEF, symptoms, rescue bronchodilator use, quality of life, exacerbations (hospitalizations, unscheduled doctor visits, days off work), safety outcomes, oropharyngeal side-effects, skin bruising	Parallel and crossover RCTs

FEV$_1$, forced expired volume in 1 second; PEF, peak expiratory flow; RCT, randomized controlled trials; ED, emergency department.

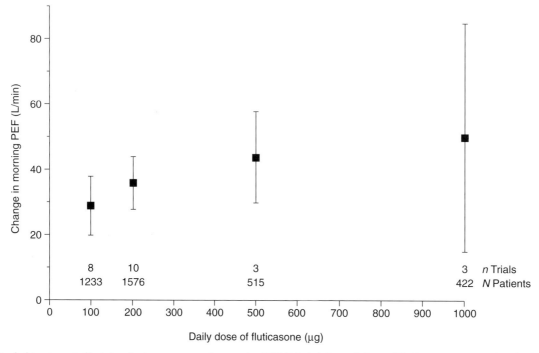

Figure 1. Pooled treatment effect sizes for improvement in morning PEF (L/min) for each dose of fluticasone compared with placebo. Squares represent weighted mean difference (WMD) across studies. Bars represent 95% confidence intervals around WMD.

µg/day (the likelihood of study withdrawal due to asthma exacerbation was a frequently reported outcome). Although the criteria for withdrawal differed between trials, there was a consistent reduction across studies for ICS-treated patients compared with placebo. Significantly fewer patients treated with either BDP or BUD were withdrawn, RR 0.26 (95% CI 0.15–0.43) and RR 0.17 (95% CI 0.09–0.33) respectively (Table 2). FP at all doses from 100 to 1000 µg/day led to a significantly reduced likelihood of trial withdrawal compared with placebo, RR 0.36 (95% CI 0.25–0.54) to RR 0.15 (95% CI 0.10–0.22). In the case of FP, these results correspond to numbers needed to treat (NNT) ranging between 2.9 (95% CI 2.4–3.4) and 2.1 (95% CI 1.8–2.4) over a 6- to 24-week treatment period (Table 2). Withdrawal rates in the context of a clinical trial cannot be considered equivalent to hospital admission rates or GP attendance rates due to exacerbation but may be a surrogate marker for these.

Oral corticosteroid (OCS) sparing effect

BDP treatment resulted in a clinically significant oral steroid sparing effect compared with placebo. End of trial mean daily prednisolone dose was 6 mg/day (95% CI 4–8 mg/day) lower in BDP-treated patients compared with placebo. Reductions in daily dose of 5 mg/day (95% CI 4–6 mg/day) in BDP-treated patients were achieved. The likelihood of discontinuing oral steroids was significantly greater for BDP-treated patients compared with placebo, RR 0.40 (95% CI 0.23–0.70). It was not appropriate to calculate NNT as trials were of varying du-

ration. It should be noted that only studies conducted in adult patients contributed to these analyses; generalization to children with oral steroid-dependent asthma therefore needs to be made with caution. Only one study assessed the role of BUD as an oral steroid sparing agent in chronic asthma.[109] However, this large trial clearly demonstrated that BUD allows a significant reduction in oral prednisolone dose and a significantly greater number of adult patients to discontinue prednisolone completely compared with placebo. FP offers unquestionable benefit over placebo in oral steroid-treated asthmatics. The NNT to allow one patient to stop oral prednisolone completely compared with placebo over a 16-week treatment period are extremely low: 1.6 (95% CI 1.4–1.8) for FP 1000–1500 µg/day and 1.2 (95% CI 1.1–1.3).

Dose–response

Within-study comparisons of beclomethasone at different doses

This review evaluated the small number of RCTs that assessed the relative efficacy of BDP at different doses in chronic asthma. Fifteen trials were included (1614 subjects).[37,61,169–181] Interpretation is complicated by the fact that a wide range of dose comparisons were made in studies, spanning less than twofold to fivefold dose differences. The majority of studies assessing different doses of BDP in non-oral steroid-treated asthmatics were crossover studies, with small patient numbers, and almost all assessed different daily dose combinations

Table 2. Efficacy of beclomethasone and budesonide versus placebo.

Inhaled corticosteroid	Outcome (difference between BDP or BUD and placebo)							
	FEV_1 (L)	FEV_1 (% predicted)	Morning PEF (L/min)	Δ Morning PEF (L/min)*	Daily asthma symptom score	Δ Daytime use rescue $β_2$-agonist (puffs/day)*	Daily use rescue $β_2$-agonist (puffs/day)	Withdrawal due to asthma exacerbation
	WMD (95% CI) n N	WMD (95% CI) n N	WMD (95% CI) n N	WMD (95% CI) n N	SMD (95% CI) n N	WMD (95% CI) n N	WMD (95% CI) n N	RR (95% CI) n N
BDP	0.34‡ (0.19–0.50) 4 11	5.9†§ (0.40–11.5) 8 215	50† (8–92) 4 111	—	1.7†§ (0.5–2.5) 4 75	—	1.7†§ (0.6–2.9) 6 343	0.26‡ (0.15–0.43) 10 1106
BUD	0.07 (−0.25 to 0.40) 4 103	3.7† (0.31–7.09) 8 217	31 (−5 to 67) 3 94	29‡ (22–36) 6 469	—	0.43† (0.06–0.80) 5 480	—	0.17‡ (0.09–0.33) 8 910

FEV_1, forced expired volume in 1 second; PEF, peak expiratory flow; WMD, weighted mean difference; SMD, standardized mean difference; RR, relative risk; 95% CI, 95% confidence interval; n, total number of trials contributing to analysis; N, total number of patients contributing to analysis.

*Change compared with baseline.

†$P < 0.05$.

‡$P < 0.01$.

§Significant heterogeneity between studies, $P < 0.05$.

—, no studies.

of BDP and could not be pooled in a meta-analysis. No significant differences between doses compared were found for most outcomes assessed by these trials; however, these are likely not to have had sufficient power to detect treatment differences. These studies do not allow any firm conclusions to be drawn regarding dose–response effect. However, when considering the parallel design studies, the following conclusions can be made. In non-oral steroid-treated asthmatics, BDP does appear to exhibit a shallow dose–response effect for a number of clinically relevant outcomes. Evidence for this comes from three large, fair-quality (Jadad score 3–4) parallel group studies, one undertaken in children[180] and two in adults.[61,172] When twofold (800 versus 400 μg/day) and fourfold (1600 versus 400 μg/day) dose differences were compared, a small improvement in favour of higher dose was evident for change in FEV_1 compared with baseline, WMD 0.09 L (95% CI 0.03–0.14 L), and percentage change in FEV_1 compared with baseline (+16% versus +7%; $P < 0.03$). BDP 800 μg/day also led to small advantages over BDP 400 μg/day for improvement in morning PEF compared with baseline [WMD 11 L/min (95% CI 4–19 L/min)], evening PEF [WMD 8 L/min (95% CI 0–16 L/min)], reduction in night-time symptoms compared with baseline [WMD 0.13 (95% CI 0.04–0.22)] and reduction in daytime β_2 agonist use [WMD 0.49 puffs/day (95% CI 0.02–0.96 puffs/day)].

Within-study comparisons of budesonide at different doses

Twenty-four studies were selected for inclusion in the review (3907 subjects).[80,81,86,102,109,117,118,182–202] In non-oral steroid-treated asthmatics, there was no evidence of a dose–response effect for FEV_1, morning PEF, symptom scores or rescue β_2-agonist use. This seemed to be the case irrespective of the estimated severity of disease. Statistically significant but very small advantages of BUD 800 μg/day over 200 μg/day were found for FEV_1 (2% predicted) and morning PEF (2 L/min) in one study only.[189] However, higher doses of inhaled BUD were found to be more effective than lower doses of BUD in the following situations. First, treatment with BUD 400 μg/day resulted in significant reductions in the fall in FEV_1 following exercise when treating ICS-naïve, symptomatic children compared with either 200 or 100 μg/day (results based on a single, high-quality study).[102] Secondly, treatment of adults with BUD 800 μg/day significantly reduced the number of exacerbations/patient/year relative to BUD 200 μg/day in a single large study.[189] Thirdly, in adults and children with suboptimally controlled, severe asthma receiving oral corticosteroids and/or high-dose ICS, improvements in FEV_1, morning PEF and rescue β_2-agonist use were apparent when high-dose BUD 800–1600 μg was compared with low-dose BUD 200 μg/day. These findings were based on two large RCTs of high methodological quality.[86,117]

Within-study comparisons of fluticasone at different doses

Twenty studies (> 6000 patients) met the inclusion criteria for this review.[81,128–130,137,142–145,149–153,157–160,164,166,167,203–208] A summary of the results is provided in Table 3. For dose comparisons over the lower to middle part of the dose range (FP 50 μg/day to FP 400–500 μg/day), no dose–response effect was apparent in non-oral steroid-treated asthmatics for FEV_1. However, a statistically significant effect was apparent for high-dose FP (800–1000 μg/day) compared with lower dose range FP (200 μg/day), although the additional benefit was relatively small: WMD 0.13 L (95% CI 0.03–0.24 L). For diary card PEF, a significant dose–response effect was seen over most parts of the dose range. This was apparent when comparing the lower and middle part of the dose range: FP 100 versus 200 μg/day led to small improvements in morning PEF (WMD 6 L/min, 95% CI 1–10 L/min) and evening PEF (6 L/min, 95% CI 2–11 L/min). Similarly, when comparing FP 100 μg/day with 400–500 μg/day, there were small benefits in morning PEF with the higher dose (WMD 8 L/min, 95% CI 1–15 L/min). Over the four- to fivefold dose comparison of 200 to 800–1000 μg/day, a greater difference favouring higher dose was seen for morning PEF (WMD 10 L/min 95% CI 3–18 L/min) and for evening PEF (WMD 8 L/min, 95% CI 1–15 L/min). With greater than 10-fold dose comparisons (FP 50–100 versus 800–1000 μg/day), the higher dose of FP produced bigger effects on morning PEF (WMD 21 L/min, 95% CI 15–29 L/min) and evening PEF (WMD 13 L/min, 95% CI 6–19 L/min). Although all daily doses of FP led to significant improvements in symptoms scores when compared with placebo, no dose–response effect was apparent when making comparisons of individual FP doses across any part of the range. The same pattern of response was present for rescue β_2-agonist requirement. Measures of health status were reported infrequently and did not cover the whole of the dose range available for FP. Where reported, however, no dose–response was apparent.

Relative oral steroid sparing effect of different doses of ICS

The evidence concerning the relative efficacy of different doses of BDP as an oral steroid sparing agent comes from two large parallel group studies of fair methodological quality.[174,179] Different doses were compared and different outcomes were reported in each study, and results could not be pooled. Different dose comparisons were made in individual studies (300 versus 1500 μg/day, 800 versus 2000 μg/day) but, throughout these ranges, no significant differences in oral prednisolone use (reduction compared with baseline or absolute daily dose) or number of patients able to reduce their oral prednisolone dose were apparent. No dose-dependent oral steroid sparing effect was apparent for BUD in oral steroid-treated asthmatics. This concerned comparisons over the dose range 1600 ver-

Table 3. Efficacy of fluticasone versus placebo.

Nominal daily dose (µg/day)	Outcome (difference between fluticasone and placebo)						
	Δ FEV$_1$ (L)*	Δ Morning PEF (L/min)*	Δ Evening PEF (L/min)*	Δ Daily asthma symptom score*	Δ Night-time awakening score*	Δ Daily use rescue β$_2$ agonist (puffs/day)*	Withdrawal due to lack of treatment efficacy
	WMD (95% CI) n N	WMD (95% CI) n N	WMD (95% CI) n N	SMD (95% CI) n N	SMD (95% CI) n N	WMD (95% CI) n N	RR (95% CI) n N
≤100	0.38[‡§] (0.24–0.51) 7 1056	29[‡] (24–33) 8 1233	18[‡] (13–23) 5 718	−0.59[‡] (−0.47 to −0.71) 7 1075	−0.25[‡] (−0.12 to −0.38) 6 895	−1.24[‡§] (−0.80 to −1.68) 7 1072	0.37[‡§] (0.28 to 0.51) 6 1003
200	0.42[‡§] (0.30–0.53) 10 1553	36[‡] (32–40) 10 1576	28[‡] (22–32) 6 942	−0.64[‡] (−0.52 to −0.75) 8 1192	−0.46[‡§] (−0.23 to −0.70) 6 884	−1.56[‡] (−1.11 to −2.00) 8 1189	0.28[‡§] (0.19–0.41) 8 1280
500	0.47[†§] (0.29–0.66) 3 515	44[‡] (37–51) 3 515	—	−0.85[‡] (−0.63 to −1.07) 2 354	−0.74[‡] (−0.52 to −0.96) 2 351	−2.70[‡] (−2.11 to −3.29) 2 351	0.23[‡§] (0.10–0.56) 3 506
1000	0.53[‡] (0.43–0.63) 3 414	50[‡§] (33–68) 3 422	41[‡] (31–51) 2 278	−0.65[‡] (−0.46 to −0.85) 3 412	—	−1.61[‡§] (−0.75 to −2.48) 3 409	0.15[‡] (0.10–0.22) 4 566

FEV$_1$, forced expired volume in 1 second; PEF, peak expiratory flow; WMD, weighted mean difference; SMD, standardized mean difference; RR, relative risk; 95% CI, 95% confidence interval; n, total number of trials contributing to analysis; N, total number of patients contributing to analysis.
*Change compared with baseline.
[†]$P < 0.001$.
[‡]$P < 0.0001$.
[§]Significant heterogeneity between studies, $P < 0.05$.
—, no studies.

sus 800 µg/day and 1600 versus 400 µg/day. Two parallel group studies assessing FP[149,151] were conducted in oral steroid-treated patients using an oral steroid sparing design. Both were large, high-quality (Jadad score 3 or 4) multicentre trials conducted in the USA, in adults with severe asthma. Treatment with, and dependence upon, oral prednisolone for asthma control at the time of enrolment was an inclusion criterion for both studies. Two nominal daily doses of FP were compared in each trial; either FP 1000 µg/day or 2000 µg/day[149] delivered via the Accuhaler DPI, and FP 1500 µg/day or 2000 µg/day delivered via MDI.[151] The mean daily baseline dose of oral prednisolone was 13.0–13.6 mg/day and 9.5–10.2 mg/day for each study respectively. A high proportion of patients (>80%) in both studies were also receiving treatment with a regular ICS (beclomethasone, triamcinolone or flunisolide) at enrolment, although this was not an inclusion criterion in either case. Reduction in daily dose of oral prednisolone was the primary outcome measure in both studies. Both trials lasted 16 weeks. Criteria for prednisolone dose reduction were established a priori in both trials and were based around maintenance of stable asthma control in relation to baseline. This was assessed using changes in FEV$_1$, PEF, rescue β$_2$-agonist use and fre-

quency of symptoms at clinic visits. The results from these studies were pooled. Significantly more patients were able to discontinue oral steroid therapy with FP 2000 µg/day compared with FP 1000–1500 µg/day, NNT 6 (95% CI 3–25). The highest dose of FP also resulted in significantly greater reductions in daily oral prednisolone requirement, WMD 2.0 mg/day (95% CI 0.1–4.0 mg/day).

Relative efficacy

Beclomethasone versus budesonide

Twenty-four studies were selected for inclusion in this review (1174 subjects).[183,209–231] The trials designed to assess the relative efficacy of inhaled BDP and BUD in non-oral steroid-treated asthmatic patients have been mainly of a two-period crossover design. Daily doses of ICS ranged from 400 µg/day or less to 1000 µg/day or more. Treatments were compared over a period of up to 5 weeks. A meta-analysis of the available data from these trials did not show any significant difference between BDP and BUD when considering FEV$_1$, morning PEF or symptoms. Only two parallel group design studies[212,224] assessed the relative efficacy of BDP and BUD in non-oral steroid-treated subjects and presented data. These studies had fundamentally different objectives from the studies of crossover design. In these studies, comparable doses of BDP and BUD required to maintain a good level of control were established using a dose-down titration design. Under the conditions of the two trials, a significantly lower dose of BUD was required to maintain control compared with BDP: WMD 444 µg/day (95% CI 332–556 µg/day). It is important to appreciate, however, that in each study, each ICS was administered using a different delivery device. In both studies, BUD delivered by the Turbohaler DPI was compared with BDP delivered by either an MDI[212] or an MDI with a large volume spacer.[224] Unfortunately, there were no studies of this design type that compared each drug delivered by identical delivery devices. Therefore, the possibility that the established nominal daily doses required to maintain control are partly or wholly a consequence of any differences in the delivery characteristics of the devices used cannot be excluded.

Oral steroid sparing effect

The relative oral steroid sparing efficacy of BDP and BUD was only assessed in one study.[223] Using an approach unique to the ICS literature, the relative oral prednisolone sparing effect of two interventions was assessed in a trial of crossover design. This study has two significant flaws. First, the minimal effective dose of prednisolone was not established for each patient either at the beginning of the study or during the 'washout' phase between treatment periods when each patient received 4–6 weeks of treatment with prednisolone. Enrolling subjects 'overtreated' with oral prednisolone could lead to an overestimate of the absolute prednisolone sparing efficacy of both BDP and BUD and lead to distortion in the assessment of their relative effects. A second problem of methodology concerns the protocol used for tapering prednisolone dose. Dose reduction was attempted at regular intervals throughout each treatment period, until the point at which asthma symptoms deteriorated to 'an unacceptable level'. However, no a priori definition for unacceptable symptoms was used. This could have led to a large degree of variation in the thresholds used by individual investigators in determining whether or not to continue dose reduction or to stop further dose reduction when assessing patients at clinic visits. Because the study was double blind and patients were randomized to each treatment sequence, these variations should have affected all patients equally. However, in a study of small size (40 subjects), this factor may have had an unpredictable effect on the overall assessment of relative efficacy of the two inhaled steroids.

Fluticasone versus beclomethasone or budesonide

Forty-two studies (>10 000 patients) were selected for inclusion.[203,205,208,232–282] The largest group of patients assessed were those in whom FP was compared with either BDP or BUD at a 1:2 nominal daily dose ratio, in non-oral steroid-treated asthmatics. FP resulted in significantly higher measurements of airway calibre compared with BDP/BUD (Table 3). It is difficult to draw conclusions concerning the relative efficacy of FP and BDP/BUD for symptom control and need for rescue β_2-agonist. Few numerical outcome data were available, different scales of measurement were used, and the possibilities for pooling results across studies were limited. However, no individual studies demonstrated a significant difference between FP and BDP/BUD at a 1:2 dose ratio or at a 1:1 dose ratio. A number of studies reported trial withdrawal as a result of an asthma exacerbation. No difference between FP and BDP/BUD at a 1:2 nominal daily dose ratio was apparent.

Oral steroid sparing effect

Little trial evidence exists regarding the relative oral steroid sparing efficacy of FP and BDP or BUD. Important design characteristics of such trials should include a prolonged run-in period to allow patients to have their prednisolone dose weaned to the minimum required to maintain asthma control prior to randomization followed by prednisolone dose reduction according to predefined criteria based around acceptable asthma control. Only one study addressed this question.[265] This study had only been published in abstract form at the time of review, and limited details regarding trial design are available.

Side-effects of treatment

Inhaled corticosteroid versus inactive placebo

Oral side-effects

There was no difference in the incidence of hoarseness or sore throat between treatment groups when either BDP or BUD was compared with placebo. Few studies reported the incidence of oropharyngeal candidiasis, so an overall assessment of relative risk was not possible. These data need to be interpreted with caution as there was little systematic recording of side-effects in these trials. In contrast, reporting of hoarseness and oral candidiasis with FP was more systematic. Compared with placebo, treatment with FP produced a significantly greater risk of hoarseness and oral candidiasis at all doses from 100 to 1000 µg/day and a greater risk of sore throat when administered at 1000 µg/day (Table 4).

Hypothalamo–pituitary axis function

The effects of BDP and BUD compared with placebo on hypothalamo–pituitary–adrenal axis (HPA) function were rarely reported. No two studies assessing BDP reported the same outcome measure, and conflicting results were found. The studies assessing HPA function by insulin and synthetic adrenocorticotropic hormone (ACTH) stress testing did not demonstrate a significant difference in response between BDP- and placebo-treated patients. Too few studies reported

Table 4. Efficacy and safety of increasing doses of fluticasone in asthma when compared with placebo.

FP dose (μg/day)	NNT (95% CI)*	NNH (95% CI)†	Oral candidiasis
	Withdrawal because of worsening asthma	Hoarseness or dysphonia	
100	2.9 (2.4–3.4)	152 (40–1139)	90 (27–746)
200	2.4 (2.2–2.8)	131 (50–417)	61 (22–255)
500	2.0 (1.7–2.3)	23 (15–52)	21 (14–46)
1000	2.1 (1.8–2.4)	17 (11–35)	23 (14–75)
2000	No studies	11 (6–100)	6 (4–17)

*NNT, number needed to treat to prevent one additional person withdrawing because of exacerbation of asthma.
†NNH, number needed to harm, or number who need to be treated to result in one additional person developing side-effects.

such outcomes to draw meaningful conclusions. Only one study assessing BUD reported the results of a dynamic stimulation test, i.e. post-synthetic ACTH (co-syntropin) infusion plasma cortisol levels.[80] This test assesses the ability of the adrenal glands to mount a cortisol secretion response. Significantly lower levels were apparent in BUD-treated adults compared with placebo; however, this was only the case in subjects treated with very high-dose BUD (3200 μg/day). At lower doses (800 and 1600 μg/day), no differences between BUD and placebo were apparent. Individual studies comparing FP with placebo assessed absolute basal plasma cortisol levels, absolute urinary free cortisol levels and stimulated plasma cortisol levels following the short ACTH stimulation test over a range of daily doses in adults and children. Significant differences between FP- and placebo-treated subjects were not found. Only two studies found statistically significant differences between FP and placebo for measures of adrenal function; both assessed FP 1000 μg/day in adults. These included change in morning plasma cortisol following 6 weeks of treatment[144] and post-ACTH infusion plasma cortisol levels following 2 years of treatment.[146]

Dose-related side-effects

Oral side-effects
Few studies comparing different daily doses of either BDP or BUD reported the incidence of oropharyngeal side-effects. A pooled estimate of relative risk according to dose could not be calculated. However, the effect of FP was assessed over a wide range of doses. A significantly greater risk of hoarseness/dysphonia was apparent for high-dose FP (800–1000 μg/day) compared with low-dose FP (50–100 μg/day), RR 0.14 (95% CI 0.03–0.77). The corresponding number needed to harm (NNH) for FP at high compared with low dose was 25 (95% CI 14–100) for a 4- to 8-week treatment period. No difference in the likelihood of hoarseness was apparent for dose comparisons over other parts of the dose range. No difference in the likelihood of sore throat/pharyngitis or oral candidiasis was apparent for any FP dose comparison.

HPA axis function
Effects of treatment on HPA function were assessed using a number of measures. These included basal measurements of HPA activity (morning plasma cortisol levels, overnight and 24-hour urinary cortisol levels) and dynamic tests of adrenocortical reserve (plasma cortisol levels following synthetic ACTH injection or infusion). Few studies comparing ICS dose reported these outcomes, and it was not possible to derive a pooled treatment effect across studies.

Beclomethasone versus budesonide: relative safety
The majority of the trials included in the review assessing the relative effects of BDP and BUD were of a two-period crossover design. Most of these did not have washout periods between treatment arms and assessed a wide range of HPA function-related measures. It was not possible to derive a pooled treatment effect across studies. Twenty-four-hour urinary free cortisol and post-synthetic ACTH test plasma cortisol levels were assessed in a single, high-quality, parallel group, dose-escalation design study undertaken in children.[210] No differences were apparent between BDP and BUD delivered by identical delivery devices (MDI).

Fluticasone versus beclomethasone or budesonide: relative safety

Oropharyngeal side-effects
When compared with BDP/BUD at a nominal daily dose ratio of 1:1, FP results in a significantly greater likelihood of hoarseness, RR 2.47 (95% CI 1.06–5.74; three studies, n = 676). No difference was apparent when FP and BDP/BUD were compared at a dose ratio of 1:2 (Table 6). No difference between FP and BDP/BUD in terms of the likelihood of oral can-

Table 5. Relative efficacy of higher versus lower dose fluticasone.

Dose comparison (µg/day)	Outcome (difference between higher dose and lower dose fluticasone)						
	Δ FEV$_1$ (L)*	Δ Morning PEF (L/min)*	Δ Evening PEF (L/min)*	Δ Daily asthma symptom score*	Δ Night-time awakening score*	Δ Daily use rescue β$_2$-agonist (puffs/day)*	Withdrawal due to lack of efficacy
	WMD (95% CI) n N	WMD (95% CI) n N	WMD (95% CI) n N	SMD (95% CI) n N	SMD (95% CI) n N	WMD (95% CI) n N	RR (95% CI) n N
50 versus 200	0.04 (−0.08 to 0.16) 2313	7 (−2 to 17) 2313	8 (−1 to 17) 2313	−0.32‡ (−0.10 to −0.54) 2313	−0.09† (−0.02 to −0.16) 2313	0.1 (−0.4 to 0.5) 2313	1.32 (0.91–1.91) 2313
100 versus 200	0.01 (−0.04 to 0.05) 7 1078	6‡ (1–10) 9 1510	7† (1–12) 5 839	0.04 (−0.08 to 0.16) 7 1092	−0.17‡ (−0.04 to −0.30) 6 921	0.24 (−0.01 to 0.49) 8 1249	0.96§ (0.68–1.38) 6 1030
200 versus 400–500	0.03 (−0.05 to 0.11) 3 527	3 (−2 to 9) 4 792	3 (−4 to 9) 2 464	0.05 (−0.04 to 0.14) 2 367	—	0.25 (−0.21 to 0.72) 2 367	1.18 (0.78–1.80) 3 530
100 versus 400–500	0.02 (−0.08 to 0.11) 2 328	8† (1–15) 593	—	—	—	—	—
200 versus 800–1000	0.13‡ (0.03–0.24) 2 291	10‡ (3–18) 3 563	8† (1–15) 2 424	0.02 (−0.07 to 0.11) 2 291	—	0.11 (−0.29 to 0.50) 2 291	1.24 (0.72–2.15) 3 448

FEV$_1$, forced expired volume in 1 second; PEF, peak expiratory flow; WMD, weighted mean difference; SMD, standardized mean difference; RR, relative risk; 95% CI, 95% confidence interval; n, total number of trials contributing to analysis; N, total number of patients contributing to analysis.
*Change compared with baseline.
†$P < 0.05$.
‡$P < 0.01$.
§Significant heterogeneity between studies, $P < 0.05$.
—, no studies.

Table 6. Relative efficacy of fluticasone versus beclomethasone or budesonide compared at a 1 : 2 nominal daily dose ratio.

Outcome (difference between FP and BDP or BUD)							
FEV$_1$ (L)	Morning PEF (L/min)	Morning PEF (L/min)*	Evening PEF (L/min)	Withdrawal due to lack of efficacy	Sore throat or pharyngitis (no. of patients)	Hoarseness (no. of patients)	Oropharyngeal candidiasis (no. of patients)
WMD (95% CI)	WMD (95% CI)	WMD (95% CI)	WMD (95% CI)	RR (95% CI)	RR (95% CI)	RR (95% CI)	RR (95% CI)
0.11† (0.10–0.20)	13‡ (5–22)	13‡ (7–17)	11† (1–20)	0.80 (0.58–1.09)	1.97 (0.95–4.12)	0.93 (0.41–2.09)	1.10 (0.64–1.90)
n = 3 N = 1107	n = 7 N = 2089	n = 4 N = 831	n = 5 N = 1698	n = 11 N = 2824	n = 6 N = 1859	n = 5 N = 1524	n = 7 N = 2748

FEV$_1$, forced expired volume in 1 second; PEF, peak expiratory flow; WMD, weighted mean difference; RR, relative risk; 95% CI, 95% confidence interval; n, total number of trials contributing to analysis; N, total number of patients contributing to analysis.
*Change compared with baseline.
†$P < 0.05$.
‡$P < 0.01$.

didiasis was seen when given at either a 1:1 or a 1:2 nominal daily dose ratio. FP was more likely to result in sore throat when compared with BDP/BUD given in a nominal dose ratio of 1:2, but there was no difference between FP and BDP/BUD when given at a dose ratio of 1:1. This discrepancy is difficult to account for. A larger number of studies assessed the 1:2 dose ratio comparison, and a more powerful meta-analysis was possible. While differences in analytical power may account for this discrepancy, this suggestion can only be speculative, especially as there was significant heterogeneity in the 1:2 dose ratio studies. Overall, the results provide evidence that FP is more likely to lead to sore throat at any given nominal dose than BDP/BUD.

Adrenal function

Accurate assessment of the relative effects of FP versus BDP/BUD on markers of adrenal function was difficult to make using the data available for this review. When comparisons of FP with BDP/BUD at a nominal daily dose ratio of 1:2 were made, a meta-analysis of the few parallel group studies[237,272] and crossover studies[241,266,269] did not find significant differences between treatment groups. The few individual studies that assessed FP versus BDP/BUD at equal nominal doses did not find any difference. It was not possible to calculate a pooled treatment effect across studies because numerical data were reported incompletely. This also meant that assessment of the relative influence of FP versus BDP/BUD across the range of ICS doses (e.g. 100 FP versus 200 BDP/BUD, 500 FP versus 1000 BDP/BUD, 1000 FP versus 2000 BDP/BUD) could not be done.

Effect modifiers

Subgroup analyses undertaken for all three drugs did not reveal any consistent variations in treatment effect that could be explained by differences in age (children or adults), duration of treatment (1 month to over 1 year) or delivery device (MDI, MDI with spacer, DPI). Subgroup analyses based upon asthma severity were also undertaken. In order to do this, trials had to be categorized according to severity. Assessment of asthma severity is a problematic area. Severity is best defined in terms of the degree of underlying airway inflammation, whereas asthma control is an estimate of the efficacy of treatment.[283] There is no agreed method for reporting asthma severity because understanding of the disease biology is incomplete and a reliable, non-invasive index of airway inflammation is not available.[284] The consensus guidelines developed by GINA provide broad bandings for disease severity based on degrees of symptom control that apply to patients before commencing treatment. An attempt was made in these reviews to categorize the included studies retrospectively according to the GINA bandings if recruits to the studies were ICS naïve, but also importantly to take into account the amounts of ICS treatment that patients were receiving based on the trial's inclusion crite-

ria. This is clearly a crude estimation of severity and, indeed, the patients enrolled in individual studies will have had asthma of heterogeneous severity. With these considerations in mind, it is probably correct to state that the great majority of patients enrolled in the studies who were not receiving oral steroids had mild to moderate disease. None of the subgroup analyses showed evidence for a difference in response between these GINA categories. Only one study, which randomized patients to different ICS doses, recruited patients judged to have moderate–severe disease.[189] Three studies recruited patients judged to have severe asthma, based on current GINA criteria. Two of these assessed BUD at 800–1600 µg/day compared with a range of doses down to 200 µg/day,[86,117] whereas one assessed FP at high dose (1000 µg/day) and very high dose (2000 µg/day).[203] Without exception, a proportion of patients in these trials was treated with oral prednisolone at the time of enrolment and throughout the study. These trials did not provide data in a form that permitted inclusion in the meta-analysis, and no additional data were forthcoming from the authors. Nevertheless, it is important to note that dose-related reductions in withdrawal rate[189] and improvement in airway function[86,117,285,285] following BUD were seen only in these studies. This suggests that patients with more severe asthma do have the potential to benefit from higher doses of ICS. In contrast, in a study of very high-dose FP (2000 µg/day) compared with high-dose FP (1000 µg/day), only marginal improvements were seen in evening PEF, and there were no significant improvements in the other efficacy measures.[203] This may have been because the plateau for the FP dose–response is reached at this level. Alternatively, patients in this study may have had severe disease because they were in some way resistant to the effects of the corticosteroids that they had received as routine therapy prior to recruitment to the trial.

Summary

ICS have an established role in the management of asthma. All three ICS reviewed here lead to statistically significant improvements in airway function, a reduced likelihood of asthma exacerbation, improvement in symptoms and a reduced need for rescue β_2-agonist. However, statistically significant differences do not necessarily mean that differences are of clinical importance. One method of providing clinical meaning is to relate change in one measure to a global measure of patient-rated change. A recent study has assessed the association of the perceptions of asthmatics to a change in their disease with a number of clinical measures, including airway function.[286] In this study, adult asthmatics were randomized to receive either Montelukast or placebo. The investigators related average minimal patient-perceivable improvement (MPPI) in a global assessment score to various control measures including airway calibre measures and rescue β_2 ago-nist use. The MPPI related to an improvement in FEV_1 of 0.23 L, PEF of 18.8 L/min and reduction in inhaled β_2

agonist use of 0.81 puffs/day. Based on these criteria, each of the ICS led to clinically worthwhile improvements in these outcomes. Symptoms are among the most commonly used asthma outcome measures in clinical research. Ideally, a symptom questionnaire or symptom scale should be able to quantify the intensity, duration and frequency of symptoms. In addition to this, such scales need to be responsive, valid and reliable. Responsiveness is the ability to detect change when one should be present. Validity refers to the extent to which the survey items cover the content area they purport to cover. Reliability is the ability to provide the same results when used repeatedly in the absence of a change in the condition measured.[287,288] In the clinical trials assessed in this review, the diary card symptom responses were scaled and scored to produce an overall 'symptom score'. Although studies to validate diary cards have been carried out recently,[289,290] these scales were not employed in the trials included in this review. Therefore, although the improvements achieve statistical significance, the conclusions are largely qualitative and are difficult to translate into clinically meaningful measures. The reductions in night-time awakening for trials comparing FP with placebo are perhaps more meaningful. Reductions in the frequency of night-time awakening ranged between 0.11/week (95% CI 0.05–0.17/week) for FP 100 µg/day to 0.18/week (95% CI 0.11–0.25/week) for FP 1000 µg/day. One study included in this analysis reported baseline frequency of sleep disturbance, with a mean of 0.05 awakenings per week.[157] If this low level, equating to one awakening per 20 weeks, was representative of other studies in the pooled analysis, then perhaps the change in scores attain greater clinical significance. These benefits appear to apply equally to children and adults and may be achieved with any hand-held delivery device. Daily nominal doses as low as 200 µg (BDP or BUD) or 100 µg (FP) are effective.

The greatest gain in asthma control appears to occur with the initiation of ICS therapy. Even the lowest doses of ICS are effective, and the efficacy dose–response curve appears to be relatively shallow. Daily nominal doses as low as 200 µg (BDP or BUD) or 100 µg (FP) are effective. Above this, there is evidence for a dose–response effect that was best seen with BUD and FP, but less clear with BDP. This difference may not be due to any intrinsic properties of BUD and FP but could be a consequence of trial size and consistency of data collection and reporting in the BUD/FP studies. Even with FP, the slope of this dose–response relationship obtained across studies was quite shallow (Fig. 1). The mean improvement in morning PEF with FP ≤ 100 µg/day compared with placebo was 29 L/min, whereas a 10-fold higher dose produced a benefit over placebo of 50 L/min, i.e. 72% greater. The between-study estimates of dose–response (i.e. from comparisons of FP versus placebo) were very similar to those from direct within-study comparisons. For example, for FP 1000 µg/day versus 200 µg/day, the improvements in morning PEF were 14 L/min (between-study) and 11 L/min (within-study). This dose–response effect was seen to a varying degree across all outcomes, but was more consistent in terms of airway function and withdrawal from the study due to lack of efficacy than asthma symptoms, night awakening or rescue medication use.

The shallow dose-related therapeutic gains are accompanied by an increased likelihood of oropharyngeal side-effects, which in contrast has a steeper dose–response profile. Oropharyngeal candidiasis is relatively rare when low doses of FP are used compared with placebo with an NNH for FP 100 µg/day of 90 (95% CI 50–417). With increasing doses, the side-effect rate progressively increases. At 2000 µg/day, the NNH drops to 6 (95% CI 4–17). The main effect of increasing FP dose appears to be a relatively sharp increase in the incidence of side-effects with little additional benefit in terms of efficacy. This is supported by the analyses directly comparing high-dose FP (800–1000 µg/day) versus lower dose FP (50–100 µg/day), in which one out 25 patients treated with high-dose FP could be expected to experience hoarseness/dysphonia (95% CI 14–100) without a reduction in the likelihood of trial withdrawal due to asthma exacerbation.

The data assembled in the review comparing BDP and BUD tend to support the suggestion that they are equipotent. However, the results require cautious interpretation for the following reasons. The majority of the trials included in this review were of a two-period crossover design. Particular strengths of the crossover design include the fact that subjects effectively act as their own controls. This has two main advantages. First, only half as many subjects are required in order to achieve the same degree of statistical power as an equivalent parallel design study. Secondly, the effect of interindividual variation in response to treatment is reduced, which may otherwise mask a true treatment effect. Unfortunately, this design also has some serious limitations when assessing the effects of relatively long-acting interventions such as ICS. Although most of the trials in this group were of fair methodological quality, only two out of 19 trials had a washout of any length between treatment periods. ICS almost certainly exert an action that persists over days if not weeks. When the performance of long-acting agents is assessed in trials of crossover design, there is always a concern that the effects of treatment administered in the first period of the trial may persist into, and 'colour', the effects of the active agent administered in the second period of the trial. This so called 'carryover' or 'sequence' effect will influence the results of the study and lead to biased judgement concerning the relative effectiveness and safety of the agents being assessed.[291] In situations in which the control intervention is inactive/placebo, this effect will tend to produce a conservative underestimate of the efficacy of the active treatment. In situations in which two active treatments (such as BDP and BUD) are studied in a trial of two-period crossover design, the results are unpredictable. It is possible that a less effective drug could falsely appear to be the more effective one if, for example, the carryover effect was strong and confined to the truly more effective drug. There are well-established statistical methods for assessing the presence or otherwise of carryover effects and excluding them. However, a commentary as to whether such tests were undertaken was rarely reported in the studies included. These considerations undermine the results of the individual trials and mean additional caution must be exercised in drawing conclusions from the meta-analysis.

The data from trials that compared FP with BDP/BUD at a 1:2 nominal daily dose ratio suggest that FP and the older corticosteroids cannot be considered equivalent with respect to clinical efficacy. The greater improvements in FEV_1 and PEF when administered at half the nominal daily dose of BDP/BUD suggest that the higher potency of FP demonstrated in laboratory studies is reflected in certain outcomes relevant to clinical practice. Although this cannot be taken to mean that FP at half daily dose is equivalent to BDP/BUD at full dose, it does suggest that clinically relevant differences in effect are unlikely to be seen when FP and BDP/BUD are used at a 1:2 daily dose ratio. A logical extension of this finding would be for even greater benefits favouring FP to be seen when given at equal nominal daily dose to BDP or BUD. This has not been clearly demonstrated. However, fewer studies made such a comparison, and an overall pooled analysis across studies was not possible. Less weight should therefore be given to these findings, and they do not undermine the more powerful analysis that was possible for the studies that compared FP with BDP/BUD at a 1:2 dose ratio.

Single-dose and short-term (< 1 week) studies have demonstrated that FP results in a significantly greater suppression of plasma cortisol than BUD when compared at equal nominal daily dose over a range of 400 to 2000 µg/day.[292–294] A recent meta-regression analysis that included these studies concluded that FP is significantly more potent than BUD in suppressing morning plasma cortisol; in other words, that FP leads to greater suppression of these levels than BUD when given at equal daily dose.[295] This effect appeared to be more pronounced at higher nominal daily doses. The absence of significant differences between FP and BDP/BUD in the individual studies that assessed the drugs at a 1:1 nominal daily dose ratio included in the Cochrane Review may be explained by issues related to the timing of cortisol measurements. In all these longer term studies, cortisol measurements were made within a 2-hour time window between 08.00h and 10.00h. In the short-term studies (not eligible for inclusion in the Cochrane Review), cortisol measurements were taken at a strictly standardized time of either 07.30h or 08.00h. Cortisol estimations over a timeframe of 2 hours have been shown to be substantially less sensitive in detecting change compared with those taken at closely controlled times, with up to threefold differences in levels occurring between 08.00h and 10.00h in healthy volunteers.[296] The greater variability introduced into estimations made over a 2-hour timeframe may have masked any true differences between FP and BDP/BUD in terms of their effects on morning cortisol levels. Twenty-four-hour urinary cortisol, a more sensitive assay of basal adrenocortical activity than morning plasma cortisol, was not reported frequently. This measurement should not be subject to the same difficulties in interpretation as plasma cortisol. In summary, firm conclusions cannot be drawn with regard to the relative effect of FP versus BDP/BUD on morning plasma cortisol or 24-hour urinary cortisol levels in randomized trials with treatment periods of 1 week or longer. These considerations should reinforce the recommendations of recent guidelines that daily doses of ICS be titrated down {National Asthma Education and Prevention Program 1995 #10400} to the lowest necessary to maintain control as assessed by FEV_1, diary card morning PEF, symptoms and rescue β_2-agonist use.

References

1 Fineman EH. The use of suprarenal cortex extract in the treatment of bronchial asthma. *J Allergy* 1933; 4:182.

2 Carey RA, Harvey AM, Howard JE, Winkenwerder WL. The effects of adrenocorticotropic hormone (ACTH) and cortisone on the course of chronic bronchial asthma. *Bull Johns Hopkins Hosp* 1950; 87:387.

3 Foulds WS, Greaves DP, Herxheimer H, Kingdom LG. Hydrocortisone in the treatment of allergic conjunctivitis, allergic rhinitis and bronchial asthma. *Lancet* 1955; 1:234–5.

4 Brockbank W, Pengelly CDR. Chronic asthma treated with powder inhalation of hydrocortisone and prednisolone. *Lancet* 1958; 1:187–8.

5 Brockbank W, Brebner H, Pengelly CDR. Chronic asthma treated with aerosol hydrocortisone. *Lancet* 1958; 2:807.

6 Langlands JHM, McNeill RS. Hydrocortisone by inhalation: effect on lung function in bronchial asthma. *Lancet* 1960; ??:404–6.

7 Morrison Smith J. Hydrocortisone hemisuccinate by inhalation in children with asthma. *Lancet* 1958; 2:1248–50.

8 Adams NP, Bestall J, Jones PW. Inhaled beclomethasone versus placebo for chronic asthma (Cochrane Review). In: *The Cochrane Library*, Issue 1. Oxford, Update Software, 2002.

9 Adams NP, Bestall J, Jones PW. Budesonide for chronic asthma in children and adults (Cochrane Review). In: *The Cochrane Library*, Issue 1. Oxford, Update Software, 2002.

10 Adams NP, Bestall J, Jones PW. Inhaled fluticasone proprionate for chronic asthma (Cochrane Review). In: *The Cochrane Library*, Issue 1. Oxford, Update Software, 2002.

11 British Thoracic Society. The British guidelines on asthma management: 1995 review and position statement. *Thorax* 1997; 52:S1–S21.

12 National Asthma Education and Prevention Program. *Global Strategy for Asthma Management and Prevention: NHBLI/WHO Workshop Report.* Bethesda, MD, National Institutes of Health, 1995.

13 National Asthma Education and Prevention Program. *Guidelines for the Diagnosis and Managment of Asthma.* Expert Panel Report No. 2. Bethesda, MD, NIH/National Heart, Lung and Blood Institute, 1997.

14 Adams NP, Bestall J, Jones PW. Inhaled beclomethasone at different doses for long-term asthma (Cochrane Review). In: *The Cochrane Library*, Issue 1. Oxford, Update Software, 2002.

15 Adams NP, Bestall J, Jones PW. Budesonide at different doses for chronic asthma (Cochrane Review). In: *The Cochrane Library*, Issue 1. Oxford, Update Software, 2002.

16 Adams NP, Bestall J, Jones PW. Inhaled fluticasone at different doses for chronic asthma (Cochrane Review). In: *The Cochrane Library*, Issue 1. Oxford, Update Software, 2002.

17 Boobis AR. Comparative physicochemical and pharmacokinetic profiles of inhaled beclomethasone dipropionate and budesonide. *Respir Med* 1998; **92**:2–6.

18 Johansson SA, Andersson KE, Brattsand R, Gruvstad E, Hedner P. Topical and systemic glucocorticoid potencies of budesonide and beclomethasone dipropionate in man. *Eur J Clin Pharmacol* 1982; **22**:523–9.

19 Stellato C, Atsuta J, Bickel CA, Schleimer RP. An *in vitro* comparison of commonly used topical glucocorticoid preparations. *J Allergy Clin Immunol* 1999; **104**:623–9.

20 Kelly HW. Establishing a therapeutic index for the inhaled corticosteroids: part I. Pharmacokinetic/pharmacodynamic comparison of the inhaled corticosteroids. *J Allergy Clin Immunol* 1998; **102**:S36–S51.

21 Phillipps GH. Structure–activity relationships of topically active steroids: the selection of fluticasone propionate. *Respir Med* 1990; **84**:19–23.

22 Thorsson L, Dahlstrom K, Edsbacker S, Kallen A, Paulson J, Wiren JE. Pharmacokinetics and systemic effects of inhaled fluticasone propionate in healthy subjects. *Br J Clin Pharmacol* 1997; **43**:155–61.

23 Adams NP, Bestall J, Jones PW. Inhaled beclomethasone versus budesonide for chronic asthma (Cochrane Review). In: *The Cochrane Library*, Issue 1. Oxford, Update Software, 2002.

24 Adams NP, Bestall J, Jones PW. Fluticasone versus beclomethasone or budesonide for chronic asthma (Cochrane Review). In: *The Cochrane Library*, Issue 1. Oxford, Update Software, 2002.

25 Bel EH, Timmers MC, Hermans J, Dijkman JH, Sterk PJ. The long-term effects of nedocromil sodium and beclomethasone dipropionate on bronchial responsiveness to methacholine in nonatopic asthmatic subjects. *Am Rev Respir Dis* 1990; **141**:21–8.

26 Bennati D, Piacentini GL, Peroni DG, Sette L, Testi R, Boner AL. Changes in bronchial reactivity in asthmatic children after treatment with beclomethasone alone or in association with salbutamol. *J Asthma* 1989; **26**:359–64.

27 Bergmann KC, Bauer CP, Overlack A. A placebo-controlled blinded comparison of nedocromil sodium and beclomethasone dipropionate in bronchial asthma. *Lung* 1990; **168**:230–9.

28 Berkowitz R, Rachelefsky G, Harris AG, Chen R. A comparison of triamcinolone acetonide MDI with a built-in tube extender and beclomethasone dipropionate MDI in adult asthmatics. *Chest* 1998; **114**:757–65.

29 Boner AL, Piacentini GL, Bonizzato C, Dattoli V, Sette L. Effect of inhaled beclomethasone dipropionate on bronchial hyperreactivity in asthmatic children during maximal allergen exposure. *Pediatr Pulmonol* 1991; **10**:2–5.

30 Anonymous. Double-blind trial comparing two dosage schedules of beclomethasone dipropionate aerosol in the treatment of chronic bronchial asthma. Preliminary report of the Brompton Hospital–Medical Research Council Collaborative Trial. *Lancet* 1974; **2**:303–7.

31 Bronsky E, Korenblat P, Harris AG, Chen R. Comparative clinical study of inhaled beclomethasone dipropionate and triamcinolone acetonide in persistent asthma. *Ann Allergy Asthma Immunol* 1998; **80**:295–302.

32 Anonymous. A controlled trial of inhaled corticosteroids in patients receiving prednisone tablets for asthma. *Br J Dis Chest* 1976; **70**:95–103.

33 Cameron SJ, Cooper EJ, Crompton GK, Hoare MV, Grant IW. Substitution of beclomethasone aerosol for oral prednisolone in the treatment of chronic asthma. *BMJ* 1973; **4**:205–7.

34 Carpentiere G, Castello F, Marino S. Effect of beclomethasone dipropionate on the bronchial responsiveness to propranolol in asthmatics. *Chest* 1990; **98**:263–5.

35 Chan KN, Silverman M. Increased airway responsiveness in children of low birth weight at school age: effect of topical corticosteroids. *Arch Dis Child* 1993; **69**:120–4.

36 Davies G, Thomas P, Broder I. Steroid-dependent asthma treated with inhaled beclomethasone dipropionate. A long-term study. *Ann Intern Med* 1977; **86**:549–53.

37 De Marzo N, Fabbri LM, Crescioli S, Plebani M, Testi R, Mapp CE. Dose-dependent inhibitory effect of inhaled beclomethasone on late asthmatic reactions and increased responsiveness to methacholine induced by toluene diisocyanate in sensitised subjects. *Pulm Pharmacol* 1988; **1**:15–20.

38 Fahy JV, Boushey HA. Effect of low-dose beclomethasone dipropionate on asthma control and airway inflammation. *Eur Respir J* 1998; **11**:1240–7.

39 Fanelli A, Maggi E, Stendardi L, Gorini M, Duranti R, Scano G. Preventive effects of beclomethasone on histamine-induced changes in breathing pattern in asthma. *Chest* 1993; **103**:122–8.

40 Fournier M, Renon D, Le Roy-Ladurie F, Pappo M, Pariente R. Bronchial tolerance to three months' inhalation of beclomethasone dipropionate. Histological and microbiological study by asthmatic patients. *Presse Med* 1990; **19**:1441–4.

41 Gaddie J, Reid IW, Skinner C, Petrie GR, Sinclair DJ, Palmer KN. Aerosol beclomethasone dipropionate in chronic bronchial asthma. *Lancet* 1973; **1**:691–3.

42 Harvey LL, Nair SV, Kass I. Beclomethasone dipropionate aerosol in the treatment of steroid-dependent asthma. A 12-week double-blind study comparing beclomethasone dipropionate and a vehicle aerosol. *Chest* 1976; **70**:345–50.

43 Hodson ME, Batten JC, Clarke SW, Gregg I. Beclomethasone dipropionate aerosol in asthma. Transfer of steroid-dependent asthmatic patients from oral prednisone to beclomethasone dipropionate aerosol. *Am Rev Respir Dis* 1974; **110**:403–8.

44 Holst PE, O'Donnell TV. A controlled trial of beclomethasone dipropionate in asthma. *NZ Med J* 1974; **79**:769–73.

45 Hoshino M, Nakamura Y, Sim JJ *et al.* Inhaled corticosteroid reduced lamina reticularis of the basement membrane by modulation of insulin-like growth factor (IGF)-I expression in bronchial asthma. *Clin Exp Allergy* 1998; **28**:568–77.

46 Katsunuma T, Hashimoto K, Akimoto K, Ebisawa M, Iikura Y. Effect of inhaled beclomethasone dipropionate on bronchial responsiveness in patients with asthma. *Ann Allergy Asthma Immunol* 1993; **70**:165–70.

47 Kerigan AT, Pugsley SO, Cockcroft DW, Hargreave FE. Substitution of inhaled beclomethasone dipropionate for ingested prednisone in steroid-dependent asthmatics. *Can Med Assoc J* 1977; **116**:867–71.

48 Kerrebijn KF. Beclomethasone dipropionate in long-term treatment of asthma in children. *J Pediatr* 1976; **89**:821–6.

49 Kerstjens HA, Brand PL, de Jong PM, Koeter GH, Postma DS. Influence of treatment on peak expiratory flow and its relation to airway hyperresponsiveness and symptoms. The Dutch CNSLD Study Group. *Thorax* 1994; **49**:1109–15.

50 Kerstjens HA, Brand PL, Hughes MD *et al.* A comparison of bronchodilator therapy with or without inhaled corticosteroid therapy for obstructive airways disease. Dutch Chronic Non-Specific Lung Disease Study Group. *N Engl J Med* 1992; **327**:1413–19.

51 Klein R, Waldman D, Kershnar H *et al.* Treatment of chronic childhood asthma with beclomethasone dipropionate aerosol: I. A double-blind crossover trial in nonsteroid-dependent patients. *Pediatrics* 1977; **60**:7–13.

52 Kraemer R, Sennhauser F, Reinhardt M. Effects of regular inhalation of beclomethasone dipropionate and sodium cromoglycate on bronchial hyperreactivity in asthmatic children. *Acta Paediatr Scand* 1987; **76**:119–23.

53 Lacronique J, Renon D, Georges D, Henry-Amar M, Marsac J. High-

dose beclomethasone: oral steroid-sparing effect in severe asthmatic patients. *Eur Respir J* 1991; **4**:807–12.

54 Laviolette M, Ferland C, Trepanier L, Rocheleau H, Dakhama A, Boulet LP. Effects of inhaled steroids on blood eosinophils in moderate asthma. *Ann NY Acad Sci* 1994; **725**:288–97.

55 Lovera J, Collins-Williams C, Bailey J. Beclomethasone dipropionate by aerosol in the treatment of asthmatic children. *Postgrad Med J* 1975; **51**:96–8.

56 Lovera J, Cooper DM, Collins-Williams C, Levison H, Bailey JD, Orange RP. Clinical and physiological assessment of asthmatic children treated with beclomethasone dipropionate. *J Allergy Clin Immunol* 1976; **57**:112–23.

57 Maestrelli P, De Marzo N, Saetta M, Boscaro M, Fabbri LM, Mapp CE. Effects of inhaled beclomethasone on airway responsiveness in occupational asthma. Placebo-controlled study of subjects sensitized to toluene diisocyanate. *Am Rev Respir Dis* 1993; **148**:407–12.

58 Martin PD, Gebbie T, Salmond CE. A controlled trial of beclomethasone dipropionate by aerosol in chronic asthmatics. *NZ Med J* 1974; **79**:773–6.

59 Matthys H, Nowak D, Hader S, Kunkel G. Efficacy of chlorofluorocarbon-free beclomethasone dipropionate 400 micrograms day^{-1} delivered as an extrafine aerosol in adults with moderate asthma. *Respir Med* 1998; **92**:17–22.

60 Messerli C, Studer H, Scherrer M. Systemic side effects of beclomethasone dipropionate aerosols (becotide, aldecine, sanasthmyl) in otherwise non steroid treated asthmatic patients. *Pneumonologie* 1975; **153**:29–42.

61 Nathan RA, Nolop KB, Cuss FM, Lorber RR. A comparison of double-strength beclomethasone dipropionate (84 microg) MDI with beclomethasone dipropionate (42 microg) MDI in the treatment of asthma. *Chest* 1997; **112**:34–9.

62 Pennings HJ, Wouters EF. Effect of inhaled beclomethasone dipropionate on isocapnic hyperventilation with cold air in asthmatics, measured with forced oscillation technique. *Eur Respir J* 1997; **10**:665–71.

63 Radha TG, Viswanathan R, Sharma AK. Beclomethasone dipropionate aerosol in asthma: a double blind study. *Ind J Med Res* 1975; **63**:1659–66.

64 Riordan JF, Dash CH, Sillett RW, McNicol MW. A comparison of betamethasone valerate, beclomethasone dipropionate and placebo by inhalation for the treatment of chronic asthma. *Postgrad Med J* 1974; **50**:61–4.

65 Ryan G, Latimer KM, Juniper EF, Roberts RS, Hargreave FE. Effect of beclomethasone dipropionate on bronchial responsiveness to histamine in controlled nonsteroid-dependent asthma. *J Allergy Clin Immunol* 1985; **75**:25–30.

66 Salmeron S, Guerin JC, Godard P et al. High doses of inhaled corticosteroids in unstable chronic asthma. A multicenter, double-blind, placebo-controlled study. *Am Rev Respir Dis* 1989; **140**:167–71.

67 Simons FE. A comparison of beclomethasone, salmeterol, and placebo in children with asthma. Canadian Beclomethasone Dipropionate–Salmeterol Xinafoate Study Group. *N Engl J Med* 1997; **337**:1659–65.

68 Smith AP, Booth M, Davey AJ. A controlled trial of beclomethasone dipropionate for asthma. *Br J Dis Chest* 1973; **67**:208–14.

69 Smith JM. A clinical trial of beclomethasone dipropionate aerosol in children and adolescents with asthma. *Clin Allergy* 1973; **3**:249–53.

70 Toogood JH, Lefcoe NM, Haines DS et al. A graded dose assessment of the efficacy of beclomethasone dipropionate aerosol for severe chronic asthma. *J Allergy Clin Immunol* 1977; **59**:298–308.

71 Trigg CJ, Manolitsas ND, Wang J et al. Placebo-controlled immunopathologic study of four months of inhaled corticosteroids in asthma. *Am J Respir Crit Care Med* 1994; **150**:17–22.

72 Turner MO, Johnston PR, Pizzichini E, Pizzichini MM, Hussack PA,

Hargreave FE. Anti-inflammatory effects of salmeterol compared with beclomethasone in eosinophilic mild exacerbations of asthma: a randomized, placebo controlled trial. *Can Respir J* 1998; **5**:261–8.

73 Vatrella A, Ponticiello A, Parrella R et al. Serum eosinophil cationic protein (ECP) as a marker of disease activity and treatment efficacy in seasonal asthma. *Allergy* 1996; **51**:547–55.

74 Ponticiello A, Vatrella A, Parrella R et al. Inhaled beclomethasone dipropionate (BDP) prevents seasonal changes in atopic asthmatics. *Monaldi Arch Chest Dis* 1997; **52**:112–17.

75 Vilsvik JS, Schaanning J. Beclomethasone dipropionate aerosol in adult steroid-dependent obstructive lung disease. *Scand J Respir Dis* 1974; **55**:169–75.

76 Vogt F, Chervinsky P, Dwek J, Grieco M. Beclomethasone dipropionate aerosol in the treatment of chronic bronchial asthma. *J Allergy Clin Immunol* 1976; **58**:316–21.

77 Wang JH, Trigg CJ, Devalia JL, Jordan S, Davies RJ. Effect of inhaled beclomethasone dipropionate on expression of proinflammatory cytokines and activated eosinophils in the bronchial epithelium of patients with mild asthma. *J Allergy Clin Immunol* 1994; **94**:1025–34.

78 Webb DR. Beclomethasone in steroid-dependent asthma. Effective therapy and recovery of hypothalamo–pituitary–adrenal function. *JAMA* 1977; **238**:1508–11.

79 Wiebicke W, Jorres R, Magnussen H. Comparison of the effects of inhaled corticosteroids on the airway response to histamine, methacholine, hyperventilation, and sulfur dioxide in subjects with asthma. *J Allergy Clin Immunol* 1990; **86**:915–23.

80 Aaronson D, Kaiser H, Dockhorn R et al. Effects of budesonide by means of the Turbuhaler on the hypothalmic–pituitary–adrenal axis in asthmatic subjects: a dose–response study. *J Allergy Clin Immunol* 1998; **101**:312–19.

81 Agertoft L, Pedersen S. Short-term knemometry and urine cortisol excretion in children treated with fluticasone propionate and budesonide: a dose response study. *Eur Respir J* 1997; **10**:1507–12.

82 Baki A, Karaguzel G. Short-term effects of budesonide, nedocromil sodium and salmeterol on bronchial hyperresponsiveness in childhood asthma. *Acta Paediatr Jpn* 1998; **40**:247–51.

83 Bel EH, Timmers MC, Zwinderman AH, Dijkman JH, Sterk PJ. The effect of inhaled corticosteroids on the maximal degree of airway narrowing to methacholine in asthmatic subjects. *Am Rev Respir Dis* 1991; **143**:109–13.

84 Boner AL, Comis A, Schiassi M, Venge P, Piacentini GL. Bronchial reactivity in asthmatic children at high and low altitude. Effect of budesonide. *Am J Respir Crit Care Med* 1995; **151**:1194–200.

85 Burke CM, Sreenan S, Pathmakanthan S, Patterson J, Schmekel B, Poulter LW. Relative effects of inhaled corticosteroids on immunopathology and physiology in asthma: a controlled study. *Thorax* 1996; **51**:993–9.

86 Busse WW, Chervinsky P, Condemi J et al. Budesonide delivered by Turbuhaler is effective in a dose-dependent fashion when used in the treatment of adult patients with chronic asthma. *J Allergy Clin Immunol* 1998; **101**:457–63.

87 Campbell LM, Watson DG, Venables TL, Taylor MD, Richardson PDI. Once daily budesonide turbohaler compared to placebo as initial prophylactic therapy for asthma. *Br J Clin Res* 1991; **2**:111–22.

88 Cockcroft DW, Swystun VA, Bhagat R. Interaction of inhaled β_2 agonist and inhaled corticosteroid on airway responsiveness to allergen and methacholine. *Am J Respir Crit Care Med* 1995; **152**:1485–9.

89 De Baets FM, Goeteyn M, Kerrebijn KF. The effect of two months of treatment with inhaled budesonide on bronchial responsiveness to histamine and house-dust mite antigen in asthmatic children. *Am Rev Respir Dis* 1990; **142**:581–6.

90 de Jong JW, van der Mark TW, Koeter GH, Postma DS. Rebound airway obstruction and responsiveness after cessation of terbutaline: effects of budesonide. *Am J Respir Crit Care Med* 1996; **153**:70–5.

91 Merkus PJ, van Essen-Zandvliet EE, Duiverman EJ, van Houwelingen HC, Kerrebijn KF, Quanjer PH. Long-term effect of inhaled corticosteroids on growth rate in adolescents with asthma. *Pediatrics* 1993; **91**:1121–6.

92 Van Essen-Zandvliet EEM, Hughes MD, Waalkens HJ, Duiverman EJ, Pocock SJ, Kerrebijn KF. Effects of 22 months of treatment with inhaled corticosteroids and/or β$_2$-agonists on lung function, airway responsiveness, and symptoms in children with asthma. *Am Rev Respir Dis* 1992; **146**:547–54.

93 Van Essen-Zandvliet EE. Long-term intervention in childhood asthma: the Dutch study results. Dutch Chronic Nonspecific Lung Disease Study Group. *Monaldi Arch Chest Dis* 1995; **50**:201–7.

94 Fuller RW, Choudry NB, Eriksson G. Action of budesonide on asthmatic bronchial hyperresponsiveness. Effects on directly and indirectly acting bronchoconstrictors. *Chest* 1991; **100**:670–4.

95 Gauvreau GM, Doctor J, Watson RM, Jordana M, O'Byrne PM. Effects of inhaled budesonide on allergen-induced airway responses and airway inflammation. *Am J Respir Crit Care Med* 1996; **154**:1267–71.

96 Gleeson JG, Price JF. Controlled trial of budesonide given by the nebuhaler in preschool children with asthma. *BMJ* 1988; **297**:163–6.

97 Greenough A, Pool J, Gleeson JG, Price JF. Effect of budesonide on pulmonary hyperinflation in young asthmatic children. *Thorax* 1988; **43**:937–8.

98 Haahtela T, Jarvinen M, Kava T *et al.* Effects of reducing or discontinuing inhaled budesonide in patients with mild asthma. *N Engl J Med* 1994; **331**:700–5.

99 Henriksen JM. Effect of inhalation of corticosteroids on exercise induced asthma: randomised double blind crossover study of budesonide in asthmatic children. *BMJ Clin Res* 1985; **291**:248–9.

100 Heuck C, Wolthers OD, Hansen M, Kollerup G. Short-term growth and collagen turnover in asthmatic adolescents treated with the inhaled glucocorticoid budesonide. *Steroids* 1997; **62**:659–64.

101 Jatakanon A, Lim S, Chung KF, Barnes PJ. An inhaled steroid improves markers of airway inflammation in patients with mild asthma. *Eur Respir J* 1998; **12**:1084–8.

102 Jonasson G, Carlsen KH, Blomqvist P. Clinical efficacy of low-dose inhaled budesonide once or twice daily in children with mild asthma not previously treated with steroids. *Eur Respir J* 1998; **12**:1099–104.

103 Jones AH, Langdon CG, Lee PS *et al.* Pulmicort Turbohaler once daily as initial prophylactic therapy for asthma. *Respir Med* 1994; **88**:293–9.

104 Juniper EF, Kline PA, Vanzieleghem MA, Ramsdale EH, O'Byrne PM, Hargreave FE. Effect of long-term treatment with an inhaled corticosteroid (budesonide) on airway hyperresponsiveness and clinical asthma in nonsteroid-dependent asthmatics. *Am Rev Respir Dis* 1990; **142**:832–6.

105 Kharitonov SA, Yates DH, Barnes PJ. Inhaled glucocorticoids decrease nitric oxide in exhaled air of asthmatic patients. *Am J Respir Crit Care Med* 1996; **153**:454–7.

106 Kivity S, Fireman E, Greif J, Schwarz Y, Topilsky M. Effect of budesonide on bronchial hyperresponsiveness and pulmonary function in patients with mild to moderate asthma. *Ann Allergy Asthma Immunol* 1994; **72**:333–6.

107 Kuo HP, Yu TR, Yu CT. Hypodense eosinophil number relates to clinical severity, airway hyperresponsiveness and response to inhaled corticosteroids in asthmatic subjects. *Eur Respir J* 1994; **7**:1452–9.

108 Lorentzson S, Boe J, Eriksson G, Persson G. Use of inhaled corticosteroids in patients with mild asthma. *Thorax* 1990; **45**:733–5.

109 Nelson HS, Bernstein IL, Fink J *et al.* Oral glucocorticosteroid-sparing effect of budesonide administered by Turbuhaler: a double-blind, placebo-controlled study in adults with moderate-to-severe chronic asthma. Pulmicort Turbuhaler Study Group. *Chest* 1998; **113**:1264–71.

110 O'Byrne P, Cuddy L, Taylor DW, Birch S, Morris J, Syrotuik J. Efficacy and cost benefit of inhaled corticosteroids in patients considered to have mild asthma in primary care practice. *Can Respir J* 1996; **3**:169–75.

111 O'Connor BJ, Ridge SM, Barnes PJ, Fuller RW. Greater effect of inhaled budesonide on adenosine 5'-monophosphate-induced than on sodium-metabisulfite-induced bronchoconstriction in asthma. *Am Rev Respir Dis* 1992; **146**:560–4.

112 Evans PM, O'Connor BJ, Fuller RW, Barnes PJ, Chung KF. Effect of inhaled corticosteroids on peripheral blood eosinophil counts and density profiles in asthma. *J Allergy Clin Immunol* 1993; **91**:643–50.

113 Osterman K, Carlholm M, Ekelund J *et al.* Effect of 1 year daily treatment with 400 microg budesonide (Pulmicort Turbuhaler) in newly diagnosed asthmatics. *Eur Respir J* 1997; **10**:2210–15.

114 Prieto L, Berto JM, Gutierrez V, Tornero C. Effect of inhaled budesonide on seasonal changes in sensitivity and maximal response to methacholine in pollen-sensitive asthmatic subjects. *Eur Respir J* 1994; **7**:1845–51.

115 Estrada Rodriguez JL, Belchi Hernandez J, Florido Lopez JF, Lopez Serrano C, Martinez Alzamora F, Ojeda Casas JA. Short-term treatment of asthma with budesonide versus placebo. *J Invest Allergol Clin Immunol* 1991; **1**:266–70.

116 Sekerel BE, Tuncer A, Saraclar Y, Adalioglu G. Inhaled budesonide reduces lung hyperinflation in children with asthma. *Acta Paediatr* 1997; **86**:932–6.

117 Shapiro G, Bronsky EA, LaForce CF *et al.* Dose-related efficacy of budesonide administered via a dry powder inhaler in the treatment of children with moderate to severe persistent asthma. *J Pediatr* 1998; **132**:976–82.

118 Swystun VA, Bhagat R, Kalra S, Jennings B, Cockcroft DW. Comparison of 3 different doses of budesonide and placebo on the early asthmatic response to inhaled allergen. *J Allergy Clin Immunol* 1998; **102**:363–7.

119 Tan WC, Koh TH, Hay CS, Taylor E. The effect of inhaled budesonide on the diurnal variation in airway mechanics, airway responsiveness and serum neutrophil chemotactic activity in Asian patients with predominant nocturnal asthma. *Respirology* 1998; **3**:13–20.

120 Toogood JH, Frankish CW, Jennings BH *et al.* A study of the mechanism of the antiasthmatic action of inhaled budesonide. *J Allergy Clin Immunol* 1990; **85**:872–80.

121 Vathenen AS, Knox AJ, Wisniewski A, Tattersfield AE. Time course of change in bronchial reactivity with an inhaled corticosteroid in asthma. *Am Rev Respir Dis* 1991; **143**:1317–21.

122 Vathenen AS, Knox AJ, Wisniewski A, Tattersfield AE. Effect of inhaled budesonide on bronchial reactivity to histamine, exercise, and eucapnic dry air hyperventilation in patients with asthma. *Thorax* 1991; **46**:811–16.

123 Wempe JB, Tammeling EP, Postma DS, Auffarth B, Teengs JP, Koeter GH. Effects of budesonide and bambuterol on circadian variation of airway responsiveness and nocturnal symptoms of asthma. *J Allergy Clin Immunol* 1992; **90**:349–57.

124 Wempe JB, Tammeling EP, Koeter GH, Hakansson L, Venge P, Postma DS. Blood eosinophil numbers and activity during 24 hours: effects of treatment with budesonide and bambuterol. *J Allergy Clin Immunol* 1992; **90**:757–65.

125 Wong CS, Wahedna I, Pavord ID, Tattersfield AE. Effect of regular terbutaline and budesonide on bronchial reactivity to allergen challenge. *Am J Respir Crit Care Med* 1994; **150**:1268–73.

126 Wongtim S, Mogmued S, Chareonlap P, Limthongkul S. Effect of inhaled corticosteroids on bronchial hyperresponsiveness in patients with mild asthma. *Asian Pac J Allergy Immunol* 1995; **13**:81–5.

127 Yates DH, Kharitonov SA, Barnes PJ. An inhaled glucocorticoid does not prevent tolerance to the bronchoprotective effect of a long-acting inhaled β$_2$-agonist [published erratum appears in *Am J*

Respir Crit Care Med 1997 Apr; 155(4):1491]. *Am J Respir Crit Care Med* 1996; **154**:1603–7.

128 Allen DB, Bronsky EA, LaForce CF *et al.* Growth in asthmatic children treated with fluticasone propionate. Fluticasone Propionate Asthma Study Group. *J Pediatr* 1998; **132**:472–7.

129 Mahajan P, Pearlman D, Okamoto L. The effect of fluticasone propionate on functional status and sleep in children with asthma and on the quality of life of their parents. *J Allergy Clin Immunol* 1998; **102**:19–23.

130 Konig P, Ford L, Galant S *et al.* A 1-year comparison of the effects of inhaled fluticasone propionate (FP) and placebo on growth in pre-pubescent children with asthma. *Eur Respir J* 1996; **9**: S294.

131 Chervinsky P, van As A, Bronsky EA *et al.* Fluticasone propionate aerosol for the treatment of adults with mild to moderate asthma. The Fluticasone Propionate Asthma Study Group. *J Allergy Clin Immunol* 1994; **94**:676–83.

132 Condemi JJ, Chervinsky P, Glodstein MF *et al.* Fluticasone propionate powder administered through Diskhaler versus triamcinolone acetonide aerosol administered thorough metered-dose inhaler in patients with persistent asthma. *J Allergy Clin Immunol* 1997; **100**:467–74.

133 Ekroos H, Lindqvist A, Saarinen T *et al.* Significant association with the decrease of bronchial hyperresponsiveness and the decrease of exhaled nitric oxide after starting inhaled fluticasone in mild asthma. *Eur Respir J* 1999; **14**:171S.

134 Ekroos HJ, Sovijarvi ARA, Lindqvist A *et al.* Short-term effect of fluticasone propionate on exhaled nitric oxide in mild asthma. *Am J Respir Crit Care Med* 1999; **159**:A628.

135 Sovijarvi ARA, Ekroos H, Lindqvist A *et al.* Short-term effect of fluticasone propionate on bronchial hyperresponsiveness to histamine diphosphate in mild asthma; significant effect within three days. *Am J Respir Crit Care Med* 1999; **159**:A629.

136 Faul JL, Leonard CT, Burke CM, Tormey VJ, Poulter LW. Fluticasone propionate induced alterations to lung function and the immunopathology of asthma over time. *Thorax* 1998; **53**:753–61.

137 Galant SP, Lawrence M, Meltzer EO, Tomasko M, Baker KA, Kellerman DJ. Fluticasone propionate compared with theophylline for mild-to-moderate asthma. *Ann Allergy Asthma Immunol* 1996; **77**:112–18.

138 Mahajan P, Okamoto L. Patient satisfaction with the Diskhaler (R) and the Diskus (R) inhaler, a new multidose powder delivery system for the treatment of asthma. *Clin Ther* 1997; **19**:1126–34.

139 Hampel F, Van Bavel J, Selner J *et al.* Inhaled fluticasone propionate administered via the Diskus or Diskhaler is safe and effective in adolescent and adult subjects with mild to moderate asthma. *Am J Respir Crit Care Med* 1996; **153**:A338.

140 Galant SP, van Bavel J, Finn A *et al.* Diskus and diskhaler: efficacy and safety of fluticasone propionate via two dry powder inhalers in subjects with mild-to-moderate persistent asthma. *Ann Allergy Asthma Immunol* 1999; **82**:273–80.

141 Hoekstra MO, Grol MH, Bouman K *et al.* Fluticasone propionate in children with moderate asthma. *Am J Respir Crit Care Med* 1996; **154**:1039–44.

142 Hofstra WB, Sterk PJ, Neijens HJ, Kuethe MC, Mulder PGH, Duiverman EJ. The effect of 24 weeks treatment with 100 mcg or 250 mcg b.d. fluticasone propionate in reducing exercise-induced bronchoconstriction in childhood asthma. *Am J Respir Crit Care Med* 1997; **155**:A267.

143 Katz Y, Lebas FX, Medley HV, Robson R. Fluticasone propionate 50 micrograms BID versus 100 micrograms BID in the treatment of children with persistent asthma. Fluticasone Propionate Study Group. *Clin Ther* 1998; **20**:424–37.

144 Lawrence M, Wolfe J, Webb DR *et al.* Efficacy of inhaled fluticasone

145 Nielsen K, Okamoto L, Shah T. Importance of selected inhaler characteristics and acceptance of a new breath-actuated powder inhalation device. *J Asthma* 1997; **34**:249–53.

146 Li JT, Ford LB, Chervinsky P *et al.* Fluticasone propionate powder and lack of clinically significant effects on hypothalamic–pituitary–adrenal axis and bone mineral density over 2 years in adults with mild asthma. *J Allergy Clin Immunol* 1999; **103**:1062–8.

147 MacKenzie CA, Weinberg EG, Tabachnik E, Taylor M, Havnen J, Crescenzi K. A placebo controlled trial of fluticasone propionate in asthmatic children. *Eur J Pediatr* 1993; **152**:856–60.

148 Nathan R, Woodring A, Baitinger L *et al.* The salmeterol/fluticasone propionate Diskus combination decreases the incidence of exacerbations compared to treatment with salmeterol or fluticasone propionate alone. *Eur Respir J* 1999; **14**:123S.

149 Nelson HS, Busse WW, deBoisblanc BP *et al.* Fluticasone propionate powder: oral corticosteroid-sparing effect and improved lung function and quality of life in patients with severe chronic asthma. *J Allergy Clin Immunol* 1999; **103**:267–75.

150 Nimmagadda SR, Spahn JD, Nelson HS, Jenkins J, Szefler SJ, Leung DY. Fluticasone propionate results in improved glucocorticoid receptor binding affinity and reduced oral glucocorticoid requirements in severe asthma. *Ann Allergy Asthma Immunol* 1998; **81**: 35–40.

151 Noonan M, Chervinsky P, Busse WW *et al.* Fluticasone propionate reduces oral prednisone use while it improves asthma control and quality of life. *Am J Respir Crit Care Med* 1995; **152**:1467–73.

152 Okamoto LJ, Noonan M, DeBoisblanc BP, Kellerman DJ. Fluticasone propionate improves quality of life in patients with asthma requiring oral corticosteroids. *Ann Allergy Asthma Immunol* 1996; **76**:455–61.

153 Noonan MJ, Chervinsky P, Wolfe J, Liddle R, Kellerman DJ, Crescenzi KL. Dose-related response to inhaled fluticasone propionate in patients with methacholine-induced bronchial hyperresponsiveness: a double-blind, placebo-controlled study. *J Asthma* 1998; **35**: 153–64.

154 O'Shaughnessy KM, Wellings R, Gillies B, Fuller RW. Differential effects of fluticasone propionate on allergen-evoked bronchoconstriction and increased urinary leukotriene E4 excretion. *Am Rev Respir Dis* 1993; **147**:1472–6.

155 Oliveri D, Chetta A, Del Donno M *et al.* Effect of short-term treatment with low-dose inhaled fluticasone propionate on airway inflammation and remodeling in mild asthma: a placebo-controlled study. *Am J Respir Crit Care Med* 1997; **155**:1864–71.

156 Overbeek SE, Rijnbeek PR, Vons C, Mulder PG, Hoogsteden HC, Bogaard JM. Effects of fluticasone propionate on methacholine dose–response curves in nonsmoking atopic asthmatics. *Eur Respir J* 1996; **9**:2256–62.

157 Pearlman DS, Noonan MJ, Tashkin DP *et al.* Comparative efficacy and safety of twice daily fluticasone propionate powder versus placebo in the treatment of moderate asthma. *Ann Allergy Asthma Immunol* 1997; **78**:356–62.

158 Mahajan P, Okamoto LJ, Schaberg A, Kellerman D, Schoenwetter WF. Impact of fluticasone propionate powder on health-related quality of life in patients with moderate asthma. *J Asthma* 1997; **34**:227–34.

159 Peden DB, Berger WE, Noonan MJ *et al.* Inhaled fluticasone propionate delivered by means of two different multidose powder inhalers is effective and safe in a large pediatric population with persistent asthma. *J Allergy Clin Immunol* 1998; **102**: 32–8.

160 Noonan M, Berger W, Thomas R *et al.* Inhaled fluticasone propionate dry powder administered via Diskus or Diskhaler is safe and

effective in pediatric patients with chronic asthma. *Eur Respir J* 1997; **10**:221S.

161 Rickard K, Srebro SH, Edwards L, Johnson MC. Inhaled fluticasone versus oral zafirlukast in asthma patients. *Eur Respir J* 1999; **??**:122S.

162 Bowers BW, Johnson M, Edwards L, Srebro S, Rickard K. The impact of fluticasone propionate and zafirlukast on patient quality of life. *Am J Respir Crit Care Med* 1999; **159**:A761.

163 Busse WW, Srebro SH, Edwards L, Johnson MC, Rickard K. Low-dose inhaled fluticasone propionate versus oral zafirlukast in asthma patients. *Am J Respir Crit Care Med* 1999; **159**:A628.

164 Sheffer AL, LaForce C, Chervinsky P, Pearlman D, Schaberg A. Fluticasone propionate aerosol: efficacy in patients with mild to moderate asthma. Fluticasone Propionate Asthma Study Group. *J Fam Pract* 1996; **42**:369–75.

165 Van Schoor J, Joos GF, Pauwels RA. The effects of inhaled fluticasone propionate on methacholine and neurokinin induced bronchoconstriction in asthmatics. *Eur Respir J* 1999; **14**:531S.

166 Wasserman SI, Gross GN, Schoenwetter WF *et al.* A 12-week dose-ranging study of fluticasone propionate powder in the treatment of asthma. *J Asthma* 1996; **33**:265–74.

167 Wolfe JD, Selner JC, Mendelson LM, Hampel F Jr, Schaberg A. Effectiveness of fluticasone propionate in patients with moderate asthma: a dose-ranging study. *Clin Ther* 1996; **18**:635–46.

168 Jadad AR, Moore RA, Carroll D *et al.* Assessing the quality of reports of randomized clinical trials: is blinding necessary? *Control Clin Trials* 1996; **17**:1–12.

169 Carmichael J, Duncan D, Crompton GK. Beclomethasone dipropionate dry-powder inhalation compared with conventional aerosol in chronic asthma. *BMJ* 1978; **2**:657–8.

170 Carpentiere G, Marino S, Castello F, Baldanza C, Bonanno CT. Dose-related effect of beclomethasone dipropionate on airway responsiveness in asthma. *Respiration* 1990; **57**:100–3.

171 Chatterjee SS, Butler AG. Beclomethasone dipropionate in asthma: a comparison of two methods of administration. *Br J Dis Chest* 1980; **74**:175–9.

172 Drepaul BA, Payler DK, Qualtrough JE *et al.* Becotide or becodisks? A controlled study in general practice. *Clin Trials J* 1989; **26**:335–44.

173 Hampel F, Lisberg E, Vanden Burgt J, Henon C, Stampone P. 50 mcg twice daily of ultrafine HFA-beclomethasone dipropionate aerosol improves asthma control in adult patients. *Am J Respir Crit Care Med* 1997; **155**:A666.

174 Hummel S, Lehtonen L. Comparison of oral-steroid sparing by high-dose and low-dose inhaled steroid in maintenance treatment of severe asthma. *Lancet* 1992; **340**:1483–7.

175 Lal S, Malhotra SM, Gribben MD, Butler AG. Beclomethasone dipropionate aerosol compared with dry powder in the treatment of asthma. *Clin Allergy* 1980; **10**:259–62.

176 Molema J, Lammers JW, van Herwaarden CL, Folgering HT. Effects of inhaled beclomethasone dipropionate on β_2-receptor function in the airways and adrenal responsiveness in bronchial asthma. *Eur J Clin Pharmacol* 1988; **34**:577–83.

177 Smith MJ, Hodson ME. Twice daily beclomethasone dipropionate administered with a concentrated aerosol inhaler: efficacy and patient compliance. *Thorax* 1986; **41**:960–3.

178 So SY, Lam WK. Twice daily administration of beclomethasone dipropionate dry-powder in the management of chronic asthma. *Asian Pac J Allergy Immunol* 1986; **4**:129–32.

179 Tarlo SM, Broder I, Davies GM, Leznoff A, Mintz S, Corey PN. Six-month double-blind, controlled trial of high dose, concentrated beclomethasone dipropionate in the treatment of severe chronic asthma. *Chest* 1988; **93**:998–1002.

180 Verberne AA, Frost C, Duiverman EJ, Grol MH, Kerrebijn KF. Addition of salmeterol versus doubling the dose of beclomethasone in children with asthma. *Am J Respir Crit Care Med* 1998; **158**:213–19.

181 Wolthers OD, Pedersen S. Short term growth during treatment with inhaled fluticasone propionate and beclomethasone diproprionate. *Arch Dis Child* 1993; **68**:673–6.

182 Bisgaard H, Pedersen S, Damkjaer Nielsen M, Osterballe O. Adrenal function in asthmatic children treated with inhaled budesonide. *Acta Paediatr Scand* 1991; **80**:213–17.

183 Boe J, Rosenhall L, Alton M *et al.* Comparison of dose–response effects of inhaled beclomethasone dipropionate and budesonide in the management of asthma. *Allergy* 1989; **44**:349–55.

184 Campbell LM, Gooding TN, Aitchison WR, Smith N, Powell JA. Initial loading (400 micrograms twice daily) versus static (400 micrograms nocte) dose budesonide for asthma management. PLAN Research Group. *Int J Clin Pract* 1998; **52**:361–8, 370.

185 Johansson SA, Dahl R. A double-blind dose–response study of budesonide by inhalation in patients with bronchial asthma. *Allergy* 1988; **43**:173–8.

186 Juniper EF, Kline PA, Vanzieleghem MA, Ramsdale EH, O'Byrne PM, Hargreave FE. Long-term effects of budesonide on airway responsiveness and clinical asthma severity in inhaled steroid-dependent asthmatics. *Eur Respir J* 1990; **3**:1122–7.

187 Kraan J, Koeter GH, van der Mark TW *et al.* Dosage and time effects of inhaled budesonide on bronchial hyperreactivity. *Am Rev Respir Dis* 1988; **137**:44–8.

188 Laursen LC, Taudorf E, Weeke B. High-dose inhaled budesonide in treatment of severe steroid-dependent asthma. *Eur J Respir Dis* 1986; **68**:19–28.

189 Pauwels RA, Lofdahl CG, Postma DS *et al.* Effect of inhaled formoterol and budesonide on exacerbations of asthma. Formoterol and Corticosteroids Establishing Therapy (FACET) International Study Group. *N Engl J Med* 1997; **337**:1405–11.

190 Pedersen S, Hansen OR. Budesonide treatment of moderate and severe asthma in children: a dose–response study. *J Allergy Clin Immunol* 1995; **95**:29–33.

191 Pedersen B, Dahl R, Karlstrom R, Peterson CG, Venge P. Eosinophil and neutrophil activity in asthma in a one-year trial with inhaled budesonide. The impact of smoking. *Am J Respir Crit Care Med* 1996; **153**:1519–29.

192 Rees TP, Lennox B, Timney AP, Hossain M, Turbitt ML, Richardson PDI. Comparison on increasing the dose of budesonide to 800 mg/day with a maintained dose of 400 mg/day in mild-to-moderate asthmatic patients. *Eur J Clin Res* 1993; **4**:67–77.

193 Campbell LM, Simpson RJ, Turbitt ML, Richardson PDI. A comparison of the cost effectiveness of budesonide 400 mug/day and 800 mug/day in the management of mild-to-moderate asthma in general practice. *Br J Med Econ* 1993; **6**:67–74.

194 Toogood JH, Baskerville J, Jennings B, Lefcoe NM, Johansson SA. Use of spacers to facilitate inhaled corticosteroid treatment of asthma. *Am Rev Respir Dis* 1984; **129**:723–9.

195 Toogood JH, Jennings B, Baskerville J, Johansson SA. Clinical use of spacer systems for corticosteroid inhalation therapy: a preliminary analysis. *Eur J Respir Dis — Suppl* 1982; **122**:100–7.

196 Tukiainen P, Lahdensuo A. Effect of inhaled budesonide on severe steroid-dependent asthma. *Eur J Respir Dis* 1987; **70**:239–44.

197 Turktas I, Gokcora N, Yavuz O, Elbek S, Cevik C, Demirsoy S. Effect of inhaled budesonide on lipid metabolism and hypothalamic–pituitary–adrenal axis function in patients with bronchial asthma. *Turk J Med Sci* 1995; **25**:183–6.

198 van der Molen T, Meyboom-de Jong B, Mulder HH, Postma DS. Starting with a higher dose of inhaled corticosteroids in primary care asthma treatment. *Am J Respir Crit Care Med* 1998; **158**:121–5.

199 Wolthers OD, Pedersen S. Growth of asthmatic children during treatment with budesonide: a double blind trial. *BMJ* 1991; **303**:163–5.

200 Wolthers OD, Juul A, Hansen M, Muller J, Pedersen S. The insulin-

like growth factor axis and collagen turnover in asthmatic children treated with inhaled budesonide. *Acta Paediatr* 1995; **84**: 393–7.

201 Wolthers OD, Pedersen S. Measures of systemic activity of inhaled glucocorticosteroids in children: a comparison of urine cortisol excretion and knemometry. *Respir Med* 1995; **89**:347–9.

202 Wolthers OD, Pedersen S. Controlled study of linear growth in asthmatic children during treatment with inhaled glucocorticosteroids. *Pediatrics* 1992; **89**:839–42.

203 Ayres JG, Bateman ED, Lundback B, Harris TAJ. High dose fluticasone propionate, 1 mg daily, versus fluticasone propionate, 2 mg daily, or budesonide, 1.6 mg daily, in patients with chronic severe asthma. *Eur Respir J* 1995; **8**:579–86.

204 Boner A, de Benedictis F, La Rosa M *et al*. Clincial trial to compare the efficacy of two doses of fluticasone propionate (FP) 200 mcg/day and 400 mcg/day, administered for 6 weeks to asthmatic children, as assessed by bronchial responsiveness to methacholine. *Am J Respir Crit Care Med* 1999; **159**:A139.

205 Dahl R, Lundback B, Malo JL *et al*. A dose-ranging study of fluticasone propionate in adult patients with moderate asthma. International Study Group. *Chest* 1993; **104**:1352–8.

206 Ind PW, Dal Negro R, Colman N, Fletcher CP, Browning DC, James MH. Inhaled fluticasone propionate and salmeterol in moderate adult asthma I: lung function and symptoms. *Am J Respir Crit Care Med* 1998; **157**:A416.

207 Ind PW, Dal Negro R, Fletcher CP, Browning DC, James MH. Inhaled salmeterol and fluticasone propionate therapy in moderate adult asthma. *Eur Respir J* 1997; **10**:1S.

208 Raphael GD, Lanier RQ, Baker J, Edwards L, Rickard K, Lincourt WR. A comparison of multiple doses of fluticasone propionate and beclomethasone dipropionate in subjects with persistent asthma. *J Allergy Clin Immunol* 1999; **103**:796–803.

209 Baran D. A comparison of inhaled budesonide and beclomethasone dipropionate in childhood asthma. *Br J Dis Chest* 1987; **81**:170–5.

210 Bisgaard H, Damkjaer Nielsen M, Andersen B *et al*. Adrenal function in children with bronchial asthma treated with beclomethasone dipropionate or budesonide. *J Allergy Clin Immunol* 1988; **81**: 1088–95.

211 Bjorkander J, Formgren H, Johansson SA, Millqvist E. Methodological aspects of clinical trials with inhaled corticosteroids: results of two comparisons between two steroid aerosols in patients with asthma. *Eur J Respir Dis — Suppl* 1982; **122**:108–17.

212 Brambilla C, Godard P, Lacronique J *et al*. A 3-month comparative dose-reduction study with inhaled beclomethasone dipropionate and budesonide in the management of moderate to severe adult asthma. *Drug Invest* 1994; **8**:49–56.

213 Dal Negro R, Micheletto C, Ciani F *et al*. Efficacy and safety of inhaled beclomethasone dipropionate dry powder in the treatment of chronic asthma: a controlled study vs. budesonide. *Eur Respir J* 1997; 351S.

214 Ebden P, Jenkins A, Houston G, Davies BH. Comparison of two high dose corticosteroid aerosol treatments, beclomethasone dipropionate (1500 micrograms/day) and budesonide (1600 micrograms/day), for chronic asthma. *Thorax* 1986; **41**:869–74.

215 Field HV, Jenkinson PM, Frame MH, Warner JO. Asthma treatment with a new corticosteroid aerosol, budesonide, administered twice daily by spacer inhaler. *Arch Dis Child* 1982; **57**:864–6.

216 Greefhorst APM. Budesonide and terbutaline delivered via Turbuhaler compared to BDP and salbutamol delivered via Rotahaler. *Eur Respir J* 1992; **5**:360S.

217 Hamalainen KM, Laurikaninen K, Leinonen M, Jager L. Comparison of two multidose powder inhalers (MDPI) in the treatment of asthma with inhaled cortisosteroids. *Eur Respir J* 1998; 61S.

218 Keelan P, Gray P, Kelly P, Frame M. Comparison of a new corticosteroid aerosol, budesonide, with beclomethasone dipropionate in the treatment of chronic asthma. *Ir Med J* 1984; **77**:244–7.

219 Micheletto C, Mauroner L, Burti E *et al*. Inhaled beclomethasone dipropionate and budesonide dry powder in chronic asthma: lung function–serum ECP relationship. *Eur Respir J* 1997; 351S.

220 Nicolaizik WH, Marchant JL, Preece MA, Warner JO. Endocrine and lung function in asthmatic children on inhaled corticosteroids. *Am J Respir Crit Care Med* 1994; **150**:624–8.

221 Pedersen S, Fuglsang G. Urine cortisol excretion in children treated with high doses of inhaled corticosteroids: a comparison of budesonide and beclomethasone. *Eur Respir J* 1988; **1**:433–5.

222 Petrie GR, Choo-Kang YFJ, Clark RA, Milledge JS, Whitfield RJ, Higgins AJ. An assessment of the acceptability of two breath-actuated corticosteroid inhalers: comparison of Turbohaler(TM) with Diskhaler(TM). *Drug Invest* 1990; **2**:129–31.

223 Rafferty P, Tucker LG, Frame MH, Fergusson RJ, Biggs BA, Crompton GK. Comparison of budesonide and beclomethasone dipropionate in patients with severe chronic asthma: assessment of relative prednisolone-sparing effects. *Br J Dis Chest* 1985; **79**:244–50.

224 Selroos O, Backman R, Forsen KO *et al*. Clinical efficacy of budesonide Turbuhaler compared with that of beclomethasone dipropionate pMDI with volumatic spacer. A 2-year randomized study in 102 asthma patients. *Allergy* 1994; **49**:833–6.

225 Springer C, Avital A, Maayan C, Rosler A, Godfrey S. Comparison of budesonide and beclomethasone dipropionate for treatment of asthma. *Arch Dis Child* 1987; **62**:815–19.

226 Stiksa G, Glennow C, Johannesson N. An open cross-over trial with budesonide and beclomethasone dipropionate in patients with bronchial asthma. *Eur J Respir Dis — Suppl* 1982; **122**:266–7.

227 Stiksa G, Glennow C. Once daily inhalation of budesonide in the treatment of chronic asthma: a clinical comparison. *Ann Allergy Asthma Immunol* 1985; **55**:49–51.

228 Svendsen UG, Frolund L, Heinig JH, Madsen F, Nielsen NH, Weeke B. High-dose inhaled steroids in the management of asthma. A comparison of the effects of budesonide and beclomethasone dipropionate on pulmonary function, symptoms, bronchial responsiveness and the adrenal function. *Allergy* 1992; **47**:174–80.

229 Svendsen UG, Frolund L, Heinig JH, Madsen F, Nielsen NH, Weeke B. [High dose inhaled steroids in the treatment of bronchial asthma. A comparison of the effects of budesonide and beclomethasone dipropionate on pulmonary function, symptoms, bronchial reactivity and adrenocortical function]. *Ugeskr Laeger* 1993; **155**:2197–202.

230 Tjwa MK. Budesonide inhaled via Turbuhaler: a more effective treatment for asthma than beclomethasone dipropionate via Rotahaler. *Ann Allergy Asthma Immunol* 1995; **75**:107–11.

231 Willey RF, Godden DJ, Carmichael J, Preston P, Frame MH, Crompton GK. Twice daily inhalation of a new corticosteroid, budesonide, in the treatment of chronic asthma. *Eur J Respir Dis — Suppl* 1982; **122**:138–42.

232 Lundback B, Alexander M, Day J *et al*. Evaluation of fluticasone propionate (500 micrograms day^{-1}) administered either as dry powder via a Diskhaler inhaler or pressurized inhaler and compared with beclomethasone dipropionate (1000 micrograms day^{-1}) administered by pressurized inhaler. *Respir Med* 1993; **87**:609–20.

233 Agertoft L, Pedersen S. A randomized, double-blind dose reduction study to compare the minimal effective dose of budesonide Turbuhaler and fluticasone propionate Diskhaler. *J Allergy Clin Immunol* 1997; **99**:773–80.

234 Barnes NC, Marone G, Di Maria GU, Visser S, Utama I, Payne SL. A comparison of fluticasone propionate, 1 mg daily, with beclomethasone dipropionate, 2 mg daily, in the treatment of severe asthma. International Study Group. *Eur Respir J* 1993; **6**:877–85.

235 Basran G, Campbell M, Knox A *et al*. An open study comparing equal doses of budesonide via Turbohaler with fluticasone propionate via

Diskhaler in the treatment of adult asthmatic patients. *Eur J Clin Res* 1997; **9**:185–97.

236 Gibson P, Rutherford C, Price M, Lindsay P. Comparison of the quality of life differences in severe asthma after treatment with beclomethasone dipropionate or budesonide and fluticasone propionate at approximately half the microgram dose. *Eur Respir J* 1998; **12**:35S.

237 Berend N. A six month comparison of the efficacy of high dose fluticasone propionate (FP) with beclomethasone dipropionate (BDP) and budesonide (BUD) in adults with severe asthma. *Eur Respir J* 1997; **10**:105S.

238 Jenkins C. High dose inhaled steroids and skin bruising. *Eur Respir J* 1998; **12**:435S.

239 Bisca N. Comparison of fluticasone propionate with beclomethasone dipropionate in moderate to severe childhood asthma. *Eur Respir J* 1997; **10**:219S.

240 Boe J, Bakke P, Rodolen T, Skovlund E, Gulsvik A. High-dose inhaled steroids in asthmatics: moderate efficacy gain and suppression of the hypothalamic–pituitary–adrenal (HPA) axis. *Eur Respir J* 1994; **7**:2179–84.

241 Bootsma GP, Dekhuijzen PN, Festen J, Mulder PG, van Herwaarden CL. Comparison of fluticasone propionate and beclomethasone dipropionate on direct and indirect measurements of bronchial hyperresponsiveness in patients with stable asthma. *Thorax* 1995; **50**:1044–50.

242 Bootsma GP, Dekhuijzen PN, Festen J, Mulder PG, Swinkels LM, van Herwaarden CL. Fluticasone propionate does not influence bone metabolism in contrast to beclomethasone dipropionate. *Am J Respir Crit Care Med* 1996; **153**:924–30.

243 Bootsma GP, Koenderman L, Dekhuijzen PN, Festen J, Lammers JW, van Herwaarden CL. Effects of fluticasone propionate and beclomethasone dipropionate on parameters of inflammation in peripheral blood of patients with asthma. *Allergy* 1998; **53**:653–61.

244 Connolly A. A comparison of fluticasone propionate 100 mcg twice daily with budesonide 200 mcg twice daily via their respective powder devices in the treatment of mild asthma. *Eur J Clin Res* 1995; **7**:15–29.

245 Dal Negro R, Micheletto C, Turco P, Pomari C. Fluticasone prop. 500 mcg, budesonide 800 mcg, and beclomethasone dip. 1000 mcg: different protection degrees against the methacholine-induced bronchoconstriction. *Am J Respir Crit Care Med* 1997; **155**:A153.

246 de Benedictis FM, Medley HV, Williams L. Long-term study to compare safety and efficacy of fluticasone propionate (FP) with beclomethasone dipropionate (BDP) in asthmatic children. *Eur Respir J* 1998; **12**:142S.

247 Fabbri L, Burge PS, Croonenborgh L *et al.* Comparison of fluticasone propionate with beclomethasone dipropionate in moderate to severe asthma treated for one year. *Thorax* 1993; **48**:817–23.

248 Payne SL, Thwaites RMA, Collins N. Estimation from clinical trial data of direct costs associated with asthma exacerbations treated in hospital. *Eur Respir J* 1997; **10**:106S.

249 Ferguson AC, Spier S, Manjra A, Versteegh FG, Mark S, Zhang P. Efficacy and safety of high-dose inhaled steroids in children with asthma: a comparison of fluticasone propionate with budesonide. *J Pediatr* 1999; **134**:422–7.

250 Manjra AI, Versteegh FGA, Mehra S, Zhang P, Mark S. Clinical equivalence of fluticasone propionate (FP) 400 mcg daily via the Diskus inhaler and budesonide (B) 800 mcg daily via the Turbuhaler in asthmatic children. *Eur Respir J* 1998; **12**:87S.

251 Fitzgerald D, Van Asperen P, Mellis C, Honner M, Smith L, Ambler G. Fluticasone propionate 750 micrograms/day versus beclomethasone dipropionate 1500 micrograms/day: comparison of efficacy and adrenal function in paediatric asthma. *Thorax* 1998; **53**:656–61.

252 Gustafsson P, Tsanakas J, Gold M, Primhak R, Radford M, Gillies E. Comparison of the efficacy and safety of inhaled fluticasone propionate 200 micrograms/day with inhaled beclomethasone dipropionate 400 micrograms/day in mild and moderate asthma. *Arch Dis Child* 1993; **69**:206–11.

253 Hoekx JC, Hedlin G, Pedersen W, Sorva R, Hollingworth K, Efthimiou J. Fluticasone propionate compared with budesonide: a double-blind trial in asthmatic children using powder devices at a dosage of 400 microg day$(^{-1})$. *Eur Respir J* 1996; **9**:2263–72.

254 Hughes GL, Edelman J, Turpin J *et al.* Randomized, open-label pilot study comparing the effects of montelukast sodium tablets, fluticasone aerosol inhaler and budesonide dry powder inhaler on asthma control in mild asthmatics. *Am J Respir Crit Care Med* 1999; **159**: A641.

255 Hughes JA, Conry BG, Male SM, Eastell R. One year prospective open study of the effect of high dose inhaled steroids, fluticasone propionate, and budesonide on bone markers and bone mineral density. *Thorax* 1999; **54**:223–9.

256 Johansson LO. A comparison of once-daily regimen of fluticasone propionate (FP) 200 mcg and budesonide (BUD) 400 mcg twice-daily regimen of fluticasone (FP) 100 mcg. *Am J Respir Crit Care Med* 1998; **157**:A404.

257 Johansson LO. A comparison of once-daily regimen of fluticasone propionate (FP) 200 mcg and budesonide (BUD) 400 mcg and twice-daily regimen of fluticasone propionate (FP) 100 mcg. *Eur Respir J* 1998; **12**:38S.

258 Joubert J, Boszormenyi G, Sanchis J, Siafakas N. A comparison of the efficacy and systemic activity of budesonide and fluticasone propionate in asthmatic patients. *Eur Respir J* 1998; **12**:37S.

259 Kemmerich B, Bruckner OJ, Petro W. Superiority of fluticasone powder from the Diskus over budesonide from the Turbuhaler in mild and moderate asthma. *Am J Respir Crit Care Med* 1999; **159**:A627.

260 Langdon CG, Capsey LJ. Fluticasone propionate and budesonide in adult asthmatics: a comparison using dry-powder inhaler devices. *Br J Clin Res* 1994; **5**:85–99.

261 Booth PC, Capsey LJ, Langdon CG, Wells NEJ. A comparison of the cost-effectiveness of alternative prophylactic therapies in the treatment of adult asthma. *Br J Med Econ* 1995; **8**:65–72.

262 Langdon CG, Thompson J. A multicentre study to compare the efficacy and safety of inhaled fluticasone propionate and budesonide via metered-dose inhalers in adults with mild-to-moderate asthma. *Br J Clin Res* 1994; **5**:73–84.

263 Leblanc P, Mink S, Keistinen T, Saarelainen PA, Ringdal N, Payne SL. A comparison of fluticasone propionate 200 micrograms/day with beclomethasone dipropionate 400 micrograms/day in adult asthma. *Allergy* 1994; **49**:380–5.

264 Lorentzen KA, Van Helmond JL, Bauer K, Langaker KE, Bonifazi F, Harris TA. Fluticasone propionate 1 mg daily and beclomethasone dipropionate 2 mg daily: a comparison over 1 yr. *Respir Med* 1996; **90**:609–17.

265 Lundback B, Sandstrom T, Ekstrom T, Hermansson BA, Alton M, Tunsater A. Comparison of the oral corticosteroid sparing effect of inhaled fluticasone propionate (FP) 750 mcg bd via the Diskhaler with budesonide (BUD) 800 mcg bd via the Turbuhaler in patients with chronic severe asthma. *Am J Respir Crit Care Med* 1998; **157**: A456.

266 Malo JL, Cartier A, Ghezzo H *et al.* Skin bruising, adrenal function and markers of bone metabolism in asthmatics using inhaled beclomethasone and fluticasone. *Eur Respir J* 1999; **13**:993–8.

267 Melaranci C. Fluticasone propionate vs beclomethasone dipropionate in pediatric patients with moderate asthma. *Am J Respir Crit Care Med* 1999; **159**:A631.

268 Murray JJ, Friedman B, Chervinsky P *et al.* Fluticasone propionate

(FP) is more effective than higher doses of beclomethasone dipropionate (BDP) in patients with moderate asthma. *Am J Respir Crit Care Med* 1998; **157**:A407.

269 Pauwels RA, Yernault JC, Demedts MG, Geusens P. Safety and efficacy of fluticasone and beclomethasone in moderate to severe asthma. Belgian Multicenter Study Group. *Am J Respir Crit Care Med* 1998; **157**:827–32.

270 Pickering CAC, Backman R, Baumgarten C, Huskisson SC. Fluticasone propionate 250 mcg bd compared to budesonide 600 mcg bd in adult asthmatics. *Eur Respir J* 1996; **9**:79S.

271 Backman R, Pickering CAC, Baumgarten C, Huskisson SC. A comparison of fluticasone propionate via Diskus (Accuhaler) inhaler and budesonide via Turbuhaler inhaler in adult asthmatics. *J Allergy Clin Immunol* 1997; **249**:249.

272 Rao R, Gregson RK, Jones AC, Miles EA, Campbell MJ, Warner JO. Systemic effects of inhaled corticosteroids on growth and bone turnover in childhood asthma: a comparison of fluticasone with beclomethasone. *Eur Respir J* 1999; **13**:87–94.

273 Gregson RK, Rao R, Murrills AJ, Taylor PA, Warner JO. Effect of inhaled corticosteroids on bone mineral density in childhood asthma: comparison of fluticasone propionate with beclomethasone dipropionate. *Osteoporos Int* 1998; **8**:418–22.

274 Ringdal N, Swinburn P, Backman R *et al.* A blinded comparison of fluticasone propionate with budesonide via powder devices in adult patients with moderate-to-severe asthma: a clinical evaluation. *Mediators Inflamm* 1996; **5**:382–9.

275 Ringdal N, Lundback B, Alton M *et al.* Comparison of the effect on HPA-axis of inhaled fluticasone propionate (FP) 1500 mcg/day via Diskus and budesonide (BUD) 1600 mcg/day via Turbuhaler in adult asthmatic patients. *Am J Respir Crit Care Med* 1998; **157**:A406.

276 Ringdal N, Lundback B, Alton M *et al.* Comparison of the effect on HPA-axis of inhaled fluticasone propionate (FP) 1500 mcg/day via Diskus and budesonide (BUD) 1600 mcg/day via Turbuhaler in adult asthmatic patients. *Eur Respir J* 1998; **12**:37S.

277 Steinmetz KO. [Vergleich der Wirksamkeit und Verträglichkeit von fluticasonpropionat-dosieraerosol und budesonid-pulverinhalat bei mittelschwerem asthma]. *Atemwegs Lungenkrankheiten* 1997; **23**:730–5.

278 Steinmetz KO, Trautmann M. Efficacy of fluticasone propionate (0.5 mg daily) via MDI and budesonide (1.2 mg daily) via Turbuhaler in the treatment of steroid-naïve asthmatics. *Am J Respir Crit Care Med* 1996; **153**:A338.

279 Steinmetz KO, Volmer T, Trautmann M, Kielhorn A. Cost effectiveness of fluticasone and budesonide in patients with moderate asthma. *Clin Drug Invest* 1998; **16**:117–23.

280 Williams J, Richards KA. Ease of handling and clinical efficacy of fluticasone propionate Accuhaler/Diskus inhaler compared with the Turbohaler inhaler in paediatric patients. *Br J Clin Pract* 1997; **51**:147–53.

281 Wolthers OD, Hansen M, Juul A, Nielsen HK, Pedersen S. Knemometry, urine cortisol excretion, and measures of insulin-like growth factor axis and collagen turnover in children treated with inhaled glucocorticosteroids. *Pediatr Res* 1997; **41**:44–50.

282 Yiallouros PK, Milner AD, Conway E, Honour JW. Adrenal function and high dose inhaled corticosteroids for asthma. *Arch Dis Child* 1997; **76**:405–10.

283 Cockcroft DW, Swystun VA. Asthma control versus asthma severity. *J Allergy Clin Immunol* 1996; **98**:1016–8.

284 Colice GL. Categorizing asthma severity and monitoring control of chronic asthma. *Curr Opin Pulm Med* 2002; **8**:4–8.

285 Shapiro G, Bronsky EA, LaForce CF *et al.* Dose-related efficacy of budesonide administered via a dry powder inhaler in the treatment of children with moderate to severe persistent asthma. *J Pediatr* 1998; **132**:976–82.

286 Santanello NC, Zhang J, Seidenberg B, Reiss TF, Barber BL. What are minimal important changes for asthma measures in a clinical trial? *Eur Respir J* 1999; **14**:23–7.

287 Bergner M, Rothman ML. Health status measures: an overview and guide for selection. *Annu Rev Public Health* 1987; **8**:191–210.

288 Guyatt GH, Feeny DH, Patrick DL. Measuring health-related quality of life. *Ann Intern Med* 1993; **118**:622–9.

289 Santanello NC, Barber BL, Reiss TF, Friedman BS, Juniper EF, Zhang J. Measurement characteristics of two asthma symptom diary scales for use in clinical trials. *Eur Respir J* 1997; **10**:646–51.

290 Wasserfallen JB, Gold K, Schulman KA, Baraniuk JN. Development and validation of a rhinoconjunctivitis and asthma symptom score for use as an outcome measure in clinical trials. *J Allergy Clin Immunol* 1997; **100**:16–22.

291 Matthews JNS. Some special designs: crossovers, equivalence and clusters. In: *An Introduction to Randomized Controlled Clinical Trials*, London, Arnold, 2000. pp. 121–37.

292 Clark DJ, Clark RA, Lipworth BJ. Adrenal suppression with inhaled budesonide and fluticasone propionate given by large volume spacer to asthmatic children. *Thorax* 1996; **51**:941–3.

293 Clark DJ, Grove A, Cargill RI, Lipworth BJ. Comparative adrenal suppression with inhaled budesonide and fluticasone propionate in adult asthmatic patients. *Thorax* 1996; **51**:262–6.

294 Wilson AM, Clark DJ, Devlin MM, McFarlane LC, Lipworth BJ. Adrenocortical activity with repeated administration of once-daily inhaled fluticasone propionate and budesonide in asthmatic adults. *Eur J Clin Pharmacol* 1998; **53**:317–20.

295 Lipworth BJ. Systemic adverse effects of inhaled corticosteroid therapy. A systematic review and meta-analysis. *Arch Intern Med* 1999; **159**:941–55.

296 Lonnebo A, Grahnen A, Jansson B, Bruden RM, Ling-Andersson A. An assessment of the systemic effects of single repeated doses of inhaled fluticasone propionate, and inhaled budesonide in healthy volunteers. *Eur J Clin Pharmacol* 1996; **49**:459–63.

CHAPTER 2.4

Anti-leukotrienes

Francine M Ducharme

Introduction

Cysteinyl leukotrienes are important inflammatory mediators that have been shown to have a critical role in asthma. They stimulate the production of airway mucus secretions, cause microvascular leakage and enhance eosinophilic migration in the airways, causing oedema and bronchopasm.[1]

In the 1990s, several anti-leukotrienes were developed as a novel therapy primarily for asthma. This new class of anti-inflammatory agents interferes directly with leukotriene production (5-lipoxygenase inhibitors) or receptors (leukotriene receptor antagonists) in the arachidonic acid pathway.[2] The 5-lipoxygenase inhibitor, zileuton (marketed by Ono in Japan and by Ultair elsewhere), blocks the conversion of the arachidonic acid into 5-HPETE prior to its transformation in cysteine LTA_4. Leukotriene receptor antagonists (montelukast, pranlukast and zafirlukast) block the receptors for the cysteinyl leukotrienes C_4, D_4 and E_4 leukotrienes. Anti-leukotriene agents have the advantage of being administered orally in a single or twice-daily dose. They are therefore promising anti-inflammatory drugs in the treatment of asthma.

There are two main ways in which the anti-leukotriene agents may be used in the treatment of asthma: as *monotherapy* or as *adjunct therapy* to inhaled glucocorticoids. Using the Cochrane Library of Systematic Reviews, these roles are examined, particularly with regard to five specific clinical questions.

Questions

Monotherapy
1. Should anti-leukotrienes be considered as monotherapy for asthma instead of inhaled glucocorticoids?

Adjunct therapy to inhaled glucocorticoids
2. What is the glucocorticoid-sparing effect of adding anti-leukotrienes to inhaled glucocorticoids in well-controlled asthmatics?

In asthmatics who are poorly controlled on their current inhaled glucocorticoid regimen, what are the relative risks and benefits of adding anti-leukotrienes compared with:

3. Placebo?
4. Doubling the dose of inhaled glucocorticoids?
5. Adding a long-acting β_2-agonist?

The efficacy of anti-leukotrienes was assessed by the relative risk (RR) of moderate exacerbations, that is those requiring systemic glucocorticoids (main outcome), and the relative risk of withdrawals due to poor asthma control; the weighted mean difference (WMD) served to compare the change from baseline in lung function (FEV_1, peak expiratory flow), use of rescue β_2-agonists and symptoms. Safety was assessed by the relative risk of overall and specific adverse events, overall withdrawals and withdrawals due to adverse events. All estimates are reported with 95% confidence intervals (CI). Homogeneity of effect sizes between studies being pooled was tested by the DerSimonian and Laird method, with $P < 0.05$ being used as the cut-off level for significance.[3] If heterogeneity was suggested, the DerSimonian and Laird random effects model was reported and applied to the summary estimates. The fail-safe N test was used to assess the robustness of the results.[4] The dose of inhaled glucocorticoids was reported in µg of chlorofluorocarbon (CFC)-propelled beclomethasone dipropionate or equivalent, where 1 µg of CFC-propelled beclomethasone = 0.5 µg of hydrofluoroalkane (HFA)-propelled beclomethasone dipropionate = 0.5 µg of fluticasone propionate = 1 µg of budesonide = 2 µg of triamcinolone or flunisolide.[5] Doses were reported ex-valve rather than ex-canister with no conversion based on delivery device used.

Anti-leukotrienes versus inhaled glucocorticoids as monotherapy

Should anti-leukotrienes be considered as monotherapy for asthma instead of inhaled glucocorticoids? Which patients are more likely to benefit from anti-leukotrienes? What is the dose of inhaled glucocorticoids equivalent to the clinical effect of anti-leukotrienes? Are there any safety issues?

Data source
The safety and efficacy of anti-leukotrienes as monotherapy were compared with inhaled glucocorticoids in a systematic review of 20 adult randomized controlled trials (RCTs), identified by August 2003.[6] Seventeen trials were published in full text,[7–23] whereas three were published as abstracts with additional unpublished data provided by authors.[24–26]

All but one trial[13] had a parallel group design, and most (11/20) were of high methodological quality. The trials were

Table 1. Characteristics of included trials comparing anti-leukotrienes with inhaled glucocorticoids as monotherapy.

Trials	Patient no.	Publication status	Mean age (years)	% Male	Baseline FEV$_1$ (mean % predicted)	% Atopy	Anti-leukotrienes Drug	Anti-leukotrienes Dose	Inhaled glucocorticoids Drug†	Inhaled glucocorticoids Dose	Duration of treatment (weeks)	Intention-to-treat analyses
Baumgartner et al.[7]	730	+	36	35	68	68	Montelukast	10 mg once daily	Beclomethasone dipropionate	200 µg twice daily	6	+
Bleecker et al.[8]	451	+	31	50	68	45	Zafirlukast	20 mg twice daily	Fluticasone propionate	100 µg twice daily	12	+
Brabson et al.[9]	440	+	35	38	73	NR	Zafirlukast	20 mg twice daily	Fluticasone propionate	100 µg twice daily	6	+
Busse et al.[10]	533	+	35	45	65	NR	Montelukast	10 mg once daily	Fluticasone propionate	100 µg twice daily	24	+
Busse et al.[11]	224	+	32	50	68	32	Zafirlukast	20 mg twice daily	Fluticasone propionate	100 µg twice daily	12	+
Hughes et al.[24]	71	–	30	48	84	87	Montelukast	10 mg once daily	Budesonide	400 µg/day	4	+
							Montelukast	10 mg once daily	Fluticasone propionate	100 µg twice daily	4	+
Israel et al.[12]	671	+	33	48	66	NR	Montelukast	10 mg once daily	Beclomethasone dipropionate	200 µg twice daily	6	+
Kanniess et al.[13]*	40	+	37	60	74	100	Montelukast	10 mg once daily	Fluticasone propionate	100 µg twice daily	4	–
Kim et al.[14]	437	+	34	40	74	57	Zafirlukast	20 mg twice daily	Fluticasone propionate	100 µg twice daily	6	+
Laitinen et al.[25]	481	–	38	51	80	54	Zafirlukast	20 mg twice daily	Beclomethasone dipropionate	200–250 µg twice daily	6	–
Laviolette et al.[15]	401	+	39	50	72	74	Montelukast	10 mg once daily	Beclomethasone dipropionate	200 µg twice daily	16	+
Malmstrom et al.[16]	638	+	35	38	65	62	Montelukast	10 mg once daily	Beclomethasone dipropionate	200 µg twice daily	12	+
Meltzer et al.[17]	522	+	36	46	66	NR	Montelukast	10 mg once daily	Fluticasone propionate	100 µg twice daily	24	+
Nathan et al.[18]	294	+	32	44	68	NR	Zafirlukast	20 mg twice daily	Fluticasone propionate	100 µg twice daily	4	–
Riccioni et al.[20]	30	+	27	57	97	100	Montelukast	10 mg once daily	Budesonide	400 µg twice daily	16	–
Riccioni et al.[21]	40	+	25	53	94	55	Montelukast	10 mg once daily	Budesonide	400 µg twice daily	16	–
Riccioni et al.[19]	24	+	33	50	93	NR	Zafirlukast	20 mg twice daily	Budesonide	400 µg twice daily	8	–
Williams et al.[22]	436	+	37	38	NR	63	Montelukast	10 mg once daily	Beclomethasone dipropionate	200 µg twice daily	37	+
Yamauchi et al.[23]	20	+	41	65	92	60	Pranlukast	450 mg once daily	Beclomethasone dipropionate	400 µg/day	4	NR
Edelman et al.[26]	400	–	35	30	93	NR	Montelukast	10 mg once daily	Fluticasone propionate	100 µg twice daily	12	NR

NR, not reported.

*Crossover trial.

†Beclomethasone was propelled by chlorofluorocarbon (CFC); no trial used hydrofluorocarbon (HFA) as propellant.

Table modified from *BMJ* 2003; 326:621, and reproduced with the permission of the *British Medical Journal*.

Patients with exacerbations requiring systemic glucocorticoids

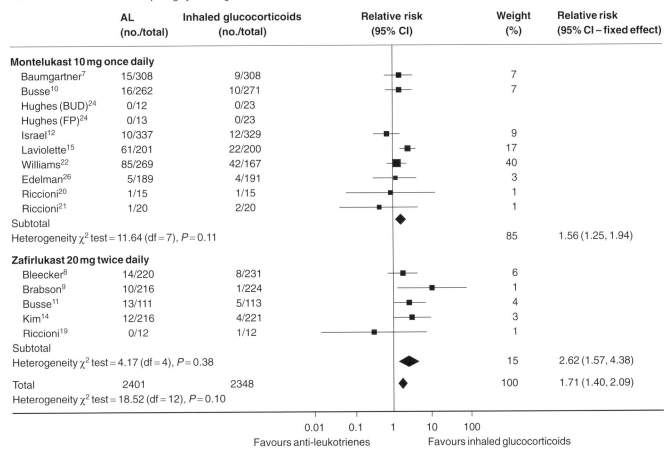

	AL (no./total)	Inhaled glucocorticoids (no./total)	Relative risk (95% CI)	Weight (%)	Relative risk (95% CI – fixed effect)
Montelukast 10 mg once daily					
Baumgartner[7]	15/308	9/308		7	
Busse[10]	16/262	10/271		7	
Hughes (BUD)[24]	0/12	0/23			
Hughes (FP)[24]	0/13	0/23			
Israel[12]	10/337	12/329		9	
Laviolette[15]	61/201	22/200		17	
Williams[22]	85/269	42/167		40	
Edelman[26]	5/189	4/191		3	
Riccioni[20]	1/15	1/15		1	
Riccioni[21]	1/20	2/20		1	
Subtotal					
Heterogeneity χ^2 test = 11.64 (df = 7), P = 0.11				85	1.56 (1.25, 1.94)
Zafirlukast 20 mg twice daily					
Bleecker[8]	14/220	8/231		6	
Brabson[9]	10/216	1/224		1	
Busse[11]	13/111	5/113		4	
Kim[14]	12/216	4/221		3	
Riccioni[19]	0/12	1/12		1	
Subtotal					
Heterogeneity χ^2 test = 4.17 (df = 4), P = 0.38				15	2.62 (1.57, 4.38)
Total	2401	2348		100	1.71 (1.40, 2.09)
Heterogeneity χ^2 test = 18.52 (df = 12), P = 0.10					

0.01　0.1　1　10　100

Favours anti-leukotrienes　　　Favours inhaled glucocorticoids

Figure 1.　Pooled relative risk of patients experiencing at least one exacerbation requiring systemic glucocorticoids comparing anti-leukotriene (AL) with inhaled glucocorticoids (ICS). Trials are stratified on the leukotriene receptor antagonist used. Hughes' trial tested two inhaled glucocorticoid preparations, 400 μg of budesonide (BUD) and 200 μg of fluticasone propionate (FP), against montelukast. To prevent over-representation of the LTRA group, the 25 participants in the montelukast group were reduced by half for the analysis. Figure modified from *BMJ* 2003; 326:621 and reproduced with the permission of the *British Medical Journal*.

relatively similar in the age and gender of participants (Table 1). Severity of airway obstruction on baseline was moderate (50% < FEV$_1$ < 80%) in 12 trials, mild (FEV$_1$ ≥ 80%) in seven trials and unspecified in the remaining trial. Duration of treatment varied between 4 and 37 weeks. Most trials compared leukotriene receptor antagonists at licensed doses with a low daily dose of inhaled glucocorticoids (i.e. 400 μg/day beclomethasone or equivalent).

Results

Adults treated with leukotriene receptor antagonists were 71% more likely to experience an exacerbation requiring systemic glucocorticoids compared with those treated with 400 μg/day beclomethasone dipropionate or equivalent (RR 1.71, 95% CI 1.4–2.1; fixed effect models) (Fig. 1). Trials were relatively homogeneous in their results with no major impact on findings of the type of leukotriene receptor antagonist, the inhaled glucocorticoid preparation, the baseline severity (mild versus

moderate) or methodological quality. Only the duration of intervention correlated with an increased protective effect of inhaled glucocorticoids. The number needed to treat (NNT) with inhaled glucocorticoids instead of leukotriene receptor antagonists to prevent one moderate exacerbation was 25 (95% CI 20–50). The robustness of this finding was supported by a fail-safe N of 110 trials, i.e. 110 additional trials with null results would be needed to reverse the current finding.[4]

The superiority of inhaled glucocorticoids was also evident within 4–6 weeks of treatment for all secondary outcomes. Patients treated with inhaled glucocorticoids had a significantly greater improvement from baseline in the change in forced expired volume in 1 second (FEV$_1$) (WMD = 120 mL, 95% CI 90–150), morning peak expiratory flow (PEF) (WMD = 19 L/min, 95% CI 15–23) and symptom-free days (WMD = 9%, 95% CI 7–13) with less requirement for rescue β$_2$-agonists (WMD = –0.28 puffs/day, 95% CI –0.20 to –0.36) than the group treated with leukotriene receptor antagonist.

Leukotriene receptor antagonist therapy was associated with an increased risk of withdrawal due to poor asthma control ($N = 12$ trials; RR $= 2.6$, 95% CI 2.0–3.4).

There was no group difference in the number of patients who experienced 'any adverse effects' ($N = 11$ trials; RR $= 0.99$, 95% CI 0.94–1.05), meeting the definition of equivalence. No group difference was noted for liver enzyme elevation, headache, oral candidiasis, nausea and death. Rare adverse effects such as the Churg–Strauss syndrome were not reported. Adverse effects typically associated with inhaled glucocorticoids (such as osteopenia and adrenal suppression) were not measured, preventing a fair comparison of the safety profile on long-term use.

Conclusion

In adult asthmatics with mild to moderate asthma, use of leukotriene receptor antagonists (LTRA) as monotherapy is safe but less effective than low-dose inhaled glucocorticoids in preventing asthma exacerbations and maintaining asthma control. Characteristics of patients who are more or less likely to benefit from LTRA have not been identified. Although the exact dose equivalence of LTRA remains elusive, 400 µg/day beclomethasone or 200 µg/day fluticasone propionate is clearly superior to 10 mg/day montelukast or 20 mg twice daily of zafirlukast. At present, the scientific evidence does not support the substitution of LTRA for inhaled glucocorticoids, which remain the first-line therapy for asthma.

Corticosteroid-sparing effect of anti-leukotrienes in well-controlled asthmatics

Question

In adult asthmatics, well controlled on their current inhaled glucocorticoid regimen, by how much can we taper the dose of inhaled glucocorticoids by adding an anti-leukotriene agent while maintaining asthma control?

Data source

A Cochrane Review considered this question.[27] Six trials[28–33] were pooled; they examined the corticosteroid-sparing effect of leukotriene receptor antagonists in adult asthmatics with no baseline airway obstruction on their current regimen of inhaled glucocorticoid (Table 2).

Only two[30,31] of the six trials had a dose optimization period prior to randomization, during which the maintenance dose of inhaled glucocorticoids was tapered over a period of 2 weeks to 3 months. Of interest, the dose optimization allowed tapering of inhaled glucocorticoids by 500–600 µg/day prior to randomization; furthermore, a similar reduction was achieved in the placebo group after randomization.[31] Licensed doses of montelukast or zafirlukast were added to doses of inhaled glucocorticoids varying from 300 to 3000 µg/day beclomethasone dipropionate or equivalent. Four trials tested montelukast 10 mg once daily and two trials examined zafirlukast 20 mg twice daily for 6–24 weeks, during which the dose of inhaled glucocorticoids was tapered to the minimum effective dose.

Results

The data from four of the six trials provided sufficient details to determine the glucocorticoid-sparing effect of leukotriene receptor antagonists.[28,30,31,33] In adults well controlled on various doses of inhaled glucocorticoids, the addition of leukotriene receptor antagonists for 12–24 weeks of treatment did not achieve a greater percentage reduction in inhaled glucocorticoids than placebo (WMD $= 3$%, 95% CI -7 to 2). When the lowest tolerated dose of inhaled glucocorticoids was considered, no meaningful group difference was observed either (WMD $= -21$ µg/day, 95% CI -65 to 23) (Fig. 2). The results were consistent across trials, although their design varied not only in the leukotriene receptor antagonist used but also in the baseline dose and the inhaled glucocorticoids used, the dose optimization period, the weaning protocol and the use of intention-to-treat analysis. The rate of complete glucocorticoids weaning was similar between groups (RR $= 1.18$, 95% CI 0.95–1.47).

To establish the overall or relative efficacy of leukotriene receptor antagonists, the level of asthma control achieved after glucocorticoid tapering must be similar among groups. Yet, patients treated with leukotriene receptor antagonists appeared to have better control than the placebo group, with a 37% reduction in rate of withdrawals due to poor asthma control ($N = 5$ trials, RR $= 0.63$, 95% CI 0.42–0.95).

There was no group difference in the rate of overall withdrawals, withdrawals due to adverse effects, elevated liver enzymes, headache or nausea. The similarity between groups in the number of overall adverse effects met our definition of equivalence ($N = 4$ trials: RR $= 0.98$, 95% CI 0.91–1.05).

Conclusion

In well-controlled patients, the addition of leukotriene receptor antagonists is probably associated with superior asthma control after inhaled glucocorticoid tapering, but there is insufficient evidence to quantify the glucocorticoid-sparing effect. Assuming similar asthma control after tapering, the maximal glucocorticoid-sparing effect of leukotriene receptor antagonists, based on the upper confidence limit for either leukotriene receptor antagonist used, would probably be about 200 µg/day beclomethasone dipropionate or equivalent. Clearly, the magnitude of glucocorticoid dose reduction achievable prior to randomization and in the placebo group without any co-treatment outweighs the reduction demonstrated to date with leukotriene receptor antagonists.

Table 2. Characteristics of trials comparing anti-leukotrienes versus placebo as add-on to tapering doses of inhaled glucocorticoids.

Trials	Design	Patient no.	Publication status	Mean age (years)	% Male	Baseline FEV$_1$ (mean % predicted)	Dose optimization prior to randomization	Anti-leukotrienes Drug	Anti-leukotrienes Dose	Inhaled glucocorticoids Drug	Intervention group dose (μg)	Control group dose (μg)	Duration of treatment (weeks)	Intention-to-treat analyses
Bateman et al.[28]	Parallel group	359	−	42	45	2.6 L	0	Z	20 mg twice daily	BDP or BUD	400–750	400–750	20	+
Kanniess et al.[29]	Crossover	50	+	40	48	93	0	M	10 mg once daily	BDP or equivalent	400	400	6	+
Laitinen et al.[30]	Parallel group	262	−	44	42	2.5 L	2 weeks–3 months	Z	20 mg twice daily	BDP or BUD	800–2000	800–2000	12	−
Lofdahl et al.[31]	Parallel group	226	+	40	43	83	≤7 weeks	M	10 mg once daily	Various§	300–3000	300–3000	12	+
Shingo et al.[32]	Parallel group	22	+	39	41	84	0	M	10 mg once daily	Various§§	1600	1350	8	+
Tohda et al.[33]	Parallel group	191	+	52	58	86	0	M	10 mg once daily	BDP	945±283	908±240	24	−

Anti-leukotrienes: montelukast (M); zafirlukast (Z).

Inhaled glucocorticoids: beclomethasone (BDP); budesonide (BUD); no trial used hydrofluorocarbon (HFA) as propellant.

Table modified from *BMJ* 2002; 324:1545–52, and reproduced with permission of the *British Medical Journal*.

§Reported use of beclomethasone dipropionate (16%), budesonide (22%), flunisoline (15%), fluticasone propionate (7%) and triamcinolone acidonide (40%). The dose reduction of ICS was not reported as μg of chloroflorocarbone-propelled beclomethasone dipropionate or equivalent (Theodore Reiss, personal communication, 2000)

§§Reported use of triamcinolone acidonide (72%), flunisoline (18%) and beclomethasone dipropionate (9%).

Lowest tolerated dose (μg) of inhaled glucocorticoids after 12–24 weeks of treatment

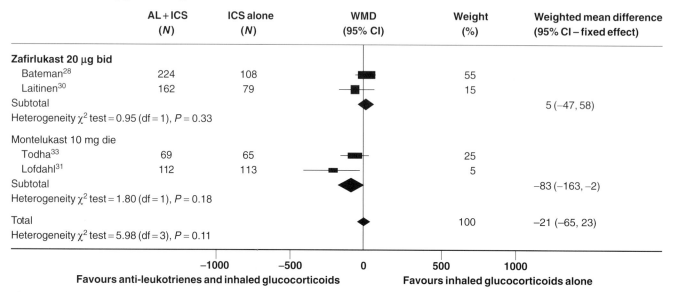

	AL + ICS (N)	ICS alone (N)	WMD (95% CI)	Weight (%)	Weighted mean difference (95% CI – fixed effect)
Zafirlukast 20 μg bid					
Bateman[28]	224	108		55	
Laitinen[30]	162	79		15	
Subtotal					5 (−47, 58)
Heterogeneity χ² test = 0.95 (df = 1), P = 0.33					
Montelukast 10 mg die					
Todha[33]	69	65		25	
Lofdahl[31]	112	113		5	
Subtotal					−83 (−163, −2)
Heterogeneity χ² test = 1.80 (df = 1), P = 0.18					
Total				100	−21 (−65, 23)
Heterogeneity χ² test = 5.98 (df = 3), P = 0.11					

−1000   −500   0   500   1000

Favours anti-leukotrienes and inhaled glucocorticoids   **Favours inhaled glucocorticoids alone**

Figure 2. Weighted mean difference of the lowest tolerated dose in μg/day inhaled glucocorticoids after tapering using anti-leukotrienes (AL) as add-on to inhaled glucocorticoids (ICS). Figure modified from *BMJ* 2002; 324:1545–52 and reproduced with the permission of the *British Medical Journal*.

Anti-leukotrienes versus placebo as add-on to inhaled glucocorticoids to improve asthma control

Question

Should anti-leukotrienes be added to inhaled glucocorticoids when asthma control is not achieved with inhaled glucocorticoids? If so, at what dose of inhaled glucocorticoids should this option be considered? What is the expected improvement in asthma control? What are the associated side-effects?

Data source

A Cochrane Review[27] addressed this issue. Seven adult trials evaluated the degree of asthma control achieved by the addition of leukotriene receptor antagonists to inhaled glucocorticoids compared with the same dose of inhaled glucocorticoids alone (Table 3).

For the seven trials[15,34–37] contributing data for the meta-analysis, the severity of airway obstruction was mild to moderate with an average FEV_1 of 64–81% of predicted at baseline in five trials, whereas it was normal in the remaining two studies. One trial[35] suddenly decreased the dose of inhaled glucocorticoids at randomization to elicit poor control. When reported, allergic triggers were identified for 46–75% of participants. Trial duration varied between 4 and 16 weeks. Five trials used licensed doses, namely montelukast 10 mg once daily and zafirlukast 20 mg twice daily; the remaining two trials used higher than licensed doses of zafirlukast (80 mg twice daily) or pranlukast (450 mg twice daily). Leukotriene receptor antagonists or placebo were added to inhaled glucocorticoids at low

dose (≤ 400 μg/day beclomethasone dipropionate or equivalent) in two trials, moderate dose (400–800 μg/day BDP equivalent) in three trials or high dose (> 800 μg/day BDP equivalent) in the remaining trial.

Results

With the addition of licensed doses of leukotriene receptor antagonists to 400–800 μg/day beclomethasone dipropionate or equivalent, a trend towards a 44% reduction in the risk of exacerbations requiring systemic glucocorticoids was observed (RR = 0.56, 95% CI 0.29–1.07). When higher than licensed doses were examined, the addition of pranlukast or zafirlukast to high doses of inhaled glucocorticoids reduced by 66% the risk of exacerbations requiring systemic glucocorticoids (RR = 0.34, 95% CI 0.13–0.88) (Fig. 3). Within each stratum, the results were homogeneous despite the different leukotriene receptor antagonists tested, baseline dose of inhaled glucocorticoids and duration of intervention.

Pooling of the five trials testing the use of licensed doses of montelukast revealed significant group differences in favour of leukotriene receptor antagonists in the improvement in FEV_1 (N = 2 trials, WMD 110 mL, 95% CI 60–150), morning PEF (N = 3 trials, WMD 7.5 L/min 95% CI 3.2–11.8) and in the reduction in β_2-agonist use (N = 2 trials, WMD = 1.5 puffs/week, 95% CI 0.35–2.5). No significant group differences were observed in symptom score, night waking or withdrawal due to poor asthma control. The intervention appeared to be safe as the addition of leukotriene receptor antagonist did not increase the risk of withdrawals due to adverse effects, or the risk of overall and specific adverse effects.

Pooling of the two trials using higher than licensed doses of

Table 3. Characteristics of trials comparing anti-leukotrienes versus placebo as add-on to inhaled glucocorticoids.

Trials	Design	Patient no.	Publication status	Mean age (years)	% Male	Baseline FEV$_1$ (mean % predicted)	Anti-leukotrienes		Inhaled glucocorticoids			Duration of treatment (weeks)	Intention-to-treat analyses
							Drug	Dose	Drug	Intervention group dose (μg)	Control group dose (μg)		
Anti-leukotrienes versus placebo as add-on to inhaled glucocorticoids													
Hultquist et al.[34]	Parallel group	352	–	38	50	72	Z	20 mg twice daily	BUD	400	400	8	+
Laviolette et al.[15]	Parallel group	393	+	40	54	72	M	10 mg once daily	BDP	400	400	16	+
Riccioni et al.[20]	Parallel group	30	+	27	47	98	M	10 mg once daily	BUD	800	800	16	–
Riccioni et al.[19]	Parallel group	24	+	33	50	92	Z	20 mg twice daily	BUD	800	800	8	–
Tamaoki et al.[35]	Parallel group	79	+	48	43	80*	P	450 mg twice daily	BDP	750	750	6	NR
Vaquerizo et al.[36]	Parallel group	639	+	43	62	81	M	10 mg once daily	BUD	800	800	16	+
Virchow et al.[37]	Parallel group	368	+	48	51	64	Z	80 mg twice daily	BDP	1598±381	1650±456	6	+
Anti-leukotrienes as add-on to inhaled glucocorticoids versus double-dose of inhaled glucocorticoids													
Nayak et al.[38]	Parallel group	394	–	39	38	67	Z	40 mg twice daily 80 mg twice daily	BDP	400	800	13	–
Price et al.[39]	Parallel group	889	+	43	40	69	M	10 mg once daily	BUD	800	1600	12	+
Ringdal et al.[40]	Parallel group	440	–	41	49	85	Z	20 mg twice daily 80 mg twice daily	BDP	400–500	800–1000	12	–
Tomari et al.[41]	Parallel group	41	+	55	41	71	P	450 mg daily	BDP	800	1600	16	+

NR, not reported.
*Reported spirometry prior to abrupt reduction by half of the maintenance dose of inhaled glucocorticoids.
Anti-leukotrienes: montelukast (M), pranlukast (P), zafirlukast (Z).
Inhaled glucocorticoids: beclomethasone (BDP); budesonide (BUD); fluticasone (F). BDP and FP were propelled by chlorofluorocarbon (CFC); no trial used hydrofluorocarbon (HFA) as propellant.
Table modified from *BMJ* 2002; 324:1545–52, and reproduced with permission of the *British Medical Journal*.

Patients with exacerbations requiring systemic steroids

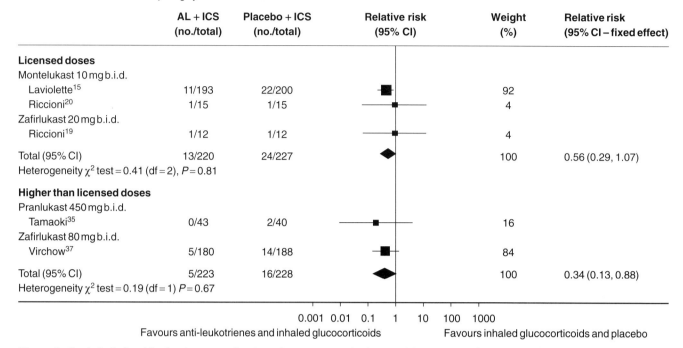

	AL + ICS (no./total)	Placebo + ICS (no./total)	Relative risk (95% CI)	Weight (%)	Relative risk (95% CI – fixed effect)
Licensed doses					
Montelukast 10 mg b.i.d.					
Laviolette[15]	11/193	22/200		92	
Riccioni[20]	1/15	1/15		4	
Zafirlukast 20 mg b.i.d.					
Riccioni[19]	1/12	1/12		4	
Total (95% CI)	13/220	24/227		100	0.56 (0.29, 1.07)
Heterogeneity χ^2 test = 0.41 (df = 2), P = 0.81					
Higher than licensed doses					
Pranlukast 450 mg b.i.d.					
Tamaoki[35]	0/43	2/40		16	
Zafirlukast 80 mg b.i.d.					
Virchow[37]	5/180	14/188		84	
Total (95% CI)	5/223	16/228		100	0.34 (0.13, 0.88)
Heterogeneity χ^2 test = 0.19 (df = 1) P = 0.67					

```
       0.001  0.01  0.1    1    10  100  1000
```
Favours anti-leukotrienes and inhaled glucocorticoids   Favours inhaled glucocorticoids and placebo

Figure 3. Pooled relative risk of patients experiencing at least one exacerbation requiring systemic glucocorticoids comparing anti-leukotrienes (AL) versus placebo as add-on to inhaled glucocorticoids (ICS). Trials are stratified on the dose and leukotriene receptor antagonist used. Figure modified from *BMJ* 2002; 324:1545–52 and reproduced with the permission of the *British Medical Journal*.

pranlukast[35] or zafirlukast[37] also revealed a significant group difference favouring leukotriene receptor antagonists in the improvement from baseline in FEV_1 (WMD 100 mL, 95% CI 10–200) and PEF (WMD 27.2 L/min, 95% CI 18.6–35.8), in the reduction in use of rescue short-acting β_2-agonists (SMD –0.43, 95% CI –0.22 to –0.63) and symptom scores (SMD –0.46, 95% CI –0.25 to –0.66). No significant group difference was observed in the change from baseline in nocturnal awakenings or withdrawals due to poor asthma control. Although there is insufficient power to conclude firmly, there was no apparent increased risk of overall or specific adverse effects.

Conclusion

In summary, when asthma control is not achieved with 400–800 μg/day beclomethasone dipropionate or equivalent, the addition of leukotriene receptor antagonists at usual doses is safe and will modestly increase asthma control, although the protective effect on asthma exacerbations remains to be confirmed. On average, this strategy should improve the FEV_1 by 110 mL, PEF by 8 L/min and reduce the use of rescue short-acting β_2-agonist by about 1.5 puffs/week. In contrast, when asthma control is not achieved on high doses of inhaled glucocorticoids, the addition to two- to four-fold the licensed dose of pranlukast or zafirlukast clearly reduces by 66% the risk of exacerbations requiring rescue glucocorticoids. However, in view of the insufficient data to conclude the safety of higher than licensed doses of leukotriene receptor antagonists, this treatment option cannot be recommended at this time.

Addition of anti-leukotrienes versus dose doubling of inhaled glucocorticoids to improve asthma control

Question

When asthma control is not achieved with low doses of inhaled glucocorticoids, a common strategy is to increase the dose of inhaled glucocorticoids. Which of the two treatment options is safest and most effective: adding anti-leukotrienes or increasing the dose of inhaled glucocorticoids? What is the dose equivalent in μg of inhaled glucocorticoids of anti-leukotrienes in this context?

Data source

A Cochrane Review[27] pooled four adult trials[38–41] comparing the addition of leukotriene receptor antagonists to inhaled glucocorticoids versus dose doubling of inhaled glucocorticoids in symptomatic patients. Licensed doses of leukotriene receptor antagonists were considered in three trials; higher than licensed doses of zafirlukast (40 mg and 80 mg twice daily) were also considered in two trials (Table 3). Participants were similar across trials in age, gender distribution and baseline airway obstruction. Trial duration was 12–16 weeks. In the intervention group, beclomethasone or budesonide was given at a dose of 400–800 μg/day while the control group received a double dose.

Patients with exacerbations requiring systemic steroids

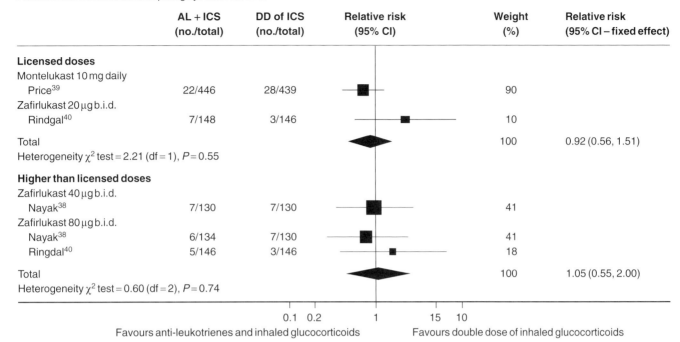

	AL + ICS (no./total)	DD of ICS (no./total)	Relative risk (95% CI)	Weight (%)	Relative risk (95% CI – fixed effect)
Licensed doses					
Montelukast 10 mg daily					
Price[39]	22/446	28/439		90	
Zafirlukast 20 µg b.i.d.					
Rindgal[40]	7/148	3/146		10	
Total				100	0.92 (0.56, 1.51)
Heterogeneity χ² test = 2.21 (df = 1), P = 0.55					
Higher than licensed doses					
Zafirlukast 40 µg b.i.d.					
Nayak[38]	7/130	7/130		41	
Zafirlukast 80 µg b.i.d.					
Nayak[38]	6/134	7/130		41	
Ringdal[40]	5/146	3/146		18	
Total				100	1.05 (0.55, 2.00)
Heterogeneity χ² test = 0.60 (df = 2), P = 0.74					

0.1 0.2   1   15 10

Favours anti-leukotrienes and inhaled glucocorticoids   Favours double dose of inhaled glucocorticoids

Figure 4. Pooled relative risk of patients experiencing at least one exacerbation requiring systemic glucocorticoids comparing anti-leukotrienes (AL) as add-on to inhaled glucocorticoids (ICS) versus double dose of inhaled glucocorticoids (DD of ICS). Trials are stratified on the dose and leukotriene receptor antagonist used. Figure modified from *BMJ* 2002; 324:1545–52 and reproduced with the permission of the *British Medical Journal*.

Results

Using licensed doses of montelukast or zafirlukast, there was no significant group difference in the risk of experiencing an asthma exacerbation requiring systemic glucocorticoids (two trials; RR 0.92, 95% CI 0.56–1.51); this finding did not meet our criteria of equivalence (Fig. 4). There was also no significant group difference in the change from baseline in morning PEF (WMD 1.56 L/min, 95% CI –5.77 to 8.89; random effect model), symptoms (SMD 0.01, 95% CI –0.09 to 0.10), use of rescue β_2-agonists (WMD –0.03 puffs/day, 95% CI –0.24 to 0.18), overall side-effects, overall withdrawals and withdrawals due to poor asthma control. The width of these confidence intervals all exceeded our definition of equivalence.

Using two- to fourfold the licensed doses of zafirlukast with 400–500 µg/day beclomethasone as opposed to doubling the dose of inhaled glucocorticoids, there was also no significant group difference in the risk of experiencing an asthma exacerbation requiring systemic glucocorticoids (N = 2 trials, RR 1.05, 95% CI 0.55–2.00); again, this finding did not meet our criteria of equivalence (Fig. 4). However, the change from baseline in FEV$_1$ reached our definition of equivalence (WMD 10 mL 95% CI –50 to 70). No significant group differences were observed in the change from baseline in morning PEF (WMD 6.05 L/min, 95% CI –1.26 to 13.36), symptoms (SMD –0.06, 95% CI –0.16 to 0.03), use of rescue β_2-agonists (WMD 0 puff/day, 95% CI –0.37 to 0.37) and in withdrawals due to poor asthma control (RR 0.72, 95% CI 0.29–1.76).

Use of higher than licensed doses of leukotriene receptor antagonist was associated with a fivefold increased risk of liver enzyme elevation (N = 3 trials, RR 4.97, 95% CI 1.45–17) but less oral candidiasis (N = 3 trials, RR 0.29, 95% CI 0.10–0.81).

Conclusion

When asthma control is not achieved with moderate to high doses of inhaled glucocorticoids, the addition of leukotriene receptor antagonists may be an alternative to doubling the dose of inhaled glucocorticoids. However, with only three trials, there are insufficient data to conclude equivalence of treatment options or to quantify the dose equivalence of anti-leukotrienes in µg/day inhaled glucocorticoids. The use of higher than licensed doses of zafirlukast is not recommended because of safety issues.

Anti-leukotrienes versus long-acting β_2-agonists as add-on to inhaled glucocorticoids

Question

In patients inadequately controlled on inhaled glucocorticoids, another option is the addition of long-acting β_2-agonists. Which of two classes of agent, anti-leukotrienes or long-acting β_2-agonists, is the safest and most effective add-on therapy to inhaled glucocorticoids? At what dose of inhaled glucocorticoids should either option be considered? Are there any characteristics that will determine a priori which patient is most likely to benefit from either option?

Data source

These questions were addressed in a recent Cochrane Review.[42] The review included seven trials, of which two trials[34,43] remained unpublished at the time of submission.[44–48] The seven included trials were quite uniform in the characteristics of enrolled participants; they all pertained to asthmatic adults with a mean age of 40 years, roughly equal gender representation and moderate airway obstruction at baseline (FEV$_1$ 66–75% of predicted) (Table 4). The proportion of participants affected by atopy, specifically allergic rhinitis, was seldom reported. Licensed doses of montelukast (10 trials) or zafirlukast (two trials) were compared with salmeterol 50 µg bid in most trials ($N=6$), while formoterol 12 µg bid was used in the remaining one. These therapies were generally added to low doses (400 µg of beclomethasone dipropionate or equivalent) for 8–12 weeks (with one trial of 48 weeks).

Results

None of the two classes of agents was clearly superior with regard to the prevention of exacerbations requiring systemic glucocorticoids, although a clinically important trend, almost reaching statistical significance, was observed in favour of long-acting β$_2$-agonist (RR 1.22, 95% CI 0.99–1.49) (Fig. 5). When reported as risk difference, patients treated with leukotriene receptor antagonists have a 2% (95% CI 0–3%) additional risk of experiencing an exacerbation compared with those treated with long-acting β$_2$-agonists. Results were relatively homogeneous across trials. There was no significant group difference, or equivalence, in the rate of withdrawals due to poor asthma control (WMD 1.11, 95% CI 0.75–1.64).

Long-acting β$_2$-agonists were more effective than leukotriene receptor antagonists in improving FEV$_1$ (WMD 90 mL, 95% CI 60–130), morning PEF (WMD 16 L/min, 95% CI 13–18), evening PEF (WMD 9 L/min, 95% CI 2–16), symptom score (SMD 0.16, 95% CI 0.08–0.24) and symptom-free days (WMD 7%, 95% CI 4–10%). Long-acting β$_2$-agonists were also superior in reducing the use of rescue fast-acting β$_2$-agonists (WMD −0.3 puffs/day, 95% CI −0.2 to −0.5).

With regard to safety, there was no group difference in the risk of withdrawals due to adverse events (RR 1.1, 95% CI 0.8–1.5), overall adverse events (RR 0.97, 95% CI 0.93–1.02), headache, cardiovascular events and oral moniliasis.

Conclusion

As expected by their nature, long-acting β$_2$-agonists were more effective than leukotriene receptor antagonists in improving

spirometry, use of rescue fast-acting β$_2$-agonists and symptoms. However, the group differences were surprisingly minor. With regard to other outcomes possibly less influenced by the nature of long-acting β$_2$-agonists, such as withdrawals due to poor asthma control, there was no significant group difference. Additional trials are needed to confirm the trend towards a 20% reduction in the risk of exacerbations requiring systemic glucocorticoids in favour of long-acting β$_2$-agonists; with only 2% fewer patients experiencing exacerbations, the apparent superiority of long-acting β$_2$-agonists appears to be quite modest. As most trials tested salmeterol 50 µg twice daily compared with montelukast 10 mg once daily, any differential effect of the long-acting β$_2$-agonist or leukotriene receptor antagonist used could not be examined. Based on current evidence, both treatment options appear to be reasonable alternatives as add-on therapy when 200 µg/day fluticasone equivalent (or equivalent) is insufficient to achieve optimal control.

Overall implications

The place of anti-leukotrienes in the therapeutic arsenal of persistent adult asthma is becoming clearer. In view of the absence of RCTs pertaining to 5-lipoxygenase inhibitors, the following conclusions apply to leukotriene receptor inhibitors, namely montelukast, pranlukast and zafirlukast.

Leukotriene receptor antagonists are mild anti-inflammatory agents with an anti-inflammatory potency equivalent to less than 400 µg/day CFC beclomethasone dipropionate or equivalent. In adults who are well controlled on very low doses of inhaled glucocorticoids, oral leukotriene receptor antagonists may serve as alternative monotherapy. In adults inadequately controlled on 400–800 µg/day CFC beclomethasone dipropionate or equivalent, the addition of leukotriene receptor antagonists brings an improvement in asthma control, but the strategy has not proved superior or equivalent to increasing the dose of inhaled glucocorticoids. As add-on therapy to inhaled glucocorticoids, long-acting β$_2$-agonists are slightly more effective than leukotriene receptor antagonists in achieving control.

In adults who are well controlled on their current regimen of inhaled glucocorticoids, careful tapering to minimal effective dose alone is the single most effective procedure in reducing the maintenance dose of inhaled glucocorticoids. Although their corticosteroid-sparing effect appears to be modest, the beneficial effect of anti-leukotrienes is suggested by the improved asthma control during steroid tapering. One must recognize that few trials were appropriately designed to assess properly the corticosteroid-sparing effect of leukotriene receptor antagonists.

Which characteristic would guide us in the selection of the best treatment strategy for our patients? The design and reporting of available RCTs are inappropriate to answer this question. Within each review, the trial participants were relatively homogeneous in their age, gender distribution, asthma

Table 4. Characteristics of trials comparing anti-leukotrienes versus long-acting β_2-agonist as add-on to inhaled glucocorticoids.

Trials	Patient no.	Publication status	Mean age (years)	% Male	Baseline FEV$_1$ (mean % predicted)	Symptoms on baseline	Anti-leukotrienes Drug	Dose	Long-acting β_2-agonists Drug†	Dose (µg)	Same inhaler as ICS	Inhaled glucocorticoids Drug	Intervention group dose (µg/day)	Control group dose (µg/day)	Duration of treatment (weeks)	Intention-to-treat analyses
Bjermer et al.[44]	1490	+	41	45	72	+	M	10 mg once daily	S	50 bid	No	FP	200	200	48	+
Fish et al.[45]	948	+	40	39	68	+	M	10 mg once daily	S	50 bid	No	Varied	545*	565*	12	+
Hultquist et al.[34]	236	–	38	48	71	+	Z	20 mg twice daily	F	12 bid	No	BUD	400	400	8	+
McCarthy et al.[43]	66	–	35	52	76	+	M	10 mg once daily	S	50 bid	Yes	FP	200	200	12	+
Nelson et al.[46]	447	+	41	40	70	+	M	10 mg once daily	S	50 bid	Yes	FP	200	200	12	+
Nelson et al.[47]	429	+	40	44	66	+	Z	20 mg twice daily	S	50 bid	NR	Varied	NR	NR	4	–
Ringdal et al.[48]	806	+	43	45	75	+	M	10 mg once daily	S	50 bid	Yes	FP	200	200	12	+

NR, not reported

*In beclomethasone equivalent (approximated from the dose and distribution of ICS in each group).

Anti-leukotrienes: montelukast (M), zafirlukast (Z).

Inhaled glucocorticoids: beclomethasone (BDP); budesonide (BUD); fluticasone (FP).

†Long-acting β_2-agonist: salmeterol (S), formoterol (F).

Patients with exacerbations requiring systemic steroids

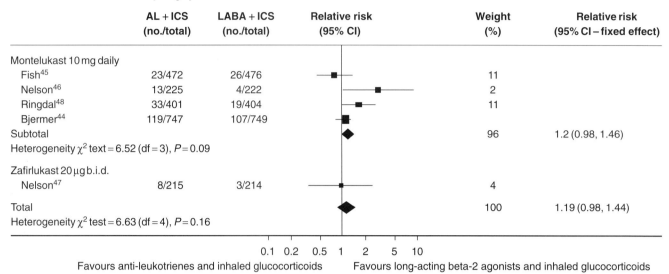

	AL + ICS (no./total)	LABA + ICS (no./total)	Relative risk (95% CI)	Weight (%)	Relative risk (95% CI – fixed effect)
Montelukast 10 mg daily					
Fish[45]	23/472	26/476		11	
Nelson[46]	13/225	4/222		2	
Ringdal[48]	33/401	19/404		11	
Bjermer[44]	119/747	107/749			
Subtotal				96	1.2 (0.98, 1.46)
Heterogeneity χ^2 text = 6.52 (df = 3), P = 0.09					
Zafirlukast 20 µg b.i.d.					
Nelson[47]	8/215	3/214		4	
Total				100	1.19 (0.98, 1.44)
Heterogeneity χ^2 test = 6.63 (df = 4), P = 0.16					

0.1 0.2 0.5 1 2 5 10

Favours anti-leukotrienes and inhaled glucocorticoids   Favours long-acting beta-2 agonists and inhaled glucocorticoids

Figure 5. Pooled relative risk of patients experiencing at least one exacerbation requiring systemic glucocorticoids comparing anti-leukotriene (AL) versus long-acting β_2-agonists (LABA) as add-on to inhaled glucocorticoids (ICS).

duration and severity of baseline airway obstruction. Asthma triggers and comorbidities, such as rhinitis, were rarely reported; when they were, they affected roughly half the participants, preventing their use as markers for response. Thus, patient attributes, if any, that may confer greater or lesser response to leukotriene receptor antagonists elude us.

Leukotriene receptor antagonists are safe agents when administered at usual licensed doses; they are not associated with an increase in adverse events such as headache and liver enzymes as originally presumed. Their use may be protective against oral candidiasis when compared with inhaled glucocorticoids. Although associated with higher efficacy, the use of two to four times the licensed doses is not recommended in view of the two- to fourfold increased risk of liver enzyme elevation, a risk that becomes more evident with an increased number of pooled trials. Randomized controlled trials are inappropriate to evaluate the causal relationship between leukotriene receptor antagonists and rare side-effects such as the Churg–Strauss syndrome, which has now been reported with all marketed leukotriene receptor antagonists.[49–51] Until now, trials have not been designed to examine appropriately the long-term safety of leukotriene receptor antagonists on bone mineralization and adrenal function, compared with inhaled glucocorticoids. For the majority of patients, safety of licensed doses of leukotriene receptor antagonists should not be of concern.

Although leukotriene receptor antagonists may be falling short of our expectations, there is increasing evidence that low doses of inhaled glucocorticoids are sufficient to prevent mortality and improve morbidity in the vast majority of asthmatics,[52] if compliance with medication, action plan, allergen avoidance and regular medical review are followed. Current evidence confirms that inhaled glucocorticoids at the lowest effective dose should remain the first choice of anti-inflammatory therapy in adults with persistent asthma. Leukotriene receptor antagonists have a mild anti-inflammatory effect that may have a role as monotherapy in very mild asthma or as add-on therapy in patients inadequately controlled on low to moderate doses of inhaled glucocorticoids.

Acknowledgements

The author was supported by a National Researcher Award from the Fonds de la Recherche en Santé du Québec, Québec, Canada.

References

1 Piper PJ. Leukotrienes and the airways. *Eur J Anaesthesiol* 1989; **6**:241–55.

2 Drazen JM, Israel E, O'Byrne PM. Treatment of asthma with drugs modifying the leukotriene pathway. *N Engl J Med* 1999; **340**:197–206.

3 DerSimonian R, Laird N. Meta-analysis in clinical trials. *Control Clin Trials* 1986; **7**:177–88.

4 Gleser LJ, Olkin I. Models for estimating the number of unpublished studies. *Stat Med* 1996; **15**:2493–507.

5 National Asthma Education and Prevention Program. *NAEPP Expert Panel Report Guidelines for the Diagnosis and Management of Asthma.* NIH publication no. 02-5075. Bethesda, MD, National Heart, Lung and Blood Institute, 2002.

6 Ducharme FM, Hicks GC. Anti-leukotriene agents compared to inhaled corticosteroids in the management of recurrent and/or chronic asthma in adults and children. In: *The Cochrane Library*, Issue 3. Oxford, Update Software, 2002.

7 Baumgartner RA, Martinez G, Edelman JM *et al.* Distribution of therapeutic response in asthma control between oral montelukast and inhaled beclomethasone. *Eur Respir J* 2003; **21**:123–8.

8   Bleecker ER, Welch MJ, Weinstein SF *et al*. Low-dose inhaled fluticasone propionate versus oral zafirlukast in the treatment of persistent asthma. *J Allergy Clin Immunol* 2000; **105**(6 Pt 1):1123–9.

9   Brabson JH, Clifford D, Kerwin E *et al*. Efficacy and safety of low-dose fluticasone propionate compared with zafirlukast in patients with persistent asthma. *Am J Med* 2002; **113**:15–21.

10 Busse W, Raphael GD, Galant S *et al*. Low-dose fluticasone propionate compared with montelukast for first-line treatment of persistent asthma: a randomized clinical trial. *J Allergy Clin Immunol* 2001; **107**:461–8.

11 Busse W, Wolfe J, Storms W *et al*. Fluticasone propionate compared with zafirlukast in controlling persistent asthma: a randomized double-blind, placebo-controlled trial. *J Fam Pract* 2001; **50**:595–602.

12 Israel E, Chervinsky PS, Friedman B *et al*. Effects of montelukast and beclomethasone on airway function and asthma control. *J Allergy Clin Immunol* 2002; **110**:847–54.

13 Kanniess F, Richter K, Bohme S, Jorres RA, Magnussen H. Montelukast versus fluticasone: effects on lung function, airway responsiveness and inflammation in moderate asthma. *Eur Respir J* 2002; **20**:853–8.

14 Kim KT, Ginchansky EJ, Friedman BF *et al*. Fluticasone propionate versus zafirlukast: effect in patients previously receiving inhaled corticosteroid therapy. *Ann Allergy Asthma Immunol* 2000; **85**:398–406.

15 Laviolette M, Malmstrom K, Lu S *et al*. Montelukast added to inhaled beclomethasone in treatment of asthma. *Am J Respir Crit Care Med* 1999; **160**:1862–8.

16 Malmstrom K, Rodriguez-Gomez G, Guerra J *et al*. Oral montelukast, inhaled beclomethasone, and placebo for chronic asthma. A randomized, controlled trial. *Ann Intern Med* 1999; **130**:487–95.

17 Meltzer EO, Lockey RF, Friedman BF *et al*. Efficacy and safety of low-dose fluticasone propionate compared with montelukast for maintenance treatment of persistent asthma. *Mayo Clin Proc* 2002; **77**:437–45.

18 Nathan RA, Bleecker ER, Kalberg C and the Fluticasone Propionate Study Group. A comparison of short-term treatment with inhaled fluticasone propionate and zafirlukast for patients with persistent asthma. *Am J Med* 2001; **111**:195–202.

19 Riccioni G, Castronuovo M, De Benedictis M *et al*. Zafirlukast versus budesonide on bronchial reactivity in subjects with mild-persistent asthma. *Int J Immunopathol Pharmacol* 2001; **14**:87–92.

20 Riccioni G, Ballone E, D'Orazio N *et al*. Effectiveness of montelukast versus budesonide on quality of life and bronchial reactivity in subjects with mild-persistent asthma. *Int J Immunopathol Pharmacol* 2002; **15**:149–55.

21 Riccioni G, D'Orazio N, Di Ilio C, Della Vecchia R., De Lorenzo A. [Effectiveness and safety of montelukast versus budesonide at various doses on bronchial reactivity in subjects with mild persistent asthma]. *Clin Ter* 2002; **153**:317–21.

22 Williams B, Noonan G, Reiss TF *et al*. Long-term asthma control with oral montelukast and inhaled beclomethasone for adults and children 6 years and older. *Clin Exp Allergy* 2001; **31**:845–54.

23 Yamauchi K, Tanifuji Y, Pan LH *et al*. Effects of pranlukast, a leukotriene receptor antagonist, on airway inflammation in mild asthmatics. *J Asthma* 2001; **38**:51–7.

24 Hughes GL, Edelman J, Turpin J *et al*. Randomized, open-label pilot study comparing the effects of montelukast sodium tablets, fluticasone aerosol inhaler, and budesonide dry powder inhaler on asthma control in mild asthmatics (abstract). *Am J Resp Crit Care Med* 1999; **159**:A641.

25 Laitinen LA, Naya IP, Binks S, Harris A. Comparative efficacy of zafirlukast and low dose steroids in asthmatics on β₂-agonists. *Eur Respir J* 1997; **10**:419–20.

26 Edelman JM for the MIAMI Study Research Group. Rescue-free days in patients with mild persistent asthma receiving montelukast sodium or an inhaled corticosteroid (abstract). *Eur Resp J* 2002; **20**(Suppl 38):113S.

27 Ducharme F, Hicks G, Kakuma R. Addition of anti-leukotriene agents to inhaled corticosteroids for chronic asthma. In: *The Cochrane Library*, Issue 1. Oxford, Update Software, 2002.

28 Bateman ED, Holgate ST, Binks SM, Tarna IP. A multicentre study to assess the steroid-sparing potential of Accolate (abstract P-0709). *Allergy* 1995; **50**(Suppl 26):320.

29 Kanniess F, Richter K, Janicki S, Schleiss MB, Jorres RA, Magnussen H. Dose reduction of inhaled corticosteroids under concomitant medication with montelukast in patients with asthma. *Eur Respir J* 2002; **20**:1080–7.

30 Laitinen LA, Zetterstrom O, Holgate ST, Binks S, Whitney JG. Effects of Accolate in permitting reduced therapy with inhaled steroids: a multicenter trial in patients with doses of inhaled steroids optimised between 800 and 2000 mcg per day (abstract P-0710). *Allergy* 1995; **50**(Suppl 26):320.

31 Lofdahl CG, Reiss TF, Leff JA *et al*. Randomised, placebo controlled trial of effect of a leukotriene receptor antagonist, montelukast, on tapering inhaled corticosteroids in asthmatic patients. *BMJ* 1999; **319**:87–90.

32 Shingo S, Zhang J, Noonan N, Reiss TF, Leff JA. A standardized composite clinical score allows safe tapering of inhaled corticosteroids in an asthma clinical trial. *Drug Inform J* 2002; **36**:501–8.

33 Tohda Y, Fujimura M, Taniguchi H *et al*. Leukotriene receptor antagonist, montelukast, can reduce the need for inhaled steroid while maintaining the clinical stability of asthmatic patients. *Clin Exp Allergy* 2002; **32**:1180–6.

34 Hultquist C, Domeij W, Kasak V, Laitinen L, O'Neill S. *Oxis Turbuhaler (formoterol), Accolate (zafirlukast) or Placebo as Add on Treatment to Pulmicort Turbuhaler (budesonide) in Asthmatic Patients on Inhaled Steroids*. AstraZeneca, 2000, SD-004CR-0216.

35 Tamaoki J, Kondo M, Sakai N *et al*. Leukotriene antagonist prevents exacerbation of asthma during reduction of high-dose inhaled corticosteroid. *Am J Respir Crit Care Med* 1997; **155**:1235–40.

36 Vaquerizo MJ, Casan P, Castillo J *et al*. Effect of montelukast added to inhaled budesonide on control of mild to moderate asthma. *Thorax* 2003; **58**:204–10.

37 Virchow JC, Prasse A, Naya I, Summerton L, Harris A. Zafirlukast improves asthma control in patients receiving high-dose inhaled corticosteroids. *Am J Respir Crit Care Med* 2000; **162**(1 Pt 1):578–85.

38 Nayak AS, Anderson P, Charous BL, Williams K, Simonson S. Equivalence of adding zafirlukast versus double-dose inhaled corticosteroids in asthmatic patients symptomatic on low-dose inhaled corticosteroids (abstract 965). *J Allergy Clin Immunol* 1998; **101**(1 Pt 2):S233.

39 Price DB, Hernandez D, Magyar P *et al*. Randomised controlled trial of montelukast plus inhaled budesonide versus double dose inhaled budesonide in adult patients with asthma. *Thorax* 2003; **58**:211–16.

40 Ringdal N, White M, Harris A. Addition of zafirlukast (Accolate) compared with a double-dose of inhaled corticosteroids in patients with reversible airways obstruction symptomatic on inhaled corticosteroids (abstract). *Am J Respir Crit Care Med* 2000; **159**(3 Pt 2):639.

41 Tomari S, Shimoda T, Kawano T *et al*. Effects of pranlukast, a cysteinyl leukotriene receptor 1 antagonist, combined with inhaled beclomethasone in patients with moderate or severe asthma. *Ann Allergy Asthma Immunol* 2001; **87**:156–61.

42 Ram FS, Ducharme FM. Anti-leukotrienes versus long-acting β₂-agonists as add-on therapy to inhaled corticosteroids in chronic asthma. In: *The Cochrane Database of Systematic Reviews* 2005; Issue 1.

43 McCarthy TP, Woodcock AA, Pavord ID, Allen DJ, Parker D, Rice L. A comparison of the anti-inflammatory and clinical effects of salmeterol 25 mcg/fluticasone propionate 50 mcg combination (sfc 50)

with fluticasone propionate (fp) plus montelukast (m) in patients with mild to moderate asthma (abstract). *Am J Respir Crit Care Med* 2003; **167**:A367.

44 Bjermer L, Bisgaard H, Bousquet J *et al.* Montelukast and fluticasone compared with salmeterol and fluticasone in protecting against asthma exacerbations in adults: one year, double-blind, randomized comparative trial. *BMJ* 2003; **327**:891.

45 Fish JE, Israel E, Murray JJ *et al.* Salmeterol powder provides significantly better benefit than montelukast in asthmatic patients receiving concomitant inhaled corticosteroid therapy. *Chest* 2001; **120**:423–30.

46 Nelson HS, Busse WW, Kerwin E *et al.* Fluticasone propionate/salmeterol combination provides more effective asthma control than low-dose inhaled corticosteroid plus montelukast. *J Allergy Clin Immunol* 2000; **106**:1088–95.

47 Nelson HS, Nathan RA, Kalberg C, Yancey SW, Rickard KA. Comparison of inhaled salmeterol and oral zafirlukast in asthmatic patients using concomitant inhaled corticosteroids. *Medscape Gen Med* 2001;**3**:3.

48 Ringdal N, Eliraz A, Pruzinec P *et al.* The salmeterol/fluticasone combination is more effective than fluticasone plus oral montelukast in asthma. *Respir Med* 2003; **97**:234–41.

49 Guilpain P, Viallard JF, Lagarde P *et al.* Churg–Strauss syndrome in two patients receiving montelukast. *Rheumatology* 2002; **41**:535–9.

50 Katsura T, Yoshida F, Takinishi Y. The Churg–Strauss syndrome after pranlukast treatment in a patient not receiving corticosteroids. *Ann Intern Med* 2003; **139**(5 Pt 1):387.

51 Green RL, Vayonis AG. Churg–Strauss syndrome after zafirlukast in two patients not receiving systemic steroid treatment. *Lancet* 1999; **353**(9154):725–6.

52 Suissa S, Ernst P. Inhaled corticosteroids: impact on asthma morbidity and mortality. *J Allergy Clin Immunol* 2001; **107**:937–44.

CHAPTER 2.5

Asthma education

Peter G Gibson and Heather Powell

Introduction

Asthma education is an important component of asthma management that underpins the effective implementation of pharmacotherapy in asthma.[1-3] Several systems to implement asthma education have been developed, which include asthma self-management programmes, written management plans and primary care-based asthma clinics.

Patient education has been defined as 'a planned learning experience using a combination of methods such as teaching, counselling, and behaviour modification techniques which influence patients' knowledge and health behaviour . . . (and) involves an interactive process which assists patients to participate actively in their health care'.[4] There is general agreement that asthma education improves patient knowledge; however, the effects on other health outcomes depend heavily on the type of education programme that is provided. Broadly, asthma education programmes can provide information about asthma or teach participants how to manage their asthma in conjunction with a doctor (self-management) or both.[4] A comprehensive asthma self-management programme is needed to improve asthma outcomes. This chapter will examine the evidence supporting educational interventions to improve asthma.

Questions

Does the provision of information about asthma improve health outcomes in adults with asthma?

Does asthma self-management education improve outcomes in adults with asthma?

What is the comparative efficacy of different components of optimal asthma self-management education?

What components of a written action plan are associated with improved health outcomes?

What is the effect of primary care-based asthma clinics?

Literature search

The Cochrane Library was searched to identify systematic reviews of randomized trials using the terms 'asthma' AND 'education'. The search identified relevant reviews that examined limited asthma education,[5] asthma self-management education programmes,[6,7] different components of asthma self-management[7-9] and different settings for the delivery of asthma education.[10]

Components of asthma education programmes

The systematic reviews of asthma education programmes in adults identified four main components of these programmes.

These were:

• Information: the provision of information about asthma and its management.

• Self-monitoring: this involves regular assessment of either symptoms or peak expiratory flow (PEF) by the participant.

• Regular medical review: the assessment of asthma control, severity and medications by a medical practitioner forms the basis of the regular medical review component.

• A written action plan: this is an individualized written plan produced for the purpose of patient self-management of asthma exacerbations. The action plan is characterized by being individualized to the patient's underlying asthma severity and treatment. The action plan also informs the patient when and how to modify medications and when and how to access the medical system in response to worsening asthma.

Interventions that provide information only are termed limited asthma education. Interventions providing two or more components are termed self-management education. Interventions using all four components are termed optimal self-management education.

Providing information about asthma

The provision of information about asthma and its treatment is one of the simplest and more economical forms of asthma education. It can easily be conducted in either a hospital or a community setting. The evidence base for examining the effects of an information-only intervention on asthma outcomes consists of 12 randomized controlled trials (RCTs) that are summarized in a Cochrane systematic review of limited (information-only) education for asthma[5] (Table 1).

Teaching modalities of asthma education

Information about asthma can be delivered to the participant in either an interactive or a non-interactive style.[5,11] Inter-

Table 1. Characteristics of Cochrane systematic reviews of asthma education.[5,6]

Limited (information-only) patient education programmes for adults with asthma[5]	Self-management intervention and regular practitioner review for adults with asthma[6]
Type of trials: randomized controlled trials *Primary comparison:* information-only education versus a usual care control group. The control comparisons (or 'usual care') varied from usual medical care and a waiting list control.	Type of trials: randomized controlled trials *Primary comparison:* the primary comparison based on the treatment of the intervention and control groups used was self-management versus usual care. 'Usual care' may have included education, self-monitoring or regular medical review. However, no control group received a written action plan.
Types of participants: participants were adults with asthma and recruited from outpatient clinics, GPs, hospital emergency departments and advertising.	*Types of participants:* 6090 adults with asthma were randomized into 36 trials. Participants were recruited from a variety of settings including hospitals, emergency departments, outpatient clinics, GPs and community settings.
Setting: the intervention was performed in hospital clinics/outpatient departments in six trials, GP clinic for one, hospital exit interview in inpatient one and combined at home and hospital in four.	*Setting:* the interventions were conducted in outpatient clinics, GP asthma clinics, community-based programmes and hospital education programmes.
Types of interventions: the type of intervention varied between trials. It included either interactive sessions (group or individual education or interactive computer sessions) or non-interactive education (provision of written material, video and/or audiocassette).	*Types of interventions:* all the interventions provided information plus components of self-management that included information, self-monitoring, regular medical review and written action plan.
Trial duration: the duration of the intervention varied among the trials and was also dependent on the style of intervention. This varied from the time taken for home reading of a booklet, a single interview with an educator or watching a video to 20 hours of instruction over a 4-week period.	*Trial duration:* duration of intervention varied from a minimum of one 45-min session to 10 hours of instruction over a 4-week period. Follow-up consisted of monthly visits or telephone follow-up for 12 months.

active learning can incorporate either individual or group sessions with an educator and may involve lectures, audiovisual presentations to encourage discussion, group discussions, demonstration of techniques, practice of skills, role playing, project- or assignment-based learning, participatory learning and a case presentation method to develop problem-solving skills.[11] Seven RCTs have conducted interactive interventions.[4,5] Individual and group interactive education lead to similar and significant improvements in symptoms; however, group programmes are simpler to administer, more cost effective and better received by patients and educators.[12]

Non-interactive interventions

Non-interactive interventions comprised written materials, audiocassette, video or non-interactive computer education that was administered without direct contact with an educator. Five RCTs have examined the effects of non-interactive methods to transfer information about asthma.[5] Overall, these studies showed a significant improvement in asthma knowledge with no significant effects on asthma morbidity. In the largest study conducted using this modality, Osman *et al.*[13] found no significant differences in asthma outcomes;

however, in the study conducted by Wilson *et al.*,[12] the non-interactive education group experienced significantly fewer symptomatic days and better asthma status.

Question: Does provision of information about asthma improve health outcomes?

There is significant variability in the results of studies that provide information about asthma as a sole intervention. When the results are pooled in a meta-analysis, the results show that education programmes that offered knowledge but no self-management skills did not reduce hospitalization rates or visits to the doctor for asthma.[5] Similarly, there was no change in medication use or improvement in lung function after information-only education. The positive outcomes from these programmes (Fig. 1) were a reduction in symptoms and in emergency department (ED) visits. Patients reported that their perception of symptoms was reduced by provision of information about asthma. There was a gradation of effect with no reduction in the more severe symptoms such as days off work or school. It is unclear whether the reduction in perceived symptoms is a true effect of the intervention on asthma symptoms or due to anticipation bias as a result of using an unblinded intervention.

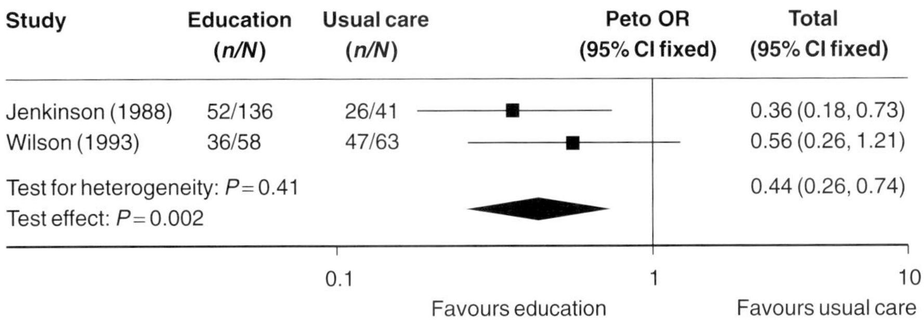

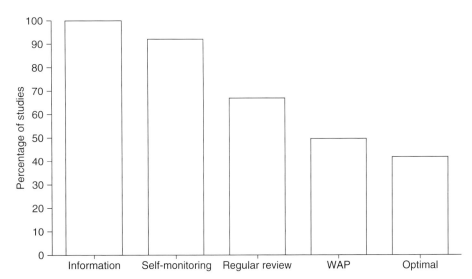

Study
Education (n/N)
Usual care (n/N)
Peto OR (95% CI fixed)
Total (95% CI fixed)
Jenkinson (1988) 52/136 26/41 0.36 (0.18, 0.73)
Wilson (1993) 36/58 47/63 0.56 (0.26, 1.21)
Test for heterogeneity: P=0.41
Test effect: P=0.002
0.44 (0.26, 0.74)
0.1
1
10
Favours education
Favours usual care

Figure 1. The effects of limited education about asthma compared with usual care on asthma symptoms (perceived disability).

100
90
80
70
60
50
40
30
20
10
0
Percentage of studies
Information
Self-monitoring
Regular review
WAP
Optimal

Figure 2. A systematic review of asthma self-management.[6] WAP, written action plan.

Asthma self-management education

Does asthma self-management education improve outcomes in adults with asthma?

The effects of an asthma self-management intervention on asthma outcomes has been evaluated in 36 RCTs involving 6090 participants[6] (Table 1). The content of the asthma self-management interventions described in the 36 studies is shown in Table 2 and Figure 2.

There were 15 studies that compared an optimal self-management programme with usual care. The optimal self-management intervention consisted of information about asthma, self-management, regular review and a written asthma action plan. The studies showed that, with a self-management programme, there was a significant reduction in the proportion of subjects reporting hospitalizations and ED visits for asthma, unscheduled doctor's visits for asthma, days lost from work due to asthma and episodes of nocturnal asthma. The effects were large enough to be of both clinical and statistical significance (Table 3 and Fig. 3). There was also a gradation of effect. Those interventions that included a written action plan consistently showed an effect, whereas less intense interventions were not always of obvious benefit. Airway function was assessed as either clinic forced expiratory volume in 1 second (FEV_1; 10 studies) or peak expiratory flow (PEF; 16 studies). There was an overall positive effect of asthma self-management, which led to an improvement in PEF ($P < 0.05$). The absolute improvement in PEF was small (14.5 L/min), and significant heterogeneity was present for both analyses (chi square 30.13, $P < 0.05$). There was no effect on clinic FEV_1.

Table 2. Asthma self-management education interventions: combinations that were examined in RCTs.

	No. of trials
Optimal self-management interventions	15
Self-monitoring, information, regular review and written action plan	
Self-monitoring, information and regular review	7
Self-monitoring and information only	10
Regular medical review	2

Table 3. Outcomes of asthma self-management.[6]

	Overall	Optimal self-management intervention	NNT
Hospitalization	0.64 (0.50–0.82)	0.58 (0.43–0.77)	21
Emergency visits	0.82 (0.73–0.94)	0.78 (0.67–0.91)	18
Unscheduled doctor visits	0.68 (0.56–0.81)	0.73 (0.58–0.91)	24
Days off work	0.79 (0.67–0.93)	0.81 (0.65–1.01)	12
Nocturnal asthma	0.67 (0.56–0.79)	0.57 (0.45–0.72)	7
PEF (L/min)	0.18 (0.07–0.29)*	0.20 (0.08–0.31)	NA

Relative risk with 95% CI. All results $P < 0.05$.
*Standardized mean difference.
NTT, number needed to treat.

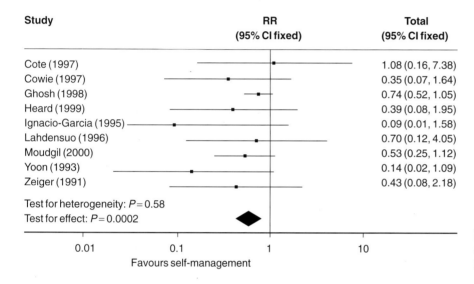

Study	RR (95% CI fixed)	Total (95% CI fixed)
Cote (1997)		1.08 (0.16, 7.38)
Cowie (1997)		0.35 (0.07, 1.64)
Ghosh (1998)		0.74 (0.52, 1.05)
Heard (1999)		0.39 (0.08, 1.95)
Ignacio-Garcia (1995)		0.09 (0.01, 1.58)
Lahdensuo (1996)		0.70 (0.12, 4.05)
Moudgil (2000)		0.53 (0.25, 1.12)
Yoon (1993)		0.14 (0.02, 1.09)
Zeiger (1991)		0.43 (0.08, 2.18)

Test for heterogeneity: $P = 0.58$
Test for effect: $P = 0.0002$

0.01   0.1   1   10
Favours self-management

Figure 3. A comparison of the effects of optimal self-management on hospitalizations for asthma.[6]

Components of asthma self-management

What is the comparative efficacy of different components of asthma self-management education?

Optimal pharmacotherapy

There is an important interaction between asthma self-management and optimal pharmacotherapy. Asthma education can improve adherence[14] and thereby facilitate the use of pharmacotherapy. Guidelines recommend that asthma education be delivered together with pharmacotherapy. When this happens, as in an optimal asthma self-management programme, then there is a significant improvement in asthma morbidity (Table 3).

Studies have attempted to identify the improvement in asthma that can be attributed to education and separate this from that attributable to therapy.[7] In four RCTs, there was optimization of pharmacotherapy prior to administration of an education programme (Table 4). In these studies, pharma-cotherapy was optimized via regular medical review and was compared with regular medical review combined with an optimal self-management programme. These trials also compared two forms of adjustment of medication, usually inhaled corticosteroids, in order to achieve improved asthma control. The usual means was by regular review by a doctor. This was contrasted with self-adjustment by the patient according to written, predetermined criteria. Overall, there was no difference in asthma outcomes between the two forms of asthma management. In particular, hospitalizations for asthma were not different between groups, and unscheduled doctor visits, disrupted days and lung function were not significantly different. These results indicate that regular medical review is an acceptable alternative to an asthma education programme, provided that the medical review includes assessment of severity, optimization of medication and instruction on management of exacerbation.

Other variations of optimal self-management have also been compared.[7] The receipt of an optimal self-management programme that did not include regular medical review led to

Table 4. Comparisons of different components of optimal self-management education for asthma.[7]

	Intervention 1	Intervention 2			Results
Regular review versus self-management *n* = 6 trials	- education - PEF self-monitoring - regular review - written action plan	- education - PEF self-monitoring - written action plan			Similar results
Optimal self-management: PEF versus symptom self-monitoring *n* = 6 trials	- education - PEF self-monitoring - regular review - written action plan	- education - symptom self-monitoring - regular review - written action plan			No difference
Modified optimal self-management *n* = 3 trials	- education - self-monitoring - regular review - written action plan	Baldwin *et al.*[17] - education - PEF self-monitoring - regular review - verbal action plan	Cote *et al.*[16] - reduced education - self-monitoring - regular review - written action plan	Kauppinen *et al.*[15] - education - self-monitoring - no regular review - written action plan	Intervention 2 was less effective

Table 5. Components of a written asthma action plan.

1. When to increase treatment
   Symptoms versus peak expiratory flow (PEF)
   PEF: % predicted versus personal best
   Number of action points: 2, 3, 4
   Presentation: 'traffic light'
2. How to increase treatment
   Increase inhaled corticosteroid
   Oral corticosteroid
   Combination
3. For how long
   Duration of treatment increase
4. When to call for help

an increase in health centre visits and sickness days in comparison with those receiving a full optimal self-management programme.[15] In a programme where the intensity of the asthma education was reduced, there was a significant increase in the proportion of subjects requiring unscheduled doctor visits.[16] Optimal self-management programmes including verbal instructions have also been compared with a written action plan with no difference reported in asthma outcomes between the two interventions.[17]

Question: What components of a written action plan are associated with improved health outcomes?

Written asthma action plans contain four essential components (Table 5). These are an instruction of when to increase treatment, how to increase treatment, the duration of the treatment increase and when to cease self-management and seek medical help.[9]

The instruction specifying when to increase treatment represents the point at which the action plan is to be activated, i.e. the action point. This may be based on symptoms or PEF values. Self-management using a written action plan based on PEF was found to be equivalent to self-management using a symptoms-based written action plan in the six studies that compared these interventions for the proportion of subjects requiring hospitalization and unscheduled visits to the doctor.[7] ED visits were significantly reduced by PEF self-management in one study,[18] but were similar to symptoms self-management in four other studies. Symptoms-based self-management reduced the number of subjects requiring a course of oral corticosteroids in one study.[19]

This is an important issue as self-monitoring of PEF involves the regular measurement of PEF and recording the best of three measurements in a diary, morning and night. Medication is then adjusted according to changes in PEF levels. In contrast, adjustment of medication can be made according to the patient's symptoms such as nocturnal asthma or an increased need for reliever medication. Both PEF and symptom self-monitoring have their limitations. Compliance with PEF monitoring in the long term is poor, and some patients are poor perceivers of their symptoms. In reviewing the six trials that compared PEF and symptom self-monitoring, no significant differences in health outcomes were found, suggesting that the use of either method is effective. This is a clinically important observation as self-monitoring can be tailored to patient preference, patient characteristics and the resources available.

Action points that use PEF can be based on PEF expressed as

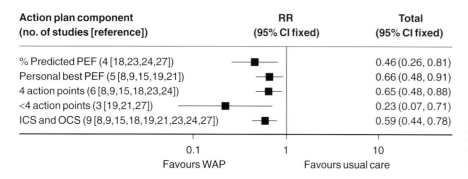

Figure 4. A comparison of the effects of action plan components on hospitalizations for asthma.[9] Reproduced with permission from the BMJ Publishing Group.

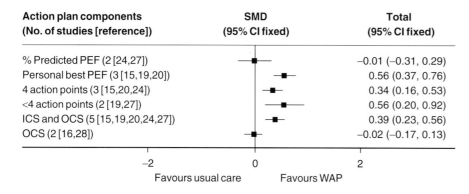

Figure 5. A comparison of the effects of action plan components on peak expiratory flow (mean) in asthma.[9] SMD, standardized mean difference. Reproduced with permission from the BMJ Publishing Group.

a percentage of the predicted PEF or as a percentage of the individual's best PEF (personal best). Action points based on personal best PEF were consistently associated with improved outcomes (Figs 4 and 5). When specifying action points, these can be further subdivided as 80% or 60% of the best value (two action points), or as 90%, 70%, 60%, 40% of the best value (four action points). A comparison of written action plans found that those using two action points gave similar results to those using four action points (Figs 4 and 5). The action points can also be presented using colour coding, where orange represents one action level and red another. This approach, termed a 'traffic light' configuration, was not obviously better than standard presentation.[9]

The instructions regarding treatment showed that action plans recommending increased inhaled corticosteroid and the commencement of oral corticosteroid were beneficial (Figs 4 and 5). The effects of increased inhaled corticosteroid alone are inconclusive at this stage. Whereas one study showed a similar effect of inhaled fluticasone 1 mg to oral prednisone,[20] other work has found that doubling the dose of inhaled corticosteroid in an asthma exacerbation may not be effective.[21]

These recommendations for action plan use are summarized in Table 6.

Asthma education in different settings

Asthma self-management education has been evaluated in several different settings. Most studies that have been con-

Table 6. Action plan variations: summary of results.[9]

Action plan variation	Result
Action point	
Symptoms versus PEF triggered	Equivalent
Standard written instruction	Consistently beneficial
Traffic light configuration	Not clearly better than standard instruction
Two or three action points	Consistently beneficial
Four action points	Not clearly better than < four points
PEF based on personal best PEF	Consistently beneficial
PEF based on % predicted PEF	Not consistently better than usual care
Treatment instruction	
Individualized WAP using ICS and OCS	Consistently beneficial
Individualized WAP using OCS only	Insufficient data to evaluate
Individualized WAP using ICS only	Insufficient data to evaluate

PEF, peak expiratory flow; WAP, written action plan; ICS, inhaled corticosteroids; OCS, oral corticosteroids.

ducted in specialist clinics or hospital-based ambulatory care clinics have shown positive results.[6] Other programmes have been conducted in primary care and emergency departments.

Primary care-based asthma clinics

A primary care-based asthma clinic is typically led by an asthma nurse and supported by a primary care physician.[19] It involves the organized recall of patients with asthma for symptom review and input from a variety of educational models. A Cochrane Review addressed the effectiveness of organized care through primary care-based asthma clinics.[10] Unfortunately, only one trial met the inclusion criteria for the review. This trial provided 11 outcome measures, two of which showed a significant effect of the intervention. More patients in the intervention group had peak flow meters [relative risk (RR) 1.30, 95% confidence interval (CI) 1.05–1.61], and fewer patients in the intervention group were likely to wake up at night as a result of their asthma (RR 0.30, 95% CI 0.16–0.81).

A subsequent study[22] examined primary care-based asthma clinics using a structured, optimal, self-management programme in children with asthma. The children who received the intervention had significantly more consultations relating to asthma, were twice as likely to use a written asthma plan, had less speech-limiting wheeze, were more likely to use a spacer and the reduction in mean FEV_1 following a cold air challenge was significantly less than in the control children. There were also non-significantly fewer ED visits for the intervention group. These results indicate that asthma self-management education can be successfully adapted to a primary care setting providing that an optimal educational strategy is used.

Asthma education in the emergency department

Asthma education programmes have targeted ED attendees in several randomized trials (Table 7).[23–32] The participants were recruited during or shortly after their ED visit with acute asthma. Six of these programmes have provided optimal asthma self-management education that has been delivered in an ambulatory care setting after discharge from the ED.[23–28] There were significant reductions in subsequent hospitalizations and ED visits following these programmes (Figs 6 and 7).

Targeting ED attendees with acute asthma is an effective management strategy to improve morbidity in asthma.

Other issues

It has been pointed out that, although patient education can be effective in reducing short- and medium-term morbidity, this is only true for the interested minority who respond to invitations to participate.[33] Many studies comment on the poor response and attendance by patients. The number of RCTs in

Table 7. Asthma education in emergency department attendees.[6]

Reference	Participants	Recruitment setting	Intervention setting/ delivery	Intervention components	Outcome
Brewin and Hughes[29]	Age > 16 years	Hospital	Hospital inpatient/nurse clinician	I, SM	Days off work, nocturnal waking, rescue medications, symptoms, knowledge
Cowie et al.[23]	Adults, adolescents	Post ED discharge	Ambulatory care/nurse clinician	I, SM, RR, AP	Hospitalizations, ED visits
Cote et al.[24]	Aged > 16 years	Hospital	Ambulatory care/specialist	I, SM, RR, AP	Hospitalizations, ED visits, days off work, knowledge, compliance, OCS
Garrett et al.[30]	Aged 2–55 years	ED	Ambulatory care/nurse/ community health worker	I, SM, RR	Hospitalizations, ED visits, days off work, nocturnal waking, PEF variability, symptoms
George et al.[31]	Aged 18–45 years	Hospital	Hospital inpatient/asthma educator	I, RR, AP	Hospitalizations, ED visits, length of stay, outpatient visits
Levy et al.[25]	Adults	ED/hospital	Ambulatory care/nurse clinician	I, SM, RR, AP	ED visits, doctor visits, PEF, rescue medications, days off work, symptoms, quality of life, ICS
Mayo et al.[32]	Aged > 18 years	Hospital	Ambulatory care/ multidisciplinary	I, SM, RR	Hospitalizations, skills, mortality, exacerbations, OCS, ICS
Sommaragua et al.[26]	Adults	Hospital	Hospital inpatient/ multidisciplinary	I, SM, RR, AP	Hospitalizations, ED visits, days off work, exacerbations, respiratory illness survey—psychological factors
Yoon et al.[27]	Aged 16–65 years	Hospital	Ambulatory care/asthma educator	I, SM, RR, AP	Hospitalizations, ED visits, days off work, lung function, knowledge, quality of life, knowledge, wheeze, ICS
Zeiger et al.[28]	Aged 6–59 years	ED/hospital	Ambulatory care/nurse clinician	I, SM, RR, AP	Hospitalizations, ED visits, nocturnal asthma, ICS, perception of asthma

ED, emergency department; I, information; RR, regular review; SM, self-monitoring; AP, written action plan; ICS, inhaled corticosteroids; OCS, oral corticosteroids; PEF, peak expiratory flow.

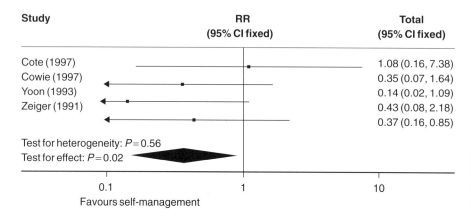

Study	RR (95% CI fixed)	Total (95% CI fixed)
Cote (1997)		1.08 (0.16, 7.38)
Cowie (1997)		0.35 (0.07, 1.64)
Yoon (1993)		0.14 (0.02, 1.09)
Zeiger (1991)		0.43 (0.08, 2.18)
		0.37 (0.16, 0.85)

Test for heterogeneity: $P = 0.56$
Test for effect: $P = 0.02$

0.1   1   10
Favours self-management

Figure 6. A comparison of the effects of optimal education in the emergency department on hospitalizations.[6] RR, relative risk.

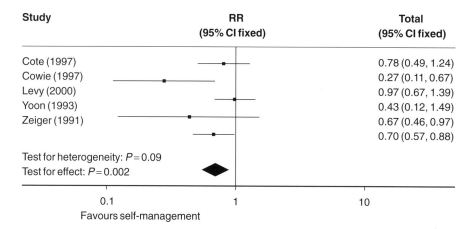

Study	RR (95% CI fixed)	Total (95% CI fixed)
Cote (1997)		0.78 (0.49, 1.24)
Cowie (1997)		0.27 (0.11, 0.67)
Levy (2000)		0.97 (0.67, 1.39)
Yoon (1993)		0.43 (0.12, 1.49)
Zeiger (1991)		0.67 (0.46, 0.97)
		0.70 (0.57, 0.88)

Test for heterogeneity: $P = 0.09$
Test for effect: $P = 0.002$

0.1   1   10
Favours self-management

Figure 7. A comparison of the effects of optimal education in the emergency department on subsequent ED visits.[6] RR, relative risk; ED, emergency department.

this area is limited and, to date, only two trials have explored the clinical, social, demographic and other relevant characteristics of attendees and non-attendees.[34,35] Overall, little is known about attendance; however, it is clear that, if non-attendance is an indicator of potential patient dissatisfaction, this could also become an issue. Average attendance rates range from 30% to 43%.[27,33,35]

Conclusion

Asthma education is a key part of asthma management. Providing information about asthma and its treatment is seen as necessary to the development of a successful therapeutic alliance between the person with asthma and their health professional. The practical results are improved understanding of asthma and reduced asthma symptoms. In common with other chronic diseases, the provision of information alone can improve knowledge but results in little behaviour change.[33,36] Thus, the effects of an information-only asthma intervention on other health outcomes are small, particularly when compared with asthma self-management programmes. In the ED setting, however, even provision of information about asthma may have a positive effect of reducing future ED visits.

Guided self-management, information and regular medical review[6] have been evaluated and shown favourable outcomes. The benefits are a clinically significant reduction in hospitalization and other measures of morbidity. Most asthma self-management programmes have been conducted in secondary or tertiary care settings. Primary care asthma clinics have been established to duplicate these results; however, it is not clear whether these results are applicable to all patients whose asthma is managed within primary care.[10]

These results support the current guideline recommendations for asthma education and self-management to be offered as part of a comprehensive programme of care for the person with chronic asthma.

• Providing information about asthma alone improves knowledge and may reduce symptoms. It does not alter other health outcomes.

• An asthma self-management programme consistently improves asthma outcomes, such as hospitalizations.

• Either symptoms or PEF can be used for monitoring.

• An effective asthma self-management programme involves information, self-monitoring, regular medical review and a written action plan.

• The best system for providing asthma education in primary care is not known.

References

1 National Institutes of Health. National Asthma Education and Prevention Program. *Expert Panel Report II: Guidelines for the Diagnosis and Management of Asthma*. Bethesda, MA, NAEPP, 1997.

2 *Australian Asthma Management Handbook 1998*. Australia, National Asthma Campaign, 1998.

3 National Heart Lung and Blood Institute and World Health Organization. *Global Initiative for Asthma: Global Strategy for Asthma Management and Prevention*. NHLBI and WHO, 1995.

4 Gibson PG, Boulet L-P. Role of asthma education. In: Fitzgerald JM, Ernst P, Boulet LP, O'Byrne PM, eds. *Evidence-based Asthma Management*. Hamilton, B C Decker, 2001.

5 Gibson PG, Powell H, Coughlan J *et al.* Limited (information only) patient education programs for adults with asthma. In: *Cochrane Database Systematic Review*, Issue 2. CD001005, 2002.

6 Gibson PG, Powell H, Coughlan J *et al.* Self-management education and regular practitioner review for adults with asthma. In: *Cochrane Database Systematic Review*, Issue 1. CD001117, 2003.

7 Powell H, Gibson PG. Options for self-management education for adults with asthma. In: *Cochrane Database Systematic Review*, Issue 1. CD004107, 2003.

8 Toelle B, Ram FSF. Written individualised management plans for asthma in children and adults. In: *Cochrane Database Systematic Review*, Issue 2. CD002171, 2004.

9 Gibson PG, Powell H. Written action plans for asthma: an evidence-based review of the key components. *Thorax* 2004; **59**:94–9.

10 Fay JK, Jones A, Ram FSF. Primary care based clinics for asthma. In: *Cochrane Database Systematic Review*, Issue 1. CD003533, 2002.

11 Wagner CW, Karpel SK. The educational aspects of asthma management. *Int Rev Asthma* 2001; **3**:73–85.

12 Wilson SR, Scamagas P, German DF *et al.* A controlled trial of two forms of self-management education for adults with asthma. *Am J Med* 1993; **94**:564–76.

13 Osman LM, Abdalla MI, Beattie JAG *et al.* (GRASSIC). Reducing hospital admission through computer supported education for asthma patients. *BMJ* 1994; **308**:568–71.

14 Bailey WC, Richards JM, Brooks CM, Soong SJ, Windsor RA, Manzella MPH. A randomised trial to improve self-management practices of adults with asthma. *Arch Int Med* 1990; **150**:1664–8.

15 Kauppinen R, Sintonen H, Tukianen H. One year economic evaluation of intensive versus conventional patient education and supervision for self-management of new asthmatic patients. *Respir Med* 1998; **92**:300–7.

16 Cote J, Bowie DM, Robichaud P, Parent J-G, Battiti L, Boulet L-P. Evaluation of two different educational interventions for adult patients consulting with an acute asthma exacerbation. *Am J Respir Crit Care Med* 2001; **163**:1415–19.

17 Baldwin DR, Pathak UA, King R, Vase BC, Pantin CFA. Outcome of asthmatics attending asthma clinics utilizing self-management plans in general practice. *Asthma Gen Pract* 1997; **5**:31–2.

18 Cowie RL, Revitt SG, Underwood MF, Field SK. The effect of a peak flow-based action plan in the prevention of exacerbations of asthma. *Chest* 1997; **112**:1534–8.

19 Charlton I, Charlton G, Broomfield J, Mullee MA. Evaluation of peak flow and symptoms only self-management plans for control of asthma in general practice. *BMJ* 1990; **301**:1355–9.

20 Levy M, Stevenson C, Maslen T. Comparison of short courses of oral prednisolone and fluticasone propionate in the treatment of adults with acute exacerbation of asthma in primary care. *Thorax* 1996; **51**:1087–92.

21 Harrison TW, Osborne J, Newton S, Tattersfield AE. Doubling the dose of inhaled corticosteroid to prevent asthma exacerbations: randomised controlled trial. *Lancet* 2004; **363**:271–5.

22 Glasgow NJ, Ponsonby AL, Yates R, Beilby J, Dugdale P. Proactive asthma care in childhood: practice based randomised controlled trial. *BMJ* 2003; **327**:659–66.

23 Cowie RL, Revitt SG, Underwood MF, Field SK. The effect of a peak flow-based action plan in the prevention of exacerbations of asthma. *Chest* 1997; **112**:1534–8.

24 Cote J, Cartier A, Robichaud P *et al.* Influence on asthma morbidity of asthma education programs based on self-management plans following treatment optimization. *Am J Respir Crit Care Med* 1997; **155**:1509–14.

25 Levy ML, Robb M, Allen J, Doherty C, Bland JM, Winter RJD. A randomized controlled evaluation of specialist nurse education following accident and emergency department attendance for acute asthma. *Respir Med* 2000; **94**:900–8.

26 Sommaragua M, Spanavello A, Migliori GB, Neri M, Callegari S, Majani G. The effects of cognitive behavioural intervention in asthmatic patients. *Monaldi Arch Chest Dis* 1995; **50**:398–402.

27 Yoon R, McKenzie DK, Bauman A, Miles DA. Controlled trial evaluation of an asthma education program for adults. *Thorax* 1993; **48**:1110–16.

28 Zeiger RS, Heller S, Mellon MH, Wald J, Falkoff R, Schatz M. Facilitated referral to asthma specialist reduces relapses in asthma emergency room visits. *Allergy Clin Immunol* 1991; **87**:1160–8.

29 Brewin AM, Hughes JA. Effect of patient education on asthma management. *Br J Nursing* 1995; **4**:81–101.

30 Garrett J, Fenwick JM, Taylor G, Mitchell E, Stewart J, Rea H. Prospective controlled evaluation of the effect of a community based asthma education centre in a multiracial working class neighbourhood. *Thorax* 1994; **49**:976–83.

31 George MR, O'Dowd L, Martin I *et al.* A comprehensive educational program improves clinical outcome measures in inner-city patients with asthma. *Arch Intern Med* 1999; **159**:1710–16.

32 Mayo PH, Richman J, Harris HW. Results of a program to reduce admissions for adult asthma. *Ann Intern Med* 1990; **112**:864–71.

33 Hilton S, Sibbald B, Anderson HR, Freeling P. Controlled evaluation of the effects of patient education on asthma morbidity in general practice. *Lancet* 1986; **1**:26–9.

34 Neville RG, Hoskins G, Smith B, Clark R. Observations on the structure, process and clinical outcomes of asthma care in general practice. *Br J Gen Pract* 1996; **46**:583–7.

35 Yoon R, McKenzie DK, Miles DA, Bauman A. Characteristics of attenders and non-attenders at an asthma education programme. *Thorax* 1991; **46**:886–90.

36 Jenkinson D, Davison J, Jones S, Hawtin P. Comparison of effects of a self management booklet and audio cassette for patients with asthma. *BMJ* 1988; **297**:267–70.

CHAPTER 2.6

Non-pharmacological and complementary interventions to manage asthma

Guy B Marks, Brett G Toelle and Cassandra A Slader

Summary for clinicians

- Allergen immunotherapy is not without important health risks, but Level A evidence exists to show that allergen immunotherapy can significantly reduce asthma symptoms and reduce the need for increased medication.
- The effectiveness of existing methods of house mite control for improving asthma control in susceptible patients remains uncertain.
- There is no conclusive evidence of benefit arising from the general application of food restriction or food supplementation as treatment for people with asthma.
- Further trials are needed to determine whether management of either symptomatic or asymptomatic gastro-oesophageal reflux improves asthma control.
- Trials of acupuncture are of insufficient quality, size and with inadequate reporting of health outcomes to show evidence of effect.
- Despite the inconsistencies in the existing data, it is unlikely that the use of isopathic homeopathy is an effective treatment for asthma.
- There is Level A evidence that relaxation therapy has a beneficial effect on lung function, but this effect may be restricted to patients who perceive their asthma to be triggered by emotions.
- Use of breathing exercises may be beneficial in reducing bronchodilator use and improving asthma-related quality of life.

Introduction

Patients who have asthma often express interest in non-pharmacological and complementary approaches to asthma management. These approaches may be added to an existing 'traditional' treatment plan or may be used instead of the more 'traditional' approach of drug therapy, individualized management plan and regular medical review.

The clinician should be armed with information about the effectiveness of various non-pharmacological and complementary approaches to asthma management. Clinicians who appear knowledgeable and supportive about effective alternative approaches are likely to be viewed by patients as a more informed and important partner in self-management decisions.

Literature search

In this chapter, we have focused on certain specific interventions that have been evaluated in randomized controlled trials (RCTs) as treatment for asthma. The broad approach to evaluating the evidence has been to seek systematic reviews, where these are available. We have summarized RCTs where there are no systematic reviews or where RCTs have been published since the last update of the systematic review.

All searches were conducted in June 2003. The Cochrane Database of Systematic Reviews was searched initially. When there was no available systematic review or the last update on the available review was prior to 2003, the following databases were also searched: Cochrane Central Register of Controlled Trials, MEDLINE, EMBASE, CINAHL (Nursing and Allied Health database) and AMED (Allied and Complementary Medicine database). For the Cochrane Databases, a simple search strategy combining the therapy descriptor(s) with the term 'asthma' was used. Table 1 shows the methodological filters, adapted from those recommended by Haynes *et al.*[1] for the purpose of identifying citations relevant to therapy (http://www.phru.nhs.uk/~casp/filters.htm).

Each search combined terms for the therapy under consideration, the term 'asthma' and the methodological filter. Searches were limited to those articles with English language abstracts in which human subjects were studied. Only those trials that measured clinically relevant outcomes (symptoms, overall 'control', medication requirement, lung function or exacerbations) were included. All hits were reviewed for their relevance to the use of the target therapy in the treatment of people with asthma.

Allergen immunotherapy

Allergen immunotherapy entails medically supervised exposure to gradually increasing doses of allergen to promote the emergence of immunological tolerance to future environmental exposures to the same allergen. Also commonly known

Table 1. Methodological filters for identifying citations relevant to therapy.

MEDLINE	randomized controlled trial.pt. OR dt.fs. OR tu.fs. OR random$.tw.
EMBASE	randomized controlled trial/ OR dt.fs. OR random$.tw.
CINAHL	dt.fs. OR tu.fs. OR random$.tw.
AMED	random$.tw.

as hyposensitization or desensitization, the application of this mode of therapy to patients with asthma has been controversial because of reports of occasional serious adverse events.

A Cochrane Review has investigated the use of allergen immunotherapy for asthma.[2] The review encompassed a range of allergen extracts including house dust mites, pollens, animal dander and mould. It has been updated twice, most recently in August 2003. The review identified 75 trials published in 80 papers.

In 28 studies in which symptoms scores were measured, the overall effect of allergen immunotherapy, compared with placebo, was a significant decrease in symptoms [standardized mean difference (SMD) −0.72, 95% confidence interval (CI) −0.99 to −0.44; Fig. 1]. Meta-analysis of a further 22 studies, in which the risk of symptom deterioration was assessed, also found evidence in favour of allergen immunotherapy over placebo [number needed to treat (NNT) for benefit 3.2, 95% CI 2.4–5.0]. There was significant heterogeneity between allergens, with the most consistent evidence of benefit being for mite and pollen allergens.

In 15 studies that reported asthma medication scores, there was an overall significant beneficial effect (SMD −0.80, 95% CI −1.13 to −0.48), and the findings from 16 studies that assessed the need to increase asthma medication also favoured immunotherapy (NNT 3.8, 95% CI 2.9–5.9).

A number of studies also measured lung function and airway hyper-responsiveness. Limitations of data presentation in studies where lung function was measured and significant heterogeneity between studies make it difficult to assess the effect of allergen immunotherapy on lung function. Allergen immunotherapy was found to be effective in improving airway hyper-responsiveness in the 15 studies that reported this outcome (SMD −0.43, 95% CI −0.71 to −0.14).

Conclusion

Allergen immunotherapy is not without important health risks, but the Cochrane Review shows that, compared with placebo, allergen immunotherapy can significantly reduce asthma symptoms and reduce the need for increased medication. Patients should be fully informed of the potential risks and the likely benefits associated with a course of allergen immunotherapy.

Allergen avoidance

The association between allergy to environmental agents, such as house dust mite, pollens, moulds and animal danders, and the presence of allergic diseases, including asthma, has been well established in many studies.[3,4] Observational studies have linked exacerbations of asthma with high levels of exposure to allergen.[5,6] Other non-randomized studies have demonstrated clinical improvements in people with asthma over a prolonged period in a low-allergen hospital environment[7] and on moving to a low-allergen alpine environment.[8–10]

A search of the Cochrane Database of Systematic Reviews using the term 'allergen avoidance' identified three relevant reviews: one dealing with house dust control measures for asthma;[11] another dealing with pet allergen avoidance;[12] and a third dealing with feather versus non-feather bedding.[13] Of these, only the review on house dust mite control measures includes a substantial body of evidence, and only this intervention is reviewed here.

House dust mite allergen avoidance

The Cochrane Review on this subject identified 29 clinical trials, including 1120 subjects in interventions lasting from 2 weeks to 1 year.[11] The house dust mite control interventions that were implemented varied substantially between the studies and included a range of alternative chemical and physical treatment methods. Most of the studies did not demonstrate that mite exposure had been substantially reduced by the test interventions.

The meta-analysis did not reveal that there was an overall beneficial effect of house dust mite control interventions, as they were implemented across the range of studies. However, among parallel group trials, there was a significant beneficial effect of the physical treatment methods on asthma symptoms with SMD of asthma symptoms −0.44 (95% CI −0.83 to −0.06, $P = 0.02$; Fig. 2). The effect was in the same direction, although not statistically significant, in the crossover studies of physical treatment methods with SMD of asthma symptoms −0.54 (95% CI −1.41 to 0.33). In contrast, the chemical treatment methods had a significant adverse effect on asthma symptoms, and the combined physical and chemical treatments had no significant effect. There were no overall beneficial effects of the interventions on lung function or medication requirement.

A recent additional, very large parallel group RCT demonstrated that impermeable mattress covers, as a stand-alone intervention, are not effective in improving asthma outcomes over a 6-month period.[14] However, the magnitude of the reduction in allergen exposure was modest in this trial.

Review: Allergen immunotherapy for asthma
Comparison: 01 Allergen immunotherapy versus placebo
Outcome: 01 Asthma symptom scores

Study	Immunotherapy (N)	Mean (SD)	Placebo (N)	Mean (SD)	Standardized mean difference (random) (95% CI)	Weight (%)	Standardized mean difference (random) (95% CI)
01 Mite immunotherapy							
Altintas (1999)	29	1.70 (1.80)	5	3.20 (1.60)		3.3	−0.82 (−1.80, 0.15)
Armentia (1995)	22	1.62 (0.55)	13	2.70 (0.42)		3.6	−2.08 (−2.94, −1.22)
Franco (1995)	24	0.30 (0.40)	25	0.30 (0.45)		4.5	0.00 (−0.56, 0.56)
Machiels (1990a)	24	3.66 (3.13)	11	5.07 (2.63)		4.0	−0.46 (−1.18, 0.26)
Mungan (1999)	10	0.59 (0.00)	11	0.88 (0.00)		0.0	Not estimable
Pichler (1997)	16	3.50 (1.75)	14	7.00 (11.25)		4.0	−0.44 (−1.17, 0.29)
Sin (1996)	7	0.29 (0.49)	8	1.75 (0.71)		2.3	−2.22 (−3.60, −0.85)
Tabar (1999)	44	2.10 (10.31)	19	6.38 (11.13)		4.6	−0.40 (−0.94, 0.14)
Torres Costa (1996)	11	0.90 (0.70)	11	1.50 (0.80)		3.6	−0.77 (−1.64, 0.10)
Subtotal (95% CI)	187		117			25.7	−0.78 (−1.27, −0.29)
Test for heterogeneity chi-squared = 22.40 df = 7 P = 0.0022							
Test for overall effect = −3.14 P = 0.002							
02 Pollen immunotherapy							
Bousquet (1985)	31	1.72 (3.01)	8	3.05 (1.75)		3.8	−0.46 (−1.25, 0.32)
Bousquet III (1989)	46	8.00 (17.25)	14	20.70 (11.00)		4.4	−0.78 (−1.40, −0.16)
Bousquet IV (1990)	39	15.20 (18.60)	18	54.80 (23.00)		4.2	−1.95 (−2.62, −1.28)
Bruce (1977)	15	4.40 (3.10)	18	4.10 (4.10)		4.1	0.08 (−0.61, 0.77)
Creticos (1996)	37	2.96 (2.31)	40	4.12 (2.52)		4.9	−0.47 (−0.93, −0.02)
Dolz (1996)	18	0.21 (0.39)	10	0.55 (0.52)		3.8	−0.75 (−1.55, 0.05)
Hill (1982)	11	6.91 (3.45)	9	4.89 (3.98)		3.5	−0.52 (−0.38, 1.42)
Kuna (1989)	12	2.57 (0.97)	12	3.75 (1.11)		3.6	−1.09 (−1.96, −0.22)
Machiels (1990b)	15	54.38 (40.69)	15	67.29 (36.38)		4.0	−0.33 (−1.05, 0.40)
Ortolani (1984)	8	1.40 (0.60)	7	4.50 (1.90)		2.4	−2.14 (−3.49, −0.79)
Reid (1986)	9	47.00 (50.90)	9	178.00 (144.90)		3.2	−1.15 (−2.17, −0.13)
Sin (1996)	9	0.33 (0.71)	7	1.43 (0.98)		2.9	−1.24 (−2.35, −0.14)
Walker (2000)	22	26.00 (204.60)	22	56.00 (103.80)		4.4	−0.18 (−0.77, 0.41)
Zenner (1999)	45	12.50 (32.87)	41	26.00 (48.66)		4.9	−0.33 (−0.75, 0.10)
Subtotal (95% CI)	317		230			53.1	−0.66 (−0.99, −0.33)
Test for heterogeneity chi-squared = 38.83 df = 13 P = 0.0002							
Test for overall effect = −3.90 P = 0.0001							
03 Other immunotherapy							
Adkinson (1997)	61	0.26 (0.21)	60	0.21 (0.17)		5.1	0.26 (−0.10, 0.62)
Alvarez (1994)	14	−81.30 (15.50)	14	−20.70 (33.20)		3.3	−2.27 (−3.25, −1.29)
Leynadier (2000)	3	0.00 (0.00)	6	0.40 (0.76)		0.0	Not estimable
Valovirta (1984)	15	29.30 (29.00)	12	35.60 (18.30)		3.9	−0.25 (−1.01, 0.52)
Vamey (1997)	13	17.10 (27.40)	15	62.10 (38.73)		3.7	−1.29 (−2.11, −0.46)
Subtotal (95% CI)	106		107			21.1	−0.83 (−1.92, 0.26)
Test for heterogeneity chi-squared = 30.12 df = 3 P < 0.00001							
Test for overall effect = −1.49 P = 0.14							
Total (95% CI)	610		454			100.0	−0.72 (−0.99, −0.44)
Test for heterogeneity chi-squared = 96.38 df = 25 P < 0.00001							
Test for overall effect = −5.14 P < 0.00001							

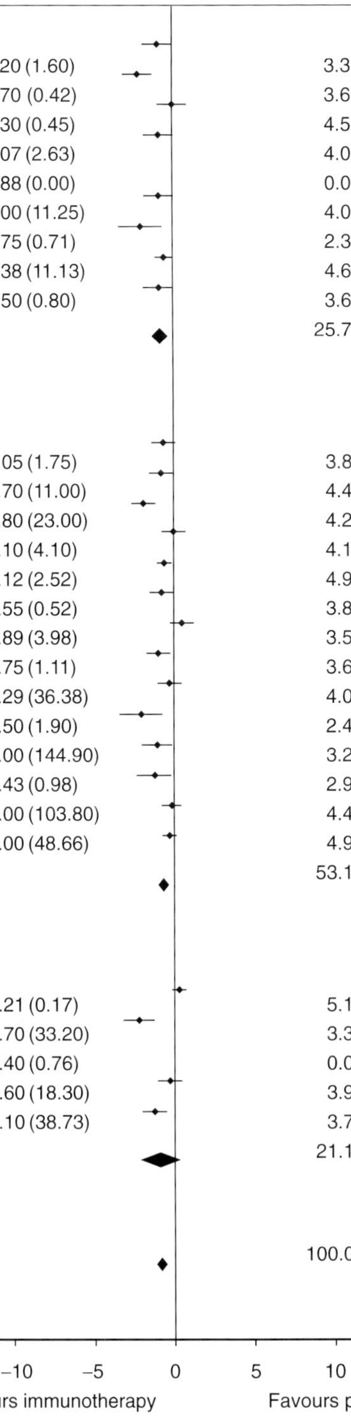

−10 −5 0 5 10

Favours immunotherapy   Favours placebo

Figure 1. The effect of allergen immunotherapy on asthma symptoms. Reproduced from Cochrane website, with permission.

Review: House dust mite control measures for asthma
Comparison: 01 House dust mite reduction vs control
Outcome: 02 Asthma symptoms score

Study	Treatment (N)	Mean (SD)	Control (N)	Mean (SD)	Standardized mean difference (random) (95% CI)	Weight (%)	Standardized mean difference (random) (95% CI)
01 Chemical methods							
Bahir (1997)	13	1.60 (1.50)	17	1.40 (1.50)		8.1	0.13 (−0.59, 0.85)
Chang (1996)	12	1.10 (1.70)	14	0.40 (0.50)		7.3	0.56 (−0.23, 1.35)
Dietemann (1993)	11	1.40 (1.24)	12	1.18 (0.36)		7.0	0.24 (−0.58, 1.06)
Reiser (1990)	23	5.50 (4.30)	23	3.30 (3.50)		9.8	0.55 (−0.04, 1.14)
Subtotal (95% CI)	59		66			25.3	0.39 (0.04, 0.75)
Test for heterogeneity chi-squared = 1.10 df = 3 P = 0.7772							
Test for overall effect = 2.16 P = 0.03							
02 Physical methods – parallel group studies							
Chen (1996)	20	0.50 (0.66)	15	0.82 (1.01)		8.6	−0.38 (−1.05, 0.30)
Cinti (1996)	10	0.30 (0.68)	10	1.00 (1.15)		6.2	−0.71 (−1.62, 0.20)
Huss (1992)	26	8.80 (10.70)	26	13.10 (11.20)		10.4	−0.39 (−0.94, 0.16)
Subtotal (95% CI)	56		51			21.6	−0.44 (−0.83, −0.06)
Test for heterogeneity chi-squared = 0.41 df = 2 P = 0.8165							
Test for overall effect = −2.24 P = 0.02							
03 Physical methods – crossover studies							
Antonicelli (1991)	9	0.16 (0.32)	9	0.26 (0.34)		6.0	−0.29 (−1.22, 0.64)
Wamer (1993)	14	0.20 (0.26)	14	0.19 (0.34)		7.9	0.03 (−0.71, 0.77)
Zwemer (1973)	12	0.70 (0.51)	12	1.40 (0.43)		6.1	−1.43 (−2.35, −0.52)
Subtotal (95% CI)	35		35			13.4	−0.54 (−1.41, 0.33)
Test for heterogeneity chi-squared = 6.17 df = 2 P = 0.0458							
Test for overall effect = −1.21 P = 0.2							
04 Combination methods							
Cloosterman (1999)	76	5.50 (6.10)	81	6.30 (6.70)		14.0	−0.12 (−0.44, 0.19)
Marks (1994)	17	0.98 (0.57)	18	0.67 (0.55)		8.6	0.54 (−0.14, 1.22)
Subtotal (95% CI)	93		99			39.7	0.14 (−0.50, 0.78)
Test for heterogeneity chi-squared = 3.06 df = 1 P = 0.0803							
Test for overall effect = 0.43 P = 0.7							
Total (95% CI)	243		251			100.0	−0.07 (−0.35, 0.22)
Test for heterogeneity chi-squared = 23.58 df = 11 P = 0.0146							
Test for overall effect = −0.47 P = 0.6							

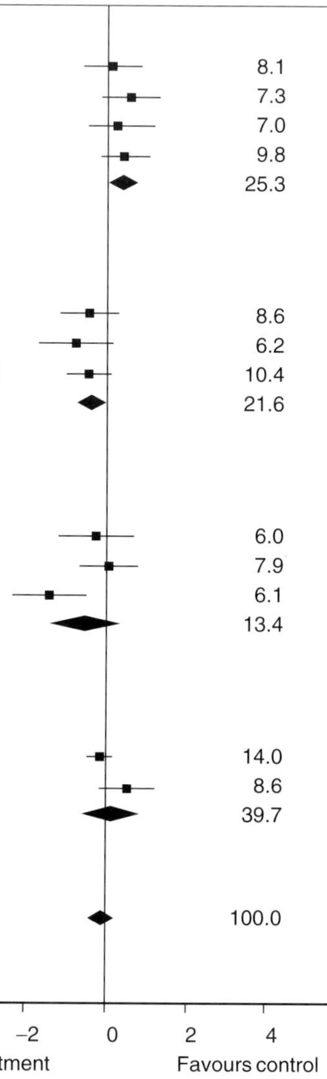

```
    −4   −2    0    2    4
Favours treatment    Favours control
```

Figure 2. The effect of house dust mite control measures on asthma symptoms. Reproduced from Cochrane website, with permission.

Conclusion

The effectiveness of existing methods of house mite control for improving asthma control in susceptible patients remains uncertain. It is likely that most trials of house dust mite control interventions failed to achieve a substantial reduction in actual mite allergen exposure.[15] Further work is required to establish a safe, feasible and effective method of reducing exposure to domestic aeroallergen, which can then be tested in a clinical trial.

Dietary interventions

Dietary factors have long been thought to play a role in the expression of asthma. Numerous theories on the role of diet have been proposed, and each has resulted in different approaches to dietary modification for the control of asthma. These theories fall into two broad categories. One approach is based on the assumption that certain foods are harmful to people with asthma or allergic disease. This approach focuses on food allergy and food chemical sensitivity. Interventions based on this model are relevant to a subgroup of people with asthma who have demonstrated adverse responses to ingestion of specific food substances. This review has not included these interventions. The alternative theories are more wide-ranging and arise from evidence that a deficiency or an imbalance in certain food types contributes to the expression of asthma. Evidence about the role of dietary fats, salt, antioxidants, vitamins, minerals and trace elements can all be included under this model, and the available evidence is summarized below.

Reduction in dietary salt

There is evidence from cross-sectional and other population studies that the presence of airway hyper-responsiveness may be linked to dietary salt intake.[16–18]

The authors of a recently updated Cochrane Review[19] identified five studies, all of short duration and with small numbers of subjects. One or more of the studies provided evidence in relation to the effect of a low-salt diet compared with either a normal-salt or a high-salt diet on lung function, inhaled corticosteroid usage, inhaled bronchodilator usage and exacerbation rate. None of the differences was significant. There were no data on symptoms. The authors state that no conclusion about the effectiveness of dietary salt reduction is possible at this stage.

Selenium supplementation

Selenium is a trace element essential for the function of the antioxidant enzyme glutathione peroxidase.[20] Relatively low selenium levels have been observed among subjects with asthma in New Zealand.[21,22]

Although a protocol for a Cochrane Systematic Review has been published, no completed review has been published. One relevant trial[23] was identified in the Cochrane Central Register of Controlled Clinical Trials. Searching the other databases identified no additional relevant trials.

A double-blind, parallel group, controlled trial was conducted among 24 adult patients with asthma who were non-atopic, that is they had negative skin prick tests and RAST and normal total serum IgE.[23] Seven of the subjects had a history of intolerance to non-steroidal anti-inflammatory drugs. The intervention comprised sodium selenite (100 µg) or placebo daily for 14 weeks. At the end of the treatment period, a blinded clinical assessment concluded that one out of 12 placebo subjects had improved, compared with six out of 12 intervention subjects ($P = 0.04$, NNT = 2.4). No significant changes in lung function were detected in this small study.

Vitamin C (ascorbic acid) supplementation

Cross-sectional and case–control studies have revealed an association between lower serum levels of vitamin C and the presence of asthma.[24,25]

A relevant Cochrane Review was identified.[26] An additional relevant RCT,[27] published since the last update of the review, was identified in the Cochrane Register of Controlled Clinical Trials. Searching the other databases did not identify any further relevant trials.

The meta-analysis identified six clinical trials of vitamin C supplementation in people with asthma (five of which included adult subjects).[26] Three of the six studies found that there were benefits from vitamin C supplementation and three did not. In general, the data were not available in a form that allowed abstraction or combination. Data on lung function were combined from two trials in 46 subjects. The weighted mean difference (WMD) in forced expired volume in 1 second (FEV_1) was 0.36 L (95% CI –0.35 to 1.08), the wide confidence interval indicating that even this meta-analysis was underpowered. A subsequently reported RCT, conducted among 158 children with asthma in Mexico City, tested the effect of vitamin C (250 mg) together with vitamin E (50 mg) versus placebo taken daily for 12 weeks. The principal finding was an abolition of the negative effect of ambient ozone on lung function in children with asthma. It is not clear how this effect would be translated into clinically relevant benefits in other settings.

Overall, the role of vitamin C supplementation in the treatment of people with asthma is not established.

Oral magnesium supplementation

Low levels of dietary magnesium have been linked to the occurrence of brittle asthma,[28] and intravenous magnesium, given in addition to standard therapy, may have beneficial effects in patients treated for acute, very severe asthma in the emergency department.[29]

There are no Cochrane Reviews examining the role of oral magnesium supplementation in subjects with stable chronic asthma. A search of the Cochrane Register of Controlled Clinical Trials revealed one relevant RCT.[30] Searching the other databases did not identify any further relevant trials.

The one available trial was a double-blind, randomized, crossover study conducted in 17 people with asthma who had been on a low-magnesium diet during a run-in period. This was followed by two 3-week periods, in random order, of daily supplementation with magnesium sulphate (400 mg) or placebo. Asthma symptom scores were significantly lower during the magnesium treatment period, the median difference from placebo being 3.8 (95% CI 0.5–7.0) symptom points per week ($P = 0.02$). However, there was no significant improvement in lung function or bronchodilator use during magnesium supplementation.

The role of magnesium supplementation in the long-term management of chronic asthma remains to be established.

Fish oil supplementation

Cross-sectional studies have revealed that children who reported consumption of fish more than once a week have a lower prevalence of asthma than those who eat fish less often.[31] It has been proposed that the mechanism underlying this association is an alteration in the synthesis of inflammatory mediators attributable to a change in the ratio of omega-3 to omega-6 fatty acids.[32]

There is one Cochrane Review examining the impact of dietary supplementation with marine fatty acids (fish oil) in subjects with asthma.[33] Search of the Cochrane Register of Controlled Clinical Trials revealed one further recently published RCT.[34] Searching the other databases did not reveal any further relevant clinical trials.

The Cochrane Review[33] identified five parallel group RCTs (124 subjects) that reported symptom scores. In these studies, there was no overall evidence of benefit with the SMD of symptom scores being −0.094 (95% CI −0.454 to 0.266), without significant heterogeneity. One crossover study (conducted in 30 subjects) also showed no effect on symptoms, whereas another crossover study showed an improvement in symptoms. Five studies (four parallel group and one crossover) showed no significant impact of the intervention on medication requirement. There was significant heterogeneity among the parallel group studies. Four parallel group studies and two crossover studies, conducted over 10–26 weeks, showed no overall effect on morning peak expiratory flow (PEF) rate. However, there was significant heterogeneity between the parallel group studies. Two studies demonstrated no significant effect on clinic lung function with WMD in FEV_1 2.08% predicted (95% CI −4.77 to 8.93%).

The additional recent study[34] was a parallel group study in which 46 subjects received omega-3 fatty acid (50 mg) or placebo for 8 weeks. Significant treatment benefits were observed for daytime wheeze, β-agonist use and morning PEF rate. There were no significant effects on sleep disturbance, FEV_1 and evening PEF rate.

Overall, we cannot be confident of any clinically important beneficial effects attributable to marine (fish oil) or omega-3 fatty acid supplementation as treatment for patients with asthma. However, the heterogeneity among the studies implies that specific subgroups of patients or modes/durations of treatment may be associated with clinical benefit. Further research is required to explore this heterogeneity.

Conclusion

There is no conclusive evidence of benefit arising from the general application of food restriction or food supplementation as treatment for people with asthma. However, the available evidence consists of a number of small trials, which, even with the application of meta-analysis, for the most part do not yield definitive results.

Gastro-oesophageal reflux

Gastro-oesophageal reflux (GOR) is commonly observed among adults with asthma.[35,36] It has been suggested that, when asthma control is not obtained with optimal standard treatment, then GOR should be considered as a potential trigger.[37]

Evidence for the effectiveness of this approach has been assessed in a Cochrane Review that was last updated in September 2002. The review evaluated the effectiveness on asthma outcomes of various treatment options for managing GOR in adults and children who have asthma.[38] The treatment options investigated include proton pump inhibitors (six studies), H_2-receptor antagonists (five studies), antireflux surgery (one study) and conservative management (one study). Studies included subjects with and without apparent reflux-associated symptoms, and their duration ranged between 1 week and 6 months. There was considerable variation in the definitions of GOR and of asthma between the studies, and this limited the synthesis of data in a meta-analysis.

Overall, there was no clear benefit demonstrated for the treatment of GOR on lung function, airway responsiveness or nocturnal asthma symptoms. One trial demonstrated an improvement in wheezing with H_2-receptor antagonist and with surgery, compared with placebo, and a further trial demonstrated an improvement in wheezing with conservative therapy.

Conclusion

Many of the trials had small sample size and insufficient assessment of the control of GOR symptoms. Further research is needed to determine whether management of either symptomatic or asymptomatic GOR improves asthma control. Studies need to be powered with sufficient subjects, well-characterized GOR and asthma outcomes and of sufficient duration that any effect or lack of effect can be reliably ascribed to the respective intervention for GOR.

Acupuncture

Acupuncture is a therapy used to treat a number of illnesses and ailments. It is most often used in China as a traditional form of medicine but, more recently, has gained fairly widespread consumer recognition in the western world as another therapeutic option. Acupuncture involves the positioning of very fine needles into the body at specific points. There is a range of traditions, and the approach may be to use standard positions or to individualize the positions for the patient.

A Cochrane Review investigated the effectiveness of acupuncture as treatment for asthma.[39] The most recent amendment to this review was in September 1999. The authors of the review identified seven trials suitable for inclusion in the review reporting data from adults and children. The method of acupuncture used differed between the trials. Five trials used needles and two trials used lasers. Additionally, six trials used identical acupuncture points for all subjects within the trial, but these points varied between trials. One trial used individualized points.

Unfortunately, the quality of the trials and the format of presentation of results did not allow for meaningful meta-analysis to be undertaken. Owing to these limitations, it is not possible to determine whether acupuncture improves lung function, decreases medication use or improves symptoms. Three trials reported PEFR with the weighted mean difference between active and sham arms after treatment being −8.4 L/min (95% CI −29.4 to 46.2 L/min).

Three additional trials have been published since the publication of the Cochrane Review.[40–42] These studies investigated both the long-term over 6 months[40] and short-term over weeks[41,42] health effects of real versus sham acupuncture. None of the studies demonstrated any clinically significant effect of 'real' acupuncture as measured by symptoms or lung function. One study, however, did show an improvement in quality of life and decreased medication use.[42]

Conclusion

Claims that acupuncture is an effective therapy for asthma are not supported by this Cochrane Review or subsequent published trials. The available trials are of insufficient quality, size and with inadequate reporting of health outcomes to show evidence of effect. It is important that future studies of the effectiveness of acupuncture address these limitations so that meaningful data can be gathered for meta-analysis.

Homeopathy

There are three forms of homeopathy—single (classical), complex and isopathy. The single or classical approach involves matching the toxic symptoms induced by a particular herb or animal at pharmacological doses with the symptoms of the patient, and then administering the selected remedy in dilute form. Complex homeopathy involves the use of medicaments containing a mixture of different herbal and homeopathic products. Isopathy is the simplest of the three forms. It is based on the treatment philosophy of 'like cures like'. Remedies are made by serial dilution of the active component, with vigorous shaking (succussion) in between each dilution step. The resulting solution is commonly diluted such that it would contain either very few or even no molecules of the active ingredient.

A Cochrane Review of homeopathy[43] included three studies.[44–46] Since its most recent substantive update (1998), an additional two RCTs[47,48] have been conducted. A placebo was administered in all of the trials. In two of the studies, the homeopathic remedy was individualized to the treatment arm.[44,48] Only two trials examined the same remedy.[45,47] The effect of homeopathy for children with asthma has been studied in two trials.[46,48] In four of the five trials, conventional treatment was continued (Table 2).[44,45,47,48]

Two studies reported statistically significant differences between placebo and the homeopathic remedy used.[44,45] The differences noted were improvements in lung function parameters (FEV$_1$, FVC and PEFR), improved symptom severity in one study[44] and decreased medication requirement in the other study.[45] No significant differences were noted in the other studies.[46–48] The Cochrane Review concluded that there 'is not enough evidence to reliably assess the possible role of homeopathy in asthma' (Table 3).

Conclusion

Despite the inconsistencies in the existing data, it is unlikely that the use of isopathic homeopathy is superior to placebo in the treatment of asthma.

Relaxation

Relaxation may be defined as the general process of reaching a state of equilibrium, free of tension. Various techniques exist to assist in the attainment of this state. Some examples include:
• Jacobsonian progressive relaxation: a routine of tensing, relaxing and attending to the sensation of each muscle group;
• autogenic training: a series of visual and sensory exercises used to gain deep relaxation;
• biofeedback training: a technique used to monitor and gain control over automatic, reflex-regulated body functions using information obtained from monitoring equipment.

A single systematic review has been published. In addition, there are eight RCTs (see Table 4). Various forms of relaxation techniques including autogenic and biofeedback training have been utilized. In several studies, a psychotherapist led relaxation training. Interventions delivered to the control arms in these studies have included 'resting quietly', 'music therapy', 'leaderless psychotherapy' and group discussion sessions. Conventional asthma medications appear to have been continued during these studies. Four of the studies have been conducted in children.[49–52]

Overall, the results of the studies do not indicate a clinically significant benefit in terms of asthma symptoms experienced or change in medication requirement. Two of the additional RCTs[49,50] indicate an improvement in lung function measures, which concurs with the conclusion of the systematic review.[57] The frequency of asthma attacks decreased significantly in two of the trials.[50,55]

Conclusion

There is a possibility that relaxation therapy has a beneficial effect on lung function. Relaxation therapy may be of most benefit for those who perceive their asthma to be triggered by emotion. It may also be of use when an acute attack is experienced.

Breathing techniques

There is a variety of breathing techniques, which are used by people with asthma. The most common are the Buteyko

Table 2. Summary of homeopathy studies.

Authors	Included in Cochrane Review	Subjects	Design	Intervention	Outcome measures
Reilly et al.[44]	Yes	28 patients with allergic asthma	Double-blind, randomized, placebo controlled	4 weeks of individualized treatment using a homeopathic preparation of house dust mite. Prescribed medications continued	Primary outcome = daily visual analogue scale for symptoms. Other outcome measures = lung function (FEV_1, FVC, PEFR) and digital symptom scores
Matusiewicz[45]	Yes	40 patients with 'steroid-dependent asthma'	Double-blind, placebo controlled (details re randomization lacking)	6 months of treatment with a standardized homeopathic formulation. Prescribed medications continued	Lung function (FVC, FEV_1, PEFR) and required daily dose of oral corticosteroid
Freitas et al.[46]	Yes	86 children with at least 'three previous asthmatic crises'	Double-blind, randomized, placebo controlled	Treatment with *Blatta orientalis*	Intensity, frequency and duration of 'asthmatic crises'
Lewith[47]	No	202 adults with asthma with a positive skin prick test to house dust mite	Double-blind, randomized, placebo controlled	16 weeks of treatment with a homeopathic preparation of house dust mite. Prescribed medications continued	Clinic-based assessments: FEV_1, quality of life and mood. Diary-based assessments: AM and PM PEFR, visual analogue scale of severity of asthma, quality of life and daily mood
White et al.[48]	No	93 children with mild to moderate asthma	Double-blind, randomized, placebo controlled	12 months of treatment with individualized homeopathic treatment determined by a homeopath. Prescribed medications continued	Primary outcome = asthma quality of life. Other outcome measures = weekly diary record of number of days of breathlessness, wheeze, cough, medication use, school days missed, PEFR

Table 3. Summary of outcome measures for homeopathy studies.

	Reilly et al.[44]	Matusiewicz[45]	Freitas et al.[46]	White et al.[48]	Lewith[47]
Symptom severity	Improved	—	—	No difference (QOL)	No difference
FVC	Slight improvement	Improvement	—	—	—
FEV_1	Slight improvement	Improvement	—	—	No difference
PEFR	No difference	Improvement	—	No difference	No difference
Steroid dose	—	Decreased	—	No change	—
Asthma exacerbations	—	—	No difference	—	—

method and yoga. Buteyko is a system of breathing exercises focusing on the nasal route of breathing, hypoventilation and avoidance of deep breaths. Yoga is an ancient Indian practice using physical postures to obtain harmony of mind, body and spirit. Through discipline of breathing and concentration during practice, tranquillity and awareness of mind are achievable.

The Cochrane Review included five studies.[58] Since its most recent substantive update, the results from an additional three studies[59–61] have been published (Table 5).

The Cochrane Review found that no reliable conclusions could be drawn concerning the use of breathing exercises for asthma in clinical practice. However, it appears that breathing exercises may be useful in decreasing bronchodilator use, and that they may have a positive impact on quality of life. Two studies have shown an improvement in PEFR (Table 6).[62,63]

Table 4. Summary of additional relaxation studies

Authors	Subjects	Design	Intervention	Outcome measures
Coen et al.[51]	20 people with asthma, aged 12–22 years	Randomized, controlled pilot study	Biofeedback-assisted relaxation for the active group over eight sessions. Prescribed medications continued	Patients monitored their symptoms and medication use. Facial muscle tension and respiratory function were measured, as well as CD4 and CD8 lymphocyte counts
Deter[53]	30 adults with asthma	Randomized, controlled study	Participants were randomized to one of three interventions: autogenic relaxation, functional relaxation or control. All sessions incorporated delivery of educational material and discussion. Prescribed medications were continued	Use of medication (reliever and corticosteroids), number of visits to the general practitioner
Hockemeyer and Smyth[49]	Young adults with asthma	Randomized, controlled trial	Participants in each group were provided with a workbook. Those randomized to the 'active' treatment received information and activities related to stress management	Lung function and perceived stress
Kern-Buell et al.[54]	16 people with mild asthma	Randomized, controlled pilot study	Those in the active group were taught biofeedback	Asthma symptoms, lung function (FEV_1, FVC), bronchodilator use, forehead muscle tension, cellular immune factors (white blood cell count, neutrophil, basophil and lymphocyte counts)
Sachs et al.[55]	86 chronic asthmatics	Controlled study	Relaxation (incorporating both functional and autogenic aspects) was taught to those with asthma. The control arm received an educational intervention. Prescribed medications were continued	Lung function, patient diary (including asthma-specific complaints, frequency of asthma attacks, sleep disturbances, morning coughing urge, medication usage), Spielberger anxiety scale, Giessen list of complaints (modified and augmented) and Ziegler coping questionnaire
Spiess et al.[56]	38 asthmatics	Randomized, controlled pilot study	Patients were taught relaxation techniques in groups in eight 2-hour sessions. The control arm received education only	Lung function, anxiety and insomnia scores, self-reported dyspnoea and the need to cough
Vazquez[52]	18 children with asthma	Controlled study	Both groups participated in an asthma self-management programme. Half were subsequently taught progressive relaxation	Anxiety scores, lung function (FEV_1, FVC)
Vazquez and Buceta[50]	27 children with mild to moderate asthma	Stratified (according to anxiety score and emotionally triggered attacks) controlled trial	Group 1 received an asthma self-management programme, Group 2 the same programme with relaxation training added, and Group 3 received only pharmacological treatment	Subjective assessment of attack intensity and duration, anxiety scores and PEFR

Table 5. Summary of additional breathing technique studies.

Authors	Subjects	Design	Intervention	Outcome measures
Manocha et al.[59]	47 patients with moderate to severe asthma completed this study	Double-blind, randomized, controlled trial	Sahaja yoga was taught to the intervention groups. Both the yoga and the control interventions required the subjects to attend a 2-hour session once a week for 4 months	Asthma-related quality of life, Profile of Mood States, level of airway hyper-responsiveness to methacholine, a diary card-based combined asthma score reflecting symptoms, bronchodilator usage and PEFR
Opat et al.[60]	28 patients with mild to moderate asthma	Randomized controlled trial	Active group was taught the Buteyko technique via video and were instructed to practise the exercises for 20 min twice daily for 4 weeks	Asthma-related quality of life, PEF, symptoms and asthma medication intake
Thomas et al.[61]	33 adults with diagnosed and currently treated asthma	Randomized controlled trial	Short physiotherapy breathing retraining was compared with an asthma nurse education control arm	Asthma Quality of Life questionnaire scores, Nijmegen questionnaire scores

Table 6. Summary of outcome measures for breathing technique studies.

	Bowler et al.[62]	Fluge et al.[64]	Girodo et al.[65]	Manocha et al.[59]	Nagarathna and Nagendra[63]	Opat et al.[60]	Thomas et al.[61]	Vedanthan et al.[66]
Symptom severity	—	—	—	No difference	—	—	—	No difference
FVC	—	No difference	–	—	—	—	—	No difference
FEV_1	No difference	No difference	—	—	—	—	—	No difference
PEFR	Improvement	—	—	No difference	Improvement	—	—	No difference
Steroid dose	Reduction	—	—	—	—	—	—	—
Bronchodilator use	Decrease	—	—	No difference	Decrease	Decrease	—	—
Asthma exacerbations	–	No difference	—	—	Decrease	—	—	—
Asthma QOL	Improvement (a non-standard questionnaire was used)	—	—	No difference (however, mood scores improved)	—	Improvement	Improvement	—

Conclusion

Use of breathing exercises may be beneficial in reducing bronchodilator use and improving asthma-related quality of life.

References

1 Haynes R, Wilczynski N, McKibbon K, Walker C, Sinclair J. Developing optimal search strategies for detecting clinically sound studies in MEDLINE. *J Am Med Inform Assoc* 1994; **1**:447–58.

2 Abramson MJ, Puy RM, Weiner JM. Allergen immunotherapy for asthma (Cochrane Review). In: *The Cochrane Library*, Issue 4. Chichester, John Wiley & Sons, 2003.

3 Britton WJ, Woolcock AJ, Peat JK, Sedgwick CH, Lloyd DM, Leeder SR. Prevalence of bronchial hyperresponsiveness in children: the relationship between asthma and skin reactivity to allergens in two communities. *Int J Epidemiol* 1986; **15**:202–9.

4 Peat JK, Woolcock AJ. Sensitivity to common allergens: relation to respiratory symptoms and bronchial hyper-responsiveness in children from three different climatic areas of Australia. *Clin Exp Allergy* 1991; **21**:573–81.

5 O'Hollaren MT, Yunginger JW, Offord KP *et al.* Exposure to an aeroallergen as a possible precipitating factor in respiratory arrest in young patients with asthma. *N Engl J Med* 1991; **324**:359–63.

6 Marks GB, Colquhoun JR, Girgis ST *et al.* Thunderstorm outflows preceding epidemics of asthma during spring and summer. *Thorax* 2001; **56**:468–71.

7 Platts-Mills TAE, Tovey ER, Mitchell EB, Moszora H, Nock P, Wilkins SR. Reduction of bronchial hyperreactivity during prolonged allergen avoidance. *Lancet* 1982; **2**:675–7.

8 Grootendorst DC, Dahlen SE, Van Den Bos JW *et al.* Benefits of high altitude allergen avoidance in atopic adolescents with moderate to severe asthma, over and above treatment with high dose inhaled steroids. *Clin Exp Allergy* 2001; **31**:400–8.

9 Peroni DG, Boner AL, Vallone G, Antolini I, Warner JO. Effective allergen avoidance at high altitude reduces allergen-induced bronchial hyperresponsiveness. *Am J Respir Crit Care Med* 1994; **149**:1442–6.

10 Piacentini GL, Vicentini L, Mazzi P, Chilosi M, Martinati L, Boner AL. Mite-antigen avoidance can reduce bronchial epithelial shedding in allergic asthmatic children. *Clin Exp Allergy* 1998; **28**:561–7.

11 Gotzsche PC, Johansen HK, Burr ML, Hammarquist C. House dust mite control measures for asthma (Cochrane Review). In: *The Cochrane Library*, Issue 4. Chichester, John Wiley & Sons, 2003.

12 Kilburn S, Lasserson TJ, McKean M. Pet allergen control measures for allergic asthma in children and adults (Cochrane Review). In: *The Cochrane Library*, Issue 4. Chichester, John Wiley & Sons, 2003.

13 Campbell F, Jones K, Gibson P. Feather versus non-feather bedding for asthma (Cochrane Review). In: *The Cochrane Library*, Issue 4. Chichester, John Wiley & Sons, 2003.

14 Woodcock A, Forster L, Matthews E *et al.* Control of exposure to mite allergen and allergen-impermeable bed covers for adults with asthma. *N Engl J Med* 2003; **349**:225–36.

15 Tovey ER, O'Meara T, Marks G. Bed covers and dust mites (letter). *N Engl J Med* 2003; **349**:1668–71.

16 Burney PGJ, Britton JR, Chinn S *et al.* Response to inhaled histamine and 24 hour sodium excretion. *BMJ* 1986; **292**:1483–6.

17 Burney PGJ, Neild JN, Twort CHC *et al.* The effect of changing dietary sodium on the bronchial response to histamine. *Thorax* 1989; **44**: 36–41.

18 Tribe RM, Barton JR, Poston L, Burney PGJ. Dietary sodium intake, airway responsiveness, and cellular sodium transport. *Am J Respir Crit Care Med* 1994; **149**:1426–33.

19 Ram FSF, Ardern KD. Dietary salt reduction or exclusion for allergic asthma (Cochrane Review). In: *The Cochrane Library*, Issue 4. Chichester, John Wiley & Sons, 2003.

20 Diplock AT, Chaudhry FA. The relationship of selenium biochemistry to selenium responsive disease in man. In: Prasad AS, ed. *Essential and Toxic Trace Elements in Human Health and Disease.* New York, Alan R Liss, 1988:211–26.

21 Stone J, Hinks LJ, Beasley R, Holgate ST, Clayton BA. Reduced selenium status of patients with asthma. *Clin Sci* 1989; **77**:495–500.

22 Flatt A, Pearce N, Thomson CD, Sears MR, Robinson MF, Beasley R. Reduced selenium in asthmatic subjects in New Zealand. *Thorax* 1990; **45**:95–9.

23 Hasselmark L, Malmgren R, Zetterstrom O, Unge G. Selenium supplementation in intrinsic asthma. *Allergy* 1993; **48**:30–6.

24 Schwartz J, Weiss ST. Dietary factors and their relation to respiratory symptoms. The Second National Health and Nutrition Examination Survey. *Am J Epidemiol* 1990; **132**:67–76.

25 Olusi SO, Ojukiku OO, Jessup WJ, Iboko MI. Plasma and white cell ascorbic acid concentrations in patients with bronchial asthma. *Clin Chim Acta* 1979; **92**:161–6.

26 Ram FSF, Rowe BH, Kaur B. Vitamin C supplementation for asthma (Cochrane Review). In: *The Cochrane Library*, Issue 2. Chichester, John Wiley & Sons, 2003.

27 Romieu I, Sienra-Monge JJ, Ramirez-Aguilar M *et al.* Antioxidant supplementation and lung functions among children with asthma exposed to high levels of air pollutants. *Am J Respir Crit Care Med* 2002; **166**:703–9.

28 Baker JC, Tunnicliffe WS, Duncanson RC, Ayres JG. Dietary antioxidants and magnesium in type 1 brittle asthma: a case control study. *Thorax* 1999; **54**:115–18.

29 Silverman RA, Osborn H, Runge J *et al.* IV magnesium sulfate in the treatment of acute severe asthma: a multicenter randomized controlled trial (comment). *Chest* 2002; **122**:489–97.

30 Hill J, Micklewright A, Lewis S, Britton J. Investigation of the effect of short-term change in dietary magnesium intake in asthma. *Eur Respir J* 1997; **10**:2225–9.

31 Hodge L, Salome CM, Peat JK, Haby MM, Xuan W, Woolcock AJ. Consumption of oily fish and childhood asthma risk. *Med J Aust* 1996; **164**:137–40.

32 Black PN, Sharpe S. Dietary fat and asthma: is there a connection? *Eur Respir J* 1997; **10**:6–12.

33 Woods RK, Thien FCK, Abramson MJ. Dietary marine fatty acids (fish oil) for asthma in adults and children (Cochrane Review). In: *The Cochrane Library*, Issue 4. Chichester, John Wiley & Sons, 2003.

34 Emelyanov A, Fedoseev G, Krasnoschekova O, Abulimity A, Trendeleva T, Barnes PJ. Treatment of asthma with lipid extract of New Zealand green-lipped mussel: a randomised clinical trial. *Eur Respir J* 2002; **20**:596–600.

35 Harding SM, Richter JE. The role of gastroesophageal reflux in chronic cough and asthma. *Chest* 1997; **111**:1389–402.

36 Field SK, Underwood M, Brant R, Cowie RL. Prevalence of gastroesophageal reflux symptoms in asthma. *Chest* 1996; **109**:316–22.

37 Harding SM. Gastroesophageal reflux and asthma: insight into the association. *J Allergy Clin Immunol* 1999; **104**:251–9.

38 Gibson PG, Henry RL, Coughlan JL. Gastro-esophageal reflux treatment for asthma in adults and children (Cochrane Review). In: *The Cochrane Library*, Issue 4. Chichester, John Wiley & Sons, 2003.

39 Linde K, Jobst K, Panton J. Acupuncture for chronic asthma (Cochrane Review). In: *The Cochrane Library*, Issue 4. Chichester, John Wiley & Sons, 2003.

40 Medici TC, Grebski E, Wu J, Hinz G, Wuthrich B. Acupuncture and bronchial asthma: a long-term randomized study of the effects of real versus sham acupuncture compared to controls in patients

with bronchial asthma. *J Altern Complement Med* 2002; **8**:737–50; discussion 751–4.

41 Shapira M-D. Short-term acupuncture therapy is of no benefit in patients with moderate persistent asthma. *Chest* 2002; **121**:1396–400.

42 Biernacki W, Peake MD. Acupuncture in treatment of stable asthma. *Respir Med* 1998; **92**:1143–5.

43 Linde K, Jobst KA. Homeopathy for chronic asthma (Cochrane Review). In: *The Cochrane Library*. Chichester, John Wiley & Sons, 2003.

44 Reilly D, Taylor MA, Beattie NG *et al.* Is evidence for homeopathy reproducible? *Lancet* 1994; **344**:1601–6.

45 Matusiewicz R. [Wirksamkeit von Engystol N bei Bronchialasthma unter kortikoidabhängiger Therapie]. *Biol Med* 1995; **24**:242–6.

46 Freitas LAS, Goldenstein E, Sanna OM. The indirect doctor–patient relationship and the homeopathic treatment of asthma in children. *Rev Homeopatia* 1995; **60**:26–31.

47 Lewith GT, Watkins AD, Hyland ME *et al.* Use of ultramolecular potencies of allergen to treat asthmatic people allergic to house dust mite: double blind randomised controlled clinical trial. *BMJ* 2002; **324**: 520.

48 White A, Slade P, Hunt C, Hart A, Ernst E. Individualised homeopathy as an adjunct in the treatment of childhood asthma: a randomised placebo controlled trial. *Thorax* 2003; **58**:317–21.

49 Hockemeyer J, Smyth J. Evaluating the feasibility and efficacy of a self-administered manual-based stress management intervention for individuals with asthma: results from a controlled study. *Behav Med* 2002; **27**:161–72.

50 Vazquez MI, Buceta JM. Psychological treatment of asthma: effectiveness of a self-management program with and without relaxation training. *J Asthma* 1993; **30**:171–83.

51 Coen BI, Conran PB, McGrady A, Nelson L. Effects of biofeedback-assisted relaxation on asthma severity and immune function. *Pediatr Asthma Allergy Immunol* 1996; **10**:71–8.

52 Vazquez I, Buceta J. Relaxation therapy in the treatment of bronchial asthma: effects on basal spirometric values. *Psychother Psychosom* 1993; **60**:106–12.

53 Deter HC. Cost–benefit analysis of psychosomatic therapy in asthma. *J Psychosom Res* 1986; **30**:173–82.

54 Kern-Buell CL, McGrady AV, Conran PB, Nelson LA. Asthma severity,

psychophysiological indicators of arousal, and immune function in asthma patients undergoing biofeedback-assisted relaxation. *Appl Psychophysiol Biofeedback* 2000; **25**:79–91.

55 Sachs G, Haber P, Spiess K, Moser G. [Effectiveness of relaxation groups in patients with chronic respiratory tract diseases]. *Wien Klin Wochenschr* 1993; **105**:603–10.

56 Spiess K, Sachs G, Buchinger C, Roggla G, Schnack C, Haber P. Effects of information and relaxation groups on lung function and psychophysical status in asthma patients — a pilot study. *Praxis Klinik Pneumol* 1988; **42**:641–4.

57 Huntley A, White AR, Ernst E. Relaxation therapies for asthma: a systematic review. *Thorax* 2002; **57**:127–31.

58 Holloway E, Ram FSF. Breathing exercises for asthma (Cochrane Review). In: *The Cochrane Library*, Issue 4. Chichester, John Wiley & Sons, 2003.

59 Manocha R, Marks GB, Kenchington P, Peters D, Salome CM. Sahaja yoga in the management of moderate to severe asthma: a randomised controlled trial. *Thorax* 2002; **57**:110–15.

60 Opat AJ, Cohen MM, Bailey MJ, Abramson MJ. A clinical trial of the Buteyko Breathing Technique in asthma as taught by a video. *J Asthma* 2000; **37**:557–64.

61 Thomas M, McKinley RK, Freeman E, Foy C, Prodger P, Price D. Breathing retraining for dysfunctional breathing in asthma: a randomised controlled trial. *Thorax* 2003; **58**:110–15.

62 Bowler S, Green A, Mitchell C, Graham T, Martin J, Antic R. Hypoventilation exercises (Buteyko Breathing) and asthma: a controlled trial. *Aust NZ J Med* 1995; **25**:457.

63 Nagarathna R, Nagendra HR. Yoga for bronchial asthma: a controlled study. *BMJ* 1985; **291**:1077–9.

64 Fluge T, Tichter J, Fabel H, Zysno E, Weller E, Wagner TO. Long-term effects of breathing exercises and yoga in patients with bronchial asthma. *Pneumologie* 1994; **48**: 484–90.

65 Girodo M, Ekstrand KA, Metiver GJ. Deep diaphragmatic breathing: rehabilitation exercises for the asthmatic patient. *Arch Physiol Med Rehabil* 1992; **73**: 717–20.

66 Vedanthan PK, Kesavalu LN, Murthy KC *et al.* Clinical study of yoga techniques in university students with asthma: a controlled study. *Allergy Asthma Proc* 1998; **19**: 3–9.

Difficult asthma

Peter A B Wark

Case scenario

A 52-year-old lady is referred to you by her primary care physician with 'steroid-dependent asthma'. She was diagnosed with asthma 10 years ago following a chest infection. She tells you her asthma was initially controlled by 'puffers' but, over the last several years, they haven't worked. She feels breathless with minimal exertion and is troubled by a dry cough that is worse at night. She has had four episodes in the last 6 months where her asthma has worsened and she has had to increase her prednisolone, although she has had no admissions to hospital. Her symptoms are so bad she has stopped work. She uses inhaled beclomethasone 1000 μg bid, salmeterol 50 μg bid, Ipratropium bromide 500 μg and salbutamol 5 mg nebulized every 4 hours, and she is currently taking 15 mg of prednisolone; it has been 2 years since she was not on a regular dose. She hates taking the prednisolone as it causes her to put on weight, makes her feel depressed and she is afraid she will develop osteoporosis. She asks you whether you can improve her asthma and get her off the prednisolone?

Introduction

Asthma is a heterogeneous disorder of variable severity with the most severe and difficult-to-treat patients forming an important group with the greatest morbidity, mortality and consumption of health resources. An international task force defined difficult-to-treat or therapy-resistant asthma in terms of chronic symptoms, episodic exacerbations, persistent variable airflow obstruction and an ongoing requirement for short-acting bronchodilators despite treatment with adequate doses of inhaled corticosteroids.[1] Even though this definition encompasses only a minority of asthmatics, they are a diverse group with multiple probable factors, both inherited and acquired, influencing their persistent symptoms and resistance to treatment. Many of these factors remain to be fully elucidated. Within this group, allergic bronchopulmonary aspergillosis (ABPA) and Churg–Strauss syndrome (CSS) will be dealt with as separate entities in the context of difficult-to-treat asthma as they have distinct and well-categorized pathologies.

Treatment-resistant asthma

Description of treatment-resistant asthma

The first step in the management of treatment-resistant asthma is confirming the diagnosis of asthma, which rests upon a consistent history and demonstrable variable airflow obstruction. This is complicated in this instance by the fact that, when most patients present for tertiary assessment, they often have a long-standing diagnosis, are on multiple medications for asthma that cannot easily be withdrawn and the symptoms of asthma are often non-specific.

A number of disorders can masquerade as asthma and may also co-exist (Table 1). In adults, chronic obstructive pulmonary disease (COPD), as a consequence of either smoking or asthma, and vocal cord dysfunction frequently co-exist with asthma and lead to similar symptoms that are poorly responsive to treatment. COPD may be particularly difficult to differentiate in elderly adult-onset asthmatics who tend as a group to have more complicated disease.[2] In children, particularly under the age of 6 years, in whom measurement of lung function is difficult, characterization of asthma is poorly defined. In this age group, viral respiratory tract infections are common and may often induce recurrent wheeze that is poorly responsive to treatment with inhaled corticosteroids; however, only a fraction of these children will have persistent asthma symptoms in later childhood.[3]

Several factors act as triggers to exacerbate asthma and predispose to a loss of asthma control (Table 2). Non-compliance with treatment remains an important factor to consider prior to escalating treatment. It is estimated that 30–55% of asthmatics do not adhere to treatment with inhaled glucocorticoids,[4] with profound implications for overall disease control; however, the incidence of non-compliance in severe asthma is unknown. In addition, issues of poor technique in using inhaled medications and access to asthma education are also likely to influence disease control and minimize medication use.[5]

Several medical conditions also worsen asthma control. Gastro-oesophageal reflux may occur in up to 60% of asthmatics,[6] and treatment of reflux in uncontrolled trials has been associated with an improvement of asthma control;[7] however, a benefit from treatment of reflux to improve asthma

Table 1. Differential diagnosis of difficult-to-treat asthma.

In children	In adults
Bronchiolitis obliterans	COPD
Vocal cord dysfunction	Vocal cord dysfunction
Bronchomalacia	Allergic bronchopulmonary aspergillosis
Inhaled foreign bodies	Churg–Strauss syndrome
Cystic fibrosis	Congestive cardiac failure
Recurrent aspiration	Cystic fibrosis/bronchiectasis
Developmental abnormalities of the upper airway	Tumours involving or impinging on the central airways
Immunoglobulin deficiencies	Inhaled foreign bodies
Ciliary dyskinesias	Tracheobronchomalacia
	Bronchial amyloid

Adapted and used with permission of *The European Respiratory Journal.*[1]

Table 2. Factors that may contribute to loss of control in asthma.

Poor compliance/adherence to treatment
Psychosocial and emotional factors
Inadequate medical facilities and asthma education or poor access to them
Ongoing exposure to allergen triggers of asthma
Exposure to occupational triggers of asthma
Gastro-oesophageal reflux
Chronic rhinosinusitis
Viral respiratory tract infections

Adapted and used with permission of *The European Respiratory Journal.*[1]

has not been shown in controlled trials.[8] Similarly, sinusitis or allergic rhinitis is often present in asthmatics, and treatment to control these conditions can improve asthma.[9] Finally, exposure to occupational triggers of asthma is particularly relevant to identify as ongoing exposure is associated with both difficult-to-control asthma and an irreversible decline in lung function.[10,11]

Therefore, before a patient is labelled with treatment-resistant asthma, they should undergo a thorough review by an asthma specialist with the diagnosis of asthma confirmed and an assessment made of the severity of their disease based on symptoms and lung function. An effort should be made to identify and then avoid triggers or conditions that exacerbate their disease. Finally, medications used to control asthma need to be optimized, ensuring compliance and adequate patient education in their use. In all, this process may take up to 12 months, with the major thoracic medicine societies providing guidelines to carry these measures out.[12–14]

Clinical patterns of treatment-resistant asthma

Three clinical patterns of treatment-resistant asthma have been described, but these have come from small highly referred groups, and a true prevalence of these patterns or their natural history is largely unknown.[15,16] First are patients who experience fatal or near-fatal asthma associated with exacerbations of their disease requiring mechanical ventilatory support despite adequate treatment and usually good symptom control between episodes. Second are patients who experience sudden severe episodes of airflow obstruction that may be life threatening and are termed brittle asthmatics.[16] In at least a proportion of these, food allergies seem to play a role.[16] Finally, there are patients with persistent symptoms and/or airflow obstruction despite adequate treatment with inhaled corticosteroids, often requiring oral corticosteroids to control their disease.[1] It is this group that most researchers have focused their attention on to find treatments that will reduce dependence on oral corticosteroids.

Treatment

Question: What is the efficacy of second-line therapeutic agents (intervention) in difficult treatment-resistant asthma (population)?

Optimization of treatment with adequate doses of inhaled corticosteroids is central to the control of all asthmatics and, for those whose symptoms persist, control with oral corticosteroids long term is often necessary. To a large extent, the treatments that will be described are second-line therapies, their primary aim being to minimize oral corticosteroid doses and therefore side-effects. The agents that have been trialled mostly target inflammation and have been used successfully in other chronic inflammatory conditions such as rheumatoid arthritis or solid organ transplantation; these are summarized in Table 3.

Literature search

Systematic reviews of randomized trials were identified from the Cochrane database and MEDLINE. Where these were unavailable, randomized controlled trials were sought.

Methotrexate

Eleven trials with 185 subjects were assessed in a systematic review;[17] there were seven crossover trials and three parallel group trials. All trials were described as randomized and, in all trials, subjects were on oral corticosteroids to control their asthma; the trials used methotrexate in doses of 7.5–15 mg per week. Most of the trials were small, all lasted at least 12 weeks, but only two lasted longer than 16 weeks. In only two of the trials were oral steroids tapered prior to commencement.[18,19] A meta-analysis demonstrated a reduction in corticosteroid dose with treatment with a weighted mean difference (WMD) in crossover trials of −2.9 mg/day [95% confidence interval (CI) −5.5 to −0.2] and parallel trials −4.1 mg/day (95% CI −6.8 to −1.3) (Fig. 1a and 1b). There was no significant improve-

Table 3. Second-line immunosuppressive therapy used in difficult-to-treat asthma.

Intervention	Systematic review	No. of RCTs	No. of subjects	Reduction in oral corticosteroids	Improvement in lung function
Methotrexate	Yes	10	185	Yes	No
Gold	Yes	3	376 (275 in one study)	Yes	No
Cyclosporin	Yes	3	98	No	No
Troleandomycin	Yes	3	90	No	No
Immunoglobulin	No	6	201	Yes	No
Hydroxychloroquine	No	2	17	No	No
Colchicine	No	2	101	No	?
Dapsone	No	0	0	?	?
Lignocaine	No	0	0	?	?

RCTs, randomized controlled trials.

ment in forced expired volume in 1 second (FEV_1) in a meta-analysis of four of the trials where results could be combined, WMD 0.12l (95% CI −0.21 to 0.45) (Fig. 1c).

Side-effects were more common with methotrexate. The development of abnormal liver function tests was increased, odds ratio (OR) 6.9 (95% CI 3.1–15.5), and five subjects needed to withdraw from trials due to hepatotoxicity. There was also an increase in gastrointestinal symptoms, OR 2.12 (95% CI 1.09–4.12). There were no reported cases of severe cytopenia or pulmonary toxicity.

Summary

Overall, methotrexate does appear to lead to a small reduction in oral corticosteroid dose, but there was no evidence of an improvement in any other disease outcomes including lung function. This was associated with an increase in abnormal liver function tests and gastrointestinal side-effects.

Gold

Three trials examined gold therapy in chronic corticosteroid-dependent asthmatics, and they were assessed in a systematic review.[20] These included 311 subjects, although 275 were from the one study. One trial administered gold parenterally and the other two orally at 3 mg bd. Trial duration varied from 22 weeks to 8 months. A meta-analysis of two of the trials demonstrated that gold treatment was associated with an increased ability to reduce oral corticosteroids, OR 0.51 (95% CI 0.31–0.31), although this effect was largely due to the findings of one trial (Fig. 2).[21] A dose reduction in oral corticosteroids was also seen with a fall in prednisone dose of 4.1 mg, significantly greater than placebo ($P = 0.01$).[22]

Only one of the trials reported an increase in FEV_1 of 6% with gold treatment;[22] in the other trials, there was no improvement in lung function or asthma exacerbations.[20]

Gold therapy was not associated with an increased risk of proteinuria, OR 1.4 (95% CI 0.6–3.3), dermatitis, OR 2.1 (95% CI 0.9–4.7), or other adverse events.[20]

Summary

In summary, gold therapy was associated with a small reduction in oral corticosteroid use and may also lead to a small increase in FEV_1; there was no significant increase in adverse events at least up to 8 months.

Cyclosporin

Three trials examined cyclosporin therapy in 98 chronic corticosteroid-dependent asthmatics and were assessed in a systematic review.[23] All trials achieved serum cyclosporin levels of 75–152 ng/mL, and the duration of treatment was 12–36 weeks. A meta-analysis of two of the trials demonstrated that cyclosporin treatment enabled asthma control at a lower dose of oral corticosteroid with a standardized mean difference (SMD) of −0.05 (95% CI −0.1 to −0.04) (Fig. 3a). One of the trials reported significant improvements in peak expiratory flow (PEF), FEV_1, forced vital capacity (FVC) and exacerbation rates.[24] This was not so clear in the other trials, with one showing a 12% increase in morning PEF[25] and the other no change in lung function but an improvement in symptoms.[26]

Side-effects were more common with cyclosporin treatment. There was a small increase in diastolic blood pressure, SMD 0.8 (95% CI 0.3–1.3), and an increase in serum creatinine, SMD 0.9 (95% CI 0.4–1.4), at meta-analysis (Fig. 3b).[23] The individual trials also reported increases in liver enzymes, nausea, vomiting, paraesthesia and hypertrichosis.

Summary

In summary, cyclosporin treatment allows a small reduction in oral corticosteroid dose, but a consistent effect on lung function has not been demonstrated. This is at the cost of an increase in side-effects, particularly renal function and diastolic blood pressure, which may have important long-term adverse effects not seen in these short-term trials.

a

Review: Methotrexate as a steroid-sparing agent for asthma in adults

Comparison: 01 Methotrexate vs placebo

Outcome: 01 Oral steroid use – parallel trials

Study	(N)	Methotrexate [mean (SD)]	(N)	Placebo [mean (SD)]	WMD (fixed) 95% CI	Weight (%)	WMD (fixed) (95% CI)
Eizurum (1991)	8	12.20 (5.12)	9	11.90 (6.12)		25.8	0.300 [−5.046, 5.646]
Kanzow (1995)	12	22.70 (13.30)	9	22.80 (8.20)		8.7	−0.100 [−9.337, 9.137]
Shiner (1990)	32	6.60 (5.97)	28	12.90 (7.14)		65.5	−6.300 [−9.658, −2.942]
Total (95% CI)	52		46			100.0	−4.058 [−6.775, −1.340]

Test for heterogeneity chi-squared = 4.97 df = −2 *P* = 0.0833

Test for overall effect *Z* = −2.93 *P* = 0.00

−10 −5 0 5 10

Methotrexate better   Placebo better

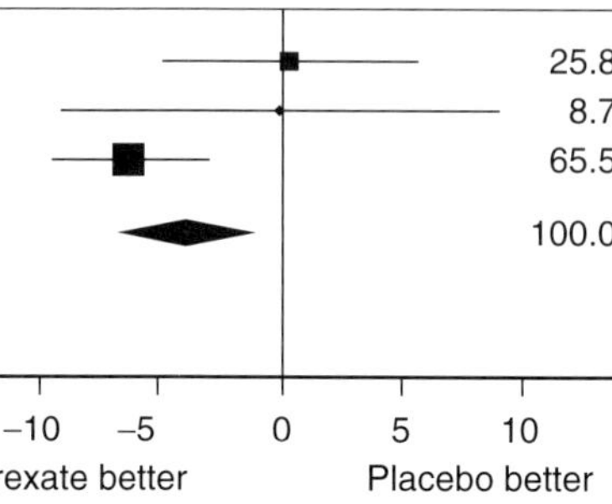

b

Review: Methotrexate as a steroid-sparing agent for asthma in adults

Comparison: 01 Methotrexate vs placebo

Outcome: 02 Oral steroid use – crossover trials

Study	(N)	Methotrexate [mean (SD)]	(N)	Placebo [mean (SD)]	WMD (fixed) (95% CI)	Weight (%)	WMD (fixed) (95% CI)
Coffey (1994)	11	20.10 (12.60)	11	24.50 (12.90)		6.3	−4.400 (−15.057, 6.257)
Dyer (1991)	10	8.37 (8.37)	10	11.97 (4.96)		19.7	−3.600 (−9.630, 2.430)
Hedman (1996)	12	7.90 (8.10)	12	12.80 (11.40)		11.4	−4.900 (−12.813, 3.013)
Mullarkey (1988)	13	16.60 (15.00)	13	26.20 (16.20)		5.0	−9.600 (−21.602, 2.402)
Stewart (1994)	21	18.40 (9.90)	21	21.45 (10.50)		18.8	−3.050 (−9.222, 3.122)
Taylor (1993)	9	14.40 (6.80)	9	12.90 (7.00)		17.6	1.500 (−4.876, 7.876)
Trigg (1993)	12	10.00 (5.30)	12	12.50 (8.80)		21.2	−2.500 (−8.312, 3.312)
Total (95% CI)	88		88			100.0	−2.863 (−5.538, −0.187)

Test for heterogeneity chi-squared = 3.42 df = 6 *P* = 0.7546

Test for overall effect *Z* = −2.10 *P* = 0.04

−10 −5 0 5 10

Methotrexate better   Placebo better

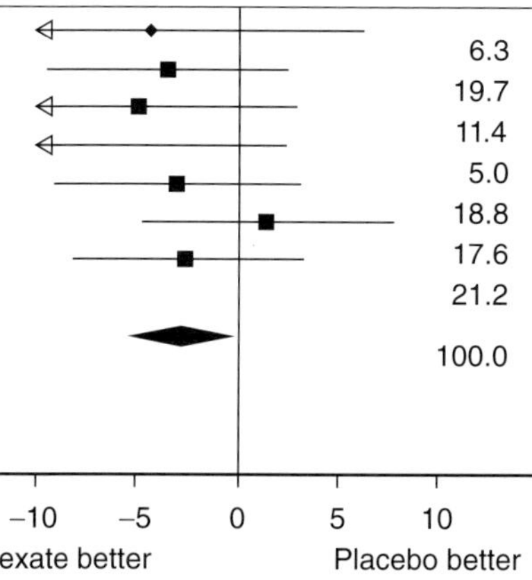

c

Review: Methotrexate as a steroid-sparing agent for asthma in adults

Comparison: 07 Methotrexate vs placebo

Outcome: 01 FEV_1 at end of trial

Study	(N)	Methotrexate [mean (SD)]	(N)	Placebo [mean (SD)]	WMD (fixed) (95% CI)	Weight (%)	WMD (fixed) (95% CI)
Coffey (1994)	11	−2.60 (1.27)	11	−2.40 (0.66)		15.3	−0.200 [−1.046, 0.646]
Hedman (1996)	12	−2.12 (0.93)	12	−1.92 (0.90)		20.3	−0.200 [−0.932, 0.532]
Kanzow (1995)	12	−1.80 (0.70)	9	−1.60 (0.50)		41.4	−0.200 [−0.713, 0.313]
Taylor (1993)	9	−1.51 (0.77)	9	−1.64 (0.72)		23.0	0.130 [−0.559, 0.819]
Total (95% CI)	44		41			100.0	−0.124 [−0.454, 0.206]

Test for heterogeneity chi-squared = 0.68 df = 3 *P* = 0.8781

Test for overall effect *Z* = −0.74 *P* = 0.50

−10 −5 0 5 10

Methotrexate better   Placebo better

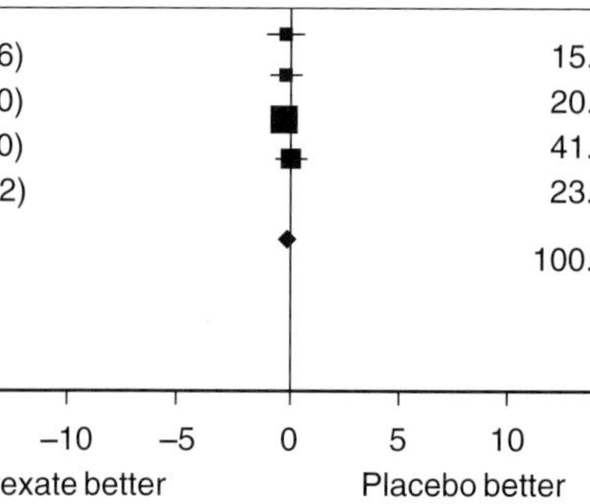

Figure 1. (a) Reduction in oral corticosteroid dose with methotrexate (data from parallel trials). (b) Reduction in oral corticosteroid dose with methotrexate (data from crossover trials). (c) FEV_1 at the completion of the trial with methotrexate and placebo (from Davies *et al.*[17] with the permission of the Cochrane Library of Systematic Reviews).

Review: Gold as an oral corticosteroid-sparing agent in stable asthma
Comparison: 01 Gold vs placebo
Outcome: 02 Treatment success (significant steroid reduction)

Study	Treatment	Control	Peto odds ratio (95% CI)	Weight (%)	Peto odds ratio (95% CI)
Bernstein	80/136	102/139		97.5	0.52 (0.32, 0.86)
Klaustermeyer	3/5	3/3		2.5	0.15 (0.01, 3.41)
Total (95% CI)	83/141	105/142		100.0	0.51 (0.31, 0.83)

Test for heterogeneity chi-squared = 0.58 df = 1 P = 0.4457
Test for overall effect Z = –2.70 P = 0.01

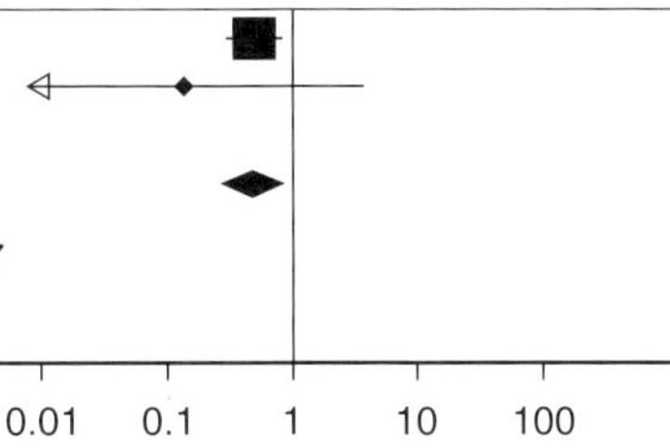

```
0.01   0.1    1    10   100
    Gold better    Placebo better
```

Figure 2. Subjects who were able to reduce oral corticosteroid dose, gold therapy compared with placebo (from Evans *et al.*[20] with the permission of the Cochrane Library of Systematic Reviews).

a
Review: Cyclosporin as an oral corticosteroid-sparing agent in stable asthma
Comparison: 01 Cyclosporin vs placebo
Outcome: 02 Dose steroids

Study	(N)	Treatment [mean (SD)]	(N)	Control [mean (SD)]	WMD (fixed) (95% CI)	Weight (%)	WMD (fixed) (95% CI)
Lock (1996)	16	2484.00 (1300.00)	20	3529.00 (1788.00)		0.0	–1045.000 (–2054.870, –35.130)
Nizankowska (1995)	17	–6.09 (4.13)	15	–4.26 (4.61)		100.0	–1.830 (–4.879, 1.219)
Total (95% CI)	33		35			100.0	–1.840 (–4.889, 1.210)

Test for heterogeneity chi-squared = 4.10 df = 1 P = 0.0429
Test for overall effect Z = –1.18 P = 0.20

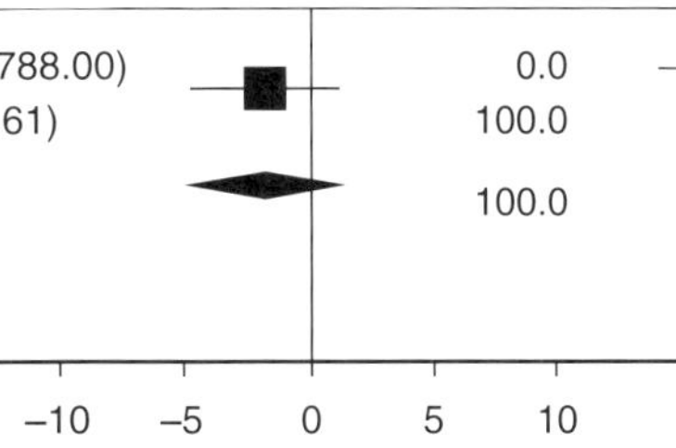

```
       -10    -5    0    5    10
    Cyolosporin better    Placebo better
```

b
Review: Cyclosporin as an oral corticosteroid-sparing agent in stable asthma
Comparison: 01 Cyclosporin vs placebo
Outcome: 05 Creatinine

Study	(N)	Treatment [mean (SD)]	(N)	Control [mean (SD)]	SMD (fixed) (95% CI)	Weight (%)	SMD (fixed) (95% CI)
Lock (1996)	19	8.28 (10.90)	20	–2.66 (7.50)		50.6	1.151 (0.468, 1.834)
Nizankowska (1995)	17	99.40 (16.30)	17	90.80 (8.80)		49.4	0.641 (–0.050, 1.333)
Total (95% CI)	36		37			100.0	0.899 (0.413, 1.385)

Test for heterogeneity chi-squared = 1.06 df = 1 P = 0.3039
Test for overall effect Z = 3.36 P = 0.00

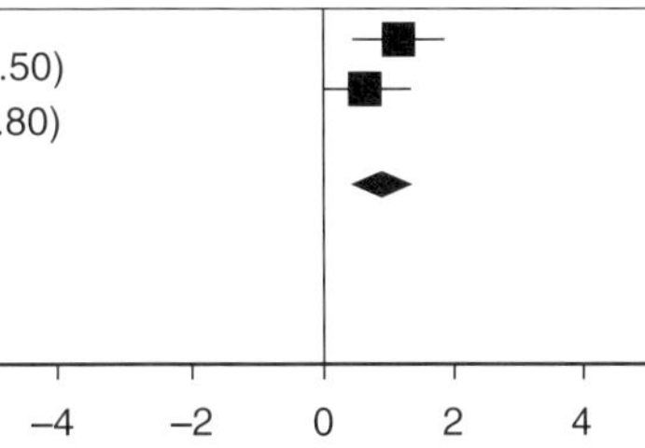

```
       -4    -2    0    2    4
    Cyolosporin better    Placebo better
```

Figure 3. (a) Reduction in oral corticosteroid dose, cyclosporin therapy compared with placebo. (b) Measurement of serum creatinine, cyclosporin therapy compared with placebo (from Evans *et al.*[23] with the permission of the Cochrane Library of Systematic Reviews).

Troleandomycin

Three parallel group studies were assessed in a systematic review examining the effect of troleandomycin 250 mg daily in 58 asthmatics dependent on oral corticosteroids.[27] Two of the three trials were in children, and in only two of the trials were corticosteroids tapered prior to treatment. The primary outcome in all trials was a reduction in oral corticosteroid dose.

A meta-analysis did not demonstrate a reduction in oral corticosteroids with treatment, SMD –0.29 (95% CI –0.75 to

0.17). None of the trials showed improvements in lung function or frequency of exacerbations. Two of the trials demonstrated an increase in corticosteroid side-effects with troleandomycin treatment, with changes in bone mineral density, fasting blood glucose plasma lipids and striae.

Summary

In summary, troleandomycin does not allow a reduction in oral corticosteroid dose nor does it improve lung function or asthma symptoms. There does appear to be an increase in the deleterious effects of corticosteroids when troleandomycin is added.

Immunoglobulin

In all, there have been five randomized double-blind, placebo, controlled trials of parenteral immunoglobulin administration in immunocompetent adults and children with asthma, although no systematic review has been performed.

Early trials of immunoglobulin were performed in children at a time when it was thought that infection played an important role in most asthmatics. These trials were in children with mild to moderate asthma, who were not dependent on oral corticosteroids. Trials by Abernathy et al.[28] and Fontana et al.[29] treated children with mild to moderate symptomatic asthma with intramuscular (IM) immunoglobulin (a dose of approximately 100 mg/kg) for 6 months. Abernathy et al.[28] did show a reduction in days requiring treatment with oral corticosteroids (56 days versus 224 days with placebo). There were no improvements in lung function, symptoms or blood eosinophils. Smith et al.[30] treated 50 mild to moderate asthmatic children with either placebo or intravenous (IV) immunoglobulin 200 mg/kg and demonstrated a reduction in frequency of use of oral corticosteroids for exacerbations and the use of short-acting β-agonists.

More recently, trials have switched to the use of higher dose intravenous (IV) immunoglobulin in keeping with its success in autoimmune disease, as well as focusing on its use in severe and treatment-resistant asthma. All these trials have used equivalent doses of 5% albumin as a placebo. Niggerman et al.[31] treated 31 children or adolescents who had symptomatic asthma and were on at least 800 μg of inhaled beclomethasone or budesonide with IV immunoglobulin up to 2 g/kg for 2 months. They failed to show any improvement in lung function or corticosteroid dose. Salmun et al.[32] focused on treating severe oral corticosteroid-dependent asthmatics aged 5–35 years. They attempted to taper corticosteroids for 3 months and then treated with IV immunoglobulin 2 g/kg every 3 weeks ($n=16$) or placebo ($n=12$) for 9 months. Overall, both groups showed an equivalent reduction in prednisone use. However, subjects who were on 5.5 mg/day or more oral prednisone had a significant reduction in prednisone dose with treatment (a reduction from 16.4 mg/day to

3 mg/day, $P<0.01$). Caution should be exercised in interpreting this as the subgroup numbered only nine in the treatment arm and eight in the placebo arm. No increase in adverse events was reported, although the trial mentions the occurrence in the treatment arm of nausea and headaches.

Kishyama et al.[33] treated severe asthmatics aged 6–66 years dependent on at least 0.1 mg/kg oral prednisone per day with 1 g/kg/month ($n=9$) or 2 g/kg/month ($n=16$) or placebo ($n=15$) for 7 months; only 30 subjects completed the trial as it was prematurely terminated due to adverse events within the treatment arms. The trial showed that IV immunoglobulin was no better than placebo in reducing oral corticosteroid dose, improving lung function or in reducing missed days from school/work or emergency department visits. However, three subjects in the high-dose immunoglobulin arm were admitted to hospital with aseptic meningitis. Severe headaches were also reported more commonly with 2 g/kg (27%) and 1 g/kg (33%) compared with placebo (16%, $P=0.02$).

Summary

In summary, it is unclear whether parenteral immunoglobulin therapy allows corticosteroid reduction in severe asthma or improves disease symptoms or lung function. Treatment at 1 g/kg or higher is however associated with the serious risk of aseptic meningitis and severe headaches. Given these side-effects and the difficulty in procuring IV immunoglobulin, its use is not justified in severe asthma.

Hydroxychloroquine

Two randomized controlled trials have examined the use of hydroxychloroquine in asthma. Roberts et al.[34] treated nine subjects dependent on oral prednisone with 400 mg/day for 2 months. They found no significant benefit with respect to reduction in prednisone dose, symptom score or PEF. No side-effects were reported.

Charous et al.[35] treated 17 milder stable asthmatics aged 18–65 years controlled on inhaled corticosteroids with hydroxychloroquine < 6.5 mg/kg/day for 30 weeks. They found that treatment led to a 10.8% increase in FEV_1, a 14.2% increase in PEF and an 18.6% reduction in β-agonist use ($P<0.05$). There was no improvement in symptom scores. It is noteworthy that these changes were not apparent until the 22nd week of treatment. No increases in adverse events were seen with treatment.

These results do not allow us to assess the effectiveness of hydroxychloroquine in severe asthma, although in milder disease, it appears to have an effect in improving lung function. Its lack of effect in the severe asthmatics may have been due to an inadequate period of treatment, and further investigations of this agent in severe asthma appear to be justified.

Colchicine

Two randomized controlled trials have assessed colchicine compared with placebo in asthma. The first trial treated 30 atopic moderately severe asthmatic children with colchicine 0.5 mg bd for 4 weeks.[36] They found an improvement in symptoms of morning chest tightness and nocturnal symptoms but no change in pulmonary function or daytime symptoms. Fish et al.[37] treated moderately severe asthmatics requiring at least 800 µg of triamcinolone with colchicine 0.6 mg bd. Seventy subjects were stabilized for 2 weeks, and then the triamcinolone was withdrawn. They then received either colchicine or placebo. Both groups demonstrated a significant deterioration in symptoms. Both trials have looked at the effect of colchicine in moderate asthma and have failed to show benefit over placebo in either symptoms or lung function.

Other treatments

Both dapsone and nebulized lignocaine have been reported as treatments for asthma in open-labelled, uncontrolled trials. But, at this stage, there are no randomized controlled trials to report.

Allergic bronchopulmonary aspergillosis

Description of the problem

Allergic bronchopulmonary aspergillosis (ABPA) is a complex condition that results from hypersensitivity to the fungus Aspergillus fumigatus (Af). ABPA was first described in the UK in 1952[38] and has been estimated to occur in 1–2% of chronic asthmatics[39] and in up to 10% of patients with cystic fibrosis.[40] In chronic asthma, ABPA is characterized by recurrent exacerbations and, at least in some patients, it leads to proximal bronchiectasis and irreversible fibrotic lung disease.[41] The criteria for diagnosis were standardized in 1977 by Patterson et al.[41,42] They require the patient to have a pre-existing diagnosis of asthma (or cystic fibrosis), immediate-type skin reactivity to Af and, at least during exacerbations or in the absence of treatment, peripheral blood eosinophilia, precipitating antibodies to Af antigen, elevated serum IgE, elevated serum IgE and IgG antibodies against Af. Radiological evidence of proximal bronchiectasis is a frequent accompaniment of ABPA, but is not now felt to be a prerequisite for diagnosis.[42,43] However, the presence of bronchiectasis along with skin test reactivity and eosinophilia is quite specific for ABPA.

The disease has been subdivided into five stages.[41] Stage I is the initial acute presentation, with eosinophilia, immediate-type skin reactivity to Af, total serum IgE > 2500 ng/mL and pulmonary infiltrates on a chest radiograph. Stage II is the disease in remission, in which there is persistent immediate-type skin reactivity and precipitating antibodies to Af antigens. In Stage III, there is an exacerbation of symptoms with all the characteristics of Stage I with a twofold rise in serum IgE and new pulmonary infiltrates. Stage IV patients have asthma where control of symptoms is dependent on chronic use of high-dose corticosteroids. Stage V patients have advanced fibrotic disease, with extensive pulmonary radiographic changes that do not reverse with treatment and irreversible or partially reversible obstructive airways disease.

The risk that patients with ABPA will develop progressive fixed airflow obstruction and some will go on to develop bronchiectasis makes it a unique and important condition to identify in the therapy-resistant asthmatic population.

Treatment

Corticosteroids

The cornerstone of treatment of ABPA has been to use systemic corticosteroids to suppress the inflammatory response provoked by Af, rather than removal of the organism. This may require prolonged treatment with high doses of corticosteroids.[44] Evidence supporting corticosteroid treatment is only from longitudinal case series that show oral corticosteroids control co-existing asthma and improve acute exacerbations where they hasten the reduction of pulmonary infiltrates.[45] Given the demonstrated efficacy of corticosteroids in asthma and their established role in ABPA, it is unlikely that a randomized controlled trial will ever be performed assessing their efficacy in ABPA; for this matter, it will be important to review the limited evidence that is available. Exacerbations can still occur while on chronic maintenance oral corticosteroid.[41,45,46] Safirstein et al.[45] retrospectively reviewed 50 ABPA patients over 5 years and found that those on < 7.5 mg of prednisone for maintenance continued to have recurrent pulmonary infiltrates, irrespective of their symptoms. Wang et al.[46] reviewed their experience over 10 years in 25 patients with ABPA. The treatment protocol involved prednisone 0.5 mg/kg/day for 2 weeks, followed by alternate-day prednisone for 3 months and then tapering the dose and ceasing. With this regime, 13 patients had no exacerbations of their disease, whereas eight patients continued to experience exacerbations, all of which were successfully treated with an increase in their corticosteroid dose.

The more widespread use of inhaled steroids in asthma is widely perceived to have had an effect on the course of subjects with ABPA and may have affected its prevalence, but no data exist examining this. A number of small studies have failed to demonstrate the efficacy of inhaled corticosteroids as maintenance treatment.[47–49] In contrast, Seaton et al.[49] reported benefit from inhaled corticosteroids used early in the course of the disease, before there was substantial damage to the airways. Patients continued maintenance inhaled corticosteroids and, over the next 15 years, they averaged one exacerbation per annum without a significant decline in lung function.

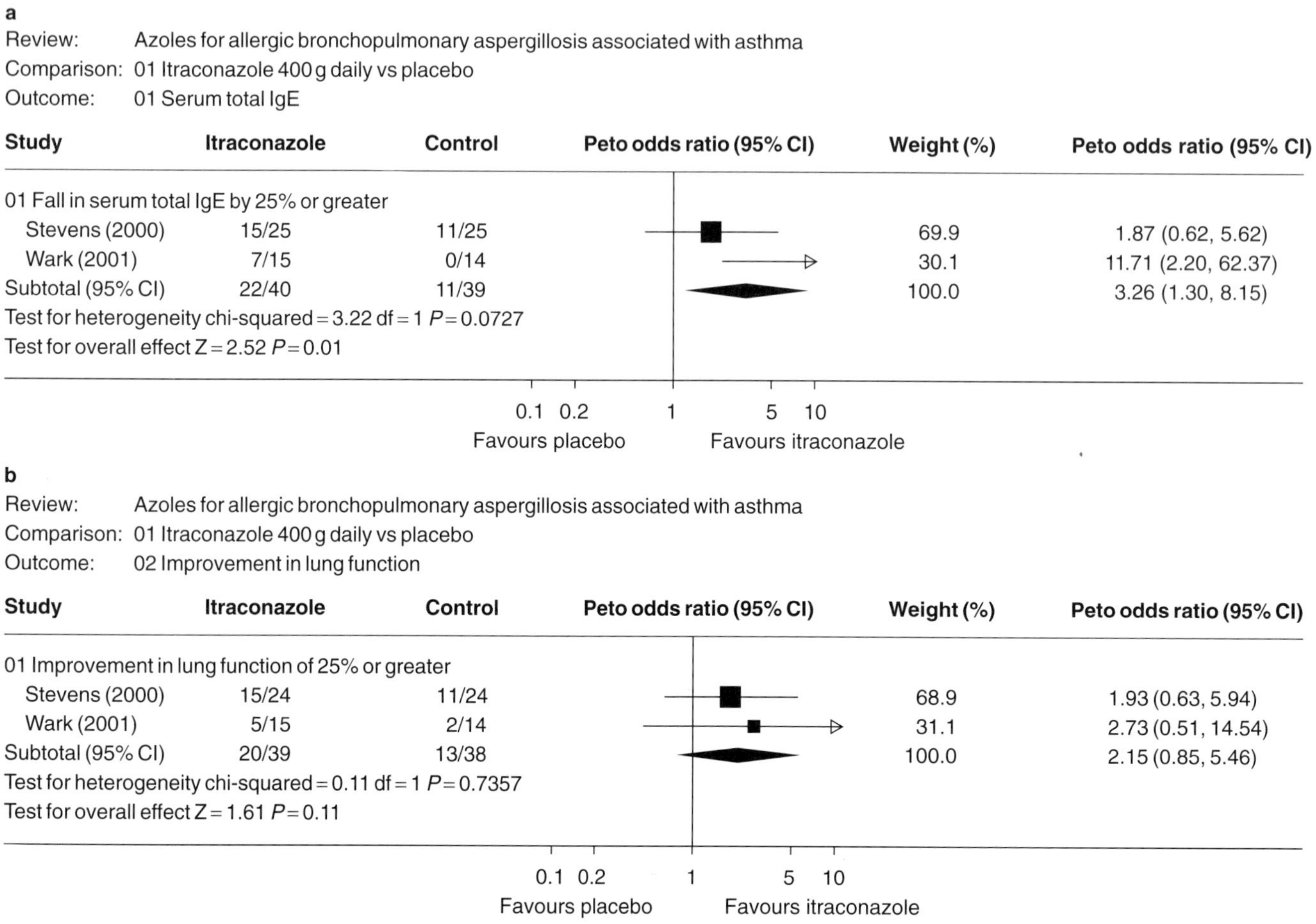

a

Review: Azoles for allergic bronchopulmonary aspergillosis associated with asthma
Comparison: 01 Itraconazole 400 g daily vs placebo
Outcome: 01 Serum total IgE

Study	Itraconazole	Control	Peto odds ratio (95% CI)	Weight (%)	Peto odds ratio (95% CI)
01 Fall in serum total IgE by 25% or greater					
Stevens (2000)	15/25	11/25		69.9	1.87 (0.62, 5.62)
Wark (2001)	7/15	0/14		30.1	11.71 (2.20, 62.37)
Subtotal (95% CI)	22/40	11/39		100.0	3.26 (1.30, 8.15)
Test for heterogeneity chi-squared = 3.22 df = 1 P = 0.0727					
Test for overall effect Z = 2.52 P = 0.01					

0.1 0.2   1   5   10
Favours placebo   Favours itraconazole

b

Review: Azoles for allergic bronchopulmonary aspergillosis associated with asthma
Comparison: 01 Itraconazole 400 g daily vs placebo
Outcome: 02 Improvement in lung function

Study	Itraconazole	Control	Peto odds ratio (95% CI)	Weight (%)	Peto odds ratio (95% CI)
01 Improvement in lung function of 25% or greater					
Stevens (2000)	15/24	11/24		68.9	1.93 (0.63, 5.94)
Wark (2001)	5/15	2/14		31.1	2.73 (0.51, 14.54)
Subtotal (95% CI)	20/39	13/38		100.0	2.15 (0.85, 5.46)
Test for heterogeneity chi-squared = 0.11 df = 1 P = 0.7357					
Test for overall effect Z = 1.61 P = 0.11					

0.1 0.2   1   5   10
Favours placebo   Favours itraconazole

Figure 4. (a) Reduction in serum IgE levels of 25% or greater in subjects with ABPA, itraconazole compared with placebo. (b) Improvement in FEV_1 of 25% or greater in subjects with ABPA, itraconazole compared with placebo (from Wark and Gibson[51] with the permission of the Cochrane Library of Systematic Reviews).

Overall, corticosteroids are useful in controlling exacerbations, but it remains unclear to what extent corticosteroids prevent relapses, loss of lung function or disease progression in ABPA.

Antifungal agents

While *Af* is known to cause persistent colonization in ABPA, it is not thought to cause invasive disease. This persistent presence may be the trigger to heightened airway inflammation and has been linked to severity of lung disease.[50] Eradication of the organism may therefore modify the disease. The only antifungal agents of known efficacy against *Af* are amphotericin B and the azoles (ketoconazole and itraconazole, but not fluconazole). Amphotericin has not been assessed in any randomized controlled trials for ABPA, and its effectiveness is limited by its toxicity and cost.

The uses of azoles in ABPA and asthma have been assessed in one systematic review of three randomized controlled trials incorporating 94 adults.[51] Two of the trials assessed oral itraconazole 400 mg/day for 16 weeks (156 subjects);[52,53] in one of the trials, subjects were dependent on oral corticosteroids.[53] A meta-analysis of the two trials showed that the addition of itraconazole led to a reduction in serum IgE (a marker of immune activation) of 25% or greater, OR 3.26 (95% CI 1.30–8.15), compared with placebo (Fig. 4a). They failed to demonstrate an improvement in lung function as measured by an increase in FEV_1 of at least 25% with itraconazole, OR 2.15 (95% CI 0.85–5.46). Individually, the outcomes of the trials were different. Stevens *et al.*[53] found that 46% of subjects treated with itraconazole achieved an improvement in one of the following outcome parameters: a 50% or more reduction in oral corticosteroid dose; a 25% or greater fall in IgE; or a 25% increase in pulmonary function tests [FEV_1, FVC, diffusion of carbon dioxide across the lung (D_LCO), FEF and peak

Table 4. American College of Rheumatology, definition of Churg–Strauss syndrome.

Clinical findings with or without pathological material; diagnosis probable when four of the six criteria are present
1. Asthma
2. Eosinophilia > 10%
3. Neuropathy, mononeuropathy or polyneuropathy
4. Pulmonary infiltrates
5. Paranasal sinus abnormality
6. Extravascular eosinophil infiltration on biopsy findings

Reproduced with the permission of *Arthritis and Rheumatism*.[57]

Table 5. Non-pulmonary organ involvement in Churg–Strauss syndrome.

Upper airway[65]	Allergic rhinitis (75%) Recurrent sinusitis Septal perforation
Neurological[56,65,66]	Peripheral neuropathy (usually mononeuritis multiplex, 65–75%) Cranial nerve palsies Cerebral haemorrhage/infarcts Seizures Psychoses
Gastrointestinal[56,65]	Abdominal pain Bloody diarrhoea Peritonitis, ascites, pancreatitis and cholecystitis (all rare) Visceral perforation
Cardiac[56,66] (leading cause of death)	Eosinophilic endomyocarditis Coronary vasculitis Valvular heart disease Pericarditis Cardiac failure
Skin	Erythematous, macular, papular or purpuric rashes
Renal (end-stage renal failure rare)	Proteinuria, microscopic haematuria and glomerular nephritis

flow] or exercise tolerance. Only 19% of the placebo group met one of these criteria for improvement (Fisher exact $P = 0.04$).[52] The primary outcome measure in Wark *et al.*[52] was a reduction in sputum inflammatory indices, and they found that itraconazole led to a 35% reduction (95% CI 20–48% reduction) in sputum eosinophils that was sustained throughout the trial, while the placebo arm showed no change (the 95% CI included a 19% fall and a 12% increase). There was a similar fall in sputum eosinophil cationic protein, a marker of eosinophil degranulation and airway inflammation. They also demonstrated that participants on itraconazole had fewer exacerbations of their chest disease requiring the use of oral corticosteroids during the period of the trial, with a mean number of exacerbations per participant of 0.4 (SD 0.5) compared with placebo 1.3 (SD 1.2), $P = 0.03$.

One trial[54] randomly assigned 10 subjects with ABPA to receive ketoconazole 400 mg daily or placebo. All were on inhaled corticosteroids and one on prednisone. The trial was conducted in a double-blind fashion. Treatment led to a 40% reduction in specific IgG antibody to *Af* ($P < 0.05$). The placebo group remained stable. Serum total IgE and specific IgE were significantly reduced after 12 months ($P < 0.05$). There was a significant improvement in symptom scores in the treatment arm, and this correlated with the change in the IgG levels. There were no significant changes in spirometry in either group over the 12 months.

There were no serious adverse events reported in the trials, although one subject withdrew due to nausea related to itraconazole.[51] Reports have emerged that, in children treated with itraconazole and high-dose inhaled corticosteroids, there was suppression of adrenal glucocorticoid synthesis in 11 out of 25 participants.[55] This also raises the possibility that the effect of itraconazole may not be specific to its antifungal action but, at least in part, may be due to an effect on corticosteroid metabolism.

Churg–Strauss syndrome

Description of the problem

Churg–Strauss syndrome (CSS) is a unique condition that almost always presents with asthma but then evolves into an eosinophilic vasculitis that can involve nearly all the major organs. The definition of CSS has been refined since its first description in 1951[56] (Table 4) to include 'a disorder that is characterized by an eosinophil rich and granulomatous inflammation involving the respiratory tract and necrotizing vasculitis affecting small–medium size vessels and usually associated with asthma and eosinophilia'.[57] In addition, subjects have elevated serum IgE, and 48–66% have elevated positive perinuclear antineutrophil cytoplasmic antibodies with antimyeloperoxidase specificity.[58]

CSS is rare, affecting 2.4–$6.8/10^6$ patient–years[59,60] but $64.4/10^6$ asthmatics.[59] While in most cases the cause of CSS is unknown, it has been associated with medication use, most recently of note the cysteinyl leukotriene receptor antagonists.[61–64] The development of CSS with the introduction of the leukotriene receptor antagonists has coincided with subsequent tapering of oral corticosteroids, and it is felt that it is the withdrawal of the steroids that has unmasked the condition rather than the medication initiating it.

Pulmonary pathology is invariably present in CSS; it begins as the earliest manifestation in the form of asthma and often persists even after the vasculitis is in remission.[58] In addition to asthma, pulmonary involvement can include migratory pulmonary infiltrates (which may be segmental or follow a peripheral distribution), non-cavitating pulmonary nodules, hilar adenopathy, alveolar haemorrhage and, rarely, pleural effusions.[58,65,66] Nearly all other major organs can be involved (Table 5) with cardiac and severe gastrointestinal involvement being the most serious and likely to lead to a fatal outcome.[58]

Treatment

Most series that have examined the treatment or prognosis of CSS include patients with polyarteritis nodosa (PAN) and, at times, there is overlap between the syndromes. While remission of the systemic vasculitis can be achieved in both conditions, patients with CSS are inevitably left with asthma, often requiring control with oral corticosteroids.

Corticosteroids have become established as the primary treatment of CSS, in most subjects controlling their asthma and vasculitis. Doses are usually commenced at 1 mg/kg/day prednisone and then tapered as tolerated.[58] Unfortunately, the requirement for oral corticosteroids is usually long term, and the high doses are associated with the usual complications of iatrogenic Cushing's disease.[58] The efficacy of oral corticosteroids has been established by retrospective case series, in which survival at 5 years with no treatment was 12% while survival with treatment with prednisone was 53% ($P < 0.05$);[67] despite the limitations of this evidence, the clinical efficacy of corticosteroids is clear.

Cyclophosphamide was introduced as a second-line agent and was found in a prospective case series of subjects with CSS and PAN to improve remission rates and reduce corticosteroid dependence.[68]

Cyclophosphamide, however, is also associated with numerous side-effects, including neutropenia, alopecia, nausea, abdominal pain, haemorrhagic cystitis and a long-term risk of carcinoma of the bladder that requires monitoring. In addition, combination treatment with corticosteroids increases the risk of opportunistic infection. Subsequent randomized controlled trials have evaluated combination treatments without a placebo. A prospective randomized controlled trial of 25 subjects with PAN or CSS compared treatment with prednisone plus cyclophosphamide 2 mg/kg/day either orally or by monthly intravenous pulse 0.6 g/m².[69] They found similar clinically efficacy, but there were more frequent side-effects with daily oral cyclophosphamide (27 events versus 14, $P < 0.05$), implying that pulse cyclophosphamide may be better tolerated. Of note in this small study, however, was the high number of side-effects in both arms (18/25 subjects experienced at least one) and one death in the intravenous pulse group due to an opportunistic infection. The French cooperative group for vasculitides have also conducted a series of randomized controlled trials involving prednisone and cyclophosphamide with and without the addition of plasma exchange. They found in a prospective randomized controlled trial that treatment with plasma exchange and prednisone

compared with prednisone alone in 78 patients neither reduced relapse rate nor improved 5-year survival.[70] Similarly, treatment with prednisone and cyclophosphamide (IV bolus) was compared with treatment with prednisone, cyclophosphamide and plasma exchange in 62 patients. The addition of plasma exchange did not improve outcomes in terms of induction of remission, relapse or survival at 5 years.[71] In a trial comparing treatment with prednisone and plasma exchange with prednisone, cyclophosphamide and plasma exchange, no differences were seen in terms of mortality at 10 years, although there were fewer relapses in the patients treated with cyclophosphamide.[72] Other second-line immunosuppressive agents have been used to treat either CSS or PAN, including azathioprine, cyclosporine A, mycophenalate, interferon α and dapsone, but their use is not widespread, and no prospective controlled trials have been performed to assess their effectiveness.

Summary

In summary, treatment for uncomplicated CSS should initially be with oral corticosteroids at high dose and then tapered according to response. Evidence would support the addition of cyclophosphamide, certainly in subjects with other major organ involvement, and it should be considered as a corticosteroid-sparing strategy in all patients. Pulse intravenous cyclophosphamide may have fewer side-effects than daily oral treatment. Even with good control of the vasculitis, there may be an ongoing requirement for oral corticosteroids to control the asthma. Plasma exchange does not appear to offer any additional benefits.

Conclusions

Patients with difficult-to-treat or therapy-resistant asthma remain a small but important group to consider in the overall management of asthma. These patients consume a disproportionate amount of time in tertiary care, have the highest morbidity and mortality of asthma subjects in general and benefit least from our treatments. The pathology underlying their disease and why it is resistant to treatment needs to be made an active area of ongoing research. This should include defining clinical phenotypes of therapy-resistant asthma as well as obtaining long-term prognostic data on them. An assessment of the pathological changes in the airways of these individuals would also be helpful in defining histology, while the use of biomarkers of airway inflammation to characterize groups and assess response to treatment should be examined. It is also necessary to identify potential genetic influences that may predispose to difficult disease or make individuals less responsive to treatment. A further definition and characterization of the problem may then allow the development of novel interventions.

At the moment, all individuals with difficult-to-control asthma should be assessed by an asthma specialist, their diagnosis confirmed and their extent of impairment measured. Every effort should be made to address and eliminate factors that will exacerbate asthma and avoid these where possible. Compliance should be regularly assessed and education optimized prior to the commencement of second-line agents. Conditions such as ABPA or CSS should be considered in these individuals, although the diagnosis may not be readily apparent. If treatment with second-line immunosuppressives is commenced, then patients will need careful follow-up to assess response but also to monitor the numerous side-effects of these agents. At this point, no one agent can be recommended, although the greatest experience is with gold and methotrexate, both of which have been shown to reduce dependence on oral corticosteroids; a similar effect has also been seen with cyclosporin. However, there is no conclusive evidence that these agents improve lung function or alter long-term outcomes.

References

1 Chung KF, Godard P, Adelroth E *et al.* Difficult/therapy-resistant asthma. *Eur Respir J* 1999; **13**:1198–208.

2 Tuuponen T, Keistinen T, Kivela SL. Hospital admissions for asthma in Finland during 1972–86 of adults aged 65 years and over. *Age Ageing* 1993; **22**:96–102.

3 Martinez FD, Wright AL, Taussig LM *et al.* Asthma and wheezing in the first six years of life. *N Engl J Med* 1995; **332**:133–8.

4 Cochrane GM. Therapeutic compliance in asthma. *Eur Respir J* 1992; **5**:122–4.

5 Gibson PG, Coughlan J, Wilson AJ *et al.* Asthma self-management education improves morbidity in adults with asthma: a systematic review. In: *The Cochrane Library*, Issue 4, 1999.

6 Gustaffsson PM, Kjellman NI, Tibbling L. Oesophageal function and symptoms in moderate and severe asthma. *Acta Pediatr Scand* 1986; **75**:729–36.

7 Harper PC, Bergner A, Kaye MD. Anti-reflux treatment for asthma. Improvements in patients with associated gastro-oesophageal reflux. *Arch Intern Med* 1987; **147**:56–60.

8 Gibson PG, Henry RL, Coughlin JL. Gastro-oesophageal reflux treatment for asthma in adults and children: Cochrane database of Systemtic Reviews. In: *The Cochrane Library*, Issue 2, 2000.

9 Coren J, Adinoff AD, Buchmeir AD, Irvin CG. Nasal beclomethasone prevents the seasonal increase in bronchial responsiveness in patients with allergic rhinitis and asthma. *J Allergy Clin Immunol* 1992; **90**:250–6.

10 Banks DE, Tarlo SM. Important issues in occupational asthma. *Curr Opin Pulm Med* 2000; **6**:37–42.

11 Yeung M, Gryzybowski S. Prognosis in occupational asthma. *Thorax* 1985; **40**:241–3.

12 British Thoracic Society. The British guidelines on asthma management. *Thorax* 1997; **52**:S1–21.

13 Boulet L-P, Becker A, Berube D, Beveridge R, Ernst P on behalf of the Canadian Asthma Consensus Group. Canadian asthma consensus report, 1999. *Can Med Assoc J* 1999; **161**:1S–5.

14 Australia National Asthma Campaign. *Asthma Management Handbook*. Melbourne, Australia NAC, 2002.

15 Turner-Warwick M. Observing patterns of airflow obstruction in chronic asthma. *Br J Dis Chest* 1971; **71**:73–86.

16 Ayres J, Miles JF, Barnes PJ. Brittle asthma. *Thorax* 1998; **53**:315–21.

17 Davies H, Olson LG, Gibson PG. Methotrexate as a steroid sparing agent for asthma in adults (Cochrane Review). In: *The Cochrane Library*, Issue 1, 2003.

18 Coffey M, Saunders G, Eschenbacher WL *et al.* The role of methotrexate in the management of steroid dependent asthma. *Chest* 1994; **105**:117–21.

19 Dyer PD, Vaughan TR, Weber RW. Methotrexate in the treatment of steroid dependent asthma. *J Allergy Clin Immunol* 1991; **88**:208–12.

20 Evans DJ, Cullinan P, Geddes DM *et al.* Gold as an oral corticosteroid sparing agent in stable asthma (Cochrane Review). In: *The Cochrane Library*, Issue 1, 2003.

21 Bernstein IL, Bernstein DI, Dubb JW *et al.* A placebo-controlled multicenter study of auronoffin in the treatment of patients with corticosteroid dependent asthma. *J Allergy Clin Immunol* 1996; **98**:317–24.

22 Nierop G, Gijzel WP, Zwinderman AH, Dijkman JH. Auronoffin in the treatment of steroid dependent asthma; a double blind study. *Thorax* 1987; **47**:349–54.

23 Evans, DJ, Cullinan P, Geddes DM *et al.* Cyclosporin as an oral corticosteroid sparing agent in stable asthma (Cochrane Review). In: *The Cochrane Library*, Issue 1, 2003.

24 Alexander A, Barnes NC, Kay AB. Trial of cyclosporin in corticosteroid-dependent chronic severe asthma. *Lancet* 1992; **339**:324–8.

25 Lock SH, Kay AB, Barnes NC. Double-blind, placebo-controlled study of cyclosporin A as a corticosteroid sparing agent in corticosteroid-dependent asthma. *Am J Respir Crit Care Med* 1996; **153**:509–14.

26 Nizankowska E, Soja J, Pinis G *et al.* Treatment of steroid dependent bronchial asthma with cyclosporin. *Eur Respir J* 1995; **8**:1091–9.

27 Evans DJ, Cullinan P, Geddes DM *et al.* Troleandomycin as an oral corticosteroid sparing agent in stable asthma (Cochrane review). In: *The Cochrane Library*, Issue 1, 2003.

28 Abernathy RS, Stem EL, Good RA. Chronic asthma in childhood: double-blind placebo controlled study of treatment with gamma globulin. *Pediatrics* 1958; **61**:980–92.

29 Fontana VJ, Kuttner AG, Wittig HJ. The treatment of infectious asthma in children with gamma globulin: a double blind controlled study. *J Pediatr* 1964; **1**:80–4.

30 Smith TF, Muldoon MF, Bain RP *et al.* Clinical results of a prospective, double-blind placebo controlled trial of intravenous gamma globulin in children with chronic chest symptoms. *Monogr Allergy* 1988; **23**:168–76.

31 Niggerman B, Leupold W, Schuster A *et al.* Prospective, double-blind, placebo-controlled, multicentre study on the effect of high-dose, intravenous immunoglobulin in children and adolescents with severe bronchial asthma. *Clin Exp Allergy* 1998; **28**:205–10.

32 Salmun LM, Barlan I, Wolf HM *et al.* Effect of intravenous immunoglobulin on steroid consumption in patients with severe asthma: a double-blind, placebo-controlled, randomised trial. *J Allergy Clin Immunol* 1999; **103**:810–15.

33 Kishyama JL, Valacer D, Cunningham-Rundles C *et al.* A multicenter, randomised, double blind, placebo controlled trial of high dose intravenous immunoglobulin for oral corticosteroid dependent asthma. *Clin Immmunol* 1999; **91**:126–33.

34 Roberts JA, Gunneberg A, Elliot JA, Thomson NC. Hydroxychloroquine in steroid dependent asthma. *Pulmon Pharmacol* 1988; **1**:59–61.

35 Charous BL, Halpern EF, Steven GC. Hydroxychloroquine improves airflow and lowers circulating IgE levels in subjects with moderate symptomatic asthma. *J Allergy Clin Immunol* 1998; **102**:198–203.

36 Adalioglu G, Turktas I, Saraclar Y, Tuncer A. A clinical study of colchicine in childhood asthma. *J Asthma* 1994; **31**:361–6.

37 Fish JE, Peters SP, Chambers CV *et al.* An evaluation of colchicine as an alternative to inhaled corticosteroids in moderate asthma. Nation-

al Heart, Lung and Blood Institute's Asthma Clinical Research Network. *Am J Respir Crit Care Med* 1997; **156**:1165–71.

38 Hinson KFW, Moon AJ, Plummer NS. Bronchopulmonary aspergillosis — a review and eight new cases. *Thorax* 1952; **7**:317–33.

39 Greenberger PA, Smith LJ, Hsu CC *et al.* Analysis of bronchoalveolar lavage in allergic bronchopulmonary aspergillosis: divergent responses of antigen specific antibodies and total IgE. *J Allergy Clin Immunol* 1988; **82**:164–70.

40 Laufer P, Fink JN, Burns WT *et al.* Allergic bronchopulmonary aspergillosis in cystic fibrosis. *J Allergy Clin Immunol* 1984; **73**:44–8.

41 Patterson R, Greenberger P, Radin R, Roberts M. Allergic bronchopulmonary aspergillosis: staging as an aid to management. *Ann Intern Med* 1982; **96**:286–91.

42 Patterson R, Greenberger G, Halwig M *et al.* Allergic bronchopulmonary aspergillosis. *Arch Intern Med* 1986; **146**:916–18.

43 Greenberger P, Miller T, Roberts M, Smith L. Allergic bronchopulmonary aspergillosis in patients with and without evidence of bronchiectasis. *Ann Allergy* 1993; **70**:333–8.

44 Rosenberg M, Patterson R, Roberts M, Wang J. The assessment of immunologic and clinical changes occurring during corticosteroid therapy for allergic bronchopulmonary aspergillosis. *Am J Med* 1978; **64**:599–606.

45 Safirstein BH, D'Souza MF, Simon G *et al.* Five year follow-up of allergic bronchopulmonary aspergillosis. *Am Rev Respir Dis* 1973; **108**:450–9.

46 Wang JL, Patterson R, Roberts M, Ghory AC. The management of allergic bronchopulmonary aspergillosis. *Am Rev Respir Dis* 1979; **120**:87–92.

47 Hilton AM, Chatterjee SS. Bronchopulmonary aspergillosis — treatment with beclomethasone dipropionate. *Postgrad Med J* 1975; **51**(Suppl):98–103.

48 British Thoracic Association. Inhaled beclomethasone dipropionate in allergic bronchopulmonary aspergillosis. *Br J Dis Chest* 1979; **73**: 349–56.

49 Seaton A, Seaton RA, Wightman AJ. Management of allergic bronchopulmonary aspergillosis without maintenance oral corticosteroids, a fifteen year followup. *QJM* 1994; **87**:529–37.

50 Wark PAB, Simpson J, Saltos N *et al.* Induced sputum eosinophils, neutrophils and bronchiectasis in allergic bronchopulmonary aspergillosis. *Eur Respir J* 2000; **16**:1095–101.

51 Wark PAB, Gibson PG. Azoles for allergic bronchopulmonary aspergillosis. *Cochrane Database Syst Rev* 2000; **3**:CD001506.

52 Wark PAB, Simpson J, Saltos N *et al.* Itraconazole reduces eosinophilic airway inflammation in allergic bronchopulmonary aspergillosis. *J Allergy Clin Immunol* 2003; **111**:952–7.

53 Stevens DA, Lee JY, Schwartz HJ *et al.* A randomised trial of itraconazole in allergic bronchopulmonary aspergillosis. *N Engl J Med* 2000; **342**:756–62.

54 Shale DJ, Faux JA, Lane DJ. Trial of ketoconazole in non-invasive pulmonary aspergillosis. *Thorax* 1987; **42**:26–31.

55 Skov M, Main KM, Sillesen IB *et al.* Iatrogenic adrenal insufficiency as a side effect of combined treatment of itraconazole and budesonide. *Eur Respir J* 2002; **20**:127–33.

56 Churg J, Strauss L. Allergic granulomatosis, allergic angiitis, and periarteritis nodosa. *Am J Pathol* 1951; **27**:277–301.

57 Jennnette JC, Falk RJ, Andrassay K *et al.* Nomenclature of of systemic vasculitides: a proposal of an international consensus conference. *Arthritis Rheum* 1994; **37**:187–92.

58 Noth I, Strek M, Leff A. Churg–Strauss syndrome. *Lancet* 2003; **361**:587–94.

59 Martin RM, Wilton LV, Mann RD. Prevalence of Churg–Strauss syndrome, vasculitis, eosinophilia and associated conditions: retrospective analysis of 58 prescription event monitoring cohort studies. *Pharmacoepidemiol Drug Safety* 1999; **8**:179–89.

60 Watts RA, Lane SE, Bentham G, Scott DG. Epidemiology of systemic vasculitis: a ten year study in the United Kingdom. *Arthritis Rheum* 2000; **43**:414–19.

61 Wechsler ME, Garpestad E, Kocher O *et al.* Pulmonary infiltrates, eosinophilia and cardiomyopathy in patients with asthma receiving zafirlukast. *JAMA* 1998; **279**:455–7.

62 Franco J, Artes MJ. Pulmonary eosinophilia associated with montelukast. *Thorax* 1999; **54**:558–60.

63 Wechsler ME, Finn D, Gunawardena E *et al.* Churg–Strauss syndrome in patients receiving montelukast as treatment for asthma. *Chest* 2000; **177**:708–13.

64 Kinoshita M, Shiraishi T, Koga T *et al.* Churg–Strauss syndrome after corticosteroid withdrawal in an asthmatic patient treated with pranlukast. *J Allergy Clin Immunol* 1999; **103**:534–5.

65 Lanham JG, Elkon KB, Pusey CD *et al.* Systemic vasculitis with asthma and eosinophilia: a clinical approach to the Churg–Strauss syndrome. *Medicine* 1984; **63**:65–81.

66 Ramakrishna G, Midthun DE. Churg–Strauss syndrome. *Ann Allergy Asthma Immunol* 2001; **86**:603–13.

67 Leib ES, Restivo C, Paulus HE. Immunosupressive and corticosteroid therapy of polyarteritis nodosa. *Am J Med* 1979; **67**:941–7.

68 Fauci AS, Katz P, Haynes BF, Wolff SM. Cyclophosphamide therapy of severe necrotising vasculitis. *N Engl J Med* 1979; **301**:235–8.

69 Gayraud M, Guillevin L, Cohen P *et al.* Treatment of good-prognosis polyarteritis nodosa and Churg–Strauss syndrome: comparison of steroids and oral or pulse cyclophosphamide in 25 patients. French co-operative study group for vasculitides. *Br J Rheumatol* 1997; **36**: 1290–7.

70 Guillevin L, Fain O, Lhote F *et al.* Lack of superiority of steroids plus plasma exchange to steroids alone in the treatment of polyarteritis nodosa and Churg–Strauss syndrome. A propective randomised trial in 78 patients. *Arthritis Rheum* 1992; **35**:208–15.

71 Guillevin L, Lhote F, Cohen P *et al.* Corticosteroids plus pulse cyclophosphamide and plasma exchanges versus corticosteroids plus pulse cyclophosphamide alone in the treatment of polyarteritis nodosa and Churg–Strauss syndrome patients with factors predicting poor prognosis. A prospective, randomised trial in sixty-two patients. *Arthritis Rheum* 1995; **38**:1638–45.

72 Guillevin L, Jarousse B, Lok C *et al.* Longterm followup after treatment of polyarteritis nodosa and Churg–Strauss angiitis with comparison of steroids, plasma exchange and cyclophosphamide to steroids and plasma exchange. A prospective randomised trial of 71 patients. The co-operative study group for polyarteritis nodosa. *J Rheumatol* 1991; **18**:567–74.

CHAPTER 2.8

Novel therapies in asthma: long-acting β₂-agonists/inhaled corticosteroids

Nicola A Marks and Philip W Ind

Introduction

New developments in asthma pharmacotherapy continue to be evaluated for clinical efficacy and safety. This chapter examines three new therapies that have undergone evaluation in randomized controlled trials (RCTs). Each therapy targets a different pathophysiological component of the asthmatic response. These therapies are:

1 long-acting β₂-agonists/inhaled corticosteroid (LABAICS) combinations;
2 anti-immunoglobulin (Ig)E monoclonal antibodies;
3 anti-interleukin (IL)-5 monoclonal antibodies.

LABAICS

Inhaled corticosteroids (ICS) remain the cornerstone of pharmacotherapy for asthma because of their multiplicity of beneficial effects, their anti-inflammatory activity and their key place in guideline recommendations. Inhaled long-acting β₂-agonists are increasingly advocated in guidelines as the next regular maintenance therapy when asthma control remains suboptimal. A Cochrane Review concluded that LABAs are effective in chronic asthma in addition to inhaled steroids.[1] A large number of studies have shown that the addition of an inhaled LABA twice daily to a regular inhaled steroid, at a range of initial doses, over a range of asthma severities in adults and adolescents is of greater benefit than doubling or more than doubling the dose of inhaled steroids. A meta-analysis has shown that the addition of inhaled salmeterol to an inhaled steroid is more effective in terms of peak expiratory flow (PEF), days and nights without symptoms and rescue salbutamol use than at least doubling the inhaled steroid dose with no increase in asthma exacerbations.[2]

These data suggesting a complementary effect of the two classes of drug, the fact that both are usually prescribed twice daily and the evidence of poor adherence to asthma medication generally have led to the production of combination inhalers delivering an inhaled steroid and LABA from the same device: Seretide[R] (salmeterol and fluticasone) and Symbicort[R] (formoterol and budesonide). Proprietary names have been used throughout for convenience. Seretide[R] is also available as Advair[TM] and Viani[TM]. Three different dose combinations

exist for each. Seretide[R] Evohaler is a pressurized metered dose inhaler (MDI) that delivers salmeterol xinafoate equivalent to salmeterol 25 μg and differing doses of fluticasone propionate 50, 125 and 250 μg per actuation of MDI (Seretide[R] Evohaler 50/25, 125/25 or 250/25). Seretide[R] Accuhaler[R] (or Diskus[R]) is a multidose breath-actuated dry powder inhaler (DPI) that delivers salmeterol 50 μg together with fluticasone 100, 250 or 500 μg at each dose. Symbicort[R] is currently available only by DPI (Turbuhaler[R] or Turbohaler[R]; a multidose, breath-actuated device). Each actuation delivers formoterol 6 μg (4.5 μg ex-actuator) with budesonide 100 μg (80 μg ex-actuator); (Symbicort[R] 100/6) or budesonide 200 μg (Symbicort[R] 200/6) or formoterol 12 μg and budesonide 400 μg (Symbicort[R] 400/12).

The combination of two agents in a single inhaler reduces the number of devices required by an individual patient, which is convenient and reduces prescription charges. It might be expected to reduce confusion over inhalers and to improve adherence with therapy, but there is little evidence supporting this. Available clinical trials (virtually all funded by pharmaceutical companies) fall into five categories;

1 comparison of individual combination preparations with individual component drugs and placebo;
2 comparison of individual combination preparations with drugs delivered concomitantly by separate inhalers;
3 study of individual combination inhalers with other comparator drugs;
4 studies of different strategies of use of combination inhalers. There is also a growing body of scientific literature examining the interaction of LABAs and corticosteroids at a cellular level (including at the β₂ receptor) *in vitro*;[3]
5 pharmacoeconomic studies of combination inhalers with comparators.

Literature search

We searched MEDLINE and the Cochrane databases for RCTs with clinical endpoints using the terms asthma, long-acting β-agonists and inhaled steroid, combination therapy (September 2004).

Comparison of combination preparations with individual component drugs and placebo

Question: What is the efficacy of individual LABAICS combination preparations compared with component LABA and ICS and placebo in asthma?

Comparison of individual combination preparations with drugs delivered concomitantly by separate inhalers

Question: What is the efficacy of individual LABAICS combination preparations compared with LABA and ICS delivered concomitantly by separate inhalers in asthma?

Seretide[R]

In four randomized, double-blind studies, Seretide[R] has been compared with salmeterol 50 μg bd and with fluticasone propionate 100, 250 and 500 μg bd delivered by Diskus inhalers. Seretide[R] was not significantly different from salmeterol and fluticasone administered concomitantly by separate inhalers over a 12-week period. Morning PEF increased by 35–43 L/min on Seretide[R] and by 33–36 L/min on the two separate drugs (Table 1). Spirometry and symptom scores improved to a very similar extent on combination as on concomitant therapy, but all studies were powered to show equivalence of morning PEF (within 15 L/min). Seretide[R] was more effective than placebo, salmeterol or fluticasone alone, with morning PEF improving by 35–54 L/min in patients taking Seretide[R] and by 15–17 L/min in patients taking fluticasone monotherapy (Table 2).[4–7]

A fixed effect meta-analysis of these clinical studies[8] examined a consistent trend in morning PEF favouring Seretide[R] over treatment with the individual constituents co-administered by separate inhalers. Whether analysed by intention to treat or per protocol, a small but consistently significant difference in morning PEF favouring the combination over concurrent therapy was demonstrated; mean over 12 weeks of 5.4 L/min [95% confidence interval (CI) 1.5–9.2]. This corresponded to a mean difference in forced expiratory volume in 1 second (FEV_1) of approximately 40 mL. Logistic regression analysis suggested an increased odds ratio (OR) of 1.42 (95% CI 1.1–1.8) for achieving an increase in morning PEF > 15 L/min above baseline compared

Table 1. Studies comparing administration of Seretide[R] (ST) and individual constituent drugs (fluticasone, FP; salmeterol, SM) and placebo (PL)

Ref. (1st author)	Duration (months)	n	Baseline ICS (μg/day)	FEV_1 (% pred.)	PEF_{AM} (L/min)	Comparison	Conclusion
Bateman[6]	3	244	400–500	76	367	ST 100/50 versus FP 100 + SM 50	Equivalent
Chapman[50]	3	371	800–1200	76	394	ST 250/50 versus FP 250 + SM 50	Equivalent
Aubier[19]	3	503	1500–2000	73	352	ST 500/50 versus FP 500 + SM 50 versus FP 500	Equivalent

Table 2. Studies comparing administration of Seretide[R] (ST) and individual constituent drugs (fluticasone, FP; salmeterol, SM) concomitantly by separate inhalers.

Ref. (1st author)	Age (years)	Duration (months)	n	Baseline ICS BDP (μg/day)	FEV_1 (% pred.)	PEF_{AM} (L/min)	Comparison	Result
Kavuru[7]	>12	3	356	200–500	85	242	ST100/50 versus FP100 versus SM 50 versus PL	ST PEF +53* FP +17 SM −2 PL −24
Shapiro[4]	39	3	349	400–800	68	371	ST 250/50 versus FP 250 versus SM 50 versus PL	ST PEF +54* +15 −12 −14

*$P < 0.05$ versus PL, FP; $P < 0.03$ versus SM.

Table 3. Studies comparing administration of LABAICS and inhaled corticosteroid alone.

Ref. (1st author)	Duration (months)	n	Baseline ICS BDP (μg/day)	FEV$_1$ (% pred.)	Baseline PEF$_{AM}$ (L/min)	Comparison	Result PEF
Jenkins[9]	6	353	800–1200	70	360	ST 250/50 bd versus	+46*
						BUD 800 bd	+20
Busse[10]	6	558	500–800	81	458	ST 100/50 bd versus	+37*
						FP 250 bd	+19
Johansson[51]	3	349				ST 100/50 bd versus	+43*
						BUD 400 bd	+33
Zetterstrom[11]	3	362	960	74	358	SB 160/4.5 iibd	+36*
						BUD 320 bd	0
						BUD 320 + FM9	+32*
Lalloo[12]	3	467	387	82	362	SB 80/4.5 bd	+16.5*
						BUD 200 bd	+7.3
Bateman[13]	3	373	400	78		SB 160/4.5 bd	+27*
						FP 250 bd	+8

*$P < 0.05 – 0.001$ versus ICS.

with concurrent therapy and an OR of 1.40 (95% CI 1.1–1.8) for an increase of 30 L/min. While these may appear to be small differences, as the authors point out, they represent an increase of 7–9% and 5–14% of patients achieving this response on the combination therapy. In addition, it raises the question of the mechanism of this additional benefit: airway co-deposition or molecular co-localization at the cellular or receptor level. A similar message probably holds true for Symbicort^R. The scientific explanation of these data is also of considerable interest as it may involve synergy of the two drugs at a receptor or molecular level or result from co-deposition within the lung.[3]

Study of individual combination inhalers with other comparator drugs

Question: what is the comparative efficacy of LABAICS combination inhaler compared with inhaled corticosteroids in asthma?

Comparison with inhaled steroids alone

Combination inhaler therapy is compared with inhaled steroid treatment alone in Table 3.

Seretide^R

Jenkins *et al.*[9] randomized 353 moderate–severe adult asthmatics on a median initial inhaled steroid dose of 1000 μg beclomethasone dipropionate (BDP) equivalent to Seretide^R 250/50 by Accuhaler one actuation bd or budesonide 800 μg by Turbohaler bd in a double-blind, double-dummy design over 24 weeks. Seretide^R was more effective than budesonide in terms of increase in morning PEF with a treatment difference of 25 L/min (95% CI 15–35, $P < 0.001$). Mean evening PEF was also significantly greater on Seretide^R with a treat-

ment difference of 16–20 L/min (95% CI 7–30, $P < 0.001$) at different time points. FEV$_1$ was significantly greater on Seretide^R at 4 and 24 weeks, and the percentage of symptom-free days (SFD) over 24 weeks was also greater ($P < 0.001$). Salbutamol-free days and nights were significantly greater on Seretide^R. Moderate–severe asthma patients symptomatic on high-dose inhaled steroids benefit more from changing to a moderate-dose combination inhaler (Seretide^R 250/50) rather than a threefold greater dose of inhaled budesonide, confirming the efficacy of adding a LABA in this situation.

Busse *et al.*[10] studied adults with moderately severe asthma who were confirmed to require fluticasone by Accuhaler 250 μg bd as minimum effective inhaled steroid dose for asthma control. A total of 558 patients were randomized to take Seretide^R 100/50 one actuation bd or fluticasone 250 μg bd double blind for 12–24 weeks. Withdrawals due to worsening asthma accounted for 5% of patients on Seretide^R and 7% on fluticasone (NS). At 24 weeks, only a further 1% in each group had withdrawn. Patients on Seretide^R had significantly higher FEV$_1$, morning and evening PEF, SFD, salbutamol reliever use and rescue-free days. In patients requiring a moderate dose of inhaled steroids, a combination inhaler effectively permitted a 60% reduction in inhaled steroid dose to fluticasone 100 μg bd without deterioration in asthma control in 95% of subjects.

Symbicort^R

Zetterstrom *et al.*[11] reported a randomized, double-blind, double-dummy comparison of Symbicort^R 160/4.5 two inhalations bd, budesonide 200 μg and formoterol 4.5 μg taken concomitantly by separate turbohalers bd and budesonide alone 200 μg bd in 362 adult asthmatics, not controlled on inhaled corticosteroids alone, over 12 weeks. Symbicort^R produced significantly greater increases in morning and evening PEF (36 and 25 L/min respectively) compared with separate

Table 4. Studies comparing administration of LABAICS and montelukast (ML), with or without inhaled corticosteroid.

Ref. (1st author)	Age (years)	Duration (months)	n	Baseline ICS (μg/day)	FEV$_1$ (% pred.)	Baseline PEF$_{AM}$ (L/min)	Comparison	Results PEF$_{AM}$	Exac. %
Calhoun[15]	37	3	423	Nil	67	374	ST 100/50 bd	+90*	0
							ML 10 od	+34	5
Pearlman[16]		3	426	Nil			ST 100/50 bd	+81*	3
							ML 10 od	+42	6
Nelson[14]	42	3	447	<600	68	395	ST 100/50 bd	+25*	2
							ML 10 + FP 100 bd	+13	6
Ringdal[17]	43	3	725	400–1000	75	369	ST	+36*	9.6
							ML 10 + FP 100 bd	+19	14.6

*$P < 0.001$.

inhaler therapy (32 and 22 L/min, $P < 0.0001$) and budesonide alone (0 and –4 L/min, $P < 0.0001$). Symbicort^R tended to produce a more rapid improvement in morning PEF than concomitant treatment, and both were significantly quicker than budesonide ($P < 0.0001$). Asthma symptoms, symptom-free days, reliever-free days and daily reliever use were significantly improved with combination treatment as Symbicort^R and by separate inhalers. There was a trend for more rapid improvement with Symbicort^R than with concomitant therapy.

Lalloo et al.[12] evaluated Symbicort^R 80/4.5 one inhalation bd compared with a higher dose of budesonide (200 μg bd) in a randomized, double-blind 12-week study of 467 patients with mild to moderate asthma not fully controlled by budesonide 100 μg bd during a 2-week run-in period. Symbicort^R produced a significantly greater increase in morning PEF (16.5 versus 7.3 L/min) and evening PEF (14 versus 4 L/min) compared with budesonide alone. There were also significant benefits of Symbicort^R over budesonide for increased asthma control days (17% versus 10%), increased SFDs (16% versus 10%) and reduced reliever β_2-agonist use (–0.33 versus –0.1 inhalations/day). Symbicort^R also reduced the risk of an exacerbation by 26% compared with higher dose budesonide ($P = 0.02$). The additional benefit of a low-dose combination inhaler over higher dose inhaled steroids in mild asthma is in line with previous evidence supporting the addition of a LABA rather than increasing the dose of an inhaled steroid.

In a similar design, Bateman et al.[13] randomized 373 patients with moderate persistent asthma who were symptomatic during a 2-week run-in on budesonide 200 μg bd to Symbicort^R 160/4.5 or fluticasone by Accuhaler 250 μg one inhalation bd. Over 12 weeks, Symbicort^R was more effective than fluticasone alone in improving morning PEF (27.4 versus 7.7 L/min, $P < 0.001$). There were also significant benefits favouring Symbicort^R over fluticasone alone for evening PEF and FEV$_1$, reliever β_2 usage and reliever-free days. Trends in SFDs, night-time awakening and asthma control days favoured Symbicort^R, but these did not achieve statistical significance. The risk of an exacerba-

tion was reduced by 32% with Symbicort^R over higher dose fluticasone ($P < 0.05$). Again, in more severe asthma, the additional benefit of a combination inhaler over higher dose inhaled steroid supports previous evidence favouring the addition of a LABA rather than increasing the dose of an inhaled steroid.

Comparison of combination therapy with leukotriene antagonists

Studies comparing the addition of LABAICS combinations and the leukotriene antagonist montelukast are summarized in Table 4.

Nelson et al.[14] randomized 447 adults with asthma symptomatic despite low-dose inhaled steroids to Seretide^R 100/50 by Accuhaler one inhalation bd or fluticasone by Accuhaler 100 μg bd plus montelukast 10 mg in a double-blind, double-dummy, multicentre study. Mean morning PEF increased more on Seretide^R (25 versus 13 L/min, $P < 0.001$) as did evening PEF (19 versus 10 L/min, $P < 0.001$) and FEV$_1$ (0.34 versus 0.20 L). Salbutamol-free days increased significantly more on Seretide^R (26% versus 19%), and total salbutamol use reduced significantly more. Fewer patients suffered an asthma exacerbation on Seretide^R than on fluticasone (2% versus 6%, $P = 0.03$). Switching patients taking low-dose inhaled steroids to a combination inhaler offered advantages over adding montelukast to low-dose fluticasone.

Calhoun et al.[15] compared the addition of Seretide^R 100/50 by Accuhaler one inhalation bd to adding montelukast 10 mg at night in 423 adult asthma patients symptomatic on inhaled β_2-agonists alone in a double-blind, double-dummy, randomized study over 12 weeks. At endpoint, mean morning PEF increased markedly on Seretide^R compared with montelukast (90 versus 34 L/min, $P < 0.001$) as did evening PEF (70 versus 31 L/min, $P < 0.001$) and FEV$_1$ (23% versus 11% baseline). Symptom score was significantly reduced as was salbutamol use. Salbutamol-free days increased significantly more on Seretide^R (53% versus 26%) as did nights without awakenings (23% versus 15.5%, $P \leq 0.001$). Fewer patients suffered an asthma exacerbation on Seretide^R than on montelukast (0%

versus 5%, $P < 0.001$). Initiating treatment with a combination inhaler in patients symptomatic on β_2-agonists alone was superior to starting montelukast, although these patients as a group were quite severe (mean baseline FEV_1 68% predicted) and would normally have been treated with an inhaled steroid beforehand in most countries.

Pearlman et al.[16] also studied patients who were symptomatic on inhaled β_2-agonists alone ($n = 432$), comparing the addition of Seretide[R] 100/50 by Accuhaler ore inhalation bd with adding montelukast 10 mg at night in a double-blind, double-dummy, randomized design over 12 weeks. At endpoint, mean morning PEF increased markedly on Seretide[R] compared with montelukast (81 versus 42 L/min, $P < 0.001$) as did evening PEF (65 versus 39 L/min, $P < 0.001$) and FEV_1 (0.61 versus 0.32 L). The percentage of SFD and salbutamol-free days increased significantly more on Seretide[R] (40% versus 27% and 53% versus 27%) as did nights without awakenings (30% versus 20%, $P \leq 0.01$). Daily rescue salbutamol use was significantly reduced by Seretide[R] (-3.6 versus -2.2 puffs, $P < 0.001$), and quality of life scores improved significantly more ($P < 0.001$) than on montelukast. Maintenance treatment with a combination inhaler in patients symptomatic on β_2-agonists alone was superior to starting montelukast in these patients as in the previous study.

Ringdal et al.[17] randomized 806 adults with asthma symptomatic despite fluticasone by Accuhaler 100 µg bd for 1 month to Seretide[R] 100/50 by Accuhaler one inhalation bd or fluticasone by Accuhaler 100 µg bd plus montelukast 10 mg in a double-blind, double-dummy, multicentre study over 12 weeks. Mean morning PEF increased more on Seretide[R] (36 versus 19 L/min, $P < 0.05$) as did evening PEF (29 versus 15 L/min, $P < 0.05$). FEV_1 increased significantly more on Seretide[R] as did SFDs, SF nights and rescue salbutamol-free days ($P < 0.05$). Exacerbations of asthma were significantly reduced on Seretide[R] (9.6% versus 14.6% on fluticasone plus montelukast, $P < 0.05$). Patients who are symptomatic despite low-dose inhaled steroids benefit more from inhaled combination therapy rather than the addition of montelukast.

Question

What is the comparative safety of LABA/ICS combination inhaler compared with other treatments in asthma?

Safety and adverse effects of these combination products have not been a major issue as the component drugs are well tolerated with relatively few adverse effects.[18–20] There is no evidence of additional or altered adverse effects with concurrent administration of the two drugs. The systemic pharmacodynamic response and development of β_2-receptor tachyphylaxis after repeated doses of salmeterol 100 µg bd was unaffected by co-administration of fluticasone 500 µg bd. Similarly, the systemic pharmacodynamic response to fluticasone was not affected by salmeterol.[21]

Side-effects consequent on the known pharmacology of LABAs and ICS are recorded in each study. Overall, these are as anticipated: headache (incidence $\leq$ 2%), throat irritation (1–4%), hoarseness (2–3%), oral candidiasis ($<$ 1–4%). In the studies, withdrawals potentially related to treatment adverse events were the same for combination products and comparators (0–3%).

Studies of different strategies of use of combination inhalers

Question

How should combination preparations be used in the management of asthma?

Seretide[R]

GOAL[22] represents an ambitious 12-month study of the extent to which the arbitrary aims of asthma control, reproduced in various guidelines, can actually be achieved in 3421 patients with initially uncontrolled asthma. Seretide[R] was compared with equal doses of fluticasone alone across three strata of patients, at different starting doses of inhaled steroid, steroid-naïve, $\leq$ 500 µg/day BDP and $>$ 500–1000 µg/day BDP. The strategy was to increase doses of fluticasone or Seretide[R] at 3-month intervals if 'total control' was not achieved over a period of seven out of eight consecutive weeks. 'Total control' comprised no day- or night-time symptoms, no exacerbations or emergency visits, no rescue β_2-agonist use, morning PEF $>$ 80% predicted every day and no adverse effects of treatment. Across each stratum, a higher success rate was obtained using Seretide[R] as opposed to fluticasone; 31% versus 19% after dose escalation and 41% versus 28% at 12 months. Using the slightly less stringent criteria for 'well-controlled' asthma, this was achieved by 63% on Seretide[R] and 50% on fluticasone after dose escalation and by 71% and 59% at the end of 12 months. Control was achieved more rapidly, with lower exacerbation rates and greater improvement in health status, on the combination therapy. At the end of the study, across all strata, 68% and 76% of patients were taking the highest doses. No attempt was made to 'step down' therapy. A large number of patients with suboptimally controlled asthma, with a range of severity, were included, but all three strata were characterized by marked reversibility (median bronchodilator response was 22% FEV_1). Guideline-defined asthma control was achievable in a majority of patients in this study, but this strategy cannot necessarily be extrapolated to everyday practice.

Symbicort[R]

A programme (Table 5) of open, randomized, parallel group studies has compared conventional twice-daily dosing with adjustable maintenance dosing with Symbicort[R] taking advantage of the four- to eightfold individual dose range

Table 5. Adjustable dosing with Symbicort[R]: randomized, open, parallel group studies.

Study	Ref. (1st author)	n	Duration (months)	Dose adjustment	Inhalations/day		Primary endpoint
					Start	End	
	Leuppi[23]	142	3	160/4.5 1, 2 or 4 bd	3.9	3.0	Success/failure
SMART CAN	FitzGerald[25]	995	5	80/4.5 1, 2 or 4 bd 160/4.5	3.9	2.5	Exacerbations
SMART	Stallberg[24]	1153	7	80/4.5 1, 2 or 4 bd	3.95	3.25	Exacerbations
ASSURE	Ind[26]	1734	3	80/4.5 1, 2 or 4 bd 160/4.5	3.8	2.65	Success/failure
SUND	Aalbers[29]	1044	1 (+6/12 ext)	160/4.5 1, 2 or 4 bd	4.0	3.4	Odds of WCAW
CAST	Canonica[27]	2358	3	80/4.5 1, 2 or 4 bd	3.86	2.95	Exacerbations
ATACO	Buhl[28]	4025	3	160/4.5 1, 2 or 4 bd	3.82	2.63	HQRL

ext, open extension; n, number of patients enrolled; WCAW, well-controlled asthma week; HQRL, health-related quality of life.

Table 6. Results of studies of adjustable dosing with Symbicort[R].

Ref. (1st author)	FEV$_1$ (% pred.)	PEF$_{AM}$ (L/min)	ICS dose (μg/day)	LABA %	Primary endpoint	Fixed bd	Adj dosing	Other Rx diff	NNT
Leuppi[23]	79	91%p	≥600	100	Success	26%	33%	↓ noct ss+	
					Failure	24%	17%	↓ β$_2$ use+	
FitzGerald[25]	93	—	582	—	Exacerbations	8.9%	4.0%	↓ cost+	21
Stallberg[24]	96	—	603	73	Exacerbations	9.5%	6.2%	↓ cost+	30
Ind[26]	—	392	672	41	Success	29%	28%	↓ PEF$_{AM/PM}$⁻	
					Failure	3%	2%	↓ β$_2$+ ↓cost+	
Aalbers[29]	84	465	735	61	WCAW	1.29	1.34	↓ β$_2$+ ↓ cost+	
Canonica[27]	85	373	626	—	Exacerbations	4.6%	4.8%	↓ cost+	
Buhl[28]	—	356	<1000	—	AQLQ	0.20	0.18	↓ cost+	

Fixed bd, twice-daily conventional regular dosing; Adj, adjustable dosing; % pred., percentage predicted; NNT, number needed to treat; ICS, inhaled corticosteroid; LABA, inhaled long-acting β$_2$-agonist; Other Rx diff, treatment difference for other endpoint; AQLQ, asthma quality of life questionnaire.

demonstrated with both formoterol (6–24 μg) and budesonide (100–800 μg) in previous studies. The results are summarized in Table 6.

Leuppi et al.[23] randomized 127 patients previously well controlled on an ICS and a LABA to fixed dosing with Symbicort[R] 160/4.5 two inhalations bd or adjustable dosing from one inhalation bd or two at night to two bd increasing if necessary to four bd. Some 72% of patients were able to reduce treatment in the adjustable arm, > 50% for > 50% of the 12 weeks of treatment with an average daily dose reduction of 23%. Asthma control was equivalent in the two groups, but nocturnal wakening and rescue β$_2$-agonist use were statistically significantly less in the adjustable group. Stallberg et al.[24] reported a significant reduction in asthma exacerbations, 6.2% on adjustable dosing compared with 9.5% on fixed Symbicort[R] dosing, a 41% reduction in combination usage and cost savings of 98 Euros over a 6-month period. Fitzgerald

et al.[25] showed that significantly fewer patients randomized to adjustable dosing experienced exacerbations, 4.0% compared with 8.9% on fixed dosing over 5 months, together with an overall reduction of 36% Symbicort[R] doses and cost saving of 141 Canadian dollars (95% CI 116–162). Ind et al.[26] showed that adjustable dosing was as effective in symptom control and in improving health-related quality of life as fixed dosing with Symbicort[R] over 12 weeks. Some 79% of patients were able to step down, and overall combination usage was reduced by 16%; reliever β$_2$-agonist usage was reduced by 0.2 inhalations daily. Treatment failure occurred in only 6% of patients with no difference between the groups. Canonica et al.[27] reported a 5% rate of asthma exacerbations in patients on fixed bd dosing and variable dosing with Symbicort[R] over 12 weeks. Secondary endpoints were equivalent in the two arms, but adjustable dosing was associated with 24% less combination usage and a cost saving of 65 Euros over 3 months. Buhl et al.[28]

showed that improvements in health-related quality of life (AQLQ, SF-36) symptom severity score and morning and evening PEF achieved during run-in on Symbicort[R] 160/4.5 bd were equivalently maintained by adjustable dosing or continued twice-daily dosing over 4 months. Adjustable dosing was associated with an overall 31% reduction in combination inhaler usage.

Aalbers et al.[29] compared fixed dosing with Symbicort[R] 160/4.5 two inhalations bd with Seretide[R] 250/50 one inhalation bd over a 4-week, double-dummy, double-blind period followed by a 6-month open extension when adjustable dosing with Symbicort[R] 160/4.5 (one and two inhalations bd combined) was compared with the two fixed dose regimens. During the 4-week, double-blind period, there were no differences between the two fixed dose combination products. During the 6-month open extension (but not in the whole study), adjustable Symbicort[R] dosing was associated with an increased chance of achieving a well-controlled asthma week (WCAW) compared with fixed dose Symbicort[R] 1.335 (95% CI 1.001–1.783) but not Seretide[R]. However, there were fewer asthma exacerbations on adjustable Symbicort[R] (35) compared with fixed dose Symbicort[R] (50) and Seretide[R] (59). Adjustable Symbicort[R] differed significantly from Seretide[R] but not from fixed Symbicort[R], and this did not differ from Seretide[R]. Other differences were minor, but adjustable dosing led to a 15% reduction in Symbicort[R] dose and lower direct and indirect health care costs.

In general, the studies show the feasibility of varying the dose of the Symbicort[R] combination inhaler according to clinical condition, particularly nocturnal symptoms, β_2-agonist use and, in some cases, PEF. Overall, adjustable dosing results in a net reduction in average daily inhalations without compromising asthma control (and in studies longer than 3 months actually improved endpoints such as exacerbations).

This approach results in inevitable drug cost savings, but pharmacoeconomic benefits (taking into account total direct and indirect costs) are potentially considerable (see below, Tables 6 and 7).

Question

How may combination inhaler preparations be used to manage asthma in the future?

To an extent, the different strategies adopted in the pharmaceutical company-sponsored studies conducted so far have focused on the different pharmacological properties of the two combination products; adjustable dosing is not so practical with Seretide[R] and has not been reported. A double-blind, controlled study of adjustable dosing would also be of interest. Gradual dose escalation (with step down at some point) needs to be compared with rapid dose adjustment, driven by symptoms, in a formal controlled clinical trial using a range of endpoints including markers of chronic inflammation and patient preference.

Definitive long-term studies of initiation of combination therapy in patients not previously taking inhaled steroids (see 4-week pilot study by Pearlman et al.[30]) are under way. It appears clear that some patients who are steroid naïve are unlikely to benefit,[31] whereas others will.[22,32] It is essential to ascertain the risk–benefit and cost–benefit of this approach.

The use of single combination inhaler therapy with Symbicort[R] (including regular maintenance and additional as required treatment, but also as required Symbicort[R] alone) requires formal evaluation as patients themselves are likely to adopt these strategies.

Pharmacoeconomic studies of combination inhalers with comparators

Question

How does the cost of LABAICS combination inhaler preparations compare with other treatments for asthma?

Table 7. Cost implications from studies of adjustable dosing with Symbicort[R].

Ref. (1st author)	n	Duration (months)	Symbicort[R] adjustable dosing (% change in drug use)	Potential savings* /patient/year (Euros)
Leuppi[23]	127	3	−23	↓
FitzGerald[25]	995	5	−36	218
Stallberg[24]	1034	7	−41	196
Ind[26]	1553	3	−16	51
Aalbers[29]	658	7	−15	↓
Canonica[27]	2063	3	−24	260
Buhl[28]	3297	3	−31	328
Michils[52]	980	4	−38	↓

n, number of patients randomized to study; ↓, reduced costs not quantified.

*total = direct + indirect costs calculated using a variety of cost assumptions and exchange rates and expressed here in Euros.

The recognition that asthma accounts for up to approximately 2% of health care spending in developed countries and the introduction of combination inhalers that have high unit cost but the potential to achieve savings overall has focused attention on pharmacoeconomic studies.

Lundback *et al.*[33] conducted an economic analysis of a multicentre, randomized, double-blind, double-dummy, parallel group comparison of 353 asthmatic patients symptomatic on BDP (or equivalent) 800–1200 µg/day who were treated with Seretide[R] 250/50 or budesonide by turbohaler 88 µg bd over 24 weeks.[9] Outcome measures included the proportion of SFD, episode-free days (EFD; no day- or night-time symptoms and no β_2-agonist use over 24 hours) and successfully treated weeks (STW, defined as morning PEF improved > 5% predicted above baseline). Seretide[R] produced a significantly higher proportion of SFD, EFD and STW throughout the study as well as increasing mean morning PEF more (406 versus 380 L/min, $P < 0.001$) and improving other outcomes. Mean total health care resources were very similar between the two study arms [19.6 versus 18.5 Swedish Kroner (SEK)]. However, the mean cost per STW was less for Seretide[R] than for budesonide, and calculating the incremental cost-effectiveness ratio (ICER), i.e. the extra cost required to achieve this additional benefit, suggested that it costs on average 32 SEK for an additional STW using Seretide[R]. Mean costs per SFD and EFD were lower with Seretide[R] than with budesonide, 51 versus 75 and 42 versus 53 SEK respectively. Cost-effectiveness analysis using a range of measures suggests that Seretide[R] is beneficial and additional costs for improved asthma control are judged to be reasonable.

Sheth *et al.*[34] carried out an economic analysis of a multicentre, double-blind, double-dummy comparison in 423 patients with symptomatic asthma treated with inhaled β_2-agonist alone randomized to receive either Seretide[R] 100/50 bd or montelukast 10 mg od with appropriate placebos over 12 weeks.[15] Effectiveness measures included proportion of SFD and proportion of patients achieving ≥ 12% increase in FEV_1 above baseline. Direct costs only were collected prospectively and analysed on an intention-to-treat basis. Seretide[R] achieved more SFD, 46.8% compared with 21.5% for montelukast ($P < 0.001$), and 71% had ≥ 12% increase in FEV_1 above baseline compared with 39% for montelukast ($P < 0.001$). Exacerbations were less on Seretide[R] than on montelukast (0% versus 11%, $P < 0.05$). Mean total (drug and non-drug) costs per patient per day were significantly greater for Seretide[R] than for montelukast (US$3.55 versus US$3.12, $P < 0.001$), although non-drug costs were significantly less (US$0.18 versus US$0.44 per day). However, mean daily costs per patient per SFD and per successfully treated patient (≥ 12% increase in FEV_1 above baseline) were significantly lower with Seretide[R] than with montelukast (US$7.63 versus US$14.89 and US$5.03 versus US$8.25). ICER calculations suggest that it costs US$1.33 per day for each extra patient achieving at least a 12% increase in FEV_1 with Seretide[R]. Sensitivity analysis suggests that results favour Seretide[R] over montelukast for increments in FEV_1 between 10% and 15%. A recent pharmacoeconomic review concludes that Seretide[R] represents a cost-effective option compared with treatment with fluticasone at the same dose, budesonide, formoterol plus budesonide and montelukast plus fluticasone in patients with uncontrolled asthma despite an inhaled steroid. Similarly, in patients with asthma not controlled on a short-acting β_2-agonist alone, Seretide[R] is cost effective compared with montelukast alone.[35]

Rosenhall *et al.*[36] examined direct and indirect costs in a 6-month extension of a previous 6-month study comparing Symbicort[R] 160/4.5 two inhalations bd with the same doses of budesonide plus formoterol in 320 adult asthma patients. Symbicort[R] resulted in a lower proportion of withdrawals compared with concomitant administration (9.2% versus 19.4% $P = 0.008$). Symbicort[R] was also associated with reduced direct (1595 SEK, $P = 0.0004$) and total health care costs (1884 SEK, $P = 0.04$) per patient per year. Conventional twice-daily dosing with Symbicort[R] was cost effective compared with concomitant administration. As we have seen, adjustable maintenance dosing with Symbicort[R] was potentially more cost effective (Tables 6 and 7).

Box points

1. Combination inhalers produce equivalent benefit, with equivalent side-effects, to their component long-acting β_2-agonist and inhaled steroid agents administered concomitantly but are more convenient and cost saving.
2. Combination inhalers produce greater benefit than either of their individual component drugs administered alone.
3. Combination inhalers produce greater benefit than inhaled steroid alone at two to three times higher dose reflecting additional benefit of the long-acting β_2-agonist component. They are also cost effective.
4. Combination inhalers produce greater benefit than addition of montelukast in patients taking low-dose inhaled steroids or on short-acting β_2-agonists alone. They are also cost effective.
5. Guideline-defined asthma control is achievable using an escalating schedule of fluticasone or Seretide[R] at 3-month intervals. Seretide[R] was more rapid and more effective.
6. Adjustable dosing with Symbicort[R] is feasible, safe and produces equivalent asthma control to conventional, fixed, twice-daily dosing. It leads to reduced combination drug usage, reduced health care costs and, in some studies, reduced asthma exacerbations.

Anti-immunoglobulin E for treatment of asthma in adults

A central mechanism of allergic inflammation in asthma is the release of proinflammatory mediators triggered by binding of the allergen to cell-bound immunoglobulin (Ig)E. Serum total IgE is frequently raised in asthmatics, and this correlates with symptoms and bronchoconstrictor response to stimuli. Omalizumab, or rhuMAb-E25, is a recombinant, humanized, monoclonal antibody. It is directed against IgE, binding free but not cell-bound IgE. It blocks IgE binding to cell membranes, thus inhibiting the release of inflammatory mediators. After a single injection, there is a dramatic reduction in circulating free IgE, and a course of injections attenuates the early and late phase reactions to inhaled allergen.

Although it is not yet licensed for treatment (except in Australia and the USA), there have been a number of studies involving children, adolescents and adults with asthma and allergic rhinitis. This section concentrates on those studies of patients with asthma, aged 16 years and above. We review studies reporting randomized, placebo-controlled trials.

Literature Search

We searched MEDLINE and the Cochrane database for RCTs with clinical endpoints, using the terms asthma, anti-IgE, anti-immunoglobulin E, monoclonal antibody, RhuMAB E25 and omalizumab (September 2004).

Initial trials

Fahy et al.[37] looked at the effects of 9 weeks of intravenous (IV) omalizumab in 19 patients with mild allergic asthma (FEV$_1$ > 70% predicted) and showed reduction in serum IgE. The allergen dose required to provoke the early asthmatic response increased, and the mean maximal falls in FEV$_1$ in the early and late asthmatic responses were reduced.

Boulet et al.[38] conducted a trial in 20 patients with mild allergic asthma (FEV$_1$ > 70% predicted) with 10 weeks of treatment with IV antibody (2 mg on day 0, then 1 mg/kg on days 7, 14 and fortnightly until day 70). Again, serum IgE was significantly reduced, and allergen PC$_{15}$ and methacholine PC$_{20}$ doses were increased in the active treatment groups compared with placebo. Skin test responses to allergens were unaffected.

Fahy et al.[39] reported a trial of aerolized anti-IgE in 33 patients with mild allergic asthma (FEV$_1$ > 70% predicted). Doses of 1 mg and 10 mg daily were compared with placebo, and treatment continued for 8 weeks. There was no significant decrease in serum IgE or change in any measures of asthma control between groups. However, one subject developed antibodies to the anti-IgE, suggesting that inhalation may be a more immunogenic route. These studies established the efficacy of IV omalizumab in blocking experimental allergen-induced asthma.

Larger scale trials (Table 8)

Question

What is the efficacy of parenteral anti-IgE antibody in adults with asthma?

Table 8. Studies examining the efficacy of anti-IgE (omalizumab).

Reference	n	Age (years)	FEV$_1$ (% pred.)	Other baseline	ICS dose (µg/day) BDP (or equivalent)	Primary endpoint	Result omalizumab	Result control	Other endpoints
Milgrom[40]	317	30	71	ASS 4/7	800 (TAA) (35 on oral also)	ASS	2.8	3.1	↓ICS dose ↓exac. PEF
Busse[41]	525	39	68	ASS 4/7	570	exac./pt	0.28	0.54	↓ASS ↓rescue med. ↑FEV$_1$ (73% versus 69%)
Solèr[42] (Buhl[44,45])	546	40	70	AQLQ 4.4	770	exac./pt pts ≥1 exac.	0.28 35	0.66 83	↓ASS ↓rescue med. ↑PEF and FEV$_1$
Holgate[53]	246	41	64	Severe asthma	1370 (FP)	dose ↓≥50%	74% pts	51%	↓rescue med. use ↓symptoms ↑AQLQ
Vignola[54]	405	38	78	Rhinitis	870	Pts with exac. Exac. rate QoL (≥1.0)	20% 0.25 58%	30% 0.4 43%	↓symptoms ↑PEF (11 L/min) ↑FEV$_1$ (73 mL)
Ayres[55]	312	38	71	Poor asthma control	2000 (66 on oral also)	ADRI-free Time until ADRI	36% 126 days	20% 75 days	Fewer exac. ↑ASS ↓rescue med.

ICS, inhaled corticosteroid; ADRI, asthma deterioration-related incidents; BDP, beclomethasone dipropionate; TAA, triamcinolone acetonide; FP, fluticasone propionate; ASS, asthma symptom score; AQLQ, asthma quality of life questionnaire; QoL, quality of life; exac., exacerbation; med., medication.

Patient groups

Milgrom *et al.*,[40] Busse *et al.*[41] and Solèr *et al.*[42] studied patients with moderate–severe asthma (FEV$_1$ 40–80% predicted). These studies included patients aged 11 years and above, including adults. Milgrom *et al.*[43] examined only children (aged 6–12 years), and this study is not included here. All patients were on daily ICS, and some also took oral steroids.

Drug delivery and dose

Milgrom *et al.*[40] gave omalizumab IV, Busse *et al.*[41] and Solèr *et al.*[42] gave it by subcutaneous (SC) injection. In Milgrom's study of 317 patients, there was a 4-week run-in, followed by omalizumab at 5.8 or 2.5 µg/kg/ng IgE/L. Half-doses were given on days 0, 4 and 7, then full doses 2-weekly for 20 weeks. Steroid dose (inhaled ± oral) was maintained for 12 weeks then reduced over 8 weeks. Follow-up continued for 10 weeks.

Busse *et al.*[41] enrolled 525 patients and employed a dose and dose interval based on body weight and baseline IgE, approximately 0.016 mg/kg/IgE (IU/mL) (range 150–750 mg per 4 weeks). There was a run-in of 4–6 weeks to switch all subjects to inhaled BDP to maintain asthma control, followed by 16 weeks of maintenance treatment, then inhaled steroid reduction over 8 weeks and 4 weeks of maintenance at the lowest possible BDP dose (or none) without worsening of symptoms.

Solèr *et al.*[42] enrolled 546 subjects in a similar study design, giving omalizumab dependent on weight and baseline IgE at ≥0.016 mg/kg/IgE IU/mL every 4 weeks. Again, there was a run-in phase to establish patients on BDP, 16 weeks of stable steroid dose, then a 12-week attempted inhaled steroid reduction phase. Buhl *et al.*[44,45] reported, in two papers, the results of an extension phase of 24 weeks in 483 of the original 546 subjects. Omalizumab was continued and the BDP dose was kept as low as possible but could be increased if required. Other asthma medication could be added at the physicians' discretion.

Outcome measures

Serum IgE

All studies showed 89–99% reduction in total free serum IgE.

Lung function

In the study by Milgrom *et al.*,[40] IV treatment resulted in a statistically significant increase in morning PEF of 30 L/min but no change in FEV$_1$. Busse *et al.*[41] reported an increase in PEF of 18.5 L/min compared with 6.9 L/min in the placebo group, and an increase in FEV$_1$ of 4.3% compared with 1.4%, but no *P*-values were given. Solèr *et al.*[42] showed small but significant differences in PEF and FEV$_1$ compared with placebo at various points in the trial. In the extension study, there were no significant differences in FEV$_1$ between the groups.[44,45]

Inhaled steroid doses

Significantly more patients in the omalizumab-treated than in the placebo groups were able to discontinue inhaled steroids completely,[41,42] and this was maintained during the extension phase.[44,45] Busse *et al.*[41] and Solèr *et al.*[42] also showed that omalizumab allowed the dose of inhaled steroid to be reduced significantly, in terms of both actual dose reduction and the number of participants achieving > 50% reduction.

Additional medication

These studies[40–42] showed a significant reduction in the use of rescue β$_2$-agonist use in the omalizumab-treated groups. The use of LABA and leukotriene inhibitors/antagonists was also reduced.[44,45]

Asthma control

All studies showed a significant improvement in asthma control. Most looked at the number of exacerbations per patient, number of patients with one or more exacerbations, time to exacerbation or length of exacerbation. Treated patients also required fewer urgent, unscheduled GP/hospital appointments. These improvements were maintained during the extension phases.

Symptom scores and quality of life

These studies[40–42] used asthma symptom scores, reporting a significant advantage in favour of omalizumab over placebo. Milgrom *et al.*[40] also reported a significant benefit in quality of life score, and Busse *et al.*[41] reported that patients and physicians rated omalizumab as more effective than normal asthma therapy alone. Buhl *et al.*[44,45] reported, after the extension phase to Solèr *et al.*'s original study,[42] on asthma-related quality of life and perceived benefit in favour of omalizumab.

Side-effects/adverse events

There were no significant side-effects such as rash, thrombocytopenia, etc. reported from the studies, and no significant differences between omalizumab and placebo groups. In these studies of IV and SC administration, no patients developed antibodies to anti-IgE. The most commonly reported side-effects were headache and injection site reactions.

Placebo effect

The studies all showed an improvement in asthma control in the placebo groups. This included measures such as improvement in asthma symptom scores, reduction in steroid usage and increase in PEF. In some cases, this could be detected in the run-in period. It is well known that patients in clinical trials generally do well, whether through intense monitoring or optimization of or adherence to treatment. The reported benefits of omalizumab significantly outweighed the placebo effect.

Patients not completing study

There were few withdrawals from the studies. Busse *et al.*[41] reported 19 (7%) from the treatment group compared with 34 (13%) from the placebo group, Solèr *et al.*[42] reported twice as many withdrawals in the placebo group, 40 (14%) versus 19 (6.9%). Milgrom et al.[40] reported three withdrawals from the treatment arm compared with five on placebo. Results were analysed on an intention-to-treat basis or as if steroid dose, symptom scores, etc. were carried forward unchanged.

Further studies

More recent trials have been published evaluating the effectiveness and safety of omalizumab, mainly using primary endpoints of reduction in steroid dose and decrease in asthma exacerbations, rather than lung function.

Patients with allergic asthma, most with persistent symptoms despite high-dose inhaled steroid (200–2000 µg/day) and best possible treatment (according to GINA 2002 guidelines) aged 12–79 years, with elevated IgE (20–1300 IU/mL) and positive skin prick tests, were treated with SC infusions of omalizumab every 2 or 4 weeks, the dose being dependent on patient weight and baseline IgE.

Patients receiving omalizumab rather than placebo had significant reductions in exacerbations, as well as in unscheduled physician and emergency room visits and hospital admissions. More treated patients were able to reduce the steroid dose, and by a greater amount, without deteriorating asthma control than patients in the placebo groups. The use of rescue medication also fell. Asthma Symptom Score and Asthma-related Quality of Life scores also showed clinically significant improvements in the treated patients. In some studies, small but significant improvements in lung function measures were also reported (morning PEF increase > 12 L/min, FEV$_1$ increase 90–115 mL).

There was no increase in serious adverse events (immune complex disease, hypersensitivity reactions, parasite infection or malignancy) in the treated group compared with placebo. There were side-effects such as urticaria and inflammation at injection sites, but omalizumab showed a similar safety and tolerability profile to placebo.

An analysis of combined studies[46] showed that patients with more severe asthma (higher initial ICS dose, lower FEV$_1$%) benefited most from omalizumab, whereas patients with a more marked placebo effect were those with more moderate asthma.

Box points

Omalizumab administered parenterally dramatically reduces free serum total IgE.

Omalizumab has beneficial effects on asthma control, when given by the IV and SC routes on a 2- or 4-weekly dosing regime, but aerolized omalizumab, shown in one study, is ineffective.

The benefits are mainly in steroid dose reduction, decrease in exacerbations, improved control and symptom score.

A small but significant improvement in lung function was reported in some of the trials.

Further research

There is scope for research to develop the use of anti-IgE therapy within clinical settings, to evaluate its appropriate places in the stepwise treatment of asthma, to determine which specific patient groups will benefit, the optimal duration of treatment and cost–benefit analyses.

Monoclonal anti-interleukin-5 antibody

Literature search

We searched MEDLINE for RCTs with clinical outcomes, using the terms anti-interleukin-5, IL-5, asthma and monoclonal antibody (August 2004).

Asthma is a chronic inflammatory disease, characterized by an eosinophilic infiltrate in the airways and reversible airflow obstruction. Eosinophils are prevalent in sputum, lavage fluid and the bronchial mucosa of asthmatics. Interleukin-5 (IL-5) is a key cytokine involved in terminal differentiation, recruitment and activation of eosinophils in bone marrow and at sites of inflammation. IL-5 levels are raised in serum and lavage fluid and in bronchial mucosal biopsies in asthmatics. Inhalation of IL-5 (by asthmatics) causes airway hyper-responsiveness (AHR) and airway eosinophilia.

The development of anti-IL-5 blocking antibodies permitted further direct evaluation of the pathophysiological importance of IL-5. Animal studies in monkeys and guinea pigs showed that anti-IL-5 could prevent eosinophilia and AHR. It is now possible to study in humans the pathological and clinical responses to two humanized, monoclonal anti-IL-5 antibodies. There have now been three double-blind trials reported in patients with asthma, looking at biological and clinical outcomes.

These randomized, placebo-controlled, parallel group studies investigated two different humanized, monoclonal antibodies. Leckie et al.[47] and Flood-Page et al.[48] used mepolizumab (SB240563) and studied n = 24 patients with mild, controlled asthma, baseline FEV$_1$ >70% predicted in both studies, while Kips et al.[49] used SCH55700 in 32 patients with severe, persistent asthma, FEV$_1$ 40–80% predicted, maintained on high-dose inhaled, with or without oral, corticosteroids.

Dosing regimes

Leckie et al.[47] and Kips et al.[49] gave single IV doses. Leckie et al.[47] used 2.5 mg/kg or 10 mg/kg, and Kips et al.[49] administered 0.03 mg/kg, 0.1 mg/kg, 0.3 mg/kg and 1.0 mg/kg to sequential groups. Flood-Page et al.[48] gave a fixed dose of 750 mg on three occasions at 4-weekly intervals.

Outcomes

Leckie et al.[47] showed that sputum eosinophils were reduced after a single dose to 0.9% in the 10 mg/kg group (compared with 12.2% in the placebo group) for up to 4 weeks, and blood eosinophils were reduced from 0.25×10^9/L to 0.04×10^9 for up to 16 weeks in the 10-mg/kg group, and to a lesser extent in the 2.5-mg/kg group. Histamine and allergen challenges at days 8 and 29, however, were unaffected by treatment at either dose.

Kips et al.[49] showed that circulating eosinophils were reduced after the two higher doses of 0.3 mg/kg and 1.0 mg/kg were administered, with a larger decrease (0.07 versus 0.23×10^9/L) at the highest dose, persisting for 30 days. No consistent changes were found in sputum eosinophils, although there was substantial variability at baseline. There was a small, significant increase from baseline in FEV_1 % predicted after 0.3 mg/kg at 24 hours only, with no significant changes at any other time point. There were no significant changes in FEV_1/FVC ratio, PEF, symptom scores or physician evaluations.

Flood-Page et al.[48] looked more closely at site of eosinophil depletion as well as clinical markers. Again, there were no significant differences in FEV_1, PEF or airway response to histamine between groups, although there was a significant increase in morning PEF during the run-in and treatment phases in all groups including placebo. Venous sampling, bone marrow aspiration and bronchoscopy were performed 2 days before the first dose and 2 weeks after the final dose.

Circulating eosinophils were reduced by 100% during the 10 weeks of treatment, returning to baseline a mean of 9 weeks (range 4–20 weeks) after the final dose. Bronchoalveolar lavage eosinophil counts reduced by 79%; however, intact eosinophil numbers were decreased by only 55% in bronchial mucosal biopsies and bone marrow eosinophils by 52%. There was no difference in intra- or extracellular eosinophil major basic protein or in airway basophils, neutrophils, macrophages, mast cells or CD3+ cells after mepolizumab compared with placebo.

Adverse effects

There were reports of headache and fatigue in the study by Kips et al.,[49] with no differences between treatment and placebo groups. No significant differences in clinical or laboratory monitoring between groups were shown. One subject developed non-neutralizing antibodies to SCH55700. Leckie et al.[47] reported no clinically significant adverse effects or development of antibodies to anti-IL-5. Flood-Page et al.[48] reported no adverse effects in any of the subjects.

Discussion

As yet, there is no evidence that anti-IL-5 is of clinical benefit in asthma, questioning the precise role of both IL-5 and eosinophils in asthma. However, the studies so far have included only small numbers of patients and were not powered to show significant clinical changes. In addition, it is possible that larger studies will show that anti-IL-5 is of benefit to particular groups of patients with asthma, or it may be of benefit in different dosing schedules or in combination with other therapies.

Box points

Interleukin-5 is involved in the recruitment and activation of eosinophils.

Anti-IL-5 reduces circulating eosinophils, but significant numbers persist in the airways, bronchial mucosa and bone marrow.

Bronchial reactivity and lung function in asthmatics does not improve following anti-IL-5 treatment when given with standard asthma treatment.

It is possible that anti-IL-5 given with other immune-modulatory drugs may improve asthma control.

References

1 Walters EH, Walters JAE, Gibson MDP. Inhaled long acting β agonists for stable chronic asthma (Cochrane Review). In: The Cochrane Library, Issue 3. Chichester, John Wiley & Sons, 2004.

2 Shrewsbury S, Pyke S, Britton M. Meta-analysis of increased dose of inhaled steroids or addition of salmeterol in symptomatic asthma (MIASMA). BMJ 2000; 320:1368–73.

3 Knox AJ. The scientific rationale of combining inhaled glucocorticoids and long acting β_2 adrenoceptor agonists. Curr Pharm Des 2002; 8:1863–9.

4 Shapiro G, Lumry W, Wolfe J et al. Combined salmeterol 50 mcg and fluticasone propionate 250 mcg in the Diskus device for the treatment of asthma. Am J Respir Crit Care Med 2000; 161:527–34.

5 Van Noord JA, Lilli H, Carrillo J, Davies P. Clinical equivalence of a salmeterol/fluticasone propionate combination product (50/500 µg) delivered via a chlorofluorocarbon-free metered-dose inhaler with the Diskus in patients with moderate to severe asthma. Clin Drug Invest 2001; 21:243–55.

6 Bateman ED, Silins V, Bogolubov M. Clinical equivalence of salmeterol/fluticasone propionate in combination (50/100 µg twice daily) when administered via a chlorofluorocarbon-free metered dose or dry powder inhaler to patients with mild-to-moderate asthma. Respir Med 2001; 95:136–46.

7 Kavaru M, Melamed J, Gross G et al. Salmeterol and fluticasone propionate combined in a new powder inhalation device for the treatment of asthma: a randomised, double-blind, placebo-controlled trial. J Allergy Clin Immunol 2000; 150:1108–16.

8 Nelson HS, Chapman KR, Pyke SD, Johnson M, Pritchard JN. Enhanced synergy between fluticasone propionate and salmeterol inhaled from a single inhaler versus separate inhalers. J Allergy Clin Immunol 2003; 112:29–36.

9 Jenkins C, Woolcock AJ, Saarelainen P, Lundback B, James MH. Salmeterol/fluticasone propionate combination therapy 50/250 µg twice daily in treating moderate to severe asthma. Respir Med 2000; 94:715–23.

10 Busse W, Koenig SM, Oppenheimer J et al. Steroid-sparing effects of fluticasone propionate 100 µg and salmeterol 50 µg administered twice daily in a single product in patients previously controlled with fluticasone propionate 250 µg administered twice daily. J Allergy Clin Immunol 2003; 111:57–65.

11 Zetterstrom O, Buhl R, Mellem H et al. Improved asthma control with budesonide/formoterol in a single inhaler, compared with budesonide alone. Eur Respir J 2001; 18:262–8.

12 Lalloo UG, Maloolepszy, Kozma D et al. Budesonide and formoterol in a single inhaler improves asthma control compared with increasing the dose of corticosteroid in adults with mild-to-moderate asthma. Chest 2003; 123:1480–7.

13 Bateman ED, Bantje TA, Joao Gomes M et al. Combination therapy with single inhaler budesonide/formoterol compared with high dose of fluticasone propionate alone in patients with moderate persistent asthma. Am J Respir Med 2003; 168:275–81.

14 Nelson HS, Busse WW, Kerwin E et al. Fluticasone propionate/salmeterol combination provides more effective asthma control than low-dose inhaled corticosteroid plus montelukast. J Allergy Clin Immunol 2000; 106:1088–95.

15 Calhoun WJ, Nelson HS, Nathan RA et al. Comparison of fluticasone propionate–salmeterol combination therapy and montelukast in patients who are symptomatic on short-acting β2-agonists alone. Am J Respir Crit Care Med 2001; 164:759–63.

16 Pearlman D, White M, Lieberman A. Fluticasone propionate/salmeterol combination compared with montelukast for the treatment of persistent asthma. Ann Allergy Asthma Immunol 2002; 88:227–35.

17 Ringdal N, Eliraz A, Pruzinec P et al. The salmeterol/fluticasone combination is more effective than fluticasone plus oral montelukast in asthma. Respir Med 2001; 97:23–41.

18 Bateman ED, Britton M, Carrillo J. Salmeterol/fluticasone combination inhaler. A new, effective and well tolerated treatment for asthma. Clin Drug Invest 1998; 16:193–201.

19 Aubier M, Pieters WR, Schlosser NJ, Steinmetz KO. Salmeterol/fluticasone (50/500 µg) in combination in a Diskus inhaler (Seretide) is effective and safe in the treatment of steroid-dependent asthma. Respir Med 1999; 93:876–84.

20 Ankherst J, Persson G, Weibull E. Tolerability of a high dose of budesonide/formoterol in a single inhaler in patients with asthma. Pulm Pharmacol Ther 2003; 16:147–51.

21 Kirby S, Falcoz C, Daniel MJ, Milleri S. Salmeterol and fluticasone propionate given as a combination. Lack of systemic pharmacodynamic and pharmacokinetic interactions. Eur J Clin Pharmacol 2001; 56:781–91.

22 Bateman ED, Boushey HA, Bousquet J et al. Can guideline-defined asthma control be achieved? The Gaining Optimal Asthma controL study. Am Rev Respir Dis 2004; 170:836–44.

23 Leuppi JD, Salzberg M, Meyer L et al. An individualized, adjustable maintenance regimen of budesonide/formoterol provides effective asthma symptom control at a lower overall dose than fixed dosing. Swiss Med Wkly 2003; 133:302–9.

24 Stallberg B, Olsson P, Jorgensen LA, Lindmarck N, Ekstrom T. Budesonide/formoterol adjustable maintenance dosing reduces asthma exacerbations versus fixed dosing. Int J Clin Pract 2003; 57:656–61.

25 FitzGerald JM, Sears MR, Boulet LP et al. Adjustable maintenance dosing with budesonide/formoterol reduces asthma exacerbations compared with traditional fixed dosing: a five-month multicentre Canadian study. Can Respir J 2003; 10:427–34.

26 Ind PW, Haughney J, Price D, Rosen J-P, Kennelly J. Adjustable and fixed dosing with budesonide/formoterol via a single inhaler in asthma patients: the ASSURE study. Respir Med 2004; 98:464–75.

27 Canonica GW, Castellani P, Cazzola M et al. Adjustable maintenance dosing with budesonide/formoterol in a single inhaler provides effective asthma symptom control at a lower dose than fixed maintenance dosing. Pulm Pharmacol Ther 2004; 17:239–47.

28 Buhl R, Creemers JP, Vondra V, Martelli NA, Naya IP, Ekstrom T. Once-daily budesonide/formoterol in a single inhaler in adults with moderate persistent asthma. Respir Med 2003; 97:323–30.

29 Aalbers R, Backer V, Kava TTK et al. Adjustable maintenance dosing with budesonide/formoterol compared with fixed-dose salmeterol/fluticasone in moderate to severe asthma. Curr Med Res Opin 2004; 20:225–40.

30 Pearlman DS, Stricker W, Weinstein S et al. Inhaled salmeterol and fluticasone: a study comparing monotherapy and combination therapy in asthma. Ann Allergy Asthma Immunol 1999; 82:257–65.

31 O'Byrne PM, Barnes PJ, Rodriguez-Roisin R et al. Low dose inhaled budesonide and formoterol in mild persistent asthma: the OPTIMA randomized trial. Am J Respir Crit Care Med 2001; 164:1392–7.

32 Price D, Dutchman D, Mawson A, Bodalia B, Duggan S, Todd P on behalf of the Flow Research Group. Early asthma control and maintenance with eformoterol following reduction of inhaled corticosteroid dose. Thorax 2002; 57:791–8.

33 Lundback B, Jenkins C, Price MJ, Thwaites RMA. Cost-effectiveness of salmeterol/fluticasone propionate combination product 50/250 µg twice daily and budesonide 800 µg twice daily in the treatment of adults and adolescents with asthma. Respir Med 2000; 94:724–32.

34 Sheth K, Borker R, Emmett A, Rickard K, Dorinsky P. Cost-effectiveness comparison of salmeterol/fluticasone propionate versus montelukast in the treatment of adults with persistent asthma. Pharmacoeconomics. 2002; 20:909–18.

35 Lyseng-Williamson KA, Plosker GL. Inhaled salmeterol/fluticasone propionate combination. A pharmacoeconomic review of its use in the management of asthma. Pharmacoeconomics 2003; 21:951–89.

36 Rosenhall I, Borg S, Andersson F, Ericsson K. Budesonide/formoterol in a single inhaler (Symbicort) reduces healthcare costs compared with separate inhalers in the treatment of asthma over 12 months. Int J Clin Pract 2003; 57:662–7.

37 Fahy JV, Fleming HE, Wong HH et al. The effect of an anti-IgE monoclonal antibody on the early and late phase responses to allergen inhalation in asthmatic subjects. Am J Respir Crit Care Med 1997; 155:1828–34.

38 Boulet L-P, Chapman KR, Cote J et al. Inhibitory effects of an anti-IgE antibody E25 on allergen-induced early asthmatic response. Am J Respir Crit Care Med 1997; 155:1835–40.

39 Fahy JV, Cockroft DW, Boulet L-P et al. Effect of aerolized anti-IgE (E25) on airway responses to inhaled allergen in asthmatic subjects. Am J Respir Crit Care Med 1999; 160:1023–7.

40 Milgrom H, Fick RB Jr, Su JQ et al. Treatment of allergic asthma with monoclonal anti-IgE antibody. RhuMAb-E25 study group. N Engl J Med 1999; 341:1966–73.

41 Busse W, Corren J, Lanier BQ et al. Omalizumab, anti-IgE recombinant humanized monoclonal antibody, for the treatment of severe allergic asthma. J Allergy Clin Immunol 2001; 108:184–90.

42 Solèr M, Matz J, Townley R et al. The anti-IgE antibody omalizumab reduces exacerbations and steroid requirement in allergic asthmatics. Eur Respir J 2001; 18:254–61.

43 Milgrom H, Berger W, Nayak A et al. Treatment of childhood asthma with anti-immunoglobulin E antibody (omalizumab). Pediatrics 2001; 108:36–46.

44 Buhl R, Solèr M, Matz J et al. Omalizumab provides long-term control in patients with moderate to severe allergic asthma. Eur Respir J 2002; 20:73–8.

45 Buhl R, Hanf G, Solèr M et al. The anti-IgE antibody omalizumab improves asthma-related quality of life in patients with allergic asthma. Eur Respir J 2002; 20:1088–94.

46 Bousquet J, Wenzel S, Holgate S, Lumry W, Freeman P, Fox H. Predicting response to omalizumab, an anti-IgE antibody, in patients with allergic asthma. Chest 2004; 125:1378–86.

47 Leckie MJ, ten Brinke A, Khan J et al. Effects of an interleukin-5 blocking monoclonal antibody on eosinophils, airway hyper-responsiveness, and the late asthmatic response. Lancet 2000; 356:2144–8.

48 Flood-Page PT, Menzies-Gow A, Kay AB, Robinson DS. Eosinophil's role remains uncertain as anti-interleukin-5 only partially depletes numbers in asthmatic airway. Am J Respir Crit Care Med 2003; 167:199–204.

49 Kips JC, O'Connor BJ, Langley SJ et al. Effect of SCH55700, a humanized anti-human interleukin-5 antibody, in severe persistent asthma Am J Respir Crit Care Med 2003; 67:1655–9.

50 Chapman KR, Ringdahl N, Backer V, Palmqvist M, Sarelainen S, Briggs M. Salmeterol and fluticasone propionate (50/250 µg) administered via combination Diskus inhaler: as effective as when given via separate Diskus inhalers. *Can Respir J* 1999; **6**:45–51.

51 Johansson G, McIvor RA, Purello D'Ambrosio F, Gratziou C, James MH. Comparison of salmeterol/fluticasone propionate combination with budesonide in patients with mild-to-moderate asthma. *Clin Drug Invest* 2001; **21**:633–42.

52 Michils A, Peche R, Verbraeken J *et al.* SURF study: real-life effectiveness of budesonide/formoterol adjustable maintenance dosing. *Allergy Clin Immunol Int* 2003; **1**:2–39.

53 Holgate ST, Chuchalin AG, Hébert J *et al.* Efficacy and safety of a recombinant anti-immunoglobulin E antibody (omalizumab) in severe allergic asthma. *Clin Exp Allergy* 2004; **34**:632–8.

54 Vignola AM, Humbert M, Bousquet J *et al.* Efficacy and tolerability of anti-immunoglobulin E therapy with omalizumab in patients with concomitant allergic asthma and persistent allergic rhinitis: SOLAR. *Allergy* 2004; **59**:709–17.

55 Ayres JG, Higgins B, Chilvers ER, Ayre G, Blogg M, Fox H. Efficacy and tolerability of anti-immunoglobulin E therapy with omalizumab in patients with poorly controlled (moderate-to-severe) allergic asthma (ETOPA). *Allergy* 2004; **59**:701–8.

PART 3

Chronic obstructive pulmonary disease

Chronic obstructive pulmonary disease — acute exacerbations

Brian H Rowe and Irvin Mayers

Case scenario

A 76-year-old woman presents to the emergency department (ED) with a 10-day history of increased cough, increased sputum production, shortness of breath and wheezing, which began after symptoms of a common cold. She has had a long history of chronic bronchitis following a 60-pack–year history of smoking. She is alert and oriented but talking in short phrases only, with a respiratory rate of 32/min and heart rate of 110/min, and her oxygen saturation is 88%. Visual examination reveals a wasted woman with a barrel chest and moderate intercostal and subcostal retractions. On auscultation, there is decreased air entry to the bases, diffuse expiratory wheezing throughout all lung fields with prolongation of the expiratory phase. The heart sounds are distant but seem normal. The remainder of the physical examination is within normal limits. You diagnose an acute exacerbation of chronic obstructive pulmonary disease (COPD) and commence bronchodilator therapy in addition to intravenous methylprednisolone.

The patient improves minimally with treatment using salbutamol and corticosteroids, and the senior house staff asks whether you would consider using antibiotics or non-invasive ventilation in this patient. Review of systems reveals that this women has had several previous episodes of acute COPD in the past 12 months presenting to the ED as a result of upper respiratory tract infections. The patient describes her COPD as being worse since receiving the flu vaccination. She uses her salbutamol puffer several times a day before and after exertion and often in the middle of the night when she awakes with coughing episodes. She does not wish to be intubated and wants to know if you can give her something else to help her breathing (she was once given aminophylline).

Background

Chronic obstructive pulmonary disease (COPD) is characterized by airflow limitation that is not fully reversible.[1] It may comprise a spectrum of diseases including chronic bronchitis, emphysema and small airways disease. COPD is one of the few major chronic diseases in which mortality has been increasing over the past decade.[2] Global mortality related to COPD is forecast to more than double over 30 years,[1] and it will be the third leading cause of death worldwide by 2020. Individuals with COPD are prone to acute exacerbations of their illness. These acute exacerbations are characterized clinically by combinations of worsening dyspnoea, cough, sputum production and sputum purulence, as well as by worsening of airflow obstruction.[3] It is difficult to predict expected exacerbation rates for individual patients; however, most patients with COPD experience one to four exacerbations per year.[4] As airflow obstruction becomes more severe, exacerbations tend to occur more frequently. Age-adjusted US data suggest that COPD exacerbations account for an average of 1.2 office visits and 0.1–0.23 hospitalizations per year per prevalent case.[5]

Patients with COPD commonly present to the emergency department (ED), or other acute care settings, with exacerbations, and disease severity is often high. For example, in a recent North American study of patients presenting to the ED with COPD symptoms, the proportion of patients admitted was over 59%, ED length of stay was nearly 6 hours, and mechanical ventilation was higher than in other acute respiratory presentations such as asthma.[6] Despite advances in treatments (e.g. corticosteroids, antibiotics, etc.) and the creation of guidelines,[1,7–9] the acute management of these patients is complicated. It is clear that COPD and acute COPD are important health care problems. Given the severe nature and importance of acute COPD as a respiratory condition, it is not surprising that there are a number of guidelines that have been developed to direct the management of this problem.[1,7–9] Management of acute COPD is aimed at relieving bronchospasm, treating infection/inflammation, maintaining adequate oxygenation and identifying the cause(s) of the exacerbation.

Formulating clinical questions

In order to address the issues of most relevance to your patient and to help in searching the literature for the evidence regarding these, you should structure your questions as recommended in Chapter 1.

Questions

1 In adults with exacerbations of COPD (population), does treatment with inhaled β-agonist alone (intervention) improve pulmonary function (outcome) compared with treatment with inhaled ipratropium bromide alone? {therapy}
2 In adults with exacerbations of COPD (population), does the addition of inhaled anticholinergic agents (ipratropium bromide) (intervention) to inhaled β-agonist improve pulmonary function (outcome) compared with treatment with β-agonists alone? {therapy}
3 In adults with exacerbations of COPD (population), does the use of intravenous aminophylline (intervention) reduce admission to hospital or improve pulmonary function (outcome)? {therapy}
4 In adults with exacerbations of COPD (population), does the use of systemic corticosteroids (intervention) reduce admission to hospital or reduce length of stay (outcome)? {therapy}
5 In adults with exacerbations of COPD (population), does the use of non-invasive ventilation (intervention) in the ED reduce complications (e.g. admissions, intubation, etc.) (outcome)? {therapy}
6 In adults with exacerbations of COPD (population), do systemic antibiotics (intervention) improve the rate of recovery (outcome)? {therapy}
7 In adults with acute COPD (population), which patients benefit (outcome) from antibiotics (intervention)? {prognosis}
8 In adult COPD patients discharged from the ED (population), does treatment with systemic corticosteroids (intervention) reduce relapse to additional care (outcome)? {therapy}
9 In adult COPD patients discharged from the ED (population), what is the role of patient education, smoking cessation and immunization (interventions) in reducing further relapses and exacerbations of COPD (outcomes)? {therapy}

General search strategy

You begin to address these questions by searching for evidence in the common electronic databases such as the Cochrane Library, MEDLINE and EMBASE looking specifically for systematic reviews and meta-analyses. The Cochrane Library is particularly rich in high-quality systematic review evidence on numerous aspects of acute asthma, as well as acute COPD.[10] When a systematic review is identified, you should search for recent updates on the Cochrane Library and also

Searching for evidence synthesis: literature search

- Cochrane Library—COPD AND (Topic)
- MEDLINE—COPD AND MEDLINE AND (systematic review OR Meta-analysis OR metaanalysis) AND adult AND (Topic)
- EMBASE—COPD AND MEDLINE AND (systematic review OR Meta-analysis OR metaanalysis) AND adult AND (Topic)

search MEDLINE and EMBASE to identify randomized controlled trials (RCTs) that became available after the publication date of the systematic review. In addition, relevant, updated and evidence-based clinical practice guidelines (CPGs) on acute COPD are accessed to determine the consensus rating of areas lacking evidence.

Critical review of the literature

Your search strategy for the Cochrane Library identified several systematic reviews addressing Question 1 outlined above.

Question

1 In adults with exacerbations of COPD, does treatment with inhaled β-agonist alone improve pulmonary function compared with treatment with inhaled ipratropium bromide alone?
- Cochrane Library—COPD AND β-agonists

The options available to physicians for the treatment of bronchospasm in acute COPD are short-acting β-agonists such as salbutamol, anticholinergic agents such as ipratropium bromide or a combination of the two. Unfortunately, few studies of bronchodilating drugs (either anticholinergic or β-agonists) have been performed on patients with acute COPD, and the studies that do explore this issue have many limitations.

Most guidelines recommend that patients with acute COPD exacerbation should initially receive treatment with short-acting β[2]-agonists such as salbutamol.[1,7–9] These agents have gained international acceptance as the treatment of choice for acute asthma and are widely used in COPD. Compared to patients with asthma, however, many patients with COPD appear to achieve limited airway reversal in the acute setting; achievable bronchodilatation (reversibility) is widely variable in COPD, even in stable disease. Nonetheless, early treatment of acute COPD has generally focused on the use of inhaled (usually via nebulizer), short-acting β[2]-agonists and anticholinergic agents because of their undisputed, generally rapid effect on relieving bronchospasm in asthma. The question for many physicians is which agents (β[2]-agonists or anticholinergic agents) are appropriate and is the combined use of bronchodilators required?

A Cochrane Review compared β[2]-agonists with anticholinergic agents (ipratropium bromide) in the treatment of acute exacerbation of COPD.[11] Surprisingly, the authors were unable to identify *any* controlled clinical trials that compare β[2]-agonists with placebo, and only a few trials involving the use of inhaled β[2]-agonists compared with anticholinergic agents in acute exacerbation of COPD. Unfortunately, none of the studies used the more modern β[2]-agonists in common use today (e.g. salbutamol). Overall, β_2-agonists and ipratropium both produce small improvements in forced expired volume in 1 second (FEV_1). Comparatively speaking, neither agent is superior at bronchodilating (FEV_1 outcomes) patients with acute exacerbation of COPD [weighted mean difference (WMD) 0.01; 95% confidence interval (CI) –0.22 to 0.23]. Side-effect data were not reported in this review, and the more important clinical outcomes, such as hospitalization, were also not reported.

In another review, five studies involving 129 patients compared the short-term effects of β_2-agonists with ipratropium bromide.[12] Once again, the authors found no difference in FEV_1 outcomes between the drugs in the treatment of exacer-

bations of COPD, at least within the first 90 min of acute treatment (WMD 0.00; 95% CI –0.19 to 0.19; Fig. 1). In practice, clinicians may select either group of agents as an initial treatment agent in acute COPD. Most clinicians employ a nebulized route of administration; however, based on a Cochrane systematic review in acute asthma that demonstrates similar outcomes (admissions and pulmonary functions) using either nebulizers or inhalers with spacer devices, it seems reasonable to substitute nebulizers in the acute setting (Table 1).[13] More recent concerns regarding transmissibility of airborne pathogens such as severe acute respiratory syndrome (SARS) may limit the use of nebulizer therapy in the future.

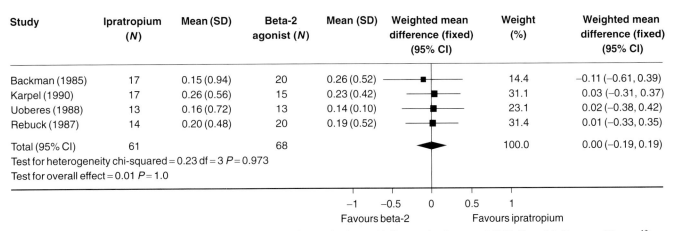

Study	Ipratropium (N)	Mean (SD)	Beta-2 agonist (N)	Mean (SD)	Weighted mean difference (fixed) (95% CI)	Weight (%)	Weighted mean difference (fixed) (95% CI)
Backman (1985)	17	0.15 (0.94)	20	0.26 (0.52)		14.4	–0.11 (–0.61, 0.39)
Karpel (1990)	17	0.26 (0.56)	15	0.23 (0.42)		31.1	0.03 (–0.31, 0.37)
Uoberes (1988)	13	0.16 (0.72)	13	0.14 (0.10)		23.1	0.02 (–0.38, 0.42)
Rebuck (1987)	14	0.20 (0.48)	20	0.19 (0.52)		31.4	0.01 (–0.33, 0.35)
Total (95% CI)	61		68			100.0	0.00 (–0.19, 0.19)

Test for heterogeneity chi-squared = 0.23 df = 3 P = 0.973
Test for overall effect = 0.01 P = 1.0

Figure 1. Change in FEV_1 at 90 min comparing ipratropium bromide alone with β_2-agonists in acute COPD (from McCrory and Brown[12]).

Table 1. Acute exacerbations of COPD — drug dosing.

Drug	Admitted (severe)	Discharged (mild–moderate)
Methylprednisolone (Solumedrol)	80–125 mg IV	NA
Prednisone	40–60 mg/dose divided bid or daily	40–60 mg/day (for outpatients: 7–10 days; tapering not required)
Methylxanthines	Not recommended	Continue oral agents if patients receiving prior to ED visit
Salbutamol	Single treatment: 2.5–5.0 mg nebulized (0.5–1.0 mL of 0.5% solution) every 20 min Inhaled: 4–6 activations via a holding chamber every 20 min	Inhaled: 1–2 activations using a holding chamber qid
Ipratropium bromide	Nebulizer: 250–500 mg qid Inhaled: 4–6 activations via a holding chamber every 20 min	Inhaled: 1–2 activations using a holding chamber qid
Antibiotics	First-line agents recommended to be started in hospital	First-line agents recommended to be continued for 7–10 days
NPPV	Respiratory failure (see text)	NA
Supplemental oxygen	Low flow titrated to Sao_2	Variable guidelines for chronic domiciliary oxygen

NPPV, non-invasive positive pressure ventilation; IV, intravenous; NA, not applicable; Sao_2, oxygen saturation; qid, four times daily; ED, emergency department.

Question

2 In adults with exacerbations of COPD, does the addition of in-haled anticholinergic agents (ipratropium bromide) to inhaled β-agonist improve pulmonary function compared with treatment with β-agonists alone?

- Cochrane Library—COPD AND ipratropium bromide

Question

3 In adults with exacerbations of COPD, does the use of intra-venous aminophylline reduce admission to hospital or improve pulmonary function?

- Cochrane Library—COPD AND aminophylline

One important clinical question in acute COPD treatment is whether there is an *additive benefit* of using ipratropium bromide with inhaled β_2-agonists, as seen in acute asthma. A meta-analysis in adults with asthma demonstrated a modest beneficial effect (reduced admissions, improved pulmonary functions) when ipratropium bromide was added to inhaled β_2-agonists in the acute setting.[14] A Cochrane systematic review has examined the issue of combining bronchodilators in exacerbations of COPD.[12] Three studies involving 118 patients, looking at short-term effects, found no advantage of adding ipratropium to β_2-agonist treatment on short-term (90 min) FEV_1 outcomes (WMD 0.02; 95% CI –0.08 to 0.12; Fig. 2). Long-term effects (24 hours) of the ipratropium bromide and β_2-agonist treatment demonstrated no additional FEV_1 changes (WMD –0.05 L; 95% CI –0.14 to 0.05). Side-effects were reported rarely, but there did not appear to be a significant change in haemodynamics or reported adverse events. Adverse drug reactions included dry mouth and tremor for ipratropium bromide-treated patients.

Overall, there was no evidence that the degree of bron-chodilation achieved with ipratropium bromide was greater than that using short-acting β_2-agonists. Contrary to their effect in acute asthma, the combination of a β_2-agonist and ipra-tropium did not appear to increase the effect on FEV_1 over either intervention used alone. Even in the setting of stable COPD, there is no evidence of additive bronchodilation.[15] Consequently, the clinician is left to decide which agent to use in the acute setting; familiarity may dictate the approach used. If bronchodilators are selected, however, clinicians should ob-serve patients for signs of toxicity (tremor and tachycardia) and use a careful approach to the use of supplemental oxygen (Table 1).

While first-line therapy in COPD has focused on the deliv-ery of inhaled bronchodilators, efforts to bronchodilate constricted airways further have focused on the use of methylxanthines, especially aminophylline. Whether the drug is effective when delivered via the intravenous route has been the subject of much debate. A Cochrane systematic review of four trials involving 169 subjects suggests that the use of intra-venous aminophylline yields no additional benefits to patients in the acute setting.[16] Mean change in FEV_1 at 2 hours was sim-ilar in aminophylline- and placebo-treated groups; however, it was transiently increased with methylxanthines at 3 days. Non-significant reductions in hospitalization and length of stay were offset by a non-significant increase in relapses at 1 week. Changes in symptom scores were not statistically or clinically significant. More concerning, methylxanthines caused more nausea/vomiting than placebo [odds ratio (OR) 4.6; 95% CI 1.7–12.6; Fig. 3]; non-significant increases in tremor, palpitations and arrhythmias were also observed. The available data do not support the use of methylxanthines for the treatment of COPD exacerbations. Potential benefits of methylxanthines on lung function and symptoms were gener-ally not confirmed at standard levels of significance, whereas the potentially important adverse events of nausea and vomiting were significantly increased in patients receiving methylxanthines.

Multiple international guidelines currently recommend methylxanthines for severe exacerbations;[1,7–9] however, the

Study	Added ipratropium (N)	Mean (SD)	Beta-2 agonist alone (N)	Mean (SD)	Weighted mean difference (fixed) (95% CI)	Weight (%)	Weighted mean difference (fixed) (95% CI)
Uoberes (1988)	13	0.14 (0.21)	13	0.14 (0.22)		35.7	0.00 (–0.17, 0.17)
Rebuck (1987)	17	0.17 (0.35)	20	0.19 (0.37)		18.1	–0.02 (–0.25, 0.21)
Shretha (1991)	30	0.24 (0.30)	25	0.19 (0.25)		46.2	0.05 (–0.10, 0.20)
Total (95% CI)	60		58			100.0	0.02 (–0.08, 0.12)

Test for heterogeneity chi-squared = 0.33 df = 2 P = 0.8464
Test for overall effect = 0.39 P = 0.7

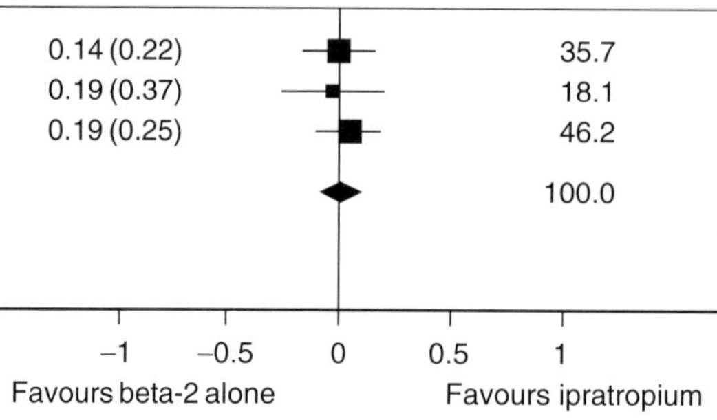

-1   -0.5   0   0.5   1
Favours beta-2 alone   Favours ipratropium

Figure 2. Change in FEV_1 at 90 min comparing ipratropium bromide combined with β_2-agonists with β_2-agonists alone in acute COPD (from McCrory and Brown[12]).

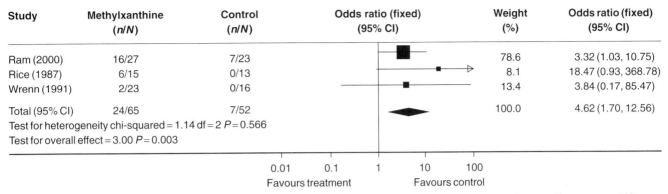

Study	Methylxanthine (n/N)	Control (n/N)	Odds ratio (fixed) (95% CI)	Weight (%)	Odds ratio (fixed) (95% CI)
Ram (2000)	16/27	7/23		78.6	3.32 (1.03, 10.75)
Rice (1987)	6/15	0/13		8.1	18.47 (0.93, 368.78)
Wrenn (1991)	2/23	0/16		13.4	3.84 (0.17, 85.47)
Total (95% CI)	24/65	7/52		100.0	4.62 (1.70, 12.56)

Test for heterogeneity chi-squared = 1.14 df = 2 P = 0.566
Test for overall effect = 3.00 P = 0.003

0.01   0.1   1   10   100
Favours treatment   Favours control

Figure 3. Adverse events (nausea/vomiting) comparing methylxanthines with standard care in COPD exacerbations (from Barr et al.[16]).

current evidence argues that methylxanthines should not be used for acute COPD exacerbations. The findings from this systematic review should be incorporated into guidelines, and attention should be focused on the use of other effective agents or examination of new agents that improve outcomes. Development of more selective methylxanthines is necessary to reduce known adverse effects; clinical trial evaluation of those agents is required to evaluate any (probably small) clinical benefits for COPD exacerbations.

Question

4 In adults with acute COPD, does the use of systemic corticosteroids reduce admission to hospital or reduce length of stay?
- Cochrane Library and MEDLINE—COPD AND corticosteroids

Systemic corticosteroids are effective and have been employed in acute asthma for many years; however, evidence of effectiveness has been less convincing in acute COPD. A Cochrane Review examined seven trials that involved over 600 adult patients in RCTs in acute COPD.[17] Four studies specifically examined patients admitted to hospital, two involved ED patients and one examined outpatients. Outcomes reported varied, and few were common to all studies. The most commonly reported airway measurement (FEV$_1$ between 6 and 72 hours after treatment) showed a significant treatment benefit for corticosteroids (WMD 120 mL; 95% CI 5–190). There were also significantly fewer treatment failures for patients treated with corticosteroids; however, the number of trials reporting this outcome was small, and there was significant heterogeneity between them. The administration of systemic corticosteroids to patients with acute COPD has been shown by others to reduce admissions,[18] decrease hospital length of stay[19] and reduce treatment failure in hospitalized patients.[17] Despite this benefit, there was an increased likelihood of an adverse drug reaction with corticosteroid treatment. There were no demonstrated differences for other outcomes including mortality, quality of life and exercise tolerance.[17]

Despite the fact that there was significant statistical hetero-

geneity for this outcome, the overall effect showed a marked benefit of corticosteroids (OR for treatment failure 0.50; 95% CI 0.32–0.79), and four of the five studies appear to point towards a benefit of corticosteroids. Although most current guidelines recommend corticosteroids, and their use is common, the evidence is strongest for admitted patients.[17] Oral corticosteroids are as effective as intravenous agents, so many physicians treating acute COPD select the intravenous route only for those too dyspnoeic to swallow or those with endotracheal tubes (Table 1). While there are limited data to support the use of methylprednisolone compared with hydrocortisone, most physicians treating acute COPD select intravenous methylprednisolone to avoid the mineralocorticoid effects of the steroid treatment. Once again, the evidence for both dosing and route of administration is anecdotal.

Question

5 In adults with exacerbations of COPD, does the use of non-invasive ventilation in the ED reduce complications (e.g. admissions, intubation, etc.)?
- Cochrane Library—COPD AND NPPV

Non-invasive positive pressure ventilation (NPPV) is a treatment approach available in many centres; however, until recently, evidence was conflicting with respect to its benefit. Eight studies were included in a Cochrane Review involving 546 enrolled patients from a variety of countries.[20] NPPV resulted in decreased mortality [relative risk (RR) 0.41; 95% CI 0.26–0.64], fewer intubations (RR 0.42; 95% CI 0.31–0.59) and fewer treatment failures (RR 0.51; 95% CI 0.39–0.67; Fig. 4). NPPV also resulted in improvements in acidosis within the first hour (WMD increased pH 0.03; 95% CI 0.02–0.04), PaCO_2 (WMD −0.40 kPa; 95% CI −0.78 to −0.03) and respiratory rate (WMD −3.08 bpm; 95% CI −4.26 to −1.89). Finally, common complications associated with treatment (RR 0.32; 95% CI 0.18–0.56) and length of hospital stay (WMD −3.24 days; 95% CI −4.42 to −2.06) were also reduced in the NPPV group.

In light of the evidence presented in this review, it appears that NPPV offers important advantages in terms of avoiding

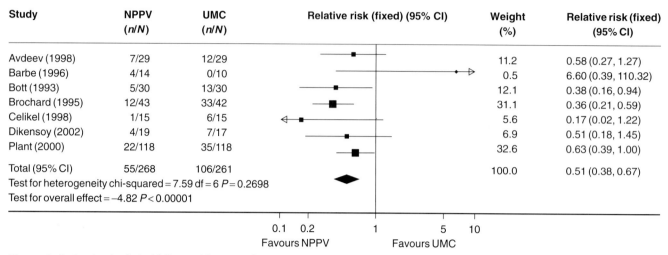

Study	NPPV (n/N)	UMC (n/N)	Relative risk (fixed) (95% CI)	Weight (%)	Relative risk (fixed) (95% CI)
Avdeev (1998)	7/29	12/29		11.2	0.58 (0.27, 1.27)
Barbe (1996)	4/14	0/10		0.5	6.60 (0.39, 110.32)
Bott (1993)	5/30	13/30		12.1	0.38 (0.16, 0.94)
Brochard (1995)	12/43	33/42		31.1	0.36 (0.21, 0.59)
Celikel (1998)	1/15	6/15		5.6	0.17 (0.02, 1.22)
Dikensoy (2002)	4/19	7/17		6.9	0.51 (0.18, 1.45)
Plant (2000)	22/118	35/118		32.6	0.63 (0.39, 1.00)
Total (95% CI)	55/268	106/261		100.0	0.51 (0.38, 0.67)

Test for heterogeneity chi-squared = 7.59 df = 6 P = 0.2698
Test for overall effect = −4.82 P < 0.00001

0.1 0.2   1   5   10
Favours NPPV   Favours UMC

Figure 4. Reduction in clinical failures with NPPV plus standard care versus standard care alone in acute COPD (from Ram *et al.*[20]).

intubation and reducing intensive care admissions. NPPV employs a full facial or nasal mask that administers ventilatory support from a flow generator. It enhances ventilation by unloading fatigued respiratory muscles and keeps collapsed alveoli open to improve ventilation–perfusion matching. Despite some variation, trials reported use for at least 6 hours/day. The expiratory pressure setting was kept constant and ranged from 2 to 6 cm H_2O, and the inspiratory pressure ranged from 9 to 30 cm H_2O. It is worth noting that all patients in these studies were treated in hospital settings and received aggressive medical management for their condition. In addition, the recent worldwide SARS outbreak and its apparent worsened spread following nebulization, NPPV and mechanical ventilation has discouraged NPPV use in some centres.[21]

Overall, NPPV should be considered for patients who have severe distress, COPD (versus non-COPD), increased Pa_{CO_2} (>38), increased respiratory rate (>25), acidosis (pH <7.38) and possibly a past history of NIPPV success.[22] There are other conditions in which this modality may be particularly helpful, such as those patients with a mixed picture of COPD/congestive heart failure.[23] The modality should not be administered to patients who are obtunded, cannot protect their airway or have other contraindications. Other relative contraindications include haemodynamic instability or difficulty controlling airway secretions. In such cases, endotracheal intubation, using rapid sequence techniques administered by a physician who is experienced at securing an airway in emergency conditions, should be employed.

Question

6 In adults with exacerbations of COPD, do systemic antibiotics improve the rate of recovery ?
 • COCHRANE DARE Database—acute COPD AND antibiotics

Worsening of pulmonary function during a COPD exacerbation is most commonly caused by respiratory infection, but can also occur secondary to environmental triggers (e.g. humidity, pollution, exposure to smoke or occupational irritants), cardiac dysfunction or progression of the underlying disease.[24] Studies using viral cultures and serology have established that viral and, to a lesser extent, mycoplasma infections are associated with approximately one-third of acute exacerbations of chronic bronchitis.[25] Three bacterial pathogens, *Streptococcus pneumoniae*, *Haemophilus influenzae* and *Moraxella catarrhalis*, are frequently implicated in flare-ups of COPD; however, these bacteria can be found in the upper respiratory tracts of healthy people and are often found in the sputum of patients with COPD during periods of clinical quiescence.[26] Moreover, a recent study also suggested that some patients acquire new strains of these three bacteria *during* COPD exacerbations.[27] Determining whether these bacteria are simply commensals or whether they are responsible for clinical deterioration is therefore often difficult. However, several clinical trials have supported the use of antibiotics for the treatment of COPD exacerbation,[3,28] suggesting that, in some patients, bacterial infection of the airways plays a causal role in provoking COPD exacerbation. In addition, this may also reflect the observation that some antibiotics have important anti-inflammatory actions.

A meta-analysis of nine randomized trials of antibiotics compared with placebo for COPD exacerbation included 1101 patients; six trials included peak expiratory flow rate (PEFR) as an outcome measure (836 patients).[28] The overall summary effect size (ES), when comparing antibiotics with placebo, was modest (ES 0.22; 95% CI 0.10–0.34; P<0.05), indicating a clinical benefit (reduction in 'clinical failures') to the antibiotic-treated group. The summary effect size for changes in PEFR was similarly modest (ES 0.19; 95% CI 0.03–0.35; P< 0.05) in favour of the antibiotic group. This translates to a difference in PEFR of nearly 11 L/min (95% CI 4.96–16.54). Subanalyses of inpatient and outpatient data provided effect sizes of 0.38 (95% CI 0.13–0.62, $P < 0.05$) and 0.17 (95% CI 0.03–0.30, $P < 0.05$) respectively. No significant heterogeneity was observed. It is critical to note that this evidence is based on trials using first-line, older and less expensive antibiotics in acute COPD such as amoxicillin, trimethoprim-sulfimethoxazole and tetracycline.

Despite this evidence, the recommendations of the various guidelines are vague, and research has demonstrated that only 51% of ED patients were prescribed antibiotics on discharge in a large international ED prospective cohort study.[28] The general approach is to recommend that the 'choice of antibiotics should reflect local patterns of antibiotic sensitivity among the three main bacterial pathogens, *Streptococcus pneumoniae*, *Haemophilus influenzae* and *Moraxella catarrhalis*'.[1] Alternatively, these guidelines recommend first-line antibiotics as a first option, and reservation of newer agents (e.g. newer macrolides, fluoroquinolones, etc.) for those patients with multiple risk factors or failure to respond in the past or during the current exacerbation. Although the antibiotic coverage in COPD is variable, the newer, heavily marketed antibiotic agents are gaining popularity among clinicians. Some argue that pathogens such as *Streptococcus pneumoniae* and *Haemophilus influenzae* have become somewhat resistant to the first-generation antibiotics *in vitro* over the past 15 years. As some guidelines point out, 'to date, however, no randomized, placebo-controlled trials have proved the superiority of the newer broad-spectrum antibiotics'.[29]

At this point in time, patients severe enough to require admission to hospital should receive antibiotics; first-line agents are indicated in most cases (Table 1). In those patients who respond to treatment or have less severe COPD exacerbations, the use of antibiotics should be reserved for patients with certain criteria (see below).[28]

Question

7 In adult patients with exacerbations of COPD, which patients benefit from antibiotics ?
• MEDLINE—COPD AND antibiotics AND prognosis

Given the evidence for systematic review summarized above, antibiotics are recommended in acute COPD. They are helpful in resolving an acute exacerbation and are valuable in decreasing the risk of further deterioration.[28] The most comprehensive outpatient study of antibiotic therapy for COPD exacerbation showed that treatment with a broad-spectrum antibiotic increased the 21-day successful recovery rate from 55% to 68% in the antibiotic-treated group ($P < 0.01$), and decreased the deterioration rate from 19% to 10% ($P < 0.05$).[3]

Moreover, the use of antibiotics was most successful in patients with type I and II exacerbations (i.e. those who had dyspnoea plus increased sputum and/or change in sputum purulence). These criteria for antibiotic use are referred to as the Anthonisen criteria and suggest that antibiotics should be reserved for those patients who have at least two of the criteria (e.g. type I and II exacerbations—patients who have dyspnoea plus increased sputum and/or change in sputum purulence; Table 2).

In the acute setting, patients should be categorized using the Anthonisen criteria. Until further evidence is available, patients with acute COPD who have type III and II criteria should receive first-line antibiotics unless contraindicated (e.g. resistance, failure, relapse, allergy, severity, etc.).

Question

8 In adult COPD patients discharged from the ED, does treatment with systemic corticosteroids reduce relapse to additional care?
• Cochrane Library—COPD AND corticosteroids AND discharge
• MEDLINE—COPD AND corticosteroids AND discharge

Approximately 20–30% of patients treated for acute COPD will relapse within 4 weeks of ED discharge, many because of unresolved inflammation and infection.[6] Guidelines variably encourage treatment with systemic corticosteroids following ED discharge for an acute exacerbation to reduce the risk of relapse.[1,7–9]

Limited evidence for this approach is found in the Cochrane systematic review of corticosteroids for acute COPD.[17] This systematic review searched for the best available evidence regarding the use of systemic corticosteroids in the treatment of COPD. The review included studies with patients from a variety of settings (admitted patients, ED patients and outpatients), with a wide range of severity and is summarized above. The authors concluded that corticosteroid treatment was indicated in the most severe admitted cases; however, their recommendations for corticosteroid therapy in the outpatient setting were tempered by a general lack of evidence.[17]

Table 2. Anthonisen criteria for classification of COPD exacerbations.

Anthonisen criteria:
Increasing dyspnoea
Increasing sputum volume
Increasing sputum purulence (thickness or tenacity)

Anthonisen classification:
Type I: all three criteria
Type II: any two criteria
Type III: any single criteria

Since that systematic review was revised, a large RCT has been published that helps to clarify the evidence for the decision.[30] In a rigorous, double-blind RCT, investigators across 10 Canadian EDs examined the effect of adding corticosteroids to standard care in 147 patients discharged after treatment for acute COPD. Patients were treated with first-generation antibiotics and bronchodilators and were randomized to oral prednisone (40 mg daily for 10 days) or placebo. The primary outcome was relapse to additional unscheduled care; the difference favoured the steroid-treated group (43% versus 27%; $P = 0.05$; Fig. 5). This represents an absolute risk reduction of 16% and a number needed to treat (NNT) of 6. In addition, the use of corticosteroids in this population significantly improved pulmonary function and dyspnoea at 10 days.

Examining the evidence, it seems appropriate to *consider* corticosteroids as the standard of care in acute COPD patients discharged from the ED. An important aspect to review in the evaluation of whether to treat patients with systemic corticosteroids is that patients with advanced COPD are often elderly and have associated comorbid conditions. Patients who receive corticosteroids are subject to bone mineral density changes, myopathies, hyperglycaemia, insomnia, hyperphagia and other associated short- and long-term side-effects and complications. While short-term corticosteroids are generally well tolerated, outpatient trials have demonstrated some impairments in quality of life associated with these agents.[30] The beneficial short-term effects of oral glucocorticoids on rate of relapse, dyspnoea and lung function should be balanced against the potential risk of short-term and long-term side-effects in the individual patient.

Small sample sizes in the RCTs performed to date prevent an examination of the relative effectiveness of various regimens, and definitive recommendation concerning dose or dosing protocol(s) cannot be provided. However, given the enhanced compliance associated with once-daily dosing and the availability of 40- or 50-mg tablets in many parts of the world, the use of fixed-dose oral corticosteroids for a short duration (7–10 days) seems appropriate for most patients discharged with an acute COPD episode (Table 1).

Clinicians assessing and treating patients with acute COPD must not lose sight of the fact that this is a chronic condition

Question

9 In adult COPD patients discharged from the ED, what is the role of patient education, smoking cessation and immunization in reducing further relapses and exacerbations of COPD?
- Cochrane Library—COPD AND education;
- Cochrane Library—COPD AND influenza immunization;
- Cochrane Library—COPD AND smoking cessation.

that requires co-ordinated, consistent and continuous care. This fact mandates that clear communication occurs between the acute setting and the primary care physician. While it is generally accepted that education is an integral aspect of all pulmonary disease care, and that respiratory rehabilitation is successful in improving important outcomes in COPD, limited research has been applied to the acute care setting. Consequently, much of the evidence in this section arises from

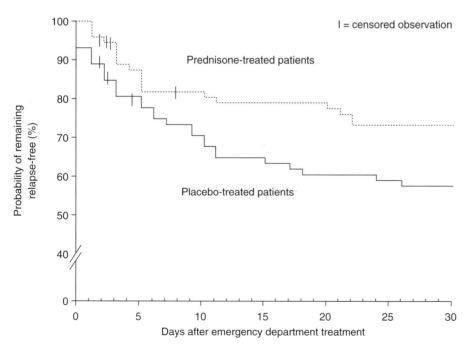

Figure 5. Comparison of prednisone (dotted line) with placebo (solid line) in patients discharged from the ED with acute COPD (from Aaron *et al.*[30]).

literature on chronic stable COPD. Certainly, encouraging smoking cessation,[31] influenza vaccination[32] and educating patients all seem like reasonable and cost-effective strategies for preventing the next attack. In addition, compliance with prescribed, evidence-based medication(s) is another important factor associated with treatment success.[33]

Influenza vaccination is considered an effective and cost-effective public health intervention to improve health. The Cochrane Review specifically addressing influenza vaccination in COPD examined all RCTs in which immunization was compared with placebo or standard care.[32] In general, the review demonstrates a reduction in exacerbations following vaccination that can be attributed to the effect over the long term. For example, the number of patients experiencing late exacerbations was significantly lower in the immunized COPD patients than in those receiving placebo (OR 0.13; 95% CI 0.04–0.45; $P = 0.002$). It is important to note that elderly patients (only a minority of whom had COPD) experienced a significant increase in the occurrence of local adverse reactions to vaccination; however, these effects were generally mild and transient. Given this evidence, future exacerbation prevention should include a recommendation to receive influenza immunization. The main barrier to the implementation of this intervention is penetration to patients and physicians.

The Cochrane Review specifically addressing smoking cessation for patients with COPD examined all RCTs in which smoking cessation was compared with placebo or standard care.[31] In general, the authors found evidence that a combination of psychosocial interventions and pharmacological interventions is superior to no treatment or to psychosocial interventions alone. Patients who have acute exacerbations of COPD and continue to smoke should be encouraged to stop smoking and seek assistance in doing so from their regular physician. Educational interventions in COPD have been studied in the stable disease state, focusing especially on self-management.[34] Pulmonary rehabilitation for patients with COPD has been shown to be effective in reducing further exacerbations and improving quality of life.[35] Referral for rehabilitation should be a *consideration* for patients with severe COPD after their exacerbation stabilizes. Overall, the role of COPD education after discharge from the ED awaits further high-quality research. Finally, compliance assessment and efforts to enhance adherence to medications and lifestyle modifications are also an important issue for patients with COPD.[33]

Conclusion

The patient mentioned above failed treatment with inhaled β-agonists *and* ipratropium bromide, systemic corticosteroids and oxygen. Intravenous antibiotics, non-invasive ventilation for 6 hours and close observation were required to prevent intubation. She required hospital admission and recovered slowly and without incident. She returned to baseline function within several weeks of the hospital admission.

COPD is a common, chronic and often debilitating disease. Despite the importance of this disease, there is surprisingly little evidence upon which to base acute therapy decisions. Many of the trials in this area are small or methodologically weak. In some cases, multiple, similar small trials have been combined appropriately in systematic reviews to produce clarity (e.g. NPPV in acute respiratory failure). This clarity is not found for some areas, and the resultant wide confidence intervals suggest insufficient sample size to demonstrate differences rather than equivalence. Moreover, in some of the important questions (e.g. the *additive* benefit of ipratropium bromide to β2-agonists), the evidence is almost completely lacking.

Overall, the area of therapy for patients presenting to the acute setting with acute COPD remains a field that is severely underdeveloped. More research is required in a variety of areas to guide better management of the in- and outpatient treatment of these complex patients. Researchers in this field must pay close attention to the conduct of their trials. For example, studies should be focused on clinically meaningful questions and designed in order to reduce the bias associated with trials (randomized, concealed allocation, multiple levels of blinding, blinded outcome assessment, etc.).

The treatment approaches outlined above to control bronchial inflammation and infection provide hope for a return to activities, reduced symptoms and improved quality of life in the subacute period following an exacerbation. Combining smoking cessation, immunization and prevention programmes with appropriate preventive medication provides patients with the best opportunity to maintain a reasonable health status and prevent an exacerbation or relapse in the future.

Summary for clinicians

- Bronchodilators (short-acting β-agonists and anticholinergics) produce small increases in FEV_1, of equal magnitude.
- There is no evidence that the combination of short-acting β-agonists and anticholinergics is more effective than either agent administered alone.
- Methylxanthines increase adverse effects, without evidence of clinical or statistical benefit.
- Oral corticosteroids increase FEV_1 and reduce treatment failure at a cost of increased likelihood of adverse effects.
- NPPV decreases the likelihood of intubation and intensive care admissions in selected patients.
- Antibiotics decrease clinical failures and increase PEFR, although the overall effect is small, and use should be reserved for patients with Anthonisen type I and II exacerbations.
- Secondary preventative measures, patient education, smoking cessation and immunization are considered important in preventing future exacerbations, but evidence for their efficacy is limited.

Acknowledgements

The authors would like to thank Mrs Diane Milette for her secretarial support. In addition, the authors would like to acknowledge the work of the Airway Review Group staff (Mr Stephen Milan and Toby Lasserson; and Mrs Karen Blackhall) and the Review Group Editor (Professor Paul Jones: 1995–2003; Dr Christopher Cates: 2003–present) at the St George's Hospital Medical School for their support with the development of reviews.

Conflicts of Interest

Dr Rowe is supported by the Canadian Institute of Health Research (CIHR; Ottawa, Canada) as a Canada Research Chair in Emergency Airway Diseases.

References

1 Pauwels R, Buist A, Calverley P et al. Global strategy for the diagnosis, management, and prevention of chronic obstructive disease. NHLBI/WHO Global initiative for chronic obstructive lung disease (GOLD) workshop summary. Am J Respir Crit Care Med 2001; 163:1256–76.

2 Stoller J. Acute exacerbations of chronic obstructive pulmonary disease. N Engl J Med 2002; 346:988–94.

3 Anthonisen N, Manfreda J, Warren P et al. Antibiotic therapy in exacerbation of chronic obstructive pulmonary disease. Ann Intern Med 1987; 106:196–204.

4 Balter M, Hyland R, Low D, Renzi P. Recommendations on the management of chronic bronchitis. A practical guide for Canadian physicians. Can Med Assoc J 1994; 151:1–23.

5 Feinleib M, Rosenberg H, Collins J et al. Trends in COPD morbidity and mortality in the United States. Am J Respir Crit Care Med 1989; 140:S9–S18.

6 Cydulka RK, Rowe BH, Clark S et al. Emergency department management of acute exacerbations of chronic obstructive pulmonary disease: the multicenter airway research collaboration. J Am Assoc Gerontol 2003; 51:908–16.

7 Anonymous. BTS guidelines for the management of chronic obstructive pulmonary disease. The COPD Guidelines Group of the Standards of Care Committee of the BTS. Thorax 1997; 52(Suppl 5):S1–28

8 O'Donnell DE, Aaron S, Bourbeau J et al. for the Canadian Thoracic Society. Canadian Thoracic Society recommendations for management of chronic obstructive pulmonary disease—2003. Can Respir J 2003; 10:11A–65A.

9 American Thoracic Society. Standards for the diagnosis and care of patients with chronic obstructive pulmonary disease. Am J Respir Crit Care Med 1995; 152:S77–S120.

10 Jadad AR, Moher M, Browman GP et al. Systematic reviews and meta-analyses on treatment of asthma: critical evaluation. BMJ 2000; 320:537–40.

11 Brown CD, McCrory D, White J. Inhaled short-acting β_2-agonists versus ipratropium bromide for acute exacerbations of chronic obstructive pulmonary disease (Cochrane Review). In: The Cochrane Library, Issue 4. Oxford, Update Software, 2003.

12 McCrory DC, Brown CD. Anticholinergic bronchodilators versus β_2-sympathomimetics for acute exacerbations of chronic pulmonary disease (Cochrane Review). In: The Cochrane Library, Issue 4. Oxford, Update Software, 2003.

13 Cates CJ, Bara A, Crilly JA Rowe BH. Holding chambers versus nebulisers for β-agonist treatment of acute asthma (Cochrane Review). In: The Cochrane Library, Issue 4. Oxford, Update Software, 2003.

14 Stoodley RG, Aaron SD, Dales RE. The role of ipratropium bromide in the emergency management of acute asthma exacerbation: a meta-analysis of randomized clinical trials. Ann Emerg Med 1999; 34:8–18.

15 Easton PA, Jadue C, Dhingra S, Anthonisen NR. A comparison of the bronchodilating effects of a β_2 adrenergic agent (albuterol) and an anticholinergic agent (ipratropium bromide), given by aerosol alone or in sequence. N Engl J Med 1986; 315:735–9.

16 Barr RG, Rowe BH, Camargo CA Jr. Methylxanthines for exacerbations of chronic obstructive pulmonary disease (Cochrane Review). In: The Cochrane Library, Issue 4. Oxford, Update Software, 2003.

17 Wood-Baker R, Walters EH, Gibson PG. Oral corticosteroids for acute exacerbations of chronic obstructive pulmonary disease (Cochrane Review). In: The Cochrane Library, Issue 4. Oxford, Update Software, 2003.

18 Bullard MJ, Liaw S-J, Tsai Y-H, Min HP. Early corticosteroid use in acute exacerbations of chronic airflow obstruction. Am J Emerg Med 1996; 14:139–43.

19 Niewoehner D, Erbland M, Deupree RH et al. Effect of systemic glucocorticoids on exacerbations of chronic obstructive pulmonary disease. Department of Veterans Affairs Cooperative Study Group. N Engl J Med 1999; 340:1941–7.

20 Ram FSF, Lightowler JV, Wedzicha JA. Non-invasive positive pressure ventilation for treatment of chronic obstructive pulmonary disease (Cochrane Review). In: The Cochrane Library, Issue 4. Oxford, Update Software, 2003.

21 Varia M, Wilson S, Sarwal S et al. Investigation of a nosocomial outbreak of severe acute respiratory syndrome (SARS) in Toronto, Canada. Can Med Assoc J 2003; 169:285–92.

22 Keenan SP, Kernerman PD, Cook DJ et al. Effect of noninvasive positive pressure ventilation on mortality in patients admitted with acute respiratory failure: a meta-analysis. Crit Care Med 1997; 25:1685–92.

23 Pang D, Keenan SP, Cook DJ, Sibbald WJ. The effect of positive pressure airway support on mortality and the need for intubation in cardiogenic pulmonary edema: a systematic review. Chest 1998; 114:1185–92.

24 O'Driscoll BR, Karla S, Wilson M et al. Double-blind trial of steroid tapering in acute asthma. Lancet 1993; 341:324–7.

25 Phillips C, Forsyth B. Role of infection in chronic bronchitis. Am J Respir Crit Care Med 1976; 113:465–74.

26 Haas H, Morris J, Samson S. Bacterial flora of the respiratory tract in chronic bronchitis: comparison of transtracheal, fiberbronchoscopic and oropharyngeal sampling methods. Am J Respir Crit Care Med 1977; 16:41–7.

27 Sethi S, Evans N, Grant BJB, Murphy TF. New strains of bacteria and exacerbations of chronic obstructive pulmonary disease. N Engl J Med 2002; 347:465–71.

28 Saint S, Bent S, Vittinghoff E, Grady D. Antibiotics in chronic obstructive pulmonary disease exacerbations. JAMA 1995; 273:957–60.

29 Snow V, Lascher S, Mottur-Pilson C. Evidence base for management of acute exacerbations of chronic obstructive pulmonary disease (Clinical Practice Guideline, Part 1). Ann Intern Med 2001; 134:595–9.

30 Aaron SD, Vandemheen K, Wells G et al. Oral prednisone for the prevention of relapse in outpatients with exacerbations of chronic obstructive pulmonary disease. N Engl J Med 2003; 348:2618–25.

31 van der Meer RM, Wagena EJ, Ostelo RWJG et al. Smoking cessation for chronic obstructive pulmonary disease (Cochrane Review). In: The Cochrane Library, Issue 4. Oxford, Update Software, 2003.

32 Poole PJ, Chacko E, Wood-Baker R, Cates CJ. Influenza vaccine for patients with chronic obstructive pulmonary disease (Cochrane Review). In: *The Cochrane Library*, Issue 4. Oxford, Update Software, 2003.

33 Haynes RB, McDonald H, Garg AX, Montague P. Interventions for helping patients to follow prescriptions for medications (Cochrane Review). In: *The Cochrane Library*, Issue 4. Oxford, Update Software, 2003.

34 Monninkhof EM, van der Valk PDLPM, van der Palen J *et al*. Self-management education for chronic obstructive pulmonary disease (Cochrane Review). In: *The Cochrane Library*, Issue 4. Oxford, Update Software, 2003.

35 Lacasse Y, Brosseau L, Milne S *et al*. Pulmonary rehabilitation for chronic obstructive pulmonary disease (Cochrane Review). In: *The Cochrane Library*, Issue 4. Oxford, Update Software, 2003.

CHAPTER 3.2

Anticholinergic bronchodilators in chronic obstructive pulmonary disease therapy

Alicia R ZuWallack and Richard L ZuWallack

Case scenario

A 74-year-old male attended his general practitioner for review of his emphysema treatment. The diagnosis had been made 10 years previously after seeing another doctor complaining of breathlessness on exercise. Over the intervening years, the breathlessness had become more severe such that he now had difficulty gardening and keeping up with his wife walking on the flat (grade 3 MRC functional limitation due to dyspnoea). He also complained of cough and clear sputum production on most days, which had been persistent over the last 3 years. Over the previous 6 months, he had gradually cut down and stopped smoking cigarettes, and was now smoking four cigars per day. Prior to this, he had smoked 30 cigarettes per day since the age of 18 years.

His current medications are budesonide 400 μg turbuhaler two puffs twice daily, although he uses this irregularly, oral theophylline 300 mg twice daily and terbutaline 500 μg turbuhaler as needed. Spirometry performed in the rooms revealed forced expiratory volume in 1 second (FEV_1) = 1.70 L (65% predicted), forced vital capacity (FVC) = 3.8 L (99% predicted) and FEV_1/FVC ratio = 45%. He demands of you whether there is any other medication that will help him, as his wife has heard of a new puffer available for emphysema.

Introduction

Botanicals with anticholinergic effects, such as *Datura stramonium*, have been used since antiquity to treat respiratory conditions.[1,2] Over the past three decades, quaternary forms of inhaled anticholinergics, such as ipratropium, have been used to treat a variety of respiratory conditions, including chronic obstructive pulmonary disease (COPD), asthma, acute bronchiolitis, bronchopulmonary dysplasia, bronchiectasis and persistent cough. Only in COPD, however, has this class of bronchodilators gained widespread acceptance as first-line therapy for individuals with daily symptoms.[3–5] Recently, a new generation of inhaled anticholinergic bronchodilator medications was ushered in with the release of tiotropium, which has prolonged and more selective activity against the M3 muscarinic receptor. The importance of this very long-acting bronchodilator has become evident over the past few years with the results of several large, controlled trials.

Pharmacology of anticholinergic bronchodilators

The lung is innervated by motor nerves derived from the vagus ganglia, which form plexa within and around the walls of the airways, but predominantly in the large, central airways more than in the small airways. Most of the efferent supply is derived from this plexus via parasympathetic–postganglionic nerves with cholinergic terminals. These terminals are found at the epithelium, submucosal glands, smooth muscle and, possibly, mast cells. Stimulation of this motor supply results in smooth muscle contraction and mucus secretion.[6]

Vagal cholinergic tone plays a much greater role in airways resistance in patients with COPD compared with normal subjects. This is because the airways are more patent in the normal lung but, in patients with chronically constricted airways, relief from vagal stimulation with an anticholinergic drug produces a perceptible improvement in airflow.[7]

At the receptor level, anticholinergics compete with endogenous acetylcholine for muscarinic receptors, thus blocking cholinergic response in the airways. Five muscarinic receptors have been identified; however, M1, M2 and M3 are the three that have been demonstrated to exist in the airways. Stimulation of the M1 receptors enhances bronchoconstriction, whereas stimulation of M3 stimulates both bronchoconstriction and mucus secretion. In contrast, M2 receptors act as presynaptic autoreceptors and feed back an inhibitory response, thereby blocking cholinergic activity.[8]

The inhaled anticholinergics, ipratropium and tiotropium, have similar pharmacological properties and mechanisms of action. Both are quaternary ammonium derivatives of *N*-isopropyl noratropine and block muscarinic receptors. Additionally, both are non-selective in stimulating all three muscarinic receptors in the smooth muscle. However, tiotropium dissociates more than 100 times more slowly from M1 and M3 receptors than ipratropium, while maintaining

Chapter 3.2

similar, relatively rapid dissociation from the M2 receptors. Therefore, tiotropium appears to have a relative selectivity for the M1 and M3 receptors[9,10]—hence its longer duration of action.

The pharmacokinetic and pharmacodynamic properties of ipratropium and tiotropium are summarized in Table 1.

Questions

1 In adults with COPD (population), is ipratropium bromide (intervention) an effective bronchodilator (outcome) compared with placebo or short-acting β-agonists? {therapy}
2 In adults with COPD (population), is the combination of ipratropium bromide and a short-acting β-agonist (intervention) more effective in producing bronchodilatation (outcome) than either agent alone? {therapy}
3 Which of ipratropium bromide or long-acting β-agonists (intervention) is a more effective bronchodilator (outcome) in adults with COPD (population)? {therapy}
4 How effective is ipratropium bromide, compared with other bronchodilators (intervention), in improving symptoms or exercise capacity (outcome) in adults with COPD (population)? {therapy}
5 Which of ipratropium bromide, β-agonists or their combination (intervention) is most effective in reducing exacerbations (outcome) in adults with COPD (population)? {therapy}
6 In adults with COPD (population), is tiotropium more effective than placebo or other bronchodilators (intervention) in improving lung function (outcome)? {therapy}
7 In adults with COPD (population), is tiotropium more effective than placebo or other bronchodilators (intervention) in improving symptoms (outcome)? {therapy}
8 Are anticholinergic bronchodilators (intervention) associated with an increased incidence of adverse effects (outcome) compared with placebo or other bronchodilators in adults with COPD (population)? {therapy}

General search strategy

This chapter will summarize efficacy and safety data from randomized controlled trials (RCTs) of inhaled forms of ipratropium and tiotropium in COPD. Unfortunately, there are no current systematic reviews available to answer all the questions above, although a number of pertinent protocols are reg-

istered with the Cochrane collaboration. For the purposes of discussion, the older generation quaternary drug, ipratropium, will be discussed separately from the newer generation drug, tiotropium. This chapter will not review the role of inhaled forms of tertiary anticholinergics such as atropine, as older data are mostly anecdotal and the newer preparations are clearly more effective drugs. Additionally, oxitropium, another anticholinergic agent with bronchodilator properties, has been used relatively little compared with ipratropium and will not be reviewed in this chapter.

Question

1 In adults with COPD, is ipratropium bromide an effective bronchodilator compared with placebo or short-acting β-agonists?

Table 2 outlines several large RCTs designed to assess the efficacy of inhaled ipratropium by comparing its bronchodilator effect with either placebo or other bronchodilators. In general, these studies prove the efficacy and safety of inhaled ipratropium as therapy for stable COPD and provide sufficient evidence to support this drug's place as an effective, first-line maintenance bronchodilator for this disease.

Bronchodilator effect

One of the first larger scale studies evaluating the efficacy of ipratropium was a 1986 multicentre trial of 261 COPD patients, which compared two inhalations (approximately 40 μg) of this anticholinergic drug with two inhalations (15 mg) of the short-acting β-agonist, metaproterenol. All patients took their test drugs four times daily. Both drugs produced significant bronchodilation compared with baseline. On day 90, ipratropium inhalation led to a statistically significant peak effect increase in mean FEV_1, from 1.04 L (predrug) to 1.39 L.[11] The ~0.35-L improvement was a significantly greater effect than that from the β-agonist (1.10 to 1.30 L or an ~0.20-L change, $P < 0.05$). The impressive bronchodilator response from ipratropium in this study may reflect its inclusion criteria, which required not only a clinical diagnosis of stable COPD with at least mild airways obstruction, but also reversibility of 15% or more in the FEV_1 following isopro-

Table 1. Pharmacological properties of the quaternary anticholinergic drugs, ipratropium and tiotropium.[17,20,49]

	Onset of action	Duration of bronchodilator effect	K_D M1	K_D M2	K_D M3	T1/2 M1	T1/2 M2	T1/2 M3
Ipratropium	3–5 min	4–6 hours	0.183	0.195	0.204	0.11	0.035	0.26
Tiotropium	5 min	≥24 hours	0.041	0.021	0.014	14.6	3.6	34.7

K_D, dissociation constant (measurement of affinity for the receptor).
T1/2, half-life (in hours) of the muscarinic receptor–drug complex.

Table 2. Randomized controlled trials of ipratropium in stable COPD: efficacy results.

Year	First author	N	IP, dose	Trial duration	Comparator (s)	Primary outcome	Results
1986	Tashkin[11]	261	IP 40 µg qid	90 days	Metaproterenol 1.5 mg qid	FEV_1 and FVC	IP resulted in higher FEV_1 and FVC than metaproterenol at most time periods of 6-hour testing at days 1, 45 and 90.
1994	Anthonisen[15]	5887	IP 36 µg bid*	5 years	PL,* no intervention (usual care)	Change in FEV_1 over 5 years	IP had no effect on the rate of decline in post-bronchodilator (isoproterenol) FEV_1 over the 5 years of the study.
1994	Anon[14]	534	IP 42 µg qid	85 days	ALB 200 µg and IP/ALB qid	FEV_1, FVC, FEF 25–75%	IP and ALB resulted in similar degrees of bronchodilation throughout the study (0.30 and 0.29 L increase in FEV_1, respectively, on day 85). IP/ALB consistently produced greater bronchodilation than either component (0.37 L increase in FEV_1 on day 85, $P < 0.001$ versus IP or ALB).
1996	Colice[13]	223	IP 500 µg tid SVN	12 weeks	ALB 2.5 mg	FEV_1	IP and ALB both led to significant, similar degrees of peak response in FEV_1 and 6-hour AUC FEV_1. Similar responses were seen in FVC and FEF 25–75%. CRQ-measured health status tended to increase more following IP than ALB, with several components also showing a clinically meaningful (i.e. 0.5 units/item or greater) change at days 43 and 85.
1996	Friedman[12]	213	IP 500 µg tid SVN	85 days	MP 15 mg	Spirometry, health status, symptoms	The median onset of action was longer for IP than for MP (5–15 min versus 5 min respectively). Both IP and MP led to similar peak increases in FEV_1 (0.34 and 0.31 L, respectively, on day 85) and 6-hour FEV_1 AUC. FVC paralleled FEV_1 results. Patients taking IP scored significantly on all four dimensions of the CRQ on day 85.
1997	Anon[50]	652	IP 500 µg tid SVN	85 days	ALB 300 µg, ALB/IP	Acute bronchodilator responses	Combined ALB/IP led to significantly greater increases in FEV_1 and FVC (peak values, 4-hour AUC) than ALB or IP. ALB/IP also led to greater improvement in evening PEF. No group differences in morning PEF, health status, diary symptoms.
1999	Friedman[32]	1067	IP 42 µg qid		ALB 240 µg qid, IB/ALB	Health care utilization	IP and IP/ALB groups had significantly fewer COPD exacerbations, patient–days of exacerbations, hospital days, antibiotic use and corticosteroid use than ALB group. IP/ALB had greater improvement in peak FEV_1 and 4-hour FEV_1 AUC.

Continued

Year	First author	N	IP, dose	Trial duration	Comparator(s)	Primary outcome	Results
1999	Mahler[22]	411	IP 36 µg qid MDI	12 weeks	SM 42 µg bid, MDI, PL	Spirometry, dyspnoea, health status	FEV_1 and FVC at multiple time points over 12 hours and FEV_1 12-hour AUC increased in IP compared with PL, but this improvement was less than that from SM. Mean TDI dyspnoea and CRQ health status scores in both IP and SM were improved compared with PL, but were not different from each other.
2000	van Noord[51]	144	IP 40 µg qid /SM 50 µg bid	12 weeks	SM 50 µg bid, PL	FEV_1, airway conductance (sGaw)	Both IP/SM and SM were significantly better than PL in multiple outcome areas. Combined IP/SM resulted in a greater increase in FEV_1, FVC and sGaw over the first 6 hours after administration than SM alone or PL.
2001	Dahl[23]	780	IP 40 µg qid MDI	12 weeks	F 12 µg QD, F 24 µg QD, PL	FEV_1 12-hour AUC at 12 weeks	The IP and both F groups had significant increases in FEV_1 AUC compared with PL; both doses of F were superior to I. Both F groups but not the I group had improvement in symptoms or health status compared with PL.
2001	Rennard[24]	405	IP 36 µg qid MDI	12 weeks	SM 42 µg MDI bid, PL	FEV_1 12-hour AUC, dyspnoea (TDI)	IP and SM both increased FEV_1 and FVC compared with PL; these effects did not wane over 12 weeks. The duration of bronchodilator action in SM was significantly longer than IP. Both treatments resulted in higher TDI over the first 6 weeks of the trial; both improved health status (CRQ) to a similar degree compared with PL.
2002	Wadbo[52]	183	IP 80 µg tid MDI	3 months	F 18 µg bid, PL	SWT (m.) at 3 months	No between-group difference in the percentage with clinically meaningful improvements in SWT; IP and F significantly improved FEV_1, FVC, PEF, dyspnoea compared with PL. F reduced daytime reliever SABA use compared with placebo.

N, total number of subjects randomized; IP, ipratropium; MDI, metered dose inhaler; F, formoterol; SWT, shuttle walk test; SABA, short-acting β-agonist; SVN, small-volume nebulizer; PL, placebo.
*Included smoking cessation intervention.

terenol inhalation. Other post-ipratropium spirometric variables, including the 6-hour FEV_1 area under the curve (AUC), peak FVC and 6-hour FVC AUC mirrored the results in FEV_1, in that all were significantly greater than baseline, and all were greater in magnitude than those associated with metaproterenol.

Two subsequent multicentre trials also showed the bronchodilator efficacy of nebulized ipratropium (0.5 mg) to be slightly greater than that of metaproterenol (15 mg)[12] or albuterol (2.5 mg).[13] A 12-week multicentre trial that was designed to evaluate the ipratropium–albuterol metered dose inhaler (MDI) combination in 534 stable COPD subjects[14] provides some insight into the effectiveness of regular dosing of ipratropium versus the more commonly used short-acting β-agonist, albuterol. In this study, standard doses of ipratropium and albuterol taken singly were each used as comparator controls. Two inhalations of ipratropium via MDI produced similar degrees of bronchodilation (an approximate 20% increase in FEV_1 at 1 hour) to albuterol.

The studies described above and others demonstrated that ipratropium was a safe and effective maintenance bronchodilator for COPD, and placed its effectiveness at a level equal to or possibly slightly greater than that of short-acting β-agonists. Based on data from the Lung Health Study in 1994, it appears that this bronchodilation resulting from ipratropium may not confer any long-term benefit in airflow limitation once the bronchodilator is withdrawn.[15] However, a retrospective analysis of data on long-term (approximately 90 days) bronchodilator effect in 1445 patients from seven clinical trials showed a small increase in predrug baseline FEV_1 (0.028 L, $P < 0.01$) and FVC (0.131 L, $P < 0.01$) with regular ipratropium use. This contrasts with results from comparator β-agonist use, which resulted in no significant changes in these variables.[16] Short-term bronchodilator responsiveness in the laboratory after 90 days of regular use was diminished following both ipratropium and β-agonists, although the effect was significantly greater in the latter.

A recent study of 456 patients with COPD demonstrated that a new ipratropium MDI with a hydrofluoroalkane (HFA) propellant had similar efficacy and safety to a conventional chlorofluorocarbon (CFC)-propelled counterpart.[17]

Question

2 In adults with COPD, is the combination of ipratropium bromide and a short-acting β-agonist more effective in producing bronchodilatation than either agent alone?

As anticholinergic and β-agonists work through different mechanisms, combined therapy may offer additive bronchodilator benefit without additive side-effects. This has been supported by several randomized trials. In the COMBIVENT trial comparing MDI forms of ipratropium, albuterol and their combination,[14] combined ipratropium and albuterol led to significantly greater bronchodilation than either agent alone. In another study of 195 COPD patients, the addition of ipratropium (0.5 mg) to albuterol nebulizer solution (2.5 mg) resulted in a 26% greater peak increase in FEV_1 and a 64% increase in the 8-hour FEV_1 AUC compared with albuterol alone.[18] Combination ipratropium–albuterol via MDI has also been shown to be more effective than albuterol MDI alone in COPD,[19] at peak effect and virtually throughout the 8-hour testing. The reason(s) behind the apparent additive effect probably reflects the differing modes of action from the two classes of bronchodilators[20] and perhaps also the submaximal dosing of each in the trial.[21]

Question

3 Which of ipratropium bromide or long-acting β-agonists is a more effective bronchodilator in adults with COPD?

The long-acting β-agonist bronchodilators, salmeterol and formoterol, are also useful maintenance bronchodilators for COPD. Trials of these bronchodilators using ipratropium as an active control provide further insight into the relative effectiveness of this anticholinergic bronchodilator in COPD. Two large placebo-controlled studies involving a total of 816 subjects, comparing four times-daily dosing of ipratropium with twice-daily dosing of salmeterol,[22,23] showed similar mean increases in the 1-hour post-drug FEV_1, which were each significantly greater than placebo and approximately 250 mL (estimated from the graph). Changes in FVC at peak activity were somewhat greater in magnitude, but again mirrored the FEV_1 results. In one study,[24] the 12-hour FEV_1 AUC of ipratropium (given twice over 12 hours) and salmeterol (given once) was not significantly different, whereas in the other, it favoured the long-acting β-agonist.[22] The FEV_1 response of both bronchodilator classes was significantly greater in patients who had previously demonstrated responsiveness to inhaled albuterol in the pulmonary function laboratory. Thus, the bronchodilator efficacy of four times-daily ipratropium was roughly equivalent to twice-daily salmeterol. Both drugs were well tolerated.

Another placebo-controlled multicentre trial compared two doses of inhaled formoterol taken twice daily with two inhalations of ipratropium four times daily for 12 weeks in 780 COPD subjects.[23] Ipratropium dosed 6 hours apart in pulmonary function testing on the last day of treatment resulted in a 0.137-L/min [95% confidence interval (CI) 0.88–1.86 L/min, $P < 0.001$] increase in the normalized 12-hour FEV_1 AUC compared with placebo. There was also a significant difference between active interventions for this primary outcome variable (formoterol 24 μg versus ipratropium mean difference = 0.057, 95% CI 0.007–0.106, $P = 0.024$; formoterol 12 μg versus ipratropium mean difference = 0.0586, 95% CI 0.037–0.136, $P = 0.001$), which places the bronchodilator efficacy of ipratropium at levels somewhat less than that of formoterol.

Question

4 How effective is ipratropium bromide, compared with other bronchodilators, in improving symptoms or exercise capacity in adults with COPD?

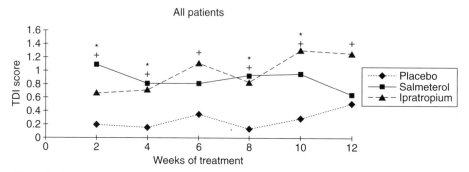

Figure 1. The effect of bronchodilator therapy on dyspnoea. Both the long-acting β-agonist salmeterol and the anticholinergic ipratropium resulted in reduced dyspnoea compared with placebo. TDI, Transition Dyspnoea Index. Higher scores mean increased dyspnoea; a one-unit change is considered to be clinically meaningful. An asterisk denotes clinical significance of salmeterol over placebo; a plus sign indicates significance of ipratropium over placebo. Adapted with permission from Mahler DA, Donohue JF, Barbee RA *et al.* Efficacy of salmeterol xinafoate in the treatment of COPD. *Chest* 1999; **115**:957–65.

Symptoms and health status

Ultimately, the usefulness of bronchodilation in COPD must be the translation of this physiologically measured effect into a reduction in distressing symptoms, such as dyspnoea, or an improvement in health status. Outcomes in these areas are usually measured by questionnaire or diary. For instance, dyspnoea can be assessed using a patient diary or a multidimensional questionnaire, such as the Baseline or Transition Dyspnea Indexes.[25] Health status is usually measured by questionnaire, such as the Chronic Respiratory Disease Questionnaire (CRQ)[26] or the St George's Respiratory Questionnaire (SGRQ).[27]

In the trials comparing ipratropium with metaproterenol and albuterol discussed previously,[12,13] the somewhat longer duration of bronchodilator response associated with the anticholinergic drug was accompanied by relatively greater improvement in several components of CRQ-measured health status. The differences between treatments (in favour of ipratropium) were not only statistically significant, but clinically meaningful (i.e. 0.5 units/item) at several time points in the dyspnoea, fatigue and mastery components. These relatively impressive health status results may reflect the higher doses of ipratropium given by small-volume nebulizer.

In the Mahler and Rennard studies comparing ipratropium with salmeterol,[22,24] the prolonged bronchodilation provided by the long-acting β-agonist was not translated into improved dyspnoea ratings for this drug compared with ipratropium. Both drugs resulted in increases (improvements) in the Transition Dyspnea Index (TDI) scores at several follow-up visits. In the Mahler study, both ipratropium and salmeterol use resulted in significant reductions in dyspnoea at several time points, as depicted in Figure 1. At all time points, the treatment–placebo differences in TDI appear to be less than 1 unit in magnitude, which is considered by some to represent the threshold for clinical meaningfulness for this instrument.[28] In the Rennard study, significance compared with placebo was lost by week 6 on account of improvement in the

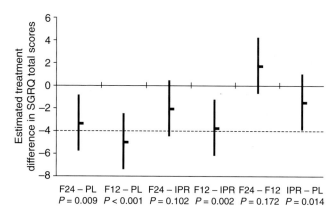

Figure 2. Comparisons of the bronchodilators, formoterol and ipratropium, on quality of life in COPD. The data represent treatment differences with standard errors. SGRQ, St George's Respiratory Questionnaire. A four-unit decrease indicates a clinically meaningful improvement in health status (health-related quality of life). F24, formoterol 24 μg (twice standard dose); F12, formoterol 12 μg (standard dose); PL, placebo; IPR, ipratropium 36 μg (standard dose). Reproduced with permission from Dahl R, Greefhorst APM, Nowak D *et al.* Inhaled formoterol dry powder versus ipratropium bromide in chronic obstructive pulmonary disease. *American Journal of Respiratory and Critical Care Medicine* 2001; **164**:778–84.

TDI score in the placebo group. There were no significant ipratropium–salmeterol differences in TDI in either study.

In both the Mahler and the Rennard studies, CRQ-assessed health status was improved compared with placebo following ipratropium and salmeterol. In the Mahler study, the mean CRQ total score at week 12 increased by 6.8 units following ipratropium, 7.1 units following salmeterol and 2.1 units following placebo (both treatments $P < 0.007$ versus placebo). These changes, although statistically significant, were below the 10-unit accepted threshold for the clinical meaningfulness of this questionnaire.[29] Similar to the dyspnoea ratings, this improvement was not significantly different in the two bronchodilator groups.

In contrast to the salmeterol studies, in the study comparing ipratropium with formoterol,[23] the favourable effect on airway calibre from the long-acting β-agonist was associated with a significant improvement in health status compared with ipratropium. Health status, measured using the SGRQ total score, is given in Figure 2. In the analysis, which used an analysis of covariance using baseline scores as covariates, the effect of ipratropium was not significantly different from that of placebo, and was significantly less than that from either dose of formoterol given once during testing. Furthermore, unlike ipratropium, the standard dose of formoterol (12 μg) led to an increase in SGRQ-measured health status that was significantly greater than placebo and the ipratropium effect.

Exercise capacity

The effect of ipratropium and other classes of bronchodilators on exercise capacity has been reviewed recently in a systematic review of the literature by Liesker and colleagues.[30] Eleven of 17 double-blind trials involving anticholinergic drugs (11 ipratropium, six oxitropium, one atropine) demonstrated an improvement in exercise capacity compared with control therapy. However, in only one of the six trials using the 6-min walk test did the improvement exceed 54 m, which is consid-

Question

5 Which of ipratropium bromide, β-agonists or their combination is most effective in reducing exacerbations in adults with COPD?

ered to be the approximate clinically meaningful threshold.[31] The importance of exacerbation frequency as an outcome variable has been appreciated over recent years. In a post hoc analysis of 1067 COPD patients by Friedman and colleagues,[32] ipratropium, either as a single agent or combined with albuterol, was associated with fewer exacerbations than albuterol alone during 85 days of follow-up: 12% for patients receiving ipratropium singly or in combination versus 18% for those receiving albuterol alone ($P < 0.05$). This resulted in lower total treatment costs.

In the Mahler study, however, salmeterol was associated with a delayed time to the first exacerbation compared with placebo or ipratropium. It appears from this study that both bronchodilators resulted in a similar reduction in exacerbation frequency compared with placebo over the first 4 weeks, but this favourable effect was sustained over the remaining 8 weeks for salmeterol alone (Fig. 3). In the Rennard study, the exacerbation rate in the first week in both the ipratropium and the salmeterol groups was decreased compared with placebo: 4.4%, 4.6% and 14.8% respectively ($P < 0.005$ for both versus

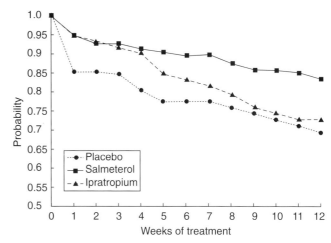

Figure 3. The effects of salmeterol and ipratropium on the frequency of exacerbations. The y-axis represents the probability of remaining in the study (dropouts usually resulted from exacerbations). Salmeterol, but not ipratropium, resulted in fewer dropouts secondary to exacerbations compared with placebo. Adapted with permission from Mahler DA, Donohue JF, Barbee RA *et al.* Efficacy of salmeterol xinafoate in the treatment of COPD. *Chest* 1999; **115**:957–65.

placebo). In the Dahl study, there were no significant differences among formoterol, ipratropium and placebo groups in number of days with additional treatment for COPD exacerbations.[33–41]

Question

6 In adults with COPD, is tiotropium more effective than placebo or other bronchodilators in improving lung function?

Since 2000, several multicentre, controlled trials have established the effectiveness of once-daily inhaled tiotropium bromide as a maintenance bronchodilator for COPD. Table 3 summarizes randomized trials of tiotropium in COPD. A study by Littner *et al.*[42] and two by Casaburi *et al.*[43,44] involving 1643 patients unequivocally demonstrated the bronchodilator effect of this medication compared with placebo. These studies, in general, express bronchodilator efficacy in three ways: as a predrug (trough) effect, a peak bronchodilator effect and as the average bronchodilator effect over 180 min after dosing. The trough effect, which reflects the degree of residual bronchodilation 24 hours following the preceding dose of the drug, is of particular importance considering the long duration of this drug's effect.

In all three studies, trough, peak and 180-min average FEV_1 and FVC responses were significantly greater than placebo. The study by Littner *et al.* showed that all four doses of tiotropium (4.5, 9, 18 and 36 μg) led to significantly greater increases in trough FEV_1 compared with placebo at days 8, 15, 22

Table 3. Randomized controlled trials of tiotropium in stable COPD: efficacy results.

Year	First author	N	Trial duration	Comparator(s)	Primary outcome	Results
2000	Littner[42]	252	4 weeks	Dose-ranging study, PL control	FEV_1, FVC, PF	Compared with PL, all doses of TIO (4.5, 9, 18, 36 µg) showed significant improvement in trough (24 hours following previous dose), peak and 6-hour FEV_1, FVC and PF. There was no significant difference in these variables among the various doses.
2000	Casaburi[43]	470	13 weeks	PL	Spirometry	Compared with PL, TIO led to significant increases in trough and average FEV_1 and FVC throughout the study. The average post-dose FEV_1 was 16% greater than baseline on day 1 and 20% greater on day 92; FVC was 17% and 19% in baseline.
2000	van Noord[46]	288	13 weeks	IP 40 µg qid MDI	Lung function, daily records	TIO led to greater increases in trough, average and peak FEV_1 and FVC compared with IP. On day 92, changes in FEV_1 were: 0.16 versus 0.03 L trough ($P = 0.0001$), 0.38 versus 0.30 L peak ($P = 0.06$) and 0.26 versus 0.18 L ($P = 0.003$) for TIO and IP respectively.
2002	Vincken[47]	555	1 year	IP 40 µg qid	Lung function, dyspnoea, health status	At 1 year, the FEV_1 was significantly greater in TIO than in IP at all time points over the 180-min testing period. The change in trough (predose) FEV_1 was + 0.12 L with TIO compared with −0.03 L with IP ($P < 0.001$). The TDI and SGRQ scores were also improved with TIO compared with IP.
2002	Donohue[48]	623	6 months	Salmeterol MDI 50 µg bid, PL	FEV_1, dyspnoea (TDI), health status (SGRQ)	First-dose TIO and SM led to similar improvements in FEV_1 over 12 hours of testing. The TIO–PL difference in trough FEV_1 at 24 weeks of 137 mL was significantly greater than the 87 mL SM–PL trough difference ($P < 0.01$). The 12-hour differences between TIO and SM appeared to increase over the course of the 6-month study. TIO was generally superior to SM in the TDI focal score and SGRQ total score.
2002	Casaburi[44]	921	1 year	PL	Lung function, dyspnoea	With chronic therapy, TIO–PL differences ranged from 0.12 to 0.15 L in trough FEV_1 and from 0.14 to 0.22 L in mean FEV_1 over 180 min. TIO was also superior in all domains and total score of the SGRQ. TIO–PL TDI focal score differences ranged from 0.8 to 1.1 units. The SGRQ total score was >4 units in 49% of TIO versus 30% of PL patients.
2003	Celli[45]	81	4 weeks	PL	IC, TGV, FEV_1, FVC	Compared with PL, TIO led to significant increases in IC at trough, peak and 3-hour IC AUC (0.22 L, 0.35 L and 0.30 L respectively) at week 4. TGV mirrored these results (−0.54 L, −0.60 L and −0.70 L respectively). FEV_1 and FVC also improved compared with PL.
2003	Donohue[53]	62	6 months	SM, PL	Spirometry	Both TIO and SM resulted in similar increases in predrug, peak and average FEV_1 and FVC on day 1. However, SM (but not TIO) was associated with small decreases in these favourable responses on day 169, suggesting tolerance to this drug.
2003	Calverley[54]	121	6 weeks	TIO dosed in PM, PL	Spirometry	Compared with PL, both morning and evening dosing of TIO improved 24-hour FEV_1 to a similar degree. Trough FEV_1 before morning and evening dosing was similar.

See footnote to Table 2 for abbreviations.

and 29. These ranged from 0.070 to 0.200 L compared with baseline, with the trough effect remaining stable from the first week after randomization to the end of the study at 4 weeks, indicating the achievement of steady-state bronchodilation by 1 week. They were not able to demonstrate significant differences among the different doses. The FVC responses paralleled the FEV_1 responses, but were generally greater in magnitude, ranging from 0.040 to 0.440 L over baseline. Similarly, peak FEV_1 and FVC responses were all significantly greater than placebo at all time periods, but were not significantly different among dose groups. In general, the peak FEV_1 and FVC responses following the first dose ranged from 0.15 L to 0.24 L and from 0.24 L and 0.47 L respectively. These did not change significantly over the 4-week study period.

The first study by Casaburi and colleagues,[43] comparing tiotropium 18 µg with placebo over 3 months, showed similar results. Approximate changes compared with baseline were: trough tiotropium 0.11 L, peak FEV_1 response 0.26 L and 3-hour average FEV_1 0.20 L. There was no demonstrable drop-off in effect over the 13 weeks of the study. The changes in FEV_1 were all significantly greater than those following placebo. Again, the FVC mirrored the FEV_1 responses but was somewhat greater in magnitude. Spirometric results in the subsequent, year-long study by Casaburi et al.[44] showed similar responses. The trough effect of approximately 0.1 L in these

placebo-controlled trials underscores the unique, prolonged duration of action of tiotropium. Representative serial FEV_1 and FVC responses to tiotropium compared with placebo are given in Figures 4 and 5.

A study by Celli and colleagues[45] showed that tiotropium not only led to increases in traditional spirometric variables compared with placebo, the drug also significantly increased the inspiratory capacity (IC) trough (0.22 L), peak (0.35 L) and 3-hour average (0.30 L) at 4 weeks in COPD patients with hyperinflation as an inclusion criterion. An increase in IC reflects a decrease in static hyperinflation. Corresponding significant decreases in thoracic gas volume (−0.54 L, −0.60 L and −0.70 L respectively) were also seen following the drug. These findings indicate that this bronchodilator causes significant lung volume reduction. To date, it is not established whether this effect is unique to this drug or (more likely) is shared by all classes of bronchodilators.

Studies comparing once-daily doses of tiotropium 18 µg with other maintenance bronchodilator regimens in COPD provide insight into the relative bronchodilator effectiveness of this drug. van Noord and associates,[46] in a study lasting 3 months, and Vincken and associates,[47] in a study lasting 1 year, compared once-daily tiotropium with ipratropium 40 µg given four times daily. In both trials, tiotropium was superior to ipratropium in FEV_1 responses at trough, peak and the average over the first 3 hours following dosing. Similar to the placebo-controlled trials, trough increases were approximately 0.12–0.16 L over baseline at the end of the study period.

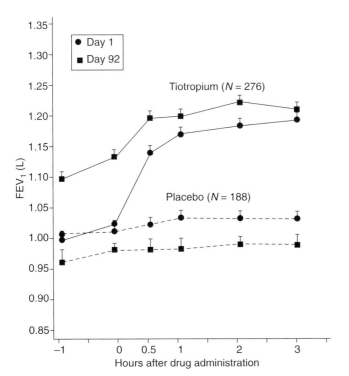

Figure 4. Serial FEV_1 responses to tiotropium compared with placebo. Reproduced with permission from Casaburi R, Briggs DD, Donohue JF, et al. The spirometric efficacy of once-daily dosing with tiotropium in stable COPD. A 13-week multicenter study. *Chest* 2000; **118**:1294–1302.

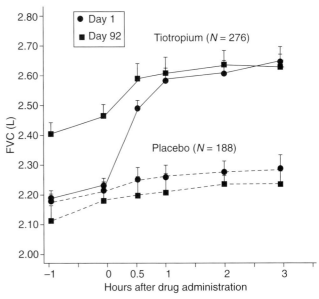

Figure 5. Serial FVC responses to tiotropium compared with placebo. Reproduced with permission from Casaburi R, Briggs DD, Donohue JF, et al. The spirometric efficacy of once-daily dosing with tiotropium in stable COPD. A 13-week multicenter study. *Chest* 2000; **118**:1294–1302.

Donohue and colleagues[48] compared tiotropium with salmeterol 50 μg inhaled twice daily via an MDI. Trough response (approximately 24 hours following tiotropium and 12 hours following salmeterol) was significantly greater following the long-acting anticholinergic: tiotropium–placebo difference = 0.137 L versus the salmeterol–placebo difference of 0.087 L at 24 weeks.

Question

7 In adults with COPD, is tiotropium more effective than placebo or other bronchodilators in improving symptoms?

Symptoms and health status

Regular tiotropium use leads to significant reductions in overall dyspnoea and improvements in respiratory-specific and generic health status, compared with placebo. In the year-long study by Casaburi *et al.*, tiotropium led to a significantly increased TDI compared with placebo, with a treatment effect ranging from 0.8 to 1.1 units. Similarly, the drug resulted in significant decreases (i.e. improvement) in all three SGRQ domains and its total score. The mean changes for the symptom domain exceeded the clinically meaningful threshold of 4 units, although the activity and impact domains as well as the total score fell short of this threshold. Forty-nine per cent of tiotropium-treated patients surpassed the clinically meaningful threshold for the total score versus 30% for placebo-treated patients.

Tiotropium also showed a significantly greater improvement in dyspnoea in trials comparing it with ipratropium[47] and salmeterol.[48] In the study by Vincken, the tiotropium–ipratropium treatment difference was 0.90 units at 12 months, and the percentage of patients achieving a clinically meaningful change was significantly greater: 31% versus 18%, $P = 0.0004$. In the study by Donohue, the tiotropium–placebo difference in TDI focal score was 1.02 units ($P = 0.01$) compared with 0.24 units ($P = 56$) for the salmeterol–placebo group. These studies found similar effects using health status outcomes. In the Vincken study, the SGRQ initially decreased (improved) in both ipratropium and tiotropium groups, but gradually returned towards baseline in the ipratropium but not the tiotropium group. At approximately 1 year, the mean change in SGRQ total score was −3.74 for tiotropium and −0.44 for ipratropium. This difference was significant, although the change did not meet the clinically meaningful threshold of 4 units. Fifty-two per cent of tiotropium-treated patients and 35% of ipratropium-treated patients achieved the clinically meaningful change at 1 year. In the Donohue study, the change in SGRQ total score at 6 months was −5.14 units versus −3.54 units in salmeterol-treated patients and −2.33 units in those given placebo. The tiotropium mean was significantly different from placebo but not from salmeterol.

Prevention of exacerbations

The two year-long trials provide data on the relationship between tiotropium use and exacerbation frequency, although in neither was the definition of exacerbation clearly defined. In the year-long study by Casaburi *et al.*, a lower proportion of patients treated with tiotropium had at least one COPD exacerbation over the year compared with the placebo group: 36% in tiotropium-treated patients versus 42% in placebo-treated patients ($P < 0.05$). This was equivalent to a 14% reduction. In the study by Vincken, similar results in favour of tiotropium were observed: 35% of tiotropium-treated patients versus 46% of ipratropium-treated patients ($P = 0.014$). Additionally, tiotropium use was associated with a prolonged time to first exacerbation and a reduced number of exacerbations per patient per year in both studies.

Question

8 Are anticholinergic bronchodilators associated with an increased incidence of adverse effects compared with placebo or other bronchodilators in adults with COPD?

In controlled trials, adverse effects attributed to ipratropium were infrequent and not severe. In the study comparing ipratropium, albuterol and the ipratropium–albuterol combination, dry mouth was the most commonly reported problem in the groups receiving the anticholinergic drug. In general, there were no significant differences between ipratropium and placebo or the comparator drugs in adverse events in the studies described above. In the Rennard study, both ipratropium and salmeterol were associated with more ear, nose and throat events (such as sore throat, upper respiratory tract infection) than placebo.[16] The most frequently reported side-effect from tiotropium was dry mouth, in general, ranging from approximately 6 to 16%.[42–44,47,48] There were no significant tiotropium–comparator differences in serious adverse events.

Conclusion

Both short-acting ipratropium and long-acting tiotropium produce significant bronchodilation compared with placebo in COPD, and both have minimal side-effects. The bronchodilator effect from this class of drugs does not appear to decline with time. For stable COPD, the efficacy of ipratropium appears to be equal to or slightly greater than that of short-acting β-agonists, although somewhat less than that of long-acting β-agonists. Ipratropium and short-acting β-agonists appear to have similar efficacy in the short-term treatment of acute exacerbations of COPD. The combination of ipratropium with a short-acting β-agonist for stable COPD produces greater bronchodilation than either agent alone, without any appreciable increase in side-effects.

However, the combination appears to add no further bronchodilation than β-agonists alone in the treatment of the exacerbation. Tiotropium has a superior bronchodilator effect over ipratropium and a longer duration than the currently available long-acting β-agonists. Associated with the bronchodilator effects are significant improvements in dyspnoea and health status. The drug also leads to a significant reduction in the frequency of exacerbations.

Summary for clinicians

- Both short-acting ipratropium and long-acting tiotropium produce significant bronchodilation compared with placebo in COPD, which does not appear to decline with time.
- The combination of ipratropium with a short-acting β-agonist for stable COPD produces greater bronchodilation than either agent alone, without any appreciable increase in side-effects.
- Associated with the bronchodilator effects of ipratropium and tiotropium are clinically significant improvements in dyspnoea and health status.
- Tiotropium has a superior bronchodilator effect over ipratropium and a longer duration than the currently available long-acting β-agonists.
- Long-term tiotropium leads to a significant reduction in the frequency of exacerbations.
- Adverse reactions to anticholinergic agents are rare, the most commonly reported being a dry mouth, which occurs in 6–16% of subjects.

References

1 Gandevia B. Historical review of the use of parasympatholytic agents in the treatment of respiratory disorders. *Postgrad Med J* 1975; **51** (Suppl 7): 3–20.

2 Witek TJ. Anticholinergic bronchodilators. *Respir Care Clinics North Am* 1999; **5**:521–36.

3 American Thoracic Society. Standards for the diagnosis and care of patients with chronic obstructive pulmonary disease (COPD). *Am J Respir Crit Care Med* 1995; **152**(Suppl): 77.

4 ERS Consensus Statement: Optimal assessment and management of chronic obstructive pulmonary disease (COPD). *Eur Respir J* 1995; **8**:1398.

5 Global Initiative for Chronic Obstructive Pulmonary Disease Workshop Report: Updated 2003. July 2003. http://www.goldcopd.com.

6 Gross NJ, Skorodin MS. Anticholinergic, antimuscarinic bronchodilators. *Am Rev Respir Dis* 1984; **129**:856–70.

7 Hansel TT, Barnes PJ. Tiotropium bromide: a novel once-daily anticholinergic bronchodilator for the treatment of COPD. *Drugs Today* 2002; **38**:585–600.

8 Barnes PJ. The pharmacological properties of tiotropium. *Chest* 2000; **117**:63s–66s.

9 Disse B, Reichl R, Speck G, Traunecker W, Rominger KL, Hammer R. Ba679BR, a new long-acting antimuscarinic bronchodilator: predicted and clinical aspects. *Life Sci* 1993; **52**:537–55.

10 Disse B, Speck GA, Rominger KL, Witek TJ, Hammer R. Tiotropium (Spiriva): mechanistical considerations and clinical profile in obstructive lung disease. *Life Sci* 1999; **64**:457–64.

11 Tashkin DP, Ashtosh K, Bleecker ER *et al.* Comparison of the anticholinergic bronchodilator ipratropium bromide with metaproterenol in chronic obstructive pulmonary disease. A 90-day multicenter study. *Am J Med* 1986; **81**(Suppl 5A):81–90.

12 Friedman M. A multicenter study of nebulized bronchodilator solutions in chronic obstructive pulmonary disease. *Am J Med* 1996; **100**(Suppl 1A):30s–38s.

13 Colice GL. Nebulized bronchodilators for outpatient management of stable chronic obstructive pulmonary disease. *Am J Med* 1996; **100**(Suppl 1A):11s–18s.

14 Anonymous. COMBIVENT Inhalation Aerosol Study Group. In chronic obstructive pulmonary disease, a combination of ipratropium and albuterol is more effective than either agent alone: an 85-day multicenter trial. *Chest* 1994; **105**:1411–19.

15 Anthonisen NR, Connett JE, Kiley JP *et al.* Effects of smoking intervention and the use of an inhaled anticholinergic bronchodilator on the rate of decline of FEV1. The Lung Health Study. *JAMA* 1994; **272**:1497–505.

16 Rennard SI, Serby CW, Ghafouri M, Johnson PA, Friedman M. Extended therapy with ipratropium is associated with improved lung function in patients with COPD. A retrospective analysis of data from seven clinical trials. *Chest* 1996; **110**:62–70.

17 Brazinsky SA, Lapidus RJ, Weiss LA, Ghafouri M, Fagan NM, Witek TJ. One-year evaluation of the safety and efficacy of ipratropium bromide HFA and CFC inhalation aerosols in patients with chronic obstructive pulmonary disease. *Clin Drug Invest* 2003; **23**:181–91.

18 Levin DC, Little KS, Laughlin KR *et al.* Addition of anticholinergic solution prolongs bronchodilator effect of B2 agonists in patients with chronic obstructive pulmonary disease. *Am J Med* 1996; **100**(Suppl 1A):40s–48s.

19 Campbell S. For COPD a combination of ipratropium bromide and albuterol sulfate is more effective than albuterol base. *Arch Intern Med* 1999; **159**:156–60.

20 Pineda R, Rennard SI. Anticholinergic bronchodilators in combination. *Exp Opin Pharmacother* 2000; **1**:1281–7.

21 Chapman KR. The role of anticholinergic bronchodilators in adult asthma and chronic obstructive pulmonary disease. *Lung* 1990; **168**(Suppl):295–303.

22 Mahler DA, Donohue JF, Barbee RA *et al.* Efficacy of salmeterol xinafoate in the treatment of COPD. *Chest* 1999; **115**:957–65.

23 Dahl R, Greefhorst APM, Nowak D *et al.* Inhaled formoterol dry powder versus ipratropium bromide in chronic obstructive pulmonary disease. *Am J Respir Crit Care Med* 2001; **164**:778–84.

24 Rennard SI, Anderson W, ZuWallack R *et al.* Use of long-acting inhaled B-2 adrenergic agonist, salmeterol xinafoate, in patients with chronic obstructive pulmonary disease. *Am J Respir Crit Care Med* 2001; **163**:1087–92.

25 Mahler D, Guyatt G, Jones P. Clinical measurement of dyspnea. In: Mahler D. ed. *Lung Biology in Health and Disease: Dyspnea.* Vol. 111. New York, Marcel Decker, 1998, pp. 149–98.

26 Guyatt GH, Feeny DH, Patrick DL. Measuring health related quality of life. *Ann Intern Med* 1993; **118**:622–9.

27 Jones PW, Quirk FH, Baveystock CM, Littlejohns P. A self-complete measure for chronic airflow limitation—the St George's Respiratory Questionnaire. *Am Rev Respir Dis* 1992; **145**:1321–7.

28 Witek TJ, Mahler DA. Minimal important difference of the transition dyspnoea index in a multinational clinical trial. *Eur Respir J* 2003; **21**:267–72.

29 Jaeschke R, Singer J, Guyatt GH. Measurement of health status. Ascertaining the minimal clinically important difference. *Control Clin Trials* 1989; **10**:407–15.

30 Liesker JJW, Wijkstra PJ, Ten Hacken NHT, Koeter GH, Postma DS, Kerstjens HAM. A systematic review of the effects of bronchodilators on exercise capacity in patients with COPD. *Chest* 2002; **121**:597–608.

31 Redelmeier DA, Bayoumi AM, Goldstein RS, Guyatt GH. Interpreting small differences in functional status: the six minute walk test in chronic lung disease patients. *Am J Respir Crit Care Med* 1997; **155**:1278–82.

32 Friedman M, Serby CW, Menjoge SS, Wilson D, Hilleman DE, Witek TJ. Pharmacoeconomic evaluation of a combination of ipratropiuml plus albuterol compared with ipratropium alone and albuterol alone in COPD. *Chest* 1999; **115**:635–41.

33 McCrory DC, Brown CD. Anticholinergic bronchodilators versus β_2-sympathomimetic agents for acute exacerbations of chronic obstructive pulmonary disease (Cochrane Review). In: *The Cochrane Library*, Issue 4. Chichester, John Wiley & Sons, 2003.

34 Backman R, Hellstrom PE. Fenoterol and ipratropium in respiratory treatment of patients with chronic bronchitis. *Curr Ther Res Clin Exp* 1985; **38**:135–40.

35 Karpel JP, Pesin J, Greenberg D, Gentry E. A comparison of the effects of ipratropium bromide and metaproterenol sulfate in acute exacerbations of COPD. *Chest* 1990; **98**:835–9.

36 Lloberes P, Ramis L, Montserrat JM *et al.* Effect of three different bronchodilators during an exacerbation of chronic obstructive pulmonary disease. *Eur Respir J* 1988; **1**:536–9.

37 Rebuck AS, Chapman KR, Abboud R *et al.* Nebulized anticholinergic and sympathomimetic treatment of asthma and chronic obstructive airways disease in the emergency room. *Am J Med* 1987; **82**:59–64.

38 Moayyedi P, Congleton J, Page RL, Pearson SB, Muers MF. Comparison of nebulized salbutamol and ipratropium bromide with salbutamol alone in the treatment of chronic obstructive pulmonary disease. *Thorax* 1995; **50**:834–7.

39 Patrick DM, Dales RE, Stark RM, Laliberte G, Dikinson G. Severe exacerbations of COPD and asthma. Incremental benefit of adding ipratropium to usual therapy. *Chest* 1990; **98**:295–7.

40 O'Driscoll BR, Taylor RJ, Horsley MG, Chambers DK, Bernstein A. Nebulized salbutamol with and without ipratropium bromide in acute airflow obstruction. *Lancet* 1989; **1**(8652):1418–20.

41 Shretha M, O'Brien T, Haddox R, Gourlay HS, Reed G. Decreased duration of emergency department treatment of chronic obstructive pulmonary disease exacerbations with the addition of ipratropium bromide to β-agonist therapy. *Ann Emerg Med* 1991; **20**:1206–9.

42 Littner MR, Ilowite JS, Tashkin DP *et al.* Long-acting bronchodilation with once-daily dosing of tiotropium (Spiriva) in stable chronic obstructive pulmonary disease. *Am J Respir Crit Care Med* 2000; **161**:1136–42.

43 Casaburi R, Briggs DD, Donohue JF, Serby CW, Menjoge SS, Witek TJ. The spirometric efficacy of once-daily dosing with tiotropium in stable COPD. A 13-week multicenter study. *Chest* 2000; **118**:1294–302.

44 Casaburi R, Mahler DA, Jones PW *et al.* A long-term evaluation of once-daily inhaled tiotropium in chronic obstructive pulmonary disease. *Eur Respir J* 2002; **19**:217–24.

45 Celli B, ZuWallack R, Wang S, Kesten S. Improvement in resting inspiratory capacity and hyperinflation with tiotropium in COPD patients with increased static lung volumes. *Chest* 2003; **124**:1743–8.

46 van Noord JA, Bantje TA, Eland ME, Korducki L, Cornelissen PJG. A randomised controlled comparison of tiotropium and ipratropium in the treatment of chronic obstructive pulmonary disease. *Thorax* 2000; **55**:289–94.

47 Vincken W, van Noord JA, Greefhorst APM *et al.* Improved health outcomes in patients with COPD during 1 year's treatment with tiotropium. *Eur Respir J* 2002; **19**:209–16.

48 Donohue JF, van Noord JA, Bateman ED *et al.* A 6-month, placebo-controlled study comparing lung function and health status changes in COPD patients treated with tiotropium or salmeterol. *Chest* 2002; **122**:47–55.

49 Massey KL, Gotz VP. Ipratropium bromide. *Drug Intell Clin Pharm* 1985; **19**:5–12.

50 Anonymous. The Combivent Inhalation Solution Study Group. Routine nebulized ipratropium and albuterol together are better than either alone in COPD. *Chest* 1997; **112**:1514–21.

51 van Noord JA, Munck DRAJ, Bantje TA, Hop WCJ, Akveld MLM, Bommer AM. Long-term treatment of chronic obstructive pulmonary disease with salmeterol and the additive effect of ipratropium. *Eur Respir J* 2000; **15**:878–85.

52 Wadbo M, Lofdahl C-G, Larsson K *et al.* Effects of formoterol and ipratropium bromide in COPD: a 3-month placebo-controlled study. *Eur Respir J* 2002; **20**:1138–46.

53 Donohue JF, Menjoge S, Kesten S. Tolerance to bronchodilating effects of salmeterol in COPD. *Respir Med* 2003; **97**:1014–20.

54 Calverley PMA, Lee A, Towse L, van Noord J, Witek TJ, Kelsen S. Effect of tiotropium bromide on circadian variation in airflow limitation in chronic obstructive pulmonary disease. *Thorax* 2003; **58**:855–60.

CHAPTER 3.3

Inhaled corticosteroids in chronic obstructive pulmonary disease

Christine Jenkins

Inhaled corticosteroids in chronic obstructive pulmonary disease (COPD)

Airway inflammation is an important pathological feature of COPD,[1,2] and so it is rational to consider using inhaled corticosteroids (ICS) to treat this disease. However, many of the early studies on the efficacy of ICS in COPD failed to demonstrate overall benefit.[3,4] Some suggested that clinical improvement correlated with certain features such as acute bronchodilator reversibility, while others failed to identify any subgroup as more responsive to ICS.[5,6] These studies tended to be short-term studies often of only a few weeks' duration and frequently focused only on a single endpoint such as forced expiratory volume in 1 second (FEV_1). Increasing awareness of the relative insensitivity of FEV_1, particularly at the end stages of COPD, along with the greater relevance and sensitivity of some functional measures, such as exercise tolerance or quality of life, resulted in studies that incorporated multiple endpoints, several of which relate more closely to the symptoms that most commonly affect COPD patients. These include cough and sputum production, frequency of reliever use, walking distance and exacerbations requiring medical intervention. Some of these endpoints, such as exacerbation frequency, necessitate longer term studies with large numbers of patients. Although these later studies have more clearly demonstrated the benefits of ICS in COPD patients than the earlier studies, the role of ICS as maintenance management for COPD is still controversial. This controversy has arisen as a result of the apparently small benefits demonstrated, the lack of clinically important effects on the rate of lung function decline, the economic cost of ICS and the potential for side-effects in this generally elderly population.

This chapter will discuss the results of randomized controlled trials (RCTs), systematic reviews and meta-analyses examining the effects of ICS in COPD. Studies included in this overview were identified by a MEDLINE search of English language papers from 1966 to November 2003. Papers were selected if they described RCTs in patients with COPD, systematic reviews or meta-analyses. These include systematic reviews on the Cochrane database. Studies were included if they were randomized, double blind and placebo controlled and contained a description of withdrawals and drop-outs in order to assess the presence of bias. The text will discuss the major studies in turn, but the table summarizes the effects of ICS on particular endpoints such as daily symptoms of cough and sputum production, exercise limitation, clinic FEV_1, mortality and health resource utilization. A brief discussion at the end of the chapter deals with recent large epidemiological studies which, although observational, have identified some interesting links between COPD outcomes and ICS use.

Early clinical trials with inhaled corticosteroids assessing lung function in patients with COPD

Initial efforts to identify the role of ICS in the management of COPD were hampered by relatively small studies with few patients, often a heterogeneous population, a single endpoint (usually FEV_1) and inconclusive results. Several of these studies deserve mention, however, as they were RCTs that compared ICS with placebo and often also with oral steroid.

In one of the earliest RCTs of ICS in patients with COPD, Weir *et al.*[7] randomized 127 patients in a double-blind, crossover trial to inhaled beclomethasone dipropionate 500 µg tds, oral prednisolone 40 mg daily or placebo for 2 weeks. Mean reversibility of FEV_1 to 10 mg of salbutamol was 18% (expressed as a percentage of the prebronchodilator value), and mean baseline FEV_1 was 1.18 L; however, 12 patients claimed to be lifelong non-smokers, raising the possibility of asthma. Despite the very short treatment period, and a carryover effect on the active treatments, this study merits comment because of the relatively large numbers for a COPD trial at that time and the clear a priori definition of a response to treatment. The authors identified a full response to treatment as an increase in FEV_1 or forced vital capacity (FVC) or an increase in mean daily peak expiratory flow (PEF) over the final week of treatment of at least 20% from baseline. A partial, smaller treatment response was also defined. The number of full responses to inhaled beclomethasone (8/34) did not differ significantly from the number responding to oral prednisolone (16/38) or placebo (3/35), although the last two differed significantly from each other. When all three treatment periods were considered, a response to prednisolone (in 39) occurred more frequently than to inhaled beclomethasone (in

26). Six-minute walk distances improved significantly with both active treatments in the steroid-responsive patients but not in those in whom there were no significant lung function changes. The authors concluded that inhaled beclomethasone dipropionate 500 µg tds was inferior to oral prednisolone 40 mg a day over 3 weeks, but superior to placebo.

In an accompanying paper,[8] these authors analysed the time course of response to oral and inhaled corticosteroids in this study, noting that the peak response occurred earlier with inhaled beclomethasone (median 9.5 days) than with oral prednisolone (median 12 days). They suggested that trials of treatment with corticosteroids in such patients should last more than 14 days. As the range of time to peak response extended to the final day of the treatment period, it is impossible to know how many more patients would have had a treatment response had the study been longer.

Auffarth et al.,[3] in a double-blind RCT in allergic smokers with COPD, assessed the effect of 8 weeks' treatment with inhaled budesonide 1600 µg daily compared with placebo. Ipratropium bromide was permitted as needed for symptom relief over the 8-week treatment period. There was a significant reduction in dyspnoea in the budesonide group but no change in symptom scores or use of reliever medication. There were no significant differences in mean spirometric values, PEF, airway hyper-responsiveness to histamine or citric acid threshold for cough. The authors noted trends in favour of budesonide despite the absence of statistically significant changes and postulated that a longer study may have demonstrated a significant difference between treatments.

In the study by Weir and Burge,[6] 105 patients, aged 49–78 years (mean 66 years) with mean FEV_1 of 1.05 L and FEV_1 mean reversibility of 6%, were randomized in a sequential placebo-controlled, blinded, parallel study to 3 weeks' placebo treatment followed by beclomethasone 750 µg or 1500 µg bd for 3 weeks. Following this, one-third remained on beclomethasone while the remainder received prednisolone 40 mg a day or placebo for 3 weeks. There were no significant differences between the two dosages of beclomethasone. More patients had a $\geq$20% improvement in FEV_1, FVC or PEF during the inhaled beclomethasone period than during the placebo period (34% versus 15%, $P < 0.001$). Mean lung function improvements were small and clinically insignificant, and there was no effect on airway hyper-responsiveness, although a small improvement in quality of life and dyspnoea was noted. There was no relationship between lung function response to inhaled or oral corticosteroids and response to bronchodilator.

In a multicentre, randomized, double-blind, placebo-controlled study of current or ex-smokers with COPD aged between 50 and 75 years and FEV_1 of 35–90% predicted, fluticasone propionate 500 µg ($n = 142$) or placebo ($n = 139$) bd were compared over a 6-month treatment period.[9] Significantly more patients in the placebo group had moderate or severe COPD exacerbations than in the fluticasone group (86%

versus 60%, $P < 0.001$). The difference between the proportion of patients with at least one exacerbation during the treatment period was not significantly different in the placebo group (37%) compared with the fluticasone group (32%), but this study was significant in identifying exacerbations as an important endpoint in COPD studies examining the effects of ICS.

Importantly, 'responders' (showing an increase in FEV_1 of more than 10%) showed no relationship to age, sex, baseline FEV_1 or smoking status. The benefit of fluticasone appeared to be dependent on the duration of COPD in responders if disease had been present for more than 10 years, but shorter durations of COPD had no effect on response status. Fluticasone had a preferential effect on cough and sputum scores, and the mean change in 6-min walk was greater on fluticasone than on placebo (27 m versus 8 m). This study marks a transition from the measurement of simple lung function measures such as FEV_1 to a range of measures that more realistically represent the potential gains that can be made if treatment is effective for COPD patients.

In a double-blind, randomized, parallel group trial of inhaled budesonide 1600 µg daily versus placebo[10] following a single-blind, 2-week treatment period with prednisolone, 79 subjects who failed to gain benefit from prednisone were randomized to budesonide 1600 µg daily or placebo for 6 months. There was no difference in the change in FEV_1 from baseline between treatment and placebo groups; both changes were clinically insignificant. The proportion of patients with 15% or more improvement in FEV_1 did not differ between treatment groups. A number of functional measures were included in this study (6-min walk test, quality of life and perception of dyspnoea), but no significant difference between the groups and no clinically important improvement was shown.

To date, there have been no long-term studies examining the dose–response to ICS in COPD. Although many different doses have been used, most studies use a single dose in comparison with placebo or oral corticosteroids. As noted above, there was no difference between 1500 and 3000 µg of beclomethasone daily over 3 weeks.[6] A high-dose study of beclomethasone dipropionate 3 mg daily used in combination with optimal use of regular salbutamol and ipratropium was undertaken in 30 patients with moderately severe, stable, carefully defined COPD.[11] It showed a small benefit in FEV_1 during a 4-week treatment period compared with placebo. A subgroup of participants had larger changes in FEV_1, but the authors concluded that the overall benefits did not justify widespread use of this level of treatment, predominantly because of the risk of adverse events.

Clinical trials examining the effect of corticosteroids on decline in FEV$_1$ in COPD

The apparent failure of ICS significantly to improve clinic lung function measures, especially FEV_1, led to studies examining other outcomes, such as exacerbation rates and exercise capacity. The recognition of the role of inflammation and the characteristic rapid decline in lung function in patients with COPD prompted studies assessing the effects of ICS on the rate of decline in FEV_1. A meta-analysis of the long-term effects of ICS in COPD,[12] published in 1999, was undertaken to answer the question 'Are ICS able to slow down the decline in lung function (FEV_1) in COPD?' A MEDLINE search of papers published from 1983 to 1996 yielded 94 references, but only five studies met the criterion of at least 24 months' duration, and only three[13–15] satisfied the additional criterion of being randomized and placebo controlled. Rigid diagnostic criteria were then applied to be certain that inclusion and exclusion criteria selected patients with symptoms compatible with the diagnosis of COPD, aged 40 years or over, with an abnormal FEV_1 and " 9% reversibility from baseline as well as previous or current smokers. The primary endpoint was prebronchodilator decline in FEV_1, measured at 2- or 3-monthly intervals, and the secondary endpoints were postbronchodilator decline in FEV_1, the number of drop-outs and number of exacerbations. The meta-analysis showed a significant beneficial effect of ICS compared with placebo on the prebronchodilator FEV_1 during 2 years of treatment but only a tendency towards an effect on the post-bronchodilator FEV_1. A daily dose of 1500 μg of budesonide was more effective than 800 μg, but only a small number of patients received the lower dose. No significant heterogeneity of response was seen in the three studies. This meta-analysis did not identify any relationship between high levels of immunoglobulin E (IgE) or FEV_1 reversibility and a better response to ICS. The authors commented that the beneficial effect on FEV_1 in patients treated with budesonide was not accompanied by a lower number of exacerbations.

One of these studies[13] compared 1600 μg of budesonide daily with or without oral prednisone 5 mg daily and placebo over 2 years in 58 patients with COPD. The rate of decline in lung function was significantly lower in the budesonide-only group compared with the placebo group, but variation was large and the differences were not statistically significant. There was a high number of withdrawals in the placebo group and no difference in exacerbation rates between the treatments. There was no significant difference between the budesonide plus prednisone group and the budesonide-alone group in clinical outcomes measured in this study.

Larger long-term studies of the effect of ICS on FEV_1 decline

Beginning in 1999, four large multicentre studies were published designed to assess the effect of ICS on the rate of FEV_1 decline in patients with COPD. The Euroscop (European Respiratory Society Study on Chronic Obstructive Pulmonary Disease) study[16] was a parallel group, randomized, double-blind study recruiting patients from 47 centres in 12 countries. Eligible patients were 30–65 years old, current smokers with minimum five pack–year intake and had an FEV_1/VC ratio < 70% and post-bronchodilator FEV_1 50–100% of predicted. Bronchodilator reversibility of < 10% predicted after 1 mg of terbutaline was required. The randomized patients had mild COPD with a mean prebronchodilator FEV_1 of 76.9% (2.54 L), mean age of 52 years, 39 pack–year average intake and average current smoking of 18 cigarettes daily. A total of 1277 subjects were randomized and 912 completed the study. During the first 6 months of the study, the FEV_1 improved (17 mL/year) in the budesonide group compared with a decline in the placebo group (81 mL/year) but, from 9 months to the end of treatment, there was no difference in the rate of decline of FEV_1 between the two groups (−57 mL/year in the budesonide group and −69 mL/year in the placebo group). More subjects in the budesonide group had skin bruising but, in the subgroup in whom bone density measurements were undertaken, there was no significant change over time and no significant treatment effect.

A 3-year, double-blind, parallel group, randomized clinical trial of budesonide versus placebo in COPD was nested into a continuing epidemiological study, the Copenhagen City Heart Study.[17] Subjects were aged 30–70 years, with FEV_1/VC ratio of < 0.7 and < 15% FEV_1 reversibility to 1 mg of terbutaline. A total of 290 patients were enrolled, and 203 patients completed the 3-year study. Budesonide 1200 μg daily was given for 6 months then 800 μg daily for 30 months. Mean age was 59 years, mean post-bronchodilator FEV_1 2.38 L and mean β-agonist reversibility 7.6% of baseline FEV_1. Most subjects (76.2%) were continuing smokers. There was no significant effect of budesonide on decline in FEV_1, being 48.1 mL/year in the placebo group and 45.1 mL/year in the budesonide group. In both treatment groups, symptoms decreased substantially (especially dyspnoea) during the study, but there were no between-treatment differences in chronic mucus secretion, exacerbations or adverse events.

A randomized, double-blind, placebo-controlled study of fluticasone was performed in patients with moderate to severe COPD (Inhaled Steroids in Obstructive Lung Disease in England — ISOLDE)[18] over 3 years. Eligible patients were aged 40–75 years with a clinical diagnosis of COPD and baseline FEV_1 after bronchodilator of less than 85% predicted normal and FEV_1/VC ratio of < 0.7. Patients were excluded if the FEV_1 improved after 400 μg of salbutamol by more than 10% predicted normal, if the life expectancy was < 5 years due to comorbidity or if they used β-blocker medication. Before the double-blind, randomized treatment phase, patients received prednisolone 0.6 mg/kg/day for 14 days to assess the acute response to oral steroid and its relationship to response to inhaled steroid. A total of 751 subjects received study treatment. During the double-blind phase, 160 patients (43%) withdrew from the fluticasone group and 195 patients (53%) from the placebo group, most commonly for frequent exacerbations of COPD. Mean FEV_1 rate of decline was 59 mL/year in the placebo group and 50 mL/year in the fluticasone group. These were not significantly different, although FEV_1 in the fluticasone group remained higher than in the placebo group throughout the treatment period. The median yearly exacerbation rate was lower in the fluticasone group (0.99/year) compared with the placebo group (1.3/year), a 25% reduction in exacerbation rate in the fluticasone group. Health status deteriorated in both treatment groups but at a significantly faster rate in the placebo-treated group, a clinically important change in score occurring at 15 months in the placebo group and 24 months in the fluticasone group. There was a significant decrease in mean cortisol concentrations in the fluticasone group compared with placebo and a slightly higher rate of inhaled steroid-related events including dysphonia, hypertension and candidiasis.

The Lung Health III Study (LHS III)[19] assessed the effect of inhaled triamcinolone on the decline in pulmonary function in a multicentre USA study enrolling 1116 patients with COPD. The participants were 40–69 years of age with FEV_1/VC ratio of less than 0.7 and FEV_1 30–90% of predicted value. All patients were current smokers or had quit within the previous 2 years. The study population had mild to moderate airflow limitation with a mean FEV_1 before bronchodilator of 64.1%. Some 90% of patients were smokers with an average

daily consumption of 24 cigarettes. There were no significant effects of treatment on the decline in FEV_1 before or after bronchodilator. The decline in FEV_1 after bronchodilator was 44.2 mL/year compared with 47.0 mL/year in the placebo group. During the study, subjects in the triamcinolone group had fewer respiratory symptoms, fewer visits to a physician because of respiratory illness and less airway reactivity at 9 months and 33 months. After 3 years' treatment, the mean bone density of neck of femur was significantly lower in the triamcinolone group.

In summary, each of these four large studies provided data indicating that ICS at moderate to high doses do not influence the rate of decline in lung function in patients with mild to severe COPD. Other important endpoints in these studies improved, e.g. baseline lung function, symptoms, airway hyper-responsiveness, health resource utilization and quality of life. There was a slight increase in some adverse events including bruising, reduction in bone mass density and reduction in mean cortisol levels in patients in the ICS groups. The characteristics and findings of these studies are summarized in Table 1.

Two recent meta-analyses have given conflicting results in relation to ICS and the rate of decline in lung function in COPD. As noted above, the first published meta-analysis[6] did

Table 1. Effects of inhaled corticosteroids on baseline lung function in stable COPD

Study	Patients (N)	Drug and dosage	Study design	Baseline FEV_1 (mean)	Duration of study	Change in FEV_1 (mean)	p value
Auffarth et al[3]	24	Budesonide 1600 µg daily or placebo	RCT	53% predicted	8 weeks	NS	NS
Weir and Burge[6]	105	Beclomethasone 1500 or 300 µg daily followed by ICS +/– prednisone 40 mg daily	RCT, parallel and sequential	1.07 L, 40% predicted	3 weeks placebo then 3 weeks BDP then 3 weeks BDP +/– prednisone	34% vs. 15% improved $FEV_1 > 20\%$ on BDP vs. placebo	<0.0005 vs. placebo
Weir et al[7]	127	Beclomethasone 1500 µg or prednisone 40 mg daily or placebo	RCT crossover study	1.19 L	3×2 weeks $+ 2 \times 2$ weeks washouts between	0.06 L; 20% increased FEV_1 in 26/107 patients	NS
Paggiaro et al[9]	281	Fluticasone 1000 µg daily or placebo	RCT	1.56 L	6 months	0.11 L FP vs. −0.04 L placebo	$p < 0.001$
Bourbeau et al[10]	79 oral steroid non-responders	Budesonide 1600 µg daily or placebo if no response to prednisone for initial 2 weeks	RCT after single blind 2 weeks prednisone	0.96 L	6 months	8 mls budesonide vs. 12 mL placebo	NS
Nishimura et al[11]	30	Beclomethasone 3000 µg daily or placebo	RCT crossover	0.97 L	2×4 weeks	11 mL BDP vs. 0 placebo	<0.001

show a small benefit in reducing the rate of the prebron-chodilator FEV_1 decline, but no effect on the post-bronchodilator FEV_1 decline. Subsequently, the three multi-centre prospective studies referred to above were unable to demonstrate an effect on decline in large numbers of patients from distinctly different subgroups, mild disease in continu-ing smokers (Euroscop), severe disease (ISOLDE) and mild to moderate COPD in smokers and non-smokers (LHS III). Fol-lowing this, a larger meta-analysis did not demonstrate any change in the rate of FEV_1 decline.[20] This study did not include two of the studies in the van Grunsven meta-analysis and, al-though the rate of decline was reduced (−5.0 mL/year), this was not significant [95% confidence interval (CI) −11.2 to 1.2, $P = 0.11$)], nor was the slightly larger change for more severe patients ($FEV_1 < 51\%$ predicted) at −11.0 mL/year reduction (95% CI −23.1 to 1.0 mL/year, $P = 0.10$).

The most recent meta-analysis suggests that there really is a small, statistically significant slowing of FEV_1 decline by ICS in COPD.[21] A comprehensive literature search for all RCTs com-paring ICS and placebo in COPD identified 82 possible trials, of which five remained after exclusion on the basis of follow-up < 1 year, inclusion of possible subjects with asthma, not a RCT with placebo or FEV_1 not the primary outcome. To the re-maining five RCTs of ≥ 2 years' duration were added the stud-ies included in the van Grusven meta-analysis,[6] giving eight trials in total ($n = 3715$ subjects). Data were abstracted from each article, and quantitative synthesis was performed using a random effects methodology and appropriate tests for hetero-geneity and bias. The analysis indicated that ICS significantly reduced the rate of decline of FEV_1 by 7.7 mL/year (95% CI 1.3–14.2, $P = 0.02$). Meta-analysis of studies with high-dose ICS (daily dose ≥ 800 μg BDP equivalent) showed a greater ef-fect on slowing the rate of FEV_1 decline (9.9 mL/year, 95% CI 2.3–17.5, $P = 0.01$), as did analysis of those patients with more severe COPD ($FEV_1 < 50\%$ predicted) where reduction in rate of FEV_1 decline was a mean of 18.3 mL/year (95% CI −1.5 to 38.0, $P = NS$).

In summary, individually, several large trials conducted in patients with varying severity of COPD showed no effect of ICS on rate of FEV_1 decline. However, the most recently pub-lished and comprehensive meta-analysis of all available RCT data indicates that there is a small, significant, dose-related and disease severity-related slowing of yearly rate of FEV_1 de-cline. Whether this is significant enough to be of clinical value and to justify long-term prescribing is a judgement that must be made in the overall context of the patient and their disease manifestations, as well as the cost-effectiveness in the particu-lar setting.

Other clinically important outcomes for COPD studies : more than lung function

Exacerbations of COPD
An enhanced understanding of the impact of COPD on quali-ty of life and activities of daily living has resulted more recent-ly in studies assessing the impact of treatment on psychosocial and physical functional measures in addition to objective measures of lung function. Lack of a clear definition of a COPD exacerbation has hampered progress in this area, but recent attempts to standardize the definition through COPD guidelines such as the Global Initiative for Obstructive Lung disease (GOLD)[9] have been helpful and are likely to result in a uniform approach to assessing exacerbations in clinical trials. Several studies have identified clinically important exacerba-tions as those that necessitate a change in treatment or prompt a patient to seek medical attention. A recent consensus state-ment included the definition of an exacerbation of COPD as a 'sustained worsening of the patient's condition from the stable state and beyond normal day-to-day variation, which is acute in onset and necessitates a change in regular medication'.[22]

Alsaeedi *et al.*[23] conducted a meta-analysis of nine random-ized trials (3976 subjects) and showed a significant benefit for ICS in reducing the rate of COPD exacerbations. Nine studies ($n = 3976$ patients) were included in the meta-analysis, which showed an overall risk reduction of about 30%: RR = 0.70 (95% CI 0.58–0.84).

Effects of ICS on inflammation in COPD
It is now well documented that airway inflammation is a fea-ture of COPD, but particular features of COPD have resulted in relatively slow progress being made in this area. Many of the studies have been performed in symptomatic patients who usually have moderate airflow limitation, which may repre-sent a more established stage of the disease. The inflammatory process appears to be most active in the small airways, which are not readily accessible to bronchoscopy and biopsy, and the airway obstruction develops as a result of peripheral airway disease, alveolar wall destruction and loss of elastic recoil. These processes may have different mechanisms, but both contribute to airflow limitation, so that it has been difficult to demonstrate clear relationships between inflammatory change and airway obstruction in COPD. The characteristic inflammation of COPD includes increased numbers of CD8+ T lymphocytes, neutrophils and mononuclear cells. Some in-vestigators have also demonstrated increased numbers of eosinophils in bronchial biopsies and higher concentrations of eosinophil cationic protein (ECP) in sputum and bron-choalveolar lavage fluid.

A MEDLINE search of COPD, ICS and airway inflamma-tion yielded only 15 titles. Of these, none was an RCT. Hand searching cross-references identified two randomized studies which are described below.

Culpitt and others[24] studied 13 patients treated with flutica-sone 500 μg or placebo bd for 4 weeks in a double-blind, crossover study. There were no clinical benefits on lung func-tion or symptom score. Induced sputum inflammatory cells, percentage neutrophils and interleukin (IL)-8 levels were unchanged. A number of cytokines thought to be active in

COPD were also unaffected by treatment. IL-8 levels were unchanged, and matrix metalloproteinase MMP-1 and MMP-9 were unaffected as was tissue inhibitor of metalloproteinase (TIMP)-1. The authors considered that inhaled corticosteroids did not affect the protease–antiprotease imbalance.

The effects of inhaled fluticasone on airway inflammation were examined in a double-blind, placebo-controlled biopsy study in 30 patients with COPD over a 3-month treatment period.[25] Subjects' mean age was 64.7 years, with a mean total of 63 pack–years of cigarette intake and mean FEV_1 of 1.28 L. Bronchoscopic bronchial biopsy was carried out at baseline and at the end of 3 months' treatment. Inhaled fluticasone had no effect on the defined primary endpoints, CD8+, CD68+ cells or neutrophils, nor on other features such as reticular basement membrane thickness. There was a reduction in the CD8:CD4 ratio in the epithelium and of the numbers of subepithelial mast cells in the fluticasone-treated group. Symptoms improved significantly during the treatment phase in the fluticasone-treated group (cough, sputum score and reliever medication use), and there was a significant reduction in exacerbation rate compared with placebo. A minority of subjects showed an improvement in FEV_1, and there was no difference between treatment groups.

In summary, there are few studies and very few consistent or impressive findings in relation to the effects of ICS on the airway pathology of COPD. The absence of an impressive effect of ICS on airway inflammation and in reducing the rate of lung function decline in patients with COPD suggests that the airway inflammatory changes are not highly responsive to ICS or, alternatively, may not be the cause of the progressive loss of lung function in this disease. The lack of effect on airway inflammation in COPD and the difficulty in linking clinical and pathological changes highlight our inadequate understanding of the pathogenesis of the disease.

Airway hyper-responsiveness

Several studies have examined the effect of ICS on airway hyper-responsiveness (AHR) in COPD. Twenty-three continuing smokers with COPD were randomized to receive either fluticasone 500 µg bd or placebo for 6 months. Patients eligible for this study had a clinical diagnosis of COPD, negative skin prick tests, an FEV_1 " 70% predicted normal and FEV_1 reversibility of less than 10% predicted after 750 µg of terbutaline. During the study period, FEV_1 showed a marked decline in the placebo group but remained stable in patients treated with fluticasone, while maximum expiratory flows improved in the fluticasone-treated group. Bronchial biopsy specimens taken at baseline and after 6 months of treatment showed only marginal (non-significant) changes in immunohistochemistry and cytokine staining. No significant changes in bronchial reactivity, maximal bronchoconstriction or EC_{50} were demonstrated, and there were no significant treatment by time interactions.

In a 6-week, randomized, placebo-controlled study of budesonide 1600 µg daily or placebo, AHR to methacholine and adenosine monophosphate (AMP) improved by 0.51 and 0.4 doubling concentrations, respectively, on budesonide, but this was not significantly different from placebo.[27] Budesonide significantly reduced serum IL-8 levels, but AMP was not different from methacholine in assessing short-term changes in AHR in the smokers with moderate to severe COPD.[27]

In the Lung Health Study,[19] those subjects taking triamcinolone had lower airway reactivity to methacholine at 9 months and 33 months compared with placebo. It seems, therefore, from these three RCTs that the effects of ICS on AHR in COPD are small and only evident after at least 6 months of treatment.

Quality of life

Health-related quality of life is known to be an important measure of disease progression and is used to assess the benefit of interventions in patients with COPD. Although generic quality of life questionnaires have been used, the most valuable (specific and sensitive) questionnaires have proved to be disease specific, and the St George's Respiratory Questionnaire (SGRQ) is the most widely used. A change of 0.5 for the chronic respiratory questionnaire (CRQ) and 4.0 for the SGRQ are thought to represent clinically important thresholds.[28,29] A number of cohort studies of patients with COPD have demonstrated poor quality of life in those with more severe disease and reduced life expectancy (SGRQ and SF 36). SGRQ total score is independently associated with mortality after adjustment for age, FEV_1 and body mass index in patients with COPD.[30]

The ISOLDE study demonstrated a reduced rate of decline in quality of life in moderately severe COPD patients treated over 3 years with fluticasone 500 µg bd compared with those receiving placebo.[18,31] A clinically important difference in quality of life score occurred more rapidly in the placebo group (approximately 15 months) compared with the fluticasone-treated group (approximately 24 months), indicating that fluticasone slowed the rate of decline of health-related quality of life in this group of patients. All SGRQ components (symptoms, activity and impacts—social and psychological effects of the disease) deteriorated faster in the placebo group. Given the larger number of drop-outs in the placebo group, this may have been an underestimation of benefit. There was a small, significant relationship between the rate of decline in SGRQ score and rate of decline in FEV_1, and worse health status was associated with lower baseline FEV_1. Patients with a high number of exacerbations had poorer quality of life, and the slower rate of decline in quality of life on fluticasone was associated with a reduced number of exacerbations.

Hospital readmission and health care resource utilization

In a 2.5-year study comparing regular short-acting β-agonists (SABA) and ICS, regular SABA and anticholinergic or regular SABA and placebo, 274 patients with moderately severe COPD were studied.[32] Compared with SABA alone, SABA and ICS resulted in significant improvements in FEV_1, AHR and symptom-free days. The cost of this was greater on regular SABA alone, but the savings in other health care costs overall in part compensated for this, and the authors concluded that adding ICS to SABA resulted in significant symptomatic and lung function benefits, which appeared to be worth this additional cost.[33] This study contained a heterogeneous population of patients, some of whom had asthma. The reduction in cost in patients taking regular SABA and ICS was more marked in those who did not smoke, who had more AHR and whose airway obstruction was more reversible, as well as in those who had a symptom-based diagnosis of asthma. The authors concluded that patients with 'an asthma profile' are more likely to benefit from ICS.

In a retrospective analysis of linked hospital and prescribing databases in Saskatchewan, the data from subjects aged over 55 years starting regular treatment for COPD with no history of asthma were analysed.[32] The cases were 846 patients with subsequent hospitalization for COPD from a cohort of 1742 subjects with a first hospitalization with a primary diagnosis of COPD. The remaining 843 cases were matched to 11 030 control person moments. There was no reduction in risk of hospitalization in patients taking ICS, even at high doses (> 800 μg daily of beclomethasone or equivalent).

Side-effects

To date, the most valuable data regarding side-effects of long-term administration of ICS come from the three large RCTs mentioned above. In the Lung Health Study,[19] after 3 years, there were no significant differences between the treatment groups in the number of subjects reporting cataracts, diabetes or myopathy. Lumbar spine bone mass density was measured at baseline, 1 year and 3 years in 328 subjects, and femoral neck bone mass density in 359 subjects. After 3 years' treatment, those on triamcinolone had a greater percentage decrease from baseline in bone density at lumbar spine and femoral neck than those taking placebo. Increased bone demineralization was evident in men and women. Those taking triamcinolone were more likely to report moderate or severe increased bruising.

In the Copenhagen study, budesonide 200 μg daily for 6 months followed by 400 μg twice daily for 13 months was well tolerated compared with placebo, and there was no specific pattern of non-severe adverse events noted.[17]

In the Euroscop study,[16] subjects were asked about corticosteroid-related side-effects at each visit, bruising area was measured, and all adverse events were recorded. Lateral thoracic and lumbar spine X-rays were obtained at baseline, and bone mineral density of the lumber spine and femoral neck was measured in 194 subjects. There were no significant changes over time and no significant effect of treatment on bone density except for a small but significant difference at the femoral trochanter in favour of budesonide. During the study, new fractures were unusual, and there was no significant difference between the treatments. Newly diagnosed hypertension, bone fractures, cataracts, myopathy and diabetes occurred in less than 5% of the subjects and were equally distributed. More subjects withdrew from the budesonide group because of non-severe adverse events (35 in the budesonide group versus 23 in the placebo group of a total 1277 subjects), predominantly due to oropharyngeal candidiasis, dysphonia and local throat irritation.

In the ISOLDE study,[18] bone density was not recorded, but morning serum cortisol concentrations and adverse events were noted. Serum cortisol concentrations were measured at randomization and every 6 months during the study. Reported adverse events were similar between treatments except for a slightly higher incidence of ICS-related side-effects in the fluticasone group (these included hoarseness, dysphonia, throat irritation and oral candidiasis). Bruising was also more common in the fluticasone-treated group. There was a significant but small decrease in mean serum cortisol concentrations in the patients taking fluticasone compared with placebo, but no more than 5% of patients on fluticasone had values below the normal range during the study at any time.

A Cochrane Review of the effect of ICS on bone metabolism in asthma and mild COPD[34] concluded from seven RCTs that there was no increased risk of bone density loss at conventional doses over 3 years (″ 1000 μg beclomethasone equivalent). However, this should be interpreted cautiously, as longer treatment periods and more severe disease in patients with limited mobility may result in different effects.

ICS withdrawal

Discontinuation of a therapy in question in a RCT is another way to assess its potential benefit.

In a 6-week, placebo-controlled, crossover study, 24 patients with moderate to severe COPD currently receiving beclomethasone were randomized to receive either beclomethasone 336 μg daily or placebo. Despite the low dose, surprisingly, there was a significant difference in favour of beclomethasone for the primary endpoint, showing a decrease in FEV_1 on placebo, but no significant differences for the other endpoints, walking distance and quality of life.[35]

In a larger and longer double-blind RCT, after 4 months' treatment with fluticasone 1000 μg daily, 244 patients with COPD were randomized to receive placebo or continue fluticasone for 6 months.[36] The hazard ratio for developing an exacerbation of COPD was 1.5 (95% CI 1.1–2.1) in the placebo group compared with the fluticasone group. In the placebo group, 21% of patients experienced rapid and frequent exacerbations compared with 4.9% in the fluticasone group. Discontinuation of fluticasone was associated with a poorer quality of life than continuing. This study does not prove that ICS are beneficial in COPD, but it does indicate that cessation after treatment may be harmful, probably because the fluticasone has a protective effect against exacerbations.

Mortality in COPD and the effect of ICS

ICS have significant benefit in reducing asthma mortality, and so it is reasonable to consider this possibility for COPD. Optimally, this information should be available from RCTs, but mortality as the primary endpoint requires a very large study, which has not yet been done. However, some recently published observational epidemiological studies shed light on the effect of ICS on mortality. While a large RCT is under way with mortality as the primary outcome, these epidemiological studies justify a brief comment.

In a population-based cohort observational study in Ontario, Canada ($n = 22\,620$), patients who received ICS therapy within 90 days of discharge from hospital had 24% fewer repeat hospitalizations for COPD and were 29% less likely to experience mortality during the 12-month follow-up period.[37] There were confounding factors, including the fact that those using ICS were slightly younger, less likely to have comorbidities and more likely to be taking other medications for COPD, specifically bronchodilators, oral corticosteroids, antibiotics and theophylline. The relative risk reduction for all-cause mortality was 29% in favour of ICS use. Receipt of other COPD medications was not associated with reduced mortality or hospital admission risk.

In a subsequent paper, linked hospital discharge data and prescribed medication data in Alberta, Canada, were used to follow all residents aged 65 years or older who had experienced at least one hospitalization for COPD between 1994 and 1998.[38] The study patients were followed for 3 years after the initial hospital admission or until death to determine whether a dose–response effect for ICS could be demonstrated in relation to mortality risk. The daily dose was divided into low dose ("500 µg daily beclomethasone or equivalent), median dose (501–1000 µg daily) or high dose (>1000 µg daily). Allowance was made for all prescriptions not dispensed, as well as indeterminate doses. ICS therapy after discharge was associated with a 25% relative reduction in risk in the all-cause mortality (0.75, 95% CI 0.68–0.82). Patients on medium- or high-dose ICS showed lower risks for mortality than those on low-dose therapy (RR 0.77, 95% CI 0.69–0.86 for low dose; RR 0.48, 95% CI 0.37–0.63 for medium dose; and RR 0.55, 95% CI 0.44–0.69 for high-dose inhaled steroids).

More recently, questions have been raised regarding the methodology used in these observational epidemiological studies.[39] There is disagreement between the authors of the two major studies (Sin and Tu versus Suissa) regarding the validity of the analysis in the Ontario study, where study subjects were deemed to be exposed to ICS if a prescription was received up to 90 days after hospital discharge. There was there-fore a group of subjects who were regarded as outcome free (as they were not yet registered as participants) for up to 90 days after discharge. This introduces the possibility of underestimating the primary endpoint (in this case, readmission or death) in the group identified as receiving inhaled steroids. Subsequent analysis indicated that about 10% of the follow-up time was affected by this. A further potential for bias existed in that subjects were identified as receiving ICS if they received one prescription within 90 days of discharge. The study does not therefore adequately relate dose or duration of exposure to ICS to the endpoints. Ideally, epidemiological data that link medication exposure and important endpoints such as hospital readmission or death should quantify the period of exposure as well as the dose of ICS, in order to provide more robust information about the protective effect of these medications.

Mortality benefit for patients receiving ICS has been assessed in a study based on data from the UK General Practice Research Database.[40] COPD patients who had been newly diagnosed between 1990 and 1999, aged ≥ 50 years old, with regular prescriptions (three prescriptions of respiratory medications over an initial 6 months) were identified, and 3-year survival was examined. A total of 1045 patients who regularly used salmeterol and/or fluticasone were compared with 3620 COPD patients who received neither drug. Cases were defined as patients who died within 1 year or more of follow-up, and each was matched with a COPD control patient within the cohort with the same data, diagnosis of COPD and similar follow-up period. COPD patients who were regular users of fluticasone and salmeterol showed significantly greater crude 3-year survival rates (78.6%) than the reference group (63.6%). Increasing age was predictive of mortality. After adjusting for confounders of age at entry, smoking, comorbidity, possible asthma and use of oral steroids, the survival observed in COPD users of salmeterol and/or fluticasone was highest in combined users (hazard ratio 0.48), followed by users of fluticasone alone (hazard ratio 0.62, 95% CI 0.45–0.85). A sensitivity analysis undertaken to determine 3-year survival rates in COPD patients who were regular users of any ICS demonstrated a class effect. Similar adjusted survival probabilities were identified for taking any ICS alone (77.9%) and any ICS plus salmeterol (82.1%).

Summary and clinical recommendations

There is Level I evidence that ICS have beneficial effects on a range of clinically important outcomes in COPD. These include symptoms, lung function, exercise capacity, FEV_1, quality of life and exacerbations. They have small positive effects in slowing the rate of lung function decline, but this is of uncertain clinical significance. It appears that patients with more severe disease may benefit more from long-term ICS use. Descriptive studies suggest that there is an effect on hospital admissions and mortality, but this has yet to be proven in RCTs. There is some weak evidence for a dose-related effect on some of these outcomes. However, randomized studies comparing different doses are needed before a firm conclusion can be drawn on the optimal dose in view of the increased risk of steroid-related adverse events at higher doses.

The weight of data favours using ICS for patients with COPD in the following circumstances:
- When patients are symptomatic due to airflow limitation, the FEV_1 is " 50% predicted, and benefit is evident to the patient.
- In patients with moderately severe disease, $FEV_1 < 50\%$ predicted who are suffering frequent exacerbations.

References

1 Turato G, Renzo Z, Miniati M *et al.* Airway inflammation in severe chronic obstructive pulmonary disease. Relationship with lung function and radiologic emphysema. *Am J Respir Crit Care Med* 2002; **166**:105–10.

2 Pesci A, Balbi B, Majori M *et al.* Inflammatory cells and mediators in bronchial lavage with patients with chronic obstructive pulmonary disease. *Eur Resp J*:1998; **12**:380–6.

3 Auffarth B, Postma DS, de Monchy JGR, van der Mark TW, Boorsma M, Koeter GH. Effects of inhaled budesonide on spirometric values, reversibility, airway responsiveness, and cough threshold in smokers with chronic obstructive lung disease. *Thorax* 1991; **46**:372–7.

4 Wardman AG, Simpson FG, Knox AJ, Page RL, Cooke NJ. The use of high-dose inhaled beclomethasone dipropionate as a mean of assessing steroid responsiveness in obstructive airways disease. *Br J Dis Chest* 1988; **82**:168–71.

5 Weir DC, Gove RI, Robertson AS, Burge PS. Response to corticosteroids in chronic airflow obstruction: relationship to emphysema and airways collapse. *Eur Resp J* 1991; **4**:1185–90.

6 Weir DC, Burge PS. Effects of high-dose inhaled beclomethasone. propionate, 750 micrograms and 1500 micrograms twice daily, and 40 mg per day oral prednisolone on lung function, symptoms, and bronchial hyperresponsiveness in patients with nonasthmatic chronic airflow obstruction. *Thorax* 1993; **48**:309–16.

7 Weir DC, Gove RI, Robertson AS, Burge PS. Corticosteroid trials in non-asthmatic chronic airflow obstruction: a comparison of oral prednisolone and inhaled beclomethasone dipropionate. *Thorax* 1990; **45**:112–17.

8 Weir DC. Time course of response to oral and inhaled corticosteroids in non-asthmatic chronic airflow obstruction. *Thorax* 1990; **45**:118–21.

9 Paggiaro PL, Dahle R, Bakran I *et al.* Multicenter randomized placebo-controlled trial of inhaled fluticasone propionate in patients with chronic obstructive pulmonary disease. *Lancet* 1998; **351**:773–80.

10 Bourbeau J, Rouleau MY, Boucher S. Randomized controlled trial of inhaled corticosteroids in patients with chronic obstructive pulmonary disease. *Thorax* 1998; **53**:477–82.

11 Nishimura K, Koyama H, Ikeda A *et al.* The effect of high-dose inhaled beclomethasone dipropionate in patients with stable COPD. *Chest* 1999; **115**:31–7.

12 Van Grunsven PM, Van Schayk CP, Derenne JP *et al.* Long-term effects of inhaled corticosteroids in chronic obstructive pulmonary disease: a meta-analysis. *Thorax* 1999; **54**:7–14.

13 Renkema TE. Effects of long-term treatment with corticosteroids in COPD. *Chest* 1996; **109**:1156–62.

14 Dompeling E, van Schayk CP, van Grusven PM *et al.* Slowing the deterioration of asthma and chronic obstructive pulmonary disease observed during bronchodilator therapy by adding inhaled corticosteroids. A four-year prospective study. *Ann Intern Med* 1993; **118**:770–8.

15 Kerstjens HAM, Brand PL, Hughes MD *et al.* A comparison of bronchodilator therapy with or without inhaled corticosteroid therapy for obstructive airways disease. *N Engl J Med* 1992; **327**:1413–19.

16 Pauwels R. Long-term treatment with inhaled budesonide in persons with mild chronic obstructive pulmonary disease who continue smoking. *N Engl J Med* 1999; **340**:1948–53.

17 Vestbo J. Long-term effect of inhaled budesonide in mild and moderate chronic obstructive pulmonary disease: a randomized controlled trial. *Lancet* 1999; **353**:1819–23.

18 Burge PS. Randomized, double-blind, placebo-controlled study of fluticasone propionate in patients with moderate to severe chronic obstructive pulmonary disease: the ISOLDE trial. *BMJ* 2000; **320**:1297–303.

19 Lung Health Study Research Group. Effect of inhaled triamcinolone on the decline in pulmonary function in chronic obstructive pulmonary disease. *N Engl J Med* 2000; **343**:1902–9.

20 Highland KB, Strange SE, Heffner JE. Long-term effects of inhaled corticosteroids on FEV1 in patients with chronic obstructive pulmonary disease. A meta-analysis. *Ann Intern Med* 2003; **138**:969–73.

21 Sutherland ER, Allmers H, Ayas NT, Venn AJ, Martin RJ. Inhaled corticosteroids reduce the progression of airflow limitation in chronic obstructive pulmonary disease: a meta-analysis. *Thorax* 2003; **58**:937–41.

22 Rodriguez-Roisin R. Towards a consensus definition for COPD exacerbations. *Chest* 2000; **117**(Suppl 2):398S–401S.

23 Alsaeedi A, Sin DD, Mc Alister FA. The effects of inhaled corticosteroids in chronic obstructive poverty disease: a systematic review of randomized placebo-controlled trials. *Am J Med* 2002; **113**:59–65.

24 Culpitt SV, Maziak W, Loukidis S, Nightingale JA, Matthews JL, Barnes PJ. Effect of high dose inhaled steroid on cells, cytokines, and proteases in induced sputum in chronic obstructive pulmonary disease. *Am J Respir Crit Care Med* 1999; **160**:1635–9.

25 Hattotuwa KL. The effects of inhaled fluticasone on airway inflammation in chronic obstructive pulmonary disease. *Am J Respir Crit Care Med* 2002; **165**:1592–6.

26 Verhoeven GT, Hegmans JPJJ, Mulder PGH, Bogaard JM, Hoogsteden HC, Prins J-B. Effects of fluticasone propionate in COPD patients with bronchial hyperresponsiveness. *Thorax* 2002; **57**:694–700.

27 Rutgers SR, Koeter GH, van der Mark TW, Postma DS. Short term treatment with budesonide does not improve hyperresponsiveness to adenosine 5′ monophosphate in COPD. *Am J Respir Crit Care Med* 1998; **157**:880–6.

28 Ferrer M, Villasante C, Alonso J *et al.* The interpretation of quality-of-life scores from the St Georges respiratory questionnaire. *Eur Respir J* 2002; **19**:405–13.

29 Jones PW. Interpreting clinically significant change in health status in asthma and COPD. *Eur Respir J* 2002; **19**:398–404.

30 Domingo-Salvany A, Lamarca R, Ferrer M *et al.* Health related quality-of-life and mortality in mild patients with chronic obstructive pulmonary disease. *Am J Respir Crit Care Med* 2002; **166**:680–5.

31 Spencer S, Calverley P, Burge P, Jones P. Health status deterioration in patients with chronic obstructive pulmonary disease. *Am J Respir Crit Care Med* 2001; **163**:122–8.

32 Bourbeau J, Ernst P, Cockcroft D, Suissa S. Inhaled corticosteroids in hospitalization due to exacerbation of COPD. *Eur Respir J* 2003; **22**:286–9.

33 Rutten-van Molken MPMH. Costs and effects of inhaled corticosteroids and bronchodilators in asthma and chronic obstructive pulmonary disease. *Am J Respir Crit Care Med* 1995; **151**:975–82.

34 Jones A, Fay JK, Stone M, Hood K, Roberts G. Inhaled corticosteroid effects on bone metabolism in asthma and mild chronic obstructive pulmonary disease. In: *The Cochrane Library*, Issue 4. Chichester, John Wiley & Sons, 2003.

35 O'Brien A, Russo-Magno P, Kraki A *et al*. Effects of withdrawal of inhaled steroids in men with severe irreversible airflow obstruction. *Am J Respir Crit Care Med* 2001; **164**:365–71.

36 van der Valk P, Monninkhof E, van der Palen J, Zielhuis G, van Herwaaden C. Effect of discontinuation of inhaled corticosteroids in patients with chronic obstructive pulmonary disease. *Am J Respir Crit Care Med* 2002; **166**:1358–63.

37 Sin DD, Jack VT. Inhaled corticosteroids and risk of mortality and readmission in elderly patients with chronic obstructive pulmonary disease. *Am J Respir Crit Care Med* 2001; **164**:580–4.

38 Sin DD, Man SFP. Inhaled corticosteroids and survival in chronic obstructive pulmonary disease: does the dose matter? *Eur Respir J* 2003; **21**:260–6.

39 Suissa S. Effectiveness of inhaled corticosteroids in chronic obstructive pulmonary disease: immortal time bias in observational studies. *Am J Respir Crit Care Med* 2003; **168**:49–53.

40 Soriano JB, Vestbo J, Pride NB *et al*. Survival in COPD patients after regular use of fluticasone propionate and salmeterol in general practice. *Eur Respir J* 2002; **20**:819–25.

Combination of inhaled corticosteroids and long-acting β_2-agonists in chronic obstructive pulmonary disease

Paul W Jones

Case scenario

A 74-year-old male with known chronic obstructive pulmonary disease (COPD) attended as an outpatient. He had been commenced on tiotropium 18 µg daily and terbutaline 500 µg turbuhaler as needed by his general practitioner. The new treatments had initially improved his symptoms but, over the last 4 months, he felt that his breathlessness was significantly restricting his daily activity. In addition, you note that he has had two 'chest infections' that required treatment with antibiotics and prednisolone. Spirometry showed that his forced expiratory volume in 1 second (FEV_1) was 1.30 L (50% predicted). He is asking what would be the advantage of adding a long-acting β_2-agonist or inhaled corticosteroid, either alone or in combination in a single inhaler?

Background

Long-acting β_2-agonists (LABA) and inhaled corticosteroids (ICS) are both recommended for use in patients with COPD, on the basis of large randomized controlled trials (RCTs). A number of recent studies have investigated the possibility that there may be an additive effect between these two agents. While the design of these studies may have been pragmatic, or even opportunistic, it has been hypothesized recently that there may be a beneficial interaction of these two classes of agent at a molecular level, as ICS increase the expression of β_2-receptors, and LABA may potentiate the molecular mechanisms of corticosteroid actions.[1] This has given rise to speculation that there may be synergism between them. There is also some evidence from trials in asthma that delivering both agents in one inhaler has a greater effect than administering the same dose of the two drugs concurrently but in different inhalers.[2] Before examining results of trials of LABA+ICS, it is very important to consider some aspects of trial design in COPD to understand where biases and limitations to generalizability could occur.

Clinical trials in COPD

Selection of trial outcomes

Most of the trials considered in this chapter were designed for new drug regulation purposes. This means that the choice of outcome was influenced by national regulatory authorities. Currently, the FEV_1 is always a primary outcome. Symptom-based co-primary endpoints are sometimes specified. Exacerbations have sometimes been predefined as a co-primary endpoint or used as a secondary endpoint, and some studies have been powered on the basis of exacerbations. Other secondary endpoints include health status (health-related quality of life), usually measured with either the St George's Respiratory Questionnaire (SGRQ) or the Chronic Respiratory Questionnaire (CRQ), and breathlessness measured using the Transitional Dyspnea Index (TDI). A variety of other outcomes may be assessed, including diary recordings, peak expiratory flow and COPD symptoms, but there is no agreed method of standardizing such measurements. The range of outcomes assessed in these trials matches quite closely the treatment objectives for COPD as recommended by the Global Initiative for Chronic Obstructive Pulmonary Disease (GOLD). Mortality, the only major outcome that is missing in the current trials, is being addressed in a large study of LABA+ICS (salmeterol plus fluticasone) that is currently under way, but will not report for another year.

FEV_1

The FEV_1 is the standard measure of treatment efficacy in COPD. It has major advantages in that there is a very large body of data using this measurement and it can be measured accurately and reliably in multicentre studies. There is no standardization of reporting, however, and values may be reported as pre- or post-bronchodilator, post-study treatment or 'trough' (a prebronchodilator measurement made in the morning before the first dose of the treatment drug). The major disadvantage with the FEV_1 is that it is a poor correlate of breathlessness during exercise[3] and impaired health.[4]

Exacerbations

Exacerbations of COPD are important because they cause hospital admissions and death, and it has been shown recently that even exacerbations that can be treated as an outpatient may have a large and prolonged impact on the patient's health.[5] There is no agreed method of identifying exacerbations, but most clinical trials use an operational definition based upon an increase in symptoms that require treatment with antibiotics and/or oral corticosteroids. Analysis of exacerbation data presents a number of challenges. For example, exacerbation frequency is often non-normally distributed. Furthermore, an exacerbation may be a predetermined reason for withdrawal. It is not possible to combine exacerbation data from trials of that type with data from those in which patients are retained in the study following an exacerbation.

Health status and breathlessness

These measurements can be made in a standardized manner and, unlike the other outcomes, there are agreed thresholds for what constitutes a clinically significant difference or change. Health status measurements have the very useful property of reflecting a wide range of effects of COPD, but this means that they can detect very readily the widely recognized benefit that patients can experience on entering the trial, regardless of treatment.

Inclusion criteria — patient selection

The standard inclusion criteria for all the trials reviewed in this chapter are a significant smoking history, absence of a history of asthma and an FEV_1 that does not return to normal following bronchodilator (in accordance with the GOLD definition of COPD). Two other criteria are often set. The first concerns a criterion for bronchodilator reversibility. This is in part historical, reflecting the old perception that COPD is an irreversible condition, and in part to avoid including asthmatic patients in COPD trials. The definition of reversibility is not based on evidence about the underlying disease, but upon the limits of between-day repeatability within an individual subject. There are a number of reasons why this entry criterion is becoming less appropriate. First, the bronchodilator response is normally distributed, with no evidence of a 'responder group', whether measured using short-acting bronchodilators[6] or following an oral corticosteroid trial.[7] Secondly, there is considerable between-day variability in response so that a patient's classification as 'responder' and 'non-responder' varies continually.[6] Thirdly, it has been reported that the correlation between the first-dose, short-term FEV_1 response to the long-acting bronchodilator tiotropium and the end-of-trial response in trough FEV_1 1 year later was $r = 0.43$.[8] In other words, only 18% of the variance between patients in the FEV_1

at 1 year was attributable to the difference in the acute response at baseline.

Another exclusion criterion may be an FEV_1 above a particular value. The value chosen is usually 50%, which coincides with a threshold between severity categories used in most COPD classification systems. Ideally, this should be the post-bronchodilator value, as this is a more repeatable measurement than the prebronchodilator value.[6] A high exacerbation frequency has also been used as an entry criterion in some studies. Patients are required to have had a minimum specified number of exacerbations requiring treatment in the year before the trial, but not in the weeks immediately prior to the trial. The potential conflict presented by the combination of these two requirements is clear. It should be noted that a criterion of low FEV_1 or high exacerbation rate may result in the inclusion of patients with similar characteristics, as patients with more severe airways obstruction have higher exacerbation rates.[9]

Run-in period

In nearly all these studies, the run-in period is short — typically 2 weeks. This is almost certainly too short to ensure that the patients are in a stable state at randomization to the study treatment, especially if there is an entry criterion that specifies severe patients with a history of frequent exacerbations. The effects of a single exacerbation on health status are large and take many weeks to recover from.[5] This is less of a problem with the FEV_1 as this changes little during a COPD exacerbation.[10] The run-in period is also used as a washout period for those patients taking ICS/LABA before entry to the study. Withdrawal from ICS may introduce a recruitment bias as ICS reduces the rate of exacerbations,[11] and withdrawal of ICS in COPD can lead rapidly to exacerbations in some patients.[12] As increasing numbers of patients have been prescribed ICS before entering these studies, patients who survive the run-in to reach the randomization stage will include, in part, patients who can withstand ICS withdrawal for 2 weeks without having an exacerbation. A recent modification of the run-in period has been adopted by one of the studies reviewed in this chapter, in which patients were given a period of treatment intensification with the long-acting LABA formoterol plus oral corticosteroid before being randomized to treatment.[13]

Trial duration

The recognition that COPD is a progressive disease and that treatments may take some time to reach full effectiveness has led to an increase in the duration of these studies in recent years, in part because of the requirements of regulatory authorities. The standard time is now 1 year in Europe, although 6-month studies are still conducted in the USA. Examination of data from recent trials shows clear justification for this approach. While the FEV_1 response occurs within days, health status and breathlessness improvements take longer to evolve (weeks or even months). Studies designed to measure the effect of treatment on exacerbations must have sufficient duration for the study to have sufficient power. Exacerbation rates reported in clinical trials in COPD are typically 1–1.5 per year. Trials of 6 months would need to be very large to have sufficient power. Furthermore, there is some evidence from published data that exacerbations may not occur at a consistent rate during a trial and that, while in some studies survival curves (for remaining within study) between treatment groups may begin to deviate from soon after the start,[13–15] this is not always the case.[16,17]

Withdrawals from COPD trials

Most patients withdraw from clinical trials because of worsening COPD. This creates a major problem because the dropouts do not occur at random. The active treatment improves the outcomes, but may also prevent some drop-outs. For that reason, there is a clear risk of a 'healthy survivor effect'. This has been documented well in the 3-year ISOLDE study in which it was shown that patients who dropped out were deteriorating faster than those who remained in the study.[17] This 'informative drop-out' rate will have its greatest effect on health status measurements as these are summative in nature. It should be noted that this may result in a conservative estimate of treatment efficacy, because the more severe patients in the placebo limb will be withdrawn, reducing the size of difference from those receiving active treatment. Currently, there is no statistical method of adjusting completely for this powerful bias.

Summary

It is clear that the inclusion criteria used for these trials, for the best of reasons, may influence the generalizability of the findings. The recent use of criteria based upon exacerbation frequency and severity of airway obstruction means that the resulting study populations are likely to be drawn from the same, more severe end of the COPD spectrum. This inclusion bias is likely to have a greater effect on the effect size and generalizability of the findings than any differences in short-term measurements of bronchodilator responsiveness. The requirement that patients receiving ICS prior to the study have to stop these in the run-in phase will bias towards exclusion of patients who need ICS to prevent exacerbations. Differential drop-out will result in a 'healthy survivor' effect particularly in placebo-treated patients. In short, the inevitable compromises that are necessary in clinical trial design will influence the results and are at least as likely to minimize treatment effects from longer term COPD trials as they are to inflate them.

Questions

1 In adults with COPD (population), is there evidence that ICS and LABA treatment (intervention) have an additive effect on the primary outcome (i.e. a proof of principle)? {therapy}

2 In adults with COPD (population), is there a difference between combination therapy and single agents (interventions) in clinical outcomes? {therapy}

3 In adults with COPD (population), does any difference between combination therapy and single agents (interventions) confer a significant advantage to the patient (outcome)? {therapy}

Literature search

There are currently six double-blind, randomized, controlled, clinical trials of LABA+ICS, but one of these[18] is very small compared with the others (18 patients versus 691–1465 patients), so will not be considered further here. All the remaining trials had four arms: LABA+ICS in one inhaler, LABA, ICS and placebo (Table 1). All used dry powder devices, and the LABA+ICS was combined in a single inhaler. All were carried out for new drug registration purposes under international good clinical practice (GCP) for clinical trials. The study populations fall into three broad groups: moderate COPD with higher reversibility;[19,20] moderate COPD with low reversibility;[15] moderate–severe COPD with moderate reversibility.[13,14]

A systematic review and meta-analysis[21] has been carried out on four of the trials available at the time (including the very small one not included here).

Abridged abstract of the Cochrane Review[21]

(Note: this was the abstract for the version of the review at the time of writing this chapter; Cochrane Reviews are updated and republished in the Cochrane Library on a regular basis.)

Main results

Four randomized trials with 2986 participants were included. No meta-analysis on clinical outcomes was possible due to different outcome assessment across studies. All studies demonstrated a reduction in exacerbation rates versus placebo. Budesonide/formoterol (BFC) was more effective than formoterol in reducing exacerbations in one study from 1.84 to 1.42 exacerbations per year. Fluticasone/salmeterol (FSC) did not significantly reduce exacerbations compared with either of its component treatments. FSC led to better quality of life compared with placebo (two studies), although there were conflicting results when compared with ICS alone (two studies). There was no significant difference between FSC and LABA (two studies). FSC led to statistically significant differences in quality of life compared with placebo, but not when compared with component ICS or LABA (one study).

Table 1. Characteristics of studies and study populations.

Study (first author)	No. of subjects	Age (years)	FEV$_1$ % predicted	FEV$_1$ reversibility (% baseline)	ICS LABA	Duration (months)
Mahler[19]	691	64	41%	20%	Fluticasone 500 Salmeterol 50	6
Hanania[20]	723	64	42%	20%	Fluticasone 250 Salmeterol 50	6
Szafranski[14]	812	64	36%	15%	Budesonide 320 Formoterol 9	12
Calverley[13]	1141	64	36%	15%	Budesonide 320 Formoterol 9	12
Tristan[15]	1465	63	46%	9%	Fluticasone 500 Salmeterol 50	12

Doses are in micrograms and were given twice daily. Age and FEV$_1$ data are means.
Note: dose of budesonide when given as monotherapy was 400 µg bd.

Reviewers' conclusions

For the primary outcome of exacerbations, BFC had a modest advantage over a component medication, formoterol, in a single trial, but FSC did not result in a significant reduction in exacerbations compared with either of its components. The combination of ICS and LABA in one inhaler was effective in improving symptoms compared with placebo and on certain clinical outcomes compared with one of the individual components alone.

The first observation about this abstract is that there is no mention of the results of the primary outcome variable. One reason for this is that numerical data (particularly standard errors, deviations or confidence intervals) were not reported in the majority of papers, in fact, in none of the 1-year studies. The Cochrane reviewers have still not been able to obtain these data from the sponsoring companies. Another problem that Cochrane reviewers face with trials of this nature is that the Cochrane analytical and data presentation software does not permit easy comparisons of four-arm studies. This is a major disadvantage because even the most casual reading of these five papers shows that LABA+ICS has an advantage over the single agents.

Question

1 In adults with COPD, is there evidence that ICS and LABA treatment have an additive effect on the primary outcome?

Spirometry results

Analysis of repeated measures data from long-term trials is complex, and results can be analysed and presented in many different ways. Graphical representation of results may contain means and distribution statistics (standard deviation, confidence intervals, etc.) made at one specific time point, but the estimates derived from modern statistical analyses do not necessarily match the raw data, as measured. Repeated measures analysis of variance was used in three of the studies reviewed here,[13–15] and the calculated means may be thought of as being averages over the study period. Another approach is an endpoint analysis, as applied in two studies.[19,20] This uses the last within-study measurement, which may be the last before withdrawal, not just measurements obtained in patients who remained until the end of the study. This is to ensure that all available data are used in the analysis. Other imputation techniques are used to account for data missed as a result of early withdrawal. The simplest and commonest is 'last number carried forward' where the last measurement obtained for a patient who withdraws from a trial is used as that patient's value at each measurement point up to the end of the study. Finally, most analyses adjust for differences at baseline due to factors such as gender, study centre, age, etc. using analysis of covariance and often report 'adjusted' estimates of the treatment effect.

Each statistical team will use a slightly different approach to analysis. It is not possible, therefore, to make precise direct quantitative comparisons of effect sizes between studies. Furthermore, this may not be possible even within a trial, using the primary analysis as published, as all these studies exhibit differential drop-out between treatment arms—with increasing imputation of data towards the end of the study. One final complication is that there is no agreed standard form of reporting FEV_1 data. In the trials reviewed here, the following were used: predose (i.e. study drug);[19,20] predose, 6 hours after reliever;[15] post-dose, 6 hours after reliever;[13] not stated.[14] The importance of specifying the timing of the measurement relative to study drug is illustrated in two of the trials, which show plots of changes in pre- and post-dose FEV_1.[19,20] Timing affected both the relative magnitude of effect and the relative ranking of effect of the component drugs, when used as monotherapy.

In an attempt to convey an indication of the effect of the treatments on the FEV_1 (the primary outcome) across the five trials, I have produced estimates in Table 2 of the changes from baseline to the end of absolute units (mL). These data must be treated as indicative values as they all needed manipulation to get them into a common format that would allow any form of comparison and data synthesis (meta-analysis is not possible with the available data). In some cases, this required measuring the final endpoint FEV_1 values from the figures with a ruler and back-calculating using percentage changes and the baseline absolute values. In one trial,[13] where the run-in consisted of a period of treatment intensification with oral corticosteroid and LABA, the FEV_1 result was presented as change from end of run-in, but only the change from beginning to end of run-in for the patients who subsequently received LABA+ICS is presented. I assumed that all treatment groups responded in the same way during that intensification phase. The precise numerical estimates contained in Table 2 will not be found in the text of the papers, for the reasons given above, but the relative sizes of effect between the treatment groups match those reported in the papers.

There appears to be a relatively consistent ranking of treatment effect. The ICS+LABA combination always produced the largest effect and, overall, the two components were jointly ranked second. In the two shorter studies, the improvement in predose (i.e. prebronchodilator) FEV_1 was greater with ICS than with LABA. This was due to a sustained slow improvement over the whole study period in the ICS group. These two studies also reported 2-hour post-dose FEV_1. The relative ranking of the ICS and LABA was now reversed. This is not unexpected. The duration of action of LABA does not extend beyond 12 hours, whereas the effect of ICS on FEV_1 is not dependent on dosing frequency in the same way. In contrast, in the Tristan study, which used the same ICS and LABA as the two 6-month studies, the relative efficacy of the single agents was the same, whether measured pre- or post-bronchodilator.[15]

The two, almost identical 6-month studies[19,20] reported FEV_1 results in subgroups categorized according to acute bronchodilator response (reversibility was determined as change > 12% and 200-mL change from baseline). The mean bronchodilator response in these two groups of patients is reported only for one study,[20] but is likely to be very similar in the other. In those classified as less reversible, the mean reversibility was 8% from baseline; in those who were more reversible, it was 30%. Meta-analysis of these data in Figure 1 shows that the mean improvement with LABA+ICS compared with placebo was higher in those with more reversibility. The weighted mean difference (WMD) was 200 mL, 95% confidence interval (CI) 150–250 mL compared with those with less reversibility: WMD 120 mL, 95% CI 70–170 mL. The difference in means was not statistically significant.

The data from these trials show very clearly that there is an additive effect of LABA and ICS on FEV_1, regardless of the study population. Precise quantification of this effect will prove difficult. There was a small difference in improvement in FEV_1 over 6 months between patients with a large acute bron-

Table 2. Relative differences in estimated FEV_1 change (mL) from baseline to end of study.

Study (first author)	Drugs	LABA+ICS	LABA	ICS	Placebo
6-month studies					
Mahler[19]	FS	182*†‡	119*	134*	−19
Hanania[20]	FS	170*†	93*	121*	4
12-month studies					
Tristan[15]	FS	114*†‡	12*	12*	−36
Szafranski[14]	BF	80*‡	38*	−11*	−57
Calverley[13]	BF	135*†‡	59*	23	2
Mean rank		1	2 =	2 =	4

These are calculated estimates derived from figures in the primary papers to show relative differences, as values for absolute change in FEV_1 were not presented in a manner that permitted direct comparison. Tests of significance are as reported from the analysis in primary papers: $P < 0.05$ *versus placebo, †versus LABA, ‡versus ICS. FS, fluticasone/salmeterol; BF, budesonide/formoterol.
Note: Calverley[13] employed an intensification period of oral steroids and LABA for 2 weeks before randomization. The changes shown here are calculated from the baseline, before treatment intensification.

chodilator response and those with much less acute reversibility, but this was not statistically significant.

Question

2 In adults with COPD, is there a difference between combination therapy and single agents in clinical outcomes?

Exacerbations

All three 1-year studies defined moderate–severe exacerbations in the same way: worsening symptoms and the need for oral corticosteroids and/or antibiotics or hospitalization.[13–15] All three studies contained an entry requirement that the patients had to have experienced one or more exacerbations requiring treatment in the preceding year. Patients were retained in the study unless judged too ill to continue. In the 6-month studies, exacerbations were defined in the same way, but patients were withdrawn after the first exacerbation that required oral or inhaled corticosteroids or hospitalization, or

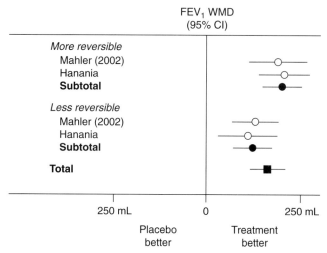

Figure 1. Meta-analysis of the effect of the combination of salmeterol plus fluticasone on predose FEV_1 in patients categorized in terms of size of acute response to bronchodilator. WMD, weighted mean difference. Bars are 95% confidence intervals.

after the third exacerbation requiring antibiotics.[19,20] Meta-analysis of the data from the 1-year studies is not yet possible because of inadequate data reporting but, for comparative purposes, the reported mean exacerbation results are presented in Table 3. There is a clear rank ordering of effect. Exacerbations were lower in the combination group than in the monotherapy groups. The exacerbation rates in the placebo group show that these populations were rather different. This is important, because treatment can only reduce exacerbations if they are occurring; however, even in the study with the lowest number of exacerbations, the size of effect in the combined group compared with placebo was of the same order of magnitude as in the other two studies (~25% reduction). It will be noted that the apparent advantage of budesonide/formoterol over its components was due to the absence of an effect of these agents on exacerbations,[13,14] unlike the study of fluticasone/salmeterol in which both components had an advantage over placebo.[15]

Question

3 In adults with COPD, does any difference between combination therapy and single agents confer a significant advantage to the patient?

Breathlessness

The 1-year trials used diary cards to collect daily symptoms, but this methodology is not standardized between studies, and clinical significance has not been established, so these data will not be considered here. The two 6-month studies used the Transition Dyspnea Index (TDI), a validated instrument for which the clinical threshold has been established.[22] Meta-analysis is not possible because distribution statistics are not available for one study,[20] but the mean results from these two, otherwise very similar, studies are conflicting (Table 4). There was a clear placebo effect in both studies, but in one, the improvement in the LABA+ICS group was approximately one TDI unit (the clinical threshold) more than either of the single agents, and this was statistically significant.[19] In contrast, in the other study, whereas the combination had a significantly

Table 3. Mean exacerbation rates (annualized).

Study (first author)	Drugs	LABA+ICS	LABA	ICS	Placebo
Tristan[15]	FS	0.97*	1.04*	1.05*	1.3
Szafranski[14]	BF	1.4*†	1.8	1.85	1.9
Calverley[13]	BF	1.38*‡	1.85	1.6	1.8
Mean rank		1	2	3	4

FS, fluticasone/salmeterol; BF, budesonide/formoterol. Tests of significance are as reported from the analyses in the primary papers: $P < 0.05$ *versus placebo, †versus LABA, ‡versus ICS.

greater effect than placebo, it was no more effective than the single agents alone.[20] There is no explanation for this difference. In one of the studies, the TDI response to LABA+ICS was reported, split by acute bronchodilator response: more reversibility group TDI 2.2, standard error (SE) 0.4; less reversible group 1.9, SE 0.4.[19] The TDI score in placebo-treated patients was 0.3, SE 0.3 (more reversible) and 0.4, SE 0.3 (less reversible). In this study, the acute bronchodilator response did not predict symptomatic benefit.

Health status

Health status was measured using two instruments, the CRQ and the SGRQ. The data are summarized in Table 5. End of study data reported from the 6-month studies are presented as in the primary papers. For the 1-year studies, data at 12 months were extracted from the figures[13,15] or text.[14] Three main patterns emerge: (a) the combination was, with one exception, the most effective treatment in each trial; (b) only the

combination treatment produced a consistent effect that was around, or above, the threshold for clinically significant improvement with these instruments (CRQ +10 units, SGRQ −4 units); (c) the component drugs given alone were less consistent in effect, as well as being less effective.

Study withdrawals

Most patients withdrew from the 1-year studies because of respiratory-related events. A previous analysis has shown that patients who are withdrawn have more severe airways obstruction, more exacerbations and a faster rate of deterioration in health status.[17] For these reasons, withdrawal may be a valid surrogate marker of overall treatment efficacy in double-blind, randomized, controlled trials. Table 6 presents the drop-out rates for the 1-year studies. A weighted mean was calculated per treatment arm. On average, 27% of LABA+ICS-treated patients withdrew, compared with 41% of placebo patients. The component arms occupied intermediate positions of 33–36%. Put another way, if withdrawal corresponds to a serious treatment failure, this occurred in approximately a quarter of patients treated with combination, a third of those receiving one of the components alone and in 40% of those in the placebo group (who just had short-acting bronchodilators).

Side-effects

There was a large difference between studies in reported adverse event rates, which included, among others, COPD-related events and those obviously linked to ICS use. One study did not report oropharyngeal side-effects.[14] There were different methods of reporting in the other four, but there was a consistent pattern: placebo 0–1%; LABA < 1–3%; ICS 2–10%; ICS+LABA 2–10%. Rates of skin bruising were not reported,[13,19,20] 'none reported'[14] or not different (6–8%)

Table 4. Change in breathlessness measured after 6 months using the Transition Dyspnea Index.

Study (first author)	LABA+ICS	LABA	ICS	Placebo
Mahler[19]	2.1*†‡	0.9	1.3	0.9
Hanania[20]	1.7*	1.6	1.7	1.0

Both studies used fluticasone and salmeterol. A change of + 1 unit is considered to be clinically significant. Tests of significance as reported from the analyses in the primary papers: P< 0.05 *versus placebo, †versus LABA, ‡versus ICS.
Note: in Hanania,[20] significance for LABA versus placebo was reported to be P= 0.023, LABA versus placebo P= 0.043 and ICS versus placebo P= 0.057.

Table 5. Changes in health status scores from baseline to end of study.

Study (first author)	Drugs	LABA+ICS	LABA	ICS	Placebo
Mean changes in CRQ scores					
Mahler[19]	FS	10.0*†‡	8.0	4.8	5.0
Hanania[20]	FS	10.0*	6.4	10.4*	5.0
Mean change in SGRQ score					
Tristan[15]	FS	−4.5	−2.4	−2.8	−2.8
Szafranski[14]	BF	−3.9*	−3.6	−1.9	0.0
Calverley[13]	BF	−7.0*†‡	−3.1*	−3.2*	+0.3
Mean rank		1	3	2	4

These are estimates derived from data or figures in the primary papers to show relative differences between treatment arms. Tests of significance as reported from the analysis in the primary papers: P< 0.05 *versus placebo, †versus LABA, ‡versus ICS. FS, fluticasone/salmeterol; BF, budesonide/formoterol; CRQ, Chronic Respiratory Questionnaire (high score is better); SGRQ, St George's Respiratory Questionnaire (low score is better). Note: Claverley[13] employed an intensification period of oral steroids and LABA for 2 weeks before randomization. The changes shown here are calculated from the baseline, before treatment intensification.

Table 6. Drop-out rates (% of those in treatment arm).

Study (first author)	Drugs	LABA+ICS	LABA	ICS	Placebo
Tristan[15]	FS	25	32	29	39
Szafranski[14]	BF	28	32	31	44
Calverley[13]	BF	29	44	40	41
Weighted mean		27	36	33	41

FS, fluticasone/salmeterol; BF, budesonide/formoterol.

between treatment arms.[15] Different measures of adrenal suppression were reported.[15,19,20] There was no evidence of suppression in any of the ICS- or combination-treated patients compared with LABA or placebo. The total number of deaths reported from four studies were: combination 11; ICS 11; LABA 19; placebo 17. One study did not report deaths.[15]

Conclusions

The five large medium-term studies reviewed here show the same pattern of efficacy of the combination of LABA+ICS, both within and between studies. Regardless of the outcome selected, the combination produced a larger and more consistent effect than either of the components when used alone. The studies offer no guide as to which combination is more effective as the studies were carried out in study populations with different characteristics, but there is little evidence to suggest that future studies will identify large differences.

The relative consistency in the pattern of results across different outcomes and across quite different study populations suggests that these results will be generalizable to a wide range of patients with moderate–severe COPD. The studies also provide some useful insights into the size of response to be expected in different groups of patients. The patients in the 6-month trials had less severe airway obstruction and a larger acute bronchodilator response than those in the 1-year trials. They also had larger improvements in prebronchodilator FEV_1. (At this point, it should be noted that there is no evidence that the patients in the 6-month trials had asthma, it is just that the triallists did not impose an entry criterion for patients with COPD with a maximum level of acute bronchodilator reversibility.) The apparent difference in the size of effect on FEV_1 between the 6-month and 1-year trials does not justify any recommendation to the effect that decisions about this therapy should be made on the basis of an acute bronchodilator response. Subgroup analysis of the 6-month trial data showed that, while there was a difference in the improvements in prebronchodilator FEV_1 between those with greater and less acute reversibility, this was not significant. These results are in agreement with a previous study[8] and show that the acute bronchodilator response is too weak as a predictor of longer term FEV_1 benefit to be reliable in clinical practice.

Furthermore, in one of the 6-month studies, the size of the improvement in dyspnoea was the same regardless of bronchodilator responsiveness.[19]

While the effect of combination treatment on the FEV_1 may have been smaller in the more severe patients, the effect on health status was comparable to that seen in the milder patients. Furthermore, one of the clear benefits of combination treatment is on exacerbation frequency. Exacerbations are more common with more severe airway obstruction, so the effect of this treatment may increase with disease severity.[9] This effect was confirmed in a subgroup analysis of the Tristan study, in which the patients were categorized into more severe and less severe using a cutpoint on baseline FEV_1 of 50% predicted.[15] The reduction in exacerbations with combination therapy in the more severe group was 30%, whereas in the milder patients, it was 10%.

This review has shown that combination therapy is better than monotherapy, but the question of clinical significance remains. This is a complex topic that has been addressed elsewhere in the context of health status measurement.[23] The studies reviewed here show that only the combination produced improvements in dyspnoea and health status that were consistently at or above the threshold for clinical significance. While these benefits were not always significantly greater than with the components, the latter usually did not produce clinically significant effects or were inconsistent between studies. It seems a little perverse to advocate the use of less effective and less consistent therapy on the basis of the differences between combination and monotherapy reported here. Continuing this argument, one might reason that, because the single components in these trials did not have a worthwhile effect, they should not be used either.

The issue of magnitude of effect on exacerbations is more controversial. The effect of the combination was to reduce the exacerbation rate by about 25%. This has led to the view being aired to the effect that: 'reducing one exacerbation in four is not very much'. This is a surprising value judgement to anyone who has talked to patients about their fear of exacerbations and the amount of distress that it causes them. Furthermore, it is not a view that is evidence based. Exacerbations carry with them the risk of hospital admission and death. A single exacerbation has a very large effect on patients' lives with a recovery period measured in months,[5] and there is an association between exacerbation frequency and health status.[24] Furthermore, there is now clear evidence that health status decline is linked to exacerbation frequency and that this decline may be prevented by reducing exacerbations.[25]

Clinical trials produce average estimates of treatment efficacy. Even if the mean effect lies above a threshold of clinical significance, more information is needed to gain an idea of the benefit to individual patients. One approach is to calculate the number of patients who need to be treated (NNT) to prevent an exacerbation or to produce one patient who has a clinically significant improvement in breathlessness or health status. Unfortunately, the data currently available do not allow such calculations, but a previous analysis of the effect of salmeterol in COPD calculated that the NNT was about five to produce one patient with a clinically significant improvement in SGRQ score compared with placebo.[23]

Differences in design of clinical trials sometimes lead to intriguing results. The two budesonide/formoterol studies recruited almost identical types of patient. The only difference between them was that one followed the standard approach of a 2-week run-in period with pretrial treatment washout before randomization,[14] whereas the other used that period to intensify the patients' therapy with a standard regime of formoterol and oral corticosteroid.[13] There were slightly fewer drop-outs in the latter study, but the more obvious differences were that the health status effects of the combination were much larger, and the FEV_1 effects were greater in all treatment groups. This poses the question as to whether treatment with ICS+LABA should begin with a course of oral corticosteroids. It is not possible to answer this at present, but further analysis of these two trials is needed.

Summary for clinicians

The results of these trials largely support current GOLD recommendations that long-acting bronchodilators should be the first-line maintenance therapy for COPD. GOLD suggests that ICS should be reserved for patients with FEV_1 less than 50% predicted. That recommendation is not strictly evidence based, but is linked to the association between degree of airway obstruction and exacerbation frequency. However, in a 3-year study, over 40% of patients with an $FEV_1 > 50\%$ predicted had one or more exacerbations per year.[9] This observation, coupled with the data from the trials reviewed here, suggests that patients who have troublesome symptoms and one or more exacerbations per year should receive an ICS in addition to LABA, regardless of the FEV_1.

Author's statement

I was co-ordinating editor of the Cochrane Airways Group until recently, but did not edit the review of LABA+ICS. I have been a principal investigator on trials of salmeterol,[26] fluticasone,[9,11] tiotropium[27] and one of the trials reviewed here.[15] I have spoken at meetings about the treatment of COPD using LABA+ICS sponsored by the makers of both the products reviewed here. I have spent much time over the last 10 years thinking about trial design, analysis, biases and data interpretation, and in editing systematic reviews. In writing this chapter, I have endeavoured to bring my background experience to this work in as impartial a manner as possible.

References

1 Barnes PJ. Scientific rationale for inhaled combination therapy with long-acting β₂ agonist and corticosteroids. *Eur Respir J* 2002; **19**:182–91.

2 Nelson HS, Chapman KR, Pyke SD, Johnson M, Pritchard JN. Enhanced synergy between fluticasone proprionate and salmeterol inhaled from a single inhaler versus separate inhalers. *J Allergy Clin Immunol* 2003; **112**:29–36.

3 Belman MJ, Botnick WC, Shin JW. Inhaled bronchodilators reduce dynamic hyperinflation during exercise in patients with chronic obstructive pulmonary disease. *Am J Respir Crit Care Med* 1996; **153**:967–75.

4 Jones PW. Health status measurement in chronic obstructive pulmonary disease. *Thorax* 2001; **56**:880–7.

5 Jones PW. Time course of recovery of health status following an infective exacerbation of chronic bronchitis. *Thorax* 2003; **58**:589–93.

6 Calverley PMA, Burge PS, Spencer S, Anderson JA, Jones PW, Investigators ftIS. Bronchodilator reversibility testing in chronic obstructive pulmonary disease. *Thorax* 2003; **58**:659–64.

7 Burge PS, Calverley PMA, Jones PW, Spencer S, Anderson JA, Group obotIS. Prednisolone response in patients with chronic obstructive pulmonary disease: results from the ISOLDE study. *Thorax* 2003; **58**:654–8.

8 Tashkin D, Kesten S. Long-term treaatment benefits with tiotropium in COPD patients with and without short-term bronchodilator responses. *Chest* 2003; **123**:1441–9.

9 Jones PW, Willits LR, Burge PS, Calverley PMA. Disease severity and the effect of fluticasone proprionate on chronic obstructive pulmonary disease exacerbations. *Eur Respir J* 2003; **21**:1–6.

10 Seemungal TA, Donaldson GC, Bhowmik A, Jeffries DJ, Wedzicha JA. Time course and recovery of exacerbations in patients with chronic obstructive pulmonary disease. *Am J Respir Crit Care Med* 2000; **161**:1608–13.

11 Burge PS, Calverley PM, Jones PW, Spencer S, Anderson JA, Maslen TK. Randomised, double blind, placebo controlled study of fluticasone propionate in patients with moderate to severe chronic obstructive pulmonary disease: the ISOLDE trial. *BMJ* 2000; **320**(7245): 1297–303.

12 van der Valk P, Monninkhof E, van der Palen J, Zielhuis G, Herwaarden C. Effect of discontinuation of inhaled corticosteroids in patients with chronic obstructive pulmonary disease: the COPE study. *Am J Respir Crit Care Med* 2002; **166**:1358–63.

13 Calverley PMA, Boonsawat W, Cseke Z, Zhong N, Peterson S, Olsson H. Maintenance therapy with budesonide and formoterol in chronic obstructive pulmonary disease. *Eur Respir J* 2003; **22**:912–19.

14 Szafranski W, Cukier A, Ramirez A *et al.* Efficacy and safety of budesonide/formoterol in the management of chronic obstructive pulmonary disease. *Eur Respir J* 2003; **21**:74–81.

15 Calverley PMA, Pauwels R, Vestbo J, Jones PW, Pride NAG. Combined salmeterol and fluticasone in the treatment of chronic obstructive pulmonary disease. *Lancet* 2003; **361**:449.

16 Vincken W, van Noord JA, Greefhorst AP *et al.* Improved health out-

comes in patients with COPD during 1 year's treatment with tiotropium. *Eur Respir J* 2002; **19**:209–16.

17 Calverley PMA, Spencer S, Willits LR, Burge PS, Jones PW. Withdrawal from treatment as an outcome in the ISOLDE study of COPD. *Chest* 2003; **124**:1350–6.

18 Dal Negro RW, Pomari C, Tognella S, Micheletto C. Salmeterol and fluticasone 50 microg/250 microg bid in combination provides a better long-term control than salmeterol 50 microg bid alone and placebo in COPD patients already treated with theophylline. *Pulmon Pharmacol Therapeut* 2003; **16**:241–6.

19 Mahler DA, Wire P, Horstman D *et al.* Effectiveness of fluticasone proprionate and salmeterol combination delivered via the diskus device in the treatment of chronic obstructive pulmonary disease. *Am J Respir Crit Care Med* 2002; **166**:1084–91.

20 Hanania NA, Darken P, Horstman D *et al.* The efficacy and safety of fluticasone proprionate (250 mcg)/salmeterol (50 mcg) combined in the Diskus inhaler for the treatment of COPD. *Chest* 2003; **124**:834–43.

21 Nannini L, Lasserson TJ, Poole P. Combined corticosteroid and long-acting β-agonist in one inhaler for chronic obstructive pulmonary disease (Cochrane Review). In: *The Cochrane Library.* Chichester, John Wiley & Sons, 2004.

22 Mahler DA, Weinberg DH, Wells CK, Feinstein AR. Measurements of dyspnea. Contents, interobserver correlates of two new clinical indices. *Chest* 1984; **85**:751–8.

23 Jones PW. Interpreting thresholds for clinically significant changes in health status in asthma and COPD. *Eur Respir J* 2002; **19**:398–404.

24 Seemungal TAR, Donaldson GC, Paul EA, Bestall JC, Jefferies DJ, Wedzicha JA. Effect of exacerbation on quality of life in patients with chronic obstructive pulmonary disease. *Am J Respir Crit Care Med* 1998; **157**:1418–22.

25 Spencer S, Calverley PMA, Burge PS, Jones PW. Impact of preventing exacerbations on deterioration of health status in COPD. *Eur Respir J* 2004; **23**:1–5.

26 Jones PW, Bosh TK. Changes in quality of life in COPD patients treated with salmeterol. *Am J Respir Crit Care Med* 1997; **155**:1283–9.

27 Casaburi R, Mahler DA, Jones PW *et al.* A long-term evaluation of once daily inhaled tiotropium in chronic obstructive pulmonary disease. *Eur Respir J* 2002; **19**:209–16.

CHAPTER 3.5

Systemic corticosteroids in stable chronic obstructive pulmonary disease

Richard Wood-Baker

Case scenario

A 64-year-old male was referred to the outpatient department by his general practitioner for investigation of breathlessness on exercise. This had been getting worse over the last 8 years, and he was now having to stop and rest when walking back from buying the paper each morning (grade 3 functional limitation on the Medical Research Council grading of dyspnoea). He denied any wheeze, but admitted to having a 'smoker's cough' with clear sputum production each morning for several years. He had begun smoking at the age of 14, but regarded himself as a 'light' smoker, as he only consumed a pack of 20 cigarettes each day. He had worked as a groundsman all his life, denied any exposure to chemical sprays and had retired last year when he found he could no longer manage all his work tasks because of breathlessness. He had been given a number of puffers by his general practitioner, which he collectively described as 'useless'.

Physical examination revealed a thin gentleman (body mass index of 19.2 kg/m^2), without digital clubbing, peripheral lymphadenopathy, central or peripheral cyanosis. The respiratory rate was 20 breaths/min, pulse 96 beats/min and blood pressure 150/90. The trachea was in the mid-line and chest expansion limited to 2 cm. The percussion note was resonant, with absence of cardiac or hepatic dullness, and breath sounds were vesicular with the occasional expiratory wheeze. Spirometry revealed a forced expiratory volume in 1 second (FEV$_1$) of 0.8 L, forced vital capacity (FVC) of 1.5 L, FEV$_1$/FVC ratio of 53% before bronchodilator and FEV$_1$ of 0.85 L, FVC of 1.9 L, FEV$_1$/FVC ratio of 45% following bronchodilator administration.

Background

Oral corticosteroids were first found to be effective in the treatment of airways disease through their activity in asthma and, as airway inflammation is characteristic of both asthma and chronic obstructive pulmonary disease (COPD), it was logical to assess their effect in COPD. There are theoretical reasons why corticosteroids may be active in COPD, as many of their actions result in suppression of the inflammatory process by inhibition of cytokine secretion [interleukin (IL)-3

to -8, tumour necrosis factor and granulocyte–macrophage colony-stimulating factor (GM-CSF)], inhibition of cyclo-oxygenase and effects on a range of inflammatory cell types. Early studies of the effect of oral corticosteroids in COPD were promising, with uncontrolled studies using the self-reporting of symptoms such as breathlessness, wheeze or exercise capacity as outcomes demonstrating positive results.[1] Whether oral corticosteroids confer a significant benefit in more rigorous studies using objective outcomes is less clear cut.

Questions

1 In adults with stable COPD (population), will treatment with oral corticosteroids (intervention) improve symptoms (outcome) when compared with placebo? {therapy}
2 In adults with COPD (population), will treatment with oral corticosteroids (intervention) improve lung function or other objective measures (outcome) when compared with placebo? {therapy}
3 In adults with COPD (population), will treatment with oral corticosteroids (intervention) affect disease progression (outcome) compared with placebo? {therapy}
4 In adults with COPD (population), can the response to oral corticosteroids (intervention) be predicted? {prognosis}

Literature search

This chapter reviews the evidence for the use of systemic corticosteroids (oral or intravenous) in the management of stable COPD. Unfortunately, a Cochrane systematic review on the topic is not available, although a relevant protocol is registered with the Cochrane Collaboration.[2] As a result, the evidence is obtained from electronic searches of commonly used databases and hand searching reference lists of articles retrieved. This is not as robust as a systematic review in its approach to literature searching, and is subject to deficiencies associated with 'journalistic reviews'.[3] In obtaining evidence for this chapter, two search strategies were used. The first was 'adrenal cortex hormones OR corticosteroids OR prednisone OR prednisolone OR cortisone OR cortisone acetate OR methyl prednisolone AND pulmonary disease, chronic obstructive OR COPD OR chronic obstructive airways disease OR COAD OR chronic airflow limitation OR CAL OR chronic bronchitis OR emphysema' run in December 2002 on EMBASE and MEDLINE. The second was 'adrenal cortex hormone* or steroid* or glucocorticoid* or corticoid* or corticosteroid* or beclomethasone or betamethasone or fluticasone or cortisone or dexamethasone or hydrocortisone or prednisolone or prednisone or methylprednisolone or methylprednisone or triamcinolone' run in August 2003 on the Cochrane Airways Group COPD trials register.

Question

1 In adults with stable COPD, will treatment with oral corticosteroids improve symptoms when compared with placebo?

While symptom control may be studied over short periods, the subjective nature of the outcomes requires strict blinding as to intervention. Of the studies retrieved that included symptoms as an outcome, only nine were adequately blinded for treatment administration and included a placebo control (Table 1). The studies used a range of outcome measures, including disease-related symptom scores, e.g. breathlessness, cough and general well-being. Self-reporting of symptoms using scales or descriptors, including breathlessness or exercise capacity, was common. Only one study[4] used a comprehensive quality of life assessment. The majority of studies failed to demonstrate a significant improvement in symptoms directly related to the COPD, particularly dyspnoea. However, when looking at the subjects' overall perception of their well-being, two studies by Mitchell et al.[5,6] found either an overall improvement in well-being score or a substantial difference in the number of subjects reporting an improvement with corticosteroids. The best measurement of well-being was performed by Brightling et al.[4] using the Chronic Respiratory Disease Questionnaire (CRQ).[7] Despite failing to find a consistent improvement in respiratory symptoms of cough, sputum production, dyspnoea or wheeze using visual analogue scales, there was a small, but statistically significant, mean improvement in the CRQ score for corticosteroid treatment when compared with placebo. This improvement did not reach a magnitude accepted as being clinically relevant (an increase greater than 0.5) for the group as a whole, although this was achieved by subjects with the highest baseline sputum eosinophil count.

Overall, randomized controlled studies have not demonstrated a consistent benefit for corticosteroid treatment on disease symptoms, including cough, sputum production, dyspnoea or wheeze. There is evidence of a positive treatment effect on subjects' quality of life, but the most rigorous study suggests that the benefit does not reach a clinically significant level in all patients.

Question

2 In adults with COPD, will treatment with oral corticosteroids improve lung function or other objective measures when compared with placebo?

A range of lung function parameters has been used to study the effect of corticosteroids in COPD, including spirometry, maximum breathing capacity, maximum voluntary ventilation, minute ventilation, mid-expiratory flow, arterial blood gases, oxygen saturation, walking tests and transfer factor. Of these, spirometric measures have been most commonly reported and the forced expiratory volume in 1 second (FEV_1) was combined in a meta-analysis by Callahan et al.[8] published in 1991. The search strategy was limited to English language studies retrieved from MEDLINE and review of the bibliographies in articles identified by the search. To be included in the analyses, a study needed to be a clinical trial, subjects had to be randomized to treatments, a placebo control treatment arm was required, investigators had to be blinded (to treatment allocation), and there needed to be objective pre- and post-treatment assessment of lung function. Studies using parenteral corticosteroids or adrenocorticotrophic hormone were excluded. Subjects had to have stable COPD, while those subjects with asthma or COPD patients having recently experienced an exacerbation of their disease were specifically excluded. Using these predetermined inclusion and exclusion criteria, 43 potential studies were identified in the literature and, following independent review by three physicians, 10 were included in the meta-analysis.

The 10 included studies were mainly performed at university hospital outpatient clinics in North America and the UK. A total of 299 subjects were included in the analysis, with drop-out rates of 0–26% in the various studies. The subjects were elderly, with a mean smoking history greater than 30 pack–years and a mean FEV_1 of less than 1.1 L in most studies, consistent with a diagnosis of COPD. A variety of treatment regimens was used; the most common active treatment was prednisolone 40 mg daily, and the most common duration of treatment was 2 weeks. The studies all reported treatment effects as change in FEV_1 compared with baseline measurements. The investigators used a 20% improvement in the FEV_1 to define a response to treatment, and then compared the proportion of responders in active and placebo treatment groups. The benefit of oral corticosteroid treatment over placebo ranged from 0 to 38% of subjects, with a weighted mean treatment effect of 10% [95% confidence interval (CI) 2–18%]. The mean effect was not altered by changing the definition of a response, nor by sensitivity analysis for study

Table 1. The effect of corticosteroids on symptoms in COPD.

Study (first author)	Subjects	Design	Interventions	Subjective outcome
Moyes[1]	55 subjects with chronic bronchitis	Double-blind parallel group	Prednisolone 5 mg tds versus 'placebo' (aminophylline 0.1 mg tds). Treatment period = 4 months. Co-intervention with tetracycline 250 mg tds	Dyspnoea (Fletcher's questions) Active: 11 better, 14 unchanged, 2 worse. Placebo: 9 better, 17 unchanged, 2 worse
Morgan[24]	7 subjects with chronic bronchitis	Double-blind crossover with 6-week washout period	Betamethasone 3.6 mg daily for 3 days then betamethasone 1.8 mg daily for 25 days versus placebo	Several subjects noted an improvement in their general sense of well-being during corticosteroids, not noted during placebo
Shim[25]	24 subjects with chronic bronchitis and >30 pack–years smoking	Double-blind crossover with 1-week washout period	Prednisolone 30 mg daily versus placebo. Treatment period = 1 week	Wheezing: active = 6 improved, placebo not reported Other symptoms not reported
O'Reilly[10]	10 males with chronic bronchitis	Double-blind crossover without a washout period	Prednisolone 10 mg tds versus placebo. Treatment period = 2 weeks	Subjective walking ability, oxygen cost diagram and rating of perceived exertion not significantly different between interventions
Mitchell[5]	43 subjects with chronic airflow limitation, breathlessness on exertion and tobacco smoking	Double-blind crossover without a washout period	Prednisolone 40 mg daily versus placebo. Treatment period = 2 weeks	Breathlessness score: active = 2.7, placebo = 2.8 (NS) Oxygen cost diagram: active = 6.7, placebo = 6.2 (NS) Well-being analogue: active = 7.6, placebo = 6.5 ($P < 0.05$)
Strain[11]	14 subjects with stable COPD	Double-blind crossover with 2-week washout period	Methylprednisolone 32 mg daily versus placebo. Treatment period = 2 weeks	Exercise tolerance: active = 4 improved, placebo = 1 improved
Eliasson[26]	16 subjects with chronic bronchitis	Double-blind crossover with 2-week washout period	Prednisolone 40 mg daily versus placebo. Treatment period = 2 weeks	Cough, sputum production and dyspnoea scores not significantly different between interventions
Mitchell[6]	33 subjects with chronic airflow limitation, breathlessness on exertion and tobacco smoking	Double-blind crossover without a washout period	Prednisolone 40 mg daily versus placebo. Treatment period = 2 weeks	Breathlessness score: active = 6 improved, placebo = 4 improved. Oxygen cost: active = 7 improved, placebo = 5 improved. General well-being: active = 8 improved, placebo = 4 improved
Syed[27]	20 subjects with chronic airflow limitation (19 chronic bronchitis) and tobacco smoking	Double-blind crossover with a 2-week washout period	Prednisolone 30 mg daily versus placebo. Treatment period = 2 weeks	Dyspnoea: active = 3 improved, placebo = 3 improved
Brightling[4]	67 subjects with chronic airflow limitation	Double-blind crossover with a 4-week washout period	Prednisolone 30 mg daily versus placebo. Treatment period = 2 weeks	Chronic Respiratory Disease Questionnaire: mean difference active versus placebo = 0.32 (95% CI 0.17–0.47, $P = 0.0001$)

quality. Publication bias was eliminated using a funnel plot and estimate of the number of negative studies needed to change the outcome. The investigators concluded that a 20% improvement in FEV_1 in patients with stable COPD would occur 10% more often in those treated with corticosteroids than by placebo. The mean increase in FEV_1 was not ascertained, and neither was it possible to determine the optimal dose or duration of treatment. A number of limitations of the study were recognized, in particular the limitation to English language studies and the variability of FEV_1 measurements affecting baseline values.

Since publication of the meta-analysis, a number of other studies have been performed which include treatment periods with both oral corticosteroids and placebo. These are often in trials involving comparison with other interventions, particularly inhaled corticosteroids (Table 2). None of these studies have found oral corticosteroids to have a statistically significant effect on lung function over placebo treatment. Whether adding these data to the studies included in the meta-analysis by Callaghan will change the overall outcome remains to be defined. Individual patient data from studies indicate that a minority of subjects may have a large increase in their FEV_1 following treatment with oral corticosteroids.[9] Whether this response is repeatable over time or any increase in FEV_1 is associated with improved symptom control remains unestablished.

A range of outcomes other than FEV_1 has been used to assess the effect of corticosteroids on lung function but, with the exception of exercise capacity, none has been assessed in a rigorous manner. As exercise limitation due to breathlessness is a common complaint among patients with COPD, any effect of corticosteroids on exercise capacity has obvious significance. Four published studies have measured exercise performance, two of which used 12-min walking distance, one a shuttle walking test and one a multistage incremental exercise test on a cycle ergometer. Although the mean exercise capacity, where reported, was higher following corticosteroid treatment than placebo, the difference only reached statistical significance in one study. O'Reilly et al.[10] found that the mean increase in walking distance compared with pretreatment was 4.6% for corticosteroid and 4.8% for placebo. Mitchell et al.,[6] defining a significant improvement as >20% increase in 12-min walking distance, found that 18% of subjects improved only during corticosteroid therapy, compared with 3% with placebo, but 39% improved during both treatment arms. Strain et al.,[11] using cycle ergometry, also found no significant difference between placebo and corticosteroid, whether measured as maximum oxygen uptake or maximal work. Only Brightling et al.[4] found a statistically significant improvement with systemic corticosteroid treatment, with a mean increase in the walking distance of 12 m. Thus, on the basis of current data, there is no clear evidence that the short-term administration of oral corticosteroids improves exercise capacity.

Question

3 In adults with COPD, will treatment with oral corticosteroids affect disease progression when compared with placebo?

The likelihood of determining any effect of corticosteroids on disease progression appears to be low, as few studies reported

Table 2. The effect of corticosteroids on FEV_1 in COPD.

Study (first author)	Subjects	Design	Interventions	Outcomes
Syed[27]	20 subjects with chronic airflow limitation (19 chronic bronchitis) and tobacco smoking	Double-blind crossover with a 2-week washout period	Prednisolone 30 mg daily versus placebo. Treatment period = 2 weeks	Post-bronchodilator FEV_1: Active: before = 0.87 ± 0.28, after = 0.91 ± 0.28; Placebo: before = 0.89 ± 0.26, after = 0.91 ± 0.26; No significant difference between treatments
Weiner[28]	44 subjects with COPD	Double-blind crossover with 4-week washout period (subjects received inhaled corticosteroids at other periods in the study)	Prednisolone 40 mg daily versus placebo. Treatment period = 6 weeks	No change in mean FEV_1 during treatment with either active or placebo medication
Brightling[4]	67 subjects with chronic airflow limitation	Double-blind crossover with a 4-week washout period	Prednisolone 30 mg daily versus placebo. Treatment period = 2 weeks	Mean FEV_1: Active: before = 1.03, after = 1.09; Placebo: before = 1.09, after = 1.08; Mean difference = 0.07 (95% CI 0.01–0.14, $P = 0.02$)

are of more than 28 days' duration. However, a small number of studies allow some assessment of long-term outcomes, including prevention of exacerbations, decline in lung function or mortality. Renkema *et al.*,[12] in a parallel group study, treated 58 COPD subjects with placebo, inhaled corticosteroids or inhaled and oral corticosteroids for 2 years. Only 5% of subjects had an increase in FEV_1 of greater than 20%, in response to an oral corticosteroid trial prior to randomization. After excluding 19% of subjects, no significant difference was found between treatment groups for disease exacerbations. Disease progression, measured as the median rate of decline in FEV_1, was lower in both active treatment groups than placebo (placebo −60 mL/year; inhaled corticosteroid −30 mL/year; combined −40 mL/year), although these differences did not reach statistical significance. Surprisingly, given the general relationship between lung function and symptoms in COPD, the rate of decline in FEV_1 was not reflected in symptom control. A composite symptom score was unchanged at 2 years in the placebo group but fell in both active treatment arms, despite the lesser decline in FEV_1. While the differences in symptom scores were statistically significant, their clinical significance is not clear.

As for all pharmacological agents, the benefits of oral corticosteroid treatment for COPD have to be weighed against the risks. This may be problematic for older drugs, where the risks associated with treatment are often not well established as a consequence of inadequate reporting of adverse drug effects in older studies. In keeping with this, few studies of systemic corticosteroids in COPD report adverse effects, despite the range of major adverse effects known to occur. These include an increased risk of infections, glucose intolerance, hypertension, development of posterior subcapsular cataracts, myopathy, cutaneous effects and psychological changes.[13] Perhaps of greatest concern are the adrenal-suppressive effects and promotion of osteoporosis. Impairment of adrenal function has been found on testing hypothalamic–pituitary–adrenal axis function in patients taking oral corticosteroids for a range of chronic diseases[14] but, despite this, low serum cortisol levels are unusual. Renkema *et al.*[12] found that morning cortisol concentrations remained within the normal range in all subjects with COPD, despite the mean concentration decreasing during corticosteroid treatment. In practice, while there is often evidence of biochemical adrenal insufficiency related to systemic corticosteroid treatment, clinical effects appear to be rare.[15] More alarming is the role that corticosteroids play in the development of osteoporosis, given the increasing prevalence and costs associated with this disease.[16] Corticosteroid-induced bone loss begins within 6–12 months of commencing treatment, characteristically occurring fastest in trabecular bone, which accounts for the ribs and vertebrae being

Table 3. The effect of corticosteroids on exercise capacity in COPD.

Study (first author)	Subjects	Design	Interventions	Outcomes
O'Reilly[10]	10 males with chronic bronchitis	Double-blind crossover without a washout period	Prednisolone 10 mg tds versus placebo. Treatment period = 2 weeks	Mean 12 MWD (m): Baseline = 792.9 Active = 869.9 (change = 4.6%) Placebo = 831.3 (change = 4.84%) No significant difference between interventions
Strain[11]	14 subjects with stable COPD	Double-blind crossover with 2-week washout period	Methylprednisolone 32 mg daily versus placebo. Treatment period = 2 weeks	Mean V_{O_2}max/work: Active = 13.9 ± 1.1/65 ± 6 Placebo = 13.0 ± 1.1/61 ± 7 No significant differences between treatments
Mitchell[6]	33 subjects with chronic airflow limitation, breathlessness on exertion and tobacco smoking	Double-blind crossover without a washout period	Prednisolone 40 mg daily versus placebo. Treatment period = 2 weeks	Change in 12 MWD: Active = 6 improved Placebo = 1 improved
Brightling[4]	67 subjects with chronic airflow limitation	Double-blind crossover with a 4-week washout period	Prednisolone 30 mg daily versus placebo. Treatment period = 2 weeks	Mean walking distance (m): Active: before = 217 ± 13, after = 230 ± 14; Placebo: before = 213 ± 12, after = 214 ± 12; Mean difference = 12 (95% CI 3–21, $P = 0.01$)

common sites of fracture. A clinically important fall in bone density has been shown to occur in those taking ≥7.5 mg of prednisolone or equivalent, and current oral corticosteroid treatment is associated with a doubling of the risk of sustaining a hip fracture. How these data apply to the COPD population is unclear. While there is clearly an increased risk of osteoporosis in patients with COPD,[17] factors other than corticosteroids, including tobacco smoking and reduced activity, may contribute. If data from asthmatics receiving oral corticosteroids are extrapolated, in whom the annual incidence of vertebral fracture is up to 42%, it seems likely that similar treatment in COPD will substantially increase the risk in a population already predisposed.

While the precise risk of morbidity from systemic corticosteroids in patients with COPD cannot be accurately defined, recent evidence from observational studies indicates that long-term oral corticosteroids may be associated with an increase in mortality. Sin and Tu[18] used a hospital discharge diagnosis of COPD in patients over 65 years of age to study the effect of inhaled corticosteroids on subsequent rehospitalization and mortality. A secondary outcome in this study revealed

that the prescription of oral corticosteroids was associated with an increased odds ratio of death (OR = 1.37, 95% CI 1.25–1.50). In a further study of 556 patients with COPD participating in an inpatient rehabilitation programme, Schols et al.[19] also found an increased risk of subsequent death in subjects receiving oral corticosteroids. The risk occurred in a dose–response manner, with a relative risk of 2.34 (95% CI 1.24–4.44) for 10 mg/day prednisolone and 4.03 (95% CI 1.99–8.15) for 15 mg/day. Interestingly, both studies showed the prescription of inhaled corticosteroids to have a protective effect on mortality, whether administered alone or in conjunction with oral corticosteroids.

Question

4 In adults with COPD, can the response to oral corticosteroids be predicted?

The minority of subjects in studies who do have a substantial improvement following corticosteroid treatment has led to a

Table 4. Predictors of a positive effect of corticosteroids in COPD.

Study (first author)	Subjects	Design	Interventions	Outcomes
Harding[21]	36 subjects with chronic bronchitis and long-standing cigarette smoking	Single-blind, sequential treatment study of placebo, inhaled steroids and oral steroids	Placebo 30 mg daily versus placebo. Treatment period = 7–10 days	FEV_1 response more likely in subjects with peripheral blood eosinophilia or variability in baseline lung function
Shim[25]	24 subjects with chronic bronchitis and tobacco smoking >30 pack–years	Double-blind crossover with a 1-week washout period	Prednisolone 30 mg daily versus placebo. Treatment period = 1 week	Significant relationship between sputum eosinophilia and FEV_1 response
Syed[27]	20 subjects with chronic airflow limitation (19 chronic bronchitis) and tobacco smoking	Double-blind crossover with a 2-week washout period	Prednisolone 30 mg daily versus placebo. Treatment period = 2 weeks	No predictive factors found
Pizzichini[20]	20 subjects with chronic airflow limitation, chronic bronchitis and cigarette smoking	Single-blind sequential treatment	Prednisolone 30 mg daily versus placebo. Treatment period = 2 weeks	Sputum eosinophilia associated with improvement in effort dyspnoea, quality of life and FEV_1, not seen in subjects without sputum eosinophilia
Davies[22]	127 subjects with COPD	Open label	Prednisolone 30 mg daily. Treatment period = 2 weeks	Subjects with >15% improvement in FEV_1 had significantly higher mean peripheral blood eosinophil count than non-responders ($P<0.001$)
Brightling[4]	67 subjects with chronic airflow limitation	Double-blind crossover with a 4-week washout period	Prednisolone 30 mg daily versus placebo. Treatment period = 2 weeks	Mean improvement with active treatment increased progressively across tertiles for sputum eosinophil count ($P=0.003$)

number of studies trying to identify factors that predict a response to systemic corticosteroids. The factors identified to date include variability in lung function measurements over time and eosinophilia, either in peripheral blood or in sputum. Both Brightling et al.[4] and Pizzichini et al.[20] found that, when subjects were divided according to the proportion of eosinophils in the sputum, those with the highest proportions had a significantly higher chance of having an increase in FEV_1 in response to oral corticosteroids. There has been debate as to whether these findings represent a subgroup of patients with co-existent asthma, where the efficacy of corticosteroids is well established, or a population of patients with COPD in whom the typical neutrophil infiltrate in the airways is accompanied by eosinophilic inflammation.[21]

Using a different approach, Davies et al.[22] studied a group of patients with COPD for 1 year following a 2-week trial of oral corticosteroids to look at the predictive value of oral corticosteroid administration on subsequent response to inhaled corticosteroids. Subjects were divided into three groups, according to whether they achieved a FEV_1 response greater than 15% to inhaled β-agonist or oral corticosteroid. Twenty three per cent of subjects had a response to both challenges and were maintained on inhaled corticosteroids over the next year, as were a proportion of the other groups. While there were no significant changes in any measures in the unresponsive group, the responsive subjects had a higher mean FEV_1 and lower mean symptom score at 1 year when compared with baseline. As a group, the responsive subjects had higher mean eosinophil counts and were more likely to be skin prick test positive than the other groups, but neither was a good predictor for individual corticosteroid responsiveness. Although a response to oral corticosteroids seemed to be a predictor of benefit from long-term treatment with inhaled corticosteroids in this study, this was not found in the ISOLDE study.[23] This discrepancy may reflect the difference in bronchodilator responsiveness between subjects in the Davis (FEV_1 change >15%) and ISOLDE (FEV_1 change <10%) studies. The conflicting evidence means that the role of short periods of treatment with oral corticosteroids to identify patients with COPD who will benefit from long-term inhaled corticosteroids remains undetermined.

Conclusion

There is evidence to indicate that short-term administration of oral corticosteroids results in about 10% of patients with stable COPD having a significant (20% of baseline) improvement in their FEV_1. Oral corticosteroids also produce a statistically significant improvement in exercise capacity and quality of life in patients with COPD. The mean change in exercise capacity and quality of life is not clinically significant, although there is considerable intrasubject variation in response. There are data to suggest that patients with COPD who have the largest responses to oral corticosteroids are predicted by the presence of blood or sputum eosinophilia. Moreover, this may represent a subgroup that will benefit from inhaled corticosteroids in the long term and explains why not all studies have shown a treatment benefit from inhaled corticosteroids. There is no evidence that treatment with oral corticosteroids improves symptoms or alters the rate of decline in lung function. Given recent observational studies reporting a dose–response association between oral corticosteroid prescription and mortality, it seems prudent to limit the exposure of patients with COPD to systemic corticosteroids, irrespective of whether this is a cause and effect relationship.

Summary for clinicians

Oral corticosteroids will improve the FEV_1 by 20% from baseline in 10% of patients with COPD following short-term administration.

Although oral corticosteroids produce a statistically significant mean improvement in exercise capacity and quality of life, these do not reach clinically significant levels.

Long-term administration of oral corticosteroids in patients with COPD does not affect the decline in FEV_1.

Acknowledgements

The author would like to acknowledge the work of the Airway Review Group staff and Editorial staff for their support over recent years.

References

1 Moyes E, Kershaw R. Long-continued treatment with tetracycline and prednisolone in chronic bronchitis: a controlled trial. Lancet 1957; 2:1187–91.
2 Stanbrook M, Kaplan A, Juurlink D, Poole P. Systemic corticosteroids for stable chronic obstructive pulmonary disease. In: The Cochrane Library, Issue 4. Chichester, John Wiley & Sons, 2003.
3 Oxman A, Cook D, Guyatt G. Users' guides to the medical literature. VI. How to use an overview. JAMA 1994; 272(17):1367–71.
4 Brightling C, Monteiro W, Ward R et al. Sputum eosinophilia and short-term response to prednisolone in chronic obstructive pulmonary disease: a randomised controlled trial. Lancet 2000; 356:1480–5.
5 Mitchell D, Gildeh P, Rahahn M, Dimond A, Collins J. Effects of prednisolone in chronic airflow limitation. Lancet 1984; 8396:193–6.
6 Mitchell D, Gildeh P, Dimond A, Collins J. Value of serial peak expiratory flow measurements in assessing treatment response in chronic airflow limitation. Thorax 1986; 41:606–10.
7 Guyatt G, Berman L, Townsend M, Pugsley S, Chambers L. A measure of quality of life for clinical trials in chronic lung disease. Thorax 1987; 42:773–8.
8 Callahan C, Dittus R, Katz B. Oral corticosteroid therapy for patients with stable chronic obstructive pulmonary disease. Ann Intern Med 1991; 114:216–23.
9 Mendella L, Manfreda J, Warren C, Anthionisen N. Steroid response in stable chronic obstructive pulmonary disease. Ann Intern Med 1982; 96:17–21.

10 O'Reilly J, Shaylor J, Fromings K, Harrison D. The use of the 12 minute walking test in assessing the effect of oral steroid therapy in patients with chronic airways obstruction. *Br J Dis Chest* 1982; **76**:374–82.

11 Strain D, Kinasewitz G, Franco D, George R. Effect of steroid therapy on exercise performance in patients with irreversible chronic obstructive pulmonary disease. *Chest* 1985; **88**:718–21.

12 Renkema TE, Schouten JP, Koeter GH, Postma DS. Effects of long-term treatment with corticosteroids in COPD. *Chest* 1996; **109**:1156–62.

13 Axelrod L. Glucocorticoid therapy. *Medicine* 1976; **55**:39–65.

14 Schlaghecke R, Kornely E, Santen R, Ridderskamp P. The effect of long-term glucocorticoid therapy on pituitary–adrenal responses to exogenous corticotrophin-releasing hormone. *N Engl J Med* 1992; **326**:226–30.

15 McEvoy C, Niewoehner D. Adverse effects of corticosteroid therapy for COPD. *Chest* 1997; **111**:732–43.

16 Reid I. Osteoporosis—emerging consensus. *Aust NZ J Med* 1997; 27:643–7.

17 Smith B, Phillips P, Heller R. Asthma and chronic obstructive airway diseases are associated with osteoporosis and fractures: a literature review. *Respirology* 1999; **4**:101–9.

18 Sin D, Tu J. Inhaled corticosteroids and the risk of mortality and readmission in elderly patients with chronic obstructive pulmonary disease. *Am J Respir Crit Care Med* 2001; **164**:580–4.

19 Schols A, Wesseling G, Kester A *et al.* Dose dependent increased mortality risk in COPD patients treated with oral glucocorticoids. *Eur Respir J* 2001; **17**:337–42.

20 Pizzichini E, Pizzichini M, Gibson P *et al.* Sputum eosinophilia predicts benefit from prednisone in smokers with chronic obstructive bronchitis. *Am J Respir Crit Care Med* 1998; **158**:1511–17.

21 Harding S, Freedman S. A comparison of oral and inhaled steroids in patients with chronic airways obstruction: features determining response. *Thorax* 1978; **33**:214–18.

22 Davies L, Nisar M, Pearson M, Costello R, Earis J, Calverley P. Oral corticosteroid trials in the management of stable chronic obstructive pulmonary disease. *Q J Med* 1999; **92**:395–400.

23 Burge P, Calverley P, Jones P, Spencer S, Anderson J, Maslen T. Randomised, double blind, placebo controlled study of fluticasone propionate in patients with moderate to severe chronic obstructive pulmonary disease: the ISOLDE trial. *BMJ* 2000; **320**:1297–303.

24 Morgan W, Rusche E. A controlled trial of the effects of steroids in obstructive airway disease. *Thorax* 1964; **39**:924–7.

25 Shim C, Stover D, Williams M. Response to corticosteroids in chronic bronchitis. *J Allergy Clin Immunol* 1978; **62**:363–7.

26 Eliasson O, Hoffman J, Trueb D, Frederick D, McCormick J. Corticosteroids in chronic obstructive pulmonary disease. A clinical trial and reassessment of the literature. *Chest* 1986; **89**:484–90.

27 Syed A, Hoeppner V, Cockcroft D. Prediction of nonresponse to corticosteroids in stable chronic airflow limitation. *Clin Invest Med* 1991; **14**:28–34.

28 Weiner P, Weiner M, Rabner M, Waizman J, Magadle R, Zamir D. The response to inhaled and oral steroids in patients with stable chronic obstructive pulmonary disease. *J Intern Med* 1999; **245**:83–9.

CHAPTER 3.6

Lung volume reduction

Tudor P Toma and Duncan M Geddes

Case scenario

The patient of Dr RWB was sent for review 2 years later. He was now able to do even less, having difficulty showering and dressing in the morning and being more reliant on his wife. Full lung function was performed, which showed forced expiratory volume in 1 second (FEV_1) = 0.82 L (42% predicted), forced vital capacity (FVC) = 2.03 L (81% predicted), ratio 41% prebronchodilator, and FEV_1 = 0.78 L, FVC = 1.96 L, ratio 40% postbronchodilator. The total lung capacity (TLC) = 7.46 L (160% predicted), residual volume (RV) = 2.12 L (237% predicted), diffusion of carbon dioxide across the lung (D_LCO) = 9.58 mL/min/mmHg (46% predicted) and lung diffusion of alveolar ventilation (D_LVA) = 3.2 mL/min/mmHg (72% predicted).

He complained that none of the medications given to him so far had made any difference to his breathlessness, but he had seen a programme on the television where someone had undergone surgery for emphysema. He wondered if he was a suitable candidate for this operation and, if so, what would be the benefits to him?

Background

Lung volume reduction surgery (LVRS) is a symptomatic treatment intended for patients with disabling breathlessness due to emphysema. LVRS was first introduced in the 1950s by Dr Otto Brantigan, who postulated that, by resecting the destroyed parts of the lungs, the elasticity of the healthy parts of the lung would be restored and the mechanics of breathing improved. His first results, published in 1959, showed symptomatic improvement in 75% of patients with benefits apparently lasting for approximately 5 years.[1,2] However, the mortality was unacceptably high at 16–19%, and there was no objective evidence of lung function benefit; the procedure was criticized and abandoned.

LVRS in its modern form resurfaced in the 1990s, after Cooper *et al.* published their results with a procedure similar to Brantigan's in 20 patients with severe emphysema. In his initial case series, Cooper *et al.* showed no mortality and a striking 82% improvement in FEV_1 6 months after surgery.[3]

This kind of surgery was revisited in the 1990s as a bridge to transplantation because of advances in the care of critically ill patients, improvement in surgical technology and a multidis-

ciplinary approach to patient care, which reduced the surgical risk. However, despite good results from initial case series, the evidence supporting LVRS was not universally accepted. Initial data were derived from observational studies, when frequent changes to patient care protocols and surgical techniques did not allow the rigorous standards required for a randomized clinical trial to be met. But the cost implications of LVRS forced its evaluation using the conventional criteria of drug-based treatments. So, a large multicentre randomized trial was set up in the USA, the National Emphysema Treatment Trial (NETT).[4] NETT is a clinical trial that compared lung volume reduction surgery with medical therapy for severe emphysema; it is one of the biggest trials of its type to be published.[5] In addition to NETT, there are several small, randomized controlled trials (RCTs) of LVRS and case series with long-term follow-up. These studies allow conclusions about the mechanisms involved, immediate effects of the procedure, the associated complications and the cost implications of LVRS to be reached. Unresolved questions remain about patient selection, surgical technique (bilateral versus unilateral, staged), perioperative management, long-term results and the possible role of new techniques.

This chapter will discuss the available evidence on LVRS from case series and small controlled trials with special emphasis on NETT. Unresolved issues and the need for further studies will be identified.

Questions

1 In subjects with COPD (population), what are the mechanisms by which LVRS (intervention) acts (outcome)? {proof of principle}

2 In subjects with COPD (population), what are the beneficial effects (outcome) from LVRS (intervention)? {therapy}

3 In subjects with COPD (population), what effect does LVRS (intervention) have on survival (outcome)? {prognosis}

4 What adverse effects (outcome) are associated with LVRS (intervention) in subjects with COPD (population)? {therapy}

5 In subjects with COPD (population), can the response (outcome) to LVRS (intervention) be predicted? {prognosis}

Literature search

A PubMed search on 25 January 2004 using the terms (lung volume reduction surgery or LVRS or lung volume reduction or lung reduction surgery) and (emphyse* or COPD or chronic obstructive pulmonary disease or pneumectomy or pneumoplasty) identified 1163 indexed articles going back to 1965. Not all are relevant to the clinical questions on LVRS. When the search is refined further, more than 500 articles with direct relevance to surgery in emphysema remain. These include one large RCT (NETT), six small RCTs (of which two are still in an abstract form and will not be discussed here) (evidence level II), three case–control studies[6–8] (evidence level III-2) and 60–70 other trial reports, most of which are case series with pre- and post-test measurements (evidence level IV) (Table 1). There is no meta-analysis or systematic review of all relevant randomized trials, although at least 56 reviews have been published, with three[9–11] meticulous systematic reviews. The one review in the Cochrane Database of Systematic Reviews, by Hensley and colleagues[12] updated to June 1999, identified only one RCT of LVRS in patients with homogeneous disease.[13] Compared with other surgical procedures, LVRS is one of the most well-documented interventions but, compared with medical treatments, the number of studies on LVRS remains small.

Question

1 In subjects with COPD, what are the mechanisms by which LVRS acts?

Several mechanisms contribute to breathlessness in COPD, and their relative importance varies from patient to patient. From the LVRS perspective, destruction of lung parenchyma causes a loss of lung elastic recoil and, as a result, the destroyed parts of the lung expand in volume and impair ventilation in the remainder. In addition, there is obstruction in the small airways caused by loss of elastic recoil in adjacent lung parenchyma, and increased lung volume that impairs respiratory muscle function.

A number of hypothetical models have been developed to explain how lung volume reduction works, despite actually removing lung tissue. According to Fessler et al.,[18] a major determinant of airflow limitation in emphysema is the ratio of residual volume to total lung capacity (RV/TLC). Their models suggest that the effects of LVRS could be almost exclusively due to improvement in the mismatch between the size of the lung and the chest wall. Loring et al.[19] suggested an alternative model for LVRS, in which increases in expiratory flow rates can result from the greater elastic recoil pressure achieved by an unchanged chest wall operating on a smaller lung.

Other possible mechanisms include:
- reduction in dynamic hyperinflation during exercise;
- improved respiratory muscle function (chiefly diaphragm);
- improved venous return;
- reduced energy expenditure of respiratory muscles;
- improved V/Q matching;
- reduced intrinsic positive end-expiratory pressure (PEEP);
- re-expansion of collapsed lung.

Mechanisms of benefit

Several observational studies have provided data on mechanisms of improvement. These have shown:
- Improved elastic recoil. Sciurba et al.[20] showed that lung reduction surgery in 20 subjects produced increases in the elastic recoil of the lung, leading to short-term improvement in dyspnoea and exercise tolerance. Sixteen patients with increased elastic recoil had a greater increase in the distance walked in 6 min than the other four patients, in whom recoil did not increase ($P = 0.002$). Furthermore, the fractional change in right ventricular area, an indicator of systolic function, increased post surgery ($P = 0.02$).

Table 1. Quality and quantity of evidence available.

Type of evidence		No. of publications
I	Evidence from a systematic review of all relevant RCTs	0
II	Evidence obtained from at least one properly designed RCT	5[5,14–17]
III-1	Evidence obtained from well-designed, pseudorandomized well-controlled trials	0
III-2	Evidence obtained from comparative studies with concurrent controls and allocation, non-randomized (cohort studies), case–control studies or interrupted time series with a control group	3[6–8]
III-3	Evidence obtained from comparative studies with historical control, two or more single arm studies or interrupted time series without a parallel control group	
IV	Evidence obtained from case series, either post-test or pre- and post-test	>60

- Reduced airflow limitation. In 12 subjects with emphysema, Gelb et al.[21] observed that the improvement in maximal expiratory airflow can be primarily attributed to increased lung elastic recoil and its secondary effect on enlarging airway diameter, which in turn caused increased airway conductance and decreased transmural pressure.
- Reduced RV. Ingenito et al.[22] measured spirometry and pulmonary mechanics pre- and postoperatively in 25 patients and observed that LVRS improves function by resizing the lung relative to the chest wall by reducing RV. LVRS did not change airway resistance, but decreased respiratory muscle contractility, which attenuates the potential benefits of LVRS that are generated by reducing RV/TLC. Among nonresponders, they found that recoil pressure increased out of proportion to reduced volume, such that no increase in vital capacity or improvement in FEV_1 occurred.
- Reduced intrinsic PEEP. Airway obstruction promotes intrinsic PEEP and concomitant dynamic hyperinflation, increasing inspiratory work in the face of decreased effectiveness of the inspiratory muscles as pressure generators.[23] In one study on homogeneous emphysema, the intrinsic PEEP decreased significantly following LVRS, together with the work of breathing.[24]
- Re-expansion of compressed lung. This phenomenon was first observed after surgery on pulmonary bullae[25] and may explain some of the spectacular improvements reported in LVRS series in which patients with bullae have been included.

Other changes that have been noted in small numbers include:
- Improvement in resting lung volumes, together with less dynamic hyperinflation during exercise.[26]
- Improvement in diaphragm strength, associated with a reduction in lung volumes and an improvement in exercise performance.[27]
- Increase in the total surface area of the diaphragm, and of the zone of apposition, but no significant change in diaphragm configuration at functional residual capacity (FRC).[28]
- A craniad displacement of the diaphragm but no change in rib cage dimensions.[29]
- Improvement in right ventricular performance, particularly during exercise.[30]
- Increased LV end-diastolic dimensions and filling and improved LV function.[31]

When lung function and ventilation improve following surgery, there are secondary benefits. LVRS seems to reduce energy expenditure of respiratory muscles, especially during exercise. This may reverse the malnourished state in end-stage emphysema. A controlled study of 60 patients with severe emphysema who were randomly assigned to receive LVRS ($n = 30$) or a 6-week respiratory rehabilitation programme ($n = 30$) observed that, despite similar energy intake, the LVRS group showed significant gain in mean weight at 3, 6 and 12 months when compared with the respiratory rehabilitation

group. Both fat mass and fat-free mass increased after surgery, but only fat-free mass had a significant improvement.[32]

Description of treatment

Preoperative assessment

Before publication of NETT, different centres had developed local protocols for patient selection and preoperative assessment.[33–36] The results of NETT have provided a validated algorithm (Fig. 1) for selection of optimal candidates for surgery (Tables 2 and 3).[37] To be reimbursed in the USA, surgery must be preceded and followed by a programme of diagnostic and therapeutic services consistent with those provided in the NETT and designed to maximize the patient's potential. The programme must include 16–20 preoperative sessions and 6–10 postoperative sessions, each lasting a minimum of 2 hours.

Anaesthetic technique

Anaesthetic protocols were developed to prevent air trapping and air leaks and offer good analgesia to promote early recovery and mobilization.[39] The anaesthetic protocols include the use of pressure-limited ventilation, lumbar epidural diamorphine, propofol infusions and intensive physiotherapy, none of which was tested in RCTs. It is not yet clear whether thoracic epidural analgesia has significant benefits over other techniques of pain relief.

Surgical technique

A number of surgical approaches and techniques exist, e.g. bilateral in one session, unilateral or staged bilateral. A survey in June 2000 of LVRS in 75 European thoracic surgical centres showed that the most commonly used technique is video-assisted thoracoscopy, which is most frequently performed bilaterally.[40]

The operation involves excision of 20–30% of the volume of each lung. The most affected portions are excised with the use of a linear stapling device fitted with buttressing material to eliminate air leakage through the staple holes.[41] The choice of buttressing material has not been shown to affect outcome. In a study of 65 patients who underwent bilateral lung volume reduction by video-assisted thoracoscopy using endoscopic staplers either without or with bovine pericardium for buttressing, Stammberger et al.[42] observed no differences between the control and treatment groups for lung function, degree of dyspnoea or arterial blood gases. Although buttressing the staple line significantly shortened the duration of air leaks and drainage time, this did not change the duration of hospital stay.

In a small randomized trial of 16 patients, Catalyurek et al.[43] observed that, if 10–20 mL of autologous venous blood was gently injected underneath the staple line, there was no air leak at the end of the operation. In comparison, using staples alone, additional sutures pledgetted with Gore-tex patches were

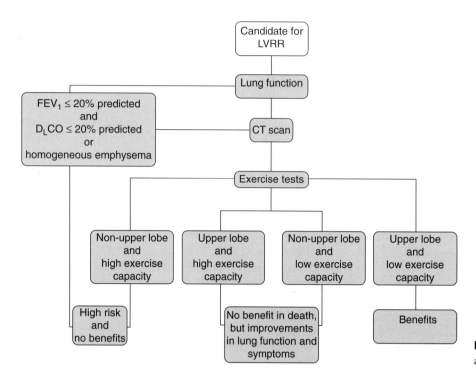

Figure 1. LVRS patient assessment algorithm.

Table 2. Inclusion criteria for LVRS (after [4,5] and http://www.cms.hhs.gov).

Assessment	Criteria
History and physical examination	Consistent with emphysema
	BMI, $\leq 31.1\,kg/m^2$ (men) or $\leq 32.3\,kg/m^2$ (women)
	Stable with $\leq 20\,mg$ of prednisone (or equivalent) qd
Radiographic	HRCT scan evidence of bilateral emphysema
Pulmonary function (pre-rehabilitation)	$FEV_1 \leq 45\%$ predicted ($\geq 15\%$ predicted if age ≥ 70 years)
	TLC $\geq 100\%$ predicted post-bronchodilator
	RV $\geq 150\%$ predicted post-bronchodilator
Arterial blood gas level (pre-rehabilitation)	$P\text{co}_2 \leq 60\,mmHg$ ($P\text{co}_2, \leq 55\,mmHg$ if 1 mile above sea level)
	$P\text{o}_2 \geq 45\,mmHg$ on room air ($P\text{o}_2 \geq 30\,mmHg$ if 1 mile above sea level)
Cardiac assessment	Approval for surgery by cardiologist if any of the following are present: unstable angina; left-ventricular ejection fraction (LVEF) cannot be estimated from the echocardiogram; LVEF $< 45\%$; dobutamine-radionuclide cardiac scan indicates coronary artery disease or ventricular dysfunction; arrhythmia (>5 premature ventricular contractions/min; cardiac rhythm other than sinus; premature ventricular contractions on ECG at rest)
Surgical assessment	Approval for surgery by pulmonary physician, thoracic surgeon and anaesthetist post-rehabilitation
Exercise	Post-rehabilitation 6-min walk of $\geq 140\,m$; able to complete 3 min unloaded pedalling in exercise tolerance test (pre- and post-rehabilitation)
Consent	Signed consents for screening and rehabilitation
Smoking	Plasma cotinine level $\leq 13.7\,ng/mL$ (or arterial carboxyhaemoglobin $\leq 2.5\%$ if using nicotine products)
	Non-smoking for 4 months prior to initial interview and throughout evaluation for surgery
Preoperative diagnostic and therapeutic programme adherence	Must complete assessment for and programme of preoperative services in preparation for surgery
Additional features	Severe upper lobe predominant emphysema (as defined by radiologist assessment of upper lobe predominance on CT scan) or severe non-upper lobe emphysema with low exercise capacity*

*Patients with low exercise capacity are those whose maximal exercise capacity is at or below 25 watts for women and 40 watts for men after completion of the preoperative therapeutic programme in preparation for LVRS.

Table 3. Exclusion criteria.

Age >75–80 years
Comorbid illness that would increase surgical mortality
Clinically significant coronary artery disease
Pulmonary hypertension (PA systolic > 45, PA mean > 35 mmHg)
Severe obesity or cachexia
Surgical constraints
Previous thoracic procedure
Pleuradesis
Chest wall deformity
Decreased inspiratory conductance
The patient presents with FEV_1 < 20% of predicted value and either
    homogeneous distribution of emphysema on CT scan or carbon
    monoxide diffusing capacity of <20% of predicted value (high-risk
    group identified October 2001 by the NETT[38])
The patient satisfies the criteria outlined above but has severe, non-
    upper lobe emphysema with high exercise capacity

FEV_1, forced expiratory volume in 1 second; PA, alveolar pressure; $Paco_2$, arterial carbon dioxide tension; Pao_2, arterial oxygen tension; RV, residual volume; TLC, total lung capacity.

needed for four cases. The authors suggest that this simple and cheap method could be used in some instances where additional staple reinforcement is necessary.

Lowdermilk et al.[44] compared the results of patients undergoing unilateral LVRS ($n = 338$) with bilateral LVRS ($n = 344$) from 1993 to 1998 at five institutions. Follow-up data were available on 671 patients between 6 and 12 months after surgery. Bilateral LVRS provided superior improvement in postoperative percentage change in FEV_1 (unilateral LVRS 23.3% ± 55.3% versus bilateral LVRS 33% ± 41%). They concluded that, although both bilateral and unilateral LVRS yield significant improvement, the results of bilateral procedures seem to be superior with regard to spirometry, lung volumes and quality of life.

Staple lung volume reduction seems to be better than laser surgery.[45] Laser bullectomy and lung reduction surgery with staples were compared in 72 patients with diffuse emphysema scored as severe on computerized tomography (CT). Patients were prospectively randomized to undergo either neodymium:yttrium aluminium garnet contact laser surgery ($n = 33$) or stapled lung reduction surgery. No significant differences were observed between the groups ($P < 0.05$) with respect to the operating time, hospital days or air leakage for more than 7 days. The mean postoperative improvement in the FEV_1 at 6 months was significantly greater for the patients undergoing the staple technique than for the laser treatment group.

A range of other surgical procedures has been combined with LVRS, but the evidence on these is limited to case reports.[46,47]

Postoperative management
Early tracheal extubation is considered to be important to minimize the risks of developing or exacerbating an air leak, although postoperative management has not been tested in the context of RCTs. Hypercapnia is a common event in the early postoperative period and should not prevent early extubation. The patient should be warm, pain free, haemodynamically stable and have a good respiratory pattern and cough.[39,48] Chest physiotherapy is usually started as early as 1 h after transfer to the recovery area. Patients receive good pain control, bronchodilators, steroids and diuretics.

Patients who develop respiratory failure and require tracheal intubation have a poor prognosis. Death can result from a variety of causes including cardiovascular, cerebrovascular and prolonged infection. The mode of death is frequently respiratory failure, with or without infection, and multiple organ failure.[39]

Question

2 In subjects with COPD, what are the beneficial effects from LVRS?

Defining what constitutes a successful outcome after LVRS is complex for a number of reasons, including our limited understanding of dyspnoea, quality of life and patient perceptions.[49] These are augmented by differences between trials in inclusion/exclusion criteria, radiomorphological reading of emphysema, surgical techniques, rehabilitation programmes and reporting. A number of reviews, including two systematic reviews, summarized the evidence available from case series[9,11,50,51] (Table 4). Case series can offer an estimate of the range of LVRS effects, but may exaggerate benefits, as poor outcomes are less likely to be reported.

Evidence from case series

Effects on dyspnoea
Case series results showed significant short-term improvements, but with a wide variation in the range of improvement, e.g.
• Improvements in the MRC dyspnoea scale by at least one point in nearly 90% of patients who had a follow-up period of more than 6 months;[56]
• A significant decrease after bilateral LVRS[57] with a mean postoperative MRC dyspnoea score of 0.8.

Effects on FEV_1
The range of reported FEV_1 improvement varies from 13%[26] to 96%.[70] But when all the data are considered, it is evident that 20–50% of patients show little short-term improvement after LVRS, with the mean data favourably skewed by individuals who have major spirometric improvement.[83]

Table 4. Results of case series (modified and updated after [9,11,50,51]).

First author/reference	Early deaths (%)	Patients (n)	FEV$_1$↑ (%)	RV↓ (%)	6MWD↑ (m)
Argenziano[52]	7.4	64	70	–	96
Bagley[53]	5	55	27	9	118
Bingisser[54]	0	20	19	59	202
Bousamra[55]	–	45	59	–	88
Brenner[56]	4.2	145	50	38	–
Cooper[57]	4	150	51	28	69
Cordova[58]		26	36	27	89
Daniel[59]	3.8	26	49	–	–
Date[60]	0	39	41	–	–
De Perrot[61]	0	18	53	–	–
Eugene[62]	2	44	51	–	–
Eugene[63]	0	28	33	–	–
Fujimoto[64]	–	–	–	–	–
Geiser[65]	0	28	17.5	18	124
Hazelrigg[66]	5.7	141	16	14	64
Keller[67]	0	25	31	14	45
Kotloff[68]	10	119	34	28	65
Kotloff[69]	4.2	80	41	28	61
Martinez[26]		17	13	59	–
McKenna[13]	2.5	79	57	–	–
Miller[70]	5.6	46	96	–	271
Mitsui[71]	6.5	65	68	50	–
Naunheim[72]	4	50	35	33	51
Norman[73]	–	14	26	73	–
Sciurba[20]	0	20	27.5	–	32
Snell[74]	5	20	54	–	125
Stammberger[75]	0	42	43	22	137
Tan[76]	20	10	33.4	27.7	52
Wakabayashi[77]	4.8	443	30	13	–
Yoshinaga[78]	0	57	42	–	–
Zenati[79]	5	20	51	46	32

Lung volumes

Variable reduction in lung volumes have been reported, e.g.
• A decrease in total lung capacity with the majority of patients experiencing a reduction of 10–15%.[51,83]
• A decrease in residual volume from 9%[53] to 73%,[73] with the majority of patients showing improvement of 20–30%.[83]

Exercise capacity

The improvements reported in exercise capacity range from 20% to 50%.[51,83] For maximum workload, oxygen consumption and minute ventilation, there is evidence of short-term increases, but long-term studies have not been reported.

Other effects

• Some case series showed significant improvements in oxygenation and decreases in carbon dioxide (Pa_{CO_2}),[57] whereas other studies have shown little change.[84]
• Liberation from oxygen was reported in 50% of the initial

150 patients operated on by the Washington University group.[57] Naunheim et al.[72] showed a similar rate of discontinuation of supplemental oxygen after unilateral LVRS.
• With regard to liberation from steroids, McKenna et al.[85] reported in their series that 85% of steroid-dependent patients were free from medication after LVRS. These results have not been confirmed in controlled trials.

Evidence from small randomized trials

Six small, randomized studies confirm short-term improvements in dyspnoea, lung function, gas exchange and exercise capacity after LVRS. There are methodological problems with each of these studies, yet they provide valuable information; two reports are still in abstract form and will not be discussed here.

Criner et al.[14] randomized 37 patients to pulmonary rehabilitation followed by surgery versus continued rehabilitation. They observed that patients undergoing LVRS achieved a statistically significant improvement in FEV_1 and Pa_{CO_2}, but the improvement in 6-min walking distance (6MWD), total exercise time and $V_{O_{2max}}$ did not reach statistical significance until crossover patients from the medically treated group were included in the analysis. Quality of life, measured by the Sickness Impact Profile, also improved post LVRS.

Pompeo et al.[15] randomized 60 patients to LVRS versus pulmonary rehabilitation but, in this study, surgically treated patients did not undergo preoperative pulmonary rehabilitation. They observed improvements in FEV_1, dyspnoea index, 6MWD, maximal incremental treadmill test and Pa_{O_2} at 6 months.

Geddes et al.[16] randomized 48 patients to intensive medical therapy (including pulmonary rehabilitation) followed by surgery versus continued medical treatment with follow-up for 12 months. Because five out of 24 (21%) surgically treated patients died after surgery, four within 90 days of LVRS, the investigators changed the selection criteria mid-study to exclude patients with $D_LCO < 30$% predicted or shuttle walking distance <150 m. They reported a statistically significant improvement in FEV_1 at all time points, improvement in exercise capacity as measured by shuttle walking distance and an improved quality of life as measured by the SF-36 at 3, 6 and 12 months.

Goldstein et al.[17] randomized patients after a 6-week programme of pulmonary rehabilitation and followed them for up to 1 year. The primary outcome was disease-specific quality of life as measured by the Chronic Respiratory Questionnaire (CRQ). The investigators observed a significant improvement in the surgical group in each of the CRQ domains of dyspnoea, fatigue, emotional function and mastery. The magnitude of this effect was also greater than the minimal clinically important difference, defined as 0.5 in all domains at each time point. In addition, they reported that LVRS had a large and significant effect in preventing treatment failure over 12 months (failure was defined as death, missing data from a treatment complication or a consistent decrease in at least two domains of the CRQ). The secondary outcomes included spirometry and exercise capacity, which improved significantly in the surgical patients through the 12-month follow-up period.

In summary (Fig. 2), four published RCTs of LVRS versus medical therapy show significantly better postoperative pulmonary function, exercise capacity and subjective health status in the surgical treatment arms than in the medical treatment arms in the short term (up to 1 year). However, it is important to note that sample sizes were small and response to surgery highly variable, with significant numbers of patients suffering complications or achieving negligible spirometric improvement after LVRS.

Evidence from the NETT

The importance of NETT in the practice of LVRS deserves spe-

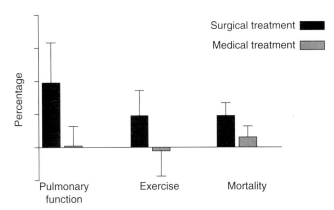

Figure 2. Summary of effects from four small randomized trials[14-17] on LVRS.

cial scrutiny. During the trial, 3777 patients were screened, and 1218 patients were finally randomized, 580 receiving bilateral LVRS (via either median sternotomy or videoscopically assisted thoracoscopic surgery) and 562 maximal medical therapy. All patients underwent 6–10 weeks of pulmonary rehabilitation before entry to the study. Before randomization, the patients performed cycle ergometry breathing 30% oxygen and standardized pulmonary function testing, and completed the disease-specific St George's Respiratory Questionnaire, a general health questionnaire and a dyspnoea questionnaire.

The primary outcomes of the trial were mortality and maximum exercise capacity 2 years after randomization. Secondary outcomes were 6-min walking distance, pulmonary function, quality of life and degree of dyspnoea.

NETT reports its results as histograms of changes from baseline, but parameters related to the degree of hyperinflation and of gas exchange are not reported in the NETT paper or its supplement. Therefore, it is difficult to make more detailed analysis and comparisons with published data. However, it seems that the achieved improvement in FEV_1 is clearly less than that reported in some case series.[86,87]

Summary of treatment effects

- Improvements in exercise capacity of more than 10 watts occurred in 28% of surgically treated patients at 6 months and were still present in 15% at 2 years compared with 4% and 3%, respectively, in the medically treated group.
- Significantly greater changes in FEV_1, health status and the degree of dyspnoea were seen in the surgically treated patients, all showing an initial improvement, with a later deterioration, compared with a steady deterioration in these variables in those undergoing medical treatment.
- The patients were stratified post hoc according to the anatomical distribution of the disease and baseline exercise capacity into four groups:
  — Predominantly upper lobe disease and low (below the sex-specific 40th percentile) baseline exercise capacity;

— Non-upper lobe disease and low baseline exercise capacity;
— Upper lobe disease and high baseline exercise capacity;
— Non-upper lobe disease and high baseline exercise capacity.

• The post hoc subgroup analysis* showed that patients with predominantly upper lobe disease and a low baseline exercise capacity in the surgical group were more likely to achieve the target increase in exercise capacity (30% versus 0%, $P < 0.001$) and the target increase in health-related quality of life at 24 months (48% versus 10%, $P < 0.001$).

• Among patients in the non-upper lobe disease and high exercise capacity, the chances of significant improvement in exercise capacity or health-related quality of life were similar.

• The results for the remaining groups (non-upper lobe disease and low exercise capacity, and upper lobe disease and high exercise capacity) distribute between these extremes. These patients had statistically significant improvements in most outcomes: health-related quality of life, spirometry and exercise capacity.

Question

3 In subjects with COPD, what effect does LVRS have on survival?

Case series

The operative mortality in these case series varied between 0% and 20% with an average of about 3.8%; the mean length of hospital stay ranged from 10.9 to 17 days.[4] However, a 1998 report to the US Congress[89] on lung volume reduction surgery and a Medicare coverage policy paper, which looked at data collected from 722 Medicare claims that used the LVRS billing code between October 1995 and January 1996, showed that mortality rates 3 and 12 months after the operation were 14.4% and 23% respectively.[4] For these patients, acute care hospitalizations and use of long-term care and rehabilitation services were greater after compared with before the operation (304 stays for 160 patients after the operation versus 197 stays for 123 patients before the operation; the inpatient stay associated with LVRS was excluded from these analyses). Average days hospitalized was greater after than before the operation

Small randomized trials

Four published randomized studies show a higher short-term

---

*NB. Together with the NETT report came a cautionary editorial,[88] which illustrated the hazards of secondary analysis of trial data when the criteria are not fully specified before the trial is conducted. The authors of this editorial concluded that the NETT data subgroup analysis has some biological plausibility but should be tested in further trials.

mortality in the surgical arms compared with the mortality in the medical arms (Fig. 2).

NETT

Results from the NETT show that:
• there was no significant difference in mortality between the two groups at the end of the trial (risk ratio for death in the surgical group = 1.01, $P = 0.90$);
• in the short term, the 90-day mortality was 7.9% in those randomized to surgery, compared with 1.9% in those undergoing medical treatment;
• among patients in the non-upper lobe disease and high exercise capacity group, mortality was higher in the surgical group than in the medical group (risk ratio = 2.06, $P = 0.02$);
• the results for the remaining groups (non-upper lobe disease and low exercise capacity, and upper lobe disease and high exercise capacity) showed no difference in mortality.

Question

4 What adverse effects are associated with LVRS in subjects with COPD?

For all the surgical LVRS techniques, air leaks of more than 7 days are reported to be the most common complication, occurring in an average of 50% of cases.[11] Although this was thought to be a complication related to the technique, the exact mechanisms of air leaks are not clear, as they now seem to appear after non-invasive lung volume procedures as well, when only lung remodelling takes place.[80] Other frequently encountered complications are pneumonia, delayed pneumothorax, ventilatory failure, wound infection and reintubation and reoperation for various indications. Colonic and gastroduodenal perforation can contribute significantly to the death of these patients, but the mechanisms remain elusive.[81,82]

Question

5 In subjects with COPD, can the response to LVRS be predicted?

Patients with homogeneous distribution of emphysema seem to have little benefit from LVRS. The review in The Cochrane Database of Systematic Reviews, by Hensley and colleagues[12] updated to June 1999, has identified only one RCT of LVRS in patients with homogeneous disease,[13] and concluded that there was insufficient evidence to support the use of LVRS for treatment of severe diffuse emphysema. Although Bloch et al.[91] observed that lung volume reduction surgery can improve lung function in severe homogeneous and, to an even greater extent, heterogeneous emphysema, early in the NETT trial, a high-risk group of patients with homogeneous disease on the CT scan and an FEV_1 and/or D_LCO below 20% predicted was identified as having an unacceptably high early death rate.[38] No further patients of this type were recruited for the NETT, and LVRS should not be applied routinely to this group.

Another group of patients who seem to have little benefit from LVRS are patients with non-upper lobe distribution with high exercise capacity. For these, NETT results suggest that LVRS is not beneficial and should not be considered. Finally, Gelb et al.[92] and Cassina et al.[93] observed limited benefit in pa-

tients with diffuse emphysema due to α_1 antitrypsin deficiency who undergo LVRS.

Other issues

Long-term outcomes

Results 3–7 years after LVRS are now emerging from the follow-up of the initial case series. None of the randomized trials provided long-term follow-up data. The evidence, based on the observational studies, suggests that, in selected patients, LVRS can achieve substantial beneficial effects with a duration of improvement of at least 5 years (Table 5). Survival is estimated to be 60–70% at 5 years in the majority of these

Table 5. Longer term follow-up studies.

First author	N	Maximum follow-up	Conclusions
Yusen[95]	200	5 years	Dyspnoea scores ↑ in 40% of patients SF-36 ↑ 69% of patients FEV_1 ↑ 58% of patients Annual Kaplan–Meier survival 63%
Flaherty[96]	89	3 years	FEV_1 ↑ 6MWD ↑ by 158 m
Bloch[91]	115	37 months	FEV_1 ↑ 37% in homogeneous ($n=27$), by 38% FEV_1 ↑ 38% in intermediately heterogeneous ($n=37$) FEV_1 ↑ 63% in markedly heterogeneous emphysema ($n=51$) at 6 months Maximal FEV_1 was reached within 6 months FEV_1 decreased in the first postoperative year by 0.16 L/year in homogeneous, by 0.19 L/year in intermediately heterogeneous and by 0.32 L/year in markedly heterogeneous emphysema ($P<0.01$ versus other morphologies) FEV_1 decline over subsequent years decelerated according to an exponential decay and was similar for all morphological types [median annual decrease of 0.09 L (9%)]
Gelb reviewed in[83]	26	7 years	A post-LVRS survival at 7 years of 15% At 1–7 years post-LVRS, this improvement was seen in 73%, 36%, 35%, 27%, 8%, 4% and 4% of patients respectively
Iwasaki[97]		6 years	A 56% survival rate at 6 years A survival advantage was observed in the patient with predominantly upper lobe disease Patients with preoperative $FEV_1 < 30%$ showed a 51.5% survival rate 5 years after LVRS Patients with preoperative $FEV_1 > 30%$ had 76.2% survival at 5 years ($P<0.05$)
Fujimoto[98]	88	5 years	At 3 years, spirometry, dyspnoea score and 6MWD were equivalent to preoperative numbers
Appleton[99]	54	5.5 years	↑ MRC scores compared with pre-LVRS BMI and post-LVRS length of stay were significantly associated with survival ↑ FEV_1 26.7% RV ↓ 27%
Munro[31]	529	6 years	↑ FEV_1 of 38%, RV ↓ by 27%, TLC ↓ by 17%, 6MWD ↑ by 24% appear to be maintained for approximately 3 years Survival status was reported in 454 cases (85.8%)

studies. However, the impact of LVRS on the mortality of patients with severe emphysema cannot be accurately determined without using an external control group. The NETT trial, the only RCT with long-term follow-up, showed no significant difference in mortality between the LVRS and the medical group at the end of 2-year follow-up (risk ratio for death in the surgical group = 1.01, $P = 0.90$).

Forced expiratory volume in 1 second peaks within 6 months postoperatively. Fessler and Wise[94] provided a detailed review of the duration of benefit following LVRS and suggested that it was probably incorrect to assume that the decline in FEV_1 will be linear over time. Whether the FEV_1 decline is most rapid in the first year and then slows down in subsequent years according to an exponential decay is not clear.

Comparative efficacy and cost

NETT included a prospective economic analysis on LVRS.[100] The analysis concluded that LVRS is expensive relative to medical therapy. The cost-effectiveness ratio for LVRS compared with medical therapy was $190 000 per quality-adjusted life year gained at 3 years and $53 000 per quality-adjusted life year gained at 10 years. The cost-effectiveness ratio in the patients with predominantly upper lobe emphysema and low exercise capacity after pulmonary rehabilitation was $98 000 per quality-adjusted life year gained at 3 years and $21 000 at 10 years, but bootstrap analysis revealed substantial uncertainty for the subgroup and 10-year estimates.

By comparison, cost-effectiveness ratios for other types of surgery compared with medical therapy include (in 2002 dollars) 8300–64 000 per quality-adjusted life year gained for coronary artery bypass surgery, $130 000–220 000 per quality-adjusted life year gained for lung transplantation, $65 000 per quality-adjusted life year gained for heart transplantation.[100]

LVRS for other obstructive diseases

The effects of LVRS in other types of obstructive lung disease are unknown. A case report describes the successful use of LVRS in a 14-year-old child with severe airflow obstruction and hyperinflation due to constrictive bronchiolitis.[101] Within days after LVRS, an improvement in symptoms and lung function occurred and persisted for >1 year. LVRS may be an option in some patients with extreme hyperinflation even if the underlying disease is not emphysema, but further studies are certainly needed in this area.

LVRS as a bridge to transplant

Transplantation after LVRS is technically possible albeit with some increase in risk of bleeding due to pleural adhesions. It has been suggested that LVRS could improve quality of life and may serve as a bridge to lung transplantation in patients with end-stage emphysema.[102–105] However, neither LVRS nor transplantation was shown to improve survival. Whether

LVRS should be used as a bridge to transplant remains controversial.

New techniques

A number of new techniques are emerging, but the evidence on these is limited to pilot studies. Results similar to surgical removal have been obtained by plication (folding) and stapling without tissue removal.[106] Swanson et al. showed in a case series of 32 patients that LVRS can be achieved by thoracoscopic lung plication of the most emphysematous lobes. They observed an improvement in mean FEV_1 of 29% after a mean follow-up period of 3.8 months and a reduction in the daily oxygen requirement in nine of 16 oxygen-dependent patients. Brenner et al.[107] described the use of a suction vacuum device, which deployed an elastomer cuff that enveloped and compressed diseased lung tissue. They only reported feasibility work from animals and suggested that this technique may reduce postoperative air leaks.

These results suggest that removal of the emphysematous lung is possibly not obligatory. As a consequence, a recent concept has emerged that reduction in lung volume can also be achieved endoscopically, without the need for surgeons or surgery, thus avoiding any trauma (hence postoperative pain) to the chest wall. This can be done either by producing controlled atelectasis in the target areas of the most diseased portions of the lung[80,108] or by reducing the degree of hyperinflation through the creation of extra-anatomical tracts between the proximal airways and the emphysematous segments.[109]

The concept of non-resectional LVRS appears to be highly promising, but the evidence is limited to a small number of short-term follow-up case studies.[80,108,110] Many unanswered questions remain, and whether or not the procedures can be helpful and can be extended to patients who have homogeneous distribution of emphysema remains to be demonstrated.

Unresolved issues

Several specific issues related to LVRS remain unresolved. These include aspects related to perioperative management, surgical technique (bilateral versus unilateral or staged) and patient selection. The classification into predominantly upper lobe and non-upper lobe emphysema is a crude simplification, which does not reflect the range of emphysema encountered in daily practice. The value of a more detailed categorization to test the role of emphysema morphology on the outcome of LVRS remains to be studied. In addition, the role of low exercise capacity needs to be confirmed by prospective studies.[88]

Conclusions

Beyond pulmonary rehabilitation and continued medical management, there are no commonly available alternatives to LVRS. The available evidence shows that, in low-risk patients with severe emphysema predominantly of the upper lobe of the lung, LVRS can improve exercise capacity and quality of life findings. For the other groups, the benefits are not so clear, and further long-term research is advocated. The best results are probably achieved when LVRS is performed in specialist centres as part of a multidisciplinary programme, where close co-ordination between physicians, surgeons, anaesthetist and intensivists, as well as physiotherapists, occupational therapists and dieticians exists. The high costs and uncertainty regarding details of the technique and the long-term cost-effectiveness of LVRS warrant further studies.

Summary for clinicians

1 Carefully selected patients with severe emphysema, who remain considerably limited by shortness of breath despite optimal medical therapy including comprehensive pulmonary rehabilitation, will benefit from LVRS with respect to relief of breathlessness, quality of life, pulmonary function and exercise capacity.

2 The survival of properly selected patients is not shortened by LVRS.

3 Patients with homogeneous disease on the CT scan and an FEV_1 and/or D_LCO below 20% predicted have an unacceptably high early mortality from LRVS.

References

1 Brantigan OC, Mueller E, Kress MB. A surgical approach to pulmonary emphysema. *Am Rev Respir Dis* 1959; **80**:194–206.

2 Cooper JD. The history of surgical procedures for emphysema. *Ann Thorac Surg* 1997; **63**:312–19.

3 Cooper JD, Trulock EP, Triantafillou AN *et al.* Bilateral pneumectomy (volume reduction) for chronic obstructive pulmonary disease. *J Thorac Cardiovasc Surg* 1995; **109**:106–16.

4 Rationale and design of the National Emphysema Treatment Trial (NETT): A prospective randomized trial of lung volume reduction surgery. *J. Thorac Cardiovasc Surg* 1999; **118**:518–28.

5 Fishman A, Martinez F, Naunheim K *et al.* A randomized trial comparing lung-volume-reduction surgery with medical therapy for severe emphysema. *N Engl J Med* 2003; **348**:2059–73.

6 Meyers BF, Yusen RD, Lefrak SS *et al.* Outcome of Medicare patients with emphysema selected for, but denied, a lung volume reduction operation. *Ann Thorac Surg* 1998; **66**:331–6.

7 Wilkens H, Demertzis S, Konig J, Leitnaker CK, Schafers HJ, Sybrecht GW. Lung volume reduction surgery versus conservative treatment in severe emphysema. *Eur Respir J* 2000; **16**:1043–9.

8 Mercer K, Follette D, Breslin E *et al.* Comparison of functional state between bilateral lung volume reduction surgery and pulmonary rehabilitation: a six-month followup study. *Int J Surg Investig* 1999; **1**:139–47.

9 Young J, Fry-Smith A, Hyde C. Lung volume reduction surgery (LVRS) for chronic obstructive pulmonary disease (COPD) with underlying severe emphysema. *Thorax* 1999; **54**:779–89.

10 Berger RL, Celli BR, Meneghetti AL *et al.* Limitations of randomized clinical trials for evaluating emerging operations: the case of lung volume reduction surgery. *Ann Thorac Surg* 2001; **72**:649–57.

11 Stirling GR, Babidge WJ, Peacock MJ *et al.* Lung volume reduction surgery in emphysema: a systematic review. *Ann Thorac Surg* 2001; **72**:641–8.

12 Hensley M, Coughlan JL, Gibson P. Lung volume reduction surgery for diffuse emphysema. *Cochrane Database Syst Rev* 2000; CD001001.

13 McKenna RJ Jr, Brenner M, Gelb AF *et al.* A randomized, prospective trial of stapled lung reduction versus laser bullectomy for diffuse emphysema. *J Thorac Cardiovasc Surg* 1996; **111**:317–21.

14 Criner GJ, Cordova FC, Furukawa S *et al.* Prospective randomized trial comparing bilateral lung volume reduction surgery to pulmonary rehabilitation in severe chronic obstructive pulmonary disease. *Am J Respir Crit Care Med* 1999; **160**:2018–27.

15 Pompeo E, Marino M, Nofroni I, Matteucci G, Mineo TC. Reduction pneumoplasty versus respiratory rehabilitation in severe emphysema: a randomized study. Pulmonary Emphysema Research Group. *Ann Thorac Surg* 2000; **70**:948–53.

16 Geddes D, Davies M, Koyama H *et al.* Effect of lung-volume-reduction surgery in patients with severe emphysema. *N Engl J Med* 2000; **343**:239–45.

17 Goldstein RS, Todd TR, Guyatt G *et al.* Influence of lung volume reduction surgery (LVRS) on health related quality of life in patients with chronic obstructive pulmonary disease. *Thorax* 2003; **58**:405–10.

18 Fessler HE, Scharf SM, Permutt S. Improvement in spirometry following lung volume reduction surgery: application of a physiologic model. *Am J Respir Crit Care Med* 2002; **165**:34–40.

19 Loring SH, Leith DE, Connolly MJ, Ingenito EP, Mentzer SJ, Reilly JJ Jr. Model of functional restriction in chronic obstructive pulmonary disease, transplantation, and lung reduction surgery. *Am J Respir Crit Care Med* 1999; **160**:821–8.

20 Sciurba FC, Rogers RM, Keenan RJ *et al.* Improvement in pulmonary function and elastic recoil after lung-reduction surgery for diffuse emphysema. *N Engl J Med* 1996; **334**:1095–9.

21 Gelb AF, Zamel N, McKenna RJ Jr, Brenner M. Mechanism of short-term improvement in lung function after emphysema resection. *Am J Respir Crit Care Med* 1996; **154**:945–51.

22 Ingenito EP, Loring SH, Moy ML, Mentzer SJ, Swanson SJ, Reilly JJ. Physiological characterization of variability in response to lung volume reduction surgery. *J Appl Physiol* 2003; **94**:20–30.

23 Milic-Emili J. Dynamic pulmonary hyperinflation and intrinsic PEEP: consequences and management in patients with chronic obstructive pulmonary disease. *Recenti Prog Med* 1990; **81**:733–7.

24 Wisser W, Tschernko E, Senbaklavaci O *et al.* Functional improvement after volume reduction: sternotomy versus videoendoscopic approach. *Ann Thorac Surg* 1997; **63**:822–7.

25 Rogers RM, DuBois AB, Blakemore WS. Effect of removal of bullae on airway conductance and conductance volume ratios. *J Clin Invest* 1968; **47**:2569–79.

26 Martinez FJ, de Oca MM, Whyte RI, Stetz J, Gay SE, Celli BR. Lung-volume reduction improves dyspnea, dynamic hyperinflation, and respiratory muscle function. *Am J Respir Crit Care Med* 1997; **155**:1984–90.

27 Criner G, Cordova FC, Leyenson V *et al.* Effect of lung volume reduction surgery on diaphragm strength. *Am J Respir Crit Care Med* 1998; **157**:1578–85.

28 Cassart M, Hamacher J, Verbandt Y *et al.* Effects of lung volume reduction surgery for emphysema on diaphragm dimensions and configuration. *Am J Respir Crit Care Med* 2001; **163**:1171–5.

29 Bellemare F, Cordeau MP, Couture J, Lafontaine E, LeBlanc P, Passerini L. Effects of emphysema and lung volume reduction surgery on transdiaphragmatic pressure and diaphragm length. *Chest* 2002; **121**:1898–910.

30 Mineo TC, Pompeo E, Rogliani P *et al.* Effect of lung volume reduction surgery for severe emphysema on right ventricular function. *Am J Respir Crit Care Med* 2002; **165**:489–94.

31 Munro PE, Bailey MJ, Smith JA, Snell GI. Lung volume reduction

surgery in Australia and New Zealand. Six years on: registry report. *Chest* 2003; **124**:1443–50.

32 Mineo TC, Ambrogi V, Pompeo E, Bollero P, Mineo D, Nofroni I. Body weight and nutritional changes after reduction pneumoplasty for severe emphysema: a randomized study. *J Thorac Cardiovasc Surg* 2002; **124**:660–7.

33 Benditt JO, Wood DE, McCool FD, Lewis S, Albert RK. Changes in breathing and ventilatory muscle recruitment patterns induced by lung volume reduction surgery. *Am J Respir Crit Care Med* 1997; **155**:279–84.

34 Tschernko EM, Gruber EM, Jaksch P *et al.* Ventilatory mechanics and gas exchange during exercise before and after lung volume reduction surgery. *Am J Respir Crit Care Med* 1998; **158**:1424–31.

35 Cleverley JR, Desai SR, Wells AU *et al.* Evaluation of patients undergoing lung volume reduction surgery: ancillary information available from computed tomography. *Clin Radiol* 2000; **55**:45–50.

36 Ingenito EP, Evans RB, Loring SH *et al.* Relation between preoperative inspiratory lung resistance and the outcome of lung-volume-reduction surgery for emphysema. *N Engl J Med* 1998; **338**:1181–5.

37 Martinez FJ, Flaherty KR, Iannettoni MD. Patient selection for lung volume reduction surgery. *Chest Surg Clin N Am* 2003; **13**:669–85.

38 National Emphysema Treatment Trial Research Group. Patients at high risk of death after lung-volume-reduction surgery. *N Engl J Med* 2001; **345**:1075–83.

39 Hillier J, Gillbe C. Anaesthesia for lung volume reduction surgery. *Anaesthesia* 2003; **58**:1210–19.

40 Hamacher J, Russi EW, Weder W. Lung volume reduction surgery: a survey on the European experience. *Chest* 2000; **117**:1560–7.

41 Cooper JD, Patterson GA. Lung-volume reduction surgery for severe emphysema. *Chest Surg Clin N Am* 1995; **5**:815–31.

42 Stammberger U, Klepetko W, Stamatis G *et al.* Buttressing the staple line in lung volume reduction surgery: a randomized three-center study. *Ann Thorac Surg* 2000; **70**:1820–5.

43 Catalyurek H, Silistreli E, Hepaguslar H, Kargi A, Acikel U. The role of autologous blood injection on postoperative air leak at lung resections. *J.Cardiovasc Surg (Torino)* 2002; **43**:135–7.

44 Lowdermilk GA, Keenan RJ, Landreneau RJ *et al.* Comparison of clinical results for unilateral and bilateral thoracoscopic lung volume reduction. *Ann Thorac Surg* 2000; **69**:1670–4.

45 Brenner M, McKenna R Jr, Gelb A *et al.* Objective predictors of response for staple versus laser emphysematous lung reduction. *Am J Respir Crit Care Med* 1997; **155**:1295–301.

46 Liopyris P, Triantafillou AN, Sundt TM III, Block MI, Cooper JD. Coronary artery bypass grafting after a bilateral lung volume reduction operation. *Ann Thorac Surg* 1997; **63**:1790–2.

47 McKenna RJ Jr, Fischel RJ, Brenner M, Gelb AF. Combined operations for lung volume reduction surgery and lung cancer. *Chest* 1996; **110**:885–8.

48 Triantafillou AN. Anesthetic management for bilateral volume reduction surgery. *Semin Thorac Cardiovasc Surg* 1996; **8**:94–8.

49 Cooper JD. Clinical trials and future prospects for lung volume reduction surgery. *Semin Thorac Cardiovasc Surg* 2002; **14**:365–70.

50 Koebe HG, Kugler C, Dienemann H. Evidence-based medicine: lung volume reduction surgery (LVRS). *Thorac Cardiovasc Surg* 2002; **50**:315–22.

51 Flaherty KR, Martinez FJ. Lung volume reduction surgery for emphysema. *Clin Chest Med* 2000; **21**:819–48.

52 Argenziano M, Thomashow B, Jellen PA *et al.* Functional comparison of unilateral versus bilateral lung volume reduction surgery. *Ann Thorac Surg* 1997; **64**:321–6.

53 Bagley PH, Davis SM, O'Shea M, Coleman AM. Lung volume reduction surgery at a community hospital: program development and outcomes. *Chest* 1997; **111**:1552–9.

54 Bingisser R, Zollinger A, Hauser M, Bloch KE, Russi EW, Weder W. Bilateral volume reduction surgery for diffuse pulmonary emphysema by video-assisted thoracoscopy. *J Thorac Cardiovasc Surg* 1996; **112**:875–82.

55 Bousamra M, Haasler GB, Lipchik RJ *et al.* Functional and oximetric assessment of patients after lung reduction surgery. *J Thorac Cardiovasc Surg* 1997; **113**:675–81.

56 Brenner M, McKenna RJ, Gelb AF *et al.* Dyspnea response following bilateral thoracoscopic staple lung volume reduction surgery. *Chest* 1997; **112**:916–23.

57 Cooper JD, Patterson GA, Sundaresan RS *et al.* Results of 150 consecutive bilateral lung volume reduction procedures in patients with severe emphysema. *J Thorac Cardiovasc Surg* 1996; **112**:1319–29.

58 Cordova F, O'Brien G, Furukawa S, Kuzma AM, Travaline J, Criner GJ. Stability of improvements in exercise performance and quality of life following bilateral lung volume reduction surgery in severe COPD. *Chest* 1997; **112**:907–15.

59 Daniel TM, Chan BB, Bhaskar V *et al.* Lung volume reduction surgery. Case selection, operative technique, and clinical results. *Ann Surg* 1996; **223**:526–31.

60 Date H, Goto K, Souda R *et al.* Bilateral lung volume reduction surgery via median sternotomy for severe pulmonary emphysema. *Ann Thorac Surg* 1998; **65**:939–42.

61 de Perrot M, Licker M, Spiliopoulos A. Muscle-sparing anterior thoracotomy for one-stage bilateral lung volume reduction operation. *Ann Thorac Surg* 1998; **66**:582–4.

62 Eugene J, Dajee A, Kayaleh R, Gogia HS, Dos SC, Gazzaniga AB. Reduction pneumonoplasty for patients with a forced expiratory volume in 1 second of 500 milliliters or less. *Ann Thorac Surg* 1997; **63**:186–90.

63 Eugene J, Ott RA, Gogia HS, Dos SC, Zeit R, Kayaleh RA. Video-thoracic surgery for treatment of end-stage bullous emphysema and chronic obstructive pulmonary disease. *Am Surg* 1995; **61**:934–6.

64 Fujimoto K, Kubo K, Haniuda M, Matsuzawa Y, Yamanda T, Maruyama Y. Improvements in thoracic movement following lung volume reduction surgery in patients with severe emphysema. *Intern Med* 1999; **38**:119–25.

65 Geiser T, Schwizer B, Krueger T *et al.* Outcome after unilateral lung volume reduction surgery in patients with severe emphysema. *Eur J Cardiothorac Surg* 2001; **20**:674–8.

66 Hazelrigg S, Boley T, Henkle J *et al.* Thoracoscopic laser bullectomy: a prospective study with three-month results. *J Thorac Cardiovasc Surg* 1996; **112**:319–26.

67 Keller CA, Ruppel G, Hibbett A, Osterloh J, Naunheim KS. Thoracoscopic lung volume reduction surgery reduces dyspnea and improves exercise capacity in patients with emphysema. *Am J Respir Crit Care Med* 1997; **156**:60–7.

68 Kotloff RM, Tino G, Palevsky HI *et al.* Comparison of short-term functional outcomes following unilateral and bilateral lung volume reduction surgery. *Chest* 1998; **113**:890–5.

69 Kotloff RM, Tino G, Bavaria JE *et al.* Bilateral lung volume reduction surgery for advanced emphysema. A comparison of median sternotomy and thoracoscopic approaches. *Chest* 1996; **110**:1399–406.

70 Miller JI Jr, Lee RB, Mansour KA. Lung volume reduction surgery: lessons learned. *Ann Thorac Surg* 1996; **61**:1464–8.

71 Mitsui K, Kurokawa Y, Kaiwa Y *et al.* Thoracoscopic lung volume reduction surgery for pulmonary emphysema patients with severe hypercapnia. *Jpn J Thorac Cardiovasc Surg* 2001; **49**:481–8.

72 Naunheim KS, Keller CA, Krucylak PE, Singh A, Ruppel G, Osterloh JF. Unilateral video-assisted thoracic surgical lung reduction. *Ann Thorac Surg* 1996; **61**:1092–8.

73 Norman M, Hillerdal G, Orre L *et al.* Improved lung function and quality of life following increased elastic recoil after lung volume reduction surgery in emphysema. *Respir Med* 1998; **92**:653–8.

74 Snell GI, Solin P, Chin W *et al*. Lung volume reduction surgery for emphysema. *Med J Aust* 1997; **167**:529–32.

75 Stammberger U, Thurnheer R, Bloch KE *et al*. Thoracoscopic bilateral lung volume reduction for diffuse pulmonary emphysema. *Eur J Cardiothorac Surg* 1997; **11**:1005–10.

76 Tan AL, Unruh HW, Mink SN. Lung volume reduction surgery for the treatment of severe emphysema: a study in a single Canadian institution. *Can J Surg* 2000; **43**:369–76.

77 Wakabayashi A. Thoracoscopic laser pneumoplasty in the treatment of diffuse bullous emphysema. *Ann Thorac Surg* 1995; **60**:936–42.

78 Yoshinaga Y, Iwasaki A, Kawahara K, Shirakusa T. Lung volume reduction surgery results in pulmonary emphysema. Changes in pulmonary function. *Jpn J Thorac Cardiovasc Surg* 1999; **47**:445–51.

79 Zenati M, Keenan RJ, Courcoulas AP, Griffith BP. Lung volume reduction or lung transplantation for end-stage pulmonary emphysema? *Eur J Cardiothorac Surg* 1998; **14**:27–31.

80 Toma TP, Hopkinson NS, Hillier J *et al*. Bronchoscopic volume reduction with valve implants in patients with severe emphysema. *Lancet* 2003; **361**:931–3.

81 Roberts JR, Bavaria JE, Wahl P, Wurster A, Friedberg JS, Kaiser LR. Comparison of open and thoracoscopic bilateral volume reduction surgery: complications analysis. *Ann Thorac Surg* 1998; **66**:1759–65.

82 Cetindag IB, Boley TM, Magee MJ, Hazelrigg SR. Postoperative gastrointestinal complications after lung volume reduction operations. *Ann Thorac Surg* 1999; **68**:1029–33.

83 Wood DE. Results of lung volume reduction surgery for emphysema. *Chest Surg Clin N Am* 2003; **13**:709–26.

84 Albert RK, Benditt JO, Hildebrandt J, Wood DE, Hlastala MP. Lung volume reduction surgery has variable effects on blood gases in patients with emphysema. *Am J Respir Crit Care Med* 1998; **158**:71–6.

85 McKenna RJ Jr, Brenner M, Fischel RJ, Gelb AF. Should lung volume reduction for emphysema be unilateral or bilateral? *J Thorac Cardiovasc Surg* 1996; **112**:1331–8.

86 Ciccone AM, Meyers BF, Guthrie TJ *et al*. Long-term outcome of bilateral lung volume reduction in 250 consecutive patients with emphysema. *J Thorac Cardiovasc Surg* 2003; **125**:513–25.

87 Russi EW, Bloch KE, Weder W. Lung volume reduction surgery: what can we learn from the National Emphysema Treatment Trial? *Eur Respir J* 2003; **22**:571–3.

88 Ware JH. The National Emphysema Treatment Trial—how strong is the evidence? *N Engl J Med* 2003; **348**:2055–6.

89 Health Care Financing Administration. Report to Congress. *Lung Volume Reduction Surgery and Medicare Coverage Policy: Implications of Recently Published Evidence*. Washington, DC, Department of Health and Human Services, 1998.

90 Calverley PM. Closing the NETT on lung volume reduction surgery. *Thorax* 2003; **58**:651–3.

91 Bloch KE, Georgescu CL, Russi EW, Weder W. Gain and subsequent loss of lung function after lung volume reduction surgery in cases of severe emphysema with different morphologic patterns. *J Thorac Cardiovasc Surg* 2002; **123**:845–54.

92 Gelb AF, McKenna RJ, Brenner M, Fischel R, Zamel N. Lung function after bilateral lower lobe lung volume reduction surgery for α_1-antitrypsin emphysema. *Eur Respir J* 1999; **14**:928–33.

93 Cassina PC, Teschler H, Konietzko N, Theegarten D, Stamatis G. Two-year results after lung volume reduction surgery in α_1-antitrypsin deficiency versus smoker's emphysema. *Eur Respir J* 1998; **12**:1028–32.

94 Fessler HE, Wise RA. Lung volume reduction surgery: is less really more? *Am J Respir Crit Care Med* 1999; **159**:1031–5.

95 Yusen RD, Lefrak SS, Gierada DS *et al*. A prospective evaluation of lung volume reduction surgery in 200 consecutive patients. *Chest* 2003; **123**:1026–37.

96 Flaherty KR, Kazerooni EA, Curtis JL *et al*. Short-term and long-term outcomes after bilateral lung volume reduction surgery: prediction by quantitative CT. *Chest* 2001; **119**:1337–46.

97 Iwasaki A, Yosinaga Y, Kawahara K, Shirakusa T. Evaluation of lung volume reduction surgery (LVRS) based on long-term survival rate analysis. *Thorac Cardiovasc Surg* 2003; **51**:277–82.

98 Fujimoto T, Teschler H, Hillejan L, Zaboura G, Stamatis G. Long-term results of lung volume reduction surgery. *Eur J Cardiothorac Surg* 2002; **21**:483–8.

99 Appleton S, Adams R, Porter S, Peacock M, Ruffin R. Sustained improvements in dyspnea and pulmonary function 3 to 5 years after lung volume reduction surgery. *Chest* 2003; **123**:1838–46.

100 Ramsey SD, Berry K, Etzioni R, Kaplan RM, Sullivan SD, Wood DE. Cost effectiveness of lung-volume-reduction surgery for patients with severe emphysema. *N Engl J Med* 2003; **348**:2092–102.

101 Bloch KE, Weder W, Boehler A, Zalunardo MP, Russi EW. Successful lung volume reduction surgery in a child with severe airflow obstruction and hyperinflation due to constrictive bronchiolitis. *Chest* 2002; **122**:747–50.

102 Shitrit D, Fink G, Sahar G, Eidelman L, Saute M, Kramer MR. Successful lung transplantation following lung volume reduction surgery. *Thorac Cardiovasc Surg* 2003; **51**:274–6.

103 Meyers BF, Patterson GA. Lung transplantation versus lung volume reduction as surgical therapy for emphysema. *World J Surg* 2001; **25**:238–43.

104 Bavaria JE, Pochettino A, Kotloff RM *et al*. Effect of volume reduction on lung transplant timing and selection for chronic obstructive pulmonary disease. *J Thorac Cardiovasc Surg* 1998; **115**:9–17.

105 Wisser W, Deviatko E, Simon-Kupilik N *et al*. Lung transplantation following lung volume reduction surgery. *J Heart Lung Transplant* 2000; **19**:480–7.

106 Swanson SJ, Mentzer SJ, DeCamp MM Jr *et al*. No-cut thoracoscopic lung plication: a new technique for lung volume reduction surgery. *J Am Coll Surg* 1997; **185**:25–32.

107 Brenner M, Gonzalez X, Jones B *et al*. Effects of a novel implantable elastomer device for lung volume reduction surgery in a rabbit model of elastase-induced emphysema. *Chest* 2002; **121**:201–9.

108 Snell GI, Holsworth L, Borrill ZL *et al*. The potential for bronchoscopic lung volume reduction using bronchial prostheses: a pilot study. *Chest* 2003; **124**:1073–80.

109 Rendina EA, De Giacomo T, Venuta F *et al*. Feasibility and safety of the airway bypass procedure for patients with emphysema. *J Thorac Cardiovasc Surg* 2003; **125**:1294–9.

110 Hwong TM, Yim AP. New treatment modalities for end-stage emphysema. *Chest Surg Clin N Am* 2003; **13**:739–53.

PART 4

Infection

CHAPTER 4.1

Bronchitis and sinusitis

Tom Fahey

Definition of the problem

Bronchitis represents a wide variety of clinical syndromes. Symptoms range from cough without sputum to an illness characterized by expectoration of mucopurulent sputum, fever, general malaise and dyspnoea.[1] Diagnostic classification is imprecise, with a diagnostic continuum starting with 'common cold' moving through 'upper respiratory tract infection or acute bronchitis' to 'lower respiratory tract infection or pneumonia'. There is considerable overlap within and between such clinical syndromes in terms of symptoms, causative agents, resolution and diagnostic labelling of illness.[1–3]

Acute sinusitis is characterized by inflammation of the paranasal sinuses lasting no more than 1 month.[4] In UK and Dutch family practice, where diagnosis is based predominantly on clinical examination, 21–28 episodes per 1000 patients occur each year.[4] However, diagnosis based on clinical examination alone is imprecise. In a Danish study in which patients were enrolled on the basis of clinical suspicion, 70% had abnormalities on computerized tomography (CT) examination, whereas 53% had acute sinusitis confirmed by purulent or mucopurulent discharge on antral puncture.[5] A Norwegian study based on general practice over a 1-year period reported an incidence of 21.7 episodes per 1000 adults per year.[6]

A literature search was conducted of The Cochrane Library, MEDLINE (post-1990), EMBASE (post-1990) and Clinical Evidence using the following Medical Subject Heading (MESH) terms 'sinusitis', 'bronchitis', 'respiratory tract infections' and 'cough'.

Description of the problem: prevalence, diagnosis and clinical course

Prevalence

Acute bronchitis is a commonly occurring respiratory illness. About 5% of adults in the USA self-report an episode of acute bronchitis each year, and up to 90% of these persons seek medical attention.[7] Chest infections are common. The overall consultation rate for acute upper respiratory infections (ICD version 10, code 465) is 772 per 10 000 person–years at risk.[8] The syndrome of acute bronchitis is thought to be preceded by and associated with a viral nasopharyngitis.[9,10] The causes of such infection are usually influenza, parainfluenza, respiratory syncitial, rhinovirus, coronavirus and adenoviruses.[1] Organisms such as *Bordetella pertussis*, *Mycoplasma pneumoniae* and *Chlamydia pneumoniae* are also responsible for chest infections. Secondary bacterial infection usually with *Streptococcus pneumoniae* or *Haemophilus influenzae* is often stated to occur, but how commonly this happens is unclear.[1,10]

In a UK-based study, 25% of sputum culture requests in individuals treated as having acute bronchitis grew recognized or potential respiratory bacterial pathogens.[11] In a more recent UK community-based study of 316 patients with lower respiratory tract infection, an aetiological diagnosis was established in 173 (55%) patients, *S. pneumoniae* (54), *H. influenzae* (31), *Moraxella catarrhalis* (7) and atypical organisms (*Chlamydia pneumoniae* 55 and *Mycoplasma pneumoniae* 23) and viruses (61) being most frequently identified.[12] Bacterial and atypical infection correlated with changes in the chest radiograph and high levels of C-reactive protein (CRP) but not with GP's assessment of whether infection was present, clinical features or chest signs, and whether or not antibiotics were prescribed or not.[12]

The infecting organisms in acute sinusitis are seldom isolated because of the invasive nature of antral puncture and low referral to ear, nose and throat specialists. The most common pathogens are *S. pneumoniae* and *H. influenzae*.[13]

Diagnosis

For bronchitis, diagnosis is usually made on clinical grounds alone, and the infecting organism is rarely sought or identified. Blood tests, such as full blood count, serology for viruses, rarely affect the immediate management of chest infections in primary care. Sputum examination and culture is seldom done, partly because the results take too long to influence management and also because bacteria are carried as normal resident flora in the upper respiratory tract, thus the aetiological role of bacterial infection when cultured from sputum samples is unclear.[10]

The predictive value of clinical findings for acute bronchitis is poor. When considering more severe illness in patients with lower respiratory symptoms, no individual clinical finding, or combinations of findings, can rule in the diagnosis of pneumonia.[14] For adults, the absence of vital sign abnormality and abnormal findings on chest auscultation substantially reduces the probability of pneumonia (< 5%).[14] Thus, for both adults and children, it is easier to rule out serious illness than rule in illness that has a poorer prognosis.[14,15]

This variability in the diagnostic utility of clinical findings has consequences in the diagnostic labelling of respiratory illness. There is evidence that diagnostic labelling bears no clear relationship to symptoms and signs of illness.[16] Furthermore, when antibiotics are prescribed, they appear to be prescribed on the basis of the diagnostic label or in the belief that a clinical feature elicited has a strong relationship to clinical outcome, when in fact this is not the case.[17]

Such diagnostic uncertainty inevitably means that other factors, such as patient's expectations and time constraints during the consultation, have a major impact on the likelihood of prescribing antibiotics.[18,19] In one UK study in which GPs prescribed antibiotics for 75% of patients presenting with acute lower respiratory tract illness, they felt that in only one-third of these cases were antibiotics definitely indicated. Other factors such as patients' expectations, time constraints and previous experience with the patient were independent factors in the decision to prescribe antibiotics.[18] Qualitative research has shown that patients presenting with acute respiratory symptoms often believe that infection is the problem and that antibiotics provide a solution.[20] Therefore, recognizing and exploring patient's understanding about the nature and cause of their illness, its likely clinical course and treatment options is essential if rational antibiotic use in acute bronchitis is to be achieved.

As it is difficult to differentiate between viral and bacterial infection on the basis of symptoms alone,[9] it is not surprising that GPs have been shown to have substantially different diagnostic and treatment thresholds for respiratory tract infection in the community.[9,16] Twelve years on from these observations, variations in diagnostic labelling and treatment thresholds of acute bronchitis persist.[21] A move towards a system of quantifying the prognostic significance of symptoms and signs, so that a more rational approach to the management of acute respiratory illness can be achieved might be a way forward in the future.[3,22]

A similar dilemma occurs when trying to make a diagnosis of acute sinusitis. Several diagnostic studies have attempted to relate the presence of symptoms and signs to a diagnosis of acute bacterial sinusitis.[5,23,24] A further complicating issue is that the reference 'gold standard' of antral puncture is not acceptable to many patients; consequently, alternative reference standards such as X-rays (opacification and fluid level) or CT scans (fluid level or mucosal thickening) of the sinuses have been used. These different reference standards produce differing estimates of acute sinusitis in patients presenting with symptoms in primary care: CT scans suggest that 63–70% of individuals have acute sinusitis, whereas for antral puncture, only 53% of patients met the diagnostic criteria of acute bacterial sinusitis.[5] A systematic review of diagnostic tests for acute sinusitis revealed that, when antral puncture is used as the

'gold standard', between 49% and 83% of symptomatic patients have acute sinusitis.[25]

These difficulties aside, there are some symptoms and signs that raise the probability of having acute bacterial sinusitis.[5,23,24] Table 1 summarizes the individual symptoms and signs and combinations with their corresponding likelihood ratios. It is apparent that no individual symptom or sign raises the probability of sinusitis to a level where antibiotic treatment can be justified.[5,23,24] Combinations of symptoms and signs yield greater diagnostic information. However, for GPs, the absence of symptoms and signs is likely to be more useful in providing reassurance to patients that the probability of acute bacterial sinusitis is low. Some studies have shown that simple blood markers of infection may have diagnostic value. Raised erythrocyte sedimentation rate (ESR) or CRP is independently associated with acute sinusitis.[5,23] Their diagnostic value is limited by the delay in obtaining results.

In a similar way to antibiotic treatment and bronchitis, other factors aside from symptoms and signs have an impact on antibiotic prescribing for acute sinusitis.[19] Patient's expectation and physician's perception of patient expectation influence whether antibiotics are prescribed or not. In terms of symptoms alone, greater emphasis is placed on individual symptoms and signs when deciding about antibiotic treatment than is warranted (Table 1). Physicians place great emphasis on the visualization of purulent nasal discharge, reporting of purulent nasal discharge or sinus tenderness.[26] Antibiotic prescribing was reported to be greater than 75% when the probability of sinusitis was intermediate (on the basis of these single findings).[26] These findings reflect the fact that antibiotics are currently prescribed when the post-test probability of sinusitis is likely to be above 40–50%.[26]

In conclusion, for both acute bronchitis and sinusitis, recognition of the relatively low prior probabilities of these conditions,[27] coupled with moderate likelihood ratios for individual symptoms and signs, should make physicians mindful that high post-test probabilities for either condition are unlikely, unless the patient presents with a combination of symptoms and signs. Acknowledgement and exploration of the patient's understanding and expectations about the clinical course and effectiveness of antibiotic treatment allows uncertainty to be shared and may help to reduce the patient's expectation of antibiotic treatment.[28]

Clinical course

The severity and duration of symptoms associated with acute bronchitis are not trivial. Impairment of daily activities can be considerable and on average last around 2–3 weeks.[29,30] Duration of cough also lasts on average between 2 and 3 weeks.[29,30] Patients usually seek medical attention between 7 and 10 days into the illness, so it is advisable to tell patients that symptoms, particularly cough, will last for at least 10 days when providing information about their likely clinical course. The clinical course of acute sinusitis can be estimated from the placebo

Table 1. Individual symptoms and signs (likelihood ratios) significantly associated with acute sinusitis (adapted from Williams[24] and Lindbaek[23]).

Symptom or sign	Frequency of presentation (%)	Positive likelihood ratio
Maxillary toothache[24]	Not reported	2.5
Purulent secretion[24]	Not reported	2.1
Poor response to decongestants[24]	Not reported	2.1
Abnormal transillumination[24]	Not reported	1.6
History of coloured nasal discharge[24]	Not reported	1.5
Purulent nasal secretion cavum nasi[23]	42	5.5
Purulent rhinorrhoea[23]	78	1.5
Worsening symptoms after initial improvement[23]	59	2.1
ESR > 10[23]	61	1.7

Combined symptoms and signs*	Positive likelihood ratio
0[24]	0.1
1[24]	0.5
2[24]	1.1
3[24]	2.6
≥4[24]	6.4
0[23]	0.1
1[23]	0.2
2[23]	0.8
3[23]	1.8
4[23]	25.2

*Combination refers to the symptoms and signs reported in each individual study.
ESR, erythrocyte sedimentation rate.

arms of randomized controlled trials (RCTs). About two-thirds of individuals with acute sinusitis are still unwell after 3–5 days, and the median duration of illness is 17 days.[13]

Descriptions of treatments

Antibiotic treatment
The aim of antibiotic treatment is to alleviate symptoms, shorten duration of illness and prevent progression or further complications. The study characteristics (participants, setting, interventions and duration of follow-up) of the randomized trials of antibiotics for acute bronchitis and acute sinusitis are summarized in Table 2.

Evidence from RCTs of antibiotic versus placebo are summarized in Tables 3 (acute bronchitis) and 4 (acute sinusitis). There is some evidence that treatment with antibiotic, on average, has some benefit for both conditions. The average duration of symptoms for acute bronchitis is reduced by about half a day, whereas the number needed to treat (NNT) for a variety of the symptoms associated with acute bronchitis varies from 6 to 33. The number needed to harm (NNH) is 16. It should be noted that the number of randomized trials that have been performed are small, so there is some uncertainty concerning efficacy and side-effects of antibiotics, reflected in the wide confidence intervals (Table 3). Similarly, the benefit of treating patients with acute sinusitis appears, on average, to be marginal. NNTs varied from 5 to 7, but the NNHs are of similar magnitude (Table 4). This evidence is based on an even smaller number of placebo-controlled randomized trials. Risk stratification, on the basis of symptoms and signs at the time of consultation, has been proposed as a more rational approach when targeting antibiotic therapy.[31] However, there is a paucity of evidence from RCTs that demonstrates clear benefits in prespecified subgroups such as the elderly or those with comorbid medical conditions.

The goal of antibiotic therapy is to treat as specifically as possible while covering the most likely organisms. In view of the prominence of *S. pneumoniae* and *H. influenzae*, these organisms should always be covered in the first instance.[2,32] Indeed, in the UK, most respiratory pathogens, with the exception of *M. catarrhalis*, remain susceptible to an aminopenicillin or macrolide.[33] Therefore, either amoxicillin or ampicillin is effective in most instances.[34] In patients with features suggestive of atypical pneumonia and those infected

Table 2. Summary of included randomized trials for acute bronchitis and acute sinusitis (adapted from Smucny *et al.*[53] and Williams *et al.*[50]).

Acute bronchitis	Acute sinusitis
Primary comparison: antibiotic versus placebo	*Primary comparison*: antibiotic versus placebo
Participants: 11 RCTs with 1018 patients aged 18–75 years with acute bronchitis/acute productive cough without underlying pulmonary disease	*Participants*: five RCTs involving 456 patients. Inclusion criteria: diagnostic confirmation of acute sinusitis by radiograph or CT scan, outcome includes clinical cure or improvement in a sample size of 30 or more adults
Setting: ambulatory care settings	*Setting*: ambulatory care settings
Interventions: variety of different broad-spectrum antibiotics including erythromycin (four RCTs), tetracyclines (five trials), trimethoprim–sulfamethoxazole (one RCT), amoxicillin–clavulanic acid (one RCT)	*Interventions*: penicillin or amoxicillin versus placebo or lincomycin (a topical decongestant)
Outcomes assessed: resolution of cough (day and night-time), productive cough, limitation in work or activities, improvement at global assessment, abnormal lung examination, adverse effects, mean number of days with cough, productive cough, days of impaired activities and days feeling ill	*Outcomes assessed*: clinical cure, clinical cure or improvement, drop-outs due to adverse effects. High rates of follow-up (>90%) achieved

Table 3. Summary of effect of antibiotics versus placebo in the treatment of acute bronchitis (adapted from Smucny *et al.*[53]).

Outcome (adults)*	Relative risk (95% CI)	NNT (95% CI)
Cough at follow-up	0.64 (0.49–0.85)	6 (3–16)
Night cough	0.76 (0.45–1.30)	15 (6–∞)
Productive cough at follow-up	0.88 (0.72–1.08)	33 (9–∞)
Limitations in activities	0.61 (0.33–1.13)	13 (6–285)
Not improved (physician assessment)	0.75 (0.56–0.97)	15 (7–∞)
Abnormal lung examination at follow-up	0.48 (0.26–0.89)	12 (6–409)

Outcome (adults)†	Relative risk (95% CI)	NNH (95% CI)
Adverse effects	1.48 (1.02–2.14)	16 (8–124)

Outcome (adults)	Weighted mean difference (95% CI)
Mean number of days with cough	−0.58 (−1.16 to −0.01)
Days of productive cough	−0.43 (−0.93 to 0.07)
Days of impaired activity	−0.48 (−0.96 to 0.01)
Days of feeling ill	−0.58 (−1.16 to 0.00)

*Outcome measured is negative; hence, relative risk >1 favours placebo, relative risk <1 favours antibiotic.
†Side-effects, relative risk >1 more side-effects with antibiotic, relative risk <1 more side-effects with placebo.

with *M. catarrhalis*, erythromycin or tetracycline are effective.[33] In those allergic to penicillin, trimethoprim or erythromycin are reasonable alternatives.[33]

Over-the-counter cough medicines

Over-the-counter (OTC) medicines represent a heterogeneous group of products, with different modes of action.[35] They include: (a) antitussives, centrally acting opioid de-rivates or peripherally acting agents; (b) mucolytics, which decrease the viscosity of bronchial secretions, making them easier to clear through coughing; (c) antihistamine–decongestant combinations, combined H1 receptor antagonists and α adrenoceptor agonists, which cause vasoconstriction of mucosal blood vessels; (d) antihistamines, H1 receptor antagonists alone; and (e) combinations of all the ingredients above. The characteristics of RCTs of OTC medicines are

Table 4. Summary of effect of antibiotics versus placebo in the treatment of acute sinusitis (adapted from Williams et al.[49]).

Outcome*	Odds ratio (95% CI)	NNT (95% CI)
Clinical cure (amoxicillin)	2.24 (1.40–3.56)	5 (3–13)
Clinical cure (penicillin)	2.22 (1.09–4.51)	6 (3–40)
Clinical cure or improvement (amoxicillin)	2.09 (1.24–3.53)	7 (4–24)
Clinical cure or improvement (penicillin)	2.06 (1.05–4.05)	6 (3–69)
Outcome†	**Odds ratio (95% CI)**	**NNH (95% CI)**
Adverse effects (amoxicillin)	2.19 (0.93–5.12)	5 (3–∞)
Adverse effects (penicillin)	2.47 (1.03–5.92)	5 (2–69)

*Outcome measured as clinical cure or clinical cure or improvement; odds ratio >1 favours antibiotic, odds ratio <1 favours placebo.
†Adverse effects calculated from results in Table 4 Lindaek et al.[13] Odds ratio >1 side-effects greater in antibiotic, odds ratio <1 side-effects greater in placebo.

Table 5. Summary of RCTs of over-the-counter cough medicine for acute cough in adults (adapted from Schroeder and Fahey[35] and, for β_2-agonists, adapted from Smucny et al.[36]).

Over-the-counter preparations[35]	β_2-agonists[36]
Primary comparison: oral over-the-counter cough preparations versus placebo	*Primary comparison*: β_2 agonist versus placebo
Participants: 15 RCTs with 2166 patients aged 16 years or over with acute cough without underlying pulmonary disease	*Participants*: five RCTs involving 418 patients. Inclusion criteria: adults with the diagnostic label of acute bronchitis who do not have underlying pulmonary disease
Setting: ambulatory care settings	*Setting*: ambulatory care settings
Interventions: variety of over-the-counter preparations including antitussives (four RCTs), expectorants (two trials), antihistamine–decongestant combinations (two RCTs), antihistamines (two RCTs) and other combinations (two RCTs)	*Interventions*: β_2 agonists in oral (three RCTs) or inhaled (two RCTs) versus placebo
Outcomes assessed: cough severity (measured by a variety of different methods including patient self-report, patient diary, patient questionnaire and recorded by microphone)	*Outcomes assessed*: cough, productive cough, night cough, mean cough at 2–7 days, side-effects (shaking, nervousness or tremor), other side-effects

summarized in Table 5. In adults, a systematic review that included 15 RCTs involving 2166 adults shows that antihistamines alone appear unlikely to produce any symptomatic relief greater than placebo. For other drugs or drug combinations, there was no evidence of a clinically important benefit.[35] Results from this systematic review, stratified by drug class, are summarized in Table 6. Despite the huge volume of sales of these products, there remains very little convincing evidence to support their efficacy in acute bronchitis or sinusitis.

Other treatments

Use of β-agonists is supported by evidence from five RCTs. The characteristics of these RCTs are summarized in Table 5.[36]

Although there is some evidence of efficacy in reducing cough symptoms, these have to be balanced against a significant increase in side-effects (Table 6).[36,37] There is insufficient evidence that steam inhalation improves clinical outcome in either condition. In people already taking antibiotics, a single RCT has shown that intranasal steroid improved the symptoms of acute sinusitis over 15 days.[37]

Effects of treatments: impact on subgroups

In otherwise healthy patients with acute cough and no other localizing features, the risk/benefit ratio does not favour the use of antibiotics. However, as the severity of illness and co-

Table 6. Summary of effect of over-the-counter cough medicines versus placebo and β_2 agonists versus placebo in the treatment of acute cough (adapted from Schroeder and Fahey[35] and Smucny et al.[36]).

Over-the-counter preparations	Results
Antitussive (five RCTs)	Two RCTs of codeine found it no more effective than placebo. Two RCTs of dextromethorphan, one associated with improved mean cough counts, the other no different from placebo. One RCT of moguisteine found no difference compared with placebo
Expectorants (two RCTs)	One RCT reported benefit, the other no difference compared with placebo
Mucolytics (one RCT)	Frequent cough reported to be less prevalent in mucolytic group
Antihistamines (two RCTs)	No difference (terfenadine) when compared with placebo
Antihistamine–decongestant combination (two RCTs)	One RCT showed lower mean severity cough scores, other RCT no different from placebo
Other drug combinations (three RCTs)	All three RCTs reported some improvement but side-effects were also greater in intervention group

β_2-agonists	Relative risk (95% CI)
Cough after 7 days	0.77 (0.54–1.09)
Productive cough after 7 days	0.66 (0.35–1.25)
Night cough after 7 days	0.85 (0.57–1.26)

Adverse outcome	Odds ratio (95% CI)
Adverse effects (shaking tremor or nervousness)	7.94 (1.17–53.94)
Adverse effects (penicillin)	0.4 (0.17–0.97)

morbid factors in each individual increases, then significant morbidity may well occur. Between 10% and 20% of patients with respiratory tract infection see their GP more than once during their illness,[2,20,38] so adequate explanation about the natural history of acute bronchitis is an important element of sharing uncertainty with patients. In some subgroups of patients (age over 60 years, persistent coughing and features suggestive of systemic illness), prognosis may well be worse and the potential benefits of antibiotic treatment may outweigh the risks.

Side-effects of treatment

Treatment with antibiotic for both bronchitis and sinusitis is not without risk. Three factors need to be considered when weighing up the risks and benefits from antibiotic treatment: benefits, side-effects and cost. A decision analysis comparing three management strategies for acute bronchitis (withholding antibiotics and treating only patients with persistent cough, screening all patients and treating only those positive for *Mycoplasma* or *Chlamydia* infection or treating all patients empirically with antibiotics) found that the most cost-effective strategy was to withhold antibiotic and treat those

individuals with persistent cough.[39] Treatment with antibiotic may alter patient expectations concerning future episodes of acute bronchitis. Observational research suggests that patient expectations may increase and influence subsequent workload among GPs.[40,41] Patient satisfaction is likely to be higher if their expectations are addressed and information given rather than antibiotic prescribed.[42] Last, bacterial resistance to antibiotics is becoming increasingly common.[33] A liberal policy of prescribing antibiotics to a patient when managing acute bronchitis or sinusitis is likely to make this situation worse.

Management of patient expectation

An observational study of the management of 1089 patients with acute respiratory illness by 115 GPs showed that, although 75% of patients received antibiotics, only in one-third of these cases did GPs feel that antibiotic was definitely indicated.[18] Other factors such as time and work constraints on the GP, prior experience with the patients and social factors had an impact on the likelihood of prescribing an antibiotic. In order to avoid unnecessary prescribing, GPs should be mindful that these other factors play an important part in the consultation and have a strong influence on antibiotic prescribing.

Adequate time, explanation and information should be given to patients presenting with acute bronchitis or sinusitis. If patients are dissatisfied with explanations given to them, they are twice as likely to reconsult during the same episode of illness.[20]

Some specific management strategies have been shown to be useful. RCTs of providing patient information leaflets (giving specific advice about the usual duration of illness, symptomatic remedies and warning signs) can reduce subsequent reconsultation for the same episode of illness.[43] In a different RCT, the same research group showed that antibiotic usage can be reduced (from 63% to 49%) when an information leaflet specifically giving advice about symptomatic treatment and antibiotics is given to patients in whom the GP judges that antibiotics are not likely to be of benefit at the time of consultation.[44] Another management strategy is to provide patients with a 'delayed' antibiotic prescription. Patients are advised to defer taking antibiotics, using them only if their symptoms get worse or they are not improving after a week. Although no direct evidence exists for using this strategy for acute bronchitis or sinusitis, there is strong evidence from RCTs that 'delayed' scripts are effective in the management of sore throat in adults.[45,46,47]

Observational studies have shown that public health strategies can be effective in changing prescription rates for antibiotics at a population level. Educational interventions directed towards health professionals (in the format of peer leader presentation) and to parents of young children and the public (by means of printed material) have produced reductions of over 11% above the natural decline in antibiotic prescribing in the USA.[48] Changes in antibiotic prescribing have an impact on antibiotic resistance. In Finland, a public health campaign aimed at curbing inappropriate prescribing of macrolide antibiotics resulted in a reduction in their use in outpatient clinics, which was followed by a reduction in the frequency of group A streptococcal isolates resistant to erythromycin from throat swabs and pus samples.[49]

Comparative efficacy and costs

There is no convincing evidence that newer antibiotics are any more effective than older broad-spectrum antibiotics such as penicillin and amoxicillin. Two systematic reviews have shown that no clinically important benefits are apparent with newer non-penicillins, amoxicillin–clavulanate or cephalosporins.[50,51] Furthermore, the superiority of antibiotics that are active against atypical organisms (*Mycoplasma pneumoniae*, *Legionella* and *Chlamydia pneumoniae*) compared with β-lactam antibiotics has not been established in patients with non-severe community-acquired pneumonia.[52]

Conclusion

Acute bronchitis and sinusitis are common reasons for seeking

medical advice. Certain symptoms and signs, particularly with sinusitis, raise the probability of bacterial infection and prolonged illness. Evidence from RCTs suggests that antibiotics are of value in patients with a higher probability of bacterial infection or comorbid conditions. For the majority of patients, the side-effects of antibiotic therapy outweigh any benefit. Therefore, it is important that patients' expectations and concerns are addressed, and that information about the self-limiting nature of both conditions is given. 'Delayed' antibiotic prescribing and patient information leaflets are useful management strategies that help to reduce unnecessary antibiotic prescribing for both conditions.

Summary

- Acute bronchitis is a diagnostic label representing a wide variety of clinical syndromes with a spectrum of illness ranging from cough without sputum to cough with mucopurulent sputum, fever, general malaise and dyspnoea.
- Acute sinusitis also represents a diagnostic label. When antral puncture is used as the 'gold standard', between 49% and 83% of symptomatic patients have confirmed acute sinusitis.
- Individual and combined symptoms and signs of illness can help to revise the probability of more serious illness or complications for both conditions.
- For both acute bronchitis and sinusitis, it is important to share information about diagnosis, prognosis and treatment with patients and to address their concerns and understanding about illness.
- Treatment with antibiotics for acute sinusitis and bronchitis is associated with marginal clinical benefits that need to be balanced against side-effects, costs, antibiotic resistance and 'medicalization' of what are frequently self-limiting conditions.

References

1 Garibaldi RA. Epidemiology of community-aquired respiratory tract infections in adults. *Am J Med* 1985; **78**:32–7.
2 Macfarlane J, Holmes W, Gard P *et al.* Prospective study of the incidence, aetiology and outcome of adult lower respiratory tract illness in the community. *Thorax* 2001; **56**:109–14.
3 Stocks N, Fahey T. Labelling of acute respiratory illness: evidence of between-practitioner variation in the UK. *Fam Pract* 2002; **19**:375–7.
4 Lindboek M, Hjortdahl P, Johnsen ULH. Use of symptoms, signs, and blood tests to diagnose acute sinus infections in primary care: comparison with computed tomography. *Fam Pract* 1996; **28**:183–8.
5 Hansen JG, Schmidt H, Rosborg J, Lund E. Predicting acute maxillary sinusitis in a general practice population. *BMJ* 1995; **311**:233–6.
6 Lindbaek M, Hjortdahl P, Holth V. Acute sinusitis in Norwegian general practice. *Eur J Gen Pract* 1997; **3**:7–11.
7 Gonzales R, Bartlett JG, Besser RE *et al.* Principles of appropriate antibiotic use for treatment of uncomplicated acute bronchitis: background. *Ann Intern Med* 2001; **134**:521–9.
8 Royal College of General Practitioners. *Morbidity Statistics from General Practice. Fourth National Study, 1991–1992.* London, HMSO, 1995.
9 Verheij T, Kaptein A, Mulder J. Acute bronchitis: aetiology, symptoms and treatment. *Fam Pract* 1989; **6**:66–9.
10 Gwaltney JM. Acute bronchitis. In: Mandell GL, ed. *Principles and*

Practice of Infectious Diseases. New York, Churchill Livingstone, 1995:606–8.

11 Johnson PH, MacFarlane JT, Humphreys H. How is sputum microbiology used in general practice? *Respir Med* 1996; **90**:87–8.

12 Macfarlane J, Holmes W, Gard P *et al.* Prospective study of the incidence, aetiology and outcome of adult lower respiratory tract illness in the community. *Thorax* 2001; **56**:109–14.

13 Lindbaek M, Hjortdahl P, Johnsen ULH. Randomised, double blind, placebo controlled trial of penicillin V and amoxicillin in treatment of acute sinus infections in adults. *BMJ* 1996; **313**:325–9.

14 Metlay J, Kapoor W, Fine M. Does this patient have community-acquired pneumonia? *JAMA* 1997; **278**:1440–5.

15 Margolis P, Gadomski A. The rational clinical examination: does this infant have pneumonia? *JAMA* 1998; **279**:308–13.

16 Verheij T, Hermans J, Kaptein A, Wijkel D, Mulder J. Acute bronchitis: general practitioner's views regarding diagnosis and treatment. *Fam Pract* 1990; **7**:175–80.

17 Mainous AGII, Hueston WJ, Eberlein C. Colour of respiratory discharge and antibiotic use. *Lancet* 1997; **350**:1077.

18 Macfarlane J, Lewis S, MacFarlane R, Holmes W. Contemporary use of antibiotics in 1089 adults presenting with acute lower respiratory tract illness in general practice in the UK: implications for developing management guidelines. *Respir Med* 1997; **91**:427–34.

19 Dosh SA, Hickner J, Mainous AGI, Ebell MH. Predictors of antibiotic prescribing for nonspecific upper respiratory infections, acute bronchitis and acute sinusitis An UPRNet study. *J Fam Pract* 2000; **49**:407–14.

20 Macfarlane J, Holmes B, MacFarlane R, Britten N. Influence of patients' expectations on antibiotic management of acute lower respiratory tract illness in general practice: a questionnaire study. *BMJ* 1997; **315**:1211–14.

21 Arroll B, Kenealy T. Antibiotics for acute bronchitis. *BMJ* 2001; **322**:939–40.

22 Stocks N, Fahey T. The treatment of acute bronchitis by general practitioners in the UK. *Aust Fam Phys* 2002; **31**:676–9.

23 Lindboek M, Hjortdahl P, Johnsen ULH. Use of symptoms, signs, and blood tests to diagnose acute sinus infections in primary care: comparison with computed tomography. *Fam Med* 1996; **28**:183–8.

24 Williams JW, Simel DL. Does this patient have sinusitis? *JAMA* 1993; **270**:1242–6.

25 Engels EA, Terrin N, Barza M, Lau J. Meta-analysis of diagnostic tests for acute sinusitis. *J Clin Epidemiol* 2000; **53**:852–62.

26 Little DR, Mann BL, Sherk DW. Factors influencing the clinical diagnosis of sinusitis. *J Fam Pract* 1998; **46**:147–52.

27 Okkes IM, Oskam SK, Lamberts H. The probability of specific diagnoses for patients presenting with common symptoms to Dutch family physicians. *J Fam Pract* 2002; **51**:31–6.

28 Butler C, Rollnick S, Kinnersley P, Jones A, Stott N. Reducing antibiotics for respiratory tract symptoms in primary care: considering 'why' and considering 'how'. *Br J Gen Pract* 1998; **48**:1865–70.

29 Verheij T, Hermens J, Kapstein A, Mulder J. Acute bronchitis: course of symptoms and restrictions in patients' daily activities. *Scand J Primary Health Care* 1995; **13**:8–12.

30 Holmes W, MacFarlane JT, Macfarlance R, Hubbard R. Symptoms, signs and prescribing for acute lower respiratory tract illness. *Br J Gen Pract* 2001; **51**:177–81.

31 Fahey T. Applying the results of clinical trials to patients in general practice: perceived problems, strengths, assumptions, and challenges for the future. *Br J Gen Pract* 1998; **48**:1173–8.

32 Woodhead MA, MacFarlane JT, McCracken JS, Rose DH, Finch RG. Prospective study of the aetiology and outcome of pneumonia in the community. *Lancet* 1987; **1**(8534):671–4.

33 Verkatesum P, Innes JA. Antibiotic resistance in common acute respiratory pathogens. *Thorax* 1995; **50**:481–3.

34 Donowitz GR, Mandell GL. Acute pneumonia. In: Mandell GL, ed. *Principles and Practice of Infectious Disease.* New York, Churchill Livingstone, 1995:619–37.

35 Schroeder K, Fahey T. Systematic review of randomised controlled trials of over the counter cough medicines for acute cough in adults. *BMJ* 2002; **324**:329–31.

36 Smuncny J, Flynn C, Becker L, Glazier R. β_2 agonists for acute bronchitis. In: *The Cochrane Review.* Chichester, John Wiley & Sons, 2004.

37 Del Mar C, Glasziou P. Upper respiratory tract infection. In: Cunnington J, ed. *Clinical Evidence.* London, BMJ Publishing, 2003:1747–56.

38 Macfarlane J, Colville A, Guion A, Macfarlane R, Rose D. Prospective study of aetiology and outcome of adult lower-respiratory-tract infections in the community. *Lancet* 1993; **341**:511–14.

39 Hueston WJ. Antibiotics: neither cost effective nor 'cough' effective. *J Fam Pract* 1997; **44**:261–5.

40 Howie JGR, Hutchison KR. Antibiotics and respiratory illness in general practice:prescribing policy and work load. *BMJ* 1978; **2**:1342.

41 Davey P, Rutherford D, Graham B, Lynch B, Malek M. Repeat consultations after antibiotic prescribing for respiratory infections: a study in one general practice. *Br J Gen Pract* 1994; **44**:509–13.

42 Hamm RM, Hicks RJ, Bemben DA. Antibiotics and respiratory infections: are patients more satisfied when expectations are met? *J Fam Pract* 1996; **43**:56–62.

43 Macfarlane J, Holmes W, MacFarlane R. Reducing reconsultations for acute lower respiratory tract illness with an information leaflet: a randomised controlled study of patients in primary care. *Br J Gen Pract* 1997; **47**:719–22.

44 Macfarlane J, Holmes W, Gard P *et al.* Reducing antibiotic use for acute bronchitis in primary care: blinded, randomised controlled trial of patient information leaflet. Commentary: More self reliance in patients and fewer antibiotics: still room for improvement. *BMJ* 2002; **324**:91.

45 Little P, Williamson I, Warner G, Gould G, Gantley M, Kinmonth AL. Open randomised trial of prescribing strategies in managing sore throat. *BMJ* 1997; **314**:722–7.

46 Little P, Gould C, Williamson I, Warner G, Gantley M, Kinmonth AL. Reattendance and complications in a randomised trial of prescribing strategies for sore throat: the medicalising effect of prescribing antibiotics. *BMJ* 1997; **315**:350–2.

47 Arroll B, Kenealy T, Kerse N. Do delayed prescriptions reduce antibiotic use in respiratory tract infections? *Br J Gen Pract* 2003; **53**: 871–7.

48 Perz JF, Craig AS, Coffey CS *et al.* Changes in antiobiotic prescribing for children after a community-wide campaign. *JAMA* 2002; **287**:3103–9.

49 Seppala H, Klaukka T, Vuopio-Varkila J *et al.* The effect of changes in the consumption of macrolide antibiotics on erythromycin resistance in group A streptococci in Finland. *N Engl J Med* 1997; **337**:441–6.

50 Williams JW, Aguilar C, Chiquette E *et al.* Antibiotics for acute maxillary sinusitis (Cochrane Review). In: *The Cochrane Library.* Oxford,Update Software, 2003.

51 de Ferranti S, Ionannidis J, Lau J, Anninger W, Barza M. Are amoxycillin and folate inhibitors as effective as other antibiotics for acute sinusitis? A meta-analysis. *BMJ* 1998; **317**:632–7.

52 Mills GD, Oehley M, Arrol B. Effectiveness of β-lactam antibiotics compared with antibiotics active against atypical pathogens in non-severe community acquired pneumonia: meta-analysis. *BMJ* 2005; **330**: 456–60.

53 Smucny J, Fahey T, Becker L, Glazier R. Antibiotics for acute bronchitis (Cochrane Review). In: *The Cochrane Library.* Chichester, John Wiley & Sons, 2004.

CHAPTER 4.2

Community-acquired pneumonia

Jihendra N Pande, Juhi Dhar and G Sowmya

Introduction

Community-acquired pneumonia (CAP) in adults is an important cause of morbidity and mortality all over the world. In industrialized countries, it is the leading cause of death from infectious diseases and the sixth most important cause of death overall.[1,2] CAP has a wide spectrum of severity ranging from relatively well patients seen in ambulatory outpatient settings to those who require urgent hospital admission to the intensive care unit. In the ambulatory setting, the diagnosis is made on the basis of clinical features alone, although radiographic demonstration of consolidation of one or more segments or lobes of the lung remains the gold standard. It is often difficult to establish the specific infectious aetiology in a given patient so that empirical antibiotic therapy is usually undertaken. In North America and Europe, *Streptococcus pneumoniae* is the most frequent cause of CAP, although a very large number of other organisms have been implicated in the aetiology of the condition.[1,3] Pneumonia caused by specific agents such as *Mycobacterium tuberculosis* or fungi needs to be differentiated from CAP of usual aetiology. Certain patient characteristics, such as advanced age, residence in a nursing home, high alcohol intake, tobacco smoking or the presence of underlying chronic lung disease or other comorbidities, influence the spectrum of causative agents, choice of antibiotic therapy and response to treatment. There is need for regular review, particularly of seriously ill and hospitalized patients, to monitor the response to treatment, detect complications, undertake further diagnostic evaluation and modify antibiotic therapy, if required. Vaccination of adults at risk with currently available vaccines against pneumococcus and influenza may be considered.

Guidelines for the diagnosis and management of CAP based on best available evidence are available in Europe and North America. These have been updated periodically with changes in prevalent microbial aetiology of CAP, availability of new diagnostic tests, emerging pattern of drug resistance and development and licensing of newer antibiotics. Similar guidelines are also available from the professional societies in many other countries. They take into account the existing health infrastructure for delivery of care, availability of resources and cost-effectiveness of various management op-

tions. Geographical differences in the prevalence of causative organisms responsible for CAP are also important in formulating these guidelines. Antibiotics continue to be the most irrationally used drugs all over the world and add to the cost of medical care, particularly in developing countries. Inappropriate use of antibiotics is also responsible for the emergence of drug resistance among several microorganisms, particularly *Strep. pneumoniae, Haemophilus influenzae* and *Staphylococcus aureus*, resulting in revision of the antibiotic guidelines for the management of CAP.

Although the currently available guidelines are based on best evidence of cost-effectiveness in general, the management of an individual patient with pneumonia is determined by several considerations ranging from patient characteristics to social factors and access to care and family support. Deviations from guidelines, however, are noted all too often and are not always justifiable. The desire to offer a wider spectrum of antibiotic cover than really required is often the root problem. There is some evidence from non-randomized studies that patients treated according to the guidelines in North America do better than those given other empirical regimens outside the suggested guidelines.[4,5] In this chapter, we summarize the existing guidelines on the management of CAP by professional societies in the UK and North America, drawing attention, whenever possible, to the evidence base supporting the various recommendations.

Definition of CAP

While radiological demonstration of consolidation on plain radiographs of the chest is the gold standard for the diagnosis of CAP, it is recognized that obtaining a chest X-ray may not always be feasible in community-based health care settings.[6] Further, routine sputum examination (Gram's stain and culture of the expectorated sputum) and white cell count are unhelpful in ruling in or ruling out the diagnosis of pneumonia suspected on clinical grounds. It is therefore recommended that CAP in ambulatory patients be diagnosed on clinical criteria, supplemented by chest radiograph, wherever feasible.[7] Relevant clinical features include cough and expectoration with fever of short duration along with increased respiratory rate and localizing findings on examination of the chest suggestive of consolidation (localized crackles, altered breath sound or bronchophony). The index of suspicion in the elderly who may present with atypical clinical features such as absence of fever, mental confusion, etc. should always be high.

The British Thoracic Society (BTS) Guidelines[7] define CAP in ambulatory setting as follows:

Symptoms of an acute lower respiratory tract illness (cough and at least one other lower respiratory tract symptom); new focal chest signs on examination; at least one systemic feature (either a symptom complex of sweating, fevers, shivers, aches and pains and/or temperature of 38°C or more); and no other explanation for the illness.

For patients admitted to hospital, demonstration of new radiological lesion on chest X-ray is essential. In this setting, the BTS defines CAP as an illness with 'symptoms and signs consistent with an acute lower respiratory tract infection associated with new radiographic shadowing for which there is no other explanation (e.g. not pulmonary oedema or infarction); the illness is the primary reason for hospital admission and is managed as pneumonia'.[7]

Diagnostic evaluation

All patients, particularly those requiring hospitalization, should have an X-ray of the chest. Blood counts and routine blood chemistry should be requested for hospitalized patients and oxygen saturation recorded by pulse oximetry. Two blood cultures should be obtained. If risk factors for unusual organisms not covered by empirical therapy are suspected, a Gram stain of the expectorated sputum and sputum culture should be undertaken. Results of sputum culture should be interpreted in light of the findings on Gram's stain. Findings may be used to broaden empirical antibiotic therapy. Routine serological testing is not recommended, but patients with severe CAP should have estimation of urinary legionella antigen. Collection of bronchoscopic samples from the lower respiratory tract may be undertaken in patients hospitalized in the intensive care unit (ICU).

Risk stratification

Clinical judgement is not reliable for assessing the severity of CAP. As a result, various severity scoring systems and predictive models have been developed to assist the clinician in identifying patients with a poor prognosis as early as possible. However, none of the existing predictive models allows unequivocal categorization into distinct risk groups, and thus clinical judgement remains important.

The BTS has developed a rule for predicting patients at high risk of death based on the assessment of four 'core risk factors' memorized as the **CURB** severity score:[7]

1 Confusion: new mental confusion (defined as an Abbreviated Mental Test score of 8 or less);[8]
2 Urea: raised >7 mmol/L (for patients being seen in hospital);
3 Respiratory rate: raised >30/min;
4 Blood pressure: low blood pressure (systolic blood pressure <90 mmHg and/or diastolic blood pressure <60 mmHg).

A prospective study in the UK including 309 adults aged 16 years and over who were admitted to hospital with CAP over a 12-month period in 1998–99 found that the number of 'core risk factors' correlated well with mortality at 30 days after admission.[9] More recently, the utility of CURB in addition to age ≥ 65 years (CURB-65) was evaluated in a larger prospective study ($n = 1068$) of patients hospitalized with CAP in the UK, New Zealand and the Netherlands.[10] This study found that information available on admission (CURB-65) allowed patients to be stratified according to increasing risk of mortality: score 0, 0.7%; score 1, 3.2%; score 2, 13%; score 3, 17%; score 4, 41.5%; and score 5, 57%. These findings were confirmed in a validation cohort. Using only clinical features (i.e. excluding blood urea estimation; CRB-65) gave a similar trend of increasing disease severity from score 0 (mortality risk 1.2%) to score 4 (mortality risk 18.2%). Based on these findings, the BTS has recommended adoption of the CURB-65/CRB-65 model for predicting disease severity.[11]

In addition to the above 'core' adverse prognostic markers, the following features are recognized as indicative of a poor prognosis:[7]
1 Hypoxaemia ($Sao_2 < 92\%$ or $Pao_2 < 8$ kPa) regardless of Fio_2;
2 Bilateral or multilobe involvement on the chest radiograph.

A complementary prediction rule for defining mortality risk has been derived and validated by the Pneumonia Patient Outcomes Research Team (PORT) in over 50 000 patients in the United States.[12] Based on demographic factors, comorbidity, physical findings and laboratory and radiographic information, patients were classified into five groups with increasing risk of death ranging from 0.6–0.7% in class I to 27.0–31.1% in class V. A limitation of this rule and others is that they were developed using mostly patients seen in hospital emergency departments or those admitted to hospital, with few patients seen and managed in the community being included.

Use of risk stratification for management of patients with CAP

The updated BTS guidelines[11] recommend the use of the CRB-65 risk score for identifying patients seen in the community who can be treated at home (score 0, low risk of death), those who should be considered for referral to hospital (score 1 or 2, higher risk of death) and those who require urgent referral

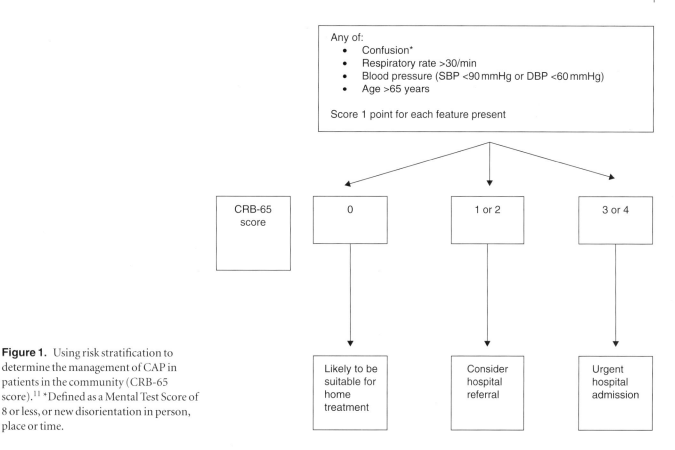

Figure 1. Using risk stratification to determine the management of CAP in patients in the community (CRB-65 score).[11] *Defined as a Mental Test Score of 8 or less, or new disorientation in person, place or time.

for hospital admission (score 3 or 4, highest risk of death) (Fig. 1).

Among those admitted to hospital for assessment, the updated BTS guidelines recommend using the CURB-65 score for making management decisions. Patients with a CURB-65 score of 0 or 1 can be considered for home treatment, those with a score of 2 can be considered for short stay inpatient care or hospitalized supervised outpatient treatment, and those with a score of 3 or more should be managed in hospital as having severe pneumonia (Fig. 2).

It should be kept in mind that a substantial proportion of patients with CAP who have a low risk of death based on a severity prediction model may still require hospitalization.[13,14] Thus, clinical judgement with careful evaluation of adverse prognostic factors is always needed.

Patients with severe CAP require admission to the ICU. The American Thoracic Society (ATS)[6] has defined severe CAP as the presence of either of two major criteria or the presence of two out of three minor criteria. The major criteria include need for mechanical ventilation and septic shock; the minor criteria include systolic blood pressure < 90 mmHg, multilobar disease, and Pao_2/Fio_2 ratio < 250. Alternatively, when using the BTS CURB-65 score, any patient with a score of 4 or 5 should be considered for ICU admission.[11]

Antibiotic therapy

Antibiotics are the cornerstone in the treatment of CAP. The choice of antibiotic therapy is influenced by the likely pathogens involved, their drug susceptibility pattern and adverse effects as well as patient characteristics such as comorbid conditions. Treatment is empirical as the isolation of the specific pathogens from individual patients is not feasible. Further, the clinical features and radiological findings do not permit aetiological diagnosis of pneumonia with a reasonable certainty.

The spectrum of pathogens causing CAP depends on the diagnostic methods used, clinical setting and the severity of illness. *Streptococcus pneumoniae* is the most frequent pathogen in CAP in all clinical settings. Among ambulatory patients, *H. influenzae* is the second most frequent pathogen followed by atypical pathogens, *S. aureus*, *Moraxella catarrhalis* and Gram-negative enteric pathogens. *Staphylococcus aureus* usually causes severe pneumonia in patients with diabetes or renal failure. A significant proportion of patients (10–20%) may have CAP caused by viruses, and no pathogens are isolated from almost half the patients with this condition. It is likely that many of them have pneumococcal pneumonia.

Legionella infection is more common among severely ill

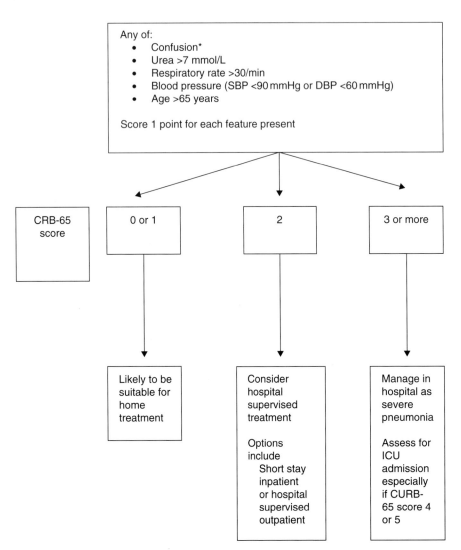

Any of:
- Confusion*
- Urea >7 mmol/L
- Respiratory rate >30/min
- Blood pressure (SBP <90 mmHg or DBP <60 mmHg)
- Age >65 years

Score 1 point for each feature present

CRB-65 score

0 or 1

2

3 or more

Likely to be suitable for home treatment

Consider hospital supervised treatment

Options include
  Short stay inpatient or hospital supervised outpatient

Manage in hospital as severe pneumonia

Assess for ICU admission especially if CURB-65 score 4 or 5

Figure 2. Using risk stratification to determine the management of CAP in patients admitted to hospital (CURB-65 score).[11] *Defined as a Mental Test Score of 8 or less, or new disorientation in person, place or time.

patients hospitalized in the ICU. *Mycoplasma pneumoniae* is frequent during outbreaks and is identified by serological testing. On the whole, atypical pathogens are isolated more frequently from hospitalized patients than from ambulatory patients with pneumonia. Risk factors for infection with specific pathogens have been identified and should be looked for before choosing empirical antibiotic therapy. Some patients with pneumonia may have mixed infection with bacteria and atypical pathogens. As atypical pathogens may take a longer time to be identified, initial microbiological findings may be misleading.

Antibiotic treatment of patients with CAP in community settings

Historically, penicillin has been the antibiotic of choice in CAP. However, its empirical use has been complicated by the worldwide emergence of penicillin resistance among *Strepto-*

coccus pneumoniae. This has led to other antibiotics replacing penicillin as first-line treatment.

One systematic review [18 randomized controlled trials (RCTs) with 1664 participants] compared the effects of the macrolide azithromycin with other macrolides (clarithromycin, erythromycin or roxithromycin; 13 RCTs), cephalosporins (cefaclor; two RCTs) and penicillins (amoxicillin plus clavulanic acid or penicillin; three RCTs).[15] Compared with all other antibiotics, azithromycin reduced clinical failures over 6–21 days by one third [random effects odds ratio (OR) 0.63, 95% confidence interval (CI) 0.41–0.95, number needed to treat (NNT) 50 to prevent one clinical failure]. Further results stratified by antibiotic class are provided in Table 1. Given the possibility of bias resulting from lack of blinding in most of the trials included in the review, the authors caution against the uncritical acceptance of these results.

A second systematic review (eight RCTs with 3131 partici-

Table 1. Systematic review of RCTs comparing the effects of azithromycin: summary estimates of findings for clinical failure with azithromycin versus comparators in patients with community-acquired pneumonia.[15]

Comparator	Type of pneumonia	Number of trials	Random effects OR (95% CI)
β-lactams	Bacterial	5	0.71 (0.29–1.76)
Macrolides	All	13	0.60 (0.36–1.00)
Macrolides	Atypical	7	0.54 (0.24–1.19)
Macrolides	Mixed	6	0.60 (0.28–1.29)
All		18	0.63 (0.41–0.95)

pants) evaluated quinolones (gatifloxacin, levofloxacin, moxifloxacin, sparfloxacin and trovafloxacin) versus high amoxicillin, macrolides and cephalosporins, finding no difference in clinical cure and improvement rates [absolute risk reduction (ARR) +1.7%, 95% CI −1.4% to +4.8%].[3] Similarly, a subsequent RCT found no difference in clinical cure rates between clarithromycin and levofloxacin (RR 1.02; 95% CI 0.93–1.12).[3]

A recent Cochrane Review draws attention to the fact that most clinical trials evaluating the efficacy of alternative antibiotics in patients with CAP were conducted in hospitalized patients.[2] Such patients have more severe disease and suffer from a number of comorbid conditions that can affect treatment responsiveness. It is therefore not known whether the results of these trials can be generalized to less severe cases of CAP treated within community settings. Limiting their selection criteria to double-blind RCTs in adult outpatients with CAP that compared one antibiotic with placebo or another antibiotic, the Cochrane Review found only three studies with 622 patients aged 12 years and older.[3] Two trials compared clarithromycin with erythromycin, finding no difference in clinical (OR 2.27; 95% CI 0.66–7.80), bacteriological (OR 0.28; 95% CI 0.03–2.57) or radiological (OR 0.91; 95% CI 0.33–2.49) outcomes. However, there were significantly more side-effects (mostly gastrointestinal) in the erythromycin group. A further trial included in the review compared clarithromycin with a sparfloxacin, finding no significant differences in clinical or bacteriological success. The authors of the review conclude that, given the current state of the evidence, it is not possible to make evidence-based recommendations about the antibiotic to be used for the treatment of CAP in ambulatory patients. This uncertainty is reflected in the different recommendations made by the British and American Thoracic Societies.

The BTS[7] recommends oral amoxicillin as the antibiotic of choice for patients being treated at home, with a macrolide (erythromycin or clarithromycin) administered to those hypersensitive to penicillin. The BTS further recommends that patients with severe pneumonia referred for hospitalization

be given the first antibiotic dose in the primary care setting as soon as possible.

In contrast, the ATS[6] recommends a macrolide as the antibiotic of choice for ambulatory patients with pneumonia (arguing that amoxicillin does not cover atypical pathogens such as chlamydia, mycoplasma and the legionella group), unless there are risk factors for drug-resistant *S. pneumoniae*, aspiration or Gram-negative organisms. In that case, the addition of a β-lactam or antipneumococcal quinolone is recommended. Whether the initial antibiotic therapy should cover atypical pathogens would depend upon the regional prevalence of these pathogens at a given time. The prevalence of drug-resistant *S. pneumoniae* also varies widely in different countries. The presence of risk factors for Gram-negative infection in CAP is more frequent and requires a β-lactam in the initial regimen.

Antibiotic treatment of patients with CAP treated in hospital

A number of trials have compared various oral or parenteral antibiotics in patients hospitalized with CAP. These studies have found either no difference between antibiotics or better clinical cure rates in people treated with quinolones. The results of these studies cannot be easily interpreted as most were too small and therefore underpowered or were designed to assess equivalence rather than superiority of one antibiotic compared with another.

One RCT assessed the efficacy of amoxicillin–clavulanate (intravenous followed by oral) versus ceftriaxone (intravenous followed by intramuscular) in 378 hospitalized patients with moderate to severe pneumonia.[16] This study found no difference in safety or efficacy between the two treatment options (RR for clinical cure 0.99, 95% CI 0.88–1.12).

A multicentre double-blind RCT with 329 hospitalized patients found no difference in clinical cure between sparfloxacin and amoxicillin at 14–21 days (RR 0.99, 95% CI 0.87–1.07).[17] Sparfloxacin produced fewer gastrointestinal effects than amoxicillin.

Another multicentre RCT with 628 participants compared the effects of moxifloxacin (intravenous followed by oral) with co-amoxiclav (intravenous followed by oral), with or without intravenous clarithromycin.[18] At 5–7 days, the clinical cure rate in patients receiving moxifloxacin (93.4%) was significantly higher than in those on co-amoxiclav (85.4%) (Δ 8.05; 95% CI 2.91–13.19, $P = 0.004$). The superiority of moxifloxacin remained after adjusting for disease severity and use of the macrolide. The rates of adverse reactions were similar in the two groups.

An open-label RCT compared intravenous and/or oral levofloxacin with intravenous ceftriaxone and/or oral cefuroxime axetil in 590 patients, 280 of whom were admitted to hospital.[19] In this study, levofloxacin significantly increased the rate of clinical cure or improvement at 5–7 days compared with the cephalosporins (96% versus 90%) with similar rates of gastrointestinal effects in the two groups. These results contrast with those of an open-label multicentre RCT with 236 participants of levofloxacin (oral or intravenous) versus intravenous azithromycin plus intravenous ceftriaxone followed by oral azithromycin given at the physician's discretion, which found no difference in clinical cure rates (RR 1.08; 95% CI 0.97–1.21).[20]

Currently, a combination of oral or parenteral amoxicillin and a macrolide for a period of 7 days is recommended for hospitalized patients with non-severe pneumonia.[7] Alternatively, a third-generation cephalosporin or a β-lactam plus β-lactamase inhibitor in combination with a macrolide can be used.[6] In regions where resistant S. pneumoniae are a concern, an antipneumococcal quinolone may be considered.

Patients with severe pneumonia should receive intravenous antibiotics at the earliest opportunity. Choices include a β-lactamase-resistant antibiotic such as co-amoxiclav, cefuroxime, cefotaxime or ceftriaxone along with clarithromycin. An intravenous antipneumococcal quinolone such as levofloxacin is an alternative recommended by the ATS.[6] For patients admitted to the ICU with risk factors for Pseudomonas infection (underlying lung disease such as bronchiectasis, undernutrition, steroid therapy, previous treatment with antibiotics), intravenous antipseudomonal β-lactam (cefepime, imipenem, meropenem, piperacillin + tazobactam) plus antipseudomonal quinolone (ciprofloxacin) are recommended by the ATS.[6]

Patients can be switched to the oral route of administration of antibiotics with clinical improvement (improvement in cough and dyspnoea), falling white cell counts and absence of fever for more than 24 hours. They should have a functional gastrointestinal tract to undertake the switch to oral therapy. Total duration of therapy should be 10 days for microbiologically undefined pneumonia, which should be extended to 2–3 weeks for patients with pneumonia caused by staphylococci, Gram-negative enteric pathogens or legionella. Treatment will also be longer if the patient develops complications such as empyema or lung abscess.

About 10% of patients do not improve with empirical treatment. These patients should be carefully evaluated by further investigation to detect unusual organisms or host factors or conditions mimicking pneumonia.

Patients should be considered fit for discharge if their vital signs are stable (afebrile for 24 hours, respiratory rate < 24/min, heart rate < 100/min, systolic blood pressure > 90 mmHg and oxygen saturation > 90% while breathing room air or back to baseline in patients with COPD) and there are no associated medical or psychological problems. Patients should have a clear mental status and should be able to take oral medications. Once these criteria are fulfilled, the risk of serious deterioration after discharge is < 1%. On the other hand, if patients are discharged when they would be considered unfit according to these criteria, the risk of death or readmission or prolonged convalescence at home is appreciably higher.[21]

Emerging antimicrobial resistance to β-lactam antibiotics and macrolides among common pathogens, namely S. pneumoniae and H. influenzae, has been noted in several parts of the world, particularly in the Americas and Europe. Its prevalence in developing countries has not been widely documented, but appears to be much lower. Patients with CAP caused by S. pneumoniae with intermediate resistance to penicillin would still respond to the currently recommended higher doses of amoxicillin, but highly resistant organisms would result in treatment failure. This has been a matter of concern in the USA. Newer macrolides, particularly clarithromycin and azithromycin, are more effective against H. influenzae, but these drugs are bacteriostatic, and drug-resistant strains are being increasingly recognized in both the USA and the European community. Both typical and atypical organisms causing CAP are currently highly susceptible to newer quinolones, particularly levofloxacin, gatifloxacin and moxifloxacin. As indicated above, several clinical trials have documented the efficacy of these agents in the management of CAP. They are acceptable alternatives for the initial treatment of CAP in those parts of the world where high levels of resistance to β-lactam antibiotics and macrolides are being documented.

Vaccination for preventing CAP

Administration of influenza and pneumococcal vaccine is recommended for patients at risk of CAP,[6,7] but these recommendations are not based on the most rigorous evidence.

The effects of influenza vaccine on the incidence of CAP have so far not been evaluated in randomized trials. However, there is evidence from prospective, observational studies that influenza vaccine may reduce the risk of pneumonia and mortality.[22]

Two recent systematic reviews have assessed the effectiveness of polysaccharide pneumococcal vaccines versus placebo or no treatment in preventing pneumonia and death in adults.[23,24] The first review[23] found that, in immunocompetent people (three RCTs with 21 152 participants), pneumococcal vaccination significantly reduced the incidence of all-cause pneumonia (RR 0.56; 95% CI 0.47–0.66), pneumococcal pneumonia (RR 0.16; 95% CI 0.11–0.23) and death due to pneumonia (RR 0.77; 95% CI 0.50–0.96). However, the review found that, in the elderly or those likely to have an impaired immune system (10 RCTs, 24 074 participants), there was no evidence that vaccination was beneficial: all-cause pneumonia (RR 1.08; 95% CI 0.92–1.27), pneumococcal pneumonia (RR 0.88; 95% CI 0.72–1.07) and death due to pneumonia (RR 0.93; 95% CI 0.72–1.20).

The second systematic review,[24] published under the aegis of the Cochrane Collaboration, evaluated and summarized the results of all randomized and quasirandomized trials in adults (Table 2), finding inconsistent results (Figs 3–6): all-cause pneumonia (14 trials; 75 008 participants; OR 0.77; random 95% CI 0.58–1.02); definitive pneumococcal pneumonia

Table 2. Cochrane Review of polysaccharide pneumococcal vaccines for preventing disease and death in adults: characteristics of included trials.[24]

Study reference	Methods	Participants	Interventions	Outcomes
25	Table of random numbers	1200 young adult gold miners in South Africa	Six valent (13 valent later) pneumococcal vaccine, group A meningococcal vaccine or saline placebo	Putative pneumococcal pneumonia, pneumococcal bacteraemia
26	'Randomly assigned' 'double-blind'	1300 adult inpatients, USA	Six valent vaccine or saline placebo	Pneumonia, death, antibody levels
27	Randomly assigned by colour codes	13 600 adults in Kaiser Permanente Health Plan, USA	12 valent vaccine or saline placebo	Pneumonia, death, antibody levels
28	Double-blind randomized using table of random numbers	103 adults with COPD, USA	14 valent vaccine or saline placebo	Antibody titres, bacteriology of sputum, respiratory infections or pneumonia and death
29	Randomized by home according to 'high-risk patient in each'	1686 adults between 55 and 85 years in France	14 valent vaccine or 'control'	Pneumonia and death
30	Assigned according to year of birth	26 295 people in northern Finland	23 valent vaccine or 'control'	Pneumonia and death
31	Patients selected 'at random' during pneumonia season	10 903 patients in 'home', USA	Type I and II pneumococcal polysaccharides administered (later I, II and III) or controls	Blood serum, pneumonia and death
32	Randomized	47 patients with bronchogenic carcinoma, Belgium	17 valent vaccine or saline placebo	Pneumonia or death
33	Randomized	2837 elderly people in Finland	14 valent vaccine and influenza vaccine or influenza vaccine alone	Pneumonia and death
34	Randomized double-blind	Outpatients at a teaching hospital in Canada	14 valent vaccine or saline placebo	Death, hospital admissions, length of hospital stay, visits to emergency departments
35	Randomized double-blind	691 non-immunocompromised adult inpatients 50 to 85 years, Sweden	23 valent vaccine or placebo	Pneumonia, pneumococcal pneumonia and death
36	Randomized double-blind	1158 adults in Papua New Guinea	14 valent vaccine or saline placebo	Pneumococcal infection
37	Randomized double-blind	2 295 high-risk patients, USA	14 valent vaccine or saline placebo	Proved infections, probable pneumococcal pneumonia, probable pneumococcal bronchitis

Review: Vaccines for preventing pneumococcal infection in adults
Comparison: 01 RCTs of Vaccination vs. Placebo
Outcome: 06 Pneumonia, all causes

Study	Vaccine (n/N)	Control (n/N)	Odds ratio (random) (95% CI)	Weight (%)	Odds ratio (random) (95% CI)
Austrian (1976, 13v)	85/1493	359/3002		9.0	0.44 (0.35, 0.57)
Austrian (1980, Grp1)	154/607	144/693		9.0	1.30 (1.00, 1.68)
Austrian (1980, Grp2)	268/6782	274/6818		9.4	0.98 (0.83, 1.17)
Davis (1987)	4/50	7/53		3.2	0.57 (0.16, 2.09)
Gaillat (1985)	3/937	12/749		3.3	0.20 (0.06, 0.70)
Honkanen (1999)	145/13980	116/12945		9.0	1.16 (0.91, 1.48)
Kaufman (1947)	99/5750	227/5153		9.1	0.38 (0.30, 0.48)
Klastersky (1986)	2/26	4/21		1.9	0.35 (0.06, 2.16)
Koivula (1997)	73/1364	69/1473		8.5	1.15 (0.82, 1.61)
Ortqvist (1998)	63/339	57/352		8.2	1.18 (0.80, 1.75)
Riley (1977)	27/2713	40/2660		7.5	0.66 (0.40, 1.08)
Simberkoff (1986)	48/1175	38/1179		7.9	1.28 (0.83, 1.97)
Smit (1977, Grp 1)	37/983	121/2036		8.3	0.62 (0.42, 0.90)
Smit (1977, Grp 2)	9/540	28/1135		5.7	0.67 (0.31, 1.43)
Total (95% CI)	1017/36739	1496/38269		100.0	0.77 (0.58, 1.02)

Test for heterogeneity chi-squared = 108.17 df = 13 $P < 0.00001$
Test for overall effect = −1.85 $P = 0.06$

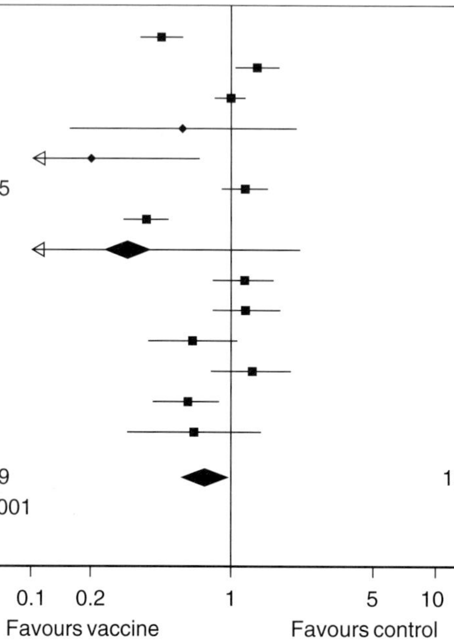

0.1   0.2   1   5   10
Favours vaccine   Favours control

Figure 3. Cochrane Review of polysaccharide pneumococcal vaccines for preventing disease and death in adults. Results for all-cause pneumonia.[24]

Review: Vaccines for preventing pneumococcal infection in adults
Comparison: 01 RCTs of Vaccination vs. Placebo
Outcome: 01 Definitive pneumococcal pneumonia

Study	Vaccine (n/N)	Control (n/N)	Odds ratio (random) (95% CI)	Weight (%)	Odds ratio (random) (95% CI)
Davis (1987)	1/50	0/53		3.7	3.24 (0.13, 81.47)
Gaillat (1985)	0/937	1/749		3.7	0.27 (0.01, 6.54)
Kaufman (1947)	8/5750	34/5153		54.2	0.21 (0.10, 0.45)
Klastersky (1986)	1/26	1/21		4.8	0.80 (0.05, 13.60)
Leech (1987)	1/92	0/97		3.7	3.20 (0.13, 79.48)
Ortqvist (1998)	1/339	5/352		8.2	0.21 (0.02, 1.77)
Riley (1977)	2/2713	14/2660		16.7	0.14 (0.03, 0.61)
Simberkoff (1986)	1/1175	1/1179		5.0	1.00 (0.06, 16.06)
Total (95% CI)	15/11082	56/10264		100.0	0.28 (0.15, 0.52)

Test for heterogeneity chi-squared = 7.22 df = 7 $P = 0.4063$
Test for overall effect = −4.02 $P = 0.0001$

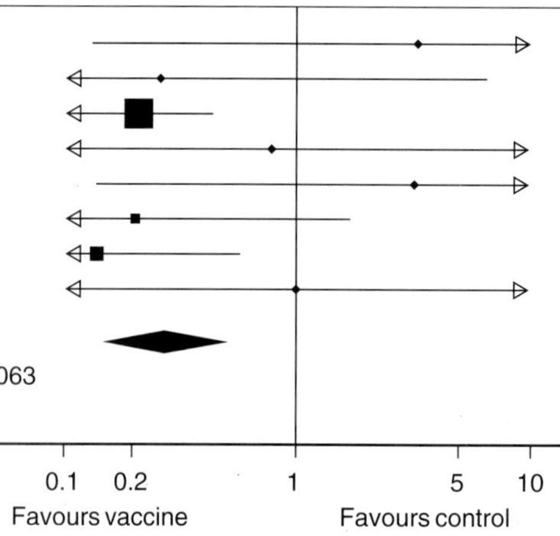

0.1   0.2   1   5   10
Favours vaccine   Favours control

Figure 4. Cochrane Review of polysaccharide pneumococcal vaccines for preventing disease and death in adults. Results for definitive pneumococcal pneumonia.[24]

Review: Vaccines for preventing pneumococcal infection in adults
Comparison: 01 RCTs of Vaccination vs. Placebo
Outcome: 08 Mortality, all causes

Study	Vaccine (n/N)	Control (n/N)	Odds ratio (random) (95% CI)	Weight (%)	Odds ratio (random) (95% CI)
Austrian (1980, Grp1)	35/607	44/693		7.4	0.90 (0.57, 1.43)
Austrian (1980, Grp2)	45/6782	47/6818		8.3	0.96 (0.64, 1.45)
Davis (1987)	14/50	13/53		3.1	1.20 (0.50, 2.88)
Gaillat (1985)	232/937	175/749		12.5	1.08 (0.86, 1.35)
Honkanen (1999)	1651/13980	1639/12945		15.5	0.92 (0.86, 0.99)
Kaufman (1947)	40/5750	98/5153		9.1	0.36 (0.25, 0.52)
Klastersky (1986)	2/26	4/21		0.8	0.35 (0.06, 2.16)
Koivula (1997)	152/1364	166/1473		12.3	0.99 (0.78, 1.25)
Ortqvist (1998)	29/339	28/352		6.1	1.08 (0.63, 1.86)
Riley (1977)	133/5946	170/6012		12.4	0.79 (0.62, 0.99)
Simberkoff (1986)	211/1175	171/1179		12.6	1.29 (1.04, 1.61)
Total (95% CI)	2544/36956	2555/35448		100.0	0.90 (0.76, 1.07)

Test for heterogeneity chi-squared = 39.40 df = 10 $P < 0.00001$
Test for overall effect = −1.19 $P = 0.2$

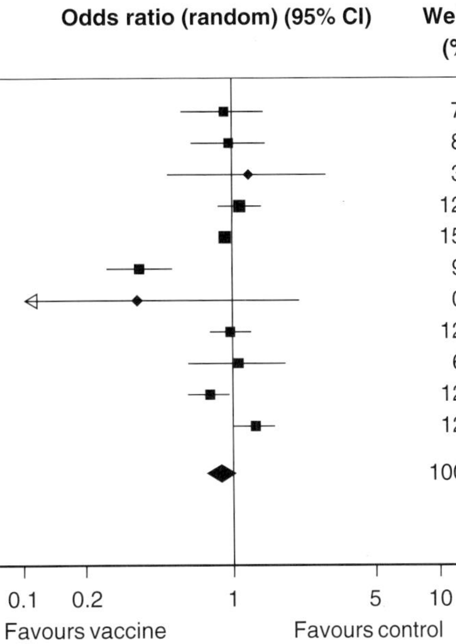

0.1   0.2   1   5   10
Favours vaccine   Favours control

Figure 5. Cochrane Review of polysaccharide pneumococcal vaccines for preventing disease and death in adults. Results for death from all causes.[24]

Review: Vaccines for preventing pneumococcal infection in adults
Comparison: 01 RCTs of Vaccination vs. Placebo
Outcome: 09 Mortality due to pneumonia

Study	Vaccine (n/N)	Control (n/N)	Odds ratio (random) (95% CI)	Weight (%)	Odds ratio (random) (95% CI)
Austrian (1980, Grp1)	23/607	30/693		15.9	0.87 (0.50, 1.52)
Austrian (1980, Grp2)	36/6782	38/6818		17.0	0.95 (0.60, 1.50)
Davis (1987)	2/50	4/53		5.8	0.51 (0.09, 2.92)
Kaufman (1947)	31/5750	98/5153		17.5	0.28 (0.19, 0.42)
Koivula (1997)	5/1364	6/1473		9.3	0.90 (0.27, 2.95)
Ortqvist (1998)	2/339	3/352		5.6	0.69 (0.11, 4.16)
Riley (1977)	23/5946	41/6012		16.4	0.57 (0.34, 0.94)
Simberkoff (1986)	16/1175	8/1179		12.5	2.02 (0.86, 4.74)
Total (95% CI)	138/22013	228/21733		100.0	0.72 (0.44, 1.19)

Test for heterogeneity chi-squared = 27.64 df = 7 $P = 0.0003$
Test for overall effect = −1.29 $P = 0.2$

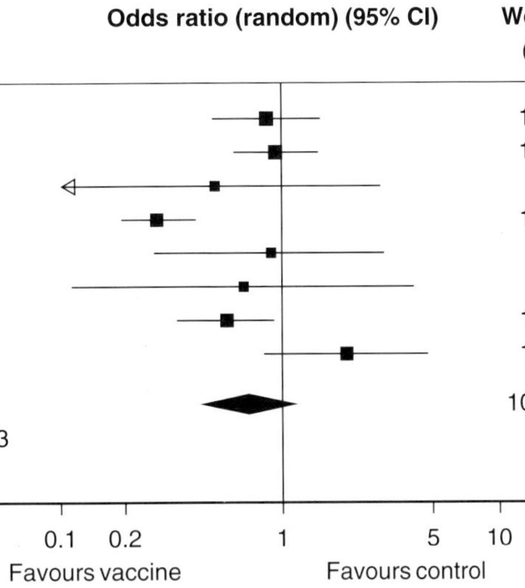

0.1   0.2   1   5   10
Favours vaccine   Favours control

Figure 6. Cochrane Review of polysaccharide pneumococcal vaccines for preventing disease and death in adults. Results for death due to pneumonia.[24]

(eight trials; 21 346 participants; OR 0.28; random 95% CI 0.15–0.52), death from all causes (11 trials; 72 402 participants; OR 0.90; random 95% CI 0.76–1.07) and death due to pneumonia (eight trials; 43 746 participants; OR 0.72; random 95% CI 0.44–1.19). The authors of the review advise cau-

tion in the interpretation of the results because of substantial heterogeneity in the study findings, the reliance on old, poor-quality trials and the possibility of publication bias. Critical evaluation of the current evidence therefore leads to the conclusion that there is no reliable basis for recommending the use of pneumococcal vaccine as an intervention for reducing the risk of pneumonia or death.

Conclusion

Community-based pneumonia is an important condition globally. A number of organisms have been implicated in the aetiology of the condition although *S. pneumoniae* appears to be the most common cause in developed countries. The severity of presentation of CAP varies widely, and various risk scores have been developed to predict patients' prognosis. Several RCTs have demonstrated the efficacy and safety of antibiotics, but the number of studies in ambulatory patients is small, making evidence-based recommendations in this group difficult. Antibiotic therapy is usually empirical with the choice of antibiotics influenced by various clinical, economic and social factors. A large number of antibiotics have been evaluated and found to have similar efficacy and safety profiles. Finally, there is currently no reliable evidence that influenza or pneumococcal vaccines reduce the incidence of CAP or death in adults at risk.

Summary for clinicians

Community-acquired pneumonia (CAP) in adults is an important cause of morbidity and mortality globally.

It has a wide spectrum of severity ranging from relatively well patients seen in ambulatory outpatient settings to those who require urgent hospital admission to the intensive care unit.

It is recommended that CAP in ambulatory patients be diagnosed on clinical criteria, supplemented by chest radiograph, wherever feasible. For patients admitted to hospital, demonstration of new radiological lesion on chest X-ray is essential.

Various disease severity scoring systems are available to assist the clinician in identifying patients with a poor prognosis as early as possible and to decide further case management. However, none of the existing predictive models allows unequivocal categorization into distinct risk groups and clinical judgement remains important.

Antibiotics are the cornerstone in the treatment of CAP with various classes of antibiotics showing similar efficacy and safety. Choice of an antibiotic remains empirical being influenced by the likely pathogens involved, their drug susceptibility pattern and adverse effects as well as patient characteristics such as comorbid conditions.

Currently, there is no reliable evidence that influenza or pneumococcal vaccines are protective against CAP either in the general population or in high-risk patients such as the elderly.

Search strategy

We searched the Cochrane Library, Issue 4, 2004, MEDLINE 1966–2004 and Clinical Evidence 2004 using the following terms: 'pneumonia'; 'community-acquired pneumonia'.

References

1 Barlett JG, Breiman RF, Mandell LA, File TM. Community-acquired pneumonia in adults: guidelines for management. *Clin Infect Dis* 1998; **26**:811–38.

2 Bjerre LM, Verheij TJM, Kochen MM. Antibiotics for community-acquired pneumonia in adult outpatients. The Cochrane Database of Systematic Reviews, Issue 2, 2004.

3 Loeb M. Community-acquired pneumonia. *Clin Evid* 2004; **12**:2062–75.

4 Dean NC, Silver MP, Bateman KA, James B, Hadlock CJ, Hale D. Decreased mortality after implementation of a treatment guideline for community-acquired pneumonia. *Am J Med* 2001; **110**:451–7.

5 Menéndez R, Ferrando D, Vallés JM, Vallterra J. Decreased mortality after implementation of a treatment guideline for community-acquired pneumonia. *Chest* 2002; **122**:612–17.

6 American Thoracic Society. Guidelines for the management of adults with community-acquired pneumonia: diagnosis, assessment of severity, antimicrobial therapy, and prevention. *Am J Respir Crit Care Med* 2001; **163**:1730–54.

7 British Thoracic Society. Guidelines for diagnosis and management of pneumonia. *Thorax* 2001; **56**(Suppl IV).

8 Qureshi KN, Hodkinson HM. Evaluation of a ten question mental test in the institutionalized elderly. *Age Aging* 1974; **3**:152–7.

9 Lim WS, Macfarlane JT, Boswell TC *et al.* Study of community acquired pneumonia aetiology (SCAPA) adults admitted to hosptital: implications for management guidelines. *Thorax* 2001; **56**:296–301.

10 Lim WS, van der Eerden MM, Laing R *et al.* Defining community acquired pneumonia severity on presentation to hospital: an international derivation and validation study. *Thorax* 2003; **58**:377–82.

11 BTS Pneumonia Guidelines Committee. BTS Guidelines for the management of community acquired pneumonia in adults — 2004 update. Published on the BTS website on 30 April 2004.

12 Fine MJ, Auble TE, Yealy DM *et al.* A prediction rule to identify low risk patients with community-acquired pneumonia. *N Engl J Med* 1997; **336**:243–50.

13 Angus DC, Marrie TJ, Obrosky DS *et al.* Severe community-acquired pneumonia: use of intensive care services and evaluation of American and British Thoracic Society Diagnostic criteria. Am J Respir Crit Care Med 2002; **166**: 717–23.

14 Roson B, Carratala J, Dorca J *et al.* Etiology, reasons for hospitalisation, risk classes and outcomes of community acquired pneumonia in patients hospitalized on the basis of conventional admission criteria. *Clin Infect Dis* 2001; **33**:158–65.

15 Contopoulos-Ioannidis DG, Ioannidis JPA, Chew P, Lau J. Meta-analysis of randomized controlled trials on the comparative efficacy and safety of azithromycin against other antibiotics for lower respiratory tract infections. *J Antimicrob Chemother* 2001; **48**:691–703.

16 Roson B, Carratala J, Tubau F *et al.* Usefulness of betalactam therapy for community-acquired pneumonia in the era of drug resistant *Streptococcus pneumoniae*: a randomised study of amoxicillin-clavulanate and ceftriaxone. *Microb Drug Resist* 2001; **7**:85–96.

17 Aubier M, Verster R, Regamey C *et al.* and the Sparfloxacin European Study Group. Once daily sparfloxacin versus high-dosage amoxicillin in the treatment of community acquired suspected pneumococcal pneumonia in adults. *Clin Infect Dis* 1998; **26**:1312–20.

18 Finch R, Schumann D, Collins O *et al.* Randomized controlled trial of sequential intravenous (i.v.), and oral moxifloxacin compared with sequential i.v. and oral co-amoxiclav with or without clarithromycin in patients with community acquired pneumonia requiring initial parenteral treatment. *Antimicrob Agents Chemother* 2002; **46**:1746–54.

19 File TM Jr, Segreti J, Dunbar L *et al.* A multicentre randomized study comparing the efficacy and safety of intravenous and/or oral lev-

ofloxaxin versus ceftriaxone and/or cefuroxime axetil in treatment of adults with community acquired pneumonia. *Antimicrob Agents Chemother* 1997; **41**:1965–72.

20 Frank E, Liu J, Kinasewitz G *et al*. A multicentre, open label, randomized comparison of levofloxacin and azithromycin plus ceftriaxone in hospitalized adults with moderate to severe community acquired pneumonia. *Clin Ther* 2002; **24**:1292–308.

21 Halm EA, Fine MJ, Kapoor WN, Singer DE, Marrie TJ, Siu AL. Instability on hospital discharge and the risk of adverse outcomes in patients with pneumonia. *Arch Intern Med* 2002; **162**:1278–84.

22 Gross PA, Hermogenes AW, Sacks HS *et al*. The efficacy of influenza vaccine in elderly persons: a meta-analysis and review of the literature. *Ann Intern Med* 1995; **123**:518–27.

23 Moore RA, Wiffen PJ, Lipsky BA. Are the pneumococcal polysaccharide vaccines effective? Meta-analysis of the prospective trials. *BMC Fam Pract* 2000. http://www.biomedcentral.com/1471-2296/1/1.

24 Dear K, Holden J, Andrews R, Tatham D. Vaccines for preventing pneumococcal infection in adults. The Cochrane Database of Systematic Reviews, Issue 3, 2003.

25 Austrian R, Douglas RM, Schiffman G *et al*. Prevention of pneumococcal pneumonia by vaccination. *Trans Assoc Am Phys* 1976; **89**:184–94.

26 Austrian R. *Surveillance of Pneumococcal Infection for Field Trials of Polyvalent Pneumococcal Vaccines*. Bethesda, MD, National Institute of Allergy and Infectious Diseases, 1980:1–84.

27 Austrian R. *Surveillance of Pneumococcal Infection for Field Trials of Polyvalent Pneumococcal Vaccines*. Bethesda, MD, National Institute of Allergy and Infectious Diseases, 1980:1–84.

28 Davis AL, Aranda CP, Schiffman G, Christianson LC. Pneumococcal infection and immunologic response to pneumococcal vaccine in chronic obstructive pulmonary disease. A pilot study. *Chest* 1987; **92**:204–12.

29 Gaillat J, Zmirou D, Mallaret MR *et al*. Clinical trial of an antipneumococcal vaccine in elderly people living in institutions. *Rev Epidemiol Sante Publ* 1985; **33**:437–44.

30 Honkanen PO, Keistinen T, Miettinen L *et al*. Incremental effectiveness of pneumococcal vaccine on simultaneously administered influenza vaccine in preventing pneumonia and pneumococcal pneumonia among persons aged 65 years or older. *Vaccine* 1999; **17**:2493–500.

31 Kaufman P. Pneumonia in old age. *Arch Intern Med* 1947; **79**:518–31.

32 Klastersky J, Mommen P, Cantraine F, Safary A. Placebo controlled pneumococcal immunization in patients with bronchogenic carcinoma. *Eur J Cancer Clin Oncol* 1986; **22**:807–13.

33 Koivula I, Sten M, Leinonen M, Makela PH. Clinical efficacy of pneumococcal vaccine in the elderly: a randomized, single-blind population-based trial. *Am J Med* 1997; **103**:281–90.

34 Leech JA, Gervais A, Ruben FL. Efficacy of pneumococcal vaccine in severe chronic obstructive pulmonary disease. *Can Med Assoc J* 1987; **136**:361–5.

35 Ortqvist A, Hedlund J, Burman LA, Elbel E, Margareta H, Leinonen M. Randomised trial of 23-valent pneumococcal capsular polysaccharide vaccine in prevention of pneumonia in middle-aged and elderly people. *Lancet* 1998; **351**:399–403.

36 Riley ID, Andrews M, Howard R *et al*. Immunization with polyvalent pneumococcal vaccine. Reduction of adult respiratory mortality in a New Guinea Highlands community. *Lancet* 1977; **1**:1338–41.

37 Simberkoff MS, Cross AP, Al-Ibrahim M, Baltch AL, Geiseler PJ, Nadler J. Efficacy of pneumococcal vaccine in high-risk patients. *N Engl J Med* 1986; **315**:1318–27.

CHAPTER 4.3
Pulmonary tuberculosis

Jimmy Volmink and Colleen Murphy

Problem definition

Tuberculosis is a disease caused by the bacterium *Mycobacterium tuberculosis*. It primarily affects the lungs (pulmonary tuberculosis) but, in a minority of cases, other organs may also be involved (extrapulmonary tuberculosis). HIV-infected patients have a particularly high risk of developing extrapulmonary disease. This chapter focuses on the pulmonary form of tuberculosis.

Epidemiology

Importance of the problem

Tuberculosis is a major cause of suffering and death in developing countries. The World Health Organization (WHO) estimates that about 8 million new cases of tuberculosis occur worldwide every year, of which 2 million are fatal; almost all of these are in low- and middle-income countries.[1] As tuberculosis affects mostly the economically active age group (15–54 years), the economic impact of the disease on families and individuals is often quite profound.[2]

Trends

In Africa and Asia, the high incidence of tuberculosis seen in the twentieth century continues to rise. This trend has been attributed to worsening poverty, collapse of health systems, a rise in drug-resistant forms of the disease and the escalating HIV epidemic. In contrast, in Europe and North America, a dramatic decline in tuberculosis rates occurred in the second half of the last century. However, since the 1980s, an increase in the number of reported cases has once again been observed in industrialized countries. Contributing factors are thought to be neglect of tuberculosis control programmes, HIV infection and immigration from high-prevalence countries.

Mode of spread

Tuberculosis is usually acquired by inhaling infected droplet nuclei originating from a patient with active pulmonary tuberculosis, which are transmitted through the air by coughing, sneezing, speaking or singing. Owing to the inefficiency of the tubercle bacillus, prolonged and intimate contact with an infectious person is necessary for transmission to occur.[3] Crowding in a poorly ventilated room is a key factor in the spread of tubercle bacilli as it increases the intensity of contact with a case. Sputum smear-positive cases of tuberculosis are the most infectious, followed by cases that are smear negative but culture positive. Patients with culture-negative pulmonary disease and those with extrapulmonary tuberculosis are generally not infectious.

Development of disease

Although one-third of the world's population is infected with *M. tuberculosis* (latent tuberculosis), most infected people will not progress to active disease. Factors influencing the risk of developing disease following infection are poorly understood.[4,5] Age seems to be important, as the incidence of tuberculosis is highest in late adolescence and early adulthood. Co-infection with HIV, which suppresses cellular immunity, is a powerful risk factor for clinical tuberculosis. Compared with HIV-negative populations, where only 5–10% will ever develop active tuberculosis,[6] those infected with HIV have a 5–8% annual risk and a 30% lifetime risk of developing clinical tuberculosis.[7] Other comorbid conditions known to increase the risk of tuberculosis include malignancies, diabetes, chronic renal failure, malnutrition and treatment with immunosuppressants.

Natural history

Before the advent of chemotherapy, tuberculosis was often fatal.[8,9] About 25% of patients died within 2 years of diagnosis and half within 5 years. Of the survivors at 5 years, about half had undergone spontaneous remission while the rest remained smear positive actively excreting tubercle bacilli in the community. The availability of chemotherapy has impacted greatly on the prognosis of tuberculosis. With adequate treatment, most patients can be cured. However, incorrect use of antituberculosis drugs may result in drug-resistant bacilli, increasing the pool of chronic infectious cases.

Clinical presentation

Pulmonary tuberculosis can manifest in primary or post-primary (secondary) forms.

Primary disease

Primary pulmonary tuberculosis results from an initial infection with tubercle bacilli. In regions of high prevalence, it is usually seen in children, typically affecting the middle and lower lung zones and their associated regional lymph nodes in the chest. The majority of cases are asymptomatic, with the only evidence of infection being the development of a positive tuberculin test 3–6 weeks after infection. In some cases, a small calcified scar (Ghon focus) can be seen on chest X-ray in later years.

Rarely, primary infection may progress rapidly to active disease. This may involve local extension into the lung parenchyma (often with cavitation and/or pleural effusion), systemic dissemination (miliary tuberculosis and tuberculous meningitis) and local complications (such as enlarged lymph nodes compressing bronchi, causing obstruction and subsequent segmental or lobar collapse, obstructive emphysema and bronchiectasis). These effects are most frequently encountered in immunocompromised persons.

Post-primary disease

This form of tuberculosis is more common and generally results from reactivation of latent infection, although in areas of high prevalence, reinfection also occurs. It is seen in adults and predominantly affects the apical and posterior segments of the upper lobes. Involvement of the lung parenchyma can vary from a few small infiltrates to extensive cavitation. Tuberculous pneumonia sometimes develops from extensive involvement of pulmonary segments or lobes.

Clinical features

Early symptoms and signs are often non-specific and insidious, consisting of fever, night sweats, weight loss, anorexia, general malaise and weakness. Most patients develop a cough, which may be non-productive initially, later being accompanied by purulent sputum. Blood flecks in the sputum are not infrequent, but frank haemoptysis can occasionally occur due to erosion of blood vessels in the wall of a cavity. Pleuritic chest pain sometimes develops in those with subpleural parenchymal lesions but can also result from muscle strain due to persistent coughing. Extensive lung involvement may produce dyspnoea and even adult respiratory distress syndrome.

Physical findings include low-grade intermittent fever, wasting and pallor. Finger clubbing may also be seen. No abnormalities may be detectable on examination of the lungs, but rales may be heard in the affected areas after coughing. More infrequently, rhonchi due to partial obstruction and amphoric breath sounds in areas with large cavities may also be detectable.

Diagnosis

Radiography

Pulmonary tuberculosis should be suspected in a patient with clinical features of the disease and an abnormal chest X-ray. The 'classic' picture is that of upper lobe disease with infiltrates and cavities but, unfortunately, no radiographic pattern can be considered pathognomonic of pulmonary tuberculosis.

Microscopy

A presumptive diagnosis can be made on finding acid-fast bacilli (AFB) on microscopic examination of at least two sputum smears. Patients with suspected tuberculosis are usually required to submit sputum specimens, preferably produced in the early morning, on three consecutive days. There is, however, evidence that two smears are as good as three in identifying culture-positive tuberculosis, with sensitivity, specificity and positive and negative predictive values for either option being almost identical at around 70%, 98%, 92% and 92% respectively.[10] The traditional method involves direct microscopy of specimens stained with a fuchsin dye, most commonly Ziehl–Neelsen. In modern laboratories, the Ziehl–Neelsen technique has been replaced by rhodamine–auromine staining and fluorescence microscopy, a method that is faster and more sensitive.[11] It is important to note that sputum microscopy usually identifies only half of patients with pulmonary tuberculosis as at least 5000 organisms/μL sputum are required to detect AFB.[12] This is particularly relevant in persons with HIV in whom lung cavitation is less common, reducing the yield of AFB and, therefore, the likelihood of diagnosing smear-positive tuberculosis.

Culture

A definitive diagnosis of pulmonary tuberculosis depends on the isolation and identification of M. tuberculosis in pure culture. Bacteriological culture is more sensitive than microscopy (about 80%) requiring only 10–100 AFB/μL for diagnosis.[13] In addition, it is able to detect viable tubercle bacilli and allows drug sensitivity testing. However, culture is more expensive, difficult to perform and time consuming. Various media are available for isolating tubercle bacilli. Lowenstein–Jensen egg medium and Kirchner broth both require up to 6–8 weeks to rule out positive growth. In modern laboratories, the use of liquid media with radiometric growth detection (e.g. BACTEC-460) and the identification of isolates by nucleic acid probes or high-pressure liquid chromatography have replaced the traditional methods of isolation on solid media and identification by biochemical tests. These new methods have decreased the time required for isolation and identification to around 3 weeks.

Tuberculin skin test

In adults, the tuberculin test is of limited value for diagnosis due to low sensitivity and specificity.[14] The test cannot distinguish between people who have been infected with M. tuberculosis and those with active disease, which is especially problematic in populations with a high prevalence of tuberculosis. In addition, positive results are found in people who have been sensitized by non-tuberculous mycobacteria or bacilli Calmette–Guerin (BCG) vaccination. False-negative reactions are common in immunosuppressed patients and in patients with overwhelming tuberculosis.

Case definition

The diagnosis of tuberculosis is concerned with recognizing active cases as these are potentially life threatening and are often responsible for the spread of the disease in the community. In order to choose the most appropriate therapy and subsequently evaluate treatment outcomes, it is also important to define various types of tuberculosis cases. Table 1 summarizes the case definitions relevant to pulmonary tuberculosis as recommended by WHO.[15]

Chemotherapy

The aims of chemotherapy for tuberculosis are to (a) achieve cure; (b) prevent death or disability from active disease or its sequelae; (c) avoid relapse of disease; (d) prevent acquired drug resistance; and (e) reduce the risk of disease transmission. Drugs chosen as first-line agents have been selected on the basis of their bactericidal activity (rapidly kills viable organisms rendering patients non-infectious), their sterilizing activity (kills all bacilli thus preventing relapses) and their low rate of induction of drug resistance. There are six drugs in this category: isoniazid, rifampicin, pyrazinamide, ethambutol, streptomycin and thioacetazone. A number of second-line drugs are reserved for patients with resistant forms of tuberculosis.

Standardized, short-course chemotherapy

Starting with the first ever randomized controlled trial (RCT) conducted in a health care setting (streptomycin versus placebo for pulmonary tuberculosis),[16] a large number of randomized trials have been carried out demonstrating the efficacy of various drug regimens in patients with tuberculosis.[17,18] Originally, treatment duration was 18–24 months, but the introduction of rifampicin in 1967 made it possible to reduce therapy to 6–9 months. The WHO currently recommends an intensive (bactericidal) phase of treatment using four first-line drugs for 2 months followed by a 4-month continuation (sterilizing) phase with two first-line drugs for all new cases of pulmonary tuberculosis.[15] The use of drug combinations rather than monotherapy reduces the likelihood of drug resistance and improves efficacy.

The evidence for short versus longer courses of antituberculosis treatment regimens has not been summarized in a systematic review. Two randomized trials in patients with smear-positive pulmonary tuberculosis compared 6-month versus 8- or 9-month regimens.[19,20] In one trial with 856 patients conducted in Africa,[19] all patients received streptomycin, isoniazid, rifampicin and pyrazinamide in the 2-month intensive phase followed by one of the following options in the continuation phase: (a) isoniazid and rifampicin for 4 months; (b) isoniazid and pyrazinamide for 4 months; (c) isoniazid alone for 4 months; or (d) isoniazid alone for 6 months. Patients were followed up for 12 months after stopping treatment. The study found that a 6-month regimen using rifampicin and isoniazid throughout was more effective (bacteriological relapse rate 2%) than a 6-month regimen with isoniazid alone in the continuation phase (bac-

Table 1. World Health Organization case definitions.[15]

Tuberculosis suspect	Symptoms or signs suggestive of tuberculosis, in particular cough of more than 2 weeks' duration
Case of tuberculosis	Tuberculosis bacteriologically confirmed or clinically diagnosed
Definite case of tuberculosis	Positive culture for *M. tuberculosis* or, where culture is not routinely available, two sputum smears positive for AFB
Pulmonary tuberculosis	Disease involving the lung parenchyma. Excludes intrathoracic, tuberculous lymphadenopathy or pleural effusion without lung involvement
Pulmonary tuberculosis, sputum smear positive	(a) two or more AFB-positive sputum smears, or (b) one AFB-positive sputum smear plus radiographic findings consistent with pulmonary tuberculosis, or (c) one AFB-positive sputum plus sputum culture positive for *M. tuberculosis*
Pulmonary tuberculosis, sputum smear negative	Case of pulmonary tuberculosis that does not meet the criteria for smear-positive tuberculosis including those without smear results
New cases	Never had treatment for tuberculosis before or who has had treatment for less than 1 month
Relapsed cases	Previously treated for tuberculosis and declared cured or treatment completed and is diagnosed with smear- or culture-positive tuberculosis

teriological relapse rate 9%, $P < 0.01$). The 8-month regimen was also effective (relapse rate 4%) but not significantly better than the 6-month isoniazid regimen.

The second trial[20] with 444 patients conducted in the UK compared the following regimens: (a) isoniazid, rifampicin, streptomycin and pyrazinamide for 2 months followed by isoniazid and rifampicin for a further 4 months; (b) as for regimen (a) but replacing streptomycin with ethambutol in the intensive phase; and (c) isoniazid, rifampicin and etham-butol for 2 months followed by isoniazid and rifampicin for a further 7 months. Results from 373 patients available at 36 months demonstrated that the 6-month and 9-month reg-imens were equally effective with relapse rates below 2.5% in all three groups. There was also no difference between regi-mens using ethambutol or streptomycin as the fourth drug in the initial phase.

Regimens less than 6 months' duration

A Cochrane systematic review, including seven RCTs with more than 2200 patients, assessed ultra short-course drug reg-imens (less than the standard 6-month course with a mini-mum of 2 months) versus longer courses for the treatment of active tuberculosis.[21] The review found consistently higher success rates for those receiving longer treatment courses, al-though relapse rates were generally low in all studies. Relapse rates ranged from 0 to 7% at 1 year (or more) for those receiv-ing longer regimes compared with 1–9% (one trial had an 18% relapse rate) for those administered shorter courses (ranging from 2 to 5 months). All regimes assessed appeared to have good sterilizing efficacy after treatment completion (ranging from 94% to 100% for drug-sensitive infections).

Intermittent short-course chemotherapy

Intermittent versus daily treatment in adults with pulmonary tuberculosis has been assessed in a Cochrane systematic re-view.[22] The review included one trial[23] with 399 participants, in which a thrice-weekly rifampicin-containing regimen used throughout treatment was compared with a daily short-course regimen (also with rifampicin). The cure rate was 99.5% for patients receiving fully intermittent therapy ver-sus 100% in those administered daily treatment [relative risk (RR) 0.99; 95% CI 0.99–1.10 95% CI]. Completion of therapy and toxicity were also similar in the two groups (RR 0.99; 95% CI 0.90–1.10 and RR 0.99; 95% CI 0.62–1.59 respectively). Disease relapse was greater for those receiving fully intermit-tent therapy, but this finding was not statistically significant (RR 4.00; 95% CI 0.66–24.10). Given the wide confidence in-terval around this estimate, larger trials should be conducted to evaluate this outcome further.

Second-line antituberculosis drugs

Second-line agents are reserved for patients with chronic tuberculosis (i.e. sputum positive at the end of standard treatment with first-line drugs) or multidrug-resistant disease (MDR-TB, i.e. bacilli resistant to at least rifampicin and isoniazid.) Currently available second-line drugs include ethionamide, cycloserine, p-aminosalicylic acid (PAS), kanamycin, amikacin and capreomycin. In general, they have lower efficacy and higher rates of intolerability and toxicity than first-line agents.

Fluoroquinolones (sparfloxacin, ofloxacin, levofloxacin, moxifloxcin and gatifloxacin) have recently emerged as a promising option; however, evidence from randomized trials remains limited. An open-label, clinical trial conducted in Tanzania randomized 200 patients with smear-positive tuberculosis to receive a regimen containing ciprofloxacin (750 mg/day) in combination with other antituberculosis agents versus a regimen without a quinolone.[24] No difference in clinical response was found between the two groups, but there was a trend towards a higher risk of relapse at 6 months with ciprofloxacin (RR 16.0; 95% CI 0.9–278.0). Data on the first 160 patients enrolled in this trial showed similar rates of adverse effects in the two groups, all of which were mild and responsive to symptomatic treatment.[25]

Adjunctive treatment

Corticosteroids

The rationale for using corticosteroids in conjunction with antituberculosis treatment is their powerful anti-inflammato-ry action, which suppresses the host immune response medi-ated through the release of lymphokines and cytokines. While widely used as an adjunct in the management of extrapul-monary forms of the disease, steroids are not generally em-ployed in the treatment of pulmonary tuberculosis. However, a recent systematic review of 11 RCTs including 1814 patients with pulmonary tuberculosis suggests a wider role for adjunc-tive steroids.[26] No meta-analysis was performed, but the re-view found that systemic steroids resulted in clinical benefits for patients with pulmonary TB in almost all studies. Pul-monary infiltrates and closure of cavities were more rapid with no major side-effects being attributable to steroid therapy.

Mycobacterium vaccae

The administration of *Mycobacterium vaccae* was advocated as immunotherapy for tuberculosis in the belief that this would enhance recognition of antigens common to all mycobacteria and accelerate destruction of tubercle bacilli, thus leading to more rapid cure.[27,28] This practice, however, is not supported by current evidence. A Cochrane systematic review with seven randomized trials and more than 2000 tuberculosis patients compared inoculation with whole, killed *M. vaccae* and placebo in patients on antituberculosis chemotherapy.[29] No effect was found either on mortality [four trials, 1741 partici-pants; Peto odds ratio (OR) 1.09, 95% CI 0.79–1.49] or the proportion of negative sputum cultures at completion of treatment (six trials, 1490 participants; Peto OR 1.09, 95% CI

0.81–1.45). Local adverse reactions were, however, more common in those receiving the vaccine (two trials, 131 participants; Peto OR 18.19, 95% CI 8.96–36.95). Ulceration and scarring were significantly greater for patients receiving the intervention (two trials, 505 participants; Peto OR 7.77, 95% CI 4.2–14.3; and three trials, 1044 participants; Peto OR 11.5, 95% CI 4.2–14.3 respectively).

Laser therapy

Low-level laser therapy has been used as an adjunct therapy for treating tuberculosis, predominantly in the former Soviet Union and India. A Cochrane Review assessing laser therapy was identified that found no randomized or quasi-randomized trials.[30] The review did, however, evaluate 29 observational studies with 3500 participants, all of which were considered to be of poor quality. There is therefore no evidence to support laser therapy as part of the armamentarium against tuberculosis.

Prevention

It has long been observed that the incidence of tuberculosis declines as socioeconomic conditions improve. Interventions aimed at reducing poverty and improving living conditions should therefore be at the forefront of efforts to eradicate the disease. With respect to health care, there is broad consensus that early diagnosis of infectious cases with the administration of appropriate treatment is the most important preventive strategy. In this section, we consider two other available options: BCG vaccination and treatment of latent tuberculosis infection (also referred to as preventive chemotherapy or chemoprophylaxis).

BCG

Bacillus Calmette–Guerin (BCG) is a live, attenuated vaccine routinely given in many countries where tuberculosis is endemic. Administered parentally to children shortly after birth, BCG is thought to protect against meningeal and miliary tuberculosis. The vaccine's efficacy in preventing pulmonary tuberculosis is, however, unclear and subject to debate. Three meta-analyses have assessed the effectiveness of BCG vaccination.[31–33] While these meta-analyses show a protective effect for meningeal and miliary TB (seven trials; RR 0.19, 95% CI 0.09–0.38)[33] and for overall TB incidence (adults[31] 13 trials; RR 0.49, 95% CI 0.34–0.70 and infants[32] four trials; RR 0.26, 95% CI 0.17–0.38), there is wide variation in the findings between individual studies. A Cochrane Review[34] currently in peer review including 14 trials has revisited the existing evidence for the effectiveness of BCG, aiming in particular to explore heterogeneity in effects across studies. The majority of the trials commenced before 1949, and all had serious methodological shortcomings. Only three trials were adequately randomized, and no trial described an adequate method of allocation concealment, a defect that, in general,

leads to an overestimate of treatment effects. Given these methodological flaws as well as the clinical heterogeneity between studies, summary statistics were not calculated. Findings from most of the individual studies included in the review, however, suggest a beneficial effect of BCG on all-cause mortality, death from TB and incidence of TB. Yet, the reviewers caution against this interpretation because of the high risk of bias and conclude that no reliable evidence exists regarding the value of BCG for preventing tuberculosis.

Treatment of latent tuberculosis

The rationale for preventive therapy is the eradication of latent infection in individuals at risk of developing clinical tuberculosis. The effects of therapies aimed at treating latent tuberculosis infection have been evaluated in two Cochrane Reviews. One review compared isoniazid regimens of 6 months or longer with placebo in HIV-negative persons.[35] Eleven high-quality randomized trials involving more than 70 000 patients followed up for at least 2 years were included in the analysis (see Table 2 for details of trial characteristics). Isoniazid chemoprophylaxis significantly reduced active tuberculosis in at-risk groups by 60% (Fig. 1) with no difference among those receiving 6-month (two trials; RR 0.44, 95% CI 0.27–0.73) versus 12-month (10 trials; RR 0.38, 95% CI 0.28–0.50) courses. Tuberculosis-related death was also reduced, but this finding was not statistically significant (two trials, 25 714 participants; RR 0.29; 95% CI 0.07–1.18). Hepatitis was the most serious adverse effect found, and this risk was significantly increased in patients receiving isoniazid (one trial, 20 874 participants; RR 5.54; 95% CI 2.56–12.00).

The second Cochrane Review sought to determine whether preventive therapy reduces the risk of active tuberculosis and death in persons with HIV infection.[36] Thirteen trials with more than 8000 patients evaluated four different drug regimens: isoniazid; isoniazid plus rifampicin; rifampicin plus pyrazinamide; and isoniazid plus rifampicin plus pyrazinamide (see Table 2 for further details of trial characteristics). Compared with placebo or no treatment, preventive therapy reduced the risk of developing active TB by 36%, with a statistically significant benefit in tuberculin-positive individuals but not in those with a negative tuberculin skin test (Fig. 2). Although the review found no difference in efficacy for different drug regimens, short-course, multidrug treatments were more likely to be discontinued because of adverse events. Overall, there was no evidence that preventive treatment reduced all-cause mortality, but there was a trend towards a lower mortality in tuberculin-positive persons (four trials; RR 0.80, 95% CI 0.63–1.02). These findings are consistent with an earlier review of isoniazid prophylaxis in HIV-positive persons.[37]

Adherence to treatment

This section focuses on evidence concerning strategies aimed at overcoming the problem of poor adherence to therapy,

Table 2. Randomized trials of drug regimens for preventing tuberculosis in HIV-positive and -negative persons: characteristics of Cochrane systematic reviews.

Systematic review (first author)	Types of participants	Intervention	Outcomes assessed

Smieja[35]	HIV-negative persons (any age) at risk of developing active TB
	Studies including patients with previous disease included if TB was inactive at time of enrolment and not previously treated with anti-TB chemotherapy
	Included trials were conducted in Czechoslovakia, East Germany, Finland, Hong Kong, Hungary, India, Kenya, Mexico, Netherlands, Philippines, Poland, Puerto Rico, Romania, United States, Yugoslavia
		Placebo versus
		  INH for 6 months or longer
		  INH for 6 months versus
		  INH for 12 months
			Active TB
			Extrapulmonary TB
			TB deaths
			All-cause death
			Hepatitis
			Hepatitis-related deaths
			Other adverse events
			Isolation of INH-resistant *Mycobacterium* TB

Woldehanna[36]	HIV-positive adults without past or current active TB, regardless of PPD status
	Included trials were conducted in Brazil, Haiti, Kenya, Mexico, Spain, Uganda, United States, Zambia
		Placebo versus
		  INH
		  INH + RIF
		  RIF + PZA
		  INH + RIF + PZA
		INH versus:
		  RIF + PZA
		  INH + RIF
		  INH + RIF + PZA
		INH + RIF versus:
		  RIF + PZA
		  INH + RIF + PZA
			Active TB
			All-cause death
			Interval to active TB
			Interval to death
			Progression to HIV disease
			Incidence of adverse drug reactions leading to discontinuation of treatment

INH, isoniazid; PPD, purified protein derivative; PZA, pyrazinamide; RIF, rifampicin.

Study	Treatment (n/N)	Control (n/N)	Relative risk (random) (95% CI)	Weight (%)	Relative risk (random) (95% CI)
Comstock (1962)	50/2480	128/2406		15.8	0.38 (0.27, 0.52)
Del Castillo (1965)	16/126	22/167		9.6	0.96 (0.53, 1.76)
Egsmose (1965)	7/325	18/301		6.1	0.36 (0.15, 0.85)
Falk (1978)	5/889	15/772		4.8	0.29 (0.11, 0.79)
Ferebee (1962)	8/8478	36/8311		7.2	0.22 (0.10, 0.47)
Ferebee (1963)	6/12339	173/12499		16.6	0.36 (0.27, 0.48)
Girling (1992)	20/100	34/99		12.1	0.58 (0.36, 0.94)
John (1994)	7/92	10/92		5.5	0.70 (0.28, 1.76)
Mount (1962)	8/1462	12/1348		5.1	0.46 (0.17, 1.22)
Thompson (1982)	58/13838	97/6990		15.7	0.30 (0.22, 0.42)
Veening (1968)	1/133	12/128		1.4	0.08 (0.01, 0.61)
Total (95% CI)	239/40262	557/33113		100.0	0.40 (0.31, 0.52)

Test for heterogeneity chi-squared = 20.94 df = 10 P = 0.0215
Test for overall effect = −7.06 P < 0.00001

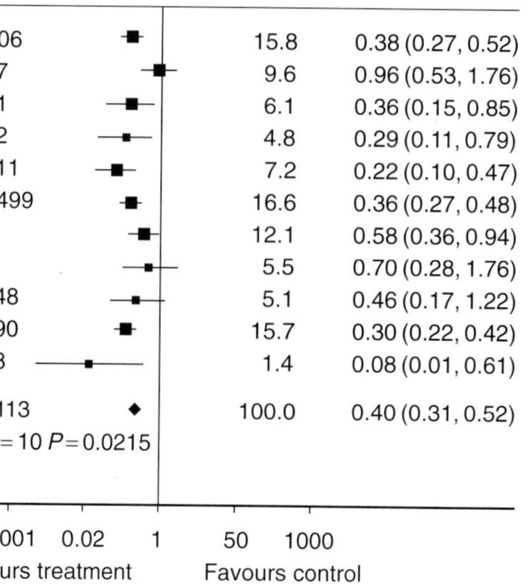

0.001 0.02 1 50 1000
Favours treatment   Favours control

Figure 1. Isoniazid versus placebo for preventing active tuberculosis in non-HIV-infected persons.

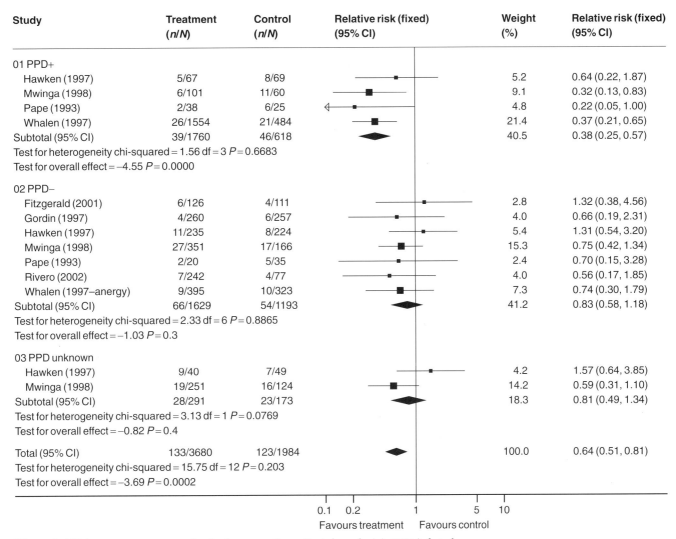

Study	Treatment (n/N)	Control (n/N)	Relative risk (fixed) (95% CI)	Weight (%)	Relative risk (fixed) (95% CI)
01 PPD+					
Hawken (1997)	5/67	8/69		5.2	0.64 (0.22, 1.87)
Mwinga (1998)	6/101	11/60		9.1	0.32 (0.13, 0.83)
Pape (1993)	2/38	6/25		4.8	0.22 (0.05, 1.00)
Whalen (1997)	26/1554	21/484		21.4	0.37 (0.21, 0.65)
Subtotal (95% CI)	39/1760	46/618		40.5	0.38 (0.25, 0.57)
Test for heterogeneity chi-squared = 1.56 df = 3 P = 0.6683					
Test for overall effect = −4.55 P = 0.0000					
02 PPD−					
Fitzgerald (2001)	6/126	4/111		2.8	1.32 (0.38, 4.56)
Gordin (1997)	4/260	6/257		4.0	0.66 (0.19, 2.31)
Hawken (1997)	11/235	8/224		5.4	1.31 (0.54, 3.20)
Mwinga (1998)	27/351	17/166		15.3	0.75 (0.42, 1.34)
Pape (1993)	2/20	5/35		2.4	0.70 (0.15, 3.28)
Rivero (2002)	7/242	4/77		4.0	0.56 (0.17, 1.85)
Whalen (1997–anergy)	9/395	10/323		7.3	0.74 (0.30, 1.79)
Subtotal (95% CI)	66/1629	54/1193		41.2	0.83 (0.58, 1.18)
Test for heterogeneity chi-squared = 2.33 df = 6 P = 0.8865					
Test for overall effect = −1.03 P = 0.3					
03 PPD unknown					
Hawken (1997)	9/40	7/49		4.2	1.57 (0.64, 3.85)
Mwinga (1998)	19/251	16/124		14.2	0.59 (0.31, 1.10)
Subtotal (95% CI)	28/291	23/173		18.3	0.81 (0.49, 1.34)
Test for heterogeneity chi-squared = 3.13 df = 1 P = 0.0769					
Test for overall effect = −0.82 P = 0.4					
Total (95% CI)	133/3680	123/1984		100.0	0.64 (0.51, 0.81)
Test for heterogeneity chi-squared = 15.75 df = 12 P = 0.203					
Test for overall effect = −3.69 P = 0.0002					

0.1 0.2   1   5 10
Favours treatment   Favours control

Figure 2. TB drug treatment versus placebo for preventing active tuberculosis in HIV-infected persons.

which has long been recognized to be a major constraint to eradicating tuberculosis.[38,39] Up to half of all tuberculosis patients do not complete treatment,[40] which often results in prolonged infectiousness, drug resistance, disease relapse and, sometimes, death. Incomplete treatment thus poses a serious risk for the individual patient as well as the community.

Many factors have been found to be associated with poor adherence to tuberculosis treatment including patient characteristics, the relationship between patient and health care provider, the treatment regimen used and the health care setting.[41] Concomitant with efforts to understand these factors better, numerous measures have been introduced in different settings in an attempt to improve adherence.[40,42,43] These interventions aim to influence the behaviour of health care

personnel, the organization of the service or the behaviour of the person with suspected or confirmed tuberculosis and can be separated into the following categories:
• Defaulter action: the action taken when patients fail to keep a prearranged appointment.
• Prompts: routine reminders to patients to keep prearranged appointments.
• Health education: provision of information about tuberculosis and the need to attend for treatment.
• Incentives and reimbursements: money or cash in kind to reimburse expenses of attending services or to improve the attractiveness of visiting the treatment centre.
• Contracts: agreements (written or verbal) to return for an appointment or course of treatment.

• Peer assistance: people from the same social group helping someone with tuberculosis keep clinic appointments and take their medication.

• Directly observed therapy (DOT): an appointed and trained agent (health worker, community volunteer, family member) directly monitors people swallowing their antituberculosis drugs.

• Staff motivation and supervision: includes training and management processes aimed at improving the way in which providers care for people with tuberculosis.

Currently, experimental research on the effects of adherence-promoting interventions is limited. Two Cochrane Reviews have summarized the results of randomized trials evaluating the effect of interventions aimed at improving adherence in people receiving curative or preventive treatment for tuberculosis.[44,45] Details of these studies, including their main results, are presented in Table 3.

One trial[46] found that reminder letters sent to patients who failed to attend clinic were of benefit even when patients were illiterate. Another[47] reported that home visits by a health worker, although more labour intensive, may be more effective than reminder letters for ensuring that defaulters complete their treatment. A further study[48] showed that prospective telephone reminders are useful for helping people to keep scheduled appointments.

Although one trial[49] found that assistance by a community health worker increased adherence to a first evaluation appointment, a subsequent study showed no impact on completion of preventive treatment at 6 months.[50] Verbal and written agreements made by people to attend for clinic follow-up seem promising; however, the evidence in favour of this intervention is currently limited to one trial in a healthy, middle-class population of students.[51]

Studies in the USA have found that monetary incentives are an effective method of improving adherence. Appointment keeping was significantly improved in homeless men[49] and in drug users[52] by offering a small payment for returning to a clinic for TB evaluation, but the results of another study[50] of monetary incentives involving homeless people were inconclusive, partly because of its small size.

The evidence for an independent effect of health education on adherence in patients with tuberculosis is weak. One trial[53] suggests some benefit, but the design of the study was flawed because individuals receiving health education were contacted or seen every 3 months, whereas those in the control group were seen only at the end of the study period. The relative contributions of health education and increased attention in this study are therefore difficult to separate. A trial[54] to examine the impact of intensive education and counselling on patients with active tuberculosis did, however, find a trend towards increased treatment completion rates for the patients who received intensive education and counselling compared with those who received routine care. Health education was found to be beneficial in another trial[55] but, unfortunately, in

this study, the effects of education were confounded by the use of a monetary incentive offered in tandem with the educational intervention. In a more recent trial[52] that aimed to disaggregate these effects, health education alone was not found to be better than routine case management for improving appointment keeping, and the impact of education combined with a monetary incentive was indistinguishable from that of the monetary incentive alone. Similarly, a small study among prisoners, comparing education versus education plus a small monetary incentive, did not demonstrate a significant difference in the rate of return to a tuberculosis clinic following release from prison.[56]

Although widely believed to improve treatment adherence and thus cure rates, directly observed therapy (DOT) of patients swallowing their medication does not appear to produce better outcomes than self-administration of treatment (SAT). Meta-analysis has found no significant differences for TB cure rates or for cure and treatment completion rates between those patients enrolled in DOT and those administering their own treatments.[45] There were no important differences in the results when the influence of different types of DOT providers was explored. Completion rates were, however, modestly higher in the one trial that allowed for patient choice of supervisor. Both trials assessing the effects of DOT on the completion of preventive treatment were negative.

An intervention directed at clinic staff rather than patients was also studied in a trial.[57] Patients attending clinics in which staff were closely supervised were more likely to complete treatment than those attending clinics where there was only routine supervision of staff.

Conclusion

Despite effective treatment being available for more than half a century, tuberculosis continues to be a major cause of morbidity and mortality. Globally, the incidence of the disease continues to rise, especially in people who are HIV positive, in whom tuberculosis is the leading cause of death. Pulmonary tuberculosis is the most common form of the disease, and cases that are sputum smear positive are highly infectious. The most important medical strategy for combating the disease consists of early diagnosis and treatment using standardized, short-course combination drug regimens. There is strong evidence from randomized trials supporting the use of currently recommended antituberculosis drug regimens. Several RCTs also support the use of various antituberculosis drug regimens for preventing active tuberculosis in people with latent infection, regardless of their HIV status. Despite the use of BCG vaccination for almost a century, its value in preventing tuberculosis is still a matter of debate. Available trials are methodologically unsound and have produced inconsistent findings. In addition, in areas of high prevalence, high levels of coverage with BCG have not resulted in demonstrable effects on the incidence of tuberculosis. One of the universal challenges faced

Table 3. Strategies to promote adherence to tuberculosis treatment.

Strategy	Study reference (first author)	Type of study	Participants	Intervention	Main findings
Contracts	Wurtele[51]	Randomized controlled trial	College students in the United States responding to newspaper invitation to participate in TB detection drive	Verbal contract versus no contract; verbal plus written contract versus no contract to return within 48 hours for skin test reading	Return for skin test reading: – verbal contract versus none: RR 1.10; 95% CI 1.03–1.18 – verbal and written contract versus none: RR 1.12; 95% CI 1.05–1.19
Defaulter action	Paramasivan[46]	Randomized controlled trial	Newly diagnosed tuberculosis patients in India admitted for 1 month for education/supervised treatment. After discharge, treatment self-administered on an outpatient basis for 4 months.	Reminder cards to patients who did not collect drugs versus no follow-up to patients who defaulted on drug collection.	Completion of treatment: RR 1.21; 95% CI 1.05–1.39
	Krishnaswami[47]	Randomized controlled trial	Adults in India with radiographic evidence of tuberculosis but negative sputum smear. Patients asked to collect drugs monthly from clinic for home self-administration	Reminder letters to patients and one home visit if patient did not return versus home visit of defaulting patients up to four times	Completion of 10- to 12-monthly drug collections: RR 1.33; 95% CI 1.02–1.71
Directly observed therapy (DOT)	Volmink[45]	Systematic review of six randomized controlled trials	People requiring treatment for clinically active tuberculosis or prevention of disease. Trials conducted in Pakistan, South Africa, Thailand, United States	Health worker, family member or community volunteer routinely watching participants taking antituberculosis drugs (DOT) versus routine self-administration of treatment (SAT) at home with intermittent clinic visits	Cure (four trials): RR 1.06; 95% CI 0.98–1.14 Cure plus completion of treatment (four trials): RR 1.06; 95% CI 1.00–1.13 Completion of preventive treatment: – DOT versus self-administration (one trial): RR 1.01; 95% CI 0.88–1.16 – own choice versus community treatment centre (one trial): RR 0.88; 95% CI 0.63–1.23

Table 3. *Continued.*

Strategy	Study reference (first author)	Type of study	Participants	Intervention	Main findings
Health education	Sanmarti[54]	Randomized controlled trial	Primary school children in Spain testing positive for tuberculin (active cases excluded)	Education of mothers during home visit from nurse versus telephone calls by nurse versus clinic visit with doctor versus leaflet alone	Completion of prophylaxis treatment: – nurse home visit versus leaflet: RR 1.33; 95% CI 1.14–1.54 – nurse telephone call versus leaflet: RR 1.31; 95% CI 1.13–1.53 – clinic visit with doctor versus leaflet: RR 1.09; 95% CI 0.91–1.69
	Liefooghe[55]	Randomized controlled trial	Newly diagnosed adults in Pakistan	One-to-one counselling and health education at follow-up versus usual care	Completion of treatment: RR 1.13; 95% CI 0.99–1.30
Monetary incentives	Tulsky[50]	Randomized controlled trial	Homeless men and women with a positive PPD test in the United States	Monetary incentive (US$5) versus routine care	Completion of preventive therapy: RR 1.68; 95% CI 0.89–3.15
Monetary incentives and health education	Malotte[52]	Randomized controlled trial	Injection drug or crack cocaine users without clear history of a positive PPD test recruited from an HIV prevention project in the United States	5- to 10-min motivational education session by nurse plus monetary incentives (US$5 or 10) versus routine care; monetary incentives only (US$5 or 10) versus routine care; education session only versus routine care	Keeping first appointment: – US$5 plus educ versus routine: RR 2.56; 95% CI 1.92–3.40 – US$10 plus educ versus routine: RR 2.79; 95% CI 2.11–3.70 – US$5 versus routine: RR 2.60; 95%CI 1.96–3.46 – US$10 versus routine: RR 2.82; 95% CI 2.13–3.74 – Educ versus routine: RR 1.04; 95% CI 0.70–1.54 Completion of treatment: RR 1.07; 95% CI 0.97–1.19
	Morisky[56]	Randomized controlled trial	New adult immigrants to the United States treated for active disease or receiving prophylaxis	Behavioural counselling in patient's language plus money to complete treatment (US$10 for cure and US$5 for prophylaxis) versus usual care, with tracing of defaulting patients	Completion of preventive treatment: RR 2.35; 95% CI 1.48–3.73

Category	Study	Study type	Population	Intervention	Outcome
	White[57]	Randomized controlled trial	Prisoners in the United States screened for TB and who agreed to antituberculosis treatment by jail physicians	Standardized TB education from medical/nursing students versus standardized TB education as above plus money (US$5) at the time of the first visit to TB clinic after release from jail	Completion of first visit to the TB clinic after release from jail: RR 1.11; 95% CI 0.46–2.67
Monetary incentives and peer education	Pilote[49]	Randomized controlled trial	Homeless people, predominantly men, in the United States testing positive for tuberculin (all receiving bus tokens)	Money (US$5) versus education by a peer from the same homeless community versus usual care	Attendance at first follow-up appointment: – money versus usual care: RR 1.58; 95% CI 1.26–0.99 – peer education versus usual care: RR 1.41; 95% CI 1.10–1.79
	Tulsky[50]	Randomized controlled trial	Homeless men and women with a positive PPD test in the United States	Money (US$5) when attending for directly observed therapy versus peer education versus usual care	Completion of preventive therapy: – money versus usual care: RR 1.68, 95% CI 0.89–3.15 – peer education versus usual care: RR 0.72; 95% CI 0.31–1.69
Peer assistance	Pilote[49]	Randomized controlled trial	Homeless people, predominantly men, in the United States testing positive for tuberculin (all receiving bus tokens)	Peer assistance with homeless community health worker versus routine care	Keeping first appointment: RR 1.41; 95% CI 1.10–1.79
	Tulsky[50]	Randomized controlled trial	Homeless men and women with a positive PPD test in the United States	Peer assistance with peer health adviser versus routine care	Completion of preventive therapy: RR 0.72; 95% CI 0.31–1.69
Prompts	Tanke[48]	Randomized controlled trial	Individuals reporting for a tuberculin skin test in the United States	Reminders using prerecorded telephone messages in participants' primary language versus no reminders	Return to read TB skin test: RR 1.05; 95% CI 1.00–1.10
Staff motivation/ supervision	Jin[58]	Cluster randomized trial	Newly diagnosed TB cases to be treated in primary health facilities in Korea	Intense staff supervision and motivation of TB clinic staff by senior medical personnel versus routine supervision	Completion of treatment: RR 1.21

by tuberculosis control programmes is how to encourage patients to complete the relatively long course of treatment for either cure or prevention of disease. However, little attention has thus far been given to evaluating interventions for improving adherence. Data from randomized trials provide little or no evidence that the widely recommended policy of directly observed therapy is better than one involving self-administration of treatment for improving adherence and cure rates. Credible methods for developing, evaluating and promoting sustainable measures to improve adherence to tuberculosis treatment are thus urgently needed.

Summary for clinicians

- Pulmonary tuberculosis remains a major cause of illness and death worldwide.
- The incidence of pulmonary tuberculosis continues to rise in developing countries and has recently also begun to increase in the developed world. An important factor fuelling this trend is the HIV pandemic.
- The definitive diagnosis of pulmonary tuberculosis depends upon isolation of *M. tuberculosis* on bacteriological culture, although a presumptive diagnosis can be made on finding acid-fast bacilli on microscopic examination of at least two sputum smears.
- There is good evidence to support currently recommended chemotherapy comprising four first-line drugs for 2 months followed by two first-line drugs for 4 months for all new cases of pulmonary tuberculosis.
- There is also sound evidence for the use of antituberculosis drug regimens for at least 6 months for the prevention of active tuberculosis in persons with latent infection.
- Many patients do not complete the relatively long courses of treatment required for cure or prevention of tuberculosis, leading to prolonged infectiousness, drug resistance, relapse and death. Few strategies for improving adherence to therapy have been rigorously evaluated to date.

Literature search

For randomized trials and systematic reviews

Database: MEDLINE (1948 to December 2003); The Cochrane Database of Systematic Reviews (Issue 1, 2004); DARE (December 2003).

Search strategy (MEDLINE)

#1 Etiology OR Incidence OR Prevalence OR Prognosis OR Diagnosis
#2 Tuberculosis
#3 #1 AND #2
#4 Randomized Controlled Trial [publication type] OR (Systematic Review) OR Meta-analysis [publication type]
#5 #3 AND #4
#6 Treatment OR Prevention OR Chemotherapy OR Adherence

#7 #5 AND #6
#8 #7 AND Human
#9 #8 NOT Animal
- Inclusion criteria: randomized controlled trials and systematic reviews focusing on treatment and preventive interventions relevant to pulmonary tuberculosis.
- Exclusion criteria: trials and systematic reviews assessing only extrapulmonary tuberculosis; non-experimental designs.

Acknowledgements

We thank Elizabeth Pienaar for help with literature searching.

References

1 Dye C, Scheele S, Dolin P *et al*. Global burden of tuberculosis: estimated incidence, prevalence and mortality by country. *JAMA* 1999; **282**:677–86.
2 Ahlburg D. *The Economic Impacts of Tuberculosis*. Geneva, World Health Organization, 2000.
3 Grzybowski S, Barnett GD, Styblo K. Contacts of cases of active pulmonary tuberculosis. *Bull Int Union Tuberc* 1975; **50**:90–106.
4 Gomez JE, McKinney JD. *M. tuberculosis* persistence, latency, and drug tolerance. *Tuberculosis* 2004; **84**:29–44.
5 Stewart GR, Roberton BD, Young DB. Tuberculosis: a problem with persistence. *Nature Rev* 2003; **1**:97–105.
6 Enarson DA, Rouillon A. The epidemiological basis of tuberculosis control. In: Davis PDO, ed. *Clinical Tuberculosis*, 1st edn. London, Chapman & Hall, 1994:19–32.
7 Selwyn PA, Hartel D, Lewis VA *et al*. A prospective study of the risk of tuberculosis among intravenous drug users with human immunodeficiency virus infection. *N Engl J Med* 1989; **320**:545–50.
8 Rutledge CJA, Crouch JB. The ultimate results in 1694 cases of tuberculosis treated at the Modern Woodmen of America Sanitorium. *Am Rev Tuberc* 1919; **2**:755–63.
9 National Tuberculosis Institute. Tuberculosis in a rural population of South India: a 5-year epidemiological study. *Bull WHO* 1974; **51**:473–88.
10 Crampin AC, Floyd S, Mwaugulu F *et al*. Comparison of two versus three smears in identifying culture-positive tuberculosis patients in a rural African setting with high HIV prevalence. *Int J Tuberc Lung Dis* 2001; **5**: 994–9.
11 Toman K. *Tuberculosis Case-finding and Chemotherapy: Questions and Answers*. Geneva, WHO, 1979.
12 Aber VR, Allen BW, Mitchison DA, Ayuma P, Edwards EA, Keyes AB. Quality control in tuberculosis bacteriology. 1. Laboratory studies on isolated positive cultures and the efficiency of direct smear examination. *Tubercle* 1980; **61**:123–33.
13 Levy H, Feldman C, Sacho H, van der MH, Kallenbach J, Koorenhof H. A reevaluation of sputum microscopy and culture in the diagnosis of pulmonary tuberculosis. *Chest* 1989; **95**:1193–7.
14 Cowie RL, Escreet BC. The diagnosis of pulmonary tuberculosis. *S Afr Med* 1980; **57**:75–7.
15 World Health Organization. *Treatment of Tuberculosis: Guidelines for National Programmes*, 3rd edn. Geneva, World Health Organization, 2003.
16 Medical Research Council. Streptomycin treatment of pulmonary tuberculosis. *BMJ* 1948; **30**:769–82.
17 Fox W, Ellard GA, Mitchison DA. Studies on the treatment of tuberculosis undertaken by the British Medical Research Council Tubercu-

losis Units, 1946–1986, with relevant subsequent publications. *Int J Tuberc Lung Dis* 1999; **3**:231–79.

18 Chan SL. Chemotherapy of tuberculosis. In: Davis PDO, ed. *Clinical Tuberculosis*, 1st edn. London, Chapman & Hall, 1994:141–56.

19 East and Central African/British Medical Research Council Fifth Collaborative Study. Controlled clinical trial of 4 short-course regimens of chemotherapy (three 6-month and one 8-month) for pulmonary tuberculosis. *Tubercle* 1983; **64**:153–66.

20 British Thoracic Society. A controlled trial of 6 months chemotherapy in pulmonary tuberculosis, final report: results during the 36 months after the end of chemotherapy and beyond. *Br J Dis Chest* 1984: **78**:330–6.

21 Gelband H. Regimens of less than six months for treating tuberculosis (Cochrane Review). In: *The Cochrane Library*, Issue 4. Chichester, John Wiley & Sons, 2003.

22 Mwandumba HC, Squire SB. Fully intermittent dosing with drugs for treating tuberculosis in adults (Cochrane Review). In: *The Cochrane Library*, Issue 4. Chichester, John Wiley & Sons, 2003.

23 Hong Kong Chest Service/British Medical Research Council. Controlled trial of four thrice weekly regimens and a daily regimen given for 6 months for pulmonary tuberculosis. *Lancet* 1981; **1**:171–4.

24 Kennedy N, Berger L, Curram J *et al.* Randomized controlled trial of a drug regimen that includes ciprofloxacin for the treatment of pulmonary tuberculosis. *Clin Infect Dis* 1996; **22**:827–33.

25 Kennedy N, Fox R, Uiso LO, Ngowi FI, Gillespie, SH. Safety profile of ciprofloxacin during long-term therapy for pulmonary tuberculosis. *J Antimicrob Chemother* 1993; **32**:897–902.

26 Smego RA, Ahmed N. A systematic review of the adjunctive use of systematic corticosteroids for pulmonary tuberculosis. *Int J Tuberc Lung Dis* 2003; **7**:208–13.

27 Stanford JL, Rook GAW, Bahr GM *et al. Mycobacterium vaccae* in immunoprophylaxis and immunotherapy of leprosy and tuberculosis. *Vaccine* 1990; **8**:525–30.

28 Stanford JL, Stanford CA. Immunotherapy of tuberculosis with *Mycobacterium vaccae* NCTC 11659. *Immunobiology* 1994; **191**:555–63.

29 de Bruyn G, Garner P. *Mycobacterium vaccae* immunotherapy for treating tuberculosis (Cochrane Review). In: *The Cochrane Library*, Issue 1. Chichester, John Wiley & Sons, 2004.

30 Vlassov VV, Pechatnikov LM, MacLehose HG. Low level laser therapy for treating tuberculosis (Cochrane Review). In: *The Cochrane Library*, Issue 1. Chichester, John Wiley & Sons, 2004.

31 Colditz GA, Brewer TF, Berkey CS *et al.* Efficacy of BCG vaccine in the prevention of tuberculosis. Meta-analysis of the published literature. *JAMA* 1994; **271**:698–702.

32 Colditz GA, Berkey CS, Mosteller F *et al.* The efficacy of bacillus Calmette-Guerin vaccination of newborns and infants in prevention of tuberculosis: meta-analyses of the published literature. *Pediatrics* 1995; **96**:29–35.

33 Rodrigues LC, Diwan VK, Wheeler JG. Protective effect of BCG against tuberculous meningitis and miliary tuberculosis: a meta-analysis. *Int J Epidemiol* 1993; **22**:1154–8.

34 Spruyt LL, Siegfried N, Matchaba PT, Volmink J. Bacillus Calmette-Guerin (BCG) vaccine for preventing tuberculosis (Cochrane review). (in peer review).

35 Smieja MJ, Marchetti CA, Cook DJ, Smaill FM. Isoniazid for preventing tuberculosis in non-HIV infected persons (Cochrane Review). In: *The Cochrane Library*, Issue 1. Chichester, John Wiley & Sons, 2004.

36 Woldehanna S, Volmink J. Treatment of latent tuberculosis infection in HIV infected persons (Cochrane Review). In: *The Cochrane Library*, Issue 1. Chichester, John Wiley & Sons, 2004.

37 Bucher HC, Griffith LE, Guyatt GH *et al.* Isoniazid prophylaxis for

tuberculosis in HIV infection: a meta-analysis of randomized controlled trials. *AIDS* 1999; **4**:501–7.

38 Fox W. The problem of self-administration of drugs: with particular reference to pulmonary tuberculosis. *Tubercle* 1958; **39**:269–74.

39 Addington WW. Patient compliance: the most serious remaining problem in the control of tuberculosis in the United States. *Chest* 1979; **76**:741–3.

40 Cuneo WD, Snider DE. Enhancing patient compliance with tuberculosis therapy. *Clin Chest Med* 1989; **10**:375–80.

41 Sumartojo E. When tuberculosis treatment fails. A social behavioral account of patient adherence. *Am Rev Respir Dis* 1993; **147**:1311–20.

42 Centers for Disease Control and Prevention. Approaches to improving adherence to antituberculosis therapy. *Morbid Mortal Wkly Rep* 1993; **42**:74–5, 81.

43 Sbarbaro JA, Sbarbaro JB. Compliance and supervision of chemotherapy of tuberculosis. *Semin Respir Infect* 1994; **9**:120–7.

44 Volmink J, Garner P. Interventions for promoting adherence to tuberculosis management (Cochrane Review). In: *The Cochrane Library*, Issue 4. Oxford, Update Software, 2000.

45 Volmink J, Garner P. Directly observed therapy for treating tuberculosis (Cochrane Review). In: *The Cochrane Library*, Issue 1. Chichester, John Wiley & Sons, 2004.

46 Paramasivan R, Parthasarathy RT, Rajasekaran S. Short course chemotherapy: a controlled study of indirect defaulter retrieval method. *Ind J Tuberc* 1993; **40**:185–90.

47 Krishnaswami KV, Somasundaram PR, Tripathy SP, Vaidyanathan B, Radhakrishna S, Fox W. A randomised study of two policies for managing default in out-patients collecting supplies of drugs for pulmonary tuberculosis in a large city in South India. *Tubercle* 1981; **61**:103–12.

48 Tanke ED, Martinez CM, Leirer VO. Use of automated reminders for tuberculin skin test return. *Am J Prev Med* 1997; **13**:189–92.

49 Pilote L, Tulsky JP, Zolopa AR, Hahn JA, Schecter GF, Moss AR. Tuberculosis prophylaxis in the homeless. A trial to improve adherence to referral. *Arch Intern Med* 1996; **156**:161–5.

50 Tulsky JP, Pilote L, Hahn JA *et al.* Adherence to isoniazid prophylaxis in the homeless: a randomized controlled trial. *Arch Intern Med* 2000; **160**:697–702.

51 Wurtele SK, Galanos AN, Roberts MC. Increasing return compliance in a tuberculosis detection drive. *J Behav Med* 1980; **3**: 311–18.

52 Malotte CK, Rhodes F, Mais KE. Tuberculosis screening and compliance with return for skin test reading among active drug users. *Am J Public Health* 1998; **88**:792–6.

53 Sanmarti L, Megias JA, Gomez MN *et al.* Evaluation of the efficacy of health education on the compliance with antituberculosis chemoprophylaxis in school children: a randomised clinical trial. *Tuberc Lung Dis* 1993; **74**:28–31.

54 Liefooghe R, Suetens C, Meulemans H, Moran MB, De Muynck A. A randomised trial of the impact of counselling on treatment adherence of tuberculosis patients in Sialkot, Pakistan. *Int J Tuberc Lung Dis* 1999; **3**:1073–80.

55 Morisky DE, Malotte CK, Choi P *et al.* A patient education program to improve adherence rates with antituberculosis drug regimens. *Health Educ Q* 1990; **17**:253–67.

56 White MC, Tulsky JP, Reilly P, McIntosh HW, Hoynes TM, Goldenson J. A clinical trial of a financial incentive to go to the tuberculosis clinic for isoniazid after release from jail. *Int J Tuberc Lung Dis* 1998; **2**:506–12

57 Jin BW, Kim SC, Mori T, Shimao T. The impact of intensified supervisory activities on tuberculosis treatment. *Tuberc Lung Dis* 1993; **74**:267–72.

CHAPTER 4.4

Influenza: vaccination and treatment

Fotini B Karassa and John P A Ioannidis

Introduction

Background

Influenza viruses can cause a highly contagious acute respiratory illness. The virus is transmitted from person to person through respiratory secretions of acutely infected individuals.[1] The incubation period can range from 1 to 7 days and usually lasts for 2 days.[2] Infected adults are contagious from the day before symptom onset until approximately 5 days after illness onset, while severely immunocompromised hosts can shed virus for weeks or months.[3]

Uncomplicated influenza typically presents with an abrupt onset of fever, severe malaise, myalgia, headache, non-productive cough, sore throat and rhinitis.[4] Not all infected people become symptomatic. The percentage of infections resulting in clinical illness can vary from 40% to 85%, depending on age and pre-existing immunity to the virus.[5] People infected with other respiratory pathogens may have symptoms identical to those of influenza.[6] Influenza is usually diagnosed clinically, although a definite diagnosis requires laboratory confirmation. Substantiation of a definitive diagnosis is not cost-effective or indicated in the vast majority of cases.

Biology

Three main types of influenza virus are known: A, B and C. Types A and B are the ones that cause significant morbidity in humans. Influenza A occurs more frequently and is more virulent than influenza B. There are several subtypes of influenza A viruses based on serological and genetic differences in two surface glycoproteins: haemagglutinin (H) and neuraminidase (N). Influenza A viruses with haemagglutinin proteins of the H1, H2 and H3 subtypes and neuraminidase proteins of the N1 and N2 subtypes have caused recorded epidemics and pandemics in humans since the early 1900s.[7] Frequent antigenic change (i.e. antigenic drift) caused by the accumulation of point mutations in the haemagglutinin and neuraminidase genes leads to the development of new strains. Antigenic shift is less common and occurs when novel subtypes of influenza appear.[7] Although an individual's immunity to the surface antigens reduces the likelihood of infection and severity of disease if infection occurs, antibody against one influenza virus type or subtype confers limited or no protection against another.[6] Antigenic drift explains the occurrence of seasonal epidemics and typically requires the incorporation of new strains in each year's influenza vaccine.

Incidence—prognosis

Influenza occurs mainly during the winter months and affects all age groups. Annual incidence varies yearly and depends partly on the underlying level of population immunity to circulating strains.[7] Each year, serological conversion with or without clinical illness occurs in approximately 10–20% of the US population, with the highest infection rates in people aged under 20 years.[8] Attack rates are higher in institutions and in areas of overcrowding.[9]

Uncomplicated influenza usually resolves within a week, although cough and fatigue may persist. Complications include otitis media, bacterial sinusitis, acute bronchitis, secondary bacterial pneumonia and, less commonly, viral pneumonia and respiratory failure.[6,7] Otitis media complicates about 1–2% of influenza-infected adults while sinusitis has been reported at 3–6% rates in various studies.[10,11] Acute bronchitis is the most common lower respiratory tract complication, occurring in about 15% of cases.[10–13] Pneumonia develops in 4–38% of adults.[13] Complications are also caused by exacerbation of underlying disease.[6,7] The risks of complications, hospitalizations and deaths from influenza are higher in people aged 65 years or older, young children and persons with underlying chronic conditions than among healthy older children and younger adults.[6,14–17] In the USA each year, over 110 000 hospital admissions[6] and over 4 million excess respiratory illnesses in persons over 20 years of age[8] are related to influenza. Estimates of the frequency of hospital admissions in the UK for high-risk patients aged 75 years or more are 1 in every 24 people with influenza.[2] In a recent study of influenza epidemics in the USA, approximately 19 000 influenza-associated pulmonary and circulatory deaths per influenza season occurred during 1976–1990, compared with approximately 36 000 deaths during 1990–1999.[14] In the UK, the number of excess deaths attributable to influenza at the time of the influenza outbreaks during non-epidemic years was estimated at 6000; this was higher in epidemic years.[2] During severe pandemics, there are often high attack rates across all age groups, and mortality is increased. Over 90% of the deaths attributed to pneumonia and influenza during recent seasonal epidemics occur among persons aged 65 years and older.[14,17] In addition, influenza seasons in which influenza A H3N2 viruses predominate are associated with higher mortality.[14]

Laboratory diagnosis

Diagnostic tests for influenza fall into four broad categories: virus isolation, detection of viral proteins or viral nucleic acid in nasopharyngeal and throat swabs and serological testing of paired sera.[7] Sensitivity and specificity of any test for influenza might vary by laboratory, type of test and type of specimen tested.[6] Among respiratory specimens for viral isolation or rapid detection, nasopharyngeal specimens are typically more effective than throat swab specimens.[18] Viral culture techniques are not helpful in treatment decisions because of their incubation time. However, culture isolates provide specific information regarding circulating influenza subtypes and strains.[6] Commercial rapid diagnostic tests are available that can be used in outpatient settings to detect influenza viruses within 30 min.[7] These rapid tests differ in the types of influenza viruses they can detect. The specificity (70–99%) and particularly the sensitivity (59–81%) of rapid tests are inferior to viral culture and vary by test.[19–23]

Options for controlling influenza

Approaches to the control of influenza include vaccination and the use of antiviral agents. At present, an inactivated vaccine and four antiviral drugs are licensed in the USA and Europe for the prevention and treatment of influenza. In 2003, a live attenuated vaccine was approved for use in the USA,[24] and other vaccines and antiviral drugs are under development.

Inactivated vaccines

Currently available inactivated influenza virus vaccines are prepared from virus grown in chick embryos; the virus is inactivated, the allantoic fluid is purified, and the material is standardized to contain 15 μg of the haemagglutinin protein of each virus.[6] Since 1948, the World Health Organization Influenza Surveillance Network has led the annual updating of influenza vaccine formulations. Currently licensed vaccines include two subtypes of the influenza A virus (H1N1 and H3N2) and an influenza B virus.[6] Because of frequent seasonal variation in the haemagglutinin and neuraminidase antigens of circulating viruses, it is necessary to administer the vaccine each autumn, shortly before the epidemic season. This schedule allows the annually reformulated influenza vaccine to include antigens detected from recent global viral surveillance, which are likely to be preponderant during the subsequent season.[6] The usual surrogate marker of immunity to influenza is the amount of serum IgG antibody against the haemagglutinin protein.[25]

Efficacy

The recommended dosages of vaccine vary per age group. Whole- and split-virus vaccines can be administered in one dose in adults.[6] Healthy school-aged children and adults almost uniformly have serum antibody responses to vaccination. Preschool children, elderly people and immunocompromised patients respond less well and unpredictably.[6,25] The relationship between antibody levels and clinical benefit is not perfect however. Furthermore, although high-risk groups may have suboptimal immunological responses, the absolute benefit at a population level (number of complications and deaths averted in these individuals) may be larger.

The reported efficacy of inactivated influenza vaccines has varied considerably since their introduction. Overall, well-defined vaccines induce protection against influenza-specific illness in 70–90% of otherwise healthy adults aged less than 65 years (Table 1) when the vaccine and epidemic viruses match antigenically.[26–29] In a meta-analysis (search date 1997; nine randomized placebo-controlled trials; 8910 healthy individuals aged 14–60 years), the efficacy of influenza vaccination for preventing serologically defined infection was 73% [95% confidence interval (CI) 67–78%]. Inactivated parenteral vaccine (three randomized placebo-controlled trials; 979 individuals) offered significant protection, as it reduced the number of influenza cases by 73% (95% CI 50–85%) when the vaccine and circulating viruses were well matched.[29] Although lost work days may also be reduced by vaccination, the benefit is less than half a day on average for each influenza episode [weighted mean difference (WMD) –0.4, 95% CI –0.8 to –0.1 days]. Hospital admissions among vaccinated healthy adults may also be decreased.[29] A recent randomized placebo-controlled trial of hospital-based health care professionals without chronic medical problems (mean age 28.4 years) demonstrated that vaccine efficacy against serologically defined infection was 88% for influenza A. Subjects who were vaccinated ($n = 181$) had fewer days of febrile respiratory illness (52 days) than control subjects (73 days for 180 subjects), but the difference was not statistically significant.[26] Another randomized controlled trial (RCT) involving 2375 healthy working adults younger than 65 years reported that vaccination can reduce lost work days by 32% and physician visits by 42%, compared with placebo, during years when the vaccine and circulating viruses are similar.[27]

As immune responses to vaccination tend to be weaker in elderly people and in persons with certain chronic diseases, these groups are particularly susceptible to influenza-related upper respiratory tract infection.[30,31] An RCT among persons aged 60 years and older (1838 non-institutionalized subjects, three-quarters of whom had no risk factors other than age) reported a 50% reduction in serologically diagnosed influenza (95% CI 39–65%). Vaccine efficacy seemed to be even lower among those aged over 70 years (Table 1). In this age subset,

Table 1. Efficacy and effectiveness of inactivated influenza virus vaccines.

Age group and outcomes	% vaccine efficacy/ effectiveness (95% CI)	Reference
Healthy adults <65 years of age		
Laboratory-confirmed influenza illness	73 (50–85)	29
	88 (47–97) for influenza A	
	89 (14–99) for influenza B	26
	50*	27
	86†	27
Lost work days	53 (–56 to 86)	26
Lost work days due to influenza-like illnesses	32†	27
Lost work days due to upper respiratory illnesses	19†	27
Health care provider visits due to influenza-like illnesses	42†	27
Health care provider visits due to upper respiratory illnesses	17†	27
Community-dwelling elderly		
Laboratory-confirmed influenza illness	50 (39–65)	32
Hospitalization		
Pneumonia or influenza	33 (27–38)	39
	32 (22–40)†	38
	29 (20–38)‡	38
Cardiac disease	19 (11–27)§	38
Cerebrovascular disease	16 (3–29)†	38
	23 (11–34)‡	38
Death (all causes)	50 (45–56)	39
	48 (43–53)†	38
	50 (45–54)‡	38
Death from cardiovascular causes	75 (14–93)	40
Elderly in nursing homes		
Upper respiratory illness	56 (39–68)	34
Pneumonia	53 (35–66)	34
Hospitalization	48 (28–65)	34
Death	68 (56–76)	34

*During the 1997–1998 influenza season when the vaccine virus differed from the predominant circulating viruses; in this season, vaccination did not reduce lost work days or physician visits.
†During the 1998–1999 influenza season.
‡During the 1999–2000 influenza season.
§During the 1998–1999 and 1999–2000 influenza seasons.

risk of influenza-specific illness did not differ significantly between vaccinated and non-vaccinated participants [relative risk (RR) 0.77, 95% CI 0.39–1.51].[32] Vaccination can also be effective in preventing secondary complications and reducing the risk of influenza-related hospitalization and death among adults aged 65 years or older (Table 1) with and without high-risk medical conditions.[33–39] Hospitalization rates may be reduced[35] by 33% (95% CI 27–38%) for pneumonia[39] and by 19% for cardiac disease (95% CI 11–27%)[38] among community-dwelling elderly persons. The risk of death from cardiovascular causes may be reduced among vaccinated patients with cardiac disease by 75% (95% CI 14–93%) during

the influenza season.[40] Vaccinated elderly people residing in nursing homes also have lower frequencies of severe influenza illness, secondary complications and deaths.[34,41,42] In a meta-analysis of 20 cohort studies (29 928 predominantly institutionalized patients with a mean age of 80 years), the vaccine efficacy was 68% (95% CI 56–76%) for preventing death.[34] Influenza vaccination of health care workers has been documented to reduce morbidity and mortality among the elderly in long-term care,[43,44] probably by decreasing rates of nosocomial transmission. Other vaccine formulations or combinations may provide even better protection.[45,46] Inactivated vaccine may also reduce exacerbations in patients with chronic obstructive pulmonary disease.[47] However, an RCT in 2032 patients with asthma (aged 3–64 years) reported that the frequency of disease exacerbations was similar in the 2 weeks after the influenza vaccination and after placebo injection (28.8% and 27.7% respectively; absolute difference 1.1%, 95% CI −1.4% to 3.6%).[48] More data are needed reliably to assess the benefits and risks of influenza vaccination for patients with certain chronic diseases.[49,50]

Vaccination of children may reduce the risk of secondary transmission of influenza within families as well as within communities. In a trial in which children were randomized to receive inactivated influenza vaccine or hepatitis A vaccine, unvaccinated household contacts of the influenza-vaccinated children had 42% fewer episodes of febrile respiratory illness.[51]

Adverse effects

The most frequent adverse effect of vaccination in healthy adults is soreness at the injection site. Evidence from a meta-analysis on parenteral vaccine recipients compared with placebo produced a pooled RR of 2.1 (95% CI 1.4–3.4).[29] Local reactions are generally mild and last up to 2 days. In published trials of influenza vaccine, about 10–64% of adults developed local tenderness and soreness at the vaccination site.[27,29,52–54] RCTs indicate that inactivated influenza vaccine in adults does not cause systemic reactions requiring medical intervention. Fever, malaise and myalgia are not significantly more frequent than with placebo.[29] The rates of adverse effects of split-, subunit and whole-virus influenza vaccines are similar among adults. Although inactivated influenza vaccines are contraindicated for people who are hypersensitive to eggs, the risk of immediate hypersensitivity reactions appears to be low. In a prospective controlled clinical trial, none of the 83 subjects with egg allergy presented significant allergic reactions.[55] The thimerosal preservative in the vaccine may rarely provoke a delayed type of hypersensitivity reaction.[56]

Inactivated influenza vaccine was considered to be potentially associated with the occurrence of Guillain–Barre syndrome during the programme of immunization against swine influenza in 1976.[57] However, studies in subsequent years did not confirm such an association.[58,59] A similar relation was reported again recently, but the calculated risk was only one additional case of Guillain–Barre syndrome per one million people vaccinated, a risk that is much lower than that of severe influenza in all age groups and particularly among people at high risk of complications.[60] Concern about the Guillain–Barre syndrome should not deter people from receiving an inactivated influenza vaccine. However, for persons known to have had the Guillain–Barre syndrome within 6 weeks after a previous influenza vaccination, avoidance of vaccination is prudent, and antiviral chemoprophylaxis is preferable.[6] Influenza vaccination is also safe in multiple sclerosis and does not seem to increase the risk of relapse.[61,62]

One quasi-randomized, double-blind, controlled trial indicated that the effectiveness of the vaccine wanes after the initial vaccination,[63] but a recent meta-analysis did not support this finding.[64]

Live attenuated vaccines

Live attenuated influenza vaccines are in use in Russia and have been newly approved in the USA for use only among healthy persons aged 5–49 years.[24] The vaccine is given intranasally by spray. Thus, attenuated virus strains replicate primarily in nasopharyngeal epithelial cells. The protective mechanisms induced by vaccination with live attenuated influenza vaccines appear to involve both serum and nasal secretory antibodies.[24]

Several trials have demonstrated the safety and efficacy of these vaccines in preventing influenza in adults.[29,65–67] A meta-analysis reported that these vaccines may reduce the number of serologically confirmed influenza cases by 79% (search date 1997; two randomized placebo-controlled trials; 427 healthy adults aged 14–60 years; 95% CI 44–92%).[29] A much larger recent trial involving 4561 healthy adults aged 18–64 years demonstrated that vaccination with live attenuated virus leads to reductions of 19–24% in the occurrence of febrile respiratory illness and reductions of 13–28% in days of work lost, compared with placebo. Days of antibiotic use were reduced by 41–45% among younger participants.[65] A recent meta-analysis of 18 randomized trials comparing attenuated live vaccines against inactivated vaccines (5000 participants aged 1–90 years) showed that the two vaccines were similarly efficacious in preventing culture-confirmed influenza illness, although modest differences cannot be excluded. The pooled odds ratio (OR) for influenza A-H3N2 was 1.50 (95% CI 0.80–2.82) and for A-H1N1 was 1.03 (95% CI 0.58–1.82). Rates of systemic reactions did not differ significantly between the two vaccine groups (OR 0.96, 95% CI 0.74–1.24).[67] A meta-analysis found that about 26% of attenuated vaccine recipients had local adverse effects; sore throat was more than twice as common with the vaccine versus placebo (RR 2.5, 95% CI 1.5–4.2).[29] Serious adverse events occurred in < 1% of healthy subjects aged 5–49 years.[24]

Cost-effectiveness of influenza vaccination

Influenza vaccination can provide substantial economic as well as health benefits. Economic studies of influenza vaccination of persons aged 65 years or older conducted in the USA and European countries have reported overall societal cost savings and substantial reductions in hospitalization and death.[13,35,68,69] Studies of younger adults have shown that vaccination can reduce both direct medical costs and indirect costs from work absenteeism.[6,27,70,71] Reductions of 34–44% in physician visits, 32–45% in lost work days[27,70] and 25% in antibiotic use for influenza-associated illnesses have been reported.[27] One cost-effectiveness analysis estimated a cost of approximately $60–4000 per illness averted among healthy persons aged 18–64 years, depending on the cost of vaccination, the influenza attack rate and vaccine effectiveness against influenza-like illness.[71] One analysis estimated that the net societal cost of vaccination of healthy, working adults aged 18–64 years may range from $11.17 to $65.59 per person, depending on the matching between circulating strains and strains included in the vaccine.[27] Another study estimated average annual savings of $13.66 per person vaccinated.[72] In the latter, 78% of all costs prevented were costs from lost work productivity,[72] whereas the first study did not include productivity losses from influenza illness,[71] and the second had a low rate of influenza-associated absenteeism from work.[27] Overall, cost utility probably improves with increasing age and among those with chronic medical conditions. In one study, among persons aged 65 years or older, vaccination resulted in net savings per quality-adjusted life year (QALY) gained and resulted in costs of $23–256/QALY among younger age groups.[6] Future studies of the relative cost-effectiveness and cost utility of influenza vaccination among adults aged less than 65 years should account consistently for year-to-year variations in influenza attack rates, illness severity and vaccine efficacy.

Policies for influenza immunization and implementation

At present, approximately 50 countries, mainly in the industrialized world, have policies for influenza immunization.[73] Policies vary from country to country. Guidelines for the annual use of inactivated influenza virus vaccine have been developed by several organizations (Table 2). They are primarily oriented towards preventing the serious consequences of the disease. Persons at increased risk of severe influenza illness and its complications as a result of age or underlying medical conditions have been the focus of recommendations from the World Health Organization and other professional organizations[2,6,74] (Table 2). In the USA, recommendations are developed by the Advisory Committee on Immunization Practices (ACIP) of the Centers for Disease Control and Prevention.[6] Recently, ACIP recommended influenza vaccination more broadly including pregnant women, persons between 50 and 64 years of age and patients with immunosuppression caused by human immunodeficiency virus (HIV) infection.[6] Excess deaths among pregnant women were documented during the influenza pandemics of 1918 and 1957, but evidence of a consistent risk was provided only recently by a survey of rates of

Table 2. Target groups for influenza vaccination.*

Recommended for:

People at high risk of complications of influenza

People ≥65 years old[†]

Residents of long-term care

Adults and children with chronic pulmonary (including asthma) or cardiovascular disease[†]

Adults and children requiring care for chronic metabolic disease (including diabetes mellitus), renal dysfunction, haemoglobinopathy or immunosuppression[†] (caused by medications or by HIV infection)

Children and adolescents (6 months–18 years old) receiving long-term aspirin therapy (a risk factor for Reye's syndrome)

Women who will be in the second or third trimester of pregnancy during the influenza season

All persons 50 to 64 years of age[§]

People who can transmit influenza to those at high risk

Health care personnel[‡] in both hospital and outpatient care settings (including emergency response workers)

Employees of long-term care facilities

Employees of residences for people at high risk

Providers of home care to people at high risk

Household members (including children) of people at high risk

May be used for:

People at high risk travelling to locations where the influenza virus may be circulating

People providing essential community services

Students and others in institutional settings

Any person wishing to prevent influenza

*These recommendations are adapted from those of the US Advisory Committee on Immunization Practices, 2003.[6]

[†]Annual immunization of these groups is currently recommended in the UK.[2] This recommendation is based on advice from the Joint Committee on Vaccination and Immunization.

[‡]There is no clear recommendation by the Joint Committee on Vaccination and Immunization for the routine immunization of this group in the UK.[13]

[§]In 2000, the US Advisory Committee on Immunization Practices broadened its influenza vaccines to include all people aged 50–64 years. This recommendation was based in part on an effort to increase the low vaccination rates among persons in this age group with high-risk conditions.[6]

hospitalization during influenza epidemics.[75] The rate of hospitalization of women in the third trimester of pregnancy was similar to that of non-pregnant women with a high-risk condition. The age recommendation was reduced from 64 years to 50 years because persons aged 50–64 years often have underlying disease, and vaccination rates in this group have been low.[6] Although limited information is available regarding the effects of influenza in HIV-infected people, influenza vaccination is highly effective in such patients and probably does not cause major changes in viral load or CD4 cell count.[76] The groups for whom vaccination is recommended now include nearly half the US population, and a similar percentage of the population would probably also be targeted in most developed countries with similar population structures. In the UK, there is no clear recommendation for healthy working age adults to be vaccinated. The Joint Committee on Vaccination and Immunization advises that there is insufficient evidence on which to base a clear recommendation about the routine immunization of all health care workers (Table 2). Since 2000, the Department of Health recommends, however, that frontline health care workers should be immunized against influenza. Social care employers were instructed to consider similar action.[2,13]

For years, only an estimated 20% of people at high risk of serious complications of influenza had been vaccinated each year.[73,77] Implementation of the recommendations has improved only recently. In 2001/02, immunization rates for individuals aged 65 years and older exceeded 65% in the USA and the UK; the goal for 2010 has been set at 90%.[2,6] Conversely, less than 40% of younger people with chronic disorders have been vaccinated in recent years.[6] Similarly, vaccination coverage of health care personnel remains low. Renewed efforts and strategies to improve immunization numbers are needed. A meta-analysis showed that organizational changes, such as separate clinics devoted to prevention, planned visits and special staff, are highly effective in improving adult immunization rates (adjusted OR 16, 95% CI 11.2–22.8).[78] If such interventions are not feasible, then a system of patient reminders should be considered (adjusted OR 2.52, 95% CI 2.24–2.82).[78] Another meta-analysis reported that reminders are effective in both academic settings (OR 3.33, 95% CI 1.98–5.58) and public health clinics (OR 2.09, 95% CI 1.42–3.07).[79]

Antiviral agents

Antiviral drugs are not a substitute for vaccination, although they may be used as adjuncts in the prevention and control of influenza.[2,6] Four agents are already licensed in many countries. The decision to prescribe an antiviral drug for the prevention or treatment of influenza as well as the choice of the specific agent must be based on the likelihood of influenza infection, the subject's age, vaccination status and comorbidity level, the willingness to pay per quality-adjusted day gained

and the accuracy and cost of diagnostic tests.[19,80] In general, testing strategies are less effective than treatment with antiviral drugs alone given the relatively low sensitivity of the tests.[19,80] Testing may be reasonable, however, when influenza likelihood is unclear, such as early in the influenza season or during seasons when influenza is uncommon.[19] For subjects older than 65 years, rapid testing before treatment is cost-effective only for those who are vaccinated or who are at low risk of complications, especially during seasons when influenza is unlikely.[80] Otherwise, empirical treatment seems to be the most cost-effective strategy.[19,80]

Ion channel blockers—efficacy

Amantadine and rimantadine are chemically related antivirals with similar mechanisms of action. They are effective only against influenza A and act by blocking an ion channel formed by the M2 protein that spans the viral membrane.[81] Both are administered orally and excreted in the urine (Table 3).

A meta-analysis (search date 1997; nine randomized placebo-controlled trials; 2438 healthy adults aged 14–60 years of whom some were vaccinated) demonstrated that amantadine prevents 63% of serologically confirmed clinical influenza A cases (95% CI 42–76%).[82] The effect in preventing serious complications of influenza is unknown. When administered within 2 days of illness onset to otherwise healthy adults, amantadine significantly reduced the duration of fever (Tables 4 and 5) by about 1 day (nine randomized placebo-controlled trials; 506 participants; WMD −1.01, 95% CI −1.29 to −0.73 days),[82] although this benefit may not be clear at a daily dose of 100 mg.[2] Furthermore, the limited existing evidence from elderly[83] and high-risk groups makes it difficult to generalize results about the efficacy of amantadine in these populations.

There is no definitive evidence about the efficacy of rimantadine in preventing influenza A in healthy adults. A meta-analysis found that this antiviral drug may prevent 72% of serologically confirmed clinical influenza cases among unvaccinated adults aged 14–60 years, but this comparison was based on a few trials and significant between-study heterogeneity was detected (three randomized placebo-controlled trials; 688 subjects; 95% CI −8% to 92%).[82] When used for the treatment of influenza A (Tables 4 and 5), rimantadine shortened the duration of fever by about 1 day in healthy adults (two randomized placebo-controlled trials; 64 adults; WMD −1.27, 95% CI −1.77 to −0.77 days).[82] No RCTs of rimantadine have involved high-risk persons.

Ion channel blockers—adverse effects

Evidence is available about the adverse effects of these drugs when used for prevention rather than treatment of influenza. A meta-analysis found that use of amantadine versus placebo for prophylaxis of influenza is associated with an increased incidence of gastrointestinal (RR 2.39, 95% CI 1.32–4.32) and central nervous system (CNS) adverse effects (RR 2.25, 95%

Table 3. Antiviral drugs for the prevention or treatment of influenza.*

Drug class	Antiviral drug	Influenza type	Route	Daily dose		Approved ages	Most common side-effects
				Adults	**Elderly**		
Ion channel blockers	Amantadine	A	Oral	200 mg[†]	≤ 100 mg	≥1 year for treatment and prophylaxis	Gastrointestinal and central nervous system symptoms
	Rimantadine	A	Oral	200 mg[‡]	100 mg	≥1 year for prophylaxis ≥13 years for treatment	Gastrointestinal symptoms
Neuraminidase inhibitors	Zanamivir	A and B	Oral inhalation	20 mg	20 mg	≥ 7 years for treatment	Possible worsening of asthma
	Oseltamivir	A and B	Oral	150 mg[§]	150 mg[§]	≥13 years for prophylaxis ≥1 year for treatment	Gastrointestinal symptoms

*The recommended daily dosage of influenza antiviral medications for treatment and prophylaxis is adapted from those of the Advisory Committee on Immunization Practices.[6]

[†]Since 1995 in the UK, the 100-mg daily dose has replaced the previously licensed dose of 200 mg/day.

[‡]A reduction in dosage to 100 mg/day is recommended for persons with creatinine clearance of <10 mL/min.

[§]A reduction in the dose of oseltamivir is recommended when used for treatment in persons with creatinine clearance of <30 mL/min. For prophylaxis, the recommended dose for adults is 75 mg/day.

CI 1.39–3.64) as well as more withdrawals due to adverse effects (RR 2.39, 95% CI 1.54–3.71). Rimantadine can cause an increased incidence of gastrointestinal adverse effects (RR 4.04, 95% CI 1.37–11.88). Amantadine is associated with more CNS adverse events (RR 2.59, 95% CI 1.54–4.35) and study withdrawals (RR 2.30, 95% CI 1.23–4.30) compared with rimantadine.[82] Amantadine stimulates catecholamine release, whereas rimantadine does not, which may account for the prominent CNS side-effects of the former in 4–39% of persons.[25,82] In healthy adults, the rate of adverse events in RCTs using amantadine 100 mg daily is lower than those in RCTs using 200 mg/day. There is little evidence about the effects of lower doses in high-risk persons. Antiviral resistance develops rapidly during treatment with either drug. Persons who develop resistance do not exhibit a prolonged illness, but they can transmit resistant virus to other persons. Viruses resistant to rimantadine show cross-reaction to amantadine and vice versa. Resistant strains have not been found to be more virulent than non-resistant viruses.[6,7]

Neuraminidase inhibitors—efficacy

The sialic acid analogues (Table 3) inhibit the neuraminidase on the viral surface.[7,25] Zanamivir is inhaled through the mouth at a high flow rate; about 78% of a dose is deposited in the oropharynx, and 10–20% of the inhaled dose is bioavailable. Absorbed drug is excreted unchanged in the urine. Oseltamivir is given orally; an estimated 75% of the dose enters the systemic circulation as oseltamivir carboxylate after conversion by hepatic enzymes.[25]

Taken prophylactically, neuraminidase inhibitors can decrease the likelihood of developing laboratory-confirmed influenza by 65% (95% CI 29–71%) in healthy adults aged 14–60 years.[84] Administration of zanamivir, in particular, may induce protection against influenza-specific illness in 69% of adults (95% CI 36–86%) and 81% of households (95% CI 62–91%).[85] A recent RCT found similar results on the protective efficacy of zanamivir (81%, 95% CI 64–90% within households)[86].

A meta-analysis (search date 2001; five randomized placebo-controlled trials; 1947 healthy adults aged 12–65 years) reported that, with zanamivir (when started within 2 days of symptom onset), the median time to alleviation of symptoms was 1.26 days sooner for the influenza-positive population (95% CI –1.93 to –0.59).[85] The time gained in returning to normal activities (Tables 4 and 5) was only half a day (95% CI –0.90 to –0.02).[13] Treating otherwise healthy adults with zanamivir may also provide a 29% (95% CI 10–44%) relative reduction in the odds of complications requiring antibiotics compared with placebo.[85] Evidence is limited for the treatment of high-risk groups including people with underlying disease and elderly people (Table 5); the median time to alleviation of symptoms was 1.99 days sooner for the influenza-positive population (95% CI –3.08 to –0.90 days), but the time gained in returning to normal activities was only 0.20 days (95% CI –1.19 to 0.79).[13,85] The results regarding complications requiring antibiotics are less conclusive in the high-risk populations,[87, 88] while insufficient evidence exists on serious complications requiring admission to hospital or causing death.

Oseltamivir given for seasonal prophylaxis led to a 74% relative reduction (95% CI 16–92%) in the odds of laboratory-confirmed influenza illness among healthy adults aged 18–65 years, a 90% relative reduction (95% CI 71–96%) within households and a 92% reduction (95% CI 39–99%)

Table 4. Eligibility criteria and summary characteristics of trials included in the meta-analyses of antiviral agents for the treatment of influenza.

Meta-analysis for the treatment of influenza with ion channel blockers[82]	Meta-analysis for the treatment of influenza with neuraminidase inhibitors[13,85]
Eligibility of trials: to be selected, trials had to be randomized or quasi-randomized and to evaluate treatment of naturally occurring influenza with amantadine and/or rimantadine	Eligibility of trials: to be selected, trials had to be randomized controlled, double-blind trials, to be published in English, to evaluate treatment of naturally occurring influenza with zanamivir and/or oseltamivir and to report at least one endpoint of relevance
Participants: apparently healthy individuals (with no known pre-existing chronic medical conditions) aged 14–60 years	Participants: three populations were considered: children aged 12 years and under; otherwise healthy individuals aged 12–65 years; and high-risk individuals (those aged 65 years and older or those having certain chronic medical conditions)
Endpoints: duration of fever (defined as a temperature greater than 37°C). Number and seriousness of adverse effects	Endpoints: primary endpoints were time to symptoms alleviated and complications requiring use of antibiotics. Secondary endpoints were time to return to normal activities and hospitalizations
Types of intervention: six studies were randomized placebo-controlled trials of amantadine. One of these used inhaled amantadine and the others oral amantadine. Another trial compared amantadine with aspirin. Two trials randomized participants to receive amantadine, rimantadine or placebo. One further trial was a placebo-controlled trial of rimantadine	Types of intervention: all included trials compared each neuraminidase inhibitor with placebo. Eight randomized controlled trials of zanamivir and nine of oseltamivir treatment met the inclusion criteria
Characteristics of study population: eight trials included only adults with laboratory-confirmed diagnosis of influenza. Mean age for participants ranged from 19 to 39 years. Unvaccinated subjects were included in two trials	Characteristics of study population. *Zanamivir trials*: four trials included mostly unvaccinated (<7%) subjects aged ≥12 years, 9–17% of whom were considered 'at risk'. One trial included only healthy, unvaccinated adults aged ≥13 years, and another was conducted exclusively in high-risk subjects aged ≥12 years, of whom 23% were vaccinated. One trial included mostly unvaccinated (2%) children, of whom 8% were considered 'at risk'. Another trial was conducted in families with 2–5 members. *Oseltamivir trials*: five trials included only high-risk subjects. Three trials were conducted in healthy, unvaccinated adults. Only one trial included healthy mostly unvaccinated (2%) children
Setting: sample size in the 10 eligible trials ranged from 14 to 355 subjects. Six studies took place during the influenza season, two studies during influenza outbreaks and one study during an influenza epidemic. One trial did not clarify the outcome period	Setting: sample size in zanamivir treatment trials ranged from 321 to 777 subjects and in oseltamivir trials from 58 to 726. Data for two zanamivir trials and five oseltamivir trials of high-risk subjects were supplied by the manufacturers
Trial duration: treatment duration ranged from 4 to 10 days. Median length of follow-up was 25.5 days (25th percentile 16 days, 75th percentile 33 days)	Trial duration: treatment duration was 5 days in all trials. Follow-up varied from 5 to 28 days. Seven out of eight zanamivir trials had a follow-up of 28 days. Four out of nine oseltamivir trials had a follow-up of 21 days or more

in a mostly vaccinated elderly population receiving residential care, compared with placebo.[85]

A meta-analysis (search date 2001; three RCTs; 937 healthy adults aged 12–65 years) that compared oseltamivir versus placebo for the treatment of influenza (Tables 4 and 5) demonstrated that the median time to alleviation of symptoms was 1.38 days sooner for the influenza-positive population (95% CI −1.96 to −0.80 days). The drug-treated group also returned to normal activities 1.64 days earlier after influenza-specific illness (95% CI −2.58 to −0.69 days).[13,85] There is also some evidence that oseltamivir treatment reduces complications. In a pooled analysis involving 3564 subjects aged 13–97 years, those with influenza-specific illness treated with oseltamivir had a significant reduction in the incidence of lower respiratory tract complications requiring antibiotics (by 55%) and in hospitalization rates (by 59%).[89]

Table 5. Summary estimates of outcome measures used in the meta-analyses of antiviral agents for the treatment of influenza.

Antiviral agent and age group	Outcome measure	Weighted median difference (days) (95% CI)	Reference
Healthy individuals aged ≤65 years			
	Duration of fever		
Oral amantadine versus placebo		−1.01 (−1.29 to −0.73)*	82
Oral rimantadine versus placebo		−1.27 (−1.77 to −0.77)*	82
Oral amantadine versus oral rimantadine		0.20 (−0.56 to 0.96)*	82
	Time to symptom alleviation		
Zanamivir versus placebo		−1.26 (−1.93 to −0.59)	13,85
Oseltamivir versus placebo		−1.38 (−1.96 to −0.80)	13,85
	Time to return to normal activities		
Zanamivir versus placebo		−0.46 (−0.90 to −0.02)	13,85
Oseltamivir versus placebo		−1.64 (−2.58 to −0.69)	13,85
High-risk subjects (those aged 65 years and older or those having certain chronic medical conditions)			
	Time to symptom alleviation		
Zanamivir versus placebo		−1.99 (−3.08 to −0.90)	13,85
Oseltamivir versus placebo		−0.45 (−1.88 to 0.97)	13,85
	Time to return to normal activities		
Zanamivir versus placebo		−0.20 (−1.19 to 0.79)	13,85
Oseltamivir versus placebo		−3.00 (−5.88 to −0.13)	13,85

*Weighted mean difference.

It is unclear whether treating elderly people and otherwise at-risk adults with oseltamivir shortens the duration of influenza symptoms (five RCTs; 1134 subjects; median time to symptom alleviation −0.45 days, 95% CI −1.88 to 0.97 days).[85] Nevertheless, oseltamivir has a significant impact on influenza-related lower respiratory tract complications, reducing the odds of such complications requiring antibiotics by 34%.[89]

Neuraminidase inhibitors — adverse effects

In clinical trials, the number, type and severity of adverse events with zanamivir have been similar to those with placebo. However, this compound has not been extensively tested in people with severe asthma or other chronic respiratory diseases. Oseltamivir has been associated with a somewhat higher rate of nausea and vomiting (a 3–7% higher rate of nausea and up to 2% higher rate of vomiting compared with placebo).[2,13,84] Because of the short period that both neuraminidase inhibitors had been available, and the lack of optimal assays to detect resistant strains, there is insufficient evidence to comment on the development of viral resistance to these agents, and determination of the full potential toxicity profile may require more extensive post-marketing experience.

Cost-effectiveness of different strategies

Economic studies have been published comparing the cost-effectiveness of different strategies for the control and management of influenza. If one considers vaccination of healthy persons aged 14–65 years, representing predominantly subjects at low risk of complications, vaccination or supportive care only are more cost-effective interventions than prophylaxis or early treatment with antiviral drugs.[71,90] A model-based cost-effectiveness analysis found that no treatment is favoured if the influenza probability is < 32% and the influenza utility is > 0.77.[19] An economic analysis estimated that, for this group of subjects, incremental cost-effectiveness ratios of zanamivir versus symptomatic treatment were £158 000/QALY gained over the duration of the influenza season, dropping to £65 000 if restricting treatment to periods when influenza is known to be circulating.[91] Another study estimated the cost-effectiveness of oseltamivir for influenza treatment in healthy Canadian adults. The conclusions were more optimistic. The base case analysis estimated a cost per QALY of £31 035 with 95% CI of £26 238 to £37 625.[92] However, results are sensitive to the percentage of patients presenting to their physician beyond 48 hours from symptom onset who get oseltamivir and the prevalence of influenza among patients presenting with influenza-like illness.

In economic analyses for influenza prevention among elderly persons, vaccination dominates any solitary antiviral prophylactic strategy in several European countries.[13,69] The cost savings from reduced medical care for elderly people outweighed the costs of vaccination strategies in the UK,[69] and the economic benefit of vaccination was mostly apparent among the elderly residential care population.[2,13] Chemoprophylaxis tended to be most cost-effective when used during the peak 4 weeks of the influenza season. Incremental costs per life–year gained were £22 329 for prophylaxis with ion channel blockers and £121 324 for prophylaxis with neuraminidase inhibitors.[69] In residential populations, the incremental cost per QALY gained for oseltamivir prophylaxis compared with vaccine was estimated at £63 234, but this figure may also be sensitive to the basic assumptions made.[2,13]

Treating early with antiviral agents high-risk persons who present with influenza-like illness during the influenza season seems to be cost-effective.[13,19,80] Amantadine treatment costs considerably less than the neuraminidase inhibitors.[13,19,80] However, the relative likelihood of influenza A is an important determinant of the cost-effectiveness of these agents. For younger patients, amantadine treatment is favoured if the likelihood of influenza A is > 67%; otherwise, neuraminidase inhibitors seem to be favoured.[80] Assuming a willingness to pay of $50 000/QALY saved, empirical treatment with neuraminidase inhibitors would be cost-effective for unvaccinated adults older than 65 years at a probability of influenza > 14%, whereas for vaccinated elderly people, it would be preferred if the likelihood of influenza was > 41%.[80] Nevertheless, there is a vast amount of uncertainty in economic studies leading to broad incremental cost-effectiveness ratios, particularly in at-risk populations,[13,69,93] where cost–benefit is highly dependent on the assumptions used to model the effects of treatment on mortality, hospitalizations and other severe complications of influenza. Given the very large potential market for these antiviral drugs, funding and potential conflicts of interest should also be considered in scrutinizing the available economic analyses.

Recommendations for the use of antiviral agents

Chemoprophylaxis is targeted at people who are at risk of serious complications, live in residential care establishments and are not protected by vaccine, but the settings need to be selected carefully.[6,94]

Treatment with antiviral drugs should be used only when influenza is known to be circulating in the community and only if this can be administered during the first 2 days after the onset of symptoms.[2] High-risk subjects in whom influenza-like illness develops should be treated.[2,80,94] Neuraminidase inhibitors may be advocated as first options in the treatment of influenza in at-risk adults.[2,80,94] Ion channel blockers have come to have limited use[2,94] either because their clinical effectiveness for the treatment of influenza A has not been convincingly proven and accepted[2] or because neuraminidase inhibitors have seemingly improved safety profiles, lower potential for inducing drug resistance and broader anti-influenza activity against both types A and B,[94] while they have

also been more intensively marketed and promoted by their manufacturers. When ability to pay is low, treatment with amantadine may still offer a low-cost alternative to the more expensive neuraminidase inhibitors.[19,80]

Conclusions

Reducing influenza to a minor medical problem may eventually require the development of better vaccines, the availability of better, rapid and cheap diagnostic methods, additions to the current antiviral options, as well as optimal and cost-effective application of all available methods. Vaccines need to be effective for more than 1 year, and antiviral agents as well as rapid diagnosis should be readily available at acceptable prices. In the interim, control of influenza could improve with prudent application of existing options and resources. Increasing current vaccination coverage of the core recommended groups should noticeably decrease the disease burden. Optimal, targeted use of antiviral agents for treatment and short-term prophylaxis in exposed, high-risk groups may produce further benefits. Co-ordinated action by practising physicians and public health authorities is important.

Summary for clinicians

Influenza virus infections cause substantial morbidity and mortality annually. Vaccination remains the primary strategy for reducing this sizeable public health burden. Inactivated vaccine effectively prevents influenza-specific illness in 70–90% of healthy adults. Although protection rates are lower among elderly persons, the vaccine efficacy is about 68% for preventing death in this age group. A live attenuated vaccine with substantial potential for control of influenza has been newly approved for use among healthy subjects. Increasing vaccination coverage of persons at risk of serious complications as well as of their contacts constitutes the most imperative current need for control of influenza. Use of rapid diagnostic tests before treatment with antiviral agents seems to be a cost-effective strategy only when influenza likelihood is low. Ion channel blockers (amantadine and rimantadine) may reduce the duration of influenza A symptoms by about 1 day. Early treatment with neuraminidase inhibitors (zanamivir and oseltamivir) can reduce the duration of uncomplicated disease (by about 1 day in healthy adults) and the likelihood of complications requiring antibiotics. However, insufficient evidence exists on the use of the antiviral agents for treating influenza in high-risk populations. Despite these shortcomings, prudent application of existing options and resources might decrease the disease burden of influenza.

References

1 Murphy BR, Webster RG. Orthomyxoviruses. In: Fields BN, Knipe DM, Howley PM et al., eds. Fields Virology, 3rd edn. Philadelphia, PA, Lippincott, 1996:1397–45.

2 National Institute for Clinical Excellence. *Technology Appraisal Guidance No 58*. London, NICE, 2003 [www.nice.org.uk/pdf/58_Flu_full-guidance.pdf (accessed 21 April 2003)].

3 Englund JA, Champlin RE, Wyde PR *et al*. Common emergence of amantadine- and rimantadine-resistant influenza A viruses in symptomatic immunocompromised adults. *Clin Infect Dis* 1998; **26**:1418–24.

4 Nicholson KG. Clinical features of influenza. *Semin Respir Infect* 1992; **7**:26–37.

5 Fox JP, Cooney MK, Hall CE, Foy HM. Influenza virus infections in Seattle families, 1975–1979. II. Pattern of infection in invaded households and relation of age and prior antibody to occurrence of infection and related illness. *Am J Epidemiol* 1982; **116**:228–42.

6 Centers for Disease Control and Prevention. Prevention and control of influenza: recommendations of the Advisory Committee on Immunization Practices (ACIP). *MMWR Morbid Mortal Wkly Rep* 2003; **52**(RR-8):1–36.

7 Cox NJ, Subbarao K. Influenza. *Lancet* 1999; **354**:1277–82.

8 Sullivan KM, Monto AS, Longini IM Jr. Estimates of the US health impact of influenza. *Am J Public Health* 1993; **83**:1712–16.

9 Kilbourne ED. *Influenza*. New York, Plenum Medical Book Co., 1987:269–70.

10 Hayden FG, Osterhaus AD, Treanor JJ *et al*. Efficacy and safety of the neuraminidase inhibitor zanamivir in the treatment of influenza-virus infections. GG167 Influenza Study Group. *N Engl J Med* 1997; **337**:874–80.

11 Treanor JJ, Hayden FG, Vrooman PS *et al*. Efficacy and safety of the oral neuraminidase inhibitor oseltamivir in treating acute influenza: a randomized controlled trial. US Oral Neuraminidase Study Group. *JAMA* 2000; **283**:1016–24.

12 Smith KJ, Roberts MS. Cost-effectiveness of newer treatment strategies for influenza. *Am J Med* 2002; **113**:300–7.

13 Turner D, Wailoo A, Nicholson K, Cooper NJ, Sutton AJ, Abrams KR. Systematic review and economic decision modeling for the prevention and treatment of influenza A and B. *NICE Assessment Report* 2002. Available at www.nice.org.uk/pdf/influenzaassrep.pdf.

14 Thompson WW, Shay DK, Weintraub E *et al*. Mortality associated with influenza and respiratory syncytial virus in the United States. *JAMA* 2003; **289**:179–86.

15 Barker WH, Mullooly JP. Impact of epidemic type A influenza in a defined adult population. *Am J Epidemiol* 1980; **112**:798–811.

16 Barker WH, Mullooly JP. Pneumonia and influenza deaths during epidemics: implications for prevention. *Arch Intern Med* 1982; **142**:85–9.

17 Simonsen L, Clarke MJ, Schonberger LB, Arden NH, Cox NJ, Fukuda K. Pandemic versus epidemic influenza mortality: a pattern of changing age distribution. *J Infect Dis* 1998; **178**:53–60.

18 Schmid ML, Kudesia G, Wake S, Read RC. Prospective comparative study of culture specimens and methods in diagnosing influenza in adults. *BMJ* 1998; **316**:275.

19 Smith KJ, Roberts MS. Cost-effectiveness of newer treatment strategies for influenza. *Am J Med* 2002; **113**:300–7.

20 Storch GA. Rapid diagnostic tests for influenza. *Curr Opin Pediatr* 2003; **15**:77–84.

21 Uyeki TM. Influenza diagnosis and treatment in children: a review of studies on clinically useful tests and antiviral treatment for influenza. *Pediatr Infect Dis J* 2003; **22**:164–77.

22 Noyola DE, Clark B, O'Donnell FT, Atmar RL, Greer J, Demmler GJ. Comparison of a new neuraminidase detection assay with an enzyme immunoassay, immunofluorescence, and culture for rapid detection of influenza A and B viruses in nasal wash specimens. *J Clin Microbiol* 2000; **38**:1161–5.

23 Atmar RL, Baxter BD, Dominguez EA, Taber LH. Comparison of reverse transcription-PCR with tissue culture and other rapid diagnos-

tic assays for detection of type A influenza virus. *J Clin Microbiol* 1996; **34**:2604–6.

24 Centers for Disease Control and Prevention. Using live attenuated influenza vaccine for prevention and control of influenza: supplemental recommendations of the Advisory Committee on Immunization Practices (ACIP). *MMWR Morbid Mortal Wkly Rep* 2003; **52**(RR-13):1–7.

25 Couch RB. Prevention and treatment of influenza. *N Engl J Med* 2000; **343**:1778–87.

26 Wilde JA, McMillan JA, Serwint J, Butta J, O'Riordan MA, Steinhoff MC. Effectiveness of influenza vaccine in health care professionals: a randomized trial. *JAMA* 1999; **281**:908–13.

27 Bridges CB, Thompson WW, Meltzer MI *et al*. Effectiveness and cost–benefit of influenza vaccination of healthy working adults: a randomized controlled trial. *JAMA* 2000; **284**:1655–63.

28 Palache AM. Influenza vaccines: a reappraisal of their use. *Drugs* 1997; **54**:841–56.

29 Demicheli V, Rivetti D, Deeks JJ, Jefferson TO. Vaccines for preventing influenza in healthy adults (Cochrane Review). In: *The Cochrane Library*, Issue 2. Oxford, Update Software, 2003.

30 Blumberg EA, Albano C, Pruett T *et al*. Immunogenicity of influenza virus vaccine in solid organ transplant recipients. *Clin Infect Dis* 1996; **22**:295–302.

31 McElhaney JE, Beattie BL, Devine R, Grynoch R, Toth EL, Bleackley RC. Age-related decline in interleukin 2 production in response to influenza vaccine. *J Am Geriatr Soc* 1990; **38**:652–8.

32 Govaert TM, Thijs CT, Masurel N, Sprenger MJ, Dinant GJ, Knottnerus JA. Efficacy of influenza vaccination in elderly individuals: a randomized double-blind placebo-controlled trial. *JAMA* 1994; **272**:1661–5.

33 Patriarca PA, Weber JA, Parker RA *et al*. Risk factors for outbreaks of influenza in nursing homes: a case–control study. *Am J Epidemiol* 1986; **124**:114–19.

34 Gross PA, Hermogenes AW, Sacks HS, Lau J, Levandowski RA. Efficacy of influenza vaccine in elderly persons: a meta-analysis and review of the literature. *Ann Intern Med* 1995; **123**:518–27.

35 Mullooly JP, Bennett MD, Hornbrook MC *et al*. Influenza vaccination programs for elderly persons: cost-effectiveness in a health maintenance organization. *Ann Intern Med* 1994; **121**:947–52.

36 Nordin J, Mullooly J, Poblete S *et al*. Influenza vaccine effectiveness in preventing hospitalizations and deaths in persons 65 years or older in Minnesota, New York, and Oregon: data from 3 health plans. *J Infect Dis* 2001; **184**:665–70.

37 Hak E, Nordin J, Wei F *et al*. Influence of high-risk medical conditions on the effectiveness of influenza vaccination among elderly members of 3 large managed-care organizations. *Clin Infect Dis* 2002; **35**:370–7.

38 Nichol KL, Nordin J, Mulloorly J, Lask R, Fillbrandt K, Iwane M. Influenza vaccination and reductions in hospitalizations for cardiac disease and stroke among the elderly. *N Engl J Med* 2003; **348**:1322–32.

39 Vu T, Farish S, Jenkins M, Kelly H. A meta-analysis of effectiveness of influenza vaccine in persons aged 65 years and over living in the community. *Vaccine* 2002; **20**:1831–6.

40 Gurfinkel EP, de la Fuente RL, Mendiz O, Mautner B. Influenza vaccine pilot study in acute coronary syndromes and planned percutaneous coronary interventions: the FLU Vaccination Acute Coronary Syndromes (FLUVACS) Study. *Circulation* 2002; **105**:2143–7.

41 Patriarca PA, Weber JA, Parker RA *et al*. Efficacy of influenza vaccine in nursing homes reduction in illness and complications during an influenza A (H3N2) epidemic. *JAMA* 1985; **253**:1136–9.

42 Monto AS, Hornbuckle K, Ohmit SE. Influenza vaccine effectiveness among elderly nursing home residents: a cohort study. *Am J Epidemiol* 2001; **154**:155–60.

43 Carman W, Elder AG, Wallace LA *et al*. Effects of influenza vaccina-

tion of health-care workers on mortality of elderly people in long-term care: a randomised trial. *Lancet* 2000; **355**:93–7.

44 Potter J, Scott DJ, Roberts MA *et al.* Influenza vaccination of health-care workers in long-term care hospitals reduces the mortality of elderly patients. *J Infect Dis* 1997; **175**:1–6.

45 Podda A. The adjuvanted influenza vaccines with novel adjuvants: experience with the MF 59-adjuvanted vaccine. *Vaccine* 2001; **19**:2673–80.

46 Treanor JJ, Mattison HR, Dammed G *et al.* Protective efficacy of combined live intranasal and inactivated influenza A virus vaccines in the elderly. *Ann Intern Med* 1992; **117**:625–33.

47 Poole PJ, Chacko E, Wood-Baker RWB, Cates CJ. Influenza vaccine for patients with chronic obstructive pulmonary disease (Cochrane Review). In: *The Cochrane Library*, Issue 3. Oxford, Update Software, 2003.

48 American Lung Association Asthma Clinical Research Centers. The safety of inactivated influenza vaccine in adults and children with asthma. *N Engl J Med* 2001; **345**:1529–36.

49 Cates CJ, Jefferson TO, Bara AI, Rowe BH. Vaccines for preventing influenza in people with asthma (Cochrane Review). In: *The Cochrane Library*, Issue 2. Oxford, Update Software, 2003.

50 Tan A, Bhalla P, Smyth R. Vaccines for preventing influenza in people with cystic fibrosis (Cochrane Review). In: *The Cochrane Library*, Issue 2. Oxford, Update Software, 2003.

51 Hurwitz ES, Haber M, Chang A *et al.* Effectiveness of influenza vaccination of day care children in reducing influenza-related morbidity among household contacts. *JAMA* 2000; **284**:1677–82.

52 Govaert TME, Dinant GJ, Aretz K, Masurel N, Sprenger MJW, Knottnerus JA. Adverse reactions to influenza vaccine in elderly people: randomised double blind placebo controlled trial. *BMJ* 1993; **307**:988–90.

53 Margolis KL, Nichol KL, Poland GA, Pluhar RE. Frequency of adverse reactions to influenza vaccine in the elderly: a randomized, placebo-controlled trial. *JAMA* 1990; **264**:1139–41.

54 Nichol KL, Margolis KL, Lind A *et al.* Side effects associated with influenza vaccination in healthy working adults: a randomized, placebo-controlled trial. *Arch Intern Med* 1996; **156**:1546–50.

55 Zeiger RS. Current issues with influenza vaccination in egg allergy. *J Allergy Clin Immunol* 2002; **110**:834–40.

56 Aberer W. Vaccination despite thimerosal sensitivity. *Contact Dermatitis* 1991; **24**:6–10.

57 Schonberger LB, Bregman DJ, Sullivan-Bolyai JZ *et al.* Guillain–Barré syndrome following vaccination in the National Influenza Immunization Program, United States, 1976–1977. *Am J Epidemiol* 1979; **110**:105–23.

58 Hurwitz ES, Schonberger LB, Nelson DB, Holman RC. Guillain–Barré syndrome and the 1978–1979 influenza vaccine. *N Engl J Med* 1981; **304**:1557–61.

59 Kaplan JE, Katona P, Hurwitz ES, Schonberger LB. Guillain–Barré syndrome in the United States, 1979–1980 and 1980–1981: lack of an association with influenza vaccination. *JAMA* 1982; **248**:698–700.

60 Lasky T, Terracciano GJ, Magder L *et al.* Guillain–Barré syndrome and the 1992–1993 and 1993–1994 influenza vaccines. *N Engl J Med* 1998; **339**:1797–1802.

61 Miller AE, Morgante LA, Buchwald LY *et al.* A multicenter, randomized, double-blind, placebo-controlled trial of influenza immunization in multiple sclerosis. *Neurology* 1997; **48**:312–14.

62 Rutschmann OT, McCrory DC, Matchar DB; Immunization Panel of the Multiple Sclerosis Council for Clinical Practice Guidelines. Immunization and MS: a summary of published evidence and recommendations. *Neurology* 2002; **59**:1837–43.

63 Hoskins TW, Davies JR, Smith AJ, Miller CL, Allchin A. Assessment of inactivated influenza-A vaccine after three outbreaks of influenza A at Christ's Hospital. *Lancet* 1979; **1**:33–5.

64 Beyer WE, de Bruijn IA, Palache AM, Westendorp RG, Osterhaus AD. Protection against influenza after annually repeated vaccination: a meta-analysis of serologic and field studies. *Arch Intern Med* 1999; **159**:182–8.

65 Nichol KL, Mendelman PM, Mallon KP *et al.* Effectiveness of live, attenuated intranasal influenza virus vaccine in healthy, working adults: a randomized controlled trial. *JAMA* 1999; **282**:137–44.

66 Mendelman PM, Cordova J, Cho I. Safety, efficacy and effectiveness of the influenza virus vaccine, trivalent, types A and B, live, cold-adapted (CAIV-T) in healthy children and healthy adults. *Vaccine* 2001; **19**:2221–6.

67 Beyer WE, Palache AM, de Jong JC, Osterhaus AD. Cold-adapted live influenza vaccine versus inactivated vaccine: systemic vaccine reactions, local and systemic antibody response, and vaccine efficacy. A meta-analysis. *Vaccine* 2002; **20**:1340–53.

68 Nichol KL, Wuorenma J, von Sternberg T. Benefits of influenza vaccination for low-, intermediate-, and high-risk senior citizens. *Arch Intern Med* 1998; **158**:1769–76.

69 Scuffham PA, West PA. Economic evaluation of strategies for the control and management of influenza in Europe. *Vaccine* 2002; **20**:2562–78.

70 Nichol KL, Lind A, Margolis KL *et al.* Effectiveness of vaccination against influenza in healthy, working adults. *N Engl J Med* 1995; **333**:889–93.

71 Demicheli V, Jefferson T, Rivetti D, Deeks J. Prevention and early treatment of influenza in healthy adults. *Vaccine* 2000; **18**:957–1030.

72 Nichol KL. Cost–benefit analysis of a strategy to vaccinate healthy working adults against influenza. *Arch Intern Med* 2001; **161**:749–59.

73 Stohr K. Preventing and treating influenza. *BMJ* 2003; **326**:1223–4.

74 World Health Organization. Influenza vaccines. *Wkly Epidemiol Rec* 2002; **77**:229–40.

75 Neuzil KM, Reed GW, Mitchel EF, Simonsen L, Griffin MR. Impact of influenza on acute cardiopulmonary hospitalizations in pregnant women. *Am J Epidemiol* 1998; **148**:1094–102.

76 Tasker SA, Treanor JJ, Paxton WB, Wallace MR. Efficacy of influenza vaccination in HIV-infected persons. A randomized, double-blind, placebo-controlled trial. *Ann Intern Med* 1999; **131**:430–3.

77 Influenza vaccination levels in selected states — behavioral risk factor surveillance system, 1987. *MMWR Morbid Mortal Wkly Rep* 1989; **38**:124–33.

78 Stone EG, Morton SC, Hulscher ME *et al.* Interventions that increase use of adult immunization and cancer screening services: a meta-analysis. *Ann Intern Med* 2002; **136**:641–51.

79 Szilagyi P, Vann J, Bordley C *et al.* Interventions aimed at improving immunization rates (Cochrane Review). In: *The Cochrane Library*, Issue 4. Oxford, Update Software, 2002.

80 Rothberg MB, Bellantonio S, Rose DN. Management of influenza in adults older than 65 years of age: cost-effectiveness of rapid testing and antiviral therapy. *Ann Intern Med* 2003; **139**:321–9.

81 Bui M, Whittaker G, Helenius A. Effect of M1 protein and low pH on nuclear transport of influenza virus ribonucleoproteins. *J Virol* 1996; **70**:8391–401.

82 Jefferson TO, Demicheli V, Deeks JJ, Rivetti D. Amantadine and rimantadine for preventing and treating influenza A in adults (Cochrane Review). In: *The Cochrane Library*, Issue 2. Oxford, Update Software, 2003.

83 Walters HE, Paulshock M. Therapeutic efficacy of amantadine HCl. *Mol Med* 1970; **67**:176–9.

84 Jefferson T, Demicheli V, Deeks J, Rivetti D. Neuraminidase inhibitors for preventing and treating influenza in healthy adults (Cochrane Review). In: *The Cochrane Library*, Issue 2. Oxford, Update Software, 2003.

85 Cooper NJ, Sutton AJ, Abrams KR, Wailoo A, Turner D, Nicholson KG. Effectiveness of neuraminidase inhibitors in treatment and pre-

vention of influenza A and B: systematic review and meta-analyses of randomised controlled trials. *BMJ* 2003; **326**:1235.

86 Monto AS, Pichichero ME, Blanckenberg SJ *et al.* Zanamivir prophylaxis: an effective strategy for the prevention of influenza types A and B within households. *J Infect Dis* 2002; **186**:1582–8.

87 Monto AS, Webster A, Keene O. Randomized, placebo-controlled studies of inhaled zanamivir in the treatment of influenza A and B: pooled efficacy analysis. *J Antimicrob Chemother* 1999; **11**:23–9.

88 Lalezari J, Camion K, Keene O. Zanamivir for the treatment of influenza A and B infection in high-risk patients: a pooled analysis of randomiized, controlled-trials. *Arch Intern Med* 2001; **161**:212–17.

89 Kaiser L, Wat C, Mills T, Mahoney P, Ward P, Hayden F. Impact of oseltamivir treatment on influenza-related lower respiratory tract complications and hospitalizations. *Arch Intern Med* 2003; **163**:1667–72.

90 Muennig PA, Khan K. Cost-effectiveness of vaccination versus treatment of influenza in healthy adolescents and adults. *Clin Infect Dis* 2001; **33**:1879–85.

91 Burls A, ClarkW, Stewart T *et al.* Zanamivir for the treatment of influenza in adults. *NICE* 2000, Supplement.

92 O'Brien BJ, Goeree R, Blackhouse G, Smieja M, Loeb M. Oseltamivir for treatment of influenza in healthy adults: pooled trial evidence and cost-effectiveness model for Canada. *Value Health* 2003; **6**:116–25.

93 Mauskopf JA, Cates SC, Griffin AD. A pharmacoeconomic model for the treatment of influenza. *Pharmacoeconomics* 1999; **16**(Suppl 1):73–84.

94 Uhnoo I, Linde A, Pauksens K, Lindberg A, Eriksson M, Norrby R; Swedish Consensus Group. Treatment and prevention of influenza: Swedish recommendations. *Scand J Infect Dis* 2003; **35**:3–11.

CHAPTER 4.5

Bronchiectasis

John Kolbe

Introduction

Bronchiectasis is a chronic condition characterized by irreversible destruction and dilatation of airways, generally associated with chronic bacterial infection. This condition is responsible for considerable morbidity and mortality, particularly in indigenous populations and in developing countries. There has been remarkably little research into the aetiology, pathophysiology, immunology and management of this condition in recent decades, and the evidence for the majority of management strategies in this condition is surprisingly poor. For most aspects of treatment, there is the need for well-designed, adequately powered studies of sufficient duration using valid and clinically relevant outcome parameters. This chapter will focus on the limited evidence for management strategies in bronchiectasis. The reader will be directed elsewhere for more comprehensive discussions of pathophysiology, aetiology and epidemiology of this condition. However, some brief introductory comments are warranted.

Pathophysiology

Bronchiectasis is characterized by chronic inflammation of the bronchial wall by polymorphonuclear leucocytes. There is also an active cell-mediated immune response with marked increases in CD8-positive T lymphocytes, antigen-progressing cells and effector macrophages.[1] The exuberant humoral immune response is reflected in the commonly associated hypergammaglobulinaemia. Cole has described a widely acknowledged 'vicious cycle' of bacteria-mediated toxicity and bacteria-provoked, host-mediated inflammatory lung damage.[2] Once 'colonization' is established, the microbes are able to subvert the normal host clearance mechanisms, modulate the respiratory environment and facilitate microbial proliferation. A variety of microbial products and host factors, including interleukin (IL)-8, are chemoattractant for neutrophils and, along with increased expression of adhesion molecules, sustain and amplify the inflammatory response. Bacterial products impair local host defences by increasing mucus production, impairing ciliary function, causing IgA breakdown and directly releasing bronchoactive substances. Neutrophil-derived myeloperoxidase contributes to the inflammatory process and tissue damage. Neutrophil elastase is capable of damaging bronchial epithelial cells, destroying components of the extracellular matrix, impairing ciliary motion, stimulating mucus secretion, cleaving immunoglobulins and complement and interfering with phagocytosis and killing of bacteria. Neutrophil elastase plays an important role in *Pseudomonas* colonization by rendering epithelial cells more susceptible to bacterial adherence.

Aetiology

Bronchiectasis should be regarded as the common outcome of a number of aetiologies and possibly a number of mechanisms. Bronchiectasis due to specific underlying conditions such as ciliary dyskinesia or immune deficiency, traction bronchiectasis associated with diffuse interstitial lung disease and bronchiectasis beyond an endobronchial obstruction will not be discussed. Cystic fibrosis (CF) in adults will be discussed in Chapter 4.6. This chapter will be devoted to 'idiopathic' bronchiectasis. This implies no specific identifiable underlying condition responsible for the bronchiectasis. It is generally surmised that this disease is a sequela of severe lower respiratory tract infection, usually in childhood, the best studied being adenovirus 21 bronchiolitis.[3,4] Pertussis and measles are frequently reported as initiating events despite a lack of supporting evidence. Bronchiectasis may be a sequela of *Mycoplasma* infection[5] or any necrotizing pneumonia, including those associated with aspiration, or may be due to *Staphylococcus*, *Klebsiella* or *M. tuberculosis*.

Airway abnormalities in this condition have been classified histologically[6] and radiologically.[7] Cylindrical bronchiectasis, defined as symmetrical dilatation of airways along a longitudinal axis, is virtually synonymous with the histological type of follicular bronchiectasis. Cystic bronchiectasis corresponds to the saccular histological type. Varicose bronchiectasis can belong to either histological type; radiological features with both morphological types can be regarded as an intermediate form of the disease. Cylindrical bronchiectasis is the most common form of 'idiopathic' bronchiectasis in Europeans;[7] in contrast, cystic/saccular disease is anecdotally believed to be more common in indigenous populations.

Epidemiology

The prevalence of bronchiectasis has not been accurately determined in any population. There are a number of reasons for this: the difficulty in distinguishing bronchiectasis clinically from other conditions because of the low specificity of symptoms and signs; the lack of sensitivity and specificity of plain chest radiographs; the lack of a simple non-invasive diagnostic test; and the impracticality of applying diagnostic tests [previously bronchography but, more recently, high-resolution computerized tomography (HRCT) scanning] to a population. There is evidence suggesting increased prevalence (and morbidity and mortality) in indigenous populations.[8] There is no convincing evidence of a genetic predisposition in these ethnic groups. The cilial structural abnormalities previously reported in Polynesians with bronchiectasis[9] are now thought to be a sequela of chronic infection rather than constituting a primary underlying abnormality.

In the late twentieth century, the apparent decline in bronchiectasis in 'developed' countries was attributed to improvements in living standards, better health care, effective anti-tuberculosis therapy, immunization against pertussis and measles and more available and effective antibiotics. As a result, bronchiectasis was regarded as 'an uncommon disease'.[10] However, the prevalence of bronchiectasis may be underestimated, the symptoms attributed to other conditions, and the health impact of this condition much greater than generally thought. In a study of 120 UK patients from primary care with the diagnosis of chronic obstructive pulmonary disease (COPD), O'Brien et al.[11] found that 29% had definite HRCT evidence of bronchiectasis. With the wider availability of HRCT scanning facilitating the diagnosis in those with milder disease, and increased immigration from countries of high prevalence to 'developed' countries, the epidemiology of bronchiectasis may be changing, and interpretation of the limited longitudinal statistics will be more difficult. The impact of various socio-economic factors on the prevalence and outcome of bronchiectasis needs to be better defined so that specific public health interventions can be subjected to randomized controlled trials (RCTs) to determine their impact on the development and progression of bronchiectasis.

Investigations

The aims of investigation are to confirm the diagnosis and to define specific causes and determine the degree of impairment and disability. Symptoms and signs are not sufficiently discriminatory; chronic cough and purulent sputum are typical but are not always present. Symptoms may be attributed to co-morbidities, e.g. smoking-related airways disease or chronic sinusitis, or be non-specific such as dyspnoea, lassitude, anorexia and weight loss. Finger clubbing is a strong pointer, but this is an inconstant finding. The auscultatory findings in bronchiectasis are variable although crackles in the early and mid-phases of inspiration and in expiration that are gravity independent and become less profuse after coughing have been reported.[12] Complications of bronchiectasis include recurrent pneumonia, haemoptysis (which may be massive), empyema, brain abscess and the development of respiratory failure and cor pulmonale.

The diagnosis of bronchiectasis is essentially radiological. In severe disease, there may be little difficulty making the diagnosis on the basis of plain chest radiographs (Fig. 1). However, at least 50% of patients with bronchiectasis have an apparently normal chest radiograph[13] and, in many others, the abnormalities are non-specific. Historically, the 'gold standard' for diagnosis was bronchography, but this unpleasant and cumbersome procedure has been replaced by HRCT scanning (Figs 2 and 3). The HRCT diagnosis is made when the internal diameter of the bronchus is greater than the diameter of the adjacent branch of the pulmonary artery. HRCT has a sensitivity of over 95% for the diagnosis of bronchographically proven bronchiectasis[14,15] and has low interobserver variation in trained radiologists.[16] Systems to 'score' the HRCT appearances have graded each lobe (including the lingula) on the basis of extent of disease, severity of bronchial dilatation, bronchial wall thickness, mucus plugging and regional inhomogeneity (on expiratory scans).[16] The discriminatory power of these abnormalities in terms of clinical features, epidemiology, pathophysiology, response to the various therapies or prognosis is not known.

HRCT evidence of bronchiectasis is not uncommon in rheumatoid disease (reportedly as high as 30%),[17,18] and there are recognized associations with other conditions including yellow nail syndrome, tracheobronchomegaly (Mounier–Kuhn syndrome) and inflammatory bowel disease (particularly ulcerative colitis,[19,20] but also Crohn's disease[21] and coeliac disease,[22] especially after colectomy).[20,21] The presence of such conditions is usually obvious, but clinicians need to be aware of the associations.

Investigations to define specific causes that would lead to important changes in management

• Quantitative assessment of immunoglobulin (Ig) levels. The more common forms of humoral immune deficiency, e.g. X-linked agammaglobulinaemia and common variable immunodeficiency, are associated with bronchiectasis. If significant hypogammaglobulinaemia is demonstrated, most clinicians would treat with Ig replacement therapy in an attempt to halt progression of the disease and prevent complications,[23,24] although an RCT of this treatment has never been carried out. IgG subclass levels are not routinely measured as the normal range is poorly defined, the role of subclass deficiency is questionable, there is no consensus on the use of Ig replacement and deficiencies are uncommon even in patients with HRCT evidence of bronchiectasis.[25] More detailed investigation of humoral immune status involving responses to im-

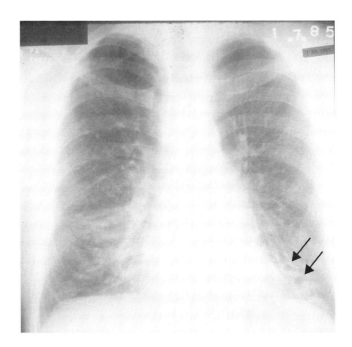

Figure 1. Chest radiograph showing dilated thick-walled bronchi (arrows).

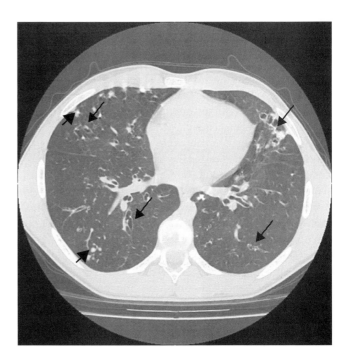

Figure 2. High-resolution CT scan of the chest showing dilated airways (long arrows) and mucus plugging (short arrows).

munizations is not justified routinely but may be useful in those with borderline levels or a history of recurrent severe infections.

• Aspergillus serology, particularly aspergillus-specific IgE.[26] The diagnosis of allergic bronchopulmonary aspergillosis has important therapeutic implications. The management of this condition is addressed elsewhere (Chapter 2.7).

• Sweat electrolyte analysis. Studies of prevalence of CF in cohorts of adult patients with bronchiectasis have yielded conflicting results. Gervais *et al.*[27] found that 16/63 (25%) patients with bronchiectasis had a sweat chloride of ≥ 60 mmol/L, and five of these had a ØF508 mutation. A higher prevalence of CF mutations was reported in unselected patients with bronchiectasis by Giroden *et al.*[28] However, King *et al.*[29] found that the prevalence of CFTR mutations in a representative cohort of adult patients with bronchiectasis was the same as in the healthy population. The difficulties of defining a diagnosis of CF are addressed elsewhere (Chapter 4.6), but those diagnosed as adults are more likely to have retained pancreatic exocrine function, less respiratory impairment, a lower rate of

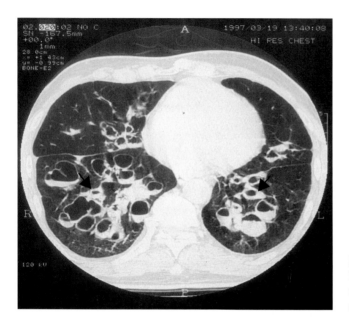

Figure 3. High-resolution CT scan of the chest showing gross bronchiectasis, mainly thin-walled dilated bronchi but also some thick-walled bronchi (arrows). Many of the airways show retained airway secretions.

Pseudomonas infection and a different profile of mutations.[30,31] As this diagnosis has implications for multiorgan involvement, different responses to treatments and issues in relation to genetic counselling, a case could be made for sweat testing of all adults diagnosed with bronchiectasis. However, the 'label' of CF may have major implications for individual patients and their families and may not always lead to important changes in management.

• Nasal and expired nitric oxide (eNO) levels. Despite increased expression of inducible nitric oxide synthetase in the airways and an earlier study reporting increased levels,[32] subsequent studies have demonstrated that eNO levels are not elevated in bronchiectasis.[33–35] Horvath *et al.*[36] reported that simultaneously low levels of nasal and expired NO differentiated patients with primary ciliary dyskinesia from other patients with bronchiectasis with a specificity of 98% and a positive predictive value of 92%.

Commonly associated conditions are rhinosinusitis and gastro-oesophageal reflux disease (GORD). Rhinosinusitis may contribute to symptoms of cough and sputum, and the upper respiratory tract may be a reservoir of infection. GORD may aggravate bronchiectasis via recurrent microaspirations or vagally mediated reflexes. The impact of treatment of these conditions on the bronchiectasis has not been studied, but reviews and consensus statements on the management of bronchiectasis stress the importance of appropriate management of these conditions.[10,37]

No studies have been undertaken to determine what baseline investigations should be undertaken in persons with 'idiopathic' bronchiectasis, nor whether these results influence management and subsequent outcome. Clinical consensus indicates that the following should be undertaken:
• Lung function testing. Bronchiectasis is characterized by airflow obstruction, particularly involving small airways. Forced expiratory volume in 1 second (FEV_1) correlates with certain HRCT features,[16] and serial measures of FEV_1 may be used to monitor disease progress and to assess response to therapies. There is an accelerated rate of decline of FEV_1 in bronchiectasis,[38] but it is not known whether FEV_1 is a powerful predictor of outcome in bronchiectasis as it is in CF and COPD. The role of more detailed testing is not clear.
• Sputum bacterial culture. Organisms frequently cultured from the sputum include *Haemophilus influenzae*, *Streptococcus pneumoniae*, *Branhamella catarrhalis*, *Staphylococcus aureus* and *Pseudomonas aeruginosa* (PA). PA infection is associated with adverse clinical features such as higher sputum volumes,[39] worse quality of life,[40] more severe and extensive bronchiectasis,[41] greater impairment of baseline lung function[42] and greater rate of decline of FEV_1.[40,42] PA may play an important role in progressive airway wall damage.[43,44]
• Sputum culture for mycobacteria. Infection by non-tuberculous mycobacteria (NTM), specifically *Mycobacterium avium-intracellulare* (MAIC), *M. malmoense* and *M. abscessus*, is increasingly recognized, but their role in inflammation and damage remains unclear. The HRCT pattern of bronchiectasis and multiple small lung nodules has a sensitivity of 80% and specificity of 87% for culture-positive MAIC[45]—other features being 'tree in bud' appearance and mosaic attenuation. For the treatment of MAIC lung disease, the reader is referred elsewhere.[46] Patients with bronchiectasis may also be infected by *Mycobacterium tuberculosis*,[47] especially in populations with a high background prevalence. Tuberculosis may not be suspected on clinical grounds with symptoms attributed to bronchiectasis.
• Assessment of functional capacity. While formal cardiopulmonary exercise testing may be undertaken, other tests such as

6-min walk distance[48] or endurance shuttle test[49] may be more appropriate.
- Assessment of health-related quality of life. This would seem to be intuitively important. Wilson *et al.*[50] have demonstrated the stability, validity and responsiveness of the St George's Respiratory Questionnaire (an instrument developed for COPD) in bronchiectasis, but no valid, responsive, disease-specific instrument exists.

Management

The overall general aims of management are to:
- reduce symptoms;
- improve health-related quality of life;
- minimize further airway damage and prevent progression of the lung disease;
- reduce morbidity (and mortality);
- prevent acute exacerbations;
- treat exacerbations that do occur promptly and effectively.

Long-term management is based on a combination of airway clearance techniques, strategies to reduce the microbial load, suppression of the excessive inflammatory response and treatment of underlying or associated conditions (Table 1). However, the evidence for these management strategies is severely limited.

A difficulty in conducting trials in bronchiectasis is that valid, responsive, objective and convenient markers of disease activity are lacking. Consequently, surrogate markers are used as outcome parameters. There is evidence of compartmentalization of the inflammatory response in bronchiectasis[51] and,

Table 1. Chronic management of bronchiectasis.

Beneficial (proven)
Likely to be beneficial
   Airway clearance techniques
   Inhaled hyperosmolar agents
   Physical training
   Treatment of comorbid conditions
Trade-off between benefits and harm
   Long-term oral antibiotics
   Nebulized antibiotics
Unknown effectiveness
   Mucolytes
   Long-term macrolide therapy
   Inhaled corticosteroids
   Non-steroidal anti-inflammatory agents
   Long-acting β-agonists
   Long-term oxygen therapy
   Surgical resection
Unlikely to be beneficial
   Methylxanthines
Likely to be ineffective (or harmful)
   DNase
   Long-term oral corticosteroids

hence, serum markers may not reflect the airway inflammatory response. Expired NO cannot be used to monitor inflammation in bronchiectasis nor to act as an outcome parameter in clinical studies.[33–35] Sputum inflammatory markers, including cytokine levels, by-products of oxidant damage and inflammatory cell products, e.g. neutrophil elastase, can be measured directly, but these assays are not widely available and nor are they likely to be used clinically. Based on the green colour of myeloperoxidase within the azurophilic granules of neutrophils, Stockley *et al.*[52] have shown that sputum colour graded visually reflects the underlying inflammatory activity and correlates cross-sectionally with markers of bronchial inflammation. The ability of this parameter to reflect airway inflammation longitudinally and to assess response to treatment has not been investigated. In bronchiectasis, FEV_1 is not a particularly responsive parameter, and assessment of rate of change in FEV_1 requires long-term studies.

Although it has been suggested that a management approach similar to that of CF can be used,[37] caution needs to be employed in extrapolating from CF to bronchiectasis as the diseases have different pathophysiology, different distribution in the lungs, different socio-economic influences and different responses to certain therapies. As in other chronic lung diseases, regular good-quality medical follow-up is considered to be an important component of management,[53] although there is no direct supportive evidence in bronchiectasis. A randomized controlled crossover trial[54] reported that clinics led by trained, experienced nurses were as safe and effective as doctor-led care. However, the nurse-led service used more resources and was more costly, largely because of increased admissions for infective exacerbations. Nevertheless, a multidisciplinary approach with nursing, physiotherapy, nutrition and social work expertise seems a logical but untested approach.

Airway clearance techniques

Impaired effectiveness of cough and reduced mucociliary clearance,[55] combined with excessive secretions having abnormal biorheological properties, lead to impaired clearance of respiratory secretions. This provides the rationale for airway clearance techniques being a mainstay of therapy in bronchiectasis.

Before proceeding further, a description of some of the clearance techniques is warranted. This list is not meant to be comprehensive, and it is acknowledged that there is no universal acceptance of some of these definitions, but it is included to assist the reader's understanding of this area.
- Postural drainage and chest percussion/vibration (PD/CP). During PD, the patient is positioned to facilitate gravitational drainage of secretions from the affected airways. CP is the technique of clapping the chest wall. Vibration applies to a fine shaking of the chest wall, usually during expiration. Percussion and vibration can be applied either manually or by mechanical techniques.

- Directed coughing. This technique mimics an effective spontaneous cough and may be assisted by the application of external pressure.
- Forced expiratory technique (FET). Also called 'huffing', this technique consists of one or two 'huffs' from mid- to low lung volume with the glottis open, followed by relaxed diaphragmatic breathing.
- Active cycle of breathing technique (ACBT). This incorporates relaxation/breathing control, FET, thoracic expansion exercises and may include PD/CP.
- Autogenic drainage. This is a three-level breathing sequence beginning at low lung volumes, then breathing at mid-lung volumes, followed by deep breathing and 'huffing'.
- Positive expiratory pressure (PEP). In this technique, the patient exhales against a pressure of 10–20 cm of H_2O, usually employing a full-face mask.
- Flutter. This technique uses a device that produces PEP with oscillations. The patient performs repeated forced expirations into the device.

PD/CP have been the traditional techniques, but ACBT is now widely advocated. Studies of airway clearance techniques have generally been small, of short duration, usually of crossover design with infrequent use of sham therapy, and a variety of outcome parameters have been employed. A recent Cochrane Review of randomized trials of airway clearance therapy for COPD and bronchiectasis[56] found that only two out of seven eligible trials included patients with bronchiectasis—a combined total of eight bronchiectasis subjects! Not surprisingly, the reviewers concluded that there was not enough evidence to support or refute the use of physical therapy in bronchiectasis. Hess[57] reached a similar conclusion after a systematic review of this subject. The question of which technique is most effective, tolerable and acceptable is far from clarified, as exemplified by the wide variety of physiotherapy techniques used for bronchiectasis in the UK.[58] Anecdotally, some patients find postural drainage unpleasant, particularly those with co-existent sinus or reflux disease.

The only mechanical form of airway clearance tested in bronchiectasis by means of an RCT is the 'Flutter' device.[59] The oscillating PEP generated by this apparatus is reported to prevent premature closure of airways and to loosen secretions, which may then be cleared by FET.[60] A randomized crossover study of 17 patients with stable bronchiectasis found that 4 weeks of daily use of the Flutter device was as effective as ACBT in terms of median weekly sputum production.[59] The majority of subjects expressed a preference for the Flutter device. However, there were no changes in pulmonary function or health-related quality of life (HRQL). Mechanical chest vibrators that use a pneumatic jacket to which is applied a rapid inflation–deflation cycle have not been subjected to RCTs.

Inhaled hyperosmolar agents

Hyperosmolar agents alter mucus rheology[61] and facilitate mucociliary clearance. Although all such agents induce a liquid flux on to the airway surface, non-ionic agents (such as mannitol) may disrupt the hydrogen bonds between mucins, whereas ionic agents may reduce the number of mucus polymer entanglements by shielding fixed charges along the mucin macromolecule.

Mannitol, an osmotic agent suitable for inhalation as a dry powder, increased mucociliary clearance in healthy subjects after a single administration.[62] In the only trial of inhaled hyperosmolar agents in bronchiectasis (a crossover study in 11 subjects), Daviskas et al.[63] found that a single administration of mannitol improved mucociliary clearance in the central and intermediate, but not peripheral, regions of the lungs. Although the use of dry powder mannitol may have advantages in terms of convenience compared with agents administered via ultrasonic nebulizers, use of individual capsules and the requirement for multiple actuations of the device use do have their drawbacks.

In in vitro experiments using the mucus-depleted bovine trachea, Wills et al.[64] have shown that the addition of salt altered the rheology of bronchiectatic sputum in a way that might allow more effective clearance. Single administrations of nebulized hypertonic saline (HS) improved mucociliary clearance in healthy subjects in a dose-dependent fashion,[65] but no studies in bronchiectasis have been undertaken. While mannitol may have an advantage over HS by maintaining an osmotic gradient in the airway for longer periods, trials of HS are certainly indicated as the cost of such treatment is likely to be lower than that of alternative osmotic agents.

All hyperosmolar agents have the potential to cause airway narrowing in subjects with underlying airway hyper-responsiveness (AHR). AHR is present in approximately one-third of patients with idiopathic bronchiectasis,[35,66,67] and reduced FEV_1 is the major determinant of AHR.[35] Prior treatment with inhaled β_2-agonist would seem to be a logical but unproven precaution. Questions remain as to whether these agents stimulate mucus secretion or increase the microbial load by adverse effects on cationic antibacterial peptides. Nevertheless, the use of hyperosmolar agents potentially represents the most important development in the management of bronchiectasis that has occurred in decades.

Mucolytics

Mucolysis implies the destruction of mucus, thus making it less viscous and easier to clear. Mucolytic agents target the hypersecretion and abnormal physicochemical characteristics of sputum produced by abnormal, inflamed and infected airways, with the aim of improving clearance of secretions. No RCTs of chronic treatment of stable bronchiectasis with mucolytics have been undertaken but, in view of the Cochrane Review suggesting benefit from the use of these agents in COPD,[68] such trials are certainly indicated.

DNase

In CF, the abnormal biorheological properties of sputum are

caused in part by high concentrations of DNA, mostly derived from degradation of neutrophils. *In vitro* studies have shown that recombinant human DNase (rhDNase) did not produce the same beneficial effects on the transportability of bronchiectatic sputum[69] as were demonstrated with CF sputum.[70] Nevertheless, in view of the central role of the neutrophil in airway inflammation, the prominence of purulent sputum production and the abnormal physical properties of bronchiectatic sputum,[63] trials of DNase in bronchiectasis seemed to be warranted. O'Donnell *et al.*,[71] in a large, 6-month, randomized, placebo-controlled trial, found that the group receiving rhDNase had more exacerbations and greater decrease in FEV_1 than the placebo group. Thus, contrary to the situation in CF, there is no role for the long-term use of DNase in the treatment of idiopathic bronchiectasis.

Physical training

Physical training may be defined as participation in a programme of regular rigorous physical activity designed to improve physical performance and/or cardiovascular function and/or muscle strength. A Cochrane Review[72] based on two RCTs available only in abstract form concluded that, compared with sham or no training, inspiratory muscle training over 8 weeks improved exercise capacity, respiratory muscle strength and quality of life. There was no information about effects on peripheral muscle strength and endurance, dyspnoea, sputum production or morbidity in terms of acute exacerbations, antibiotic use or hospitalization. There is no evidence on the effects of other types of physical training. The effects of a comprehensive rehabilitation programme, which includes patient education, strategies for managing breathlessness and adapting to chronic illness, stress management, relaxation techniques and nutritional advice, as well as physical training,[73] have not been investigated in stable bronchiectasis. Considering the magnitude of the benefits that accrue from pulmonary rehabilitation in COPD, systematic evaluation in stable bronchiectasis is warranted.

Long-term antibiotics

As infection, neutrophilic inflammation and their sequelae are integral to the vicious cycle of airway damage in bronchiectasis, prophylactic long-term antibiotics might have a role in reducing symptoms, improving HRQL, reducing frequency of exacerbations and inhibiting progression of disease. A double-blind, randomized, placebo-controlled trial of amoxicillin 3 mg twice daily for 32 weeks found that antibiotic use was associated with reduced sputum volume and improved symptoms but no change in the frequency of exacerbations.[74] There are no studies that address the issue of whether long-term antibiotics modify disease progression nor are there any studies of potential adverse effects of such a strategy, e.g. whether it leads to the development of microbial resistance or encourages infection by other bacteria such as PA.

For those chronically infected with PA, there are no oral antibiotics suitable for long-term use, and inhaled antibiotics are an appealing alternative because a suitable antibiotic can be delivered in high concentration directly to the site of infection, thus avoiding high systemic concentrations and reducing the risk of systemic toxicity. Orriols *et al.*,[75] in a small study of persons with bronchiectasis and chronic PA infection, found that 12 months of treatment with inhaled ceftazidime or tobramycin was associated with reduced hospital admissions but no differences in lung function, use of oral antibiotics or emergence of resistant bacteria. Lin *et al.*[76] found that nebulized gentamicin 40 mg bid for 3 days reduced the level of neutrophil enzymes in sputum, sputum production and frequency of nocturnal desaturation and improved peak expiratory flow. In an 8-week, placebo-controlled, double-blind, randomized, multicentre trial, high-dose, non-pyogenic, preservative-free, pH-adjusted tobramycin solution designed for inhalation (TOBI) was administered twice daily for 4 weeks followed by 2 weeks off drug to patients with bronchiectasis and chronic PA infection.[77] The primary efficacy endpoints were microbiological; at week 4, the density of PA had decreased in the tobramycin group and, at week 6, PA was eradicated in 35% of tobramycin patients but in none of the placebo group. However, tobramycin resistance developed in 11% in the tobramycin group (versus 3% in the placebo group), and there was no change in FEV_1. While there is some evidence that nebulized antipseudomonal therapy in 'idiopathic' bronchiectasis produces short- and medium-term improvements, longer term trials to determine the effect on the clinical course and to address safety concerns, particularly in terms of the development of microbiological resistance, are required.

Based on the immune-modulating properties of macrolide antibiotics,[78–80] their effects on PA,[81] the benefits of their use in diffuse pan-bronchiolitis[82] and preliminary evidence suggesting benefit in adult CF,[83,84] there is a clear rationale for investigating the role of these agents in bronchiectasis. Tsang *et al.*[85] reported that patients who received erythromycin (500 mg bd) plus physiotherapy in an 8-week, double-blind, placebo-controlled study had significant improvements in FEV_1 and sputum volume, but not in inflammatory cytokines, compared with the placebo group. In a double-blind, placebo-controlled, parallel group study of 25 children with bronchiectasis and AHR, the group receiving roxithromycin for 12 weeks had reduced airway responsiveness to methacholine but there was no change in FEV_1.[86] Further long-term studies of this promising therapy are required to assess both effectiveness and adverse effects. Before embarking on long-term macrolide therapy, infection by NTM needs exclusion because macrolide use may result in the NTM acquiring resistance to this class of antibiotics, thereby making eradication almost impossible.

Anti-inflammatory agents

The presence of marked airway inflammation, albeit neutrophilic rather than eosinophilic, a high prevalence of

AHR[35,66,67] and the possible beneficial effects of 'anti-inflammatory' therapies in CF[87,88] provide a rationale for investigating their use in bronchiectasis. There are no randomized trials of long-term use of oral corticosteroids in stable bronchiectasis.[89] A Cochrane Review of the role of inhaled steroids[90] could identify only two small short-duration trials[91,92] and concluded that there was insufficient evidence to recommend the widespread use of inhaled corticosteroids in bronchiectasis. Although these limited studies suggest that there may be a steroid-responsive component of the airway inflammation, larger studies of longer duration are indicated.

No RCTs of non-steroidal anti-inflammatory agents in bronchiectasis have been conducted but, considering their proven benefit of slowing the rate of decline of FEV_1 in CF[93] and preliminary evidence in bronchiectasis,[94,95] such studies would seem justified. A Cochrane Review[96] was unable to identify any RCTs of leukotriene receptor antagonists in bronchiectasis.

Bronchodilators

As airflow obstruction that may be partly reversible[97] to aerosol β_2-agonists and/or anticholinergic agents is common in bronchiectasis, and as a substantial proportion have AHR,[35,66,67] there would seem to be a rationale for long-term bronchodilator use. Certain bronchodilators may have additional beneficial effects, e.g. salmeterol reduces *P. aeruginosa*-induced epithelial damage.[98] No studies of long-term use of short-acting β_2-agonists (SABAs) in bronchiectasis have been reported. A Cochrane Review[99] was unable to identify any RCTs investigating the effectiveness of long-acting β_2-agonists (LABAs) in bronchiectasis. Cochrane Reviews on anticholinergic therapy[100] and oral methylxanthines[101] each failed to identify RCTs that met the inclusion criteria.

Long-term oxygen therapy

There are no trials of long-term oxygen therapy in bronchiectasis. Clinicians have tended to use criteria based on studies in COPD for the administration of oxygen in bronchiectasis.

Resectional surgery

Surgical resection for bronchiectasis has declined dramatically. There is general acceptance of the role of surgery for resection of local bronchiectasis distal to an obstructing lesion and for life-threatening haemorrhage from an identified site (although the need for resectional surgery for haemoptysis has reduced dramatically because of the safety and effectiveness of bronchial artery embolization[102]). However, the role of resectional surgery is less certain for limited disease in conjunction with poorly controlled bronchopulmonary suppuration, despite optimal medical therapy.

A recent Cochrane Review[103] found no randomized or controlled clinical trials of surgical versus non-surgical treatment, and thus it is not possible to provide an unbiased estimate of benefit from surgery compared with non-surgical treatment. Although improvement in symptoms even with relatively long postoperative follow-up has been reported,[104–107] some evidence[108] and the anecdotal experience of many clinicians are less favourable, with higher than usual surgical morbidity, less than expected impact on symptoms and the development of progressive bronchiectasis in sites seemingly previously unaffected. No studies have been undertaken to assess whether certain HRCT features are predictive of a suboptimal result from resectional surgery.

Lung transplantation

Evidence from the international database[107] indicates that bronchiectasis is an infrequent indication for lung transplantation; the reasons for this are not clear but are likely to be multiple and complex.

Acute exacerbations of bronchiectasis

Exacerbations of bronchiectasis are the major reason for hospitalization and contribute substantially to the morbidity and health care costs. Exacerbations are presumed to be on the basis of infection, but data on the specific organisms responsible and their relationship to those chronically infecting the airways are limited, making a logical antibiotic choice difficult. There is no evidence on the role or impact of sputum cultures and sensitivity testing. Even the identification of an exacerbation is problematic. In the largest prospective study of subjects with bronchiectasis,[71] an exacerbation was defined as four out of nine symptoms, many of which were highly subjective, such as increased wheeze, malaise/fatigue/lethargy, decreased exercise tolerance or changes in chest sounds, although others, such as change in sputum production, fever, increased dyspnoea, reduced pulmonary function or new radiographic abnormalities, tend to be those used clinically.

Although clinicians are required to manage patients with such exacerbations and do so with a combination of antibiotics, bronchodilators, airway clearance techniques and possibly nebulized hypertonic saline and systemic steroids, the evidence supporting such management is extremely limited (Table 2).

In a randomized, double-blind, placebo-controlled trial of 88 subjects with bronchiectasis, Olivieri et al.[110] compared high-dose oral bromhexine (30 mg three times per day) plus antibiotics with placebo plus antibiotics in the treatment of acute exacerbations of bronchiectasis. Bromhexine was well tolerated, and use was associated with greater improvements in 'difficulty in expectoration' sputum volume and quality and cough score, but there was no change in FEV_1. On the basis of this one trial, the widespread use of bromhexine for exacerbations of bronchiectasis cannot be recommended.

Issues for which good-quality RCTs are lacking include:
• Antibiotic choice. Ip et al.[111] reported that antibiotics effec-

Table 2. Management of exacerbations of bronchiectasis.

Beneficial
Likely to be beneficial
    Antibiotics
    Airway clearance techniques
    Bronchodilators
    Treatment of comorbid conditions
Trade-off between benefits and harm
    Systemic corticosteroids
Unknown effectiveness
    Inhaled hyperosmolar agents
    Mucolytes
Unlikely to be beneficial
    DNase
Likely to be ineffective (or harmful)

tively controlled the upsurge in inflammatory activity associated with acute exacerbations, thus providing some theoretical support for the use of these agents. In a randomized, double-blind trial in bronchiectatics with infective exacerbations, 34% of whom had PA, ciprofloxacin (500 mg bd) was reported to produce a 'better clinical response' than amoxicillin (1 mg tds), but the lack of reporting of clinically relevant outcome parameters means that relative effectiveness of these antibiotics could not be reliably assessed.[112] Appropriately designed comparative studies of antibiotic therapy in infective exacerbations have not been undertaken. Clinicians have taken the pragmatic approach to extrapolate the results of studies in COPD and community-acquired pneumonia to antibiotic choice in bronchiectasis. Although this may be appropriate, there is no evidence to support such an approach.

• Antibiotic duration. Although it is generally assumed that, in view of the underlying structural damage in bronchiectasis, a longer course of antibiotic therapy (10–14 days) is indicated, there is no supportive evidence.

• Intensification of airway clearance techniques. This is an integral component of the management of exacerbations, although no RCTs have been carried out.

• The role and effectiveness of bronchodilators (β_2-agonists, anticholinergics, methylxanthines). This has not been examined during exacerbations by means of RCTs.

• Hyperosmolar agents. The use of neither nebulized HS nor inhaled mannitol in exacerbations has been studied.

• DNase. Given the lack of response to DNase in stable bronchiectasis, and the lack of efficacy in exacerbations of CF, it would seem unlikely that DNase will have an important role.

• Systemic steroids. These are not infrequently used, and clinical experience suggests that there is often a steroid-responsive component to the airway inflammation during exacerbations, but no clinical trials have been undertaken.[89]

• Treatment of co-existent conditions such as gastro-oesophageal reflux and rhinosinusitis. This seems to be self-evident and is unlikely ever to be subjected to an RCT.

Conclusions

Despite the morbidity and mortality associated with this condition, there is a common theme running through this chapter; namely that, for virtually all aspects of management of bronchiectasis, both chronic and acute, there is a lack of evidence. There is the need for well-designed, adequately powered studies of sufficient duration using valid and clinically relevant outcome parameters to address most aspects of the assessment and treatment of this condition. However, the possibilities of exciting new therapies and the resurgence of research interest in this condition are reasons for optimism.

Summary

• Bronchiectasis remains an important cause of morbidity and mortality worldwide, especially in developing countries and in indigenous populations.
• It is likely to be underdiagnosed and undertreated in 'developed' countries.
• There is limited knowledge of the aetiology, pathophysiology and epidemiology of this condition.
• The evidence for most aspects of management of this condition is limited, and few of the treatment strategies are based on evidence from RCTs.
• There is the need for well-designed, adequately powered studies of sufficient duration using valid and clinically relevant outcome parameters to address most aspects of the assessment and treatment of this condition.
• The possibilities of exciting new therapies and the resurgence of research interest in this condition are reasons for optimism.

Acknowledgements

The author would like to thank Drs Tam Eaton and Adrian Harrison for their constructive input and Ms Michelle Ryan and Barbara Semb for preparation of the manuscript.

References

1 Lapa de Silva JR, Jones JAH, Cole PJ, Poulter LW. The immunological component of the cellular inflammatory infiltrate in bronchiectasis. *Thorax* 1989; **44**:668–73.

2 Cole P. Bronchiectasis. In: Brewis RAL, Corrin B, Geddes DM, Gibson GJ, eds. *Respiratory Medicine*. 2nd edn. Saunders, 1995:1289–93.

3 Becroft DMO. Histopathology of fatal adenovirus infection of the respiratory tract in young children. *J Clin Pathol* 1967: **20**: 561–9.

4 Becroft DMO. Bronchiolitis obliterans, bronchiectasis and other sequelae of adenovirus type 21 infection in young children. *J Clin Pathol* 1971; **24**:72–82.

5 Whyte KF, Williams GR. Bronchiectasis after mycoplasma pneumonia. *Thorax* 1984; **39**:390–1.

6 Whitwell F. A study of the pathology and pathogenesis of bronchiectasis. *Thorax* 1952; **7**:213–39.

7 Reiff DB, Wells AU, Carr DH, Cole PJ, Hansell DM. CT findings in bronchiectasis: value in distinguishing between idiopathic and specific types. *AJR* 1995; **165**:261–7.

8 Kolbe J, Wells AU. Bronchiectasis: a neglected cause of respiratory morbidity and mortality. *Respirology* 1996; **1**:221–5.

9 Wakefield St J, Waite D. Abnormal cilia in Polynesians with bronchiectasis. *Am Rev Respir Res* 1980; **121**:1003–9.

10 Barker AF. Medical progress: bronchiectasis. *N Engl J Med* 2002; **346**:1383–93.

11 O'Brien C, Guest PJ, Hill SJ, Stockley RA. Physiological and radiological characterisation of patients diagnosed with chronic obstructive pulmonary disease in primary care. *Thorax* 2000; **55**:635–42.

12 Nath AR, Capel LH. Lung crackles in bronchiectasis. *Thorax* 1980; **35**:694–9.

13 Currie DC, Cooke JC, Morgan DA *et al*. Interpretation of bronchograms and chest radiographs in patients with chronic sputum production. *Thorax* 1987; **42**:278–84.

14 Grenier P, Maurice F, Mussel D *et al*. Bronchiectasis: assessment by thin section CT. *Radiology* 1986; **161**:95–9.

15 Joharjy JA, Bashi SA, Abdullah AK. Value of medium thickness CT in the diagnosis of bronchiectasis. *AJR* 1987; **149**:113–17.

16 Roberts HR, Wells AU, Milne DG *et al*. Airflow obstruction in bronchiectasis: correlation between computed tomography features and pulmonary function tests. *Thorax* 2000; **55**:198–204.

17 Remy-Jardin M, Remy J, Cortet B, Mauri F, Delcambre B. Lung changes in rheumatoid arthritis: CT findings. *Radiology* 1994; **193**:375–82.

18 Carter B, Perez T, Roux N *et al*. Pulmonary function tests and high resolution computed tomography of the lungs in patients with rheumatoid arthritis. *Ann Rheum Dis* 1997; **56**:596–600.

19 Kraft SC, Earle RH, Roesler M *et al*. Unexplained bronchopulmonary disease with inflammatory bowel disease. *Arch Intern Med* 1976; **136**:454–9.

20 Butland RJ, Cole P, Citron KM, Turner-Warwick M. Chronic bronchial suppuration and inflammatory bowel disease. *Q J Med* 1981; **197**:63–75.

21 Eaton TE, Lambie N, Wells AU. Bronchiectasis following colectomy for Crohn's disease. *Thorax* 1998; **53**:529–31.

22 Mahadeva R, Flower C, Shneerson J. Bronchiectasis in association with coeliac disease. *Thorax* 1998; **53**:527–9.

23 Haeney M. Intravenous immune globulin in primary immunodeficiency. *Clin Exp Immunol* 1994; **97**(Suppl):11–15.

24 Skull S, Kemp A. Treatment of hypogammaglobulinaemia with intravenous immunoglobulin. *Arch Dis Child* 1996; **74**:527–30.

25 Hill SL, Mitchell JL, Burnett D, Stockley RA. IgG subclasses in the serum and sputum from patients with bronchiectasis. *Thorax* 1998; **53**:463–8.

26 Eaton T, Garrett J, Milne D, Frankel A, Wells AU. Allergic bronchopulmonary aspergillosis in the asthma clinic. A prospective evaluation of CT in the diagnostic algorithm. *Chest* 2000; **118**:66–72.

27 Gervais R, Lafitte J-J, Dunmur V *et al*. Sweat chloride and ØF508 mutation in chronic bronchitis or bronchiectasis. *Lancet* 1993; **342**:997.

28 Giroden E, Cazeneune C, Lebargy F *et al*. CFTR gene mutations in adults with disseminated bronchiectasis. *Eur J Hum Genet* 1997; **5**:149–55.

29 King PT, Forshaw K, Du Sart D, Freezer NJ, Holmes PJ, Holdsworth SR. Prevalence of cystic fibrosis mutations in adult bronchiectasis. *Am J Respir Crit Care Med* 2003; **167**:A994.

30 Penketh ARL, Wise A, Mearns MB *et al*. Cystic fibrosis in adolescents and adults. *Thorax* 1987: **42**:912–30.

31 Gan K, Guess WP, Bakker W *et al*. Genetic and clinical features of patients diagnosed with cystic fibrosis after the age of 16 years. *Thorax* 1995; **50**:1301–4.

32 Kharitonov S, Wells AU, O'Connor B *et al*. Elevated levels of exhaled nitric oxide in bronchiectasis. *Am J Respir Crit Care Med* 1995; **151**:1889–93.

33 Ho LP, Innes JA, Greening AP. Exhaled nitric oxide is not elevated in the inflammatory airways diseases of cystic fibrosis and bronchiectasis. *Eur Respir J* 1998; **12**:1290–4.

34 Tsang KW, Leung R, Fung PC *et al*. Exhaled and sputum nitric oxide in bronchiectasis. Correlation with clinical parameters. *Chest* 2002; **121**:88–94.

35 Moody A, Fergusson W, Wells A, Milne D, Kolbe J. Prevalence of airway hyperresponsiveness and predictors of responsiveness in idiopathic bronchiectasis. *Respiratory* 2002; **7**:A35.

36 Horvath I, Loukides S, Wodehouse T *et al*. Comparison of exhaled and nasal nitric oxide and exhaled carbon monoxide levels in bronchiectatic patients with and without primary ciliary dyskinesia. *Thorax* 2003; **58**:68–72.

37 Chang AB, Grimwood K, Mulholland EK, Torzillo PJ, for the Working Group on Indigenous Pediatric Respiratory Health. Bronchiectasis in indigenous children in remote Australian communities. *Med J Aust* 2002; **177**:200–4.

38 King PT, Freezer NJ, Holdsworth SR, Holmes PW. Long-term prospective study of outcome in adult bronchiectasis. *Am J Respir Crit Care Med* 2003; **167**:A223.

39 Pujana I, Gallego L, Martin G, Lopez F, Conduela J, Cisterna R. Epidemiological analysis of sequential *Pseudomonas aeruginosa* isolates from bronchiectasis patients without cystic fibrosis. *J Clin Microbiol* 1999; **37**:2071–3.

40 Wilson CB, Jones PW, O'Leary CJ, Hansell DM, Cole PJ, Wilson R. Effect of spectrum of bacteriology on the quality of life to patients with bronchiectasis. *Eur Respir J* 1997; **10**:1754–60.

41 Mishiel KA, Wells AU, Rubens MB, Cole PJ, Hansell DM. Effects of airway infection by *Pseudomonas aeruginosa*: a computed tomography study. *Thorax* 1997; **52**:260–4.

42 Evans SA, Turner SM, Bosch BJ, Hardy CC, Woodhead MA. Lung function in bronchiectasis the influence of *Pseudomonas aeruginosa*. *Eur Respir J* 1996; **9**:1601–4.

43 Amitani R, Wilson R, Rutman A *et al*. Effects of human neutrophil elastase and *Pseudomonas aeruginosa* proteinases on human respiratory epithelium. *Am J Respir Cell Mol Biol* 1991; **4**:26–32.

44 Tsang KWT, Rutman A, Tanaka A *et al*. Interaction of *Pseudomonas aeruginosa* with human respiratory mucosa *in vitro*. *Eur Respir J* 1994; **7**:1746–53.

45 Swensen SJ, Hartman TE, Williams DE. Computed tomographic diagnosis of *Mycobacterium avium–intracellulare* complex in patients with bronchiectasis. *Chest* 1994; **105**:49–52.

46 Wallace RJ Jr, Glassroth J, Griffith DE, Olivier KN, Cooke JL, Gordin F. Diagnosis and treatment of disease caused by non-tuberculous mycobacteria. *Am J Respir Crit Care Med* 1997; **156**(Suppl):S1–S25.

47 Chan CH, Ho AK, Chan RC, Cheung H, Cheng AF. Mycobacteria as a cause of infective exacerbation in bronchiectasis. *Postgrad Med J* 1992; **68**:896–9.

48 Redelmeier DA, Bayoumi AM, Goldstein RS, Guyatt GH. Interpreting small differences in functional status: the six minute walk test in chronic lung disease patients. *Am J Respir Crit Care Med* 1997; **155**:1278–82.

49 Singh SL, Morgan MDL, Scott S, Walters D, Hardman AE. Development of a shuttle walking test of disability in patients with chronic airways obstruction. *Thorax* 1992; **47**:1019–24.

50 Wilson CB, Jones PW, O'Leary CJ, Cole PJ, Wilson R. Validation of the St George's Respiratory Questionnaire in bronchiectasis. *Am J Respir Crit Care Med* 1997; **156**:536–41.

51 Angill J, Agusti C, De Celis R *et al*. Bronchial inflammation and colonisation in patients with clinically stable bronchiectasis. *Am J Respir Crit Care Med* 2001; **164**:1628–32.

52 Stockley RA, Bayley D, Hill SL, Hill AT, Croaks S, Campbell EJ. Assessment of airway neutrophils by sputum colour: correlation with airway inflammation. *Thorax* 2001; **56**:366–72.

53 Kolbe J. Psychosocial influences on adherence to self-management plans. *Dis Man Health Outcomes* 2002; **10**:551–70.

54 Sharples LD, Edmunds J, Bilton D *et al*. A randomised controlled cross-over trial of nurse practitioner versus doctor led outpatient care in a bronchiectasis clinic. *Thorax* 2002; **57**:661–6.

55 Currie DC, Pavia D, Agnew JE *et al*. Impaired tracheobronchial clearance in bronchiectasis. *Thorax* 1987; **42**:126–30.

56 Jones AP, Rowe BH. Bronchopulmonary hygiene physical therapy for chronic obstructive pulmonary disease and bronchiectasis (Cochrane Review). In: *The Cochrane Library*, Issue 1. Oxford, Update Software, 2003.

57 Hess DR. The evidence for secretion clearance techniques. *Respir Care* 2001; **46**:1276–93.

58 O'Neill B, Bradley JM, McArdle N, MacMahon J. The current physiotherapy management of patients with bronchiectasis: a UK survey. *Int J Clin Pract* 2002; **56**:34–5.

59 Thompson CS, Harrison S, Ashley J, Day K, Smith DL. Randomised cross-over study of the Flutter device and the active cycle of breathing technique and non-cystic fibrosis bronchiectasis. *Thorax* 2002; **57**:446–8.

60 Girard JP, Terki N. The Flutter VRP1: a new personal pocket therapeutic device used as an adjunct to drug therapy in the management of bronchial asthma. *J Invest Allergol Clin Immunol* 1994; **4**:23–7.

61 King M. Mucoactive therapy: what the future holds for patients with cystic fibrosis. *Pediatr Pulmol* 1997; **24**:122–3.

62 Daviskas E, Anderson SD, Brannan JD, Chan HK, Eberl S, Bautovich G. Inhalation of dry powder mannitol increases muco-ciliary clearance. *Eur Respir J* 1997; **10**:2449–54.

63 Daviskas E, Anderson SD, Eberl S, Chan H-K, Bautovich G. Inhalation of dry power mannitol improves clearance of mucus in patients with bronchiectasis. *Am J Respir Crit Care Med* 1999; **159**:1843–8.

64 Wills P, Hall R, Chan W-M, Cole PJ. Sodium chloride increases the ciliary transportability of cystic fibrosis and bronchiectasis sputum on the mucus-depleted bovine trachea. *J Clin Invest* 1997; **99**:9–13.

65 Daviskas E, Anderson SD, Jonda I *et al*. Inhalation of hypertonic saline enhances muco-ciliary clearance in asthmatic and healthy subjects. *Eur Respir J* 1996; **9**:725–32.

66 Bahous J, Carter A, Pincau L *et al*. Pulmonary function tests and airway responsiveness to methacholine in chronic bronchiectasis of the adult. *Bull Eur Physiopathol Respir* 1984; **20**:375–80.

67 Pong J, Chan HS, Sung JY. Prevalence of asthma, atopy and bronchial hyperreactivity in bronchiectasis: a controlled study. *Thorax* 1989; **44**:948–51.

68 Poole PJ, Black, PN. Mucolytic agents for chronic bronchitis [systematic review]. *Cochrane Airways Group Cochrane Database Syst Rev* 2003; **1**.

69 Wills PJ, Wodehouse T, Corkery K, Mallon K. Short term recombinant human DN'ase in bronchiectasis. *Am J Respir Crit Care Med* 1996; **154**:413–17.

70 Shah S, Capon DJ, Hellmiss R, Marsters SA, Baker CL. Recombinant human DNase I reduces the viscosity of cystic fibrosis sputum. *Proc Natl Acad Sci USA* 1990; **87**:9188–92.

71 O'Donnell AE, Barker AF, Ilowite JS, Fick RB. Treatment of idiopathic bronchiectasis with aerosolised recombinant human DN'ase I. *Chest* 1998; **113**:1329–34.

72 Bradley J, Moran F, Greenstone M. Physical training for bronchiectasis (Cochrane Review). In: *The Cochrane Library*, Issue 1. Oxford, Update Software, 2003.

73 Young P, Fergusson W, Drewse M, Kolbe J. Improvements in outcomes for chronic obstructive pulmonary disease attributable to a hospital-based respiratory rehabilitation programme. *Aust NZ J Med* 1999; **29**:59–65.

74 Currie DC, Garbett ND, Chan KL *et al*. Double-blind randomized study of prolonged higher-dose oral amoxycillin in purulent bronchiectasis. *Q J Med* 1990; **76**:799–816.

75 Orriols R, Roig J, Ferrer J *et al*. Inhaled antibiotic therapy in non-cystic fibrosis patients with bronchiectasis and chronic bronchial infection by *Pseudomonas aeruginosa*. *Respir Med* 1999; **93**:476–80.

76 Lin HC, Chen HF, Wong CH, Liu CY, Yu CT, Kuo HP. Inhaled gentamicin reduces airway neutrophil activity and mucus hypersecretion in bronchiectasis. *Am J Respir Crit Care Med* 1997; **155**:2024–9.

77 Barker AF, Cough L, Fiel SB *et al*. Tobramycin solution for inhalation reduces sputum *Pseudomonas aeruginosa* density in bronchiectasis. *Am J Respir Crit Care Med* 2000; **162**:481–5.

78 Jaffe A, Bush A. Anti-inflammatory effects of macrolides in lung disease. *Pediatr Pulmon* 2001; **31**:464–73.

79 Takizawa H, Desaki M, Ohtashi T *et al*. Erythromycin modulates IL-8 expression in normal and inflamed human bronchial epithelial cells. *Am J Respir Crit Care Med* 1997; **156**:266–71.

80 Khan AA, Slifer TR, Araujo FG *et al*. Effect of clarithromycin and azithromycin on production of cytokines by human monocytes. *Int J Antimicrob Agents* 1999; **11**:121–32.

81 Wozniak DJ, Kayser R. Effects of subinhibitory concentrations of macrolide antibiotics on *Pseudomonas aeruginosa*. *Chest* 2004; **125**:625–69.

82 Hoiby H. Diffuse panbronchiolitis and cystic fibrosis: East meets West. *Thorax* 1994; **49**:531–2.

83 Wolter J, Seeney S, Bell S, Bowler S, Mosel P, McCormack J. Effect of long term treatment with azithromycin on disease parameters in cystic fibrosis: a randomised trial. *Thorax* 2002; **57**:212–16.

84 Equi A, Balfour-Lynn IM, Bush A, Rosethal M. Long term azithromycin in children with cystic fibrosis: a randomised, placebo-controlled, crossover trial. *Lancet* 2002; **360**:978–84.

85 Tsang KW, Ho P-I, Chen K-N *et al*. A pilot study of low-dose erythromycin in bronchiectasis. *Eur Respir J* 1999; **13**:361–4.

86 Koh YY, Lee MH, Sun YH, Sung KW, Chae JH. Effect of roxithromycin on airway responsiveness in children with bronchiectasis: a double-blind, placebo-controlled study. *Eur Respir J* 1997; **10**:994–9.

87 Auerbach HS, Williams M, Kilpatrick JA, Colten HR. Alternate-day prednisone reduces morbidity and improves pulmonary function in cystic fibrosis. *Lancet* 1985; **2**:686–8.

88 Eigen H, Rosenstein BJ, Fitzsimmons S, Schidlow DV and the Cystic Fibrosis Foundation Prednisone Trial Group. A multicentre study of alternate-day prednisone therapy in patients with cystic fibrosis. *J Pediatr* 1995; **126**:515–23.

89 Lasserton T, Holt K, Greenstone M. Oral steroids for bronchiectasis (stable and acute exacerbations) (Cochrane Review). In: *The Cochrane Library*, Issue 1. Oxford, Update Software, 2003.

90 Kolbe J, Wells A, Ram FSF. Inhaled steroids for bronchiectasis (Cochrane Review). In: *The Cochrane Library*, Issue 1. Oxford, Update Software, 2003.

91 Elborn JS, Johnston B, Allen F, Clarke J, McGarry J, Varghere G. Inhaled steroids in patients with bronchiectasis. *Respir Med* 1992; **86**:121–4.

92 Tsang KW, Ho P, Lam W *et al*. Inhaled fluticasone reduces sputum inflammatory indices in severe bronchiectasis. *Am J Respir Crit Care Med* 1998; **158**:723–7.

93 Konstan MW, Byard PJ, Happel CL, Davies PB. Effect of high-dose ibuprofen in patients with cystic fibrosis. *N Engl J Med* 1995; **332**:848–54.

94 Tamachi J, Chiyotani A, Kobayashi K, Sakai N, Kanemura T, Takizama T. Effect of indomethacin on bronchorrhoea in patients with chronic bronchitis, diffuse panbronchiolitis or bronchiectasis. *Am Rev Respir Dis* 1992; **145**:548–52.

95 Llewellyn-Jones CG, Johnson MM, Mitchell JL *et al. In vivo* study of indomethacin in bronchiectasis: effect on neutrophil function and lung secretion. *Eur Respir J* 1995; **8**:1479–87.

96 Corless JA, Warburton CJ. Leukotriene receptor antagonists for non-cystic fibrosis bronchiectasis (Cochrane Review). In: *The Cochrane Library*, Issue 1. Oxford, Update Software, 2003.

97 Hassan JA, Saadiah S, Roslan H, Zainudin BM. Bronchodilator response to inhaled β$_2$ agonist and anticholinergic drugs in patients with bronchiectasis. *Respirology* 1999; **4**:423–6.

98 Dowling RB, Rayner CFJ, Rutman A *et al.* Effect of salmeterol on *Pseudomonas aeruginosa* infection in respiratory mucosa. *Am J Respir Crit Care Med* 1997; **155**:326–36.

99 Sheikh A, Nolan D, Greenstone K. Long-acting β$_2$ agonists for bronchiectasis (Cochrane Review). In: *The Cochrane Library*, Issue 1. Oxford, Update Software, 2003.

100 Lasserton T, Holt K, Evans D, Greenstone M. Anticholinergic therapy for bronchiectasis (Cochrane Review). In: *The Cochrane Library*, Issue 1. Oxford, Update Software, 2003.

101 Steele K, Lasserson JA, Greenstone M. Oral methyl-xanthines for bronchiectasis (Cochrane Review). In: *The Cochrane Library*, Issue 1. Oxford, Update Software, 2003.

102 Yoon W, Kim JK, Kim YH, Chung TW, Kang HK. Bronchial and non-bronchial systemic artery embolization for life-threatening haemoptysis: a comprehensive review. *Radiographics* 2002; **22**:1395–409.

103 Corless JA, Warburton CJ. Surgery versus non-surgical treatment for bronchiectasis (Cochrane Review). In: *The Cochrane Library*, Issue 1. Oxford, Update Software, 2003.

104 Agasthian T, Deschamps C, Trostek VF, Allen MS, Pairolero PC. Surgical management of bronchiectasis. *Am Thorac Surg* 1996; **62**:976–80.

105 Arhour M, Al-Kattan K, Ropay MA, Saja KF, Hajjar W, Al-Frayi AR. Current surgical therapy for bronchiectasis. *World J Surg* 1999; **23**:1096–104.

106 Fujimoto T, Hillejan L, Stamatis G. Current strategy for surgical management of bronchiectasis. *Am Thorac Surg* 2001; **72**:1711–15.

107 Mazieres J, Murris M, Didier A *et al.* Limited operation for severe multi-segmental bilateral bronchiectasis. *Am Thorac Surg* 2003; **75**:382–7.

108 Annest JS, Kratz JM, Crawford FA. Current results of treatment of bronchiectasis. *J Thorac Cardiovasc Surg* 1982; **83**:546–50.

109 Hosenpud JD, Bennett LE, Keck BM, Boueck MM, Novick RJ. The registry of the International Society for Heart and Lung Transplantation: seventeenth official report—2000. *J Heart Lung Transplant* 2000; **19**:909–31.

110 Olivieri D, Ciaccia A, Marangio E, Marisco S, Todisco T, Del Vita M. Role of bromhexine in exacerbations of bronchiectasis. *Respiration* 1991; **58**:117–121.

111 Ip M, Shum D, Lauder I, Lam WK, So SY. Effect of antibiotics on sputum inflammatory contents in acute exacerbations of bronchiectasis. *Respir Med* 1993; **87**:449–54.

112 Chan TH, Ho SS, Lai CK *et al.* Comparison of oral ciprofloxacin and amoxycillin in treating infective exacerbations of bronchiectasis in Hong Kong. *Chemotherapy* 1996; **42**:150–6.

CHAPTER 4.6

Adult cystic fibrosis

John Kolbe

Introduction

Cystic fibrosis (CF) is the commonest fatal autosomal-recessive disease among Caucasians. It is a multisystem disease affecting children and, increasingly so, adults, such that CF is now an important cause of morbidity and mortality from a chronic lung disease in young adults. It is therefore appropriate that a section of a book on adult respiratory medicine should be devoted to this subject. Recent advances in CF research have not only had implications for the management of CF, but have substantially increased our understanding of respiratory disease generally. Therefore, the importance and relevance of this condition to respiratory medicine and science is much greater than the number of clinical cases might suggest.

CF is an autosomal-recessive disease due to mutations of the CF gene, which resides on the long arm of chromosome 7. The CF gene spans approximately 250 kb of DNA, contains 27 exons and encodes 180 kDa of transmembrane glycoprotein—cystic fibrosis transmembrane conductance regulator (CFTR).[1] CFTR acts as a phosphorylation-regulated, chloride channel but has other functions including the regulation of other ion channels and possibly exocytotic and endocytotic events. In the airways, CFTR is located in the apical cell membrane of respiratory epithelial and glandular acinar (and ductal) cells. CFTR is also functionally important in the paranasal sinuses, salivary glands, apocrine sweat glands, small intestine, pancreas, biliary system, uterine cervix and Wolffian duct structures, all of which may be clinically involved in CF.

The most common mutation is designated ØF508 to indicate a 3-bp deletion that results in the loss of phenylalanine at the 508 position in the functional, ATP-binding region of the protein. ØF508 is responsible for up to 80% of mutations in CF patients, although the frequency varies in different ethnic groups. Most of the clinically significant mutations result in the mutated CFTR being abnormally folded or processed and thus not reaching either the Golgi apparatus or the apical cell membrane. Some other mutations result in dysfunctional CFTR reaching the plasma membrane where it is refractory to regulatory influences or exhibits conduction abnormalities. A large number (over 900) of other 'mutations'

have been identified, but many do not cause the CF phenotype.

While genotypic variation provides some rationale for the different phenotypes of CF, there is substantial overlap between genotypes, and there is also considerable variation between patients belonging to the same genotypic group. The genotype–phenotype correlations appear to be highest for pancreatic exocrine disease (e.g. homozygosity for the ØF508 mutation almost always confers pancreatic insufficiency) and much lower for pulmonary disease.[2,3] Certain mutations are associated with a milder phenotype such as retention of pancreatic exocrine function and milder lung disease.[4–6] The substantial clinical variation within a single genotype may be due to postnatal environmental influences,[7] differences in CFTR splicing or so-called 'modifier' genes,[8–10] genes other than those coding for CFTR that may modify the clinical course. The 5T variant in the intron 8 polythymidine tract (IV5 805T) has been shown to downregulate CFTR expression,[11] and interactions with other polymorphisms in the CFTR gene may explain some of the variability of associated phenotypes.

Epidemiology

CF mutations are most prevalent in northern and central Europeans and their descendants, with a gene frequency of about 1 in 25 and consistent with an observed frequency of disease of about 1 in 2500 live births. CF is rare in native Americans, Asians, Polynesians and Africans. Heterozygotes have no stigmata of CF, but an excess prevalence of CF mutations has been reported in association with bronchiectasis[12,13] and chronic pancreatitis.[14]

Previously, CF was regarded solely as a disease of childhood, but the situation has changed quite dramatically in recent decades. The greater than 70% mortality rate of CF babies under 1 year of age observed in 1938[15] contrasts markedly with a median life expectancy of 40 years for British CF children born in 1990.[16] In 1978, the median age at death was 24 years and is now 32 years.[17] Nevertheless, the clinical course of this disease is highly variable. Far from being entirely a paediatric condition, CF patients are now surviving to attend adolescent and adult clinics—from 1969 to 1990, the proportion of CF adults increased fourfold.[18] In many centres, the number of adult patients equals or exceeds the number attending paediatric clinics.

While some of the improved survival may be due to diagnosis of milder forms of the disease, there is a consensus that improved management has also contributed to better survival. Although CF is a multisystem disease, respiratory complications are the major cause of morbidity and mortality. Exacerbations of respiratory disease are the major reason for hospital admissions and the major contributor to health care costs, while more than 90% of CF patients die of their lung disease.[16,18] The degree of pulmonary impairment is the major determinant of survival—a forced expiratory volume in 1 second (FEV_1) less than 30% predicted indicated a 2-year mortality rate of around 50%. The relative risk of death was 2.0 [95% confidence interval (CI) 1.9–202] for each 10% decrement in predicted FEV_1. On average, FEV_1 declines in CF by about 2% per year, but this decline tends to occur in a stepwise fashion.[19] Infection by *Pseudomonas aeruginosa* (PA) or *Burkholderia cepacia*, the development of pneumothorax or massive haemoptysis are regarded as indicators of a poorer prognosis.[3] The better survival of males compared with females is a well-recognized but unexplained phenomenon. Others have found that body wasting (% ideal body weight) was also an independent predictor of mortality.[20] In the USA, Medicaid status (used as a proxy for low socio-economic status) was associated with an adjusted risk of death 3.65 times higher than for those not receiving Medicaid,[7] indicating that adverse environmental factors impact on outcome in CF. Age at diagnosis has not been demonstrated as a clear determinant of outcome.

Survival benefits in CF need to be matched by reasonable levels of psychosocial adjustment and quality of life. While some adults adjust well, complete their education/training, establish careers and engage in long-term relationships, this is not always the case, and a significant proportion of adult CF patients have a variety of serious and debilitating psychosocial problems. However, Blair *et al.*[21] found that, in spite of their illness, most adolescents and young adults still living in the parental home were in 'robust psychological health' and differed only from their peers in that they were less likely to be in employment. While mothers of CF patients were more likely to be emotionally distressed, on the whole, families of CF patients functioned at a healthy adaptive level.

Pathogenesis

CF is a disease that effects the epithelial lining of various organs, and the physiological consequences of CF mutations are dependent on the normal function of CFTR in the individual organs, e.g. salt-absorbing, volume-absorbing or volume-secreting functions. In airways, it is not clear whether the major pathophysiological impact occurs in the airway epithelial cells or in glandular elements (although the latter are not present in bronchioles where initial pathological abnormalities seem to occur). CF airway epithelial cells demonstrate abnormal apical membrane-conductive chloride permeability and increased Na^+-dependent volume absorption. Abnormal CFTR function leads to abnormalities in the volume (isotonic volume depletion theory[22]) and/or ion concentration of airway surface lining fluid (hypotonic salt hypothesis[23]). The former theory postulates that the isotonic absorption of water from the apical cell membrane leads to depletion of the volume of airway surface (periciliary) liquid, 'dehydration' of the mucus layer, impaired mucus clearance by cough and ciliary mechanisms, airway obstruction and predisposition to bacterial colonization. The latter theory proposes that the pathogenesis of the lung disease is primarily due to the deactivation of cationic antibacterial peptides, such as B defensins, by the less hypotonic fluid, thus promoting bacterial colonization. Whatever the mechanism, the result is obstruction, infection and inflammation of small airways.

A vicious cycle of inflammation and infection of the airways is associated with the recruitment of large numbers of neutrophils. The lungs are normal at birth, although careful morphometric studies have demonstrated dilation of submucosal gland acinar and ductal lumens. Studies based on bronchoalveolar lavage of infants have demonstrated that airway inflammation is present at a very young age and in association with clinically mild disease.[24] Such inflammation appears to follow respiratory infections, which may be asymptomatic.[25] Dakin *et al.*[26] have shown that the presence of bacteria in bronchoalveolar lavage fluid of infants was associated with a marked increase in the number of inflammatory cells and in the levels of interleukin (IL)-8. There is no evidence of defective humoral or cellular immune responses in CF. On the contrary, there is evidence that the inflammatory response to any degree of stimulation is exaggerated in CF; the magnitude of neutrophil influx in the airways, normalized to bacterial counts, was greater in CF than in non-CF persons.[27] Neutrophil (and bacterial) elastases overwhelm antiproteases, stimulate the complement cascade, interfere with cilial function, stimulate mucus secretion and contribute directly to the destruction of structural components of airway walls. Increased levels of a wide variety of inflammatory mediators including leukotrienes, complement products, tumour necrosis factor (TNF)-α and IL-1β along with neutrophil products such as elastase and cathepsin G have been reported in CF. There is also compelling evidence of oxidant damage, via the production of hypochlorous acid.[28] Even those who are clinically stable and those with mild disease have large numbers of bacteria within their lower airways, accompanied by neutrophil influx and uninhibited elastase activity.

Respiratory disease in CF can be regarded as a form of progressive bronchiectasis, bronchiolectasis and obliterative bronchiolitis, along with peribronchiolar and peribronchial fibrosis. The distribution of disease differs from that of 'idiopathic' bronchiectasis being more severe in the upper rather than the lower lobes. The disease is characterized by abnormally viscid purulent secretions, chronic infection especially by *Staphylococcus aureus* and PA, recurrent 'infective' exacerbations, progressive damage to airways and parenchyma, worsening airflow obstruction, leading eventually to respiratory failure and death. This lung disease can be viewed as having a number of components, which may (artificially) be separately managed, viz. the fundamental underlying defect, retention of secretions, infection, inflammation and airflow obstruction (see section on Treatment).

The course of CF lung disease may be punctuated by the development of complications such as pneumothorax or haemoptysis, the development of other associated conditions, such as allergic bronchopulmonary aspergillosis (ABPA), and the acquisition of highly drug-resistant bacteria such as *Stenotrophomonas maltophilia* and *B. cepacia* or unusual infections such as by non-tuberculous mycobacteria mainly *Mycobacterium avium-intracellulare* (MAIC).[29] The risk of pneumothorax increases with age, and up to 20% of CF adults have at least one pneumothorax.[30] Recurrent episodes are common. Detection of a pneumothorax can be difficult on clinical grounds, and symptoms may be erroneously attributed to a CF exacerbation. Moderate or large pneumothoraces almost always require intercostal tube drainage and, if surgical pleurodesis is required, the fact that the patient may be a future lung transplant candidate needs to be taken into account. The risk of haemoptysis increases with age, is more common in those with coagulation abnormalities associated with biliary cirrhosis or hypersplenism, often occurs in association with an exacerbation and may be massive. Bleeding is generally from anastomoses between hypertrophied bronchial arteries and branches of the pulmonary artery. It may arise from any lobe and can be difficult to localize even at bronchoscopy. Bronchial artery embolization is now an effective and safe treatment for large or recurrent bleeds.[31,32] ABPA is reported to occur in 1–10% of CF adults,[33] but this is a probable underestimate as a much higher proportion have positive serology, and the diagnosis of ABPA is problematic in CF, although diagnostic criteria have been suggested.[34] Culture of *B. cepacia* has relevance because of its resistance to many antibiotics, the propensity for person-to-person spread and the poor outcome of some patients temporally associated with acquisition of *B. cepacia*. Infection by this organism is regarded as an indication for segregation of the patient in some clinics[35] and may preclude attendance at CF meetings. Acquisition has been linked to a rapid decline in lung function and death in some patients ('cepacia syndrome').[36] However, not all *B. cepacia* are equal; they can be divided into different genetic groups called genomovars. Genomovars II and III have been associated with the 'cepacia syndrome', and genomovar III includes the highly transmissible strain that may be linked to expression of the cable pilus.[37] Infection by non-tuberculous mycobacteria, particularly MAIC, is increasing (and is found in up to 20%), although the role it plays in the cycle of inflammation and damage remains unclear.[29] Single culture-positive, smear-negative sputum specimens for MAIC are of uncertain clinical

importance, and the American Thoracic Society criteria for diagnosis of disease and indications for treatment[38] are not necessarily applicable in the context of CF lung disease. There is no evidence that provides guidance as to which CF patients would benefit most from antimycobacterial therapy. *Mycobacterium tuberculosis* is found occasionally, the diagnosis often being delayed as a result of clinical and radiological features being attributed to the CF.

Chronic PA infection, which is a feature of CF lung disease, has an important role in the epithelial surface damage, neutrophil recruitment and progressive airway damage, and adversely influences prognosis. The abnormal composition of airway secretions is generally regarded as the most important host factor that predisposes to PA infection by interfering with phagocytosis by macrophages and neutrophils and, possibly, by adversely affecting the action of anti-microbial peptides that are sensitive to osmolality. CFTR mutations may increase PA adherence to airway epithelial cells, as intracellular retention of CFTR R domains leads to alterations in the degree of sialylation of epithelial cell glycolipids and thus allows the binding of PA via bacterial pili. The CFTR protein also serves as a receptor for epithelial cell internalization of PA, which is a critical factor in the innate clearing of this organism. Thus, the abnormality in CF is specific for chronic PA infection, explaining the high prevalence in this condition.

Longitudinal studies of CF patients have shown that most harbour the same *P. aeruginosa* isolate for many years,[39,40] but additional strains can be acquired over time. PA strains found early in infection resemble those from the environment, being relatively susceptible to antibiotics and possessing a colonial non-mucoid appearance. An important feature of PA is the tendency of this microbe to change within months to years to an antibiotic-resistant, mucoid phenotype as a result of the production of a polysaccharide known as both alginate and mucoid exopolysaccharide. Once a particular clone has infected the lung, DNA macrorestriction studies demonstrate subclonal variation, which may result from sequence alterations in restriction recognition sites, genomic rearrangements and incorporation of extrachromosomal DNA, for example from bacteriophages. These hypermutable strains are unique to CF patients and are able to adapt promptly to their environment by not only switching genes on and off, but also by an increased frequency of mutation events. One such mutation triggers conversion to the mucoid phenotype, which is positively selected for under the environmental stresses of nutritional limitation and hypoxia found within the CF bronchiolar mucus. The excessive alginate contributes to the resistance to the host innate immune mechanisms, e.g. alginate reduces chemotaxis of polymorphonuclear leucocytes, scavenges hypochlorite produced by phaghocytic cells, inhibits opsonic and non-opsonic phagocytosis, enhances adherence properties of the bacteria and decreases sensitivity to antibiotics and reactive intermediates produced by leucocytes. This inability of the host immune response to eliminate

PA further contributes to the inflammatory response in the lungs.

Another survival strategy is the formation of biofilms. This is under quorum sensing control, which involves sensing cell density and the production of soluble factors that regulate other genes. A dense matrix protects the bacterial microcolonies from phagocytosis and also interferes with antibiotic activity.

CF patients can acquire PA in their respiratory tracts at any time, although most studies indicate that 70–80% of patients are infected by their teenage years and, with progression of the lung disease, PA may be the only organism cultured. Once established, PA infection is seldom eradicated. Over time, the prevalence of chronic PA infection has increased and has been temporally associated with the development of regional centres specializing in CF.[41] Most clinical isolates are considered to originate in the environment, although the precise mechanism is not known, and many patients harbour a number of different strains.[39] The issue of person-to-person transmission of PA remains controversial. Two recent large longitudinal studies from CF centres in Canada[40] and Britain,[42] one spanning almost two decades, have found no evidence to support person-to-person transmission of PA. Epidemiological evidence for shared strains was confined to siblings living within the same household. (The sharing of strains within families may be related to either common source exposure or the high contact density between siblings within the same household.) Nevertheless, evidence of person-to-person transmission of PA is increasing, and acquisition of transmissible strains of PA is associated with increased treatment requirements.[43] When molecular typing was employed, cross-infection of PA between patients was reported from two major British CF clinics[44,45] and for Danish CF patients attending a summer camp in Spain.[46] This included well-documented cases of superinfection in those previously colonized with their own strain of the organism.[47] Since then, additional reports from Australia have provided compelling evidence for the large-scale spread of a transmissible strain of PA within and between CF clinics.[48,49] The sharing of a limited number of strains by unrelated CF patients from geographically disperse regions and the failure to demonstrate an environmental reservoir strongly suggests that cross-infection within clinics has taken place. It is yet to be conclusively proven that transmissible strains are more virulent than others and that their acquisition is not merely a marker of increased clinic exposure (or other factors) related to severe disease. However, PA acquisition adversely influences prognosis.[3] Epidemic strains are more frequently multiresistant and more difficult to treat, with patients requiring longer periods of hospitalization than those having sporadic PA isolates.[43] A study from Denmark reported a decrease in PA infection after the introduction of cohort isolation.[50] Others[51] have reported a slower initial acquisition of PA among patients who were segregated from PA-infected patients, in comparison with patients from another clinic that did not have a policy of segregation. Thus, the acquisition of PA by CF patients can be influenced by treatment settings and infection control procedures. However, it needs to be borne in mind that cohorting strategies are not without adverse psychological consequences.[35] Large, long-term, longitudinal molecular epidemiological studies using appropriate technology[39] are required to determine the rate and circumstances of PA acquisition/transmission and to ensure that future infection control guidelines are evidence based.

Diagnosis

In the case of most adult CF patients, the diagnosis was made many years before by the paediatric service. Traditionally, the diagnosis of CF has depended on the demonstration of abnormal sweat electrolytes — specifically, a sweat chloride of >60 mmol/L (i.e. evidence of abnormal CFTR function). With the discovery of the CF gene and the defining of the common mutations, one might have expected the diagnosis of CF to be made with greater confidence and security. Paradoxically, this has not been the case. The spectrum of disease is much wider than previously and includes milder phenotypes. The large number of mutations and the ability to test for only a small proportion of these in clinical practice (testing for >20 mutations is usually available to clinicians), the appreciation that some mutations may be associated with intermediate (40–60 mEq/L)[52] or normal sweat chloride levels,[4,53] the fact that some patients, particularly those diagnosed as adults, may have milder disease and lack some typical features has actually made the diagnosis of CF more difficult. Those presenting as adults are less likely to be ∅F508 homozygous, are more likely to be pancreatic sufficient, have less severe impairment of lung function and have a better prognosis.[5] A consensus statement on behalf of the CF Foundation[54] proposed that the diagnosis of CF could be made on the diagnosis of characteristic phenotypic features, a history of CF in a sibling or a positive newborn screening test, plus evidence of a CFTR abnormality as supported by elevated sweat chloride concentrations, identification of mutations to cause CF or *in vivo* demonstration of characteristic abnormalities of ion transport across nasal or airway epithelium (usually by measurement of nasal potential difference). In the majority of cases, the diagnosis will still be confirmed by an abnormal concentration of chloride in sweat obtained by pilocarpine iontophoresis and not by the identification of two CF mutations. A substantial proportion of those diagnosed as adults may have unidentified mutations.[55] While the above statement represents a clinically useful definition, it does not cover all clinical situations, leading to the concept that 'cystic fibrosis is not an "all or none" disease'.[56] In adults, the diagnosis of CF is generally entertained because of a compatible phenotype, and the concepts of genetic pre-CF, electrical or chemical pre-CF and subclinical CF[56] are not usually applicable. The diagnosis of CF does have clinical relevance in terms of multiorgan involvement, e.g. in relation to fertility or the subsequent development of pancreatic insufficiency or diabetes, the likelihood of response to, and access to, certain therapies and the possible need for genetic counselling. Nevertheless, there will continue to be a small number of difficult and taxing diagnostic dilemmas.

Management

Management of adult CF should be comprehensive and multidisciplinary but individualized and, when possible, preventive. Expert consensus[57,58] has recommended that care of adult CF patients should take place in specialist centres with expertise, experience and a multidisciplinary approach to management. Although a randomized controlled trial (RCT) has never been undertaken, there is some evidence that outcome is better for patients managed in specialized clinics,[59,60] but this may relate to the intensity of care delivered. In an overview of care in the UK, Walters et al.[61] found evidence that adults with CF attending special CF clinics received more intensive care and had more direct access to care and that patients had better symptom control and were more satisfied with the service than those attending general clinics. However, care based solely in specialized centres may have problems in terms of travel distance, and a model of shared care and mechanisms for disseminating expertise to local clinicians may need to be developed for local circumstances.

Clear transition pathways from paediatric to adult care are increasingly being recognized as important.[62] This should be based on a close working relationship between the paediatric and adult CF teams with the actual patient transfer merely being part of a prolonged transition process involving planning and education. Such a process needs to address adolescent developmental issues such as risk taking, body image, sexuality, peer relationships and autonomy, as well as educational and vocational goals, in the context of a chronic illness involving a number of management strategies. Also to be taken into account are the parents/caregivers with regard to their changing role, issues of guilt associated with an inherited disease and overprotectiveness. One aim is to promote the patient's independence while maintaining family connections and support. For the patients, the adult clinic raises issues such as different styles of management, different pathways of access, a different and often sicker mix of patients and the need to assume greater responsibility for their own care.

The overall aims of management are to:
• control and minimize chronic bronchopulmonary infection and inflammation;
• prevent deterioration in lung function;
• maintain nutrition, growth and development;
• maintain physical activity, health-related quality of life and a knowledgeable realistic attitude in the face of progressive multisystem involvement.

In this review, only the respiratory aspects of care will be addressed in detail. This in no way suggests that non-respiratory aspects of care are not important. Furthermore, respiratory physicians often assume a lead role in the care of adults with CF and need to be aware of the evidence base for non-respiratory management and be comfortable in the management of both respiratory as well as non-respiratory aspects of an individual patient's disease. However, space precludes an in-depth review of the non-respiratory aspects of care.

A feature of CF management is the degree of variation in treatment strategies between different centres. This is due in part to the paucity of good-quality scientific evidence to support many individual treatments. Cheng et al.[63] reviewed all 506 RCTs in CF between 1966 and 1997. Over that time, there was a 30-fold increase in the number of RCTs published in a 5-year period, but the median sample size decreased from 30 to 19 over the period. Only 8.7% were multicentre trials, raising concerns about the generalizability of any results. Sixty per cent of abstracts presented at meetings did not reach full publication. While this may be due to methodological or other shortcomings, there is also the possibility of publication bias with studies showing no group differences being less likely to be published. The absence of a single, universally applicable, readily measured, responsive outcome parameter in CF means that a variety of parameters have been used. Furthermore, the difficulties of conducting studies in CF should not be underestimated. Mortality is not usually an appropriate outcome. Other measures include pulmonary function (including the rate of decline), frequency of pulmonary exacerbations, inflammatory and microbiological markers and health-related quality of life (HRQL) measures. Certain outcome parameters, such as FEV_1, show substantial spontaneous variation over time, and the clinical course may be punctuated by acute exacerbations. Only recently has a validated, disease-specific HRQL instrument been developed.[64] Other outcomes may be relatively insensitive to change. Because of carryover effects, a crossover design may not be appropriate in many cases. To be adequately powered, studies of CF may require large numbers of subjects. This information merely serves to emphasize the need for large, well-designed, adequately powered, multicentre RCTs using appropriate outcome parameters and addressing all aspects of management of CF.

The improvement in survival in CF over the last three decades has been attributed to an earlier, more aggressive approach with multiple strategies. Treatment of CF tends to be increasingly complex, expensive, time-consuming, is often 'preventive' and, in some cases, is not without significant adverse effects and/or has a major impact on patients' daily activity. Consequently, there is increasing interest in the issue of adherence to health management plans in CF.[65] Different types of non-adherence have been described,[66] and failure to differentiate between these may be a partial explanation as to why predictive factors explain only a small proportion of the variance in adherence.[65] Health care professionals have tended to categorize patients inappropriately as being adherent or non-adherent. Such a classification obscures the fact that a patient's level of adherence varies over time, and the adherence to one aspect of management may differ greatly from adherence to another strategy. For example, in CF, adherence to pancreatic enzyme supplements is greater than to physiotherapy.[67] On the other hand, non-adherence to certain aspects of management may be predictive of non-adherence to other aspects, and an individual's previous non-adherent behaviour may influence subsequent management decisions, e.g. listing for transplantation. Non-adherence is more likely when long-term treatment is required, if treatment is preventive, if treatment is perceived as difficult or when the regimen is complex—factors clearly relevant to the management of CF. For most treatments, the minimal level of adherence to produce the desired benefit is unknown. Disease severity and general CF knowledge are poorly associated with adherence,[67–69] consistent with findings in other chronic diseases.[70] However, there is some evidence that accurate knowledge about a specific therapy may be associated with improved adherence.[71,72] The impact on adherence of the type, complexity and multiplicity of individual treatments, of transfer to an adult CF service, the changing role of family members and caregivers, the influence of a multidisciplinary team and social, economic and psychological factors is largely unknown. The limited studies of adherence in adults with CF are largely descriptive, and the reliability, validity and generalizability of much of the information is doubtful. If the understanding of, and ability to predict, adherence is to be improved, longitudinal studies of adherence behaviour with effective, valid and relevant measurement tools are required. Rather than attributing blame or taking a judgemental approach, the clinician should attempt to understand the influences on an individual's level of adherence and use these insights to modify management strategies accordingly.[70]

There are no data on what should constitute an initial (or annual) assessment of the adult CF patient, nor how this information influences management or outcome. However, such an assessment may include:

• Pulmonary function tests. In CF, there is progressive airflow obstruction, and serial measurements of spirometric lung volumes are regarded as a minimum, especially as FEV_1 is the most important determinant of prognosis.[19] Expiratory flow volume curves demonstrate reduced flows at mid- and low lung volumes, indicative of small airway obstruction. Plethysmographic lung volumes demonstrate static hyperinflation. Exercise tolerance may be assessed by cardiopulmonary exercise testing, but this has not been formally compared with other measures that may be more readily used and repeated in the clinic such as a 6-min walk distance[73] or endurance shuttle test.[74] However, it is not clear whether these additional tests influence management or outcome in any meaningful way. Oxygen saturation can be monitored non-invasively by pulse oximetry, but arterial blood gas examination may be indicated in those with reduced oxygen saturations or severely impaired

lung function. Elevated $Paco_2$ generally only occurs with FEV_1 <30% predicted. Although nocturnal hypoxaemia is regarded as a contributing factor to pulmonary hypertension, the usefulness of a single assessment of overnight oxygen saturations is not clear, particularly in view of the variability that occurs in other forms of severe lung disease.[75]

• Sputum microbiology. Sputum cultures to determine chronic infection by *H. influenzae*, *S. aureus*, PA or *B. cepacia* are certainly clinically relevant (see earlier). Cultures may reveal other highly resistant bacteria such as *Stenotrophomonas maltrophilia* or *Alicaligenes xylosoxidans*.

• Fungal cultures may reveal *Aspergillus fumigatus*. Patients should also have skin or serological testing for *Aspergillus*,[33,34] as a proportion will fulfil criteria for allergic bronchopulmonary aspergillosis.

• Mycobacterial culture—for *Mycobacterium avium-intracellulare* complex[29] and *M. tuberculosis*.

• Chest radiograph. Chest radiographic scoring systems have been developed and, although they allow quantitative assessment of the radiological abnormality that may be used longitudinally in clinical studies, they are more frequently used clinically in paediatric than in adult clinics. Discernible radiological changes seldom occur between serial films even during exacerbations, but complications such as mucus plugging, atelectasis or pneumothorax may be demonstrated. High-resolution computerized tomographic (HRCT) scans allow more accurate assessment of the severity and distribution of bronchiectasis[76] (Fig. 1) and may also be useful in the assessment of complications. The role of serial high-resolution CT (HRCT) scanning has not been clarified, although it is

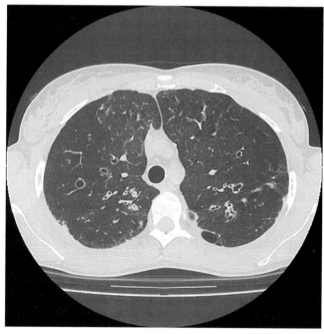

Figure 1. HRCT image demonstrating bronchiectasis in the upper lobes.

recognized that progressive structural changes demonstrable on HRCT can occur without change in lung function tests.[77]

• Liver function tests. Biliary cirrhosis may a feature of CF but is symptomatic in less than 5% and is the cause of death in about 2% of patients.[78] Tests should include serum bilirubin, liver enzymes and assessment of synthetic function.

• Assessment of pancreatic function. Pancreatic insufficiency is present in over 90% of persons with CF. However, in those with known pancreatic insufficiency who are on replacement therapy, measurement of faecal fat is not indicated unless there are concerns about ongoing significant fat malabsorption, e.g. unexplained weight loss or ongoing intestinal symptoms. Faecal elastase measurements can be used to determine the adequacy of pancreatic function in those considered to be pancreatic sufficient.

• Fat-soluble vitamins. Because of a degree of persistent fat malabsorption despite supplements, fat-soluble vitamin levels may be low, and serum levels need to be checked periodically to ensure adequacy of supplements.

• Bone densitometry. Metabolic bone disease is increasingly being recognized in CF[79] and may be influenced by vitamin D and calcium levels, levels of physical activity, corticosteroid therapy, sex hormone levels, pro-inflammatory cytokines and the disease itself. Low bone mineral density is associated with low body mass index (BMI) and impaired lung function. Although rarely symptomatic, osteopenia may be a problem in conjunction with transplantation with the development of rib fractures and distortion of the thorax by kyphosis, with these problems being further aggravated by high-dose steroid therapy. While bisphosphonate therapy (intravenous pamidronate) has been shown to increase bone mineral density in CF patients, such treatment was commonly associated with bone pain in those not using oral corticosteroids.[80]

The following sections will focus on the chronic management of CF in adults (see Table 1). Trials conducted solely in children will not generally be included unless of particular importance. Many of the trials conducted in CF include both adults and children—these trials will be included but, where possible, information on the age range of subjects or proportion of adult subjects will be provided. This is not to suggest that management of CF in childhood is not relevant to adult respiratory physicians; quite the opposite, as the patient's condition when they transfer from paediatric to adult services is in part determined by their management in childhood years, and will therefore have a major influence on their subsequent progress and prognosis.

Pharmacological correction of the underlying defect

A logical approach to therapy would be pharmacological manipulation of the underlying biochemical defect. Because of the different classes of mutation responsible for the CF phenotype, individual strategies may not be applicable to all patients.

Table 1. Chronic management of cystic fibrosis.

Beneficial
  Nebulized DNase

Likely to be beneficial
  Multidisciplinary management in specialized clinics
  Airway clearance techniques
  Physical training
  Nebulized hypertonic saline
  Nebulized anti-pseudomonal antibiotics
  Macrolide antibiotics (azithromycin)
  Long-acting b-agonists

Trade-off between benefit and harm
  Cohorting of patients
  Nebulized high-dose tobramycin
  Long-term anti-staphylococcal antibiotics
  Oral corticosteroids
  Non-steroidal anti-inflammatory agents (ibuprofen)
  Non-invasive ventilation
  Lung transplantation

Unknown effectiveness
  Gene therapy
  Other inhaled hyperosmolar agents
  Leukotriene antagonists
  Long-term oxygen therapy

Unlikely to be beneficial
  Nebulized *N*-acetylcysteine
  Pseudomonas vaccination
  Inhaled corticosteroids
  Oral theophylline

In this regard, the mechanisms of action of pharmacological agents can be divided broadly into drugs that increase trafficking of the mutant CF protein to the apical membrane and are applicable to the most common CF mutation, ∅F508 (a class II mutation), drugs that increase chloride secretion and drugs that reduce sodium reabsorption across the apical membrane.

The conformational change that occurs in CFTR as a result of the ∅F508 mutation makes it vulnerable to degradation within the endoplasmic reticulum of the epithelial cells. Low temperature induced an increased proportion of CFTR to insert into the apical cell membrane, and a search for chemical 'chaperones' with similar properties found that glycerol seemed to be promising *in vitro*. However, an open parallel group study of glycerol showed no effect on the nasal potential difference of CF subjects.[81] In a randomized, parallel group pilot study in 18 ∅F508 patients, an analogue of butyrate (which upregulates CFTR messenger RNA), sodium 4-phenylbutyrate, partially restored nasal epithelial CFTR function.[82] RCTs of other chaperone molecules are awaited.

The defective outward-rectifying chloride channel regulation in CF can be overcome *in vitro* by topical adenosine triphosphate (ATP) or uridine triphosphate (UTP). UTP also has effects on ciliary beating and goblet cell degranulation. Knowles et al.[83] found, in nine CF subjects, that superfusion of UTP had beneficial effects on chloride secretion and epithelial potential difference in the nose. Bennett et al.,[84] in a study of 14 adult CF subjects, showed that aerosolized UTP/amiloride improved mucociliary clearance from the peripheral airways, compared with vehicle control subjects. However, the effect was modest and of short duration. Clinical trials of more potent and longer acting analogues are required. Another strategy would be to stimulate alternative chloride channels, e.g. calcium-dependent channels, but there are no published trials of such treatments.

Amiloride inhibits several epithelial sodium transport processes including the sodium channel, which is responsible for the increased sodium absorption in CF airway epithelium as a result of the abnormal regulation by defective CFTR. Placebo-controlled, crossover studies of nebulized amiloride have shown conflicting results.[85–87] A 25-week, double-blind, crossover North American study[85] showed a reduction in decline of forced vital capacity (FVC), but not FEV_1, in 18 CF adult subjects receiving aerosolized amiloride (5×10^{-3} M) four times per day. However, a 6-month, double-blind, placebo-controlled, crossover UK study using aerosolized amiloride (3.8×10^{-3} M) four times daily[86] showed no effect in terms of lung function, body weight, exacerbation rate or other parameters. In a French multicentre, randomized, double-blind, placebo-controlled trial involving 137 subjects aged >5 years (although the intention was to recruit 550 subjects) with an FEV_1 >50% predicted, the use of nebulized amiloride three times daily for 6 months was not associated with benefit in terms of lung function or any of the other secondary endpoints. Post hoc analysis failed to identify a subgroup responsive to amiloride.[87] Overall, the lack of effectiveness of amiloride therapy means that its widespread use cannot be recommended.

Sodium absorption through the basolateral sodium–potassium–adenosine triphosphatase (Na^+/K^+-ATPase) channel is increased in CF and can be inhibited by cardiac glycosides such as oubain and digoxin. However, double-blind, placebo-controlled crossover studies showed no effect on nasal potential difference for either topically applied oubain or oral digoxin given to CF patients over 2 weeks,[88] suggesting that current Na^+/K^+-ATPase inhibitors are unlikely to be therapeutically useful in CF. Combining a sodium channel blocker with a chloride channel opener, thus mimicking 'normal' conditions, would intuitively seem like an attractive option, but is one that has yet to be subjected to clinical trials.

A variety of strategies have been investigated to activate mutant CFTR although, because of the different classes of mutations, a number of different strategies will be needed (allele-specific therapy). There are no published studies using such agents. Key advances in the management of CF in the next decade or two are likely to occur in this general area, and RCTs

of agents showing promise in in vitro studies or in animal models will be eagerly awaited. Furthermore, the role of some of these pharmacological treatments may be to augment other treatments.

Gene therapy

The ultimate treatment option may be gene replacement therapy, which aims to deliver a copy of a normal CF gene to defective cells. Crystal and colleagues[89] demonstrated 'proof of concept' by demonstrating the feasibility of CFTR cDNA transfection and expression of CFTR in the lung by means of adenoviral vector systems. A phase II, double-blind, randomized, placebo-controlled clinical trial of maxillary sinus delivery of an adeno-associated CFTR viral vector/gene construct in 23 CF subjects, with the other maxillary acting as control, provided little evidence of efficacy.[90] Although viruses (adenovirus and adeno-associated virus) are attractive vectors because of their ability to enter cells, the immunological and inflammatory defence mechanisms to combat viral invasion of the human airway have limited the use of these vectors. Newer viral vectors and receptor-directed molecular conjugates are being investigated. Non-viral cationic liposome plasmid complexes are an alternative method of transferring cDNA that is non-immunogenic and non-inflammatory and which overcomes the lack of expression of transgenes in non-replicating cells. Studies using liposomal methodology have shown CFTR protein expression in rats and have corrected chloride channel ion transport defects in transgenic mice[91] and CF patients.[92] However, their relative lack of transfection efficiency and the lack of understanding of intracellular biopharmaceuticals currently limit this methodology. Cationic polymers have chemical and biological properties that may make them more efficient in mediating gene transfer than lipids,[92] but have not yet been trialled in CF. Thus, despite a prodigious amount of research, multiple technical barriers still exist, and none of the current strategies has shown sufficient promise to be subjected to large clinical trials. Nevertheless, it is hard not to be optimistic that safe and effective gene-based therapies will emerge in the not too distant future.

Reduction in the mucus burden

Airway clearance techniques

Airway clearance techniques have been the mainstay of treatment for CF for many decades and are based on the fact that excessive production of abnormal mucus overwhelms the normal clearance mechanism and leads to airway obstruction, infection and inflammation. A variety of methods have been used to clear secretions in CF, some physical, either 'manual' or using a variety of devices, and some chemical (see next section).

Chest physiotherapy has been regarded by many patients as unpleasant, uncomfortable and time-consuming, and thus adherence has been a major issue.[93,94] While some of these concerns may have been applicable to older techniques, e.g. postural drainage and chest percussion (PD/CP), more recent self-administered techniques are considered to be more acceptable, cause less interference with usual activities and provide the patient with more independence. For a more detailed description of some of the chest physiotherapy techniques, see Chapter 4.5 on Bronchiectasis.

The first issue with respect to chest physiotherapy is whether it produces benefit when compared with no chest physiotherapy. This issue was addressed in a Cochrane Review.[95] One hundred and twenty trials were identified, of which six crossover trials (five published) with only 66 participants were eligible for inclusion; the majority were excluded because of the lack of a control group. Five studies were of a single treatment; the other involved treatments twice a day for 2 days. Two studies showed that physiotherapy increased the amount of expectorated secretions and, in three studies, the clearance of inhaled radioactive tracer was increased by physiotherapy compared with a control period. While physiotherapy may have beneficial acute effects, there is no evidence of the long-term benefit (or otherwise) of these treatments. This subject has been reviewed by Hess,[96] who concluded '. . . there is a dearth of high-level evidence to support any secretion clearance technique'. Despite this extraordinary paucity of information on the long-term effectiveness, chest physiotherapy is now such an integral component of management that RCTs addressing this issue are unlikely to take place because of ethical concerns with respect to the control group. Balanced against this is the evidence that chest physiotherapy is not necessarily an entirely benign therapy; complications include hypoxaemia,[97,98] increased oxygen consumption,[99] gastro-oesophageal reflux[100] and increased intracranial pressure.[101] However, most clinicians would argue that the presumed benefits of therapy outweigh any negative effects.

The other major issue with respect to chest physiotherapy in CF is whether one method is clearly superior.[102] The number of diverse techniques currently in use argues strongly against this. Most comparative studies of chest physiotherapy have had small numbers of subjects, included patients with a variety of conditions, used crossover designs, few used sham therapy (although this is not always possible), few were controlled, and most were limited to short-term outcomes such as sputum weight or volume following a single session. Most studies showed a wide spectrum of individual responses, and the lack of statistical difference between techniques in many studies can be attributed to lack of statistical power. The study by Reisman et al.[103] in 1988 established PD/CP as the standard for chest physiotherapy in CF. McIlwaine et al.[104] conducted one of the few long-term trials of chest physiotherapy in CF. They undertook a single-centre, long-term (1 year), randomized, parallel group study of positive expiratory pressure (PEP) using a PEP mask versus PD/CP in 36 CF patients aged 6–17 years, matched by age, gender and baseline FEV_1. FEV_1 showed

a 6% improvement in the PEP group compared with a 2% decline in the PD/CP group ($P = 0.04$), and similar improvements occurred in other pulmonary function parameters. There were no differences in number of hospitalizations. These results are encouraging but whether the apparently more effective PEP technique leads to a reduction in the rate of progression of lung disease in CF in the longer term is unknown.

Devices to assist in the removal of secretions are gaining popularity because of convenience of use, acceptability to patients and effectiveness. The Flutter device causes a variable (oscillating) PEP in the airway, which it is believed causes the airway walls to vibrate, loosen mucus and promote its clearance, as well as possible beneficial effects on the rheological properties of the secretions.[105] Konstan et al.[106] demonstrated that short-term use of a Flutter device led to the production of more sputum than did directed coughing or a shortened form of PD/CP. However, in a longer term (1 year), randomized, parallel group study of 40 stable CF patients aged 7–17 years, in which a Flutter device was compared with PEP, the Flutter group had a greater mean annual rate of decline in FEV_1 (−11% versus −1%; $P = 0.08$), a significant decline in Huang scores, increased hospitalizations (18 versus 5; $P = 0.03$) and increased antibiotic use.[107] Thus, the Flutter device was not only less effective but was also associated with greater health care costs. The authors comment that it was not until 6–9 months into the study that the unsatisfactory results in the Flutter group began to be apparent. This study demonstrated that results of short-term interventions do not necessarily predict longer term outcomes and that future studies of chest physiotherapy techniques in CF should be of sufficient duration. Studies should also measure a variety of clinically relevant outcome parameters including HRQL and take into account patient preferences, tolerability and acceptability of treatment. Future studies should also examine the most effective form of chest physiotherapy in conjunction with other treatments to improve clearance of secretions, such as DNase and hyperosmolar agents.

Physical training

Exercise tolerance in CF declines as the disease progresses, and a lower functional capacity is an adverse prognostic factor.[108] Physical training, defined as participation in a programme of regular vigorous physical activity designed to improve physical performance and/or cardiovascular function and/or muscle strength, is already encouraged for most adults with CF. Such training has a number of potential benefits for CF patients: alleviation of the reduced exercise tolerance and dyspnoea; enhanced performance at work and during recreational and sporting activities; improved clearance of secretions; improved appetite; better control of diabetes; delayed onset of osteoporosis; and increased feelings of well-being. Exercise might have other potential beneficial effects; Hebestreit et al.[109] demonstrated that moderate-intensity exercise partially blocked the amiloride-sensitive sodium conductance in the respiratory epithelium that would be expected to increase the water content of the airway mucus in the CF lung.

A recent Cochrane Review of this subject[110] identified six trials involving 184 patients and concluded that exercise tolerance was improved by physical training during an acute hospital admission. The largest study was conducted entirely in children by Selvadurai et al.,[111] who randomized 66 children admitted to hospital for acute exacerbations of CF into three groups: aerobic training aimed at improving cardiovascular function group, resistance training (to improve muscle strength) group and a control group. Those who received aerobic training had significantly better peak aerobic capacity, activity levels and quality of life than children in the other two groups. Children who received resistance training had better weight gain, lung function and leg strength than children in the other groups. All changes persisted for 1 month after discharge. The authors concluded that a combination of aerobic and resistance training may be the best programme for CF patients. This evidence in children and the fact that inpatient training programmes are generally encouraged for adult CF patients suggest that this practice should continue but does not obviate the need for RCTs in adults.

The only published long-term controlled trial of an outpatient or home exercise programme in CF was by Schneiderman-Walker et al.[112] Sixty-five CF patients, aged 7–19 years with mean predicted FEV_1 of 88%, were randomized to an exercise group (a minimum of 20 min of aerobic exercise, three times per week) or a control group (usual activity). There was no difference in the rate of decline in FEV_1, maximum minute ventilation, maximum work capacity or weight, although there was a reduced rate of decline in FVC in the exercise group (−0.03 versus −2.4; $P = 0.02$). Thus, there is no convincing evidence to support the use of unsupervised exercise programmes in order to slow the rate of decline of lung function, although other potential benefits were not examined. Additional long-term studies in adults are required to determine the efficacy of exercise programmes, the best type of exercise, the intensity and pattern of the programme, as well as studies in subjects with more severe impairment of lung function and whether the effects of exercise may be additive to those of physiotherapy[113] or other strategies.

DNase

In CF, the abnormal biorheological properties of airway secretions contribute to the vicious cycle of obstruction, inflammation and infection and consequent damage to the airways. Two macromolecules contribute in major ways to the physical properties of airway secretions: mucus glycoproteins and DNA. DNA, a viscous polyanion, makes up about 10% of the dry weight of airway secretions in CF and is derived mainly from lysed neutrophils. Deoxyribonuclease I is the human enzyme that is normally responsible for the digestion of extracellular DNA but, in CF sputum, it is overwhelmed by the

quantity of DNA. The availability of recombinant human deoxyribonuclease (rhDNase) and in vitro evidence that it reduced the viscosity of CF sputum[114] provided the basis for the trialling of nebulized rhDNase as a treatment for CF. In a study of the effect of the short-term (7 days) use of rhDNase in 13 patients aged 18–36 years with a wide spectrum of lung function, Robinson et al.[115] found that patients who achieved a ≥10% improvement in FEV_1 had no greater change in mucociliary clearance than non-responders. This and an earlier study[116] raised doubts as to whether the benefits of rhDNase are simply due to improvements in mucociliary clearance or whether other, as yet unknown, mechanisms are more important.

A Cochrane Review[117] concluded that rhDNase therapy was associated with an important improvement in lung function after 6 months of treatment. Although the conclusion of effectiveness was based on several trials involving 1710 subjects, the largest and longest RCT was that by Fuchs et al.[118] In a double-blind, placebo-controlled study, 968 adults and children with CF and mean baseline FEV_1 of 61% predicted were randomized to receive rhDNase once daily, rhDNase twice daily or placebo for 24 weeks as outpatients. Compared with placebo, rhDNase once and twice daily reduced the age-adjusted risk of exacerbations requiring parenteral antibiotic therapy by 28% and 37%, respectively, and improved FEV_1 by 5.8% and 5.6% respectively. Thirty per cent of those who received rhDNase had ≥ 10% improvement in FEV_1 (compared with 15% in those who received placebo). Once-daily (but not twice-daily) therapy was associated with reduced dyspnoea, improved well-being and reduced CF symptoms. A subsequent 12-week, multicentre, double-blind, placebo-controlled study in 420 subjects with more advanced lung disease (baseline FEV_1 of 22%) by McCoy et al.[119] reported similar findings (mean percentage change in FEV_1 from baseline of 9.4% compared with 2.1% for placebo). An increased risk of voice alteration ($RR = 2.4$, 95% CI 1.5–3.9) was the only adverse effect attributable to rhDNase.[117]

The clinical studies of rhDNase showed a wide variation in the response. In none of these studies could the responding subgroup be defined. Consequently, some authorities have required demonstration of a physiological response to rhDNase before funding long-term treatment.[120] An improvement in FEV_1 of ≥ 10% is generally regarded as being a clinically significant response and renders the patient eligible for ongoing treatment. Others have advocated more formal, randomized, double-blind, placebo-controlled n-of-1 trials to define acute responders.[121] Such approaches to identify responders are supported by data indicating that early improvement is a good predictor of longer term benefit.[122] Given the lack of response to DNase in acute exacerbations,[123] it is suggested that such individual assessments should be undertaken when the patient is clinically stable. Assessment of individual DNase responses allows CF patients, who already have a plethora of treatments, to avoid the burden of additional and ineffective treatment, as well as directing limited health care resources to those most likely to benefit.

The study by Fuchs et al.[118] was a landmark study in CF, being the first large multicentre trial in CF that addressed a specific treatment question in a methodologically sound way. Acknowledging the insights to be gained from meta-analysis, the power and influence of the results of a large, adequately powered study, using clinical relevant outcome parameters, cannot be underestimated. While some lament the lack of longer term studies,[117] so convincing were the results of the 25-week studies and so widespread is the use of rhDNase[124] that longer term, randomized, placebo-controlled trials are unlikely to be performed. In lieu of such trials, Shah et al.[125] reported an open label extension of a phase II trial[126] in a cohort of 52 subjects aged 16–55 years with a mean FEV_1 of 1.47 L. FEV_1 was improved by 13.3% in the first month and was then maintained at a mean of 7.1% above baseline for the subsequent 23 months. A steady increase in weight of the subjects was noted during the trial. Thus, there is some evidence supporting the long-term effectiveness of rhDNase.

It has been said that 'the studies of DNase are of insufficient duration and size to identify the effect on mortality'.[117] The use of mortality as a primary endpoint may be impractical unless very large long-term international studies are contemplated. Such a study would need to recruit patients with severely impaired lung function. As such, it would need to recruit a substantial proportion of eligible patients in a number of countries. The study by McCoy et al.,[119] which demonstrated the effectiveness of rhDNase in subjects with severely impaired lung function, enrolled and randomized approximately 44% of the potentially eligible CF population (FVC <40% predicted) in the USA.

There are a number of practical issues related to the use of rhDNase. To prevent degradation of the protein, rhDNase must be protected from excessive heat and strong light. It is recommended that it be stored in a refrigerator at 2–8°C in a foil pouch. Only a recommended jet nebulizer system should be used. Ultrasonic devices should not be used as they may cause thermal degradation of rhDNase. Also, many battery-powered compressors have insufficient power to nebulize rhDNase. rhDNase should not be combined with any other medications in the nebulizer, as changing the characteristics of the solution might alter the rhDNase protein.

In the Cochrane Review,[117] no eligible studies comparing rhDNase with another mucolytic, were found. However, Suri et al.,[127] in an open crossover trial in 48 children in which subjects were randomized to 12 weeks of daily rhDNase, alternative-day rhDNase and twice-daily 7% hypertonic saline, found that the improvements in FEV_1 were 16%, 14% and 3% respectively. These results indicated that daily and alternate-day DNase produced a significantly greater improvement in FEV_1 than hypertonic saline and that alternate-day use of rhDNase may be just as effective as daily use (but much cheaper). However, these conclusions need to be con-firmed by further adequately powered, methodologically sound RCTs.

Actin can bind to DNA and can potentially inhibit the enzymatic activity of rhDNase. Compared with wild-type rhDNase, actin-resistant DNase variant had enhanced capacity to improve the physical properties of CF sputum and cough transportability of airway secretions in vitro.[128] This new preparation has not yet been subjected to clinical trials.

Other mucolytic agents

Mucolytic drugs that aim to reduce sputum viscosity may provide benefit in CF by assisting the removal of secretions. The most commonly prescribed agent is N-acetylcysteine (NAC), which depolymerizes mucus in vitro by breaking disulphide bridges between macromolecules. NAC may be taken either orally or by inhalation, and differences between these two methods of administration have not been formally studied. After oral ingestion, NAC is reduced to cysteine, a precursor of the potent antioxidant glutathione, and these antioxidant properties could be useful in reducing airway damage and slowing the decline of lung function in CF. NAC is prescribed to a significant minority of CF patients[124] but in a systematic review Duijvestijn and Brand[129] were able to identify only three RCTs of nebulized NAC in CF, and these demonstrated no benefits in terms of lung function. In six RCTs of oral NAC with a total of 181 subjects, there was a tendency to benefit in terms of lung function, but the effect was small (2%, 95% CI −0.3 to 4.9) and of doubtful clinical significance. Studies were of 3 months' duration or shorter. Thus, there is no evidence to support the widespread long-term use of NAC either nebulized or oral. Other mucolytic agents have not been studied.

Hyperosmolar agents

In CF, the isotonic volume depletion theory[22] states that altered CFTR results in defects in electrolyte transport and increased water reabsorption across the respiratory epithelium. This reduced volume of airway surface liquid may alter the physical properties of the mucus and prevent its normal clearance. In studies using the mucus-depleted bovine trachea model, the application of sodium chloride improved mucociliary clearance of CF mucus.[130] Robinson et al.[131] argued that hypertonic saline (HS) may induce an osmotic flow of water into the mucus layer, rehydrating secretions and thereby improving mucus rheology. HS may also break the ionic bonds within the mucus gel, reducing cross-linking and entanglements and thus lowering viscosity and elasticity. With chronic infection, the mucin macromolecules develop fixed negative charges, causing increased repulsion. The addition of HS, by increasing the ionic concentration of the mucus, causes a conformational change by shielding the negative charges and reducing repulsion. Using the mucus-depleted bovine trachea model, Shiburya et al.[132] found that the addition of hypertonic sodium chloride improved mucociliary clearance but did not change the viscoelastic properties of CF sputum. This suggests an effect other than a direct effect on the physical properties of sputum. Hyperosmolar solutions also increase ciliary beat frequency,[133] possibly via activation of sensory nerves and the release of neuropeptides.[133,134] Hyperosmolar stimuli may also act as secretagogues,[134,135] but it is unclear whether the increased volume of secretions might be advantageous or not. Any long-term improvements in mucociliary clearance may reduce bacterial load, reduce the vicious cycle of infection and inflammation and potentially reduce the decline in lung function. However, this treatment is not without potential adverse effects. HS may theoretically interfere with the function of cationic antibacterial peptides such as defensins, and thus increase the airway microbiological load. Also, airway hyper-responsiveness (AHR) is well recognized in CF,[136] and HS has the potential to cause airway narrowing in this patient group. As HS is easy and inexpensive to produce, short and then longer term RCTs of HS in CF are certainly justified to determine effectiveness and assess adverse effects.

A Cochrane Review of nebulized HS for CF[137] was based on nine trials that met inclusion criteria and concluded that, in short-term trials, HS increased lung clearance compared with control and that, when 3–7% saline was used in a volume of 10 mL twice a day, HS led to a significant increase in FEV_1 in comparison with placebo. However, of the nine trials, two were published only as abstracts, one compared HS with daily and alternate-day rhDNase and controls,[127] and two were studies of lung clearance after single administration.[131,138] In a randomized, crossover study of CF adults aged 18–28 years with mean FEV_1 of 61% predicted, Robinson et al.[138] demonstrated that a single administration of 7% HS produced improved isotope clearance from the lungs, compared with isotonic saline. In a subsequent study, Robinson et al.[131] demonstrated that HS (3–12%) improved clearance in a dose-dependent fashion, although there was no statistically significant difference between clearance due to 7% and 12% HS. In a randomized, parallel group, unblinded study by Eng et al.,[139] 58 patients (aged 7–25 years, FEV_1 36–70% predicted) received 10 mL of either 6% hypertonic or isotonic saline, nebulized bd for 2 weeks. In those receiving HS, there were improvements in FEV_1 [15% versus 3%, weighted mean difference (WMD) 12.2, 95% CI 4.3–20.1], in exercise tolerance and in symptoms of quality of sleep and 'feeling of chest cleared'. The study by Suri et al.,[127] which compared nebulized HS with daily or alternate-day rhDNase, demonstrated only a small (3%) improvement in FEV_1 with HS. However, a low volume (5 mL) of 7% HS was used, and it is possible that this lower volume of HS was responsible for the modest response.

The results of long-term studies, such as the large RCT currently being undertaken in Australia, of the effectiveness of HS and assessment of adverse effects, including impact on airway bacteriology, are eagerly awaited. Notwithstanding the results of Suri et al.,[127] studies comparing the alternate, supplementary or complementary effects of rhDNase and HS are required. The long-term effects of HS on morbidity, on mucosal inflammation, on AHR and the rate of decline in FEV_1 have yet to be studied.

Other inhaled osmotic agents may also have a role in management as they also induce an influx of water into the airway lumen and improve hydration of secretions. Non-ionic osmotic agents have the theoretical advantage of not impairing the antimicrobial effect of defensins in the airways. Using the mucus-depleted bovine trachea model, Wills et al.[140] reported that mannitol improved tracheal mucus velocity of CF sputum. In a study of 12 adult subjects with CF by Robinson et al.,[141] mannitol and HS both improved lung clearance of radiolabelled particles to a similar degree. Despite premedication with β-agonist bronchodilator, both mannitol and HS produced an immediate fall in FEV_1 of 7% and 6%, respectively, although FEV_1 returned to baseline by the end of the study. A dry powder preparation may have advantages in terms of rapidity of administration, portability and duration of action. Results of RCTs investigating the long-term effectiveness of non-ionic hyperosmolar agents are eagerly awaited.

Control of infection

Nebulized antipseudomonal antibiotics

The most common bacteria causing chronic infection in older CF patients is PA and, based on its purported role in airway inflammation and damage, antipseudomonal antibiotics would seem to be a logical component of treatment. Delivery of the antibiotic by inhalation is appealing because a suitable antibiotic can be delivered in high concentration directly to the site of infection, thus avoiding high systemic concentrations and reducing the risk of systemic toxicity. Nebulized antipseudomonal antibiotics may be used to eradicate PA in the early stages of colonization, to provide long-term suppression of PA and to treat exacerbations. Based on the consequences of chronic PA infections, early treatment of PA infection to prevent chronic infection holds the promise of reducing morbidity and reducing the rate of decline of lung function. Treatments, using oral, nebulized or intravenous antibiotics, have not been subject to RCTs, although there are proponents of early treatment.[50]

In a Cochrane Review of the use of nebulized antipseudomonal antibiotics for long-term suppression of PA, Ryan et al.[142] included 10 trials: two were published only in abstract form, two studies involved the use of gentamicin, two studies used gentamicin plus carbenicillin, and one used ceftazidime. There were large variations in study design often with small subject numbers, short duration, uncertain delivery of antibiotics, different antibiotics, different doses, the frequent absence of a taste-masked placebo and a variety of outcome measures were studied. The authors concluded that lung function was generally better in the antibiotic groups than in the control groups, but a pooled estimate of effect was not possible. In three trials, the rate of hospitalization was reduced in the groups using nebulized antibiotics [odds ratio (OR) = 0.69, 95% CI 0.5–0.96]. There was also evidence of reduced courses of antibiotics in the treated group (OR = 0.62, 95% CI 0.45–0.87). Similar conclusions were reached by Mukhopadhyay et al.[143] after a meta-analysis.

The study by Ramsey et al.[144] contained 68% of subjects included in the Cochrane Review. In a multicentre, double-blind, placebo-controlled trial, 520 CF subjects (mean age 21 years) with PA infection and baseline FEV_1 of 50% predicted received either a high-dose, preservative-free, pH-adjusted formulation of tobramycin designed for efficient jet nebulization (TOBI) or a taste-masked placebo. The active treatment consisted of 200 mg of tobramycin/day in three cycles, with each cycle consisting of 28 days of drug administration and then 28 days during which drug was not administered. At 20 weeks, the tobramycin group had an increase in FEV_1 of 10% (compared with a 2% decline in the placebo group) and a significant fall in PA density (compared with an increase in the placebo group). The tobramycin group was 26% less likely to be hospitalized than the placebo group. In a separate publication, an improvement in HRQL was reported in association with tobramycin use.[145] Inhaled tobramycin was not associated with any detectable ototoxicity or nephrotoxicity. However, there was an increase from 25% to 32% in the proportion of patients with PA resistant to tobramycin. Improvements occurred in the subgroup of patients using rhDNase, suggesting a possible additive effect. In the open label extension of this trial, Moss[146] found that improvements in FEV_1 were maintained at 2 years, and days in hospital were reduced by 25–33%. The response to tobramycin could not be predicted by PA susceptibility. Thus, while there were certainly benefits from the use of high-dose tobramycin, these benefits must be balanced against the cost of the preparation, the possible loss of effectiveness and the potential adverse effects of increasing resistance of PA to tobramycin or the acquisition of other drug-resistant bacteria with prolonged use.

Smaller RCTs have been conducted using other nebulized antibiotics. A placebo-controlled study of 40 patients receiving either nebulized colistin (1 megaunit) or placebo twice daily for 30 days showed that the FEV_1 declined in both groups, although the decline was less in the colistin treatment arm.[147] In a randomized, placebo-controlled, crossover trial of nebulized gentamicin over 6 months in 20 patients, Hodson et al.[148] found significant objective and subjective improvements in the treatment group. In a three-period, partially blinded, placebo-controlled, 4-month, crossover study of 18 CF subjects aged 13–41 years, Stead et al.[149] compared ceftazidime 1 mg twice daily with gentamicin 80 mg plus carbenicillin 1 mg twice daily, with 'placebo' (3.5% saline). Both antibiotic regimens demonstrated benefits in terms of FEV_1 compared with 'placebo'. Hodson et al.[150] compared 4 weeks of twice-daily nebulized tobramycin (300 mg) with nebulized colistin (80 mg) in a randomized, parallel group study of 115 CF patients ≥6 years of age. Tobramycin produced a significant

6.9% improvement in FEV_1 from baseline whereas, in the colistin group, FEV_1 was not different from baseline. There was an associated improvement in HRQL in the tobramycin group. In both groups, there was a significant decrease in PA density. Hence, high-dose nebulized tobramycin appears to be superior to nebulized colistin in terms of improvement in lung function. Results also suggest that the improvement in lung function with nebulized antibiotics is not directly related to the reduction in PA density.

Further trials are warranted to address issues such as optimal dose, frequency of administration and frequency of intermittent treatment, as well as changes in microbiological profiles and resistance patterns. Research is also required into delivery systems for nebulized therapy to increase efficiency of nebulization, reduce treatment time, enhance drug delivery to the lung and reduce drug wastage.

Intravenous antipseudomonal antibiotics

Because of the role of PA-associated inflammation in the progressive airway damage in CF, intermittent suppression of the chronic PA infection by a policy of intravenous (IV) antipseudomonal antibiotics at regular intervals, irrespective of symptoms, may theoretically reduce morbidity and increase patient survival. The Danish CF Centre has used intermittent antibiotic therapy (2 weeks of intravenous antibiotics every 3 months) for patients chronically infected by PA irrespective of their clinical state since 1976[151] and has attributed the improved outcome of their patients in terms of reduced deaths and improved 5-year survival in recent years to this policy.[152] However, this conclusion was based on comparison with historical controls and is confounded by other changes in management that took place over that time and that are likely to have influenced survival.

In the Cochrane Review that addressed the issue of elective versus symptomatic intravenous antibiotic therapy for cystic fibrosis,[153] Breen and Aswani identified two trials involving 79 patients, but neither trial demonstrated significant differences in outcome measures between intervention and comparison groups.[154,155] Elborn et al.[155] undertook a multicentre 3-year trial of parallel group design in which 60 subjects over the age of 8 years were stratified by age, radiographic score and treatment centre, and were randomized to receive either elective IV antibiotics every 3 months or IV antibiotics only when symptoms indicated. Patients in the symptomatic group received a mean of three antibiotic treatments per year, while the elective group received four treatments per year. There were no significant differences in lung function between the groups, but there was a statistically non-significant higher death rate in the elective group (4 versus 0), all due to cardiopulmonary failure secondary to overwhelming pulmonary infection, which in three was associated with B. cepacia infection. Although these results need to be viewed with caution because the study may not have been sufficiently powered, there is no good-quality evidence to support the use of elective IV antibiotic therapy.

Nevertheless, many units have a 'low threshold' policy for the use of IV antibiotic therapy for those chronically infected with PA.

Oral antibiotics

Sheldon et al.,[156] in a 1-year, randomized, double-blind study of 31 adults with CF chronically infected with PA, administered ciprofloxacin (or placebo) for 10 days every 3 months. Although there were symptomatic and lung function improvements associated with the use of ciprofloxacin, there was no reduction in hospital admissions for acute exacerbations. Because of concerns about the adverse effects of ciprofloxacin and the emergence of resistant organisms, long-term use of oral ciprofloxacin cannot be recommended.

Vaccination

Vaccination aims to elicit a long-term protective immune response by the administration of a safe preparation of an organism or a purified or recombinant component. Once an immune response has been induced, it cannot readily be reversed. Vaccines that prevent infection with PA may theoretically improve outcome in CF, but an exuberant humoral immune response to vaccination could be detrimental. A Cochrane Review of this subject[157] found only one suitable trial. This was undertaken in the 1980s and included 17 vaccinated patients followed for 10 years. There was no difference between the vaccinated group and control subjects.

Long-term oral antistaphylococcal antibiotic therapy

A pathogenic role for S. aureus (and non-typeable H. influenzae) in the development of CF lung disease is inferred. Recent bronchoalveolar lavage (BAL) studies in infants have highlighted the association between infection and inflammation,[25] and infection by S. aureus occurs in 25–30% during the first decade of life. Some centres start patients on antistaphylococcal antibiotics from diagnosis while, in others, treatment is from the first infection by S. aureus. An antibiotic that is active against S. aureus (mostly flucloxacillin) is usually chosen with the aim of reducing infection and inflammation in the developing lung and slowing progression of bronchiectasis.

In a systematic review of trials of antistaphylococcal antibiotics in CF, McCaffery et al.[158] concluded that such treatment consistently achieves sputum clearance of S. aureus and is likely to be of clinical benefit. However, the trials were heterogeneous, and a total of 19 antibiotics were used. This conclusion was based mainly on a 2-year study of 38 subjects by Weaver et al.,[159] who found that long-term use of prophylactic antistaphylococcal antibiotic treatment reduced the frequency of sputum S. aureus isolates, reduced cough frequency and reduced the number of antibiotic courses and hospital admissions. The review by McCaffery et al.[158] suggested that long-term antibiotic use led to the development of resistant strains, although this was less of a problem with flucloxacillin. In a

Cochrane Review of prophylactic antibiotics for cystic fibrosis, Smyth and Walters[160] concluded that 'anti-staphylococcal antibiotic prophylaxis may be of benefit when commenced early in infancy and continued up to three years of age' but there was 'insufficient evidence . . . to say whether use in older children or adults or for periods of over 3 years is beneficial'. Those caring for adolescent or adult patients require additional evidence from RCTs to assist them with decisions as to whether to continue antistaphylococcal therapy whether or not PA infection has occurred. Although not seen in the study by Weaver et al.,[159] the use of these antibiotics may increase the rate at which subjects acquire PA. A study of CF patients in the European Register of Cystic Fibrosis[161] showed that PA acquisition in the group receiving continuous antistaphylococcal therapy was significantly higher than in those receiving no or only intermittent therapy. This effect was greatest in the 0–6 years age group. This raises concerns that benefits associated with the suppression of S. aureus may be offset by the detrimental effect of PA acquisition.

Control of inflammation

Oral corticosteroids

Corticosteroids are potent, non-specific, anti-inflammatory agents, which have been demonstrated in asthma to reduce both inflammation and AHR. Although closely related to infection, the inflammatory response in the airways in CF occurs early in life,[24–26] may be present even in those without clinical manifestations and contributes to the progressive lung damage in CF. That the humoral response may be detrimental is suggested by the study by Wheeler et al.,[162] in which CF children with low serum IgG had better respiratory status than those with normal or high IgG levels. Up to half of CF patients have measurable AHR, which seems to be independent of the presence of atopy.[163,164] Although not a universal finding, airway responsiveness was related to baseline FEV_1,[136] suggesting that changes in airway geometry and increased inner wall area amplify the response of the airway to constrictor agents.[165] Thus, it seems logical that anti-inflammatory therapy including oral and inhaled steroids should be trialled in CF.

In a Cochrane Review of oral steroids in CF, Cheng et al.[166] identified three trials[167–169] involving 354 subjects aged 1–19.5 years with mild to moderate lung disease. They concluded that oral corticosteroids at a prednisone-equivalent dose of 1–2 mg/kg slowed the progression of lung disease but that this benefit was outweighed by the occurrence of adverse effects, particularly cataracts and growth retardation.

The most comprehensive and detailed trial was that by Eigen et al.,[169] who undertook a multicentre, randomized, double-blind, placebo-controlled trial involving 285 CF subjects aged 6–14 years with baseline FEV_1 of >60% predicted. Subjects received prednisone 2 mg/kg or 1 mg/kg on alternate days or placebo. An excess of adverse events resulted in the high-dose prednisone (2 mg/kg on alternate days) being discontinued prematurely 3 years after accrual of patients commenced, and low-dose prednisone (1 mg/kg on alternate days) was discontinued a year later. At 48 months, there had been a decline in the FEV_1 of the placebo group from 79% to 73% predicted but no change in FEV_1 in the 1-mg/kg group. Interestingly, there was no difference between the change in FEV_1 in the 2-mg/kg and placebo groups. An adverse effect on growth was evident in the 2-mg/kg group by 6 months but not until 24 months in the 1-mg/kg group. At 24 months, the mean change in height Z-scores was + 0.02% for the placebo group, –0.1% for the 1-mg/kg group and –0.3% for the 2-mg/kg group. Lai et al.[170] examined the growth patterns of these children during the 6–7 years after discontinuation of steroids. Although there was evidence of catch-up growth 2 years after discontinuation of steroids, the Z-scores for height in boys remained significantly lower in those who received steroids compared with those who received placebo; at 18 years, height in those who received 1 mg/kg was 170.7 cm compared with 174.5 cm in the placebo group. In girls, there was no significant difference in height between those who received steroids or placebo. Eigen et al.[169] reported that, during the first 24 months, cataracts were seen more often in subjects in the 2-mg/kg prednisone group ($n = 11$) compared with the 1-mg/kg group ($n = 3$) but, curiously, seven in the placebo group developed cataracts. Abnormalities in glucose metabolism were seen more often in the 2-mg/kg group than in the 1-mg/kg group ($P < 0.05$), but there was no difference between the 1-mg/kg and placebo groups. Hospitalization rate was virtually the same in the three groups.

Therefore, although use of oral steroids may provide benefit in terms of maintaining lung function and slowing the progression of lung disease, these benefits need to be balanced against adverse effects, particularly growth retardation, cataracts and glucose intolerance. There was no evidence of benefit from steroids in terms of hospitalization, and effects on HRQL were not assessed. In view of the relatively well-maintained lung function at baseline, it is unlikely that an effect on survival could be demonstrated except with long-term follow-up. Hence, long-term oral corticosteroids are not generally recommended in CF (in the absence of ABPA).

Inhaled corticosteroids

While it is unlikely that further RCTs of long-term oral corticosteroids at the above doses could be justified, good-quality RCTs of inhaled corticosteroids (ICS) seem more appropriate. ICS may be indicated for the treatment of AHR, to decrease airway inflammation and to reduce the progressive decline in FEV_1. In a Cochrane Review of ICS for CF, Dezateux et al.[171] identified nine trials, which included 266 subjects aged 7–45 years. Four of these were only available in the form of abstracts. The studies were heterogeneous with respect to inclusion criteria, age of subjects, severity of lung disease, presence of AHR and chronic infection with PA. Trials also differed in

design, as well as in the type, dose and duration of inhaled steroids. Even data on lung function could not be combined for analysis. The authors concluded that current evidence is insufficient to establish whether there is a beneficial (or detrimental) effect of inhaled steroids.

The UK trial[172] was a double-blind, placebo-controlled, randomized sequence, crossover trial of dry powder fluticasone (400 mg/day) in 23 children (mean age 10.3 years) with baseline FEV_1 of 64% predicted. No significant benefit was shown for the use of fluticasone in any of the clinical outcomes, although levels of IL-8 but not other inflammatory markers were reduced. The response to inhaled steroids was not predicted by atopic status, baseline FEV_1 or concomitant use of rhDNase. The Danish trial[173] was a placebo-controlled, parallel group, double-blind, single-centre trial of 3 months of budesonide dry powder (800 μg bd) in 55 stable CF subjects (mean age 20 years and baseline FEV_1 of 63% predicted) chronically infected with PA. After 3 months, the FEV_1 had fallen by 32 mL in the budesonide group compared with 187 mL in the placebo group, while at the conclusion of the trial the changes were +2 and –98 mL, respectively, with neither comparison being statistically significantly different. There was a substantial drop-out rate, and only 42 subjects completed the trial. However, those on budesonide had a reduction in responsiveness to histamine (compared with the placebo group) and, although the magnitude of the change is not likely to be clinically significant, there was a correlation between pretrial histamine responsiveness and response to inhaled steroids.

Thus, while there is some 'proof of concept', current evidence does not support the effectiveness of inhaled steroids in CF, which contrasts with the widespread use of these agents in CF.[124]

Non-steroidal anti-inflammatory agents

As chronic inflammation, particularly in association with chronic PA, plays a major role in progressive pulmonary deterioration, and as ibuprofen attenuates the inflammatory response in a rat model of chronic PA endobronchial infection and inflammation,[174] clinical trials of ibuprofen in CF to assess efficacy and adverse effects were a logical step. In a Cochrane Review, Dezateux and Crighton[175] identified three trials involving 145 subjects and concluded that, although there was preliminary evidence to suggest that non-steroidal anti-inflammatory drugs may prevent progression of pulmonary disease in persons with mild CF lung disease, routine use was not recommended.

Two trials of ibuprofen in CF children with mild lung disease were from the same centre and included some of the same patients. The first of these trials[176] focused on pharmacokinetics and was a 3-month dose evaluation study. The second study,[177] the largest assessing the role of non-steroidal anti-inflammatory agents in CF, was a randomized, double-blind, placebo-controlled parallel group study in 85 subjects, aged

5–39 years of age, with mild/moderate lung disease (FEV$_1$ ≥60% predicted). Subjects took either ibuprofen or placebo for a period of 4 years. The primary outcome variable, FEV$_1$, declined significantly more slowly in the patients assigned to ibuprofen than in those assigned to placebo (annual rate of change –2.17 ± 0.57% versus –3.6 ± 0.55%, $P = 0.02$). Those using ibuprofen also had a slower rate of decline in FVC, higher percentage ideal body weight and better chest radiograph score, but there was no difference in the frequency of hospitalization. The beneficial effect was particularly evident in those less than 13 years of age at the time of initiating therapy. Ibuprofen was well tolerated. However, a feature of this study was that the doses of ibuprofen were individually adjusted to achieve plasma concentrations within a certain range. The requirement for this complex pharmacokinetic adjustment has meant that, despite its apparent effectiveness, the use of ibuprofen has not become widespread.

The current evidence for the generalizability of the effectiveness of non-steroidal anti-inflammatory drugs (NSAIDs) in CF is limited. In a small, randomized, double-blind, placebo-controlled study of 41 CF subjects aged 5–37 years with chronic PA infection, Sordelli et al.[178] found that those who received piroxicam (5–20 mg based on weight) for 12–19 months had a trend towards reduced days in hospital. Further long-term studies are required to confirm the effectiveness of NSAIDs, to determine whether this is a property of ibuprofen alone or a class effect, whether the beneficial effects can be achieved without complex pharmacokinetic monitoring and whether there are clinical subgroups for whom the drugs may be more effective such as those with mild lung disease in whom only minor structural damage has occurred.

Macrolide therapy

Macrolide antibiotics are ineffective against PA but are known to have immunomodulatory properties, mediated by inhibition of neutrophil chemotaxis,[179] reduction of neutrophil elastase, suppression of pro-inflammatory cytokines such as IL-1, IL-6, IL-8[180] and TNF-α[181] and reduced activity of alveolar macrophages.[181–184] Macrolides may also have effects directly relevant to PA—they reduce airway adhesion of PA, disrupt the integrity of the protective biofilm, inhibit flagella synthesis and motility, suppress virulence factors and impair the transformation of non-mucoid PA to the more virulent mucoid phenotype.[184–186]

Diffuse panbronchiolitis (DPB), a condition with a high prevalence in Japan but rare elsewhere, has a number of similarities to CF; in both, there is chronic productive cough, exertional dyspnoea, airflow obstruction, frequent mucoid PA colonization, marked neutrophil airway inflammation and bronchiectasis.[187] Macrolide treatment for DPB has had a dramatic effect on outcome, increasing the 10-year survival from 12–22% to >90% in those colonized with PA.[183,188] These effects seem to be a class effect of macrolides, having been demonstrated with clarithromycin, roxithromycin and azithromycin.[183,189] Of the newer macrolides, an azalide, azithromycin, has shown the greatest in vitro activity against virulence factors of PA[190] and also has benefits in terms of safety, tolerability, oral bioavailability, marked accumulation in the lungs and sputum and a long duration of action.

Initial, open, non-randomized studies reported improvements in lung function with macrolides (azithromycin).[191] In a prospective, randomized, placebo-controlled trial of azithromycin (250 mg/day for 3 months) in 60 stable CF adults (mean age 28 years, mean FEV$_1$ of 56% predicted, 88% with mucoid PA), Wolter et al.[192] found that the use of azithromycin was associated with fewer courses of intravenous antibiotics, better maintenance of lung function, reduction in mean C-reactive protein levels and improved quality of life scores. There was no change in sputum microbiology. The drug was well tolerated, and no significant adverse effects were observed apart from an urticarial response in one patient on azithromycin. Despite randomization, there were baseline differences between the groups in terms of gender, lung function and weight. Statistical analysis adjusted for baseline differences, and the authors stated that the differences would have biased the results in favour of a reduced effect of azithromycin.

Equi et al.[193] undertook a 15-month, randomized, double-blind, placebo-controlled, crossover trial of azithromycin in 41 CF children (aged 8–18 years). The median relative difference in FEV$_1$ between azithromycin and placebo groups was 5.4% (95% CI 0.8–10.5). However, there was no difference between the groups in terms of exercise tolerance, quality of life or sputum microbiology.

The North American CF Foundation-sponsored multicentre, randomized, placebo-controlled, double-blind trial of 6 months of azithromycin (weight-adjusted dose) in CF patients (mean age 20 years, FEV$_1$ of 69% predicted, chronically infected with PA) found that those on azithromycin had significant improvements in FEV$_1$ (44.4% versus –1.8%, $P = 0.001$), a 40% reduction in exacerbations, reduced hospitalization (16% versus 30%, $P = 0.05$), improved weight gain and improvements in HRQL. The improvements in lung function occurred by day 28 and were sustained throughout the trial. There was no change in sputum microbiology. A high proportion of subjects were using TOBI and/or rhDNase, suggesting that the effect of azithromycin may be additive to these other treatments (NACFF website). Furthermore, the magnitude of impact of azithromycin on lung function and reduction in hospitalization compared favourably with those obtained in phase III studies of rhDNase[118] and high-dose inhaled tobramycin (TOBI).[144]

Despite these promising results, further studies are needed to define the most appropriate dose and dosing schedule of azithromycin, whether this is a class effect of all macrolides and to determine the impact of long-term treatment on disease progression and the microbiological environment.

Other treatments

Bronchodilatory therapy

Wheeze and airflow obstructions are well-recognized features of CF lung disease.[194] Longitudinal studies have demonstrated a high prevalence of bronchodilator responsiveness, although this is inconsistent over time and may relate in part to exacerbations of lung disease[187,188] but, seemingly, not to atopy or history of wheeze.[195,196] Others have found that bronchodilator responsiveness increases as lung function deteriorates and the airways become more structurally damaged.[197] Those with AHR are most likely to have bronchodilator responsiveness.[197]

Cropp[198] suggested that most patients with CF are likely to benefit from bronchodilators. Unfortunately, there is very little evidence on which to determine the extent of benefit, the most appropriate dose or the effect of drug combinations with respect to long-term use. Acute studies have demonstrated that some but not all CF patients have a greater response to combined SABAs and antimuscarinic agents than either used alone,[199,200] but few long-term studies have been performed. In a double-blind, placebo-controlled, crossover trial of albuterol (by metered dose inhaler), 180 mg bd, in 21 CF patients,[201] there was no significant difference in spirometric lung volumes between the two groups, although there was a non-statistically significant reduction in days of hospitalization in the albuterol group. Concerns have been expressed with regard to the possibility of bronchodilators paradoxically worsening pulmonary function by making airways more compressible[202,203] or by causing non-homogeneous lung emptying,[204,205] but this seems to be clinically relevant only infrequently. Nevertheless, the use of bronchodilators is widespread,[124] probably because patients perceive benefit.

Because of their duration of action, long-acting β-sympathomimetic agents (LABAs) may be more useful in CF. Hordvik et al.[206] undertook a randomized, double-blind, double-dummy, placebo-controlled, crossover (24-week periods) trial of salmeterol (100 μg bd) versus nebulized albuterol (2.5 mg bd) in 19 subjects. There was a significant decrease from baseline in FEV_1 with albuterol compared with salmeterol (−6.5% versus 1.7%, $P = 0.002$). More rescue medication was required while on albuterol, as well as more antibiotic interventions, and subjects had higher symptom scores. Importantly, there was no correlation between the acute bronchodilator response and long-term response to LABA. This supports other data that a recommendation for long-term bronchodilator therapy should not be based upon a single acute bronchodilator response. Also, there was no relationship between response to LABA and the baseline impairment of lung function. Thus, while there is information supporting the use of LABAs in CF, future studies of LABAs are required to address issues including optimal dose, the impact on other physiological variables, as some of the benefits may not be reflected in FEV_1, and the benefits of co-administration with inhaled steroids and/or long-acting antimuscarinic agents (tiotropium).

Theophylline

The role of long-term oral theophylline has not been fully evaluated. The lack of clinical trials in the last decade, the modest effects of these agents in asthma, the potential adverse effects including behavioural and sleep effects and the need to monitor blood levels make it unlikely that theophylline would have a major clinical role. The newer phosphodiesterase 4 inhibitors have not been trialled in CF.

Leukotriene antagonists

Leukotriene (Lt) B_4 is a potent neutrophil chemoattractant that inhibits neutrophil apoptosis and induces release of elastase and oxygen free radicals. There is evidence that it is involved in CF lung pathophysiology,[207] but there are no published trials of 5-lipoxygenase inhibitors or Lt B_4 antagonists in CF.

Cysteinyl leukotrienes (C_4, D_4, E_4) are also involved in the pathophysiology of CF lung disease[207] and, although an open study of leukotriene receptor antagonists in CF was promising,[208] no longer term methodologically robust RCTs have been undertaken.

Influenza vaccination

Observational studies have suggested adverse effects in terms of lung function and disease progression in CF patients following influenza A virus infections.[200,210] Johansen and Hoiby[211] found that the majority of patients are first infected with PA during the winter months and speculated that respiratory viral infections may 'pave the way' for chronic infection by PA. Many units recommend annual influenza vaccination to their CF patients.

Currently available influenza vaccines give 70–80% protection and need to be repeated each year because the principal surface antigen (haemagglutinin) of influenza A and B undergoes frequent change. Commonly used influenza vaccines contain two influenza A viruses or virus particles and one influenza B virus particle (trivalent vaccine) to increase effectiveness. A Cochrane Review of this subject[212] included four trials involving 179 subjects, 80% of whom were children aged 1–16 years. There was no study comparing a vaccine with placebo or whole-virus vaccine with a subunit or split-virus vaccine. Two studies compared an intranasal applied live virus vaccine with an intramuscular inactivated virus vaccine, and the other studies compared a split-virus with a subunit vaccine and a virosome with a subunit vaccine (all intramuscular). The incidence of adverse effects was high but depended on the type of vaccine, being highest for the split-virus vaccine. Although limited by statistical power, there were no differences in outcomes demonstrated between the study vaccinations. Thus, there is no evidence of benefit from annual influenza vaccination to CF subjects, and any potential benefit in individual patients needs to be balanced against possible side-effects.

Long-term oxygen therapy (LTOT)

As severe lung disease develops, CF patients may develop hypoxaemia, particularly during sleep. Pulmonary hypertension in adults with CF is strongly correlated with hypoxaemia and is associated with increased mortality.[213] Nocturnal oxygen desaturation can be improved by nocturnal oxygen therapy,[214,215] although this may be accompanied by increases in Pa_{CO_2}.[215,216] However, studies of LTOT in CF have failed to demonstrate improved survival. Zinman et al.[217] undertook a double-blind, randomized trial of 28 subjects with advanced CF and an awake Pa_{O_2} of <65 mmHg (8.7 kPa). Supplemental oxygen flow rates, via nasal prongs, were adjusted to increase Pa_{O_2} to ≥70 mmHg (9.3 kPa). After 3 years, the group receiving oxygen was not different in terms of number of deaths, frequency of hospitalization or progression of disease. However, school or work attendance was better in the oxygen group. Thus, while there is some evidence to support the use of LTOT in CF, larger long-term studies of LTOT with more relevant outcome measures including HRQL are required.

Bilevel ventilatory support

CF patients with advanced lung disease develop hypoxaemia and hypercapnia. These are poor prognostic factors[19] and are more likely to occur during rapid eye movement (REM) sleep. Bilevel non-invasive ventilation has been used in CF as a bridge to transplantation[218] and for the relief of symptoms such as morning headache as part of palliative care management. Gozal[216] showed that non-invasive ventilation was more effective than oxygen therapy in controlling Pa_{CO_2} during sleep. In a study of 13 adult CF subjects with mean predicted FEV_1 of 32% and nocturnal oxygen desaturation, Milross et al.[219] found that bilevel ventilatory support attenuated the REM-associated fall in O_2 saturation and rise in Pa_{CO_2}; these effects were attributed to improvements in alveolar ventilation. Thus, bilevel ventilation may be useful in certain circumstances in which RCTs are unlikely ever to be performed and where n-of-1 trials of therapy may be more relevant. There are no reported RCTs of the effect of long-term, non-invasive ventilation on the development of chronic daytime hypoxaemia and hypercapnia and subsequently on mortality or morbidity in CF patients with severe lung disease.

Transplantation

As the major cause of death among patients with CF is end-stage respiratory disease, lung transplantation is a therapeutic option to be considered in many patients.[220] Bilateral sequential lung transplantation is the procedure of choice in most centres. While criteria for assessment and transplantation will vary between units, patients are generally considered for transplant assessment when they have a life expectancy of less than 2 years, i.e. when the FEV_1 falls below 30% predicted.[19]

Liou et al.[221] reported that only those with FEV_1 <30% predicted had improved 5-year survival after lung transplantation. More recently, Mayer-Hamblett et al.[222] developed and validated predictors for 2-year mortality using the largest available data set. However, the model was no better at predicting 2-year mortality than FEV_1 criteria alone. Both methods had high negative predictive values and low positive predictive values, i.e. both can predict reasonably well who will survive 2 years, but neither can predict well who will die within 2 years. Thus, choosing the correct time to list a CF patient for transplantation is difficult, and other factors, including the rate of deterioration of the overall status of the patient, the rate of decline in FEV_1 and waiting time for donor availability, need to be taken into account. In general, it is far better to refer the patient to the transplant team for assessment too early rather than too late. In the latter situation, the patient may be too sick to survive the waiting time or to undergo intensive rehabilitation and preparation for surgery. Death on the waiting list for transplantation is more likely for CF patients than for other potential recipients. With increasing experience, the previous strict contraindications have been relaxed, although factors such as active infection with Aspergillus spp., mycobacteria or panresistant bacteria, the presence of gross malnutrition, high-dose steroid therapy and non-adherence with therapy are still regarded as relative and, in some cases, absolute contraindications. However, in most centres, the scarcity of donor organs is the limiting factor.

CF is now the single commonest condition for which bilateral lung transplantation is undertaken.[220] Although there are no RCTs of this treatment, the major benefit from transplantation is considered to be the improvement in quality of life, with many patients able to return to employment or education. However, those transplanted with an FEV_1 <30% predicted had improved 5-year survival.[221] The outcome for transplantation in CF is similar to that for lung transplantation generally, viz. approximately 70% survival at 1 year, 60% at 2 years and falling to 50% at 5 years.[220] The group from Sydney have reported 1- and 7-year survivals post transplant of 92% and 56%, respectively, in the first 100 CF patients transplanted at their institution.[223] While CF does not recur in the transplanted lung, those who have undergone lung transplantation have had the usual problems of infection and rejection as well as increased likelihood of problems associated with glucose intolerance, metabolic bone disease and inconstant drug absorption. While acute rejection occurs most commonly in the first 3 months after transplantation, the most serious late complication is that of obliterative bronchiolitis.

Nutritional supplements

Although this article has focused on respiratory aspects of management of adult CF, maintenance of nutrition is such an important aspect of management that brief mention will be made. Malnutrition may be a problem in CF adults and is associated with a poorer outcome. Malnutrition is multifactorial, and causes include reduced intake due to nausea and anorexia, malabsorption, caloric loss as in diabetes, increased energy requirements due to the chronic inflammatory process in the lungs,[224] the increased work of breathing and the increased energy requirements associated with the basic defect of CF.[225] Despite the presumed importance of maintenance of nutritional status in CF and the widespread use of both oral caloric supplements and enteral tube feeding, the evidence supporting their use is lacking. In a Cochrane Review, Smyth and Walters[226] found only two trials (involving 29 patients) of oral caloric supplements. These demonstrated no differences in outcome between the intervention and comparison groups. In another Cochrane Review, Conway et al.[227] found no suitable trials of enteral tube feeding in CF. The need for good-quality RCTs is obvious, but it is doubtful whether placebo-controlled trials will ever be conducted for ethical reasons given the accepted and widespread use of these treatments. Clinicians must balance the potential benefits of such treatments against possible adverse effects and the negative impact of further treatments on an individual patient's quality of life.

Treatment of exacerbations

Exacerbations are the commonest reason for admission in CF and are a major contributor to the cost of treatment, yet the quality of information guiding this aspect of management is poor (see Table 2).

Antibiotics

In mild and moderate disease, much of the morbidity from CF

Table 2. Management of respiratory exacerbations of cystic fibrosis.

Beneficial
    Once-daily use of aminoglycosides

Likely to be beneficial
    Intravenous anti-pseudomonal antibiotics
    Airway clearance techniques
    Exercise therapy
    Inhaled bronchodilators

Trade-off between benefit and harm
    Home intravenous therapy
    Parenteral corticosteroids
    Oxygen therapy
    Non-invasive ventilation

Unknown effectiveness
    Use of >1 intravenous antibiotic
    Nebulized hyperosmolar agents

Unlikely to be beneficial
    Nebulized DNase
    Nebulized amiloride

---

is associated with acute 'infective' exacerbations, although the precise role of various microorganisms is not clear. Such episodes are characterized by increased respiratory symptoms (cough, sputum production, shortness of breath and sometimes haemoptysis), decline in lung function and non-specific symptoms (fever, lassitude, anaemia and sometimes weight loss), but new infiltrates on the chest radiograph are uncommon. Although there is some evidence that viruses may play a role in some episodes, it is generally assumed that most exacerbations are due to bacteria. While most would argue that morbidity associated with exacerbations is reduced by antibiotic use, most decisions regarding when to treat, which antibiotics to use, by what route and for how long are largely empirical but partly based on patient's age, the colonizing organisms, antibiotic sensitivity profiles and the severity of the exacerbation.

Because of greater total body clearance and volume of distribution,[228] antibiotic dosages in CF need to be higher than in non-CF persons. Furthermore, it is presumed to be necessary to achieve therapeutic levels in the airway wall and mucus-filled lumen as well as in the lung parenchyma. In those not colonized by PA, antibiotic choice tends to be based on results of sputum culture or on extrapolations of data from community-acquired pneumonia or chronic obstructive pulmonary disease (COPD) studies. No RCTs of antibiotic therapy of exacerbations have been conducted in this group.

In those chronically colonized by PA, this organism is generally assumed to play a role in exacerbations, although the lack of correlation between quantitative PA cultures and clinical outcome argues somewhat against this. The effectiveness of antibiotics against PA is compromised by the intrinsic resistance of this microorganism. Although results of sputum culture may be considered to guide antibiotic therapy, data on resistance patterns are complex because of multiple strains of PA being present in many individual patients[39] and the inability to reliably identify individual strains on the basis of phenotypic characteristics. There is no evidence in CF relating clinical outcome to the appropriateness of antibiotic therapy based on the results of sensitivity testing of sputum cultures. Smith et al.,[229] in an analysis of exacerbations of CF occurring during a large RCT, found no correlation between in vitro sensitivity of PA and response to antibiotic therapy.

Oral antibiotics with activity against PA are currently limited to the quinolones, specifically ciprofloxacin. Ciprofloxacin use is limited by concerns about cartilage toxicity in young children (although subsequent studies have not justified the concern[230]), the rapid emergence of resistance[231] and other adverse effects including tendonitis and tendon rupture.[232]

The conventional approach for more severe exacerbations has been to admit the patient to hospital for a 10- to 14-day course of intravenous antibiotics, which includes antipseudomonal therapy in those with chronic PA infection. Although there has been a tendency to ascribe the improved outcome in CF to the use of more effective antibiotics, Geddes,[233] in a review of antimicrobial therapy, concluded that 'empiricism is still ahead of science and more studies are needed to both justify current practice and to make future changes logical'. Indeed, the role of antipseudomonal antibiotics in the treatment of CF exacerbations has been questioned, with some justification. In an earlier double-blind trial of intravenous tobramycin versus placebo by Weintzen et al.,[234] the placebo group fared badly, but they had worse baseline disease. In a randomized trial of 31 courses of ceftazidime versus placebo in 26 patients, Gold et al.[235] found no significant differences between the groups in terms of clinical or lung function parameters. Regelmann et al.[236] conducted a double-blind, placebo-controlled trial in which patients ($n = 12$) were randomized to receive either parenteral tobramycin and ticarcillin or placebo. For the first 4 days of the study, when all patients received bronchodilator aerosols and chest physiotherapy but no antibiotics, FEV_1 improved by 6.6% predicted, and there were also improvements in weight. During the subsequent 14 days, the group receiving antibiotics had greater increases in FEV_1 (16% versus 0%), and this improvement correlated with reduction in PA sputum density. Although the sputum bacterial density in the antibacterial group had returned to pretreatment levels within 2 weeks of cessation of antibiotic therapy, they entered the follow-up period with better lung function, and a greater time elapsed before they returned for medical care. This trial provided support for the use of bronchodilators, chest physiotherapy combined with antipseudomonal therapy. Wolter et al.[237] found that PA sputum colony counts did not change during or after IV antibiotic therapy (ceftazidime plus tobramycin for 12 days) despite clinical improvement, and there was no relationship between colony counts and clinical or lung function criteria. This study raised inconsistencies about the role of PA and anti-PA antibiotics, and this issue certainly warrants further critical bacteriological and clinical evaluation.

The use of two antibiotics with different pharmacological activities is generally considered to enhance the likelihood of therapeutic success; there may be advantages in terms of wider range of modes of action, possible synergy and reduced rate of emergent resistance. In vitro, double antibiotic combination therapy appears to be more effective than monotherapy.[238] On the other hand, monotherapy has advantages in terms of lower cost, ease of administration (particularly on an outpatient basis), reduced drug toxicity and may obviate the need for drug monitoring. The use of single versus combination intravenous antibiotic therapy for exacerbations of CF has been the subject of a Cochrane Review by Elphick and Tan.[239] They identified nine studies with 386 patients that compared a single agent with a combination of the same antibiotic plus one other. There was considerable variation in the antibiotics used. Eight of the studies compared a β-lactam antibiotic (penicillin-related or third-generation cephalosporin) with a β-lactam–aminoglycoside combination, whereas three compared an aminoglycoside alone with a β-lactam–aminoglycoside combination. Three of the trials were available only in abstract form. Although there was considerable heterogeneity among the trials, the meta-analysis did not demonstrate any significant differences between monotherapy and combination therapy in terms of lung function, symptom scores or adverse effects. There was some evidence that single therapy was associated with an increase in resistant strains of PA at 2–8 weeks of follow-up (OR 2.54, 95 CI 1.13–5.68), but longer term effects are not known. The authors of the meta-analysis indicated that these results should be interpreted with caution as all but two of the trials were published between 1977 and 1988, were small single-centre studies and most had serious methodological flaws. Of the two trials published since 1988, one is available only as an abstract. The other trial by Smith et al.[240] compared azlocillin plus placebo with azlocillin plus tobramycin in 76 CF patients with exacerbations of their lung disease. No difference was seen between the groups in terms of clinical evaluation, sputum DNA levels or spirometric lung volumes. Time to readmission for a pulmonary exacerbation was significantly longer in the azlocillin plus tobramycin group, although emergence of tobramycin-resistant organisms was greater.

Thus, there is insufficient evidence to determine whether combination therapy is superior to monotherapy. Furthermore, there is no clear evidence from RCTs of clear superiority of any single antibiotic or combination over any other(s). Considering the frequency with which antibiotics are used in CF, there is certainly the need for further well-designed, sufficiently powered RCTs of antibiotic therapy in CF exacerbations.

The majority of those receiving combination antibiotic therapy receive an aminoglycoside. These agents demonstrate concentration-dependent killing and post-antibiotic effect,[241] which suggest that these agents could be given in higher concentrations with extended dosing intervals. The efficacy of once-daily dosing has been demonstrated in non-CF patients, but these results could not simply be extrapolated to the CF population because of more rapid plasma clearance in CF patients.[242] In a Cochrane Review of once-daily versus multiple-daily dosing with intravenous aminoglycosides in CF, Tan and Bunn[243] concluded from three trials involving 175 subjects that once-daily dosing did not differ from thrice-daily dosing in terms of effects on lung function and nutrition, or in terms of ototoxicity or nephrotoxicity. Although these results need to be interpreted with caution because of the relatively small subject numbers, there is evidence to support the use of once-daily aminoglycosides in CF, which has advantages in terms of convenience and cost.

Home IV antibiotics have been considered in CF in an effort to ensure that treatment interferes as little as possible with the patient's normal lifestyle and quality of life and in an effort to reduce health care costs. Although the question of the effectiveness of home IV therapy has been subjected to a Cochrane Review,[244] this is based on a single study.[245] Wolter et al.[237] undertook a prospective, randomized trial in adults (17 subjects,

31 admissions) presenting with exacerbations of CF. The antibiotic regimen used was ceftazidime 2 mg/12-hourly and daily tobramycin. Patients were randomized such that they were discharged after 2–4 days or remained in hospital. After 10 days of therapy, there were no differences in terms of improvement in lung function, exercise tolerance, sputum weight or body weight. Patients who remained in hospital were less fatigued and had a greater degree of mastery, perhaps related to the unfamiliarity of IV treatment in the home environment. Patients discharged early noted less disruption to their family life, personal life and sleeping pattern. The total cost for the home therapy arm was approximately half that of the hospital therapy arm. Thus, home IV in CF patients is a feasible and cost-effective form of therapy that is not associated with clinical compromise and is associated with both advantages and disadvantages in terms of quality of life factors. It is important to reinforce the fact that, in this study, the home IV group had an initial (2–4 days) period of hospitalization and did not receive all treatment in the home environment.

Chest physiotherapy

This is an integral component of regular management of CF and, thus, it is logical to continue (or intensify) such therapy during an acute exacerbation. There remains considerable doubt as to the most appropriate method of clearing respiratory secretions. Homnick et al.[246] undertook an open, comparative trial with alternate assignment of either the Flutter device or standard chest physiotherapy in 22 CF patients aged 8–44 years who were hospitalized for acute pulmonary exacerbation. There were no differences between the groups in terms of improvements in clinical scores and lung function. Gondor et al.[247] randomized 23 patients, aged 5–21 years, admitted to hospital for 2 weeks' treatment of pulmonary exacerbation, to either Flutter device or standard chest physiotherapy (PD/CP). Although lung function was better in the Flutter group at 1 week, there were no differences between the groups in terms of lung function and exercise tolerance at 2 weeks. However, both studies were grossly underpowered, and future comparative studies of sputum clearance techniques need to be of sufficient size to demonstrate any real differences in clinically relevant outcomes.

As mentioned above, a recent Cochrane Review[110] concluded that exercise tolerance, in the short term during an acute admission, was improved by physical training. Thus, there is some evidence supporting the use of exercise training during periods of hospitalization.

DNase

In view of the pathophysiology of acute exacerbations and the benefits associated with long-term use of rhDNase, there are good theoretical reasons to consider the use of rhDNase in acute exacerbations. Wilmott et al.[123] undertook a multicentre, double-blind, placebo-controlled study of 80 patients, mean age 20 years and baseline FEV_1 of 40% predicted, presenting with an exacerbation of CF. Subjects were randomized to receive 2.5 mg of aerosolized rhDNase twice daily for 14 days or placebo. There were no statistically significant differences in the mean change in FEV_1 or dyspnoea score between the two groups at 2 weeks. Thus, there is no evidence to support the addition of rhDNase to a regimen of antibiotics and chest physiotherapy for acute exacerbations.

Other treatments that are often part of the treatment regimen for acute exacerbations include the following.

Bronchodilators

In view of the worsening of airflow obstruction and some evidence suggesting increased bronchodilator responsiveness during exacerbations,[195,196] bronchodilators are commonly used in the management of acute exacerbations. Hordvik et al.,[248] in a 2-day double-blind, placebo-controlled, randomized crossover study of 24 hospitalized patients, found that albuterol (salbutamol, 0.5 mL of 0.5% solution via nebulizer, three times per day) improved pulmonary function in the majority (75%), and there was a mean increase in FEV_1 of 14.8%; in no patient was bronchodilator therapy detrimental. However, pulmonary function declined overnight. Therefore, in a placebo-controlled, three-way, random crossover, double-blind trial of 18 hospitalized CF patients, Hordvik et al.[249] found that salmeterol (four puffs: 42 μg bid) compared favourably with nebulized albuterol (improvements in FEV_1 of 22.7% and 14.9% respectively) and produced a bronchodilator effect that persisted overnight. Higher dose salmeterol was more effective than standard dose. These improvements may be due to bronchodilation or enhanced clearance of mucus.

Oral corticosteroids

Whether short courses of oral steroids are useful for respiratory exacerbations of CF (in the absence of ABPA) has not been subjected to appropriately designed RCTs, but these agents are commonly used.

Hyperosmolar agents

There are no RCTs of nebulized hypertonic saline, inhaled mannitol or other hyperosmolar agents in acute exacerbations. However, these agents would seem to have enormous potential, and RCTs of these agents in acute exacerbations would seem to be a high priority.

Amiloride

Lung function was unaffected when amiloride was added to inpatient treatment of pulmonary exacerbations in an RCT involving 27 CF patients[250] and, thus, there is no indication to add this therapy to the treatment regimen.

Oxygen therapy

There are no RCTs of oxygen therapy as part of the management of acute exacerbations. Considering that the use of oxygen in those who are (transiently) hypoxaemic is widespread and is associated with a very low rate of adverse effects, it is unlikely that such trials will be undertaken. However, those with severe lung disease and chronic hypoxaemia are at risk of hypercapnia and acute respiratory acidosis with supplemental oxygen therapy.[215,216]

Non-invasive ventilation (NIV)

Madden et al.[251] reported their experience with NIV in 113 adult CF subjects with chronic respiratory failure during episodes of acute deterioration in respiratory function, found it to be effective and recommended its use, particularly for those who had been accepted, or were being evaluated, for transplantation. There are no clear indications for the use of this therapy, and use in persons who are not transplant candidates will depend on a number of factors but, first and foremost, the wishes of the patient and their family. There are no RCTs of NIV in acute or chronic respiratory failure in CF, and many clinicians will be tempted to extrapolate from the COPD recommendations.

Intensive care unit (ICU) admission

Criteria for admission to ICU will vary between centres, but the outcome following ICU admission is dependent on the primary indication for admission. Sood et al.[252] reviewed the outcome of all CF patients admitted to the University of North Carolina ICU. Some 86% of those admitted for haemoptysis or pneumothorax were alive 1 year after ICU discharge. Of those who required assisted ventilation, 55% survived the ICU admission and, of those not transplanted, only 7% were alive at 1 year. Hence, the decision regarding ICU admission depends on the clinical indication, the overall philosophy of management at the time and the wishes of the patient and their family.

References

1 Riordan JA, Rommens JM, Kerem B et al. Identification of the cystic fibrosis gene: cloning and characterisation of complementary DNA. Science 1989; 245:1066–73.

2 Zielenski J. Genotype and phenotype in cystic fibrosis. Respiration 2000; 67:117–33.

3 Hamosh A, Corey M. Correlation between genotype and phenotype in patients with cystic fibrosis. The Cystic Fibrosis Genotype–Phenotype Consortium. N Engl J Med 1993; 329:1308–13 (see also ref. 5).

4 Gan KH, Veeze HJ, van den Ouwland MW et al. A cystic fibrosis mutation associated with mild lung disease. N Engl J Med 1995; 333:95–9.

5 The Cystic Fibrosis Genotype–Phenotype Consortium. Correlation between genotype and phenotype in patients with cystic fibrosis. N Engl J Med 1993; 329:1308–13 (see also ref. 3).

6 Gan K, Guess WP, Bakker W et al. Genetic and clinical features of patients diagnosed with cystic fibrosis after the age of 16 years. Thorax 1995; 50:1301–4.

7 Schechter MS, Shelton BJ, Margolis PA, Fitzsimmons SC. The association of socio-economic status with outcomes in cystic fibrosis patients in the United States. Am J Respir Crit Care Med 2001; 163:1331–7.

8 Mahadeva R, Sharples L, Ross-Russell RI, Webb AK, Bilton D, Lomas DA. Association of α-1-antichymotrypsin deficiency with milder lung disease in patients with cystic fibrosis. Thorax 2001; 56:53–8.

9 Grasemann H, Storm van's Gravesande K, Buscher R et al. Endothelial nitric oxide synthase variants in cystic fibrosis lung disease. Am J Respir Crit Care Med 2003; 167:390–4.

10 Arkwright PD, Pravica V, Geraghty PJ et al. End-organ dysfunction in cystic fibrosis: association with angiotensin I converting enzyme and cytokine gene polymorphisms. Am J Respir Crit Care Med 2003; 167:384–9.

11 Friedman KJ, Heim RA, Knowles MR, Silverman LM. Rapid characterisation of the variable length polythymidine tract in the cystic fibrosis (CFTR) gene: association of the 5T allele with selected CFTR mutations and its incidence in atypical non-pulmonary disease. Hum Mutat 1997; 10:108–15.

12 Gervois R, Lafitte J-J, Dunmur V et al. Sweat chloride and ∅F508 mutation in chronic bronchitis or bronchiectasis. Lancet 1993; 342:997.

13 Giroden E, Cazeneune C, Lebargy F et al. CFTR gene mutations in adults with disseminated bronchiectasis. Eur J Hum Genet 1997; 5:149–55.

14 Shorer N, Schwarz M, Malone G et al. Mutations of the cystic fibrosis gene in patients with chronic pancreatitis. N Engl J Med 1998; 339:645–52.

15 Anderson DH. Cystic fibrosis of the pancreas and its relation to celiac disease. A clinical and pathologic study. Am J Child 1938; 56:344–99.

16 Elborn JS, Shale DJ, Britton JR. Cystic fibrosis: current survival and population estimates to the year 2000. Thorax 1991; 46:881–5.

17 Epidemiologic Registry of Cystic Fibrosis Advisory Board. CRCF Annual Report 1998. North Ryde, NSW.

18 Fitzsimmons SC. The changing epidemiology of cystic fibrosis. J Pediatr 1993; 122:1–9.

19 Kerem E, Reisman J, Carey M et al. Prediction of mortality in patients with cystic fibrosis. N Engl J Med 1992; 326:1187–91.

20 Sharma R, Florea VC, Bolger AP et al. Wasting as an independent predictor of mortality in patients with cystic fibrosis. Thorax 2001; 56:746–50.

21 Blair E, Cull A, Freeman CP. Psychosocial functioning of young adults with cystic fibrosis and their families. Thorax 1994; 49:798–802.

22 Matsui H, Grubb BR, Tarron R et al. Evidence for periciliary liquid layer depletion, not abnormal ion composition, in the pathogenesis of cystic fibrosis airway disease. Cell 1998; 95:1005–15.

23 Smith JJ, Travis SM, Greenberg EP, Welsh MJ. Cystic fibrosis airway epithelia fail to kill bacteria because of abnormal airway surface fluid. Cell 1996; 85:229–36.

24 Konstan MW, Hilliard KA, Norwell TM, Berger M. Bronchoalveolar lavage findings in cystic fibrosis patients with stable, clinically mild lung disease suggests ongoing infection and inflammation. Am J Respir Crit Care Med 1994; 150:448–54.

25 Armstrong DS, Grimwood K, Carlin JB et al. Lower airway inflammation in infants and young children with cystic fibrosis. Am J Respir Crit Care Med 1997; 156:1197–204.

26 Dakin Cj, Numa AH, Wang H, Morton JR, Vertzyas CC, Henry RL. Inflammation, infection, and pulmonary function in infants and young children with cystic fibrosis. Am J Respir Crit Care Med 2002; 165:904–10.

27 Muhlebach MS, Noah TL. Endotoxin activity and inflammatory markers in the airways of young patients with cystic fibrosis. Am J Respir Crit Care Med 2002; 165:911–15.

28 Van der Vliet A, Nguyen MN, Shigenoga MK, Eiserich JP, Marelich GP, Cross CE. Myeloperoxidase and protein oxidation in cystic fibrosis. *Am J Physiol Lung Cell Mol Physiol* 2000; **279**:L537–46.

29 Torrens JK, Dawkins P, Conway SP, Moya E. Non-tuberculous mycobacteria in cystic fibrosis. *Thorax* 1998; **53**:182–5.

30 Spector ML, Stern RC. Pneumothorax in cystic fibrosis: a 26 year experience. *Ann Thorac Surg* 1989; **47**:204–7.

31 Antonelli M, Midulla F, Tancredi G *et al*. Bronchial artery embolization for the management of nonmassive hemoptysis in cystic fibrosis. *Chest* 2002; **121**:796–801.

32 Barben J, Robertson D, Olinsky A, Ditchfield M. Bronchial artery embolization for hemoptysis in young patients with cystic fibrosis. *Radiology* 2002; **224**:124–30.

33 Becker JW, Burke W, McDonald G *et al*. Prevalence of allergic bronchopulmonary aspergillosis and atopy in adult patients with cystic fibrosis. *Chest* 1996; **109**:1536–40.

34 Greenberger PA. Allergic bronchopulmonary aspergillus. *J Allergy Clin Immunol* 2002; **110**:685–92.

35 Duff AJA. Psychological consequences of segregation resulting from chronic *Burkholderia cepacia* complex infection in adults with CF. *Thorax* 2002; **57**:758.

36 Ledson MJ, Gallagher MJ, Jackson M, Hart CA, Walshaw MJ. Outcome of *Burkholderia cepacia* colonisation in an adult cystic fibrosis centre. *Thorax* 2002; **57**:142–5.

37 Pitt TL, Kaufmann ME, Patel PS *et al*. Type characteristics and antibiotic susceptibility of *Burkholderia* (*Pseudomonas*) *cepacia* isolates from patients with cystic fibrosis in the UK and the Republic of Ireland. *J Microbiol* 1996; **44**:203–10.

38 Wallace RJ Jr, Glassroth J, Griffith DE, Olivier KN, Cook JL, Gordon F. Diagnosis and treatment of disease caused by nontuberculous mycobacteria. *Am J Respir Crit Care Med* 1997; **156**:S1–S25.

39 Al Samarrai T, Zhong N, Lamont I *et al*. A fast, highly discriminating and inexpensive method for computer-assisted typing of *Pseudomonas aeruginosa*. *J Clin Microbiol* 2000; **38**:4445–52.

40 Speert DP, Campbell ME, Henry DA *et al*. Epidemiology of *Pseudomonas aeruginosa* in cystic fibrosis in British Columbia, Canada. *Am J Respir Crit Care Med* 2002; **166**:988–93.

41 Pedersen SS, Jensen T, Pressler T, Hoiby N, Rosendal K. Does centralised treatment of cystic fibrosis increase the risk of *Pseudomonas aeruginosa* infection? *Acta Pediatr Scand* 1986; **75**:840–5.

42 Tubbs D, Lenney W, Alcock P, Campbell CA, Gray J, Pantin C. *Pseudomonas aeruginosa* in cystic fibrosis: cross-infection and the need for segregation. *Respir Med* 2001; **95**:147–52.

43 Jones AM, Dodd ME, Doherty CJ, Govan JRW, Webb AK. Increased treatment requirements of patients with cystic fibrosis who harbour a highly transmissible strain of *Pseudomonas aeruginosa*. *Thorax* 2002; **57**:924–5.

44 Cheng K, Smyth RL, Govan JR *et al*. Spread of β-lactam resistant *Pseudomonas aeruginosa* in a cystic fibrosis clinic. *Lancet* 1996; **348**:639–42.

45 Jones AM, Govan JR, Doherty CJ *et al*. Spread of a multiresistant strain of *Pseudomonas aeruginosa* in an adult cystic fibrosis clinic. *Lancet* 2001; **358**:557–8.

46 Ojeniyi B, Frederiksen B, Hoiby N. *Pseudomonas aeruginosa* cross infection among patients with cystic fibrosis during a winter camp. *Pediatr Pulmonol* 2000; **29**:177–81.

47 McCallum SJ, Corkill J, Gallagher M, Ledson MJ, Hart CA, Walshaw MJ. Superinfection with a transmissible strain of *Pseudomonas aeruginosa* in adults with cystic fibrosis chronically colonised by *Pseudomonas aeruginosa*. *Lancet* 2001; **358**:558–60.

48 Anthony M, Rose B, Beard Pegler M *et al*. Genetic analysis of *Pseudomonas aeruginosa* isolates from the sputa of Australian adult cystic fibrosis patients. *J Clin Microbiol* 2002; **40**:2772–8.

49 Armstrong D, Bell S, Robinson M *et al*. Evidence for spread of a clonal strain of *Pseudomonas aeruginosa* among cystic fibrosis clinics. *J Clin Microbiol* 2003; **41**:2266–7.

50 Fredericksen B, Koch C, Hoiby N. Changing epidemiology of *Pseudomonas aeruginosa* infection in Danish cystic fibrosis patients (1974–1995). *Pediatr Pulmonol* 1999; **28**:159–66.

51 Farrell PM, Shen G, Splaingard M *et al*. Acquisition of *Pseudomonas aeruginosa* in children with cystic fibrosis. *Pediatrics* 1997; **100**:E2.

52 Lebecque P, Leal T, de Boeck C, Jaspers M, Cuppens H, Cassiman J-J. Mutations of the cystic fibrosis gene and intermediate sweat chloride levels in children. *Am J Respir Crit Care Med* 2002; **165**:757–61.

53 Veeze HJ, Gan HK, Heijerman HG. A cystic fibrosis mutation associated with mild lung disease. *N Engl J Med* 1995; **333**:1644.

54 Rosenstein BJ, Cutting GR for the Cystic Fibrosis Foundation Consensus Panel. The diagnosis of cystic fibrosis: a consensus statement. *J Pediatr* 1998; **132**:589–95.

55 McWilliams T, Wilsher ML, Kolbe J. Cystic fibrosis diagnosed in adulthood. The Green Lane Hospital experience. *NZ Med J* 2000; **113**:6–8.

56 Bush A, Wallis C. Time to think again: cystic fibrosis is not an 'all or none' disease. *Pediatr Pulmonol* 2000; **30**:139–44.

57 British Paediatric Association Working Party on Cystic Fibrosis. Cystic fibrosis in the United Kingdom 1977–85: an improving picture. *BMJ* 1988; **297**:1599–602.

58 Royal College of Physicians. *Cystic Fibrosis in Adults: Recommendations for Care of Patients in the United Kingdom*. London, Royal College of Physicians of London, 1990.

59 Hill DJ, Martin AJ, Davidson GP *et al*. Survival of cystic fibrosis patients in South Australia. Evidence that cystic fibrosis center care leads to better survival. *Med J Aust* 1985; **143**:230–2.

60 Mahadeva R, Webb K, Westerbeek RC *et al*. Clinical outcome in relation to care in centers specialising in cystic fibrosis: cross sectional study. *BMJ* 1998; **316**:1771–5.

61 Walters S, Britton J, Hodson ME. Hospital care for adults with cystic fibrosis: an overview and comparison between special cystic fibrosis clinics and general clinics using a patient questionnaire. *Thorax* 1994; **49**:300–6.

62 Phelan PD, Bowes G. Management of cystic fibrosis in Melbourne, Australia. *Thorax* 1991; **46**:383–4.

63 Cheng K, Smyth RL, Motley J, O'Hea U, Ashby D. Randomised controlled trials in cystic fibrosis (1966–1997) categorised by time, design and intervention. *Pediatr Pulmonol* 2000; **29**:1–7.

64 Gee L, Abbott J, Conway SP, Etherington C, Webb AK. Development of a disease specific health related quality of life measure for adults and adolescents with cystic fibrosis. *Thorax* 2000; **55**:946–54.

65 Kettler LJ, Sawyer SM, Winefield HR, Greville HW. Determinants of adherence in adults with cystic fibrosis. *Thorax* 2002; **57**:459–64.

66 Donovan JL, Blake DR. Patient non-compliance: deviance or reasoned decision-making? *Soc Sci Med* 1992; **34**:507–13.

67 Abbott J, Dodd M, Bilton D, Webb AK. Treatment compliance in adults with cystic fibrosis. *Thorax* 1994; **49**:115–20.

68 Conway SP, Pond MN, Hamnett T *et al*. Compliance with treatment in adult patients with cystic fibrosis. *Thorax* 1996; **51**:29–33.

69 Conway SP, Pond MN, Watson A *et al*. Knowledge of adult patients with cystic fibrosis about their illness. *Thorax* 1996; **51**:34–8.

70 Kolbe J. The influence of socioeconomic and psychological factors on patient adherence to self-management strategies. Lessons learned in asthma. *Dis Manage Health Outcomes* 2002; **10**:551–70.

71 Henley LD, Hill ID. Errors, gaps, and misconceptions in the disease-related knowledge of cystic fibrosis patients and their families. *Pediatrics* 1990; **85**:1008–13.

72 Levers CE, Brown RT, Drotar D *et al*. Knowledge of physician prescriptions and adherence to treatment among children with cystic fibrosis and their mothers. *J Dev Behav Pediatr* 1999; **20**:335–43.

73 ATS Statement: guidelines for the six minute walk test. *Am J Respir Crit Care Med* 2002; **166**:111–17.

74 Revill SM, Morgan MD, Singh SJ, Williams J, Hardman AE. The endurance shuttle walk: a new field test for the assessment of endurance capacity in chronic obstructive pulmonary disease. *Thorax* 1999; **54**:213–22.

75 Lewis CA, Eaton TE, Fergusson W *et al.* Home overnight pulse oximetry in COPD patients: more than one recording may be needed. *Chest* 2003; **123**:1127–33.

76 Reiff DB, Wells AU, Carr DH, Cole PJ, Hansell DM. CT findings in bronchiectasis: value in distinguishing between idiopathic and specific types. *AJR* 1995; **165**:261–7.

77 De Jong PA, Nakano Y, Lequin MH, Woods R, Pare PD, Tiddens HAWM. Progression of mucus and bronchiectasis on high-resolution CT despite stable lung function tests in children with cystic fibrosis. *Am J Respir Crit Care Med* 2003; **167**:A323.

78 Sokol RJ, Durie PR. Recommendations for management of liver and biliary tract disease in cystic fibrosis. Cystic Fibrosis Foundation Hepatobiliary Consensus Group. *J Pediatr Gastroenterol Nutr* 1999; **28**:S1–S13.

79 Haworth CS, Selby PC, Horrocks AW, Mawer EB, Adams JE, Webb AK. A prospective study of change in bone mineral density over one year in adults with cystic fibrosis. *Thorax* 2002; **57**:719–23.

80 Brenckmann C, Papaioannou A. Biphosphonates for osteoporosis in people with cystic fibrosis (Cochrane Review). In: *The Cochrane Library*, Issue 1. Oxford, Update Software, 2003.

81 Chadwick S, Browning JE, Stern M *et al.* Nasal application of glycerol in ØF508 cystic fibrosis patients. *Thorax* 1998; **53**:A60.

82 Rubenstein RC, Zeithlin PL. A pilot clinical trial of oral sodium 4-phenylbutyrate (Buphenyl) in ØF508 homozygous cystic fibrosis patients. *Am J Respir Crit Care Med* 1998; **157**:484–90.

83 Knowles MR, Clarke LL, Boucher RL. Activation by intracellular nucleotides of chloride secretion in the airway epithelia of patients with cystic fibrosis. *N Engl J Med* 1991; **325**:533–8.

84 Bennett WD, Olivier KN, Zeman KL, Hohnekner KW, Boucher RC, Knowles MR. Effect of uridine 5′-triphosphate plus amiloride on mucociliary clearance in adult cystic fibrosis. *Am J Respir Crit Care Med* 1996; **153**:1796–801.

85 Knowles MR. Church NL, Waltner WE *et al.* A pilot study of aerosolised amiloride for the treatment of lung disease in cystic fibrosis. *N Engl J Med* 1990; **322**:1189–94.

86 Graham A, Hasani A, Alton EWFW *et al.* No added benefit from nebulised amiloride in patients with cystic fibrosis. *Eur Respir J* 1993; **6**:1243–8.

87 Pons G, Marchand MC, d'Athis P *et al.* French multicenter randomised double-blind placebo-controlled trial on nebulised amiloride in cystic fibrosis patients. *Pediatr Pulmonol* 2000; **30**:25–31.

88 Peckham DG, Conn A, Chotai C, Lewis S, Knox AJ. Effect of oral digoxin, topical oubain and salbutamol on trans-epithelial nasal potential difference in patients with cystic fibrosis. *Clin Sci* 1995; **89**:277–84.

89 Crystal RG. The gene as a drug. *Nature Med* 1995; **1**:15–17.

90 Wagner JA, Nepomuceno IB, Messner AH *et al.* A phase II double-blind, randomized, placebo-controlled clinical trial of tgAAVCF using maxillary sinus delivery in patients with cystic fibrosis with antrostomies. *Hum Gene Therapy* 2002; **13**:1349–59.

91 Alton EWFW, Middleton PG, Caplen NJ *et al.* Non-invasive liposome-mediated gene delivery can correct the ion transport defect in cystic fibrosis mutant mice. *Nature Genet* 1993; **5**:135–42.

92 Bragonzi A, Conese M. Non-viral approach toward gene therapy of cystic fibrosis lung disease. *Curr Gene Therapy* 2002; **2**:295–305.

93 Muszynshi-Kwan AT, Perlman R, Rivington-Law BA. Compliance with and effectiveness of chest physiotherapy in cystic fibrosis: a review. *Physiother Can* 1988; **40**:28–30.

94 Passero M, Remor B, Solomon J. Patient reported compliance with cystic fibrosis therapy. *Clin Pediatr* 1981; **20**:264–6.

95 Van der Schans C, Prasad A, Maine E. Chest physiotherapy compared to no chest physiotherapy for cystic fibrosis (Cochrane Review). In: *The Cochrane Library*, Issue 1. Oxford, Update Software, 2003.

96 Hess DR. The evidence for secretions clearance techniques. *Respir Care* 2001; **46**:1276–93.

97 Connors AF Jr, Hammon WE, Martin RJ, Rogers RM. Chest physical therapy: the immediate effect on oxygenation in acutely ill patients. *Chest* 1980; **78**:559–64.

98 Pryor J, Webber BA, Hodson ME. Effect of chest physiotherapy on oxygen saturation in patients with cystic fibrosis. *Thorax* 1990; **45**:77.

99 Horiuchi K, Jordan D, Cohen D, Kemper MC, Weissman C. Insights into the increased oxygen demand during chest physiotherapy. *Crit Care Med* 1997; **25**:1347–51.

100 Button BM, Heine RG, Catto-Smith AG, Phelan PD. Postural drainage in cystic fibrosis: is there a link with gastro-oesophageal reflux. *J Paediatr Child Health* 1998; **34**:330–4.

101 Ersson V, Carlson H, Mellstrom A, Ponten U, Hedstrond U, Kobsson S. Observations on intra-cranial dynamics during respiratory physiotherapy in unconscious neurosurgical patients. *Acta Anaesthesiol Scand* 1990; **34**:99–103.

102 Williams MT. Chest physiotherapy and cystic fibrosis. Why is the most effective form of treatment still unclear? *Chest* 1994; **106**:1872–80.

103 Reisman JJ, Rivington-Law B, Corey ML *et al.* Role of conventional physiotherapy in cystic fibrosis. *J Pediatr* 1988; **113**:632–6.

104 McIlwaine PM, Wong LT, Peacock D, Davidson AGF. Long term comparative trial of conventional postural drainage and percussion versus positive expiratory pressure physiotherapy in the treatment of cystic fibrosis. *J Pediatr* 1997; **131**:570–4.

105 Girard JP, Terki N. The Flutter VRP1: a new personal pocket therapeutic device used as an adjunct to drug therapy in the management of bronchial asthma. *J Invest Allergol Clin Immunol* 1994; **4**:23–7.

106 Konstan MW, Stern RC, Doershuk CF. Efficacy of the Flutter device for airway mucus clearance in patients with cystic fibrosis. *J Pediatr* 1994; **124**:689–93.

107 McIlwaine PM, Wong LT, Peacock P, Davidson GA. Long term comparative trial of positive expiratory pressure versus oscillating positive expiratory pressure (flutter) physiotherapy with the treatment of cystic fibrosis. *J Pediatr* 2001; **138**:845–50.

108 Nixon PA, Orsenstein DM, Kelsey SF, Doershuk CF. The prognostic value of exercise testing of patients with cystic fibrosis. *N Engl J Med* 1992; **327**:1785–8.

109 Hebestreit A, Kersting U, Basler B, Jeschke R, Hebestreit H. Exercise inhibits epithelial sodium channels in patients with cystic fibrosis. *Am J Respir Crit Care Med* 2001; **164**:443–6.

110 Bradley J, Moran F. Physical training for cystic fibrosis (Cochrane Review). In: *The Cochrane Library*, Issue 1. Oxford, Update Software, 2003.

111 Selvadurai HC, Blimkie CJ, Meyers N, Mellis CM, Cooper PJ, Van Asperen PP. Randomised controlled study of in-hospital exercise training programs in children with cystic fibrosis. *Pediatr Pulmonol* 2002; **33**:194–200.

112 Schneiderman-Walker J, Pollock SL, Carey M *et al.* A randomised-controlled trial of a 3 year home exercise program in cystic fibrosis. *J Pediatr* 2000; **136**:304–10.

113 Baldwin DR, Hill AL, Peckham DG, Knox AJ. Effect of addition of exercise to chest physiotherapy on sputum expectoration and lung function in adults with cystic fibrosis. *Respir Med* 1994; **88**:49–53.

114 Shah S, Capon DJ, Hellmiss R, Marsters SA, Baker CL. Recombinant human DNase I reduces the viscosity of cystic fibrosis sputum. *Proc Natl Acad Sci USA* 1990; **87**:9188–92.

115 Robinson M, Hemming AL, Moriaty C, Ebert S, Bye PTP. Effect of a short course of rhDNase on cough and mucociliary clearance in patients with cystic fibrosis. *Pediatr Pulmonol* 2000; **30**:16–24.

116 Laube BL, Auci RM, Shields DE *et al.* Effects of rhDN'ase on airflow obstruction and mucociliary clearance in cystic fibrosis. *Am J Respir Crit Care Med* 1996; **153**:752–60.

117 Kearney CE, Wallis CE. Deoxyribobonuclease for cystic fibrosis (Cochrane Review). In: *The Cochrane Library*, Issue 1. Oxford, Update Software, 2003.

118 Fuchs HJ, Borowitz DS, Christiansen DH *et al.* Effect of aerosolised recombinant human DNase on exacerbations of respiratory symptoms and on pulmonary function in patients with cystic fibrosis. *N Engl J Med* 1994; **331**:637–41.

119 McCoy K, Hamilton S, Johnson C for the Pulmozyme Study Group. Effects of 12-week administration of dornase α in patients with advanced cystic fibrosis lung disease. *Chest* 1996; **110**:889–95.

120 Ledson M J, Wahbi Z, Convery RP, Cowperthwaite C, Heaf DP, Walshaw MJ. Targeting of dornase α therapy in adult cystic fibrosis. *J R Soc Med* 1998; **91**:360–4.

121 Bollert FGE, Paton JY, Marshall TG, Calvert J, Greening AP, Innes JA on behalf of the Scottish Cystic Fibrosis Group. Recombinant DN'ase in cystic fibrosis: a protocol for targeted introduction through n-of-1 trials. *Eur Respir J* 1999; **13**:107–13.

122 Davies J, Trindale M-T, Wallis C, Rosenthal M, Crawford O, Bush A. Retrospective review of the effect of DNase in children with cystic fibrosis. *Pediatr Pulmonol* 1997; **23**:243–8.

123 Wilmott RW, Amin RS, Colin AA *et al.* Aerosolised recombinant human DNase in hospitalised cystic fibrosis patients with acute pulmonary exacerbations. *Am J Respir Crit Care Med* 1996; **153**:1914–17.

124 Konstan MW, Butler SM, Schidlaw DV *et al.* Patterns of medical practice in cystic fibrosis. Part II. Use of therapies. *Pediatr Pulmonol* 1999; **28**:248–51.

125 Shah PL, Scott SF, Geddes DM, Hodson ME. Two years experience with recombinant human DNase I in the treatment of pulmonary disease in cystic fibrosis. *Respir Med* 1995; **89**:499–502.

126 Ranasinha C, Assoufi B, Shah S *et al.* Efficacy and safety of short term administration of aerosolised recombinant human DNase I in adults with stable stage cystic fibrosis. *Lancet* 1993; **342**:199–302.

127 Suri R, Metcalf C, Lees B *et al.* Comparison of hypertonic saline and alternate-day or daily recombinant human deoxyribonuclease in children with cystic fibrosis: a randomised trial. *Lancet* 2001; **358**:1316–21.

128 Zahm, J-M, Debordeaux C, Maurer C *et al.* Improved activity of an actin-resistant DNase I variant on the cystic fibrosis airway secretions. *Am J Respir Crit Care Med* 2001; **163**:1153–7.

129 Duijvestijn YCM, Brand PLP. Systematic review of N-acetylcysteine in cystic fibrosis. *Acta Paediatr* 1999; **88**:38–41.

130 Wills P, Hall R, Chan W-M, Cole PJ. Sodium chloride increases the ciliary transportability of cystic fibrosis and bronchiectasis sputum on the mucus-depleted bovine trachea. *J Clin Invest* 1997; **99**:9–13.

131 Robinson M, Hemming A, Reqnis J *et al.* Effect of increasing doses of hypertonic saline on mucociliary clearance in patients with cystic fibrosis. *Thorax* 1997; **52**:900–3.

132 Shiburya Y, Wills PJ, Cole PJ. Effect of osmolality on muco-ciliary transportability and rheology of cystic fibrosis and bronchiectasis sputum. *Respirology* 2003; **8**:121–5.

133 Winters SL, Yeates DB. Roles of hydration, sodium and chloride in regulation of canine mucociliary transport system. *J Appl Physiol* 1997; **83**:1360–9.

134 Price AM, Webber SE, Widdicombe JG. Osmolality affects ion and water fluxes and secretion in the ferret trachea. *J Appl Physiol* 1993; **74**:2788–94.

135 Peatfield AC, Richardson PS, Wells UM. The effect of airflow on mucus secretion into the trachea of the cat. *J Physiol* 1986; **380**:429–39.

136 Eggleston P, Rosenstein BJ, Stackhouse CM, Alexander MF. Airway hyper-reactivity in cystic fibrosis. Clinical correlates and possible effects on the course of the disease. *Chest* 1988; **94**:360–5.

137 Wark PAB, McDonald V. Nebulised hypertonic saline for cystic fibrosis (Cochrane Review). In: *The Cochrane Library*, Issue 1. Oxford, Update Software, 2003.

138 Robinson M, Regnis J, Bailey DL, King M, Bautovich G, Bye PTP. The effects of hypertonic saline, amiloride and cough on mucociliary clearance in patients with cystic fibrosis. *Am J Respir Crit Care Med* 1996; **153**:1503–9.

139 Eng PA, Morton J, Douglass JA, Riedler J, Wilson J, Robertson CF. Short-term efficacy of ultrasonically nebulised hypertonic saline in cystic fibrosis. *Pediatr Pulmonol* 1996; **21**:77–83.

140 Wills PJ, Chan WM, Hall RL, Cole PJ. Ciliary transportability of sputum is governed by its osmolality. In: Baum GL, Priel Z, Roth Y, Liron N, Ortfield EJ, eds. *Cilia, Mucus and Microciliary Interactions*. New York, Marcel Dekker, 1998:281–4.

141 Robinson M, Daviskas E, Ebert S *et al.* The effect of inhaled mannitol on bronchial mucus clearance in cystic fibrosis patients: a pilot study. *Eur Respir J* 1999; **14**:678–85.

142 Ryan G, Mukhopadhyay S, Singh M. Nebulised anti-pseudomonal antibiotics for cystic fibrosis (Cochrane Review). In: *The Cochrane Library*, Issue 1. Oxford, Update Software, 2003.

143 Mukhopadhyay S, Singh M, Cater JI, Ogston S, Franklin M, Oliver RE. Nebulised antipseudomonal antibiotic therapy in cystic fibrosis: a meta-analysis of benefits and risks. *Thorax* 1996; **51**:364–8.

144 Ramsey BW, Pepe MS, Quan JM *et al.* Intermittent administration of inhaled tobramycin in patients with cystic fibrosis. *N Engl J Med* 1999; **340**:23–30.

145 Quittner AL, Buu A. Effects of tobramycin solution for inhalation on global ratings of quality of life in patients with cystic fibrosis and *Pseudomonas aeruginosa* infection. *Pediatr Pulmonol* 2002; **33**:269–76.

146 Moss RB. Administration of aerosolised antibiotics in cystic fibrosis patients. *Chest* 2001; **120**:1075–85.

147 Jensen T, Pedersen SS, Garne S, Heilmann C, Hoiby N, Koch C. Inhalation therapy in cystic fibrosis patients with chronic *Pseudomonas aeruginosa* lung infection. *J Antimicrob Chemother* 1987; **19**:831–8.

148 Hodson ME, Penketh ARL, Batten JC. Aerosol carbenicillin and gentamicin treatment of *Pseudomonas* infections in patients with cystic fibrosis. *Lancet* 1981; **ii**:1137–9.

149 Stead RJ, Hodson ME, Button JC. Inhaled ceftazidime compared with gentamicin and carbenicillin in older patients with cystic fibrosis infected with *Pseudomonas aeruginosa*. *Br J Dis Chest* 1987; **81**:272–9.

150 Hodson ME, Gallagher CG, Goven JR. A randomised clinical trial of nebulised tobramycin or colistin in cystic fibrosis. *Eur Respir J* 2002; **20**:658–64.

151 Pedersen SS, Jensen T, Hoiby N, Koch N. Management of *Pseudomonas aeruginosa* in Danish cystic fibrosis patients. *Acta Paediatr Scand* 1987; **76**:955–61.

152 Friederiksen B, Lanng S, Koch C, Hoiby N. Improved survival in the Danish center-treated cystic fibrosis patients: results of aggressive treatment. *Pediatr Pulmonol* 1996; **21**:153–8.

153 Breen L, Aswani N. Elective versus symptomatic intravenous antibiotic therapy for cystic fibrosis (Cochrane Review). In: *The Cochrane Library*, Issue 1. Oxford, Update Software, 2003.

154 Brett MM, Simmonds EJ, Ghoneim ATM, Littlewood JM. The value of serum IgG titres against *Pseudomonas aeruginosa* in the management of early pseudomonal infection in cystic fibrosis. *Arch Dis Child* 1992; **67**:1086–8.

155 Elborn JS, Prescott RJ, Stack BHR *et al*. Elective versus symptomatic antibiotic treatment in cystic fibrosis patients with chronic *Pseudomonas* infection of the lungs. *Thorax* 2000; **55**:355–8.

156 Sheldon CD, Assoufi BK, Hodson ME. Regular three monthly oral ciprofloxacin in adult cystic fibrosis patients infected with *Pseudomonas aeruginosa*. *Respir Med* 1993; **87**:587–93.

157 Keagan MT, Johansen HK. Vaccines for preventing infection with *Pseudomonas aeruginosa* in people with cystic fibrosis (Cochrane Review). In: *The Cochrane Library*, Issue 1. Oxford, Update Software, 2003.

158 McCaffery K, Oliver RE, Franklin M, Mukhopadhpyay S. Systematic review of anti-staphylococcal antibiotic therapy in cystic fibrosis. *Thorax* 1999; **54**:380–3.

159 Weaver LT, Green MR, Nicholson K *et al*. Prognosis in cystic fibrosis treated with continuous flucloxacillin from the neonatal period. *Arch Dis Child* 1994; **70**:84–9.

160 Smyth A, Walters S. Prophylactic antibiotics for cystic fibrosis (Cochrane Review). In: *The Cochrane Library*, Issue 1. Oxford, Update Software, 2003.

161 Ratjen F, Gomes G, Paul K, Posselt HG, Wagner TO, Harms K. Effect of continuous anti-staphylococcal therapy on the rate of *P. aeruginosa* acquisition in patients with cystic fibrosis. *Pediatr Pulmonol* 2001; **31**:13–16.

162 Wheeler WB, Williams RN, Matthews WJ, Colten HR. Progression of cystic fibrosis lung disease as a function of serum immunoglobulin G levels: a 5 year longitudinal study. *J Pediatr* 1984; **104**:695–9.

163 Burdon JG, Cade JF, Sutherland PW, Pain MC. Cystic fibrosis and bronchial hyperactivity: concomitant defects or cause and effect? *Med J Aust* 1980; **2**:77–8.

164 Tobin MJ, Maguire D, Keen D, Tempony E, Fitzgerald MX. Atopy and bronchial reactivity in older patients with cystic fibrosis. *Thorax* 1980; **35**:807–13.

165 Mareno RH, Hogg JC, Pare PD. Mechanics of airway narrowing. *Am Rev Respir Dis* 1986; **133**:1171–80.

166 Cheng K, Ashby D, Smyth R. Oral steroids for cystic fibrosis (Cochrane Review). In: *The Cochrane Library*, Issue 1. Oxford, Update Software, 2003.

167 Auerbach HS, Williams M, Kilpatrick JA, Colten HR. Alternate-day prednisone reduces morbidity and improves pulmonary function in cystic fibrosis. *Lancet* 1985; **2**:686–8.

168 Greally P, Hussain PJ, Vergani D, Price JF. Interleukin-1α, soluble interleukin-2 receptor, and IgG concentrations in cystic fibrosis treated with prednisolone. *Arch Dis Child* 1994; **71**:35–9.

169 Eigen H, Rosenstein BJ, Fitzsimmons S, Schidlow DV and the Cystic Fibrosis Foundation Prednisone Trial Group. A multicentre study of alternate-day prednisone therapy in patients with cystic fibrosis. *J Pediatr* 1995; **126**:515–23.

170 Lai HC, Fitzsimmons SC, Allen DB *et al*. Risk of persistent growth impairment after alternate-day prednisone treatment in children with cystic fibrosis. *N Engl J Med* 2000; **342**:851–9.

171 Dezateux C, Walters S, Balfour-Lynn I. Inhaled corticosteroids for cystic fibrosis (Cochrane Review). In: *The Cochrane Library*, Issue 1. Oxford, Update Software, 2003.

172 Balfour-Lynn I, Klein NJ, Denwiddie R. Randomised controlled trial of inhaled corticosteroids (fluticasone propionate) in cystic fibrosis. *Arch Dis Child* 1997; **77**:124–30.

173 Bisgaard H, Pedersen SS, Nielsen KG *et al*. Controlled trial of inhaled budesonide in patients with cystic fibrosis and chronic bronchopulmonary *Pseudomonas aeruginosa* infection. *Am Rev Respir Crit Care Med* 1997; **156**:1190–6.

174 Konstan MW, Vargo KM, Davis PB. Ibuprofen attenuates the inflammatory response to *Pseudomonas aeruginosa* in a rat model of chronic pulmonary infection. *Am Rev Respir Dis* 1990; **141**:186–92.

175 Dezateux C, Crighton A. Oral non-steroidal anti-inflammatory drug therapy for cystic fibrosis (Cochrane Review). In: *The Cochrane Library*, Issue 1. Oxford, Update Software, 2003.

176 Konstan MW, Hoppel CL, Choi B, Davis PB. Ibuprofen in children with cystic fibrosis (CF): pharmacokinetics and adverse effects: a randomised, double-blind, placebo-controlled, 3 month dose-escalation study in children with cystic fibrosis. *J Pediatr* 1991; **118**:956–64.

177 Konstan MW, Byard PJ, Hoppel CL, Davis PB. Effect of high-dose ibuprofen in patients with cystic fibrosis. *N Engl J Med* 1995; **332**:848–54.

178 Sordelli DD, Macri CN, Mailkie AJ, Cerquetti MC. A preliminary study of the effect of anti-inflammatory treatment in cystic fibrosis patients with *Pseudomonas aeruginosa* lung infection. *Int J Immunopathol Pharmacol* 1994; **7**:109–17.

179 Vilbragrasa V, Besto L, Cortijo J *et al*. Effects of erythromycin on chemo-attractant-activated human polymorphonuclear leukocytes. *Gen Pharmac* 1997; **29**:605–9.

180 Takizawa H, Desaki M, Ohtashi T *et al*. Erythromycin modulates IL-8 expression in normal and inflamed human bronchial epithelial cells. *Am J Respir Crit Care Med* 1997; **156**:266–71.

181 Khan AA, Slifer TR, Araujo FG *et al*. Effect of clarithromycin and azithromycin on production of cytokines by human monocytes. *Int J Antimicrob Agents* 1999; **11**:121–32.

182 Morikawa K, Watabe H, Aroahe M *et al*. Modulatory effect of antibiotics on cytokine production by human monocytes *in vitro*. *J Antimicrob Agents Chemother* 1996; **40**:1366–70.

183 Black PN. Anti-inflammatory effects of macrolide antibiotics. *Eur Respir J* 1959; **10**:971–2.

184 Jaffe A, Bush A. Anti-inflammatory effects of macrolides in lung disease. *Pediatr Pulmonol* 2001; **31**:464–73.

185 Molinari G, Guzman CA, Pesce A *et al*. Inhibition of *Pseudomonas aeruginosa* virulence factors by subinhibitory concentrations of azithromycin and other macrolide antibiotics. *J Antimicrob Chemother* 1993; **31**:681–8.

186 Fisher JJ, Bauman U, Gudowius P *et al*. Azithromycin reduces epithelial adherence of *P. aeruginosa* in patients with cystic fibrosis (abstract). *Pediatr Pulmonol* 1999; **Suppl 19**:265.

187 Koyama H, Geddes DM. Erythromycin and diffuse panbronchiolitis. *Thorax* 1997; **52**:915–18.

188 Hoiby H. Diffuse panbronchiolitis and cystic fibrosis: East meets West. *Thorax* 1994; **49**:531–2.

189 Peckham DG. Macrolide antibiotics and cystic fibrosis: do the macrolides have a role in the treatment of cystic fibrosis? *Thorax* 2002; **57**:189–90.

190 Ichimaya T, Takeoka K, Hiramatsu K, Hirai K, Yamasaki T, Nasu M. The influence of azithromycin on the biofilm formation of *Pseudomonas aeruginosa in vitro*. *Chemotherapy* 1996; **42**:186–91.

191 Jaffe A, Francis J, Rosenthal M *et al*. Long term azithromycin may improve lung function with cystic fibrosis. *Lancet* 1998; **351**:420.

192 Wolter J, Seeney S, Bell S, Bowler S, Mosel P, McCormack J. Effect of long term treatment with azithromycin on disease parameters in cystic fibrosis: a randomised trial. *Thorax* 2002; **57**:212–16.

193 Equi A, Balfour-Lynn IM, Bush A, Rosethal M. Long term azithromycin in children with cystic fibrosis: a randomised, placebo-controlled, crossover trial. *Lancet* 2002; **360**:978–84.

194 de Sant'Agnese PA. Pulmonary manifestations of fibrocystic disease of pancreas. *Dis Chest* 1955; **27**:654–67.

195 Hordvik NL, Konig P, Morris D, Kreutz C, Barbero GJ. A longitudinal study of bronchodilator responsiveness in cystic fibrosis. *Am Rev Respir Dis* 1985; **131**:889–93.

196 Pattishall EN. Longitudinal response of pulmonary function to bronchodilators in cystic fibrosis. *Pediatr Pulmonol* 1990; **9**:80–5.

197 Van Haren EHJ, Lanimers JWJ, Fester J, van Herwaarden CLA. Bronchial vagal tone and responsiveness to histamine, exercise and bronchodilators in adult patients with cystic fibrosis. *Eur Respir J* 1992; **5**:1083–8.

198 Cropp G. Effectiveness of bronchodilators in cystic fibrosis. *Am J Med* (Suppl) 1996; **100**:19–28.

199 Weintraub SJ, Eschenbacker WL. The inhaled bronchodilators ipratropium bromide and metaproteronal in adults with cystic fibrosis. *Chest* 1989; **95**:861–4.

200 Sanchez I, Halbrow J, Cherniak V. Acute bronchodilator response to a combination of β-agonists and anti-cholinengic agents in patients with cystic fibrosis. *J Pediatr* 1992; **120**:486–8.

201 Konig P, Poehler J, Barberro GS. A placebo-controlled double-blind trial of the long-term effects of albuterol administration in patients with cystic fibrosis. *Pediatr Pulmonol* 1998; **25**:32–7.

202 Zach MS, Oberwalder SB, Forche G, Polgar G. Bronchodilators increase airway instability in cystic fibrosis. *Am Rev Respir Dis* 1985; **131**:537–43.

203 Eber E, Oberwalder B, Zach M. Airway obstruction and airway wall instability in cystic fibrosis: the isolated and combined effects of theophylline and sympathomimetics. *Pediatr Pulmonol* 1988; **4**:205–12.

204 Landau LI, Phelan PD. The variable effect of bronchodilating agent on pulmonary function in cystic fibrosis. *J Pediatr* 1973; **82**:863–8.

205 Zinman R, Wohl MEB, Ingram RH Jr. Non-homogeneous lung emptying in cystic fibrosis patients; volume history and bronchodilator effects. *Am Rev Respir Dis* 1991; **143**:1257–61.

206 Hordvik NL, Sammut PH, Judy CG, Colombo JL. Effectiveness and tolerability of high-dose salmeterol in cystic fibrosis. *Pediatr Pulmonol* 2002; **34**:287–96.

207 Lammers J-W. Leukotines and cystic fibrosis. *Clin Exp Allergy Rev* 2001; **1**:175–7.

208 Morice AH, Kastelik JA, Aziz I. Montelukast sodium in cystic fibrosis. *Thorax* 2001; **56**:244–5.

209 Wang EEL, Prober CG, Manson B, Corey M, Levison H. Association of respiratory viral infections with pulmonary deterioration in patients with cystic fibrosis. *N Engl J Med* 1984; **311**:1653–8.

210 Conway SP, Simmonds EJ, Littlewood JM. Acute severe deterioration in cystic fibrosis associated with influenza A virus infection. *Thorax* 1992; **47**:112–14.

211 Johansen HK, Hoiby N. Seasonal onset of initial colonisation and chronic infections with *Pseudomonas aeruginosa* in patients with cystic fibrosis in Denmark. *Thorax* 1992; **47**:109–11.

212 Tan A, Bhalla P, Smyth R. Vaccines for preventing influenza in people with cystic fibrosis (Cochrane Review). In: *The Cochrane Library*, Issue 1. Oxford, Update Software, 2003.

213 Fraser KL, Tullis DE, Sasson Z *et al*. Pulmonary hypertension and cardiac function in adult cystic fibrosis: role of hypoxaemia. *Chest* 1999; **115**:1321–8.

214 Hazinski TA, Hansen TN, Simon JA, Tooley WH. Effect of oxygen administration during sleep on skin surface oxygen and carbon dioxide tensions in patients with chronic lung disease. *Pediatrics* 1981; **67**:626–30.

215 Speir S, Rivlin J, Hughes D, Levison H. The effect of oxygen on sleep, blood gases, and ventilation in cystic fibrosis. *Am Rev Respir Dis* 1984; **129**:712–18.

216 Gozal D. Nocturnal ventilatory support in patients with cystic fibrosis: comparison with supplemental oxygen. *Eur Respir J* 1997; **10**:1999–2003.

217 Zinman R, Corey M, Coates AL *et al*. Nocturnal home oxygen in the treatment of hypoxemic cystic fibrosis patients. *J Pediatr* 1989; **114**:368–77.

218 Caronia CG, Silver P, Nimkoff L, Gorvoy J, Quinn C, Sagy M. Use of bilevel positive airway pressure (BiPAP) in end-stage patients with cystic fibrosis awaiting lung transplantation. *Clin Pediatr* 1998; **37**:555–9.

219 Milross MA, Piper AJ, Norman M *et al*. Low-flow oxygen and bilevel ventilatory support. *Am J Respir Crit Care Med* 2001; **163**:129–34.

220 Hosenpud JD, Bennett LE, Keck BM, Boueck MM, Novick RJ. The registry of the International Society for Heart and Lung Translantation: seventeenth official report—2000. *J Heart Lung Transplant* 2000; **19**:909–31.

221 Liou TG, Adler FR, Cahill BC *et al*. Survival effect of lung transplantation among patients with cystic fibrosis. *JAMA* 2001; **286**: 2683–9.

222 Mayer-Hamblett N, Rosenfeld M, Emerson J, Goss CH, Aitken ML. Developing cystic fibrosis lung transplant referral criteria using predictors of 2-year mortality. *Am J Respir Crit Care Med* 2002; **166**:1550–5.

223 Morton JM, Santos J, Malouf MA *et al*. Lung transplantation for cystic fibrosis: outcome of the first 100 patients at St Vincents. *Am J Respir Crit Care Med* 2003; **167**:A245.

234 Ionescu AA, Nixon LS, Luzio S *et al*. Pulmonary function, body composition, and protein catabolism in adults with cystic fibrosis. *Am J Respir Crit Care Med* 2002; **165**:495–500.

225 Shepherd RW, Holt TL, Vasques-Velasquez L, Coward WA, Prentice A, Lucas A. Increased energy expenditure in young children with cystic fibrosis. *Lancet* 1988; **i**:1300–3.

226 Smyth R, Walters S. Oral calorie supplements for cystic fibrosis (Cochrane Review). In: *The Cochrane Library*, Issue 1. Oxford, Update Software, 2003.

227 Conway SP, Morton A, Wolfe S. Enteral tube feeding for cystic fibrosis (Cochrane Review). In: *The Cochrane Library*, Issue 1. Oxford, Update Software, 2003.

228 Smith A, Cohen M, Ramsey B. Pharmacotherapy. In: Yankaskas JR, Knowles MR, eds. *Cystic Fibrosis in Adults*. Philadelphia, Lippincott-Raven Publishers, 1999:345–64.

229 Smith AL, Fiel SB, Mayer-Hamblett N, Ramsey B, Burns JL. Susceptibility testing of *Pseudomonas aeruginosa* isolates and clinical response to potential antibiotic administration. Lack of assocation in cystic fibrosis. *Chest* 2003; **123**:1495–502.

230 Burkhardt JE, Waltespiel JN, Schaad UB. Quinolone arthropathy in animals versus children. *Clin Invest Dis* 1997; **25**:1196–204.

231 Shalit I, Stutman HR, Marks MI, Chartrend SA, Hilman BL. Randomised study of two dosage regimens of ciprofloxacin for treating chronic bronchopulmonary infection in patients with cystic fibrosis. *Am J Med* 1987; **82**:189–95.

232 Van der Linden PD Sturkenboom MCJM, Herings RMC, Leufkens HGM, Stricker BHCh. Fluoroquinalones and risk of Achilles tendon disorders: case–control study. *BMJ* 2002; **334**:1306–7.

233 Geddes DM. Antimicrobial therapy against *Staphylococcus aureus*, *Pseudomonas aeruginosa*, and *Pseudomonas cepacia*. *Chest* 1998; **94**:1405–45.

234 Weintzen R, Prestidge CB, Kramer RI *et al*. Acute pulmonary exacerbations in cystic fibrosis: a double-blind trial of tobramycin and placebo-therapy. *Am J Dis Child* 1980; **134**:1134–8.

235 Gold R, Carpenter S, Heurter H, Corey M, Levison H. Randomised trail of ceftazidime versus placebo in the management of acute respiratory exacerbations in patients with cystic fibrosis. *J Pediatr* 1987; **111**:907–13.

236 Regelmann WE, Elliott GR, Warwich WJ, Clawson CC. Reduction of sputum *Pseudomonas aeruginosa* density by antibiotics improves lung function in cystic fibrosis more than do bronchodilators and chest physiotherapy alone. *Am Rev Respir Dis* 1990; **141**:914–21.

237 Wolter JM, Bowler SD, McCormack JG. Are anti-pseudomonal antibiotics really beneficial in acute respiratory exacerbations of cystic fibrosis? *Aust NZ J Med* 1999; **29**:15–21.

238 Lang BJ, Aaron SD, Ferris W, Herbert PC, Macdonald NE. Multiple combination bactericidal antibiotic testing for patients with cystic fibrosis infected with multi-resistant strains of *Pseudomonas aeruginosa. Am J Respir Crit Care Med* 2000; **162**:2241–5.

239 Elphick HE, Tan A. Single versus combination intravenous antibiotic therapy for people with cystic fibrosis (Cochrane Review). In: *The Cochrane Library*, Issue 1. Oxford, Update Software, 2003.

240 Smith AL, Doershuk C, Goldmann D *et al.* Comparison of a β-lactam alone versus β-lactam and an amino-glycoside for pulmonary exacerbation in cystic fibrosis. *J Pediatr* 1999; **134**:413–21.

241 Spivey JM. The post antibiotic effect. *Clin Pharm* 1992; **11**:865–75.

242 de Groot R, Smith AL. Antibiotic pharmacokineics in cystic fibrosis. Differences and clinical significance. *Clin Pharm* 1987; **13**:228–53.

243 Tan K, Bunn H. Once daily versus multiple daily dosing with intravenous aminoglycosides for cystic fibrosis (Cochrane Review). In: *The Cochrane Library*, Issue 1. Oxford, Update Software, 2003.

244 Merco T, Asencio O, Bosque M, de Gracia J, Serra C. Home intravenous antibiotics for cystic fibrosis (Cochrane Review). In: *The Cochrane Library*, Issue 1. Oxford, Update Software, 2003.

245 Wolter JM, Bowler SD, Nolan PJ, McCormack JG. Home intravenous therapy in cystic fibrosis: a prospective randomised trial examining clinical quality of life and cost aspects. *Eur Respir J* 1997; **10**:896–900.

246 Homnick DN, Anderson K, Marks JH. Comparison of the Flutter device to standard chest physiotherapy in hospitalised patients with cystic fibrosis : a pilot study. *Chest* 1998; **114**:993–7.

247 Gondor M, Nixon PA, Mutich R, Rebovich PL, Qrenstein DM. Comparison of Flutter device and chest physical therapy in the treatment of cystic fibrosis pulmonary exacerbation. *Pediatr Pulmonol* 1999; **28**:255–60.

248 Hordvik NL, Sammut PH, Judy CG, Strizek SJ, Colombo JL. The effects of albuterol on the lung function of hospitalised patients with cystic fibrosis. *Am J Respir Crit Care Med* 1996; **154**:156–60.

249 Hordvik NL, Sammut PH, Judy CG, Colombo JL. Effects of standard and high doses of salmeterol on lung function of hospitalised patients with cystic fibrosis. *Pediatr Pulmonol* 1999; **27**:43–53.

250 Bowler IM, Kelman B, Worthington D *et al.* Nebulised amiloride in respiratory exacerbations of cystic fibrosis: a randomised controlled trial. *Arch Dis Child* 1995; **73**:427–30.

251 Madden BP, Kariyawasam H, Siddiqi AJ, Machin A, Pryor JA, Hodson ME. Noninvasive ventilation in cystic fibrosis patients with acute on chronic respiratory failure. *Eur Respir J* 2002; **19**:310–13.

252 Sood N, Paradowski LJ, Yankaskas JR. Outcomes of intensive care unit care in adults with cystic fibrosis. *Am J Respir Crit Care Med* 2001; **163**:335–8.

CHAPTER 4.7

Antibiotics in chronic obstructive pulmonary disease, bronchiectasis and cystic fibrosis

Ian A Yang, Samuel T Kim and Scott C Bell

Introduction

Respiratory infection is the cause of the majority of exacerbations of chronic obstructive pulmonary disease (COPD, including chronic bronchitis), bronchiectasis and cystic fibrosis (CF). However, despite international guidelines, the optimal antibiotic regime to treat acute exacerbations is not yet fully defined, and clinical practice frequently differs between centres. This chapter summarizes the current evidence for use of antibiotics in the management of acute exacerbations of these chronic airway diseases.

Aims

The primary clinical question of this systematic review was: how effective is antibiotic therapy in the management of acute exacerbation of COPD, bronchiectasis or CF?

Questions

The specific questions for each of these diseases were:
1 Do antibiotics work in acute exacerbations?
2 Which antibiotics work in acute exacerbations?
3 When should antibiotics be given in acute exacerbations?
4 Does maintenance antibiotic therapy work in clinically stable patients?

Methods

Literature search

A search of medical literature databases from 1966 to March 2003 was undertaken for randomized controlled trials (RCTs) or meta-analyses of antibiotic therapy in COPD, bronchiectasis or CF. The MEDLINE search strategy used was (Lung Diseases, Obstructive OR Cystic Fibrosis OR Bronchiectasis) AND Antibiotics, limited to meta-analysis or RCT and English language articles. A similar search strategy was used for the Cochrane Database of Systematic Reviews, ACP Journal Club, Database of Abstracts of Reviews of Effectiveness and Cochrane Central Register of Controlled Trials. A full list of articles is available from the authors on request.

Inclusion criteria for studies

We included randomized, double-blind, controlled trials of antibiotic versus placebo, or antibiotic versus antibiotic, which reported clinical outcomes after at least 3 days of treatment. The potential relevance of each article was determined independently by two reviewers based on the title and abstract and, where necessary, the full text.

Exclusion criteria for studies

- trials that were not randomized;
- trials that were not double blind;
- trials in which outcomes for the disease of interest (COPD, bronchiectasis or CF) were not reported separately from other diseases (e.g. asthma, lower respiratory tract infection).

Outcome measures

All outcome measures were considered. The primary outcomes extracted were:
- clinical response;
- bacteriological response;
- duration of exacerbation;
- symptoms;
- health-related quality of life;
- lung function;
- radiological response;
- inflammatory markers;
- adverse side-effects.

Intention-to-treat analysis, when reported, was preferred over efficacy-valid (per protocol) analysis.

Statistical analysis

Comparisons between antibiotic versus placebo, and antibiotic versus antibiotic (based on comparisons between classes of antibiotics), were performed. Where data were available and appropriate to pool, trials were combined using the Cochrane Review statistical software, *Review Manager* 4.2.3. Categorical outcomes were summarized using an odds ratio (OR), with calculation of the 95% confidence interval (CI). Continuous outcomes were summarized using weighted mean difference (WMD). Weighting was performed according to sample size. A random effects model was applied to take into account any heterogeneity between study designs and settings. Testing for heterogeneity between studies was performed in *Review Manager*.

Search results

A total of 689 articles were retrieved from the search. Of these, 28 were duplicates and 371 either did not study antibiotics in the diseases of interest (e.g. studied lower respiratory tract infections, acute bronchitis) or had studied other airway diseases (e.g. asthma). There were 188 COPD studies, 12 bronchiectasis studies and 87 CF studies.

Chronic obstructive pulmonary disease

Infection in acute exacerbations of COPD

Acute exacerbation is a frequent cause of morbidity and mortality in COPD. Bacteria, particularly *Haemophilus influenzae*, *Streptococcus pneumoniae* and *Moraxella catarrhalis*, cause about 50% of exacerbations. In the remaining, the causes include viruses, air pollution, heart failure, pulmonary embolism and pneumothorax, although in some cases no cause is identifiable.[1] Repeated respiratory infections accelerate the decline in lung function[2] and may therefore worsen prognosis. Of concern, antibiotic resistance to β-lactam antibiotics is increasing in respiratory pathogens in acute exacerbations of COPD (*H. influenzae*, *Strep. pneumoniae* and *M. catarrhalis*), as is penicillin resistance in *Strep. pneumoniae*.

Use of antibiotics in acute exacerbations of COPD

Antibiotics are commonly prescribed by clinicians in the management of acute exacerbations of COPD. The GOLD 2001 guidelines[1] recommend that antibiotics are only effective when patients with worsening dyspnoea and cough also have increased sputum volume and purulence (evidence level B — RCTs, limited body of evidence, based on the study by Anthonisen *et al.*[3]). The guidelines recommend that the choice of antibiotic should reflect local patterns of antibiotic sensitivity among common pathogens. However, the exact role of bacteria in acute exacerbations of COPD is still controversial. Currently unresolved issues include which subgroups of patients benefit the most from antibiotics, which antibiotics should be used and whether antibiotic resistance is of clinical importance.

Search results for COPD

In all, 188 COPD articles were retrieved, and a further nine relevant studies were found from reference lists, bringing the total to 197 potentially relevant COPD articles. Of these, 24 were excluded for the reasons given in Table 1.

Of the remaining 173 articles, there were three systematic reviews (including one meta-analysis), 13 trials of antibiotic versus placebo and 157 trials of antibiotic versus antibiotic.

Table 1. Reasons for exclusion of COPD articles.

Reason	No. of studies
Not a randomized trial of antibiotics	11
Clinical outcomes not reported	2
COPD outcomes not reported separately from other diseases	7
Outcomes reported for exacerbations rather than for patients	3
Outcomes reported for one organism only	1
Total number of excluded COPD articles	24

Do antibiotics work in acute exacerbations of COPD?

Results

Thirteen randomized, double-blind trials of antibiotic versus placebo in 1536 patients in acute exacerbations of COPD were identified (Table 2). Virtually all studied older antibiotics. The Jadad score of study quality[4] was satisfactory except in one letter to the editor.[5] There was much variability in study design, particularly in the antibiotics used, exclusion of pneumonia, use of oral steroids, clinical setting, sample size and outcomes assessed. This variability precluded statistical pooling of results. The 1995 meta-analysis by Saint *et al.*[6] analysed nine of these trials,[3,7–14] of which three studies reported a benefit with antibiotics. Pooling showed a small but statistically significant benefit with antibiotics, equivalent to 0.22 standard deviations of outcome measure. There was an average improvement in peak expiratory flow rate (PEFR) of 11 L/min over placebo.

In our systematic review, we considered the nine studies analysed by Saint *et al.*[6] together with three additional studies not included by them[5,15,16] and one published after their meta-analysis.[17] Overall, five out of 13 studies reported a benefit from antibiotics, including three of the four largest studies. The largest trial was a multicentre study of amoxicillin/clavulanic acid versus placebo in 369 patients with acute exacerbations of COPD, first published by Allegra *et al.* in 1991[16] and subsequently reanalysed.[18] In their per protocol analysis, clinical success or improvement occurred in 86% of patients taking antibiotic, compared with 51% taking placebo (*P* < 0.001). If one assumes that drop-outs were clinical failures, intention-to-treat analysis would still have shown clinical benefit in 80% of patients randomized to antibiotic versus 46% randomized to placebo.[18] Thus, although the 13 placebo-controlled trials varied considerably in study design, we conclude that antibiotics provide a small benefit overall (at least in some patients), based on the results of the meta-analysis[6] together with the largest recent study.[16]

Discussion

Placebo-controlled antibiotic studies were assessed to answer

Table 2. Randomized, placebo-controlled studies of antibiotic in acute exacerbations of COPD.

First author	Date	Ref.	No.	Disease	Antibiotic versus placebo	Jadad score	ITT or PP*	Exclude pneumonia	Oral steroids	Baseline FEV$_1$ or PEFR	Sputum purulence	Bacteriology	Outcome
Elmes	1957	7	88	CB	Oxytetracycline	5	PP	No	Not stated	Not reported	Not reported	Done	Trend to shorter exacerbations
Berry	1960	8	58	CB	Oxytetracycline	5	ITT	No	Not stated	Not reported	60%	Done	Benefit in moderate exacerbations
Fear	1962	9	62	CB	Oxytetracycline	5	ITT	No	Not stated	Not reported	Not reported	Not done	Trend to shorter exacerbations
Elmes	1965	10	56	CB	Ampicillin	5	ITT	No	Not permitted	PEFR	78%	Done	No benefit
Petersen	1967	12	43	CB	Chloramphenicol	4	ITT	No	Not stated	FEV$_1$, PEFR	74%	Not done	No benefit
Pines	1968	11	30	CB	Penicillin+streptomycin	5	ITT	No	Not stated	PEFR	100%	Not done	Benefit in severe exacerbations
Pines	1972	15	259	CB	Tetracycline or chloramphenicol	5	ITT	No	Not stated	PEFR	100%	Done	Benefit in moderate exacerbations
Nicotra	1982	13	40	CB	Tetracycline	4	ITT	Yes	Used as needed	FEV$_1$, PEFR	Not reported	Done	No benefit
Anthonisen	1987	3	173	COPD	Cotrimoxazole or amoxicillin or doxycycline	4	ITT	No	Used as needed	PEFR	60%	Not done	Benefit in type I or 2 exacerbations
Manresa	1987	5	19	CB	Cefaclor	2	ITT	Yes	Not stated	PEFR	Not reported	Done	No benefit
Allegra	1991	16	369	COPD	Amoxicillin/clavulanic acid	4	PP	Yes	Not stated	FEV$_1$	45%	Not done	Benefit for patients with low stable FEV$_1$
Jorgensen	1992	14	278	CB	Amoxicillin	4	ITT	Yes	Excluded	PEFR	33%	Not done	No benefit
Sachs	1995	17	61	COPD	Amoxicillin or cotrimoxazole	4	ITT	No	Used in all	PEFR	38%	Done	No benefit

Jadad score of study quality: at least 3 out of the maximum score of 5 indicates satisfactory quality of study design for RCTs.

*ITT, intention to treat; PP, per protocol.

this clinical question. The placebo-controlled trials varied markedly in their study design. For example, pneumonia was not excluded in some studies, while use of oral steroids was permitted in others.[19] There was a wide range of clinical outcomes, including cure/improvement, duration of exacerbation, symptom scores, days off work and PEFR. Nevertheless, we concluded that there is probably a small benefit overall from the use of antibiotics in acute exacerbations of COPD, at least in some patients. This is in agreement with the meta-analysis by Saint et al.,[6] which found a small benefit when primary outcomes were pooled, and also recent systematic reviews.[20,21] In clinical practice, there is now widespread empirical use of antibiotics in acute exacerbations of COPD.[22]

Placebo-controlled trials, together with prospective cohort studies, are still warranted[19,23] to help us to understand better the role of bacteria and the use of antibiotics in COPD. Taking a recent study as an example,[18] clinical improvement occurs more often in those taking antibiotics, supporting the importance of bacteria. However, some patients on antibiotics deteriorate, potentially due to non-susceptible bacteria, excessive bacterial load, non-bacterial causes, complications and comorbidities. Conversely, fewer patients on placebo improve, but in those that do improve, bacterial clearance by host defences or resolution of other non-bacterial causes may be important. Placebo-controlled trials may also help to address unanswered questions such as: are antibiotics effective in milder exacerbations and how can non-bacterial exacerbations be identified?

Which antibiotics work in acute exacerbations of COPD?

Results
Of the 158 antibiotic comparator trials (antibiotic versus antibiotic) in acute exacerbations of COPD:
- three were non-English language;
- two studied maintenance antibiotic therapy;
- 23 studied older antibiotics no longer used in respiratory disease;
- 18 compared the same antibiotic in different doses or durations, and generally demonstrated equivalence;
- 34 compared antibiotics within the same class, in open label, single-blind or double-blind studies. Almost all studies showed equivalence.
- 33 open label or single-blind studies compared antibiotics from different classes. As these studies were not double blind, quantitative analysis was not performed. Older antibiotics were generally shown to be equivalent, and macrolides were equivalent to penicillins. In the non-blinded studies of quinolones versus β-lactams, nearly half showed greater clinical efficacy with the quinolone.
- Finally, 44 double-blind studies of antibiotics from different classes were analysed quantitatively (Table 3). All studied oral

antibiotics. We classified antibiotics as older (traditional antibiotics such as cotrimoxazole, amoxicillin, older macrolides, tetracyclines) or newer (broad-spectrum antibiotics such as amoxicillin/clavulanic acid, cephalosporins, newer macrolides, quinolones),[24] and made the comparisons accordingly.

Older antibiotics
There were no differences in results for amoxicillin versus tetracyclines,[25–27] macrolides versus tetracycline[28] and amoxicillin versus trimethoprim[29] or cotrimoxazole.[30,31] There was a trend towards benefit of cotrimoxazole over tetracycline,[32–35] although this only reached significance in one crossover study.[36]

Cephalosporins versus cotrimoxazole
No clinical differences were observed in two studies of cephalosporins versus cotrimoxazole.[37,38] There was a trend to better bacterial eradication with cotrimoxazole, but the sample sizes were small.

Cephalosporins versus penicillins
No differences were found in five studies testing cephalosporins versus amoxicillin[39,40] or amoxicillin/clavulanic acid.[41–43]

Macrolides versus tetracyclines
No differences were observed in clinical efficacy of roxithromycin versus doxycycline in one study, although roxithromycin was better tolerated.[28]

Macrolides versus β-lactams
There were no differences detected in clinical or bacteriological outcomes in seven studies comparing newer macrolides versus amoxicillin,[44–46] amoxicillin/clavulanic acid[47–49] or cefuroxime.[42] In a published meta-analysis of azithromycin versus other antibiotics (four double-blind, nine non-double-blind studies), the rate of clinical failures was similar.[50]

Quinolones versus β-lactams
Seven studies compared quinolones versus β-lactams, either amoxicillin,[51,52] amoxicillin/clavulanic acid[53–57] or cefuroxime.[58] Clinical efficacy at follow-up was similar (Fig. 1). In contrast, bacteriological eradication at end of therapy was superior for quinolones (OR 2.3, $P = 0.0006$) (Fig. 2), due to higher eradication when compared with amoxicillin[52] or cefuroxime[58] but not amoxicillin/clavulanic acid.[54–56] Similarly, bacterial eradication at follow-up was higher for quinolones (OR 1.8, $P = 0.008$) (Fig. 3), mostly due to the superiority of quinolones over amoxicillin.[51]

Quinolones versus macrolides
Nine studies compared quinolones versus macrolides.[59–67] Although clinical efficacy was similar (Fig. 4), the bacteriological

Table 3. Double-blind studies of antibiotic versus antibiotic in acute exacerbations of COPD.

Comparison: test versus comparator	Total no. of studies*	Clinical benefit of test antibiotic			Bacterial eradication of test antibiotic		
		Studies, patients	Time point	Results OR (95% CI)	Studies, patients	Time point	Results OR (95% CI)
Cotrimoxazole versus tetracyclines	5†	3 studies, $n=370$	End therapy	1.58 (0.95–2.64)	2 studies, $n=244$	End therapy	1.65 (0.45–6.03)
Amoxicillin versus tetracyclines	3	1 study, $n=46$ 1 study, $n=58$	End therapy Follow-up	1.24 (0.27–5.68) 0.36 (0.08–1.52)	1 study, $n=87$	Follow-up	1.04 (0.45–2.43)
Macrolides versus tetracyclines	1	1 study, $n=62$	End therapy	1.07 (0.30–3.85)	1 study, $n=12$	End therapy	2.54 (0.09–75.8)
Amoxicillin versus cotrimoxazole (or trimethoprim)	3‡	1 study, $n=37$	End therapy	4.67 (0.82–26.6)			
Cephalosporins versus cotrimoxazole	2	1 study, $n=57$ 1 study, $n=39$	End therapy Follow-up	0.40 (0.14–1.17) 1.25 (0.28–5.59)	1 study, $n=24$ 1 study, $n=16$	End therapy Follow-up	0.09 (0.01–1.00) 0.06 (0.00–1.36)
Cephalosporins versus penicillins	5	4 studies, $n=457$ 1 study, $n=40$	End therapy Follow-up	1.45 (0.76–2.75) 2.20 (0.58–8.28)	3 studies, $n=188$ 1 study, $n=30$	End therapy Follow-up	0.99 (0.53–1.85) 1.50 (0.32–6.99)
Macrolides versus β-lactams	7	5 studies, $n=1238$ 7 studies, $n=1407$	End therapy Follow-up	1.16 (0.86–1.56) 1.10 (0.82–1.48)	6 studies, $n=541$ 3 studies, $n=308$	End therapy Follow-up	1.30 (0.87–1.92) 0.61 (0.36–1.05)
Quinolones versus β-lactams	8	5 studies, $n=1526$ 6 studies, $n=2523$	End therapy Follow-up	1.00 (0.70–1.37) 0.95 (0.76–1.19)	5 studies, $n=622$ 3 studies, $n=695$	End therapy Follow-up	**2.30 (1.43–3.71)** **1.84 (1.18–2.87)**
Quinolones versus macrolides	9	7 studies, $n=3190$ 6 studies, $n=2826$	End therapy Follow-up	1.21 (0.93–1.57) 1.15 (0.93–1.44)	6 studies, $n=1190$ 5 studies, $n=880$	End therapy Follow-up	**2.36 (1.19–4.71)** **1.71 (1.24–2.36)**
Telithromycin versus amoxicillin/clavulanate	1	1 study, $n=320$ 1 study, $n=320$	End therapy Follow-up	1.21 (0.70–2.09) 1.13 (0.69–1.85)	1 study, $n=94$	End therapy	1.14 (0.50–2.59)
Cefdinir versus loracarbef	1	1 study, $n=326$	End therapy	1.11 (0.60–2.07)	1 study, $n=470$	End therapy	0.78 (0.44–1.41)

*Total number of studies does not necessarily equal the number of studies cited for each result, because of variable use of outcomes in individual studies.
†Including one crossover study.
‡Including two crossover studies.
Amoxicillin and ampicillin were considered to be equivalent.
OR > 1 indicates benefit in favour of the test antibiotic (first listed) against the comparator (second listed).
OR < 1 indicates benefit in favour of the comparator antibiotic.
Statistically significant OR in bold.

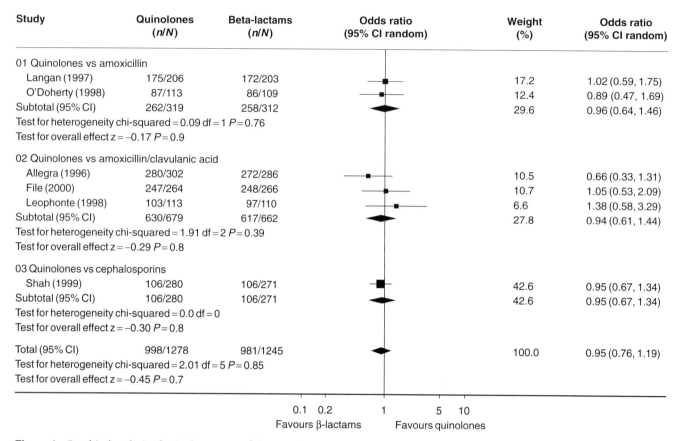

Figure 1. Graphical analysis of quinolones versus β-lactams for clinical outcomes at follow-up.

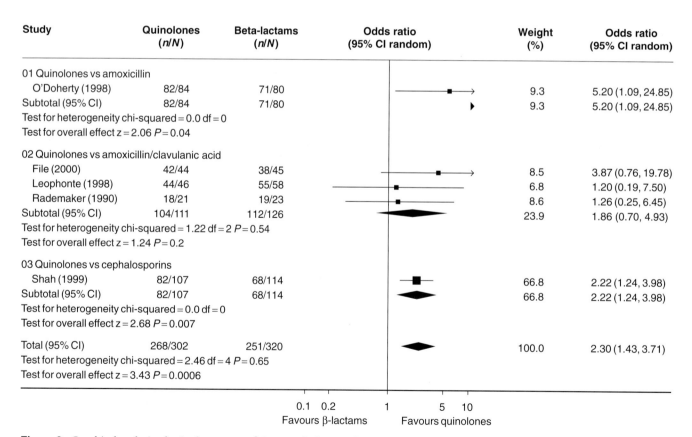

Figure 2. Graphical analysis of quinolones versus β-lactams for bacteriological eradication at end of therapy.

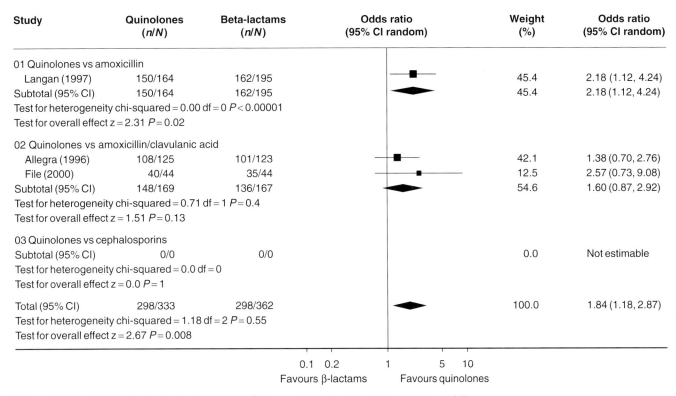

Figure 3. Graphical analysis of quinolones versus β-lactams for bacteriological eradication at follow-up.

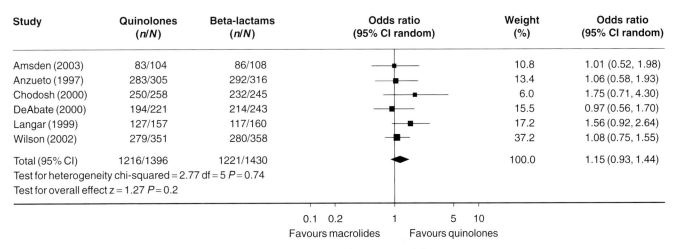

Figure 4. Graphical analysis of quinolones versus macrolides for clinical outcomes at follow-up.

eradication rate was superior for quinolones at end of therapy (OR 2.4, $P = 0.01$) (Fig. 5) and follow-up (OR 1.7, $P = 0.001$).

Other comparisons of newer antibiotics

One study of telithromycin (a ketolide) versus amoxicillin/clavulanic acid showed equivalent efficacy and greater tolerability with telithromycin.[68] A study of loracarbef versus cefdinir also showed equivalence.[69]

Pooled analysis of discontinuation due to adverse drug effects was possible for the newer agents (macrolides versus β-lactams, quinolones versus β-lactams, quinolones versus macrolides), as a result of the larger numbers of studies. No differences in rates of discontinuation were observed.

Discussion

Antibiotic comparator studies were assessed to answer this clinical question. To ensure evidence of the highest quality and relevance, we analysed randomized, double-blind trials of antibiotics currently marketed for use in respiratory infections. We found no statistically significant differences in clinical suc-

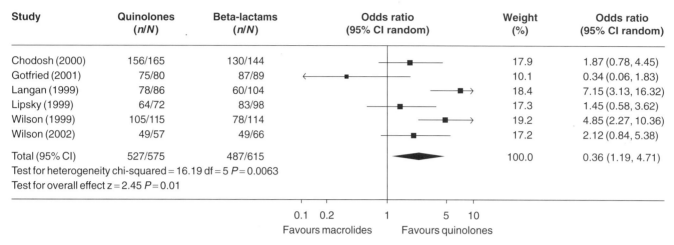

Study	Quinolones (n/N)	Beta-lactams (n/N)	Odds ratio (95% CI random)	Weight (%)	Odds ratio (95% CI random)
Chodosh (2000)	156/165	130/144		17.9	1.87 (0.78, 4.45)
Gotfried (2001)	75/80	87/89		10.1	0.34 (0.06, 1.83)
Langan (1999)	78/86	60/104		18.4	7.15 (3.13, 16.32)
Lipsky (1999)	64/72	83/98		17.3	1.45 (0.58, 3.62)
Wilson (1999)	105/115	78/114		19.2	4.85 (2.27, 10.36)
Wilson (2002)	49/57	49/66		17.2	2.12 (0.84, 5.38)
Total (95% CI)	527/575	487/615		100.0	0.36 (1.19, 4.71)

Test for heterogeneity chi-squared = 16.19 df = 5 P = 0.0063
Test for overall effect z = 2.45 P = 0.01

0.1　0.2　　　1　　　5　10
Favours macrolides　　　Favours quinolones

Figure 5. Graphical analysis of quinolones versus macrolides for bacteriological eradication at follow-up.

cess between different antibiotic classes. Whereas there were relatively small numbers of trials of older agents, the newer antibiotics were studied in large multicentre trials, resulting in pooled subject groups ranging from >500 (macrolides versus penicillins) to >3000 (quinolones versus macrolides), giving relatively small 95% confidence intervals. As most studies for registration purposes show equivalence,[70,71] our pooled results were not unexpected. The endpoint of 'cure/improvement with no further need for antibiotics' may be too insensitive to detect real differences, and other outcomes may be more sensitive, e.g. symptom scores, quality of life, rate of improvement and time to next exacerbation.[72]

In contrast, we found that bacterial eradication was significantly higher with quinolones (OR >2 at end of therapy) than some β-lactams, and higher with quinolones than macrolides, although this apparent superiority did not translate into greater clinical efficacy. These results suggest that clinical resolution of an acute exacerbation is likely to depend on factors other than, or in addition to, bacterial eradication, e.g. reduction in airway inflammation and airflow obstruction.[73] The relationship between clinical and bacteriological outcomes helps us to understand better bacterial and non-bacterial factors in exacerbations. Both clinical and bacteriological cure occurs commonly with broad-spectrum antibiotics. Conversely, it is rare to observe both clinical and bacteriological failure.[73] However, clinical success may occur with bacteriological failure, possibly indicating that bacteria were not the main cause of symptoms in those patients, or bacterial load was reduced sufficiently.[70] When clinical failure has occurred despite bacterial eradication, it is possible that non-bacterial causes are persisting, or complications and comorbidities have occurred.

Methodological issues in antibiotic comparator studies of COPD

A number of methodological issues should be addressed:

1 Inclusion criteria: the majority of COPD patients had chronic bronchitis, with sputum purulence during the acute exacerbation. These included patients therefore had the greatest likelihood of improvement with antibiotics, as reflected by clinical success rates of >90% for quinolones, macrolides and amoxicillin/clavulanic acid in recent studies.

2 Severity of COPD: many studies did not measure baseline lung function, making it difficult to stratify results by disease severity.[23,74]

3 Concomitant therapy: additional therapy such as steroids,[74] bronchodilators and physiotherapy were rarely controlled for.

4 Funding source: we did not stratify by funding source, as others have found no difference based on this factor.[50]

5 Year of publication: with the emergence of antibiotic resistance, the results for first-line antibiotics from older studies may not be clinically applicable now. Current studies use amoxicillin/clavulanic acid as the gold standard comparator or, alternatively, newer quinolones or macrolides.

A recent editorial has highlighted areas of potential improvement in study design of antibiotic trials in acute exacerbations of COPD,[74] which include many of the issues described above. In particular, there has been a call not just to plan equivalence trials, but also to consider populations at risk of treatment failure and newer, more useful outcomes such as future need for antibiotics and time free from exacerbation.

When should antibiotics be given in acute exacerbations of COPD?

Results

Anthonisen *et al.*[3] studied oral antibiotics (cotrimoxazole, amoxicillin or doxycycline) versus placebo in 173 COPD patients. They categorized exacerbations based on the number of cardinal symptoms present: type 1 (increased dyspnoea, sputum volume and sputum purulence), type 2 (two cardinal symptoms) and type 3 (one cardinal symptom, with a minor symptom). In type 1 exacerbations (severe), the success rate was greater with antibiotic therapy (63%) than with placebo (43%). The benefit was not as marked in type 2 exacerbations (moderate), and there was no benefit in type 3 (mild) exacerbations. Similarly, Berry et al.[8] observed that oxytetracycline had greater clinical benefit in moderately severe, but not mild, exacerbations. Finally, retrospective stratification by Allegra et al.[18] showed that the greatest benefit from amoxicillin/clavulanate occurred in those patients with severe impairment of forced expiratory volume in 1 second (FEV_1) at baseline. So, while not prospectively randomized for severity factors, these studies support the notion that antibiotics are of greater benefit in more severe exacerbations or patients with more severe COPD.

Discussion

No studies have prospectively randomized or stratified patients based on severity, although several studies have retrospectively stratified their data.[3,8,18] The greatest benefit from antibiotics is obtained in patients with a more severe exacerbation or with more severe baseline disease. Possible mechanisms include greater bacterial burden, antibiotic resistance and larger effects of bacterial infection on airway inflammation in already compromised patients. However, these factors should be confirmed in future trials. Sputum purulence is likely to be an important predictive factor for success with antibiotics. In a prospective cohort study, purulent exacerbations of chronic bronchitis were mainly bacterial and benefited from antibiotics, whereas mucoid exacerbations did not require antibiotics.[75] Which exacerbated patients are infected and who will clearly benefit from antibiotics remain questions that need to be resolved in future studies.[23]

Does maintenance antibiotic therapy work in COPD?

In a Cochrane systematic review,[76] nine trials of maintenance antibiotic therapy for COPD were analysed, all of which were performed before 1970 using older antibiotics. There was a small but statistically significant reduction in days of illness (WMD of 2 days less with maintenance antibiotic therapy) and a slightly reduced chance of an exacerbation (relative risk 0.9). However, the authors cautioned against maintenance antibiotic therapy for COPD because of concerns about antibiotic resistance, adverse effects and lack of recent studies.[76]

In summary, the role of bacterial infection in acute exacerbations of COPD remains controversial.[23] Table 4 presents the main evidence for and against the role of bacteria, in terms of results from culture of sputum in COPD patients, involvement of airway inflammation, benefit from antibiotics and results of this systematic review. On balance, the evidence is in favour of an important role for bacteria in acute exacerbations of COPD, including evidence of the effectiveness from RCTs and subgroups of COPD patients with type I exacerbations.

Bronchiectasis

Infection in bronchiectasis

Bronchiectasis is a common chronic lung disease characterized by a 'vicious cycle' of infection, inflammation and irreversible tissue destruction in the airway.[77] The interrelationship between these processes has not yet been clearly defined. Clinical decision making about antibiotic therapy in bronchiectasis is complicated by the presence of bacterial colonization or persistence and new in vivo infection due to either different bacterial strains or even viruses.[78] In studies of different prospective cohorts of patients,[79–82] the microbiological flora is highly variable.

Table 4. Evidence for and against the role of bacteria in acute exacerbations of COPD.

	Supports role of bacteria	Against role of bacteria
Sputum culture	Bacteria cultured in sputum in 50% of exacerbations, new strain is association with exacerbations	Bacteria may be cultured during stable phase (colonization)
Bacteria and airway inflammation	Antibiotic treatment of exacerbations reduces airway inflammation	Inflammation is also present during stable phase (i.e. not only in exacerbation)
Antibiotics	Antibiotics improve clinical outcomes in exacerbations	At least half of exacerbations resolve spontaneously
This systematic review	At least small benefit from antibiotics (versus placebo) in exacerbations Greatest benefit in more severe exacerbations (type I) when bacteria more likely to be present	Bacteriological effectiveness of quinolones not translated to superior clinical effectiveness

Use of antibiotics in acute exacerbations of bronchiectasis

Along with chest physiotherapy to assist drainage of secretions, antibiotics have been the key therapy for bronchiectasis. Short courses of antibiotics result in clinical improvements and have been shown to reduce the levels of inflammatory mediators in the sputum.[78] Long-term antibiotic therapy has been suggested to be beneficial in bronchiectasis by reducing microbial load and thus attenuating inflammation in the lung to allow tissue repair.[78] In clinical practice, exacerbations respond well to broad-spectrum antibiotics effective against *Pseudomonas aeruginosa*, *H. influenzae* and *S. aureus* in conventional doses.[83] However, unlike COPD or CF, there are no published consensus guidelines to guide antibiotic therapy in bronchiectasis.

Despite the lack of large-scale RCTs, short-term therapy with low-dose macrolide antibiotics has been used most commonly for diffuse panbronchiolitis, bronchiectasis and CF.[84] Similar to the situation in CF, nebulized antibiotics have been used increasingly in moderate to severe bronchiectasis to treat chronic *P. aeruginosa* infection.[85] Currently unresolved issues in bronchiectasis include the role for long-term use of broad-spectrum antibiotics, such as doxycycline and macrolides, and the identification of subgroups of patients who would benefit the most from nebulized antibiotics.

Search results for bronchiectasis

Twelve studies of patients with bronchiectasis were retrieved. One study by Orriols *et al.*[86] was excluded due to lack of double blinding. There was one Cochrane systematic review protocol of the use of antibiotics in bronchiectasis.[87] The 10 remaining studies were RCTs of short-term antibiotic therapy in bronchiectasis with a total of 430 patients (Table 5). The studies used antibiotics either during an acute exacerbation or during clinical stability.

Do antibiotics work in acute exacerbations of bronchiectasis?

Despite their widespread acceptance in clinical practice, there are no published RCTs comparing antibiotics with placebo in acute exacerbations of bronchiectasis.

Which antibiotics work in acute exacerbations of bronchiectasis?

Results

Four studies with a total of 150 patients examined antibiotic treatment during an acute exacerbation of bronchiectasis (Table 5). These studies compared quinolones with β-lactam drugs.[88–91] Three studies demonstrated quinolones to be superior to oral amoxicillin in improving sputum purulence,

Table 5. Randomized controlled trials of antibiotics in bronchiectasis.

First author, ref. no.	Date	Study design	No. of patients (*n* = 430)	Exacerbation or stable disease	Antibiotic 1	Antibiotic 2	Duration of intervention
Lam*[89]	1986	RCT, DB	32	Exacerbation	Ofloxacin 200 mg tds	Amoxicillin 1 g tds	10 days
Lam*[90]	1989	RCT, DB	41	Exacerbation	Ofloxacin 200 mg tds	Amoxicillin 1 g tds	10 days
Chan[88]	1996	RCT, DB	42	Exacerbation	Ciprofloxacin 500 mg bd	Amoxicillin 1 g tds	7 days
Tsang[91]	1999	RCT, DB	35	Exacerbation	Levofloxacin 300 mg bd	Intravenous ceftazidime 1 g tds	10 days
MRC[94]	1957	RCT, DB	122	Stable	Oxytetracycline 250–500 mg daily OR penicillin 2–3 g daily	Placebo	12 months
Currie[95]	1990	RCT, DB	38	Stable	Amoxicillin 3 gm BD	Placebo	32 weeks
Koh[96]	1997	RCT, DB	25	Stable	Roxithromycin 4 mg/kg bd	Placebo	12 weeks
Tsang[97]	1999	RCT, DB	21	Stable	Erythromycin 500 mg bd	Placebo	8 weeks
Barker[98]	2000	RCT, DB	74†	Stable	Nebulized TOBI 300 mg bd	Placebo	4 weeks
Couch[99]	2001	RCT, DB	74†	Stable	Nebulized TOBI 300 mg bd	Placebo	14 days

*Different cohorts of hospitalized adult bronchiectasis patients.[89,90]

†Same patient cohort but different therapy duration in Barker *et al.*[98] and Couch.[99] Total number of patients has been adjusted accordingly.

cough and dyspnoea, leucocyte count and overall clinical scores.[88–90] One study showed that oral quinolone (levofloxacin) was as effective as a parenteral β-lactam antibiotic (intravenous ceftazidime) in terms of improving 24-hour sputum volume, sputum purulence, cough and dyspnoea score.[91]

Discussion

Limited study of antibiotic choice has been undertaken; thus, very little pooling of data from individual studies was possible due to heterogeneity of outcomes between studies. These studies have reported changes in lung function (FEV_1), sputum volume, leucocyte counts and *P. aeruginosa* culture density as their primary study endpoints. Clinical parameters to define the onset of pulmonary exacerbations are not well defined in these studies, and future research in this area would benefit from the application of criteria for an exacerbation, as has been undertaken in some studies of COPD[3] and CF.[92,93]

When should antibiotics be given in acute exacerbations of bronchiectasis?

There is currently no evidence to indicate whether a specific subgroup of patients benefits more from antibiotics in acute exacerbations. Further, there is no study that has addressed the timing of antibiotic therapy, i.e. given electively or symptomatically based on conventional clinical parameters of exacerbation (e.g. symptom-directed therapy).

Does maintenance antibiotic therapy work in bronchiectasis?

Results

Six studies with a total of 280 patients have addressed maintenance antibiotic therapy in clinically stable patients with bronchiectasis[94–99] (Table 5). Four studies compared oral antibiotics with placebo. The MRC 1957 study compared the prolonged use of either oxytetracycline or penicillin with placebo over 12 months. Oxytetracycline was more effective than penicillin or placebo in reducing 24-hour sputum volume, cough, dyspnoea and days confined to bed. However, the long-term benefits of either penicillin or oxytetracycline in bronchiectasis could not be established.[94] A trial of 38 patients randomized to either amoxicillin or placebo for 32 weeks showed improvement in the amoxicillin group. There was reduction in the severity of exacerbations and frequency of *H. influenzae* in the sputum cultures, although there was a trend towards increased bacterial resistance.[95]

Two studies examined the use of macrolide antibiotics as maintenance antibiotic therapy in bronchiectasis. The first study recruited 25 children with bronchiectasis and bronchial hyper-responsiveness (BHR) to methacholine.[95] This demonstrated a reduction in BHR and sputum volume after 12 weeks of therapy with roxithromycin, but there were no significant changes in lung function (FEV_1). The second study examined

21 adults with mild to moderate bronchiectasis, defined to include up to four affected lobes.[96,97] This showed significant improvements in FEV_1 and sputum volume in the erythromycin group when compared with placebo.

Nebulized tobramycin (TOBI®) has been compared with placebo using 4 weeks of nebulized TOBI at 300 mg bd, with follow-up reported at 14 days[98,99] and 4 weeks in the same cohort of 74 patients.[98,99] Nebulized TOBI resulted in greater improvement in the subjective perception of general health and reduction in sputum *P. aeruginosa* colony density. However, there was no significant improvement in lung function, with more reported side-effects of dyspnoea, wheezing and chest tightness in the TOBI group. There was a concerning trend towards the greater isolation of tobramycin-resistant *P. aeruginosa* strains in the tobramycin-treated patients.

Discussion

The major studies of bronchiectasis encompass patients with diverse aetiology and vary widely in sample size.[79–82] There are only a limited number of placebo-controlled trials in stable bronchiectasis. Overall, there was a lack of large-scale prospective data, particularly in relation to nebulized and macrolide antibiotics.

Decisions regarding timing, duration and combination of antibiotic therapy for pulmonary exacerbation and long-term treatment of clinically stable patients with bronchiectasis are not well supported by RCTs. Wide variations in antibiotic prescription may be due to the heterogeneous aetiology of bronchiectasis and limited understanding of the pathogenesis of acute pulmonary exacerbations. Data registries of patients with bronchiectasis may facilitate a more co-ordinated approach to clinical research. Use of prolonged maintenance antibiotic therapy in bronchiectasis is currently being reviewed by the Cochrane Collaboration.[87]

Methodological issues for antibiotic studies in bronchiectasis

In this review, we have elected to include published studies and have not included studies reported in abstract form, whereas the Cochrane Reviewers have included studies from publications and conference proceedings where further data have been obtained from the authors. Similarly, this review has only included data from studies of crossover design, where first-cycle data are available in the manuscript. Some methodological issues that need to be considered include the following.

Clinical setting

Only one study in bronchiectasis, by Koh *et al.*,[96] recruited children with bronchiectasis. The remaining studies involved adult patients.

Inclusion criteria

Studies used clinical criteria for the diagnosis of bronchiectasis and specifically excluded patients with CF. Limited information was available on definitions of clinical stability in these studies[96] and infective exacerbations. One study specifically excluded patients with asthma using methacholine challenge test and lack of >20% diurnal variation in PEFR.[96]

The definition of an infective exacerbation included: a change in sputum colour,[88] a deterioration in other symptoms such as dyspnoea, wheezing, fever or chest pain[91] and/or radiological infiltrates.[98] In an attempt to distinguish exacerbation of bronchiectasis from its stable disease phase, the concept of so-called 'steady-state' bronchiectasis was used in two studies (defined as '<10% alteration in 24-hour sputum volume'),[91,97] but this was not utilized in other published studies.

Study size
The majority of studies did not describe whether sample size calculation had been performed, and it is not clear whether reported studies were adequately powered to assess significant differences between therapeutic arms.

Single versus multicentre studies
All studies recruited patients from a single clinical setting.

Severity of bronchiectasis
The majority of studies reported baseline lung function, although disease stratification was not performed. Quantification of the disease severity based on a formal radiological scoring system was used in only one study by Tsang et al.[97] using simplified high-resolution computerized tomography (HRCT) criteria based on the number of lobes affected.

Year of publication
The studies reviewed were performed from the 1970s to 2003 during a period of advances in survival and the development of new antibiotics and other therapies. All antibiotics included in the studies were antibiotics often used in the current era.

Cystic fibrosis

Infection in cystic fibrosis
Cystic fibrosis is the most common lethal autosomal-recessive disease of Caucasian populations. Clinical manifestations are protean but commonly include chronic respiratory infection and bronchiectasis, pancreatic insufficiency, biliary cirrhosis, male infertility and undernutrition. *Haemophilus influenzae* and *S. aureus* frequently cause early infection in CF airways.[73,100] With increasing age, the prevalence of *P. aeruginosa* infection increases. More than 80% of young adults with CF will have evidence of chronic *P. aeruginosa* infection.[101] Once established, chronic *P. aeruginosa* infection is unable to be eradicated with currently available therapies including antibiotics. Common pathogens in patients with CF include *Burkholderia cepacia*, *Stenotrophomonas maltophilia*, *Achromobacter xylosoxidans*, non-tuberculous mycobacteria and methicillin-resistant *S. aureus*.[101,102] Chronic bacterial infec-

tion results in a vigorous inflammatory response that leads to damage and destruction of airway and lung parenchyma.[102]

Use of antibiotics in acute exacerbations of cystic fibrosis
Survival of people with CF has improved dramatically during the past 40 years, and most children currently born with CF are now expected to live well into adult life.[103] Factors that are thought to have influenced improved patient survival include the development of newborn screening programmes, improved airway clearance techniques, nutritional support and CF specialist centre-based care.[104] Potent antipseudomonal antibiotics and increasingly aggressive administration of antibiotic therapy may have contributed to improved patient survival.

A recent consensus statement from the European CF Society and a state of the art review have addressed many of the current therapeutic approaches (and controversies) for chronic pulmonary infection in patients with CF.[105,106] Despite this, there remain many unresolved issues regarding administration of antibiotic therapy in CF. Clinically important issues include:

1 What is the optimal antibiotic therapy (duration and antibiotic combination choice)?

2 Is there a role for elective antibiotic therapy compared with therapy administered for symptomatic exacerbation of symptoms?

3 Is maintenance antibiotic therapy advantageous or does it enhance the development of more resistant bacteria?

4 Does antibiotic resistance influence outcome of treatment (both short term and long term)?

Therapeutic approaches for airway infection are currently under investigation, including multicentre studies of treatment of initial *P. aeruginosa* isolates from airway secretions in young children with CF and administration of intravenous aminoglycoside antibiotics.

Search results for cystic fibrosis
Eighty-seven CF studies were retrieved. Of these, 64 were antibiotic studies in CF. Twenty-seven studies were excluded because data have been published in conference abstract form only or involved single-blinded studies or crossover studies, and first-cycle data have not been available within the publications.

Seven were Cochrane systematic reviews on CF:
- Elective versus symptomatic intravenous antibiotic therapy in CF;[107]
- Single versus combination antibiotic therapy for people with CF;[108]
- Prophylactic antibiotic therapy for CF;[109]
- Macrolide antibiotic therapy for CF;[110]
- Once-daily versus multiple-daily dosing with intravenous aminoglycoside for CF;[111]
- Home intravenous antibiotics for CF;[112]

- Nebulized antipseudomonal antibiotic therapy for CF.[113]
Three were systematic reviews on CF.
- Systematic review of antistaphylococcal antibiotic therapy for CF, Database of Abstracts of Review of Effectiveness;[114]
- Nebulized antipseudomonal antibiotic therapy in CF, Database of Abstracts of Review of Effectiveness;[115]
- Nebulized antipseudomonal antibiotic therapy in CF: a meta-analysis of risk and benefits.[116]

Twenty-seven studies were double-blind RCTs that we included for analysis.

Do antibiotics work in acute exacerbations of CF?

Results
Only two placebo-controlled trials, with a total of 56 patients, have been performed in acute exacerbations of CF. Both these studies addressed hospitalized patients admitted with pulmonary exacerbation based on clinical symptoms, examination and laboratory findings such as chest radiograph (CXR) changes, elevated erythrocyte sedimentation rate (ESR) and leucocyte count. Wientzen et al.[117] studied intravenous tobramycin versus placebo in children with a mean age of 10 years (range 9 months to 25 years) and showed that global clinical response was more likely in the intravenous tobramycin group (12/12, 100%) compared with the placebo group (7/12, 58%). In addition, improvement in pulmonary function was more common in the tobramycin group (4/6, 67%) compared with the placebo group (0/7, 0%). However, there was no significant difference in quantitative sputum culture of either P. aeruginosa or S. aureus between groups.

Gold et al.[118] enrolled adults with CF with a mean age of 18 years and compared intravenous ceftazidime versus placebo. There was no significant difference in the percentage of patients who improved their global clinical scores in the intravenous ceftazidime group (16/16, 100%) compared with the placebo group (12/16, 75%). Following 14 days of treatment, there were no significant differences in improvements in pulmonary function or clinical symptom score in either group. However, there was a two or greater log reduction in colony counts of P. aeruginosa in the ceftazidime group (5/8, 62.5%) compared with the placebo group (1/9, 11%). Pooled data analysis was not feasible because of the small number of studies. Overall, single intravenous antibiotic therapy was more effective than placebo in pulmonary exacerbations of CF.

Discussion
This review highlights the limited number of placebo-controlled trials to guide treatment of pulmonary exacerbations in CF. Both the placebo-controlled trials support the use of single antibiotic therapy for a pulmonary exacerbation, yet no studies have compared the use of combination (β-lactam and aminoglycoside) therapy with placebo in patients with CF. Ethical concerns have almost certainly prevented further stud-

ies of this type, which are unlikely to be undertaken in the future. Placebo-controlled trials may be useful in answering questions such as: are antibiotics required in mild exacerbations of CF in the outpatient setting? To date, there have been no prospective placebo-controlled trials of the use of quinolone monotherapy in acute pulmonary exacerbations of CF.

Which antibiotics work in acute exacerbations of CF?
This analysis is divided into two groups: single intravenous antibiotic versus single intravenous antibiotic therapy; and combination intravenous antibiotic therapy.

Single intravenous antibiotic versus single intravenous antibiotic therapy
Two studies have compared the efficacy of single antibiotic versus single antibiotic therapy. Pooling of data was not possible because of the limited number of studies remaining and the heterogeneous nature of the therapy, namely azlocillin versus carbenicillin in 26 patients with a median age of 12 years (range 5–24 years),[119] and ceftazidime against aztreonam in 22 adult patients.[120] In the study by Huang et al.,[119] there was greater improvement in the global clinical score after 10 days of azlocillin compared with carbenicillin, although there was no significant difference in improvement in lung function. In the study by Salh et al.,[120] the patients in the aztreonam group had a greater improvement in FEV_1 and reduction in sputum weight compared with ceftazidime.

Combination intravenous antibiotic therapy
Nine RCTs have compared antibiotic monotherapy with either double/multiple or specific antibiotic combinations. We analysed these studies in two subgroups according to the various antibiotic combinations reported (Table 6).

Double intravenous versus single intravenous antibiotic therapy
Six randomized, controlled, double-blind studies with 291 patients compared the use of single antibiotic with a double antibiotic combination in exacerbations of CF (Table 6). In all studies, the added antibiotic was an aminoglycoside. One of these studies included treatment specifically directed towards S. aureus by comparing flucloxacillin–tobramycin combination against piperacillin.[123]

The antibiotic regimens were diverse with one study on ticarcillin–tobramycin combination,[121] two studies on ceftazidime–aminoglycoside combination[124,125] and one study each on azlocillin,[126] oxacillin[122] or flucloxacillin–tobramycin combination.[123] The duration of therapy between the studies was comparable with contemporary clinical practice, i.e. between 7 and 14 days. However, all these studies involved a small number of patients, ranging from 17[123] to 76 patients.[126] These studies included CF patients of mixed paediatric and

Table 6. Randomized controlled trials of antibiotic combinations in acute pulmonary exacerbations of CF.

First author, ref. no.	Date	Study type*	Study design	No. of patients (n = 291)	Antibiotic 1	Antibiotic 2[†]	Duration of intervention
McLaughlin[121]	1983	2a	RCT, DB	51	Ticarcillin + tobramycin or azlocillin + tobramycin	Tobramycin	10 days
Hyatt[122]	1981	2a	RCT, DB	24	Oxacillin + carbenicillin + sisomicin	Oxacillin	14 days
Macfarlane[‡123]	1985	2a	RCT, DB	17	Flucloxacillin + piperacillin + tobramycin	Flucloxacillin + tobramycin	14 days
Padoan[124]	1997	2a	RCT, DB	40	Ceftazidime + sisomicin	Ceftazidime	14 days
Master[125]	2001	2a	RCT, DB	83	Ceftazidime + tobramycin	Tobramycin	10 days
Smith[126]	1999	2a	RCT, DB	76	Azlocillin + tobramycin	Azlocillin	14 days

*Study type refers to antibiotic subgroups, i.e. 2a = double intravenous versus single intravenous antibiotic therapy; 2b = either double or multiple OR specific antipseudomonal combinations.
[†]Antibiotic 2 includes saline placebo unless specified otherwise.
[‡]Study included antibiotics specifically directed at *S. aureus*.

Review: EBM in antibiotic therapy in CF (meta-analysis)
Comparison: 01 Single antipseudomonal vs double antipseudomonal
Outcome: 02 Clinical score

Study or subcategory	(N)	Double IV [mean (SD)]	(N)	Single IV [mean (SD)]	SMD (fixed) (95% CI)	Weight (%)	SMD (fixed) (95% CI)
Hyatt (1981)	14	5.14 (3.88)	9	2.78 (4.15)		26.14	0.57 (−0.29, 1.43)
Padoan (1987)	20	9.20 (3.90)	20	8.60 (3.20)		49.77	0.16 (−0.46, 0.79)
Master (2001)	12	0.70 (5.30)	9	−2.80 (4.70)		24.09	0.66 (−0.23, 1.56)
Total (95% CI)	46		38			100.00	0.39 (−0.05, 0.83)

Test for heterogeneity: chi-squared = 1.04, df = 2 (P = 0.59), I^2 = 0%
Test for overall effect: z = 1.75 (P = 0.08)

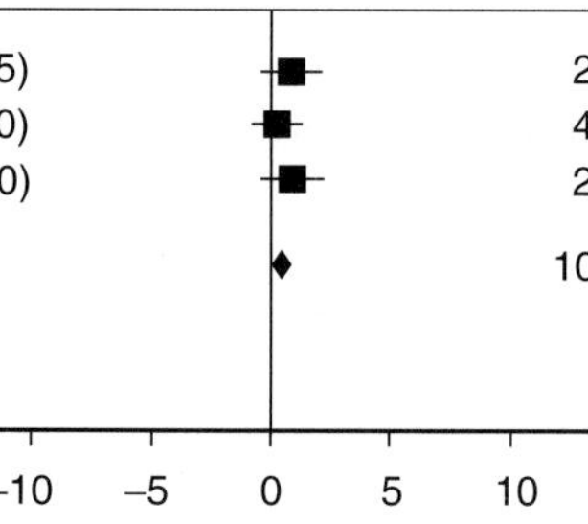

−10 −5 0 5 10
Favours double IV Favours single IV

Figure 6. Clinical score improvement between double and single intravenous antibiotic therapy.

adult population, although one study specifically addressed the paediatric population, defined as older than 6 years but less than 12 years.[123]

Pooled data analysis was limited by heterogeneous outcomes and interventions between the different studies. For example, McLaughlin *et al.*[121] included three intervention arms, ticarcillin–tobramycin, azlocillin–tobramycin and azlocillin–placebo, in CF patients aged 11 years and older with specific emphasis on sputum *P. aeruginosa* and *S. aureus* culture density and overall bacteriological response.

We were able to pool clinical outcomes from three studies for clinical score, and only two studies for lung function. In

terms of improvement in clinical scores (Fig. 6), there was no difference between the single and double antibiotic group [standardized mean difference (SMD) 0.39, 95% CI −0.05 to 0.83, P = 0.08].[122,124,125] Ten to 14 days after completion of therapy, the analysis showed no statistically significant difference (P = 0.70 and 0.73) in improvements in spirometry (FEV$_1$ and FVC) in the double intravenous group compared with the single intravenous group (Fig. 7).[121,126]

Smith *et al.*[126] compared azlocillin–tobramycin combination with azlocillin alone in 76 patients (age 17 years in the tobramycin group) and showed no significant differences between the two groups in terms of clinical benefit. Reduced *P.*

Review: EBM in antibiotic therapy in CF (meta-analysis)
Comparison: 01 Single antipseudomonal vs double antipseudomonal
Outcome: 04 FEV_1 post-therapy 10–14 days

Study or subcategory	(N)	Double IV [mean (SD)]	(N)	Single IV [mean (SD)]	WMD (fixed) (95% CI)	Weight (%)	WMD (fixed) (95% CI)
McLaughlin (1983)	36	46.30 (19.20)	30	50.90 (19.80)		71.33	−4.60 (−14.06, 4.86)
Smith (1999)	15	52.00 (25.00)	12	46.00 (14.00)		28.67	6.00 (−8.93, 20.93)
Total (95% CI)	51		42			100.00	−1.56 (−9.55, 6.43)

Test for heterogeneity: chi-squared = 1.38, df = 1 ($P = 0.24$), $I^2 = 27.6\%$
Test for overall effect: z = 0.38 ($P = 0.70$)

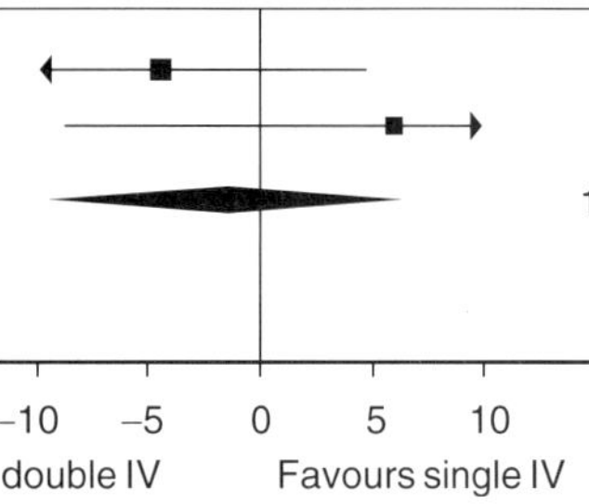

```
        -10   -5   0   5   10
      Favours double IV   Favours single IV
```

Figure 7. Mean lung function (FEV_1) post-therapy between double and single intravenous antibiotic therapy.

Review: EBM in antibiotic therapy in CF (meta-analysis)
Comparison: 01 Single antipseudomonal vs double antipseudomonal
Outcome: 06 FVC post-therapy 10–14 days

Study or subcategory	(N)	Double IV [mean (SD)]	(N)	Single IV [mean (SD)]	WMD (fixed) (95% CI)	Weight (%)	WMD (fixed) (95% CI)
McLaughlin (1983)	15	67.00 (22.00)	12	69.00 (11.00)		38.53	−2.00 (−14.75, 10.75)
Smith (1999)	36	72.70 (20.40)	30	73.70 (21.20)		61.47	−1.00 (−11.10, 9.10)
Total (95% CI)	51		42			100.00	−1.39 (−9.30, 6.53)

Test for heterogeneity: chi-squared = 0.01, df = 1 ($P = 0.90$), $I^2 = 0\%$
Test for overall effect: z = 0.34 ($P = 0.73$)

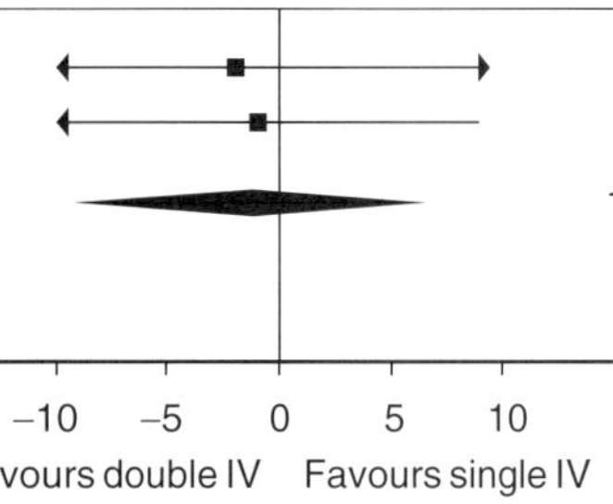

```
        -10   -5   0   5   10
      Favours double IV   Favours single IV
```

Figure 8. Mean lung function (FVC) post therapy between double and single intravenous antibiotic therapy.

aeruginosa sputum density and increased tobramycin resistance in the tobramycin group were observed.

Thus, based on limited pooling and descriptive analysis of clinical outcomes between the six double-blind studies, it can be concluded that there are no obvious differences between double against single intravenous antibiotic therapy.

Specific antipseudomonal combinations
Three RCT studies of specific antibiotic combinations were identified,[127–129] but these were either pseudorandomized or single-blinded trials.

Discussion
Combination intravenous antibiotics (e.g. β-lactam and aminoglycoside) are usually administered for acute exacerbations in patients with CF. The optimal choice of the specific antibiotic combination and duration of therapy cannot be defined from the published RCTs in CF.

It is worth comparing the current results with those published in the Cochrane Review on the same subject. A comparison of single versus combination intravenous antibiotics for CF identified 27 trials with a total of 386 patients and included 10 trials for analysis.[108] Nine studies analysed by the Cochrane Reviewers focus on the comparison of a single agent (i.e. mostly a β-lactam) with a combination of the same antibiotic and one other (i.e. aminoglycoside). The included studies in our review are distinct from that of the Cochrane Review, which included data from trials currently in progress, those published in conference abstract forms[130–132] and a crossover study after access to first-cycle data provided by the authors.[132]

In the Cochrane Review, single antibiotic therapy was associated with an increased number of patients with resistant *P. aeruginosa* at follow-up. The reviewers concluded that there was insufficient evidence to support single antibiotic therapy over combination treatment. In the current review, clinical scores and changes in lung function were not different between treatment groups, highlighting the need for further study. In addition, further study of the long-term effects of single antipseudomonal antibiotics compared with combination antibiotic therapy is warranted but cannot be supported at present by the available literature.

The interpretation of antibiotic studies in CF is compromised by the lack of a uniform definition of a pulmonary exacerbation. Recent studies examining the role of aerosolized medications including recombinant deoxyribonuclease (DNase)[9] and tobramycin (TOBI®)[93] have applied strict criteria for the definition of pulmonary exacerbations. Unfortunately, these definitions have rarely been applied to the RCTs examining antibiotics for pulmonary exacerbations in CF. Conventionally, the endpoints for antibiotic studies have included changes in spirometry, clinical and radiological scores and requirements for hospitalization. Recently, two CF-specific quality of life tools have been validated that are sensitive and applicable to clinical trials in CF.[133] Future studies examining the efficacy of antibiotics should include rigorous definition of a pulmonary exacerbation and include the use of quality of life tools as an outcome measure.

Increasing numbers of clinical trials involving patients with CF in North America are supported and/or sponsored by a Clinical Trials Network co-ordinated from the University of Washington in Seattle. This is likely to result in improved planning of study design and incorporation of clinically meaningful outcomes. An example of this is the recent multicentre study of azithromycin in children and adults with CF.[134]

When should antibiotics be given in acute exacerbations of CF?

Few placebo-controlled trials have examined whether intravenous antibiotic therapy is best administered regularly (elective treatment, not dictated by clinically defined symptoms), as is standard clinical practice in CF centres in Denmark, or dictated by symptoms and reduced lung function.

Two published studies were identified. In a multicentre RCT of 60 CF patients by Elborn et al.,[135] comparing elective and symptomatic antibiotic therapy, there were no differences in clinical scores, lung function, weight or radiological score between the treatment groups over the 3-year period. There was a non-significant trend towards higher mortality in the elective antibiotic group. In a single-centre study of 19 CF patients by Brett et al.,[136] no differences between the groups were noted.

A Cochrane Review has recently compared antibiotics administered for symptomatic pulmonary exacerbations with antibiotics administered at regular intervals (elective), with three trials identified involving a total of 79 patients, including one in abstract form.[137] It concluded that there was no benefit from elective treatment; however, study recruitment in the larger study by Elborn et al. was lower than required at the initial power calculations, and the elective antibiotic group only received on average one extra course of antibiotics compared with the symptomatic group.[107]

Does maintenance antibiotic therapy work in CF?

Studies have examined the use of antibiotic therapy in clinically stable patients with CF including nebulized antibiotic therapy, antistaphylococcal antibiotics and the use of macrolide antibiotic therapy.

Nebulized antibiotic therapy

Seven published RCTs of nebulized antibiotic therapy in CF have been included in this analysis (Table 7). In contrast to the recent Cochrane systematic review,[113] our review excluded

Table 7. Randomized controlled trials of nebulized antibiotic therapy in CF.

First author, ref. no.	Date	Study design	No. of patients ($n=814$)	Antibiotic 1	Antibiotic 2	Duration of intervention
Jensen[145]	1987	RCT, DB	40	Colistin 1 million units bd	Isotonic saline bd	3 months
Stead[146]	1987	RCT, crossover	18	Ceftazidime 1 g bd OR carbenicillin 1 g bd + gentamicin 80 mg bd	Placebo OR gentamicin 80 mg bd alone	4 months
MacLusky[147]	1989	RCT, DB	28	Tobramycin 80 mg tds	Placebo	Mean 32 months
Wiesemann[143]	1998	RCT, DB	22	Tobramycin 80 mg bd	Placebo	12 months
Ramsey[148]	1993	RCT, DB, crossover	71	Tobramycin 600 mg tds	Placebo	3 months
Ramsey[93]	1999	RCT, DB	520	Nebulized TOBI 300 mg daily	Colistin 80 mg bd	6 months
Hodson[144]	2002	RCT, DB	115	Nebulized TOBI bd (dose undefined)	Colistin bd (dose undefined)	4 weeks

crossover studies with no published first-cycle data[138,139] and conference abstracts with unpublished data.[140–142] Two recent large-scale prospective trials[143,144] are included in this analysis.

The consistent therapeutic endpoints in these studies were frequency of pulmonary exacerbations requiring intravenous antibiotics, changes in sputum *P. aeruginosa* culture-forming unit (CFU) density, mean lung function and side-effect profile with emphasis on auditory and renal toxicity. The age range of selected patients varied between the studies with the youngest group (10 ± 8 years old) in the study by Wiesemann *et al.*,[143] but all studies have enrolled patients older than the minimum age of 6 years with similar gender distribution. Baseline lung function was highly variable but tended to be better in the smaller studies by Wiesemann *et al.* (FEV$_1$ 79 ± 33% predicted)[143] and MacLusky *et al.* (FEV$_1$ 70 ± 22% predicted)[147] and poorer in the multicentre US study by Ramsey *et al.* (FEV$_1$ 50 ± 16%).[93] The duration of therapy ranged from 4 weeks to 32 months.

There were wide variations in dosing regimens and administration of nebulized antibiotics, e.g. tobramycin dose ranged from 80 mg bd[147] to 600 mg tds[143] and gentamicin 80 mg bd.[146] Owing to the diverse methodological differences between studies, pooling was not feasible. Therefore, a descriptive summary of the effects on nebulized antibiotic therapy is provided.

Nebulized tobramycin versus placebo
Four studies have made direct comparison of nebulized tobramycin against placebo.[93,143,147,149] Nebulized tobramycin led to improvement in pulmonary function (change in FEV$_1$ of 7% compared with 0.4%) and reduction in bacterial load in the treatment arms after relatively short therapy duration of 4 weeks.[143] Although no objective benefit was demonstrated on the lowest dose of 80 mg bd,[143] nebulized tobramycin produced no significant deterioration in lung function or clinical status at 80 mg tds (9/15 compared with 11/12 in the normal saline placebo who deteriorated). However, over a third of these patients subsequently developed tobramycin-resistant strains of *P. aeruginosa*.[147] The largest published studies of nebulized tobramycin by Ramsey *et al.*[93,148] demonstrated significant improvements in pulmonary function (average increase of 10% in FEV$_1$ at 5 months in the treatment group compared with a 2% decline in the placebo group). There were also significant improvements in clinical status including reduced severity of pulmonary exacerbations, decreased hospitalization frequency and improved quality of life scores.

Nebulized colistin versus placebo
Jensen *et al.*[145] demonstrated that there were no significant differences in the mean lung function in either intervention arm (mean % FEV$_1$ change of 11 ± 6 in nebulized tobramycin, 17 ± 11 in placebo) after 90 days of treatment. However, 11/20 in the placebo group completed the study compared with 18/20 in the nebulized colistin group, with four patients requiring hospitalization for intravenous antibiotic therapy in the placebo group.

Nebulized gentamicin or nebulized ceftazidime versus placebo
In a small single-centre study, combinations of nebulized gentamicin and carbenicillin or nebulized ceftazidime were found to be superior to placebo after 3 months of therapy, but no difference was noted between the different antibiotic regimens in improvement of lung function, sputum scores or hospitalization frequency.[145,146]

Nebulized colistin versus nebulized tobramycin
A multicentre study by Hodson *et al.*,[144] involving 16 CF centres in the UK and Ireland, demonstrated a significant decrease in the sputum bacterial load and *P. aeruginosa* density in both treatment arms, yet nebulized tobramycin resulted in a greater improvement in lung function (6.7% compared with 0.4% in the nebulized colistin group).

There are differences between selection of relevant studies in our review and the Cochrane Review,[113] which included 11 trials with a total of 758 patients, as a result of differences in review criteria. Despite these differences, our results were consistent with the findings of the Cochrane Review. Nebulized antibiotics are effective when administered to clinically stable patients with chronic *P. aeruginosa*. Nebulized colistin or tobramycin may be used as treatment of patients with CF that leads to improved lung function and possibly reduced hospitalization. Direct comparison of therapies has been subjected to limited study. Future studies should examine comparison between available antibiotics, particularly as some antibiotics are not currently approved for administration in some countries because of cost. Studies of the long-term effects on bacterial resistance of nebulized antibiotics are also required.

Use of antistaphylococcal antibiotic therapy
Of six studies that have examined the use of prophylactic antistaphylococcal antibiotics, only two satisfied our criteria for inclusion (Table 8).

Stutman *et al.*[150] has examined the role of low-dose cephalexin therapy in stable CF children. Their results showed that the sputum culture isolation rate for *S. aureus* was substantially lower for the cephalexin group (6% compared with 30% for placebo), but with increased risk of culture isolation for *P. aeruginosa* (26% versus 13%). There were no statistically significant differences in other major clinical outcomes, such as changes in lung function, between groups at the end of the study. Loening-Baucke *et al.*[151] found similar results, although their cephalexin group had decreased frequency of respiratory illnesses requiring antibiotics and hospitalizations in those initially colonized with *H. influenzae* (10/17 patients) and/or *S. aureus* (13/17 patients).

The current review provided similar results to that pub-

Table 8. Randomized controlled trials of prophylactic antistaphylococcal antibiotics in CF.

First author, ref. no.	Date	Study design	No. of patients (*n* = 136)	Antibiotic 1	Antibiotic 2	Duration of intervention
Loening-Baucke*[151]	1979	RCT, DB, crossover	17	Cephalexin	Placebo	2 years
Stutman[150]	2002	RCT, DB	119	Cephalexin 80–100 mg/kg/day	Placebo	7 years

*Only first-cycle analysis in crossover study by Loening-Baucke *et al.*[151] included.

Table 9. Randomized controlled trials of macrolide antibiotics in CF.

First author, ref. no.	Date	Study design	No. of patients (*n* = 286)	Antibiotic 1	Antibiotic 2	Duration of intervention
Wolter[155]	2002	RCT, DB	60	Azithromycin 250 mg daily	Placebo	3 months
Equi[156]	2002	RCT, DB, crossover	41	Azithromycin 500 mg daily (if weight <45 kg, 250 mg daily)	Placebo	6 months, 2 months washout, 15 months follow-up
Saiman[134]	2003	RCT, DB	185	Azithromycin 500 mg Mon/Wed/Fri (if weight >45 kg, 250 mg Mon/Wed/Fri)	Placebo	6 months

lished in the recent Cochrane Systematic Review, which included four studies[150,152–154] with 303 patients all under the age of 7 years.[109] It concluded that there were no differences in improvement in lung function, nutrition, hospitalization, additional antibiotic use, adverse side-effects or *P. aeruginosa* isolation despite a trend towards reduced *S. aureus* isolation. In addition, the Systematic Review by the NHS Centre for Reviews and Dissemination also concluded that no definite recommendation could be made for the long-term use of antistaphylococcal antibiotics[114] based on the heterogeneity of the studies and short follow-up duration. The two relevant studies included in this review support their consensus.

Use of macrolide antibiotic therapy
Three RCTs have studied a total of 286 patients examining the role of azithromycin in clinically stable patients with CF (Table 9). These studies were different in patient population, study design and treatment regimens. Baseline lung function was highest in the US study[134] and lowest in the Australian study.[155] One study was a crossover RCT over 15 months with two 6-month treatment periods and a 2-month washout period.[156] Compared with the Cochrane Review, we were able to include the multicentre US study of azithromycin that involved 23 CF centres over a 6-month treatment period.[134]

Pooling of data was only possible for changes in lung function (FEV$_1$ and FVC, Figs 8 and 9). As reported FEV$_1$ and FVC were not at completion of treatment periods in one study, we have not included these data in the meta-analysis.[156]

The azithromycin group had greater mean percentage improvements in FEV$_1$ (WMD 4.60. 95% CI 2.00–7.19, P=0.00001) and FVC at the completion of the therapy (WMD 5.53, 95% CI 3.33–7.33, P=0.0003).[134,155] The relative changes in lung function were a 3.6% increase in FEV$_1$ % predicted mean excess of azithromycin over placebo (Australian study), 5.4% (UK study) and 6.2% (US study).

There was a significant reduction in C-reactive protein in the study by Wolter *et al.*[155] and reduced frequency of intravenous antibiotic therapy. Equi *et al.*[156] found that up to 40% of patients had fewer oral antibiotic courses while on the macrolide arm. Frequency of hospitalization was decreased and quality of life improved in two of the three studies. In general, therapy was well tolerated in all studies.

Discussion
Nebulized antibiotics (tobramycin and colistin) and oral azithromycin result in improved lung function and reduced treatment requirement including need for hospitalization and intravenous antibiotic therapy. The studies in this section highlight an important limiting factor of short-term antibiotic studies in CF. Recurrent and/or long-term treatment is often required, and the outcomes defined in a short-duration clinical trial may not reflect risks to the patient if long-term treatment is administered, such as the development of increased antibiotic resistance of existing airway flora or superinfection with more resistant organisms. This has been demonstrated in the long-term study of cephalexin in children with CF.[134]

Review: EBM in antibiotic therapy in CF (macrolides in CF)
Comparison: 03 Macrolide in CF
Outcome: 01 Mean FEV_1% predicted improvement post therapy

Study or subcategory	(N)	Azithromycin [mean (SD)]	(N)	Placebo [mean (SD)]	WMD (fixed) (95% CI)	Weight (%)	WMD (fixed) (95% CI)
Wolter (2002)	30	1.61 (8.84)	30	−1.17 (5.85)		46.79	2.78 (−1.01, 6.57)
Saiman (2003)	87	4.40 (13.60)	98	−1.80 (10.70)		53.21	6.20 (2.64, 9.76)
Total (95% CI)	117		128			100.00	4.60 (2.00, 7.19)

Test for heterogeneity: chi-squared = 1.66, df = 1 (P = 0.20), I^2 = 39.8%
Test for overall effect: z = 3.47 (P = 0.0005)

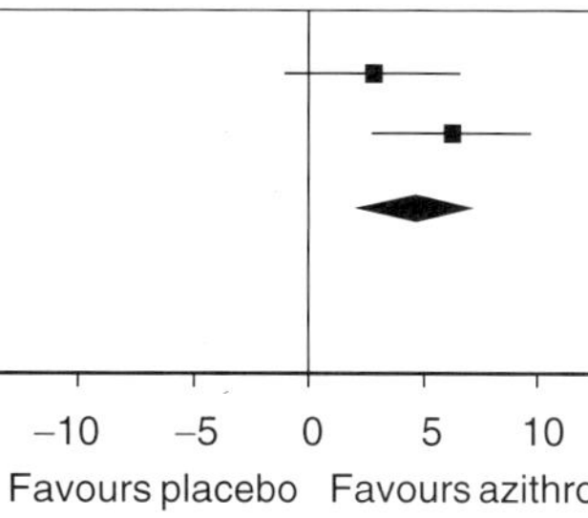

```
        -10    -5     0     5    10
     Favours placebo   Favours azithromycin
```

Figure 9. Mean FEV_1% improvement with macrolide antibiotics in CF at completion of therapy.

There is a difficult balance between performing clinical trials for new therapies (e.g. antibiotics) in a timely fashion, and yet carefully assessing the potential long-term consequences in a disease where lifelong therapies may be required. The current evidence suggests a role for long-term nebulized and macrolide antibiotics in clinically stable CF patients. More study of antistaphylococcal antibiotic therapy is warranted.

Methodological issues for antibiotic studies in CF

Clinical setting
In most studies in CF, a mixed population of children and adults with CF has been recruited. These studies may not be directly relevant for adult patients with advanced lung disease. None of the studies has specifically addressed antibiotic therapy in patients with resistant bacteria such as *B. cepacia*, *Stenotrophonomas maltophilia* or methicillin-resistant *S. aureus*.

Inclusion criteria
In CF, inclusion criteria for studies have been based on clinical features, abnormal sweat electrolytes and, in some, the presence of CFTR mutations. A clinical definition of pulmonary exacerbation has been used in most of the studies; however, specific details of exacerbations are not always reported.

Study size
The majority of studies did not provide a description of sample size calculation, so it is often unclear whether the study was adequately powered to assess a significant difference between treatments.

Single versus multicentre
Most studies have recruited patients from a single clinical setting, except for several of the recent larger studies, e.g. nebulized antibiotic[93,144] and azithromycin studies.[134]

Funding source
Funding source was not usually described in the studies.

Year of publication
The studies reviewed were performed over the past 30 years. During this period of significant advances in survival, the development of new antibiotics and other therapies has occurred. Earlier studies included antibiotics that are not available in the current era. For example, no studies of carbipenem antibiotics (imipenem or meropenem) or fourth-generation cephalosporins (cefipime) were identified in this review. This is despite the frequent use of such drugs for the treatment of pulmonary exacerbations.[93,144]

Conclusions for bronchiectasis and CF
Given the extent of antimicrobial therapy for infective exacerbations, there are remarkably few randomized controlled studies that have examined the efficacy of antimicrobial therapy. Ethical concerns of study design are likely to prevent the undertaking of placebo-controlled RCTs to provide supportive evidence. However, the prevailing literature evidence favours antibiotic therapy in acute pulmonary exacerbations in bronchiectasis and CF.

Implications for clinical practice
This analysis highlights the need for further prospective studies of the effect of short-term antibiotic therapy, e.g. in mild exacerbations of COPD. Studies are also required of long-term antibiotic therapy, e.g. nebulized and macrolide antibiotics in clinically stable patients with bronchiectasis and CF, on disease progression, quality of life and the altered microbiological flora due to the development of resistant bacteria. Improved understanding of the evidence for current antimicrobial strategies will enable more judicious use of antibiotics in patients with COPD, bronchiectasis and CF patients.

Review: EBM in antibiotics therapy in CF (macrolides in CF)
Comparison: 03 Macrolide in CF
Outcome: 03 Mean FEV% predicted improvement post therapy

Study or subcategory	(N)	Azithromycin [mean (SD)]	(N)	Placebo [mean (SD)]	WMD (fixed) (95% CI)	Weight (%)	WMD (fixed) (95% CI)
Wolter (2002)	30	4.28 (6.46)	30	−1.82 (6.06)	—■—	48.13	6.10 (2.93, 9.27)
Saiman (2003)	87	3.70 (11.80)	98	−1.30 (9.00)	—■—	51.87	5.00 (1.95, 8.05)
Total (95% CI)	117		128		◆	100.00	5.53 (3.33, 7.73)

Test for heterogeneity: chi-squared = 0.24, df = 1 ($P = 0.62$), $I^2 = 0\%$
Test for overall effect: z = 4.93 ($P < 0.00001$)

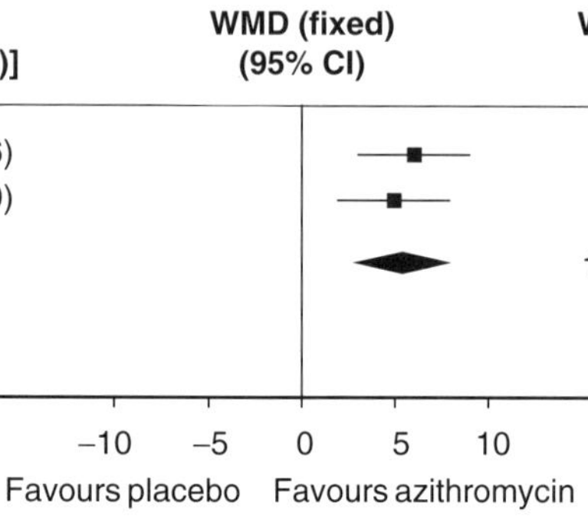

```
        -10   -5    0    5    10
   Favours placebo   Favours azithromycin
```

Figure 10. Mean FVC % improvement with macrolide antibiotics in CF at completion of therapy.

Summary for the clinician

COPD

Do antibiotics work in exacerbations of COPD?
Yes, antibiotics provide a small benefit overall.

Which antibiotics work in exacerbations of COPD?
Different classes of antibiotics have similar clinical effectiveness.

Bacterial eradication may be more effective for quinolones than β-lactams or macrolides, but this does not appear to result in improved clinical effectiveness.

When should antibiotics be given in acute exacerbations of COPD?
Antibiotics produce greater benefit in:
• exacerbations with increased dyspnoea, sputum purulence and sputum volume;
• exacerbations in patients with severe disease.

Does maintenance antibiotic therapy work in COPD?
Only a small benefit was observed, in studies performed before the emergence of antibiotic resistance.

Bronchiectasis

Do antibiotics work in acute exacerbations of bronchiectasis?
There are no placebo-controlled trials to address this question.

Which antibiotics work in acute exacerbations of bronchiectasis?
There are limited studies to support the choice of specific antibiotics.

Oral quinolones may be superior to oral β-lactams, and as effective as intravenous third-generation cephalosporin.

When should antibiotics be given in acute exacerbations of bronchiectasis?
There is no evidence to indicate whether specific subgroups of patients benefit to a greater degree from antibiotics during an acute exacerbation.

Does maintenance antibiotic therapy work in bronchiectasis?
Oral antibiotics (β-lactam, tetracycline or macrolide) are more effective than placebo. Short-term prophylactic nebulized antibiotic therapy with tobramycin is not associated with improved health status.

Cystic fibrosis

Do antibiotics work in acute exacerbations of CF?
Antibiotic therapy is effective in acute pulmonary exacerbations of CF.

Which antibiotics work in acute exacerbations of CF?
Specific antibiotic choice is diverse. There is no convincing evidence that single antipseudomonal antibiotic is more effective than combination antipseudomonal antibiotics.

When should antibiotics be given in acute exacerbations of CF?
Regular elective antibiotics and antibiotics for clinically defined pulmonary exacerbation appear to be equally effective, although more research in this area is required.

Does maintenance antibiotic therapy work in CF?
A small lung function benefit was observed in patients with CF receiving antistaphylococcal maintenance antibiotic therapy; however, infection with bacterial flora with increased antibiotic resistance may occur. Short-term use of macrolides and nebulized aminoglycosides is effective in clinically stable patients with CF.

Acknowledgements

We wish to thank Chris Parker and Lyn Waller, Medical Librarians at The Prince Charles Hospital, for designing the comprehensive medical literature search and for obtaining archived publications. We are also grateful for helpful assistance in providing relevant outcome data for nebulized antibiotic therapy

(Professor Bonney Ramsey and Dr Nicole Hamblett), for azithromycin in CF (Dr Mark Rosenthal) and for providing additional details about Allegra 1991 (Professor Francesco Blasi) and Barker *et al.* 2000 (Dr Alan Barker). Ian Yang was supported by the Thoracic Society of Australia and New Zealand/Allen & Hanbury Respiratory Research Fellowship, NHMRC Programme Grant (with Professor Philip Thompson), The Prince Charles Hospital Foundation and The Prince Charles Hospital Clinical Research Fellowship. Samuel Kim was supported by the NHMRC Postgraduate Medical Scholarship and The Prince Charles Hospital, Queensland Health. Scott Bell was supported by an NHMRC project grant (245513).

Contributions

Ian Yang and Samuel Kim selected the articles for inclusion. Ian Yang (COPD), Samuel Kim (bronchiectasis/CF) and Scott Bell (CF/bronchiectasis) extracted data from the included articles. All authors drafted and approved the final version of this chapter.

Conflict of interest

None declared. The funding sources had no role in the preparation of this chapter.

References

1 Pauwels RA, Buist AS, Calverley PM *et al.* Global strategy for the diagnosis, management, and prevention of chronic obstructive pulmonary disease. NHLBI/WHO Global Initiative for Chronic Obstructive Lung Disease (GOLD) Workshop Summary. *Am J Respir Crit Care Med* 2001; **163**:1256–76.

2 Kanner RE, Anthonisen NR, Connett JE. Lower respiratory illnesses promote FEV(1) decline in current smokers but not ex-smokers with mild chronic obstructive pulmonary disease: results from the lung health study. *Am J Respir Crit Care Med* 2001; **164**:358–64.

3 Anthonisen NR, Manfreda J, Warren CP *et al.* Antibiotic therapy in exacerbations of chronic obstructive pulmonary disease. *Ann Intern Med* 1987; **106**:196–204.

4 Jadad AR, Moore RA, Carroll D *et al.* Assessing the quality of reports of randomized clinical trials: is blinding necessary? *Control Clin Trials* 1996; **17**:1–12.

5 Manresa F, Blavia R, Martin R *et al.* Antibiotics for exacerbations of chronic bronchitis. *Lancet* 1987; **2**:394–5.

6 Saint S, Bent S, Vittinghoff E *et al.* Antibiotics in chronic obstructive pulmonary disease exacerbations. A meta-analysis. *JAMA* 1995; **273**:957–60.

7 Elmes PC, Fletcher CM, Dutton AAC. Prophylactic use of oxytetracycline for exacerbations of chronic bronchitis. *BMJ* 1957; **2**:1272–5.

8 Berry DG, Fry F, Hindley CP *et al.* Exacerbations of chronic bronchitis: treatment with oxytetracycline. *Lancet* 1960; **1**:137–9.

9 Fear EC, Edwards G. Antibiotic regimes in chronic bronchitis. *Br J Dis Chest* 1962; **56**:153–62.

10 Elmes PC, King TK, Langlands JH *et al.* Value of ampicillin in the hospital treatment of exacerbations of chronic bronchitis. *BMJ* 1965; **5467**:904–8.

11 Pines A, Raafat H, Plucinski K *et al.* Antibiotic regimens in severe and acute purulent exacerbations of chronic bronchitis. *BMJ* 1968; **2**:735–8.

12 Petersen ES, Esmann V, Honcke P *et al.* A controlled study of the effect of treatment on chronic bronchitis. An evaluation using pulmonary function tests. *Acta Med Scand* 1967; **182**:293–305.

13 Nicotra MB, Rivera M, Awe RJ. Antibiotic therapy of acute exacerbations of chronic bronchitis. A controlled study using tetracycline. *Ann Intern Med* 1982; **97**:18–21.

14 Jorgensen AF, Coolidge J, Pedersen PA *et al.* Amoxicillin in treatment of acute uncomplicated exacerbations of chronic bronchitis. A double-blind, placebo-controlled multicentre study in general practice. *Scand J Primary Health Care* 1992; **10**:7–11.

15 Pines A, Raafat H, Greenfield JS *et al.* Antibiotic regimens in moderately ill patients with purulent exacerbations of chronic bronchitis. *Br J Dis Chest* 1972; **66**:107–15.

16 Allegra L, Grassi C, Grossi E *et al.* The role of antibiotics in the treatment of chronic bronchitis exacerbation: follow-up of a multicenter study. *Ital J Chest Dis* 1991; **45**:138–48.

17 Sachs AP, Koeter GH, Groenier KH *et al.* Changes in symptoms, peak expiratory flow, and sputum flora during treatment with antibiotics of exacerbations in patients with chronic obstructive pulmonary disease in general practice. *Thorax* 1995; **50**:758–63.

18 Allegra L, Blasi F, de Bernardi B *et al.* Antibiotic treatment and baseline severity of disease in acute exacerbations of chronic bronchitis: a re-evaluation of previously published data of a placebo-controlled randomized study. *Pulmon Pharmacol Therapeut* 2001; **14**:149–55.

19 Hirschmann JV. Antibiotics for common respiratory tract infections in adults. *Arch Intern Med* 2002; **162**:256–64.

20 Bach PB, Brown C, Gelfand SE *et al.* Management of acute exacerbations of chronic obstructive pulmonary disease: a summary and appraisal of published evidence. *Ann Intern Med* 2001; **134**:600–20.

21 Russo RL, D'Aprile M. Role of antimicrobial therapy in acute exacerbations of chronic obstructive pulmonary disease. *Ann Pharmacother* 2001; **35**:576–81.

22 Anthonisen NR. Bacteria and exacerbations of chronic obstructive pulmonary disease. *N Engl J Med* 2002; **347**:526–7.

23 Sohy C, Pilette C, Niederman MS *et al.* Acute exacerbation of chronic obstructive pulmonary disease and antibiotics: what studies are still needed? *Eur Respir J* 2002; **19**:966–75.

24 Akalin HE. The place of antibiotic therapy in the management of chronic acute exacerbations of chronic bronchitis. *Int J Antimicrob Agents* 2001; **18**(Suppl 1):S49–55.

25 Allan GW, Fallon RJ, Lees AW *et al.* A comparison between ampicillin and tetracycline in purulent chronic bronchitis. *Br J Dis Chest* 1966; **60**:40–3.

26 Bennion-Pedley J. Treatment of acute exacerbations of chronic bronchitis in general practice. *Br J Clin Pract* 1969; **23**:280–3.

27 Welton FJ. Experiences with antibiotic trials in chronic bronchitis. *Public Health* 1970; **84**:95–101.

28 De Vlieger A, Druart M, Puttemans M. Roxithromycin versus doxycycline in the treatment of acute exacerbations of chronic bronchitis. *Diagn Microbiol Infect Dis* 1992; **15**(4 Suppl):123S–127S.

29 Gove RI, Cayton RM. A double-blind comparison of amoxycillin with trimethoprim in acute exacerbations of chronic bronchitis. *J Antimicrob Chemother* 1985; **15**:495–9.

30 Anonymous. Trimethoprim–sulphamethoxazole in chronic bronchitis. *Practitioner* 1969; **203**:817–19.

31 Chodosh S, Eichel B, Ellis C *et al.* Trimethoprim–sulfamethoxazole compared with ampicillin in acute infectious exacerbations of chronic bronchitis: a double-blind, crossover study. *J Infect Dis* 1973; **128**(Suppl):710–18.

32 Anonymous. A comparison of trimethoprim–sulphamethoxazole

compound and tetracycline in exacerbations of chronic bronchitis. A double-blind multi-centre trial on in-patients. *Br J Dis Chest* 1972; **66**:199–206.

33 Huddy RB, Jones DM, Lee HY. Tetracycline and co-trimoxazole in acute exacerbations of chronic bronchitis. *Br J Dis Chest* 1973; **67**:241–5.

34 Pines A, Raafat H, Greenfield JS *et al*. The management of purulent exacerbations of chronic bronchitis. A comparison of co-trimoxazole and tetracycline. *Practitioner* 1972; **208**:265–7.

35 Renmarker K. A comparative trial of co-trimoxazole and doxycycline in the treatment of acute exacerbations of chronic bronchitis. *Scand J Infect Dis* 1976; **8**(Suppl):75–8.

36 Anonymous. A further comparative trial of co-trimoxazole in chronic bronchitis. *Practitioner* 1972; **209**:838–40.

37 Anderson G, Williams L, Pardoe T *et al*. Co-trimoxazole versus cefaclor in acute or chronic bronchitis. *J Antimicrob Chemother* 1981; **8**:487–9.

38 Cooper J, McGillion FB. Treatment of acute exacerbations of chronic bronchitis. A double-blind trial of cotrimoxazole and cephalexin. *Practitioner* 1978; **221**:428–32.

39 Law MR, Holt HA, Reeves DS *et al*. Cefaclor and amoxycillin in the treatment of infective exacerbations of chronic bronchitis. *J Antimicrob Chemother* 1983; **11**:83–8.

40 Trigg CJ, Wilks M, Herdman MJ *et al*. A double-blind comparison of the effects of cefaclor and amoxycillin on respiratory tract and oropharyngeal flora and clinical response in acute exacerbations of bronchitis. *Respir Med* 1991; **85**:301–8.

41 Landau Z, Schlaffer F, Pitlik S. Cefuroxime axetil vs. augmentin for the treatment of acute bronchitis and exacerbation of chronic obstructive pulmonary disease. *Isr J Med Sci* 1992; **28**:797–9.

42 Langan C, Clecner B, Cazzola CM *et al*. Short-course cefuroxime axetil therapy in the treatment of acute exacerbations of chronic bronchitis. *Int J Clin Pract* 1998; **52**:289–97.

43 Periti P, Novelli A, Schildwachter G *et al*. Efficacy and tolerance of cefodoxime proxetil compared with co-amoxiclav in the treatment of exacerbations of chronic bronchitis. *J Antimicrob Chemother* 1990; **26**(Suppl E):63–9.

44 Aldons PM. A comparison of clarithromycin with ampicillin in the treatment of outpatients with acute bacterial exacerbation of chronic bronchitis. *J Antimicrob Chemother* 1991; **27**(Suppl A):101–8.

45 Bachand RT Jr. Comparative study of clarithromycin and ampicillin in the treatment of patients with acute bacterial exacerbations of chronic bronchitis. *J Antimicrob Chemother* 1991; **27**(Suppl A):91–100.

46 Mertens JC, van Barneveld PW, Asin HR *et al*. Double-blind randomized study comparing the efficacies and safeties of a short (3-day) course of azithromycin and a 5-day course of amoxicillin in patients with acute exacerbations of chronic bronchitis. *Antimicrob Agents Chemother* 1992; **36**:1456–9.

47 Hoepelman IM, Mollers MJ, van Schie MH *et al*. A short (3-day) course of azithromycin tablets versus a 10-day course of amoxycillin–clavulanic acid (co-amoxiclav) in the treatment of adults with lower respiratory tract infections and effects on long-term outcome. *Int J Antimicrob Agents* 1997; **9**:141–6.

48 Zachariah J. A randomized, comparative study to evaluate the efficacy and tolerability of a 3-day course of azithromycin versus a 10-day course of co-amoxiclav as treatment of adult patients with lower respiratory tract infections. *J Antimicrob Chemother* 1996; **37**(Suppl C):103–13.

49 Gris P. Once-daily, 3-day azithromycin versus a three-times-daily, 10-day course of co-amoxiclav in the treatment of adults with lower respiratory tract infections: results of a randomized, double-blind comparative study. *J Antimicrob Chemother* 1996; **37**(Suppl C):93–101.

50 Contopoulos-Ioannidis DG, Ioannidis JP, Chew P *et al*. Meta-analysis of randomized controlled trials on the comparative efficacy and safety of azithromycin against other antibiotics for lower respiratory tract infections (comment). *J Antimicrob Chemother* 2001; **48**:691–703.

51 Langan CE, Cranfield R, Breisch S *et al*. Randomized, double-blind study of grepafloxacin versus amoxycillin in patients with acute bacterial exacerbations of chronic bronchitis. *J Antimicrob Chemother* 1997; **40**(Suppl A):63–72.

52 O'Doherty B, Daniel R. Treatment of acute exacerbations of chronic bronchitis: comparison of trovafloxacin and amoxicillin in a multicentre, double-blind, double-dummy study. Trovafloxacin Bronchitis Study Group. *Eur J Clin Microbiol Infect Dis* 1998; **17**:441–6.

53 Allegra L, Konietzko N, Leophonte P *et al*. Comparative safety and efficacy of sparfloxacin in the treatment of acute exacerbations of chronic obstructive pulmonary disease: a double-blind, randomised, parallel, multicentre study. *J Antimicrob Chemother* 1996; **37**(Suppl A):93–104.

54 File T, Schlemmer B, Garau J *et al*. Gemifloxacin versus amoxicillin/clavulanate in the treatment of acute exacerbations of chronic bronchitis. The 070 Clinical Study group. *J Chemother* 2000; **12**:314–25.

55 Leophonte P, Baldwin RJ, Pluck N. Trovafloxacin versus amoxicillin/clavulanic acid in the treatment of acute exacerbations of chronic obstructive bronchitis. *Eur J Clin Microbiol Infect Dis* 1998; **17**:434–40.

56 Rademaker CM, Sips AP, Beumer HM *et al*. A double-blind comparison of low-dose ofloxacin and amoxycillin/clavulanic acid in acute exacerbations of chronic bronchitis. *J Antimicrob Chemother* 1990; **26**(Suppl D):75–81.

57 Schmidt EW, Zimmermann I, Ritzerfeld W *et al*. Controlled prospective study of oral amoxicillin/clavulanate vs ciprofloxacin in acute exacerbations of chronic bronchitis. *J Antimicrob Chemother* 1989; **24**(Suppl B):185–93.

58 Shah PM, Maesen FP, Dolmann A *et al*. Levofloxacin versus cefuroxime axetil in the treatment of acute exacerbation of chronic bronchitis: results of a randomized, double-blind study. *J Antimicrob Chemother* 1999; **43**:529–39.

59 Anzueto A, Niederman MS, Haverstock DC *et al*. Efficacy of ciprofloxacin and clarithromycin in acute bacterial exacerbations of complicated chronic bronchitis: interim analysis. Bronchitis Study Group. *Clin Therapeut* 1997; **19**:989–1001.

60 DeAbate CA, Mathew CP, Warner JH *et al*. The safety and efficacy of short course (5-day) moxifloxacin vs. azithromycin in the treatment of patients with acute exacerbation of chronic bronchitis. *Respir Med* 2000; **94**:1029–37.

61 Langan CE, Zuck P, Vogel F *et al*. Randomized, double-blind study of short-course (5 day) grepafloxacin versus 10 day clarithromycin in patients with acute bacterial exacerbations of chronic bronchitis. *J Antimicrob Chemother* 1999; **44**:515–23.

62 Lipsky BA, Unowsky J, Zhang H *et al*. Treating acute bacterial exacerbations of chronic bronchitis in patients unresponsive to previous therapy: sparfloxacin versus clarithromycin. *Clin Therapeut* 1999; **21**:954–65.

63 Wilson R, Kubin R, Ballin I *et al*. Five day moxifloxacin therapy compared with 7 day clarithromycin therapy for the treatment of acute exacerbations of chronic bronchitis. *J Antimicrob Chemother* 1999; **44**:501–13.

64 Wilson R, Schentag JJ, Ball P *et al*. A comparison of gemifloxacin and clarithromycin in acute exacerbations of chronic bronchitis and long-term clinical outcomes. *Clin Therapeut* 2002; **24**:639–52.

65 Gotfried MH, DeAbate CA, Fogarty CM *et al*. Comparison of 5-day, short-course gatifloxacin therapy with 7-day gatifloxacin therapy

and 10-day clarithromycin therapy for acute exacerbation of chronic bronchitis. *Clin Therapeut* 2001; **23**:97–107.

66 Chodosh S, DeAbate CA, Haverstock D *et al.* Short-course moxifloxacin therapy for treatment of acute bacterial exacerbations of chronic bronchitis. The Bronchitis Study Group. *Respir Med* 2000; **94**:18–27.

67 Amsden GW, Baird IM, Simon S *et al.* Efficacy and safety of azithromycin vs levofloxacin in the outpatient treatment of acute bacterial exacerbations of chronic bronchitis. *Chest* 2003; **123**:772–7.

68 Aubier M, Aldons PM, Leak A *et al.* Telithromycin is as effective as amoxicillin/clavulanate in acute exacerbations of chronic bronchitis. *Respir Med* 2002; **96**:862–71.

69 Paster RZ, McAdoo MA, Keyserling CH *et al.* A comparison of a five-day regimen of cefdinir with a seven-day regimen of loracarbef for the treatment of acute exacerbations of chronic bronchitis. *Int J Clin Pract* 2000; **54**:293–9.

70 Wilson R. Bacteria, antibiotics and COPD. *Eur Respir J* 2001; **17**:995–1007.

71 Miravitlles M. Exacerbations of chronic obstructive pulmonary disease: when are bacteria important? *Eur Respir J* 2002; **36**(Suppl):9s–19s.

72 Wislon S, Miller R, Collins N *et al.* Factors associated with frequent admission to hospital for patients with chronic airflow limitation. *Aust Fam Phys* 2001; **30**:822–4.

73 Rosenfeld M, Gibson RL, McNamara S *et al.* Early pulmonary infection, inflammation, and clinical outcomes in infants with cystic fibrosis. *Pediatr Pulmonol* 2001; **32**:356–66.

74 Miravitlles M, Torres A. No more equivalence trials for antibiotics in exacerbations of COPD, please. *Chest* 2004; **125**:811–13.

75 Stockley RA, O'Brien C, Pye A *et al.* Relationship of sputum color to nature and outpatient management of acute exacerbations of COPD. *Chest* 2000; **117**:1638–45.

76 Black P, Staykova T, Chacko E *et al.* Prophylactic antibiotic therapy for chronic bronchitis [Systematic Review]. *Cochrane Database Syst Rev* 2003; **1**.

77 Barker AF. Bronchiectasis. *N Engl J Med* 2002; **346**:1383–93.

78 Evans DJ, Greenstone M. Long-term antibiotics in the management of non-CF bronchiectasis—do they improve outcome? *Respir Med* 2003; **97**:851–8.

79 Angrill J, Agusti C, de Celis R *et al.* Bacterial colonisation in patients with bronchiectasis: microbiological pattern and risk factors. *Thorax* 2002; **57**:15–19.

80 Palwatwichai A, Chaoprasong C, Vattanathum A *et al.* Clinical, laboratory findings and microbiologic characterization of bronchiectasis in Thai patients. *Respirology* 2002; **7**:63–6.

81 Pasteur MC, Helliwell SM, Houghton SJ *et al.* An investigation into causative factors in patients with bronchiectasis. *Am J Respir Crit Care Med* 2000; **162**(4 Pt 1):1277–84.

82 Wilson CB, Jones PW, O'Leary CJ *et al.* Systemic markers of inflammation in stable bronchiectasis. *Eur Respir J* 1998; **12**:820–4.

83 Stockley RA. Bronchiectasis—new therapeutic approaches based on pathogenesis. *Clin Chest Med* 1987; **8**:481–94.

84 Garey KW, Alwani A, Danziger LH *et al.* Tissue reparative effects of macrolide antibiotics in chronic inflammatory sinopulmonary diseases. *Chest* 2003; **123**:261–5.

85 Cole PJ. The role of nebulized antibiotics in treating serious respiratory infections. *J Chemother* 2001; **13**:354–62.

86 Orriols R, Roig J, Ferrer J *et al.* Inhaled antibiotic therapy in non-cystic fibrosis patients with bronchiectasis and chronic bronchial infection by *Pseudomonas aeruginosa*. *Respir Med* 1999; **93**:476–80.

87 Greenstone M, Sullivan P, Brady C. Prolonged high-dose antibiotics for purulent bronchiectasis [Protocol]. *Cochrane Database Syst Rev* 2003; **1**.

88 Chan TH, Ho SS, Lai CK *et al.* Comparison of oral ciprofloxacin and amoxycillin in treating infective exacerbations of bronchiectasis in Hong Kong. *Chemotherapy* 1996; **42**:150–6.

89 Lam WK, Chau PY, So SY *et al.* A double-blind randomized study comparing ofloxacin and amoxycillin in treating infective episodes in bronchiectasis. *Infection* 1986; **14**(Suppl 4):S290–2.

90 Lam WK, Chau PY, So SY *et al.* Ofloxacin compared with amoxycillin in treating infective exacerbations in bronchiectasis. *Respir Med* 1989; **83**:299–303.

91 Tsang KW, Chan WM, Ho PL *et al.* A comparative study on the efficacy of levofloxacin and ceftazidime in acute exacerbation of bronchiectasis. *Eur Respir J* 1999; **14**:1206–9.

92 Fuchs HJ, Borowitz DS, Christiansen DH *et al.* Effect of aerosolized recombinant human DNase on exacerbations of respiratory symptoms and on pulmonary function in patients with cystic fibrosis. The Pulmozyme Study Group. *N Engl J Med* 1994; **331**:637–42.

93 Ramsey BW, Pepe MS, Quan JM *et al.* Intermittent administration of inhaled tobramycin in patients with cystic fibrosis. Cystic Fibrosis Inhaled Tobramycin Study Group. *N Engl J Med* 1999; **340**:23–30.

94 MRC. Prolonged antibiotic treatment of severe bronchiectasis. *BMJ* 1957; **Aug 3**:255–9.

95 Currie DC, Garbett ND, Chan KL *et al.* Double-blind randomized study of prolonged higher-dose oral amoxycillin in purulent bronchiectasis. *Q J Med* 1990; **76**:799–816.

96 Koh YY, Lee MH, Sun YH *et al.* Effect of roxithromycin on airway responsiveness in children with bronchiectasis: a double-blind, placebo-controlled study. *Eur Respir J* 1997; **10**:994–9.

97 Tsang KW, Ho PI, Chan KN *et al.* A pilot study of low-dose erythromycin in bronchiectasis. *Eur Respir J* 1999; **13**:361–4.

98 Barker AF, Couch L, Fiel SB *et al.* Tobramycin solution for inhalation reduces sputum *Pseudomonas aeruginosa* density in bronchiectasis. *Am J Respir Crit Care Med* 2000; **162**(2 Pt 1):481–5.

99 Couch LA. Treatment with tobramycin solution for inhalation in bronchiectasis patients with *Pseudomonas aeruginosa*. *Chest* 2001; **120**(3 Suppl):114S–17S.

100 Armstrong DS, Grimwood K, Carlin JB *et al.* Lower airway inflammation in infants and young children with cystic fibrosis. *Am J Respir Crit Care Med* 1997; **156**(4 Pt 1):1197–204.

101 Cystic Fibrosis Foundation. *Patient Registry Annual Data Report, 2000.* Bethesda, MD, Cystic Fibrosis Foundation, 2001.

102 Davis PB, Drumm M, Konstan MW. Cystic fibrosis. *Am J Respir Crit Care Med* 1996; **154**:1229–56.

103 Elborn JS, Shale DJ, Britton JR. Cystic fibrosis: current survival and population estimates to the year 2000. *Thorax* 1991; **46**:881–5.

104 Noone PG, Knowles MR. Standard therapy of cystic fibrosis lung disease. In: Yankaskas JR, Knowles MR, eds. *Cystic Fibrosis in Adults.* Philadelphia, Lippincott-Raven, 1999:145–74.

105 Doring G, Conway SP, Heijerman HG, *et al.* Antibiotic therapy against *Pseudomonas aeruginosa* in cystic fibrosis: a European consensus. *Eur Respir J* 2000; **16**:749–67.

106 Gibson RL, Burns JL, Ramsey BW. Pathophysiology and management of pulmonary infections in cystic fibrosis. *Am J Respir Crit Care Med* 2003; **168**:918–51.

107 Breen L, Aswani N. Elective versus symptomatic intravenous antibiotic therapy for cystic fibrosis [Systematic Review]. *Cochrane Database Syst Rev* 2003; **1**.

108 Elphick HE, Tan A. Single versus combination intravenous antibiotic therapy for people with cystic fibrosis [Systematic Review]. *Cochrane Database Syst Rev* 2003; **1**.

109 Smyth A, Walters S. Prophylactic antibiotics for cystic fibrosis [Systematic Review]. *Cochrane Database Syst Rev* 2003; **1**.

110 Southern KW, Barker PM, Solis A. Macrolide antibiotics for cystic fibrosis [Systematic Review]. *Cochrane Database Syst Rev* 2003; **1**.

111 Tan K, Bunn H. Once daily versus multiple daily dosing with intra-

venous aminoglycosides for cystic fibrosis [Systematic Review]. *Cochrane Database Syst Rev* 2003; **1**.

112 Marco T, Asensio O, Bosque M *et al.* Home intravenous antibiotics for cystic fibrosis [Systematic Review]. *Cochrane Database Syst Rev* 2003; **1**.

113 Ryan G, Mukhopadhyay S, Singh M. Nebulised anti-pseudomonal antibiotics for cystic fibrosis [Systematic Review]. *Cochrane Database Syst Rev* 2003; **1**.

114 NHS Centre for Reviews and Dissemination. Systematic review of antistaphylococcal antibiotic therapy in cystic fibrosis. *Database of Abstracts of Reviews of Effectiveness* 2003; **1**.

115 NHS Centre for Reviews and Dissemination. Nebulised antipseudomonal antibiotic therapy in cystic fibrosis. *Database of Abstracts of Reviews of Effectiveness* 2003; **1**.

116 Mukhopadhyay S, Singh M, Cater JI *et al.* Nebulised antipseudomonal antibiotic therapy in cystic fibrosis: a meta-analysis of benefits and risks (comment). *Thorax* 1996; **51**:364–8.

117 Wientzen R, Prestidge CB, Kramer RI *et al.* Acute pulmonary exacerbations in cystic fibrosis. A double-blind trial of tobramycin and placebo therapy. *Am J Dis Child* 1980; **134**:1134–8.

118 Gold R, Carpenter S, Heurter H *et al.* Randomized trial of ceftazidime versus placebo in the management of acute respiratory exacerbations in patients with cystic fibrosis. *J Pediatr* 1987; **111**(6 Pt 1):907–13.

119 Huang NN, Palmer J, Keith H *et al.* Comparative efficacy and tolerance study of azlocillin and carbenicillin in patients with cystic fibrosis: a double blind study. *J Antimicrob Chemother* 1983; **11**(Suppl B):205–14.

120 Salh B, Bilton D, Dodd M *et al.* A comparison of aztreonam and ceftazidime in the treatment of respiratory infections in adults with cystic fibrosis. *Scand J Infect Dis* 1992; **24**:215–18.

121 McLaughlin FJ, Matthews WJ Jr, Strieder DJ *et al.* Clinical and bacteriological responses to three antibiotic regimens for acute exacerbations of cystic fibrosis: ticarcillin–tobramycin, azlocillin–tobramycin, and azlocillin–placebo. *J Infect Dis* 1983; **147**:559–67.

122 Hyatt AC, Chipps BE, Kumor KM *et al.* A double-blind controlled trial of anti-*Pseudomonas* chemotherapy of acute respiratory exacerbations in patients with cystic fibrosis. *J Pediatr* 1981; **99**:307–14.

123 Macfarlane PI, Hughes DM, Landau LI *et al.* The role of piperacillin therapy in pulmonary exacerbations of cystic fibrosis: a controlled study. *Pediatr Pulmonol* 1985; **1**:249–55.

124 Padoan R, Cambisano W, Costantini D *et al.* Ceftazidime monotherapy vs. combined therapy in *Pseudomonas* pulmonary infections in cystic fibrosis. *Pediatr Infect Dis J* 1987; **6**:648–53.

125 Master V, Roberts GW, Coulthard KP *et al.* Efficacy of once-daily tobramycin monotherapy for acute pulmonary exacerbations of cystic fibrosis: a preliminary study. *Pediatr Pulmonol* 2001; **31**:367–76.

126 Smith AL, Doershuk C, Goldmann D *et al.* Comparison of a β-lactam alone versus β-lactam and an aminoglycoside for pulmonary exacerbation in cystic fibrosis. *J Pediatr* 1999; **134**:413–21.

127 Penketh AR, Hodson ME, Batten JC. Ticarcillin compared with carbenicillin in the treatment of exacerbations of bronchopulmonary infection in cystic fibrosis. *Br J Dis Chest* 1983; **77**:179–84.

128 Schaad UB, Desgrandchamps D, Kraemer R. Antimicrobial therapy of *Pseudomonas* pulmonary exacerbations in cystic fibrosis. A prospective evaluation of netilmicin plus azlocillin versus netilmicin plus ticarcillin. *Acta Paediatr Scand* 1986; **75**:128–38.

129 Whitehead A, Conway SP, Etherington C *et al.* Once-daily tobramycin in the treatment of adult patients with cystic fibrosis. *Eur Respir J* 2002; **19**:303–9.

130 Costantini D, Padoan R, Brenza A *et al.* Clinical evaluation of car-

benicillin and sisomycin alone or in combination in CF patients with pulmonary exacerbations. *Proceedings of the 11th International Cystic Fibrosis Conference* (abstract) 1982:227.

131 Huang NN, Palmer J, Braverman S *et al.* Theapeutic efficacy of ticarcillin and carbenicillin in patients with cystic fibrosis: a double-blind study. *23rd Cystic Fibrosis Club Abstract* 1982:124.

132 Tan KH, Hyman-Taylor, P, Mulheran, M, Knox, A, Smyth, A. Once-daily tobramycin monotherapy in cystic fibrosis. *Pediatr Pulmonol* 2002; **33**:406–7.

133 Quittner AL, Sweeny S, Watrous M *et al.* Translation and linguistic validation of a disease-specific quality of life measure for cystic fibrosis. *J Pediatr Psychol* 2000; **25**:403–14.

134 Saiman L, Marshall BC, Mayer-Hamblett N *et al.* Azithromycin in patients with cystic fibrosis chronically infected with *Pseudomonas aeruginosa*: a randomized controlled trial. *JAMA* 2003; **290**:1749–56.

135 Elborn JS, Prescott RJ, Stack BH *et al.* Elective versus symptomatic antibiotic treatment in cystic fibrosis patients with chronic *Pseudomonas* infection of the lungs. *Thorax* 2000; **55**:355–8.

136 Brett MM, Simmonds EJ, Ghoneim AT *et al.* The value of serum IgG titres against *Pseudomonas aeruginosa* in the management of early pseudomonal infection in cystic fibrosis. *Arch Dis Child* 1992; **67**:1086–8.

137 De Boeck SK, Vandeputte S. Meropenem versus ceftazidime plus tobramycin for pulmonary disease in CF patients (abstract). *Neth J Med* 1999; **54**(Suppl):S39.

138 Carswell F, Ward C, Cook DA *et al.* A controlled trial of nebulized aminoglycoside and oral flucloxacillin versus placebo in the outpatient management of children with cystic fibrosis. *Br J Dis Chest* 1987; **81**:356–60.

139 Kun P, Landau LI, Phelan PD. Nebulised gentamicin in children and adolescents with cystic fibrosis. *Aust Paediatr J* 1984; **20**:43–5.

140 Nathanson I, Cropp GJA, Li P, Neter P. Effectiveness of aerosolised gentamicin in cystic fibrosis. *Cystic Fibrosis Club Abstracts* 1985:Abstract 145.

141 Day A, Williams J, McKeown C, Bruton A, Weller PH. Evaluation of inhaled colomycin in children with cystic fibrosis. *Proceedings of the 10th International Cystic Fibrosis Congress* 1988:Abstract 106.

142 Hodson ME, Gallagher CG, Govan JRW *et al.* Randomised UK/Eire clinical trial of the efficacy and safety of tobramycin 300 mg/5 ml nebulised solution or nebulised colistin in CF patients. *Pediatr Pulmonol* 2000; **20**:248–9.

143 Wiesemann HG, Steinkamp G, Ratjen F *et al.* Placebo-controlled, double-blind, randomized study of aerosolized tobramycin for early treatment of *Pseudomonas aeruginosa* colonization in cystic fibrosis. *Pediatr Pulmonol* 1998; **25**:88–92.

144 Hodson ME, Gallagher CG, Govan JR. A randomised clinical trial of nebulised tobramycin or colistin in cystic fibrosis. *Eur Respir J* 2002; **20**:658–64.

145 Jensen T, Pedersen SS, Garne S *et al.* Colistin inhalation therapy in cystic fibrosis patients with chronic *Pseudomonas aeruginosa* lung infection. *J Antimicrob Chemother* 1987; **19**:831–8.

146 Stead RJ, Hodson ME, Batten JC. Inhaled ceftazidime compared with gentamicin and carbenicillin in older patients with cystic fibrosis infected with *Pseudomonas aeruginosa*. *Br J Dis Chest* 1987; **81**:272–9.

147 MacLusky IB, Gold R, Corey M *et al.* Long-term effects of inhaled tobramycin in patients with cystic fibrosis colonized with *Pseudomonas aeruginosa*. *Pediatr Pulmonol* 1989; **7**:42–8.

148 Ramsey BW, Dorkin HL, Eisenberg JD *et al.* Efficacy of aerosolized tobramycin in patients with cystic fibrosis. *N Engl J Med* 1993; **328**:1740–6.

149 Ramsey B, Burns J, Smith A. Safety and efficacy of tobramycin solution for inhalation in patients with cystic fibrosis: the results of two

phase II placebo controlled clinical trials. *Pediatr Pulmonol* 1997; **Suppl 14**:137–8.

150 Stutman HR, Lieberman JM, Nussbaum E *et al.* Antibiotic prophylaxis in infants and young children with cystic fibrosis: a randomized controlled trial. *J Pediatr* 2002; **140**:299–305.

151 Loening-Baucke VA, Mischler E, Myers MG. A placebo-controlled trial of cephalexin therapy in the ambulatory management of patients with cystic fibrosis. *J Pediatr* 1979; **95**:630–7.

152 Schlesinger EMW, von der Hardt H, Schirg E, Rieger CHL. Effect of longterm continuous anti-staphylococcal antibiotic treatment in young children with cystic fibrosis (abstract). *9th International Cystic Fibrosis Congress* 1984; **4**:14.

153 Chatfield S, Owen G, Ryley HC *et al.* Neonatal screening for cystic fibrosis in Wales and the West Midlands: clinical assessment after five years of screening. *Arch Dis Child* 1991; **66**:29–33.

154 Weaver LT, Green MR, Nicholson K *et al.* Prognosis in cystic fibrosis treated with continuous flucloxacillin from the neonatal period. *Arch Dis Child* 1994; **70**:84–9.

155 Wolter J, Seeney S, Bell S *et al.* Effect of long term treatment with azithromycin on disease parameters in cystic fibrosis: a randomised trial. *Thorax* 2002; **57**:212–16.

156 Equi A, Balfour-Lynn IM, Bush A *et al.* Long term azithromycin in children with cystic fibrosis: a randomised, placebo-controlled crossover trial. *Lancet* 2002; **360**:978–84.

PART 5

Respiratory failure/sleep-disordered breathing

CHAPTER 5.1

Respiratory rehabilitation

Yves Lacasse, François Maltais and Roger S Goldstein

Definition of problem

Less than 10 years ago, the effectiveness of respiratory rehabilitation in chronic obstructive pulmonary disease (COPD) was still the subject of debate.[1,2] The views expressed included the notion that exercise was of no value, as patients with COPD were so limited by their irreversible airflow obstruction. There was also an incomplete appreciation of randomized controlled trials (RCTs) demonstrating important improvements in health-related quality of life among those subjects assigned to the treatment groups.

A recent guideline by the American Thoracic Society defined pulmonary rehabilitation as 'a multidisciplinary program of care for patients with chronic respiratory impairment that is individually tailored and designed to optimize physical and social performance and autonomy'.[3] To establish the influence of respiratory rehabilitation on health-related quality of life and exercise capacity in patients with COPD, we recently published a meta-analysis of RCTs addressing this subject.[4] Rehabilitation included systemic exercise for at least 4 weeks, treated patients being compared with control patients who were offered only conventional community care. This chapter: (a) defines respiratory rehabilitation in practical terms; (b) provides the underlying physiological rationale for this treatment modality in COPD; (c) summarizes the findings of our Cochrane Review; and (d) comments on strategies to extend the benefits of respiratory rehabilitation.

Description of treatment

Pulmonary rehabilitation comprises a variety of interventions, typically grouped into three main categories: exercise training, education and psychological support. As most rehabilitation programmes incorporate various combinations of these components, it is often difficult to quantify the relative contribution of each to the global improvement documented among those treated. In a typical rehabilitation programme, patients participate in a programme of set exercise rehabilitation two or three times a week for 6–12 weeks, at the same time being encouraged to incorporate simpler breathing and stretching exercises as part of their daily routine. For the majority of patients, a supervised outpatient programme offers the best combination of efficacy and cost-effectiveness.[5–8] More disabled patients, those with active comorbidities, those who live far from an outpatient facility or those requiring specific resources such as nutritional supplementation or training for home ventilation should be directed to an inpatient programme.

Home-based exercise programmes are also effective in improving exercise tolerance and quality of life,[9–15] although the magnitude of these improvements may be smaller compared with programmes in which exercise training is closely supervised.[6] Home-based exercise programmes are well suited for highly motivated, self-directed individuals for whom compliance with exercise does not require close supervision. Once patients become disabled to the point of being housebound, home-based programmes are of limited value,[16] and such individuals should be referred to a closely supervised inpatient programme.

Exercise training

Although, in most of the reported controlled studies of exercise in COPD, exercise training was part of a more comprehensive pulmonary rehabilitation programme, the results do not differ from studies in which exercise training was the only treatment intervention, as neither education nor psychological support, in isolation, improves exercise tolerance.[17,18] Thus, exercise training is the cornerstone for rehabilitation programmes targeted to improve dyspnoea and exercise performance.[19]

Evidence from several RCTs supports the use of lower extremity exercise training for patients with COPD.[4,20] In most circumstances, simple aerobic exercises such as walking, cycle ergometry or treadmill training are recommended.[10,15,19,21–23] As training is specific to the muscle groups used, it is also recommended that upper extremity training be included in pulmonary rehabilitation.[18] Arm exercises generally include either weightlifting or arm ergometry. Unsupported arm exercises may be more effective than supported exercises.[24] Muscle strengthening is usually incorporated into the training regimen, with upper and lower extremity exercise at low or moderate intensity depending on the objectives of the programme.[25–29] Such exercises can be performed alone or in combination with aerobic training.[29,30]

Education and psychological support

Education and psychological support are important to the

overall success of rehabilitation, although their exact contribution is more difficult to define. Education improves knowledge, coping and self-management, actively engaging patients to maintain strategies that reduce dyspnoea, maintain good lifestyle habits and participate in the decision making when acute exacerbations occur. In an RCT of disease-specific self-management in COPD, Bourbeau and colleagues[31] reported important between-group differences of 40% fewer hospital admissions and 41% fewer emergency room visits among those tutored and supported in self-management, versus control subjects who received usual care.

Rationale for use of treatment

Physiological rationale

The benefits of pulmonary rehabilitation are mediated through a combination of physiological and psychological changes that result from the rehabilitation process. There are no expected changes in lung mechanics other than the small changes associated with optimization of pharmacological therapy, which occur at the time of assessment or enrolment in the rehabilitation programme.

Peripheral muscle dysfunction commonly contributes to exercise intolerance among patients with COPD,[32–34] with muscle wasting and weakness being present in up to 25% of patients referred for pulmonary rehabilitation.[35] The perception of leg fatigue limiting exercise is very common. As with healthy individuals, in COPD, leg fatigue is inversely proportional to muscle strength. Therefore, for any given power output, leg fatigue occurs more readily in weak than in strong individuals.[36] In fact, quadriceps strength is a significant determinant of exercise capacity independently of lung function.[32,36] In addition to muscle weakness and wasting, poor peripheral muscle aerobic capacity and reduced muscle endurance are common in patients with COPD.[37–39] Exercise training will improve peripheral muscle mass and strength,[30] reduce muscle fatigability[40] and increase aerobic capacity.[38,41] In fact, exercise training is the most appropriate approach to peripheral muscle dysfunction in COPD.

Other important physiological effects of rehabilitation in COPD[42] include reduced ventilatory demand leading to less dynamic hyperinflation and less dyspnoea, improved ventilatory muscle function, improved cardiac function and improved nutritional status.

Non-physiological rationale

Non-physiological effects of pulmonary rehabilitation include improvements in anxiety and depression,[43] as well as increased coping and motivation. The mechanisms of dyspnoea desensitization have been difficult to quantify, but a study has shown that it does occur following exercise training.[44] The overall impact of rehabilitation among patients with moderate and severe COPD has been an improvement in exercise and

functional activity resulting in an improvement in health status and a reduction in health care utilization.[31,45]

Acute effects of respiratory rehabilitation in COPD: meta-analysis

Literature search

In 1996, we published a meta-analysis of respiratory rehabilitation in COPD that was not conducted under the patronage of the Cochrane Collaboration.[20] We reported its update in 2001, in which we included the 14 trials from the original meta-analysis.[4] Additional trials were identified with assistance from the Cochrane Airways Group COPD trial registry, which was searched for original articles, published in any language, using the following strategy: [exp, lung diseases, obstructive] and [exp, rehabilitation or exp, exercise therapy] and [research design or longitudinal studies or evaluation study or randomized controlled trial]. We reviewed the reference lists of relevant articles and retrieved additional citations. Abstracts presented at international meetings such as the American Thoracic Society, 1980–2000, the American College of Chest Physicians, 1980–2000, and the European Respiratory Society, 1987–2000, were also hand searched. We contacted the authors of studies included in the meta-analysis and experts in the field of respiratory rehabilitation in order to uncover unpublished material.

Summary of methods for the meta-analysis

We included only RCTs comparing rehabilitation with conventional community care, in order to study the overall effect of rehabilitation without partitioning its components. In the trials, more than 90% of patients had COPD defined according to a clinical diagnosis of COPD plus either the best recorded forced expiratory volume in 1 second (FEV_1)/forced vital capacity (FVC) ratio being <0.7 or the best recorded FEV_1 being <70% predicted. We included inpatient, outpatient or home-based rehabilitation programmes provided that they were of at least 4 weeks' duration and provided that they included exercise therapy, with or without other modalities, delivered to patients whose exercise limitation was attributable to COPD.

The main outcome measures were health-related quality of life and exercise capacity. We defined maximal exercise capacity as the peak capacity measured following an incremental exercise test, and defined functional exercise capacity according to the results of timed walk tests. We chose to analyse maximal and functional exercise separately because the two measures (incremental cycle ergometry and timed 6- or 12-min walk tests) correlated only moderately and probably represented different constructs.[46,47]

Throughout the analysis, we used weighted mean differences (WMD) that we determined from the difference between the pre- and postintervention changes in the treatment and control groups. For each outcome, we limited the analysis to trials in which the same measure was used. The WMD were combined according to a random effects model.[48] Homogeneity across studies was tested for each outcome. Given the low sensitivity of the test of homogeneity, we declared heterogeneity when $P < 0.10$. Whenever possible, the common effect was related to the minimal clinically important difference (MCID) for each outcome. The MCID has been defined as the smallest difference in score corresponding to the smallest difference perceived by the average patient that would mandate (in the absence of troublesome side-effects or excessive cost) a change in patient management.[49]

Findings

Twenty-three randomized controlled trials were included in the meta-analysis.[7,9,10,13,15,21–23,25,27,45,50–61] With only one exception, all the trials that met the inclusion criteria of the meta-analysis were parallel group trials, summarized in Table 1. The primary results of the meta-analysis are summarized in Table 2. The levels of evidence and grades of recommendations are according to Cook et al.[62]

Dyspnoea and health-related quality of life

Among the 23 trials included in the meta-analysis, 13 measured health-related quality of life, using a total of eight different strategies. Only three of these strategies, the Transitional Dyspnea Index,[63] the Chronic Respiratory Disease Questionnaire (CRQ)[64] and the St George's Respiratory Questionnaire,[65] have proved to be valid and responsive. The analysis was restricted to the CRQ, as it represented the most widely used questionnaire among the trials included. For each domain of the CRQ, the common effect size exceeded the MCID (0.5 point on the seven-point scale).[49] The boundary of the confidence intervals (CIs) suggested that the smallest effect exceeded the MCID for dyspnoea (Fig. 1), fatigue and mastery domains, whereas for the emotional function domain, it included the MCID, leaving the importance of the effect uncertain for this domain.

Functional exercise capacity

Fifteen trials including 300 actively treated and 280 control subjects were available. Limiting the meta-analysis to the 10 trials (235 actively treated and 219 control subjects) in which the 6-min walk test was used as an outcome, the common effect (WMD) was 49 m (95% CI 26–72; homogeneity $P = 0.08$; Fig. 2). Our estimate of the MCID of the walk test (50 m; 95% CI 37–71 m) was derived from a study in which COPD participants rated their walking ability through subjective comparisons with one another.[66] As the inferior limit of the CI around the common effect was beyond the limit of the CI for the MCID of the walking test, the clinical significance of the result obtained from the meta-analysis remains uncertain.

Maximal exercise capacity

Maximal exercise capacity was measured in 15 trials (265 participants received active rehabilitation and 243 participants served as control subjects). Limiting the meta-analysis to the 14 trials that used the incremental cycle ergometer test as the outcome (255 treated participants and 233 control subjects), the common effect (WMD) was 5.46 W (95% CI 0.49–10.23 W). We found this number difficult to interpret, notwithstanding it reaching statistical significance.

Additional studies

Subsequent to our submitting the above meta-analysis to the Cochrane Library, we identified five additional randomized trials of respiratory rehabilitation for which incomplete information was available.[67–71] Each of these trials reported benefits in either quality of life or exercise capacity among the treatment group compared with control subjects. We anticipate including these results in the next update submitted to the Cochrane Library.

Summary

This meta-analysis showed that respiratory rehabilitation was effective in reducing dyspnoea and fatigue as well as improving patients' sense of control (mastery) over their condition. The magnitude of these improvements was beyond the MCID of the outcome measures used. Given that the management of patients with COPD is largely symptomatic,[72] outcome measures that include health-related quality of life are of primary importance to trials of respiratory rehabilitation.

Rehabilitation programmes included in the meta-analysis differed in several aspects, including their clinical settings, duration and composition. For instance, the contribution of educational activities and psychological support in addition to exercise training remains uncertain. This information would be of utmost importance to physicians and allied health professionals who prescribe rehabilitation and those who allocate the resources. We addressed this issue in a systematic overview of the literature.[17] Since the publication of this review, further evidence from RCTs has been published to define better the types and intensity of exercise,[30] as well as the influence of the programme components.[73] Sometimes, the evidence even took the form of systematic reviews.[74] Such questions were too specific to be addressed directly in this meta-analysis that aimed at investigating the overall effect of rehabilitation in COPD (and not the effect of its components). Nevertheless, homogeneity among study results suggested that less sophisticated rehabilitation programmes may also be effective in improving quality of life, although the between-study comparison from which this conclusion follows is relatively weak.

Other treatment modalities

Inspiratory muscle training

A few studies have evaluated whether inspiratory muscle training represented a useful addition to general exercise training. In some reports, maximal inspiratory pressure and

Table 1. Summary of the characteristics of the trials included in the meta-analysis.

Reference (first author)	Rehabilitation programme				Outcome measures		Methodological quality	
	Setting	Components*	Duration	Sample size†	Exercise capacity‡	Quality of life§	Concealed randomization	Blinded assessment of outcomes
McGavin (1977)[9]	Home-based	LLE	Continuous	Rehab.: 12 Control: 12	12-min WT; ICET	Interviews;	Yes	No
Cockcroft (1981)[50]	Inpatient	LLE, ULE	6 weeks	Rehab.: 18 Control: 16	12-min WT; ITT	Interviews; POMS; Eysenck	Yes	Yes
Booker (1984)[51]	Home-based	LLE; BE, PD; Edu, Psy	9 weeks	Rehab.: 32 Control: 37	6-min WT	Anxiety/depression scale	N/A	Yes
Jones (1985)[52]	Home-based	LLE, ULE	10 weeks	Rehab.: 8 Control: 6	12-min WT; ICET; SSCET	Daily diary; Lubin; Affectometer	Yes	12-min WT, SSCET: Yes; ICET: No
Busch (1988)[13]	Home-based	LLE; BE	18 weeks	Rehab.: 6 Control: 6	ICET; multistep stage test	CRQ (dyspnoea domain only)	Yes	No
Lake (1990)[21]	Outpatient	LLE, ULE	8 weeks	Rehab.: 7 Control: 7	6-min WT; ICET; IAET	Bandura scale of well-being	Yes	ICET: Yes; 6-min WT: No
Simpson (1992)[27]	Outpatient	LLE, ULE	8 weeks	Rehab.: 14 Control: 14	6-min WT; ICET; SSCET	CRQ	Yes	CRQ: Yes; Others: No
Weiner (1992)[23]	Outpatient	LLE, ULE; IMT, BE	6 months	Rehab.: 12 Control: 12	12-min WT; ICET; SSCET;	Not measured	Yes	Yes
Goldstein (1994)[53]	Inpatient	LLE, ULE; BE; Edu, Psy	8 weeks	Rehab.: 38 Control: 41	6-min WT; ICET; SSCET	CRQ; BDI/TDI	Yes	Yes
Reardon (1994)[22]	Outpatient	LLE, ULE; BE; Edu, Psy	6 weeks	Rehab.: 10 Control: 10	ITT	BDI/TDI	Yes	Yes
Vallet, (1994)[54]¶	Inpatient	LLE; BE	8 weeks	Rehab.: 10 Control: 10	ICET	Not measured	Yes	No
Wijkstra (1994)[10]	Home-based	LLE, ULE; IMT, BE; Edu, Psy	12 weeks	Rehab.: 28 Control: 15	6-min WT; ICET	CRQ	Yes	No
Guell (1995)[55]	Outpatient	LLE; BE, PD	6 months	Rehab.: 29 Control: 27	6-min WT; ICET	CRQ	Yes	Yes
Strijbos (1996)[15]	Outpatient	LLE; BE; PD; Edu, Psy	12 weeks	Rehab.: 15 Control: 15	4-min WT; ICET	Interview	No	Yes

Table 1. Continued.

Reference (first author)	Rehabilitation programme				Outcome measures		Methodological quality	
	Setting	Components*	Duration	Sample size†	Exercise capacity‡	Quality of life§	Concealed randomization	Blinded assessment of outcomes
Bendstrup (1997)[56]	Outpatient	LLE, ULE, IMT	12 weeks	Rehab.: 16 Control: 16	6-min WT	CRQ; Activities of daily living: York QLQ	Unclear	NA
Cambach (1997)[57]	Community-based	LLE, ULE, Edu, IMT	12 weeks	Rehab.: 15 Control: 8	6-min WT; ICET	CRQ	Adequate	No
Clark (1996)[25]	Home-based	LLE, ULE	12 weeks	Rehab.: 32 Control: 16	ICET, ITT	Not measured	Unclear	NA
Emery (1998)[58]	Outpatient	LLE, ULE, Edu, Psy	10 weeks	Rehab.: 25 Control: 25	ICET	SIP	Adequate	Yes
Engstrom (1999)[59]	Outpatient	LLE, ULE, Edu, IMT	52 weeks	Rehab.: 26 Control: 24	6-min WT, ICET	SIP, SGRQ	Adequate	HRQL: Yes WT: No
Troosters (2000)[7]	Outpatient	LLE, ULE	24 weeks	Rehab.: 37 Control: 33	6-min WT, ICET	CRQ	Adequate	No
Griffiths (2000)[45]	Outpatient	LLE, ULE, Edu, Psy, NS, SmC	6 weeks	Rehab.: 93 Control: 91	Shuttle walk test	CRQ, SF-36, SGRQ	Adequate	Yes
Hernandez (2000)[60]	Home-based	LLE	12 weeks	Rehab.: 20 Control: 17	ICET, Shuttle walk test	CRQ, BDI/TDI	Adequate	Yes
Ringbaek (2000)[61]	Outpatient	LLE, ULE	8 weeks	Rehab.: 7 Control: 7	6-min WT, ICET, IAET	Bandura scale of well-being	Adequate	ICET: Yes; 6-min WT: No

*LLE, lower limb exercise; ULE, upper limb exercise; IMT, inspiratory muscle training; BE, breathing exercises; PD, postural drainage; Edu, education; Psy, psychological support.

†Number of patients who were accounted for in the analysis.

‡WT, walk test; ICET, incremental cycle ergometer test; ITT, incremental treadmill test; SSCET, steady-state cycle ergometer test; SSTT, steady-state treadmill test; IAET, incremental arm ergometer test.

§POMS: Profile of Mood State (Lorr–McNair Mood questionnaire); Eysenck, Eysenck personality questionnaire; Lubin, Lubin depression adjective check list; CRQ, Chronic Respiratory Disease Questionnaire; BDI/TDI, Baseline Dyspnea Index/Transitional Dyspnea Index.

¶The data from eight patients (five in the treatment group and three in the control group) were excluded because of an $FEV_1 \geq 70\%$ of predicted value.

Table 2. Primary results of the meta-analysis.

Outcomes	No. of trials	No. of patients	Treatment effect (95% CI) (WMD)		Homogeneity (*P*-value)	Level of evidence*
Dyspnoea	9	277 treated/ 242 controls	1.0 CRQ units	0.8–1.2	0.53	Level I+ (grade A)
Fatigue	8	273 treated/ 240 controls	0.9 CRQ units	0.7–1.1	0.48	Level I+ (grade A)
Emotional function	8	273 treated/ 240 controls	0.7 CRQ units	0.4–1.0	0.17	Level II+ (grade B)
Mastery	8	273 treated/ 240 controls	0.9 CRQ units	0.7–1.2	0.87	Level I+ (grade A)
Maximal exercise capacity	14	255 treated/ 233 controls	5.4 W	0.5–10.2	0.14	Level I+ (grade A)
Functional exercise capacity	10	235 treated/ 219 controls	49 m	26–72	0.08	Level II– (grade B)

*The levels of evidence are graded according to Cook *et al.*[62]

Review:　　Meta-analysis of respiratory rehabilitation in chronic obstructive pulmonary disease
Comparison:　03 Rehabilitation vs usual care
Outcome:　　04 QoL, CRQ-dyspnoea

Study or subcategory	N	Rehab [mean (SD)]	N	Usual care [mean (SD)]	WMD (fixed) (95% CI)	Weight (%)	WMD (random) (95% CI)
Busch (1988)	7	−0.60 (10.40)	7	1.30 (5.20)		1.41	−1.90 (−10.51, 6.71)
Cambach (1997)	14	6.00 (6.00)	8	0.00 (4.00)		5.97	6.00 (1.81, 10.19)
Goldstein (1994)	40	3.40 (5.70)	39	0.10 (6.50)		14.39	3.30 (0.60, 6.00)
Gosselink (2000)	34	4.00 (6.40)	28	−0.10 (6.60)		9.88	4.10 (0.84, 7.36)
Griffiths (2000)	93	5.00 (6.40)	91	−0.90 (5.00)		38.14	5.90 (4.24, 7.56)
Güell (1995)	29	6.00 (7.00)	27	−0.50 (5.50)		9.71	6.50 (3.21, 9.79)
Hernandez (2000)	20	5.40 (5.70)	17	1.50 (6.00)		7.29	3.90 (0.11, 7.69)
Simpson (1992)	12	6.00 (5.70)	10	0.00 (4.20)		6.10	6.00 (1.86, 10.14)
Wijkstra1 (1994)	28	4.30 (5.10)	15	−0.20 (6.60)		7.12	4.50 (0.66, 8.34)
Total (95% CI)	277		242			100.00	5.06 (4.04, 6.09)

Test for heterogeneity: chi-squared = 7.03, df = 8 (*P* = 0.53), I^2 = 0%
Test for overall effect: z = 9.69 (*P* < 0.00001)

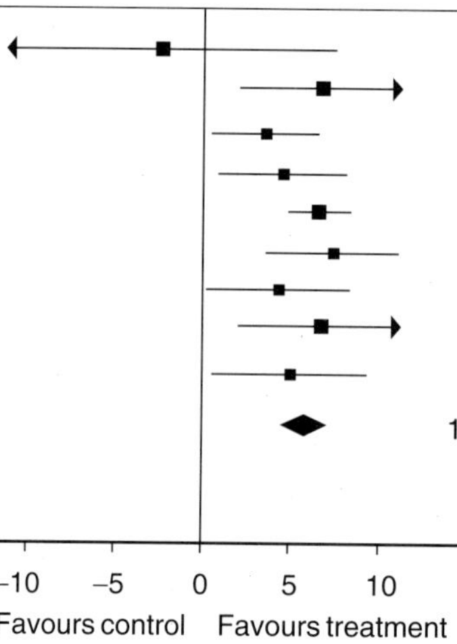

−10　−5　0　5　10
Favours control　Favours treatment

Figure 1. The effect of respiratory rehabilitation in chronic obstructive pulmonary disease on dyspnoea as measured by the Chronic Respiratory Questionnaire: meta-view. The results are presented as the domain total score (five items graded on a seven-point scale; maximal score = 35), as opposed to the treatment effect values in Table 2 that are presented as item scores (from Lacasse *et al.*,[4] copyright Cochrane Library, reproduced with permission).

exercise capacity improved, compared with exercise training alone,[75,76] whereas in others, the addition of inspiratory muscle training was not associated with any further improvements in exercise capacity or health status.[77,78] To be included in a rehabilitation programme, the benefits of inspiratory muscle training should extend beyond improvements in measures of respiratory muscle function to include improvements in dyspnoea or exercise capacity, or an improved handling of increased respiratory loads similar to those experienced by patients during a respiratory exacerbation. A meta-analysis of trials in which inspiratory muscle training was added to general exercise training reported that additional improvements in functional exercise capacity did not reach statistical significance.[79]

Review: Meta-analysis of respiratory rehabilitation in chronic obstructive pulmonary disease
Comparison: 03 Rehabilitation vs usual care
Outcome: 05 Functional exercise capacity

Study or subcategory	N	Rehab [mean (SD)]	N	Usual care [mean (SD)]	WMD (random) (95% CI)	Weight (%)	WMD (random) (95% CI)
Booker (1984)	32	21.00 (85.00)	37	5.00 (90.00)		13.84	16.00 (−25.33, 57.33)
Cambach (1997)	12	51.00 (89.00)	7	46.00 (79.00)		6.53	5.00 (−72.21, 82.21)
Engström (1999)	26	38.00 (90.00)	24	−2.00 (102.00)		10.62	40.00 (−13.50, 93.50)
Goldstein (1994)	36	32.00 (102.00)	41	−11.00 (99.00)		12.76	43.00 (−2.04, 88.04)
Gosselink (2000)	34	58.00 (125.00)	28	3.00 (104.00)		9.85	55.00 (−2.00, 112.00)
Güell (1995)	29	91.00 (67.00)	27	8.00 (67.00)		15.81	83.00 (47.88, 118.12)
Lake (1990)	7	108.60 (79.00)	7	−35.00 (50.00)		7.64	143.60 (74.34, 212.86)
Ringbaek (2000)	17	10.47 (85.09)	19	−18.52 (77.50)		10.64	28.99 (−24.40, 82.38)
Simpson (1992)	14	36.00 (102.00)	14	7.00 (120.00)		5.91	29.00 (−53.50, 111.50)
Wijkstra1 (1994)	28	9.00 (87.00)	15	−28.00 (141.00)		6.40	37.00 (−41.29, 115.29)
Total (95% CI)	235		219			100.00	48.95 (26.00, 71.89)

Test for heterogeneity: chi-squared = 15.52, df = 9 (P = 0.08), I^2 = 42.0%
Test for overall effect: z = 4.18 (P < 0.0001)

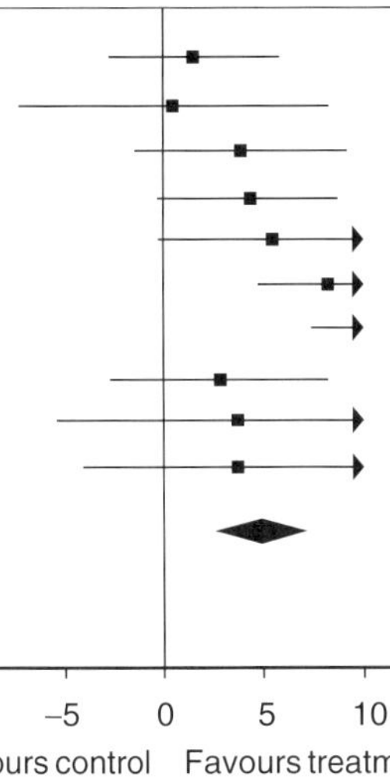

```
        -10    -5     0     5     10
        Favours control   Favours treatment
```

Figure 2. The effect of respiratory rehabilitation in chronic obstructive pulmonary disease on functional exercise capacity as measured by the 6-min walk test: meta-view (from Lacasse et al.,[4] copyright Cochrane Library, reproduced with permission).

Nutritional and anabolic hormone supplementation

The addition of nutritional supplementation, either alone or in combination with anabolic medications, to exercise training has been evaluated in a number of trials[35,80,81] and summarized in a meta-analysis.[82] Anabolic medications and nutritional support may result in increases in muscle mass, when compared with exercise training alone.[35,80,81] However, the clinical relevance of this effect is questionable as any additional benefits, in terms of exercise tolerance, were modest. Therefore, further studies are recommended to elucidate the possible role of nutritional supplementation and anabolic medications in respiratory rehabilitation.

Supplemental oxygen during exercise training

The administration of supplemental oxygen during exercise training has been shown to improve laboratory measures of maximal exercise capacity[83,84] and, in theory, might enable patients with COPD to train at higher intensities than they would otherwise achieve while breathing ambient air. As with healthy volunteers, the physiological benefits of training are higher in patients with COPD when they train at a higher power output.[85] However, the results of two RCTs in which supplemental oxygen has been added during exercise training have been disappointing. In one study, 24 patients with COPD (mean FEV_1 34% predicted) and exercise-induced O_2 desaturation[86] were randomly allocated to breathe either room air or oxygen at 4 L/min during exercise training. After 10 weeks, the intensity of walking, stair-climbing, weightlifting and health status increased in both groups with no significant between-group differences. In another study, 25 patients (mean FEV_1 30% predicted) with a ≥4% fall in arterial saturation from baseline to 90% or below were randomized to a similar training protocol with or without supplemental oxygen during exercise training.[87] After 6 weeks of training, dyspnoea improved in those trained with oxygen, but there was no difference between groups with respect to their functional exercise capacity (shuttle walking distance) or health status.

In a more recent trial, 30 patients with non-hypoxaemic COPD (both at rest and during exercise) were randomized to received either oxygen at 3 L/min or compressed air at 3 L/min during a closely supervised 7-week exercise training programme.[88] In this study, subjects underwent high-intensity exercise training. The authors noted that the training intensity reached was 20% higher in those receiving supplemental oxygen compared with the control subjects who received compressed air. Improvements in constant power endurance time and in physiological responses to training were greater among those who received supplemental oxygen. Both groups reached significant and clinically important improvement in the disease-specific respiratory questionnaire, except in the domain of mastery, in which the improvement was greater among the oxygen group. The authors concluded that supplemental oxygen might enable normoxic patients with COPD to train at higher intensities and therefore to obtain additional physiological benefits from exercise training. Whether this approach will be of benefit during activities of daily living, whether it is practical and cost-effective and whether it would also apply to patients with COPD who experience exercise-induced desaturation remains unclear.

Ventilatory support during exercise training

Evidence from acute, short-term physiological studies has shown that mechanical ventilatory support during exercise may decrease dyspnoea and improve exercise tolerance among patients with COPD.[83,89–93] In one community study of normocapnic COPD patients, nasal positive pressure ventilation (NIPPV) for 2 hours/day plus exercise training improved functional exercise (shuttle walking distance) and quality of life, compared with control subjects who received only rehabilitation.[94] The role of NIPPV during exercise for hypercapnic patients with COPD remains unanswered, although a meta-analysis of NIPPV for stable hypercapnic patients with COPD has shown no effect.[95] Widespread use of ventilatory support during rehabilitation requires larger clinical trials in order to identify whether it will be a useful adjunct to exercise training.

Maintenance programmes

Respiratory rehabilitation is an accepted therapeutic intervention that has been shown in a variety of well-designed RCTs, in which valid, reproducible and interpretable outcome measures were used, to improve functional exercise capacity and health-related quality of life.[12,19,20,31,53] However, the benefits of rehabilitation diminish with time. Ries et al.[19] noted that the initial improvements in exercise gained during rehabilitation diminished over the subsequent 18 months. Wedzicha et al.[16] reported that, at 1 year, no significant improvements in health status or exercise tolerance remained. Foglio et al.[96] noted (in asthmatics and patients with COPD) that, 12 months post rehabilitation, only 52% of subjects had clinically relevant improvements in health status. Griffiths et al.[45] attributed the loss of effect following rehabilitation to poor self-management practices and a lack of adherence to treatment protocols after discharge.

The explanation as to why some patients do not adhere to medical advice includes many contributing variables.[45,97] Patient factors include knowledge, health beliefs and attitude towards their condition. The interaction with the health care provider will probably influence the patient's adherence, as will the presence of anxiety or depression. A previous history of non-adherence is often predictive of future behaviour. Practitioner factors include the quality of the explanation and the amount of individual attention given to the patient. Regimen factors are important as the demands made on the patient, such as the number and frequency of medications prescribed or the complexity and duration of an exercise programme, may be quite unrealistic. External factors, such as the presence of a stable social support network, family cohesiveness, positive environmental attitudes and interpersonal re-

sources, may all have a bearing on compliance with medical advice. Although the determinants of poor compliance are often complex, with many of the socio-demographic variables still to be defined, an improved understanding of this issue will assist health care providers in identifying those individuals at high risk.

Patient factors

Not everyone improves in a similar way following rehabilitation. Ketalaars and colleagues[98] used hierarchical cluster analysis to define patients in whom long-term benefits of rehabilitation were sustained 9 months after completion of an inpatient programme. Complete data sets were obtained from 77 patients with similar pulmonary function characteristics. In one group ($n = 44$), health status was moderate on admission, improved with rehabilitation and subsequently deteriorated at follow-up. In the second group ($n = 33$), health status reflected severe impairment on admission with little improvement after rehabilitation and no further change at follow-up. The second group would be unlikely to improve further even if additional resources were allocated for maintenance. This information is important in developing strategies for aftercare at home that aim to maintain the benefits of rehabilitation.

Programme location

The immediate benefits of rehabilitation are not site specific. Excellent improvements have been reported among inpatient,[53] outpatient[45,99] and community-based programmes.[12] However, programme location may influence the longer term patient adherence. Strijbos and colleagues[15] described 41 subjects who completed an 18-month study in which they were randomized to enrol in a hospital outpatient pulmonary rehabilitation programme or a home-based programme. Each programme offered supervision twice a week for 12 weeks. Similar improvements in both groups were noted at 3 and 6 months. However, only those who underwent the home-based programme experienced a sustained improvement at 18 months. A possible explanation is that an initial familiarity with exercising at home might enable subjects to continue their exercises at home more readily and therefore extend its duration of benefit. This conclusion was supported by the patient's diary cards, which reflected greater participation during the unsupervised home period.

Programme duration

In our meta-analysis of rehabilitation, we noted consistent modest improvements in nearly all the programmes evaluated. In a post hoc analysis, the magnitude of the improvement appeared to be influenced by the programme duration. This hypothesis was tested prospectively by Troosters et al.[7] and Guell et al.[100] Troosters et al.[7] reported on 100 patients randomized to 6 months of outpatient rehabilitation versus control subjects. Sixty-two patients were evaluated at 6 months and 49 at 18 months. The between-group differences in 6-min walk and health status noted at 6 months were sustained at 18 months, at which time they still remained above the MCID. In a subsequent study by Guell and colleagues,[100] 60 subjects received 12 months of outpatient rehabilitation versus usual care. Between-group differences in dyspnoea, health status and functional exercise were evident by the third month and continued with somewhat diminished magnitude into the second year of follow-up. In this study, the number needed to treat (NNT) to achieve a significant benefit in health status for a 2-year period was approximately three. In support of the importance of programme duration in contributing to the effects of rehabilitation, Green and colleagues[101] noted lesser improvements following rehabilitation among 23 subjects randomized to 4 weeks of rehabilitation versus 21 subjects randomized to a 7-week programme.

Exercise maintenance

In a retrospective report of 51 patients who completed outpatient pulmonary rehabilitation, Vale and colleagues[102] noted that 19 individuals had participated in a structured, weekly, postrehabilitation exercise maintenance programme, whereas 32 had not. In both groups, functional exercise capacity (12-min walk) and health-related quality of life (CRQ) decreased at the time of follow-up (11.0±6.1 months), although these measures remained above the baseline. There were no between-group differences attributable to the postrehabilitation exercise maintenance programme.

Programme repeat

Foglio et al.[103] reported a pilot study in which 61 stable patients (26 COPD, 35 asthma) who completed rehabilitation were randomized to receive a repeat programme 12 months later and again at 24 months, or just to receive a 24-month repeat. Only 36 subjects completed this study. Although subsequent yearly interventions resulted in comparable short-term gains in exercise capacity and health status, there were no additive long-term benefits from a standard annual programme repeat.

Enhanced follow-up

Brooks and colleagues[97] reported on an RCT of enhanced aftercare versus usual aftercare among 109 individuals with COPD who completed pulmonary rehabilitation. Those receiving enhanced follow-up were enrolled in monthly hospital group sessions and also received telephone contact 2 weeks after each visit to the centre. All subjects were seen in follow-up every 3 months. At 6 months, the distance walked in 6 min was slightly greater in the enhanced follow-up group compared with control subjects. At 1 year, this difference had disappeared. Health-related quality of life did not differ between groups. When asked (self-reported compliance) 'Are you doing any regular exercises at home?', the percentage of subjects who continued to exercise declined in both groups with

no between-group difference. Brooks et al.[97] noted that individuals complied differently with different exercises. Good compliance was noted with breathing exercises and with aerobic exercise, but compliance with interval training and muscle strengthening was poor in both groups. This raises important issues regarding the best content for a maintenance programme, an area in which little information is available. When asked why they discontinued exercise, many individuals identified a respiratory exacerbation as the trigger after which they dropped out of the programme. Conceivably, it might be possible to maintain function following an exacerbation by applying additional resources soon after clinical recovery, thereby preventing the patients discontinuing their exercise programme.

Ries and colleagues[99] reported on 172 individuals randomized to 1 year of maintenance treatment or usual care following 8 weeks of pulmonary rehabilitation. During the maintenance programme, patients received weekly telephone calls in addition to their monthly visits to the centre. Subjects adhered well to the trial with 138 subjects completing their 12-month assessment and 131 subjects completing their 24-month assessment. However, when compared with the control group, there were only minimal improvements in maximal treadmill exercise, 6-min walk test and health status during the 12-month maintenance period and, by 24 months, these differences had disappeared.

Summary

Although there is good evidence that rehabilitation improves health-related quality of life and functional exercise capacity, these improvements diminish with time, almost certainly because of reduced patient compliance. Although longer programmes will extend the clinical benefits of rehabilitation, programme enhancements with regular facility visits and phone calls have resulted in only minimal gains. Conceivably, an abbreviated period of rehabilitation, provided for those who have completed an initial rehabilitation programme, might be of value in improving compliance with exercise activities and extending the duration of the benefit obtained by the patient.

Implications for research

There are now strong arguments that respiratory rehabilitation will improve quality of life, to the extent of there being no need for additional RCTs comparing respiratory rehabilitation with conventional community care for patients with COPD. However, several interesting issues remain to be explored. These include the value of various components of rehabilitation, programme length, the required degree of supervision, the intensity of training and the best approach to maintaining programme adherence. An improved understanding of these issues will be of value to those who receive, fund and provide respiratory rehabilitation.

Summary for clinicians

- Respiratory rehabilitation is defined as 'a multidisciplinary program of care for patients with chronic respiratory impairment that is individually tailored and designed to optimize physical and social performance and autonomy'. It is usually composed of a variety of components grouped into three main categories: exercise training, education and psychological support.
- The results of a meta-analysis of respiratory rehabilitation, including at least 4 weeks of exercise training, show clear benefit especially in the domains of dyspnoea, fatigue and mastery for patients with COPD.
- Trials of adjuncts to respiratory rehabilitation such as inspiratory muscle training and nutritional supplementation have shown limited effects. These modalities should therefore be considered on an individual basis, when indicated. The application of supplemental oxygen or mechanical ventilatory support during exercise training requires further investigation.
- The benefits of rehabilitation diminish with time. Strategies to maintain these benefits, especially following an acute exacerbation, remain a challenge for clinicians.
- Rehabilitation is a cost-effective approach to the management of COPD and should be included as part of the standard of care.

References

1 Celli BR. Is pulmonary rehabilitation an effective treatment for chronic obstructive pulmonary disease? Yes. *Am J Respir Crit Care Med* 1997; **155**:781–3.

2 Albert RK. Is pulmonary rehabilitation an effective treatment for chronic obstructive pulmonary disease? No. *Am J Respir Crit Care Med* 1997; **155**:784–5.

3 American Thoracic Society. Pulmonary rehabilitation. *Am J Respir Crit Care Med* 1999; **159**:1666–82.

4 Lacasse Y, Brosseau S, Milne S *et al*. Pulmonary rehabilitation for chronic obstructive pulmonary disease (Cochrane Review). In: *The Cochrane Library*. Oxford, Update Software, 2002.

5 Brooks D, Lacasse Y, Goldstein RS. Pulmonary rehabilitation programs in Canada: national survey. *Can Respir J* 1999; **6**:55–63.

6 Puente-Maestu L, Sanz ML, Sanz P, Cubillo JM, Mayol J, Casaburi R. Comparison of effects of supervised versus self-monitored training programmes in patients with chronic obstructive pulmonary disease. *Eur Respir J* 2000; **15**:517–25.

7 Troosters T, Gosselink R, Decramer M. Short- and long-term effects of outpatient rehabilitation in patients with chronic obstructive pulmonary disease: a randomized trial. *Am J Med* 2000; **109**:207–12.

8 Goldstein RS, Gort EH, Guyatt GH, Feeny D. Economic analysis of respiratory rehabilitation. *Chest* 1997; **112**:370–9.

9 McGavin CR, Gupta SP, Lloyd EL, McHardy GJ. Physical rehabilitation for the chronic bronchitic: results of a controlled trial of exercises in the home. *Thorax* 1977; **32**:307–11.

10 Wijkstra PJ, van Altena R, Kraan J, Otten V, Postma DS, Koeter GH. Quality of life in patients with chronic obstructive pulmonary disease improves after rehabilitation at home. *Eur Respir J* 1994; **7**:269–73.

11 Strijbos JH, Postma DS, van Altena R, Gimeno F, Koeter GH. Feasibility and effects of a home-care rehabilitation program in patients with chronic obstructive pulmonary disease. *J Cardiopulm Rehabil* 1996; **16**:386–93.

12 Wijkstra PJ, Ten Vergert EM, van Altena R *et al*. Long term benefits of rehabilitation at home on quality of life and exercise tolerance in patients with chronic obstructive pulmonary disease. *Thorax* 1995; **50**:824–8.

13 Busch AJ, McClements JD. Effects of a supervised home exercise program on patients with severe chronic obstructive pulmonary disease. *Phys Ther* 1988; **68**:469–74.

14 Debigare R, Maltais F, Whittom F, Deslauriers J, LeBlanc P. Feasibility and efficacy of home exercise training before lung volume reduction. *J Cardiopulm Rehabil* 1999; **19**:235–41.

15 Strijbos JH, Postma DS, van Altena R, Gimeno F, Koeter GH. A comparison between an outpatient hospital-based pulmonary rehabilitation program and a home-care pulmonary rehabilitation program in patients with COPD. A follow-up of 18 months. *Chest* 1996; **109**:366–72.

16 Wedzicha JA, Bestall JC, Garrod R, Garnham R, Paul EA, Jones PW. Randomized controlled trial of pulmonary rehabilitation in severe chronic obstructive pulmonary disease patients, stratified with the MRC dyspnoea scale. *Eur Respir J* 1998; **12**:363–9.

17 Lacasse Y, Guyatt GH, Goldstein RS. The components of a respiratory rehabilitation program: a systematic overview. *Chest* 1997; **110**:1077–88.

18 ACCP/AACVPR Pulmonary Rehabilitation Guidelines Panel. American College of Chest Physicians. Pulmonary rehabilitation: joint ACCP/AACVPR evidence-based guidelines. *Chest* 1997; **112**:1363–96.

19 Ries AL, Kaplan RM, Limberg TM, Prewitt LM. Effects of pulmonary rehabilitation on physiologic and psychosocial outcomes in patients with chronic obstructive pulmonary disease. *Ann Intern Med* 1995; **122**:823–32.

20 Lacasse Y, Wong E, Guyatt GH, King D, Cook DJ, Goldstein RS. Meta-analysis of respiratory rehabilitation in chronic obstructive pulmonary disease. *Lancet* 1996; **348**:1115–19.

21 Lake FR, Henderson K, Briffa T, Openshaw J, Musk AW. Upper-limb and lower-limb exercise training in patients with chronic airflow obstruction. *Chest* 1990; **97**:1077–82.

22 Reardon J, Awad E, Normandin E, Vale F, Clark B, ZuWallack RL. The effect of comprehensive outpatient pulmonary rehabilitation on dyspnea. *Chest* 1994; **105**:1046–52.

23 Weiner P, Azgad Y, Ganam R. Inspiratory muscle training combined with general exercise reconditioning in patients with COPD. *Chest* 1992; **102**:1351–6.

24 Martinez FJ, Vogel PD, Dupont DN, Stanopoulos I, Gray A, Beamis JF. Supported arm exercise vs unsupported arm exercise in the rehabilitation of patients with severe chronic airflow obstruction. *Chest* 1993; **103**:1397–402.

25 Clark CJ, Cochrane L, Mackay E. Low intensity peripheral muscle conditioning improves exercise tolerance and breathlessness in COPD. *Eur Respir J* 1996; **9**:2590–6.

26 Clark CJ, Cochrane LM, Mackay E, Paton B. Skeletal muscle strength and endurance in patients with mild COPD and the effects of weight training. *Eur Respir J* 2000; **15**:92–7.

27 Simpson K, Killian K, McCartney N, Stubbing DG, Jones NL. Randomised controlled trial of weightlifting exercise in patients with chronic airflow limitation. *Thorax* 1992; **47**:70–5.

28 Spruit MA, Gosselink R, Troosters T, De Paepe K, Decramer M. Resistance versus endurance training in patients with COPD and peripheral muscle weakness. *Eur Respir J* 2002; **19**:1072–8.

29 Ortega F, Toral J, Cejudo P *et al*. Comparison of effects of strength and endurance training in patients with chronic obstructive pulmonary disease. *Am J Respir Crit Care Med* 2002; **166**:669–74.

30 Bernard S, Whittom F, LeBlanc P *et al*. Aerobic and strength training in patients with chronic obstructive pulmonary disease. *Am J Respir Crit Care Med* 1999; **159**:896–901.

31 Bourbeau J, Julien M, Maltais F *et al*. Reduction of hospital utilization in patients with chronic obstructive pulmonary disease: a disease-specific self-management intervention. *Arch Intern Med* 2003; **163**:585–91.

32 Gosselink R, Troosters T, Decramer M. Peripheral muscle weakness contributes to exercise limitation in COPD. *Am J Respir Crit Care Med* 1996; **153**:976–80.

33 Gosker HR, Wouters EF, van der Vusse GJ, Schols AM. Skeletal muscle dysfunction in chronic obstructive pulmonary disease and chronic heart failure: underlying mechanisms and therapy perspectives. *Am J Clin Nutr* 2000; **71**:1033–47.

34 Maltais F, LeBlanc P, Jobin J, Casaburi R. Peripheral muscle dysfunction in chronic obstructive pulmonary disease. *Clin Chest Med* 2000; **21**:665–77.

35 Schols AM, Soeters PB, Mostert R, Pluymers RJ, Wouters EF. Physiologic effects of nutritional support and anabolic steroids in patients with chronic obstructive pulmonary disease. A placebo-controlled randomized trial. *Am J Respir Crit Care Med* 1995; **152**(4 Pt 1):1268–74.

36 Hamilton AL, Killian KJ, Summers E, Jones NL. Muscle strength, symptom intensity, and exercise capacity in patients with cardiorespiratory disorders. *Am J Respir Crit Care Med* 1995; **152**(6 Pt 1):2021–31.

37 Maltais F, Simard AA, Simard C, Jobin J, Desgagnes P, LeBlanc P. Oxidative capacity of the skeletal muscle and lactic acid kinetics during exercise in normal subjects and in patients with COPD. *Am J Respir Crit Care Med* 1996; **153**:288–93.

38 Sala E, Roca J, Marrades RM *et al*. Effects of endurance training on skeletal muscle bioenergetics in chronic obstructive pulmonary disease. *Am J Respir Crit Care Med* 1999; **159**:1726–34.

39 Saey D, Debigare R, LeBlanc P *et al*. Contractile leg fatigue after cycle exercise: a factor limiting exercise in patients with chronic obstructive pulmonary disease. *Am J Respir Crit Care Med* 2003; **168**:425–30.

40 Mador MJ, Kufel TJ, Pineda LA *et al*. Effect of pulmonary rehabilitation on quadriceps fatiguability during exercise. *Am J Respir Crit Care Med* 2001; **163**:930–5.

41 Maltais F, LeBlanc P, Simard C *et al*. Skeletal muscle adaptation to endurance training in patients with chronic obstructive pulmonary disease. *Am J Respir Crit Care Med* 1996; **154**(2 Pt 1):442–7.

42 O'Donnell DE, McGuire M, Samis L, Webb KA. The impact of exercise reconditioning on breathlessness in severe chronic airflow limitation. *Am J Respir Crit Care Med* 1995; **152**(6 Pt 1):2005–13.

43 Toshima MT, Blumbert E, Ries AL, Kaplan RM. Does rehabilitation reduce depression in patients with chronic obstructive pulmonary disease? *J Cardiopulm Rehabil* 1992; **12**:261–9.

44 Belman MJ. Exercise in patients with chronic obstructive pulmonary disease. *Thorax* 1993; **48**:936–46.

45 Griffiths TL, Burr ML, Campbell IA *et al*. Results at 1 year of outpatient multidisciplinary pulmonary rehabilitation: a randomised controlled trial. *Lancet* 2000; **355**:362–8.

46 McGavin CR, Gupta SP, McHardy GJ. Twelve-minute walking test for assessing disability in chronic bronchitis. *BMJ* 1976; **1**: 822–3.

47 Cahalin L, Pappagianopoulos P, Prevost S, Wain J, Ginns L. The relationship of the 6-min walk test to maximal oxygen consumption in transplant candidates with end-stage lung disease. *Chest* 1995; **108**:452–9.

48 Shadish WR, Haddock CK. Combining estimates for effect size. In: Cooper H, Hedges LV, eds. *The Handbook of Research Synthesis*. New York, Russel Sage Foundation, 1994: 261–81.

49 Jaeschke R, Singer J, Guyatt GH. Measurement of health status. Ascertaining the minimal clinically important difference. *Control Clin Trials* 1989; **10**:407–15.

50 Cockcroft AE, Saunders MJ, Berry G. Randomised controlled trial of rehabilitation in chronic respiratory disability. *Thorax* 1981; **36**:200–3.

51 Booker HA. Exercise training and breathing control in patients with chronic airflow limitation. *Physiotherapy* 1984; **70**:258–60.

52 Jones DT, Thomson RJ, Sears MR. Physical exercise and resistive breathing training in severe chronic airways obstruction — are they effective? *Eur J Respir Dis* 1985; **67**:159–66.

53 Goldstein RS, Gort EH, Stubbing D, Avendano MA, Guyatt GH. Randomised controlled trial of respiratory rehabilitation. *Lancet* 1994; **344**:1394–7.

54 Vallet G, Varray A, Fontaine JL, Prefaut C. [Value of individualized rehabilitation at the ventilatory threshold level in moderately severe chronic obstructive pulmonary disease]. *Rev Mal Respir* 1994; **11**:493–501.

55 Guell R, Morante F, Sangenis M *et al*. Effects of respiratory rehabilitation on the effort capacity and on the health-related quality of life of patients with chronic obstructive pulmonary disease. *Eur Respir J* 1995; **8**(Suppl.):356.

56 Bendstrup KE, Ingemann JJ, Holm S, Bengtsson B. Out-patient rehabilitation improves activities of daily living, quality of life and exercise tolerance in chronic obstructive pulmonary disease. *Eur Respir J* 1997; **10**:2801–6.

57 Cambach W, Chadwick-Straver RV, Wagenaar RC, van Keimpema AR, Kemper HC. The effects of a community-based pulmonary rehabilitation programme on exercise tolerance and quality of life: a randomized controlled trial. *Eur Respir J* 1997; **10**:104–13.

58 Emery CF, Schein RL, Hauck ER, MacIntyre NR. Psychological and cognitive outcomes of a randomized trial of exercise among patients with chronic obstructive pulmonary disease. *Health Psychol* 1998; **17**:232–40.

59 Engstrom CP, Persson LO, Larsson S, Sullivan M. Long-term effects of a pulmonary rehabilitation programme in outpatients with chronic obstructive pulmonary disease: a randomized controlled study. *Scand J Rehabil Med* 1999; **31**:207–13.

60 Hernandez MT, Rubio TM, Ruiz FO, Riera HS, Gil RS, Gomez JC. Results of a home-based training program for patients with COPD. *Chest* 2000; **118**:106–14.

61 Ringbaek TJ, Broendum E, Hemmingsen L *et al*. Rehabilitation of patients with chronic obstructive pulmonary disease. Exercise twice a week is not sufficient! *Respir Med* 2000; **94**:150–4.

62 Cook D, Guyatt GH, Laupacis A *et al*. Clinical recommendations using levels of evidence for antithrombotic agents. *Chest* 1995; **108**(Suppl.):227S–230S.

63 Mahler DA, Weinberg DH, Wells CK, Feinstein AR. The measurement of dyspnea. Contents, interobserver agreement, and physiologic correlates of two new clinical indexes. *Chest* 1984; **85**:751–8.

64 Guyatt GH, Berman LB, Townsend M, Pugsley SO, Chambers LW. A measure of quality of life for clinical trials in chronic lung disease. *Thorax* 1987; **42**:773–8.

65 Jones PW, Quirk FH, Baveystock CM, Littlejohns P. A self-complete measure of health status for chronic airflow limitation. The St George's Respiratory Questionnaire. *Am Rev Respir Dis* 1992; **145**:1321–7.

66 Redelmeier DA, Bayoumi AM, Goldstein RS, Guyatt GH. Interpreting small differences in functional status: the Six Minute Walk test in chronic lung disease patients. *Am J Respir Crit Care Med* 1997; **155**:1278–82.

67 Finnerty JP, Keeping I, Bullough I, Jones J. The effectiveness of outpatient pulmonary rehabilitation in chronic lung disease: a randomized controlled trial. *Chest* 2001; **119**:1705–10.

68 Flicker M, Wanke T, Zwick H. [Training results exemplified by 3 patient groups]. *Prax Klin Pneumol* 1988; **42**:628–33.

69 Lewczuk J, Piszko P, Kowalska-Superlak M, Jagas J, Wojciak S, Wrabec K. [The impact of 2-year rehabilitation on exercise tolerance

and transcutaneous oxygen saturation during exercise in patients with chronic obstructive pulmonary disease]. *Pol Arch Med Wewn* 1998; **100**:331–6.

70 Moros Garcia JSM, Cisneros Lanuza MT, Rubio Obanos MT, Samperiz Legarre AL, Escolar Castellon F, Moros Garcia MT. Rehabilitacion de la discapacidad en la enfermedad pulmonar obstructiva cronica [Rehabilitation of disability in COPD]. *Rehabilitacion (Madr)* 1996; **30**:194–200.

71 Sudo E, Ohga E, Matsuse T, Teramoto S *et al*. [The effects of pulmonary rehabilitation combined with inspiratory muscle training on pulmonary function and inspiratory muscle strength in elderly patients with chronic obstructive pulmonary disease]. *Nippon Ronen Igakkai Zasshi* 1997; **34**:929–34.

72 American Thoracic Society. Standards for the diagnosis and care of patients with chronic obstructive pulmonary disease. *Am J Respir Crit Care Med* 1995; **152**(Suppl.):77–120.

73 Watson PB, Town GI, Holbrook N, Dwan C, Toop LJ, Drennan CJ. Evaluation of a self-management plan for chronic obstructive pulmonary disease. *Eur Respir J* 1997; **10**:1267–71.

74 Ferreira IM, Brooks D, Lacasse Y. Nutritional supplementation in stable chronic obstructive pulmonary disease. In: *The Cochrane Library*. Oxford, Update Software, 2001.

75 Dekhuijzen PN, Folgering HT, van Herwaarden CL. Target-flow inspiratory muscle training during pulmonary rehabilitation in patients with COPD. *Chest* 1991; **99**:128–33.

76 Wanke T, Formanek D, Lahrmann H *et al*. Effects of combined inspiratory muscle and cycle ergometer training on exercise performance in patients with COPD. *Eur Respir J* 1994; **7**:2205–11.

77 Berry MJ, Adair NE, Sevensky KS, Quinby A, Lever HM. Inspiratory muscle training and whole-body reconditioning in chronic obstructive pulmonary disease. *Am J Respir Crit Care Med* 1996; **153**(6 Pt 1):1812–16.

78 Larson JL, Covey MK, Wirtz SE *et al*. Cycle ergometer and inspiratory muscle training in chronic obstructive pulmonary disease. *Am J Respir Crit Care Med* 1999; **160**:500–7.

79 Lotters F, van Tol B, Kwakkel G, Gosselink R. Effects of controlled inspiratory muscle training in patients with COPD: a meta-analysis. *Eur Respir J* 2002; **20**:570–6.

80 Burdet L, de Muralt B, Schutz Y, Pichard C, Fitting JW. Administration of growth hormone to underweight patients with chronic obstructive pulmonary disease. A prospective, randomized, controlled study. *Am J Respir Crit Care Med* 1997; **156**:1800–6.

81 Martins Ferreira I, Verreschi IT *et al*. The influence of 6 months of oral anabolic steroids on body mass and respiratory muscles in undernourished COPD patients. *Chest* 1998; **114**:19–28.

82 Ferreira IM, Brooks D, Lacasse Y, Goldstein RS. Nutritional support for individuals with COPD: a meta-analysis. *Chest* 2000; **117**:672–8.

83 O'Donnell DE, Sanii R, Giesbrecht G, Younes M. Effect of continuous positive airway pressure on respiratory sensation in patients with chronic obstructive pulmonary disease during submaximal exercise. *Am Rev Respir Dis* 1988; **138**:1185–91.

84 Dean NC, Brown JK, Himelman RB, Doherty JJ, Gold WM, Stulbarg MS. Oxygen may improve dyspnea and endurance in patients with chronic obstructive pulmonary disease and only mild hypoxemia. *Am Rev Respir Dis* 1992; **146**:941–5.

85 Casaburi R, Patessio A, Ioli F, Zanaboni S, Donner CF, Wasserman K. Reduction in exercise lactic acidosis and ventilation as a result of exercise training in patients with obstructive lung disease. *Am Rev Respir Dis* 1991; **143**:9–18.

86 Rooyackers JM, Dekhuijzen PN, van Herwaarden CL, Folgering HT. Training with supplemental oxygen in patients with COPD and hypoxaemia at peak exercise. *Eur Respir J* 1997; **10**:1278–84.

87 Garrod R, Paul EA, Wedzicha JA. Supplemental oxygen during pulmonary rehabilitation in patients with COPD with exercise hypoxaemia. *Thorax* 2000; **55**:539–43.

88 Emtner M, Porszasz J, Burns M, Somfay A, Casaburi R. Benefits of supplemental oxygen in exercise training in nonhypoxemic chronic obstructive pulmonary disease patients. *Am J Respir Crit Care Med* 2003; **168**:1034–42.

89 Keilty SE, Ponte J, Fleming TA, Moxham J. Effect of inspiratory pressure support on exercise tolerance and breathlessness in patients with severe stable chronic obstructive pulmonary disease. *Thorax* 1994; **49**:990–4.

90 Maltais F, Reissmann H, Gottfried SB. Pressure support reduces inspiratory effort and dyspnea during exercise in chronic airflow obstruction. *Am J Respir Crit Care Med* 1995; **151**:1027–33.

91 Bianchi L, Foglio K, Pagani M, Vitacca M, Rossi A, Ambrosino N. Effects of proportional assist ventilation on exercise tolerance in COPD patients with chronic hypercapnia. *Eur Respir J* 1998; **11**:422–7.

92 Dolmage TE, Goldstein RS. Proportional assist ventilation and exercise tolerance in subjects with COPD. *Chest* 1997; **111**:948–54.

93 Hernandez P, Maltais F, Gursahaney A, LeBlanc P, Gottfried SB. Proportional assist ventilation may improve exercise performance in severe chronic obstructive pulmonary disease. *J Cardiopulm Rehabil* 2001; **21**:135–42.

94 Garrod R, Mikelsons C, Paul EA, Wedzicha JA. Randomized controlled trial of domiciliary noninvasive positive pressure ventilation and physical training in severe chronic obstructive pulmonary disease. *Am J Respir Crit Care Med* 2000; **162**(4 Pt 1):1335–41.

95 Wijkstra PJ, Lacasse Y, Guyatt GH *et al*. A meta-analysis of nocturnal noninvasive positive pressure ventilation in patients with stable COPD. *Chest* 2003; **124**:337–43.

96 Foglio K, Bianchi L, Bruletti G, Battista L, Pagani M, Ambrosino N. Long-term effectiveness of pulmonary rehabilitation in patients with chronic airway obstruction. *Eur Respir J* 1999; **13**:125–32.

97 Brooks D, Krip B, Mangovski-Alzamora S, Goldstein RS. The effect of postrehabilitation programmes among individuals with chronic obstructive pulmonary disease. *Eur Respir J* 2002; **20**:20–9.

98 Ketelaars CA, Abu-Saad HH, Schlosser MA, Mostert R, Wouters EF. Long-term outcome of pulmonary rehabilitation in patients with COPD. *Chest* 1997; **112**:363–9.

99 Ries AL, Kaplan RM, Myers R, Prewitt LM. Maintenance after pulmonary rehabilitation in chronic lung disease: a randomized trial. *Am J Respir Crit Care Med* 2003; **167**:880–8.

100 Guell R, Casan P, Belda J *et al*. Long-term effects of outpatient rehabilitation of COPD: a randomized trial. *Chest* 2000; **117**:976–83.

101 Green RH, Singh SJ, Williams J, Morgan MD. A randomised controlled trial of four weeks versus seven weeks of pulmonary rehabilitation in chronic obstructive pulmonary disease. *Thorax* 2001; **56**:143–5.

102 Vale F, Reardon JZ, ZuWallack RL. The long-term benefits of outpatient pulmonary rehabilitation on exercise endurance and quality of life. *Chest* 1993; **103**:42–5.

103 Foglio K, Bianchi L, Ambrosino N. Is it really useful to repeat outpatient pulmonary rehabilitation programs in patients with chronic airway obstruction? A 2-year controlled study. *Chest* 2001; **119**:1696–704.

CHAPTER 5.2

Non-invasive ventilation in acute respiratory failure

Peter Wark

Introduction

Definitions of acute respiratory failure and its aetiology

Acute respiratory failure (ARF) is an inability to maintain adequate gas exchange, resulting in significant hypoxaemia with or without hypercapnia and systemic acidosis. The condition is best defined on arterial blood gases and subdivided into: type I or hypoxic failure with a $Pao_2 < 50mmHg$ (8.0 kPa) and normal or low $Paco_2$; and type II or hypercapnoeic failure with a $Pao_2 < 50mmHg$ and a $Paco_2 > 55mmHg$ (6.0 kPa). ARF can occur in an individual with no pre-existing lung disease and is acute, or in the context of prior lung disease where it may be on a background of chronic respiratory failure.

Excluding respiratory failure that results from impaired respiratory drive as a consequence of drugs or a neurological event and cardiac failure, parenchymal lung disease accounts for most ARF. The most prevalent cause is community-acquired pneumonia (CAP), which accounts for 500 000 admissions to hospital per year in the USA,[1] with 10% of all those hospitalized with CAP developing ARF,[2] the presence of which is associated with more severe disease, an increased risk of mechanical ventilation and death.[3] Other causes of ARF include chest trauma, aspiration pneumonitis, pulmonary thromboembolic disease and acute lung injury as a result of systemic multiorgan disease. In the context of pre-existing lung disease, conditions that result in ARF are the leading cause of death. Exacerbations of chronic obstructive pulmonary disease (COPD) account for 500 000 admissions in the US per year,[4] with up to 20% of all admissions complicated by ARF,[5] which is an independent risk factor for death and mechanical ventilation.[5] Individuals who do require invasive ventilation may have prolonged intensive care unit (ICU) admissions and a mortality rate of 20–33%.[6,7] Acute exacerbations of asthma that present to hospital result in ARF in up to 46% of subjects, although most respond to initial treatment and no more than 8% deteriorate and require invasive mechanical ventilation.[8,9] ARF is the leading cause of death in cystic fibrosis (CF), with those requiring mechanical ventilation having mortality rates of up to 70%.[10] In patients with fibrotic lung disease,[11] restrictive thoracic cage disorders and neuromuscular disorders, complications resulting in ARF are the leading cause of death and hospitalization.[12]

Definitions of non-invasive ventilatory support

The nomenclature used to describe ventilatory modes is confusing due to a lack of standardization between the manufacturers. Ventilators that are used extend from standard ICU ventilators that separate inspiratory and expiratory gas mixtures and monitor inspiratory pressures and minute volumes (described as ICU ventilators for simplicity) to less sophisticated machines with single tubing and limited monitoring facilities.[13] Negative pressure devices will not be discussed, as they are now used rarely and largely only in settings of chronic respiratory failure or in the treatment of neonates. Machines used for non-invasive ventilation (NIV) are either pressure support (or assist-control) ventilators (PSV) or volume-assist ventilators.[13] PSV are the most commonly used machines in which most clinical experience has been gained. These ventilators offer bilevel pressure support ventilatory assistance, where an inspiratory pressure is set and is triggered internally by inspiratory effort or by determining the end of inspiration and then followed by a lower expiratory pressure. While the addition of positive end-expiratory pressure (PEEP) is not essential, it does reduce the work of breathing, increases oxygenation and helps to eliminate exhaled air and CO_2 rebreathing.[14] These ventilators can vary in terms of their inspiratory triggers, response times and times to reach set pressures, but all compensate for leak. Depending on the models, they can deliver bilevel support initiated spontaneously or assisted (also called spontaneous/timed) where the machine initiates a preset number of some or all of the breaths.

Volume assist-control ventilators (VCV) deliver a set tidal volume to the patient irrespective of pressure. Few comparative studies have been done between the modes. Volume-assist ventilators may be more effective at correcting alveolar hypoventilation but are probably less well tolerated.[13] Most VCV ventilators do not have an intrinsic ability to deliver PEEP. Oxygen can be entrained into all NIV machines but, in most PSV used for NIV, the flow rate will vary with inspiratory flow and an Fio_2 of >50% cannot be delivered reliably. If a higher Fio_2 is required, ICU ventilators, VCV or the Respironics Vision® (at the time of writing, the only PS NIV machine with internal oxygen enrichment) need to be used.[13]

Machines are also available that deliver continuous positive airway pressure (CPAP). This increases the recruitment of underventilated lung units, reduces the work of breathing and

Table 1. Study characteristics of NIV for ARF in COPD.

Study (first author)	No. of subjects	Ventilator used	Outcomes
ICU based			
Brochard (1995)[45]	85	PSV	1, 2, 3, 5
Celikel (1998)[48]	30	PSV	1, 4, 5
Kramer (1995)[49]	31	BiPAP	1, 5
Ward based			
Avdeev (1998)[50]	58	BiPAP	1, 2, 3, 5
Bott (1993)[44]	60	VCV	1, 2, 3, 5
Dikensoy (2002)[51]	34	BiPAP	1, 2, 3, 4, 5
Plant (2000)[46]	236	VPAP II	1, 2, 3, 4, 5
Emergency room based			
Barbe (1996)[52]	24	BiPAP	1, 2, 3

Ventilators used: BiPAP®, a bilevel PSV; PSV refers to ICU standard ventilator on pressure-assist/control settings; VCV, volume-assist/control ventilator; VPAP II ®, a bilevel PSV.

Outcomes: 1, treatment failure; 2, death; 3, intubation; 4, complications of treatment; 5, length of stay.

permits a higher Fio_2.[13] CPAP is generally employed to correct type I respiratory failure and is particularly helpful in cardiac failure. The treatment of cardiac failure is outside the scope of this chapter and will not be dealt with here.

By definition, NIV is performed without the need for endotracheal intubation and is usually delivered by either face or nasal mask. Both mask types have been used successfully in ARF with no general advantage of one over another.[13] The choice of mask should be individualized to maximize comfort and reduce leak. Ventilators used for NIV are increasingly being used in tracheotomized patients, especially in weaning from ventilation, but will not be reviewed here, as this is not NIV support.

Management of ARF with NIV

In recent years, the use of NIV has greatly increased and has been prompted by a need to find ways to provide ventilatory support without the need for endotracheal intubation and to do so outside an ICU setting. This has proved most advantageous in patients with pre-existing respiratory disease where invasive ventilation was associated with prolonged admission in the ICU and a high rate of nosocomial complications. The limitation with NIV is that it does not provide airway protection where this is compromised and is ill-suited to individuals with multiorgan dysfunction and haemodynamic instability. None of the randomized controlled trials (RCTs) reported here have been blinded, because of the difficulty, if not impossibility, of a realistic placebo treatment.

ARF and COPD

The prevalence of ARF during exacerbations of COPD and the morbidity and mortality associated with invasive ventilation in COPD have resulted in this being the most thoroughly investigated application of NIV in ARF. There are eight prospective RCTs of 558 subjects with acute exacerbations of COPD that are summarized in Table 1 and have undergone systematic review.[15,16] The review was confined to trials of NIV in subjects with COPD and evidence of hypercapnoea where NIV was compared with usual medical care, which could include respiratory stimulants, oxygen and bronchodilators. Excluded were studies of pneumonia, weaning from invasive ventilation and the use of CPAP. Most of the individual trials excluded subjects with a reduced level of consciousness and who were acutely confused, haemodynamically unstable or judged to require immediate intubation. The review reported outcomes that took into account a number of potential confounders: disease severity by comparing those with a lower initial pH due to respiratory acidosis (pH < 7.30) with those with pH 7.35–7.30; and the location of the intervention by comparing ICU with a ward setting.

Outcomes are summarized in Table 2. Treatment failure was defined as a combination of mortality, need for intubation and intolerance to allocated treatment. NIV resulted in a significantly lower risk of treatment failure: relative risk (RR) 0.51 [95% confidence interval (CI) 0.38–0.67] (Fig. 1) with the number needed to treat (NNT) being 5 (95% CI 4–7). In terms of mortality, treatment with NIV was associated with significantly lower mortality: RR 0.41 (95% CI 0.26–0.64) with a NNT of 8 (95% CI 6–13) (Fig. 2). NIV led to a significant reduction in intubation (RR 0.42; 95% CI 0.31–0.59) with a NNT of 5 (95% CI 4–7) to prevent one intubation (Fig. 3). In addition, treatment with NIV led to a significant reduction in length of stay: weighted mean difference (WMD) −3.24 days; 95% CI −4.42 to −2.06 days (Fig. 4). The benefits seen for treatment failure, mortality and intubation were independent of

Table 2. Effects of non-invasive (NIV) positive pressure ventilation as an adjunct to usual medical care, compared with usual care alone for subjects with ARF and COPD: overall results of the review for dichotomous outcome measures.

Outcome	No. of patients	Relative risk (95% CI)	Number needed to treat (95% CI)
Treatment failure	529	0.51 (0.38–0.67)	5 (4–7)
Mortality	523	0.41 (0.26–0.64)	8 (6–13)
Intubation	546	0.42 (0.31–0.59)	5 (4–7)
Complications	143	0.32 (0.18–0.56)	3 (2–4)

Adapted with permission from Lightowler et al.[15]

Review: Non-invasive positive pressure ventilation for treatment of respiratory failure due to exacerbations of chronic obstructive pulmonary disease

Comparison: 01 NPPV + usual medical care vs usual medical care — Overall

Outcome: 01 Treatment failure

Study	NPPV (n/N)	UMC (n/N)	Relative risk (fixed) (95% CI)	Weight (%)	Relative risk (fixed) (95% CI)
Avdeev (1998)	7/29	12/29		11.2	0.58 (0.27, 1.27)
Barbe (1996)	4/14	0/10		0.5	0.60 (0.39, 110.32)
Bott (1993)	5/30	13/30		12.1	0.38 (0.16, 0.94)
Brochard (1995)	12/43	33/42		31.1	0.36 (0.21, 0.59)
Celikel (1998)	1/15	6/15		5.6	0.17 (0.02, 1.22)
Dikensoy (2002)	4/19	7/17		6.9	0.51 (0.18, 1.45)
Plant (2000)	22/118	35/118		32.6	0.63 (0.39, 1.00)
Total (95% CI)	55/268	106/261		100.0	0.51 (0.38, 0.67)

Test for heterogeneity chi-squared = 7.59 df = 6 P = 0.2698

Test for overall effect = − 4.82 P < 0.00001

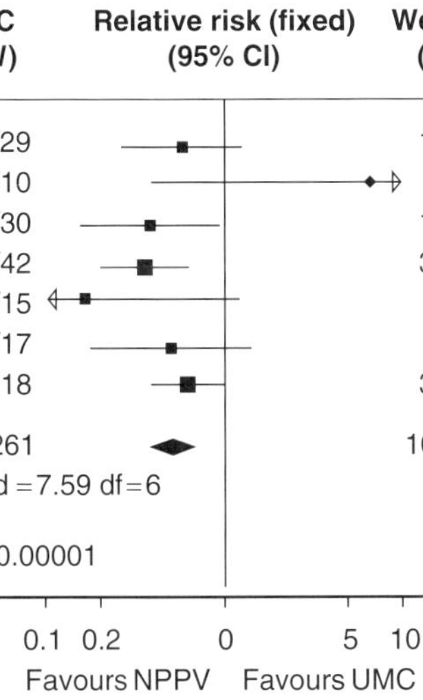

0.1 0.2   0   5   10

Favours NPPV   Favours UMC

Figure 1. Acute exacerbations of COPD, NIV and usual medical care versus usual medical care alone; treatment failure. Reproduced with the permission of Ram et al.[16]

Review: Non-invasive positive pressure ventilation for treatment of respiratory failure due to exacerbations of chronic obstructive pulmonary disease

Comparison: 01 NPPV + usual medical care vs usual medical care — Overall

Outcome: 02 Mortality

Study	NPPV (n/N)	UMC (n/N)	Relative risk (fixed) (95% CI)	Weight (%)	Relative risk (fixed) (95% CI)
Avdeev (1998)	3/29	9/29		15.6	0.33 (0.10, 1.11)
Barbe (1996)	0/10	0/10		0.0	Not estimable
Bott (1993)	3/30	9/30		15.6	0.33 (0.10, 1.11)
Brochard (1995)	4/43	12/42		21.1	0.33 (0.11, 0.93)
Celikel (1998)	0/15	1/15		2.6	0.33 (0.01, 7.58)
Dikensoy (2002)	1/17	2/17		3.5	0.50 (0.05, 5.01)
Plant (2000)	12/118	24/118		41.6	0.50 (0.26, 0.95)
Total (95% CI)	23/262	57/261		100.0	0.41 (0.26, 0.64)

Test for heterogeneity chi-squared = 0.82 df = 5 P = 0.9755

Test for overall effect = − 3.96 P = 0.0001

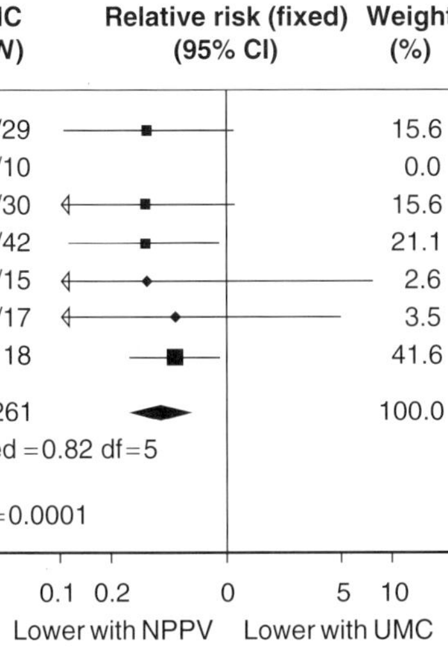

0.1 0.2   0   5   10

Lower with NPPV   Lower with UMC

Figure 2. Acute exacerbations of COPD, NIV and usual medical care versus usual medical care alone; mortality. Reproduced with the permission of Ram et al.[16]

Review: Non-invasive positive pressure ventilation for treatment of respiratory failure due to
exacerbations of chronic obstructive pulmonary disease

Comparison: 01 NPPV + usual medical care vs usual medical care—Overall

Outcome: 03 Intubation

Study	NPPV (n/N)	UMC (n/N)	Relative risk (fixed) (95% CI)	Weight (%)	Relative risk (fixed) (95% CI)
Avdeev (1998)	5/29	8/29		8.8	0.63 (0.23, 1.68)
Barbe (1996)	0/10	0/10		0.0	Not estimable
Bott (1993)	0/30	2/30		2.8	0.20 (0.01, 4.00)
Brochard (1995)	11/43	31/42		34.7	0.35 (0.20, 0.60)
Celikel (1998)	1/15	2/15		2.2	0.50 (0.05, 4.94)
Dikensoy (2002)	2/17	7/17		7.7	0.29 (0.07, 1.18)
Kramer (1995)	1/11	8/12		8.6	0.14 (0.02, 0.92)
Plant (2000)	18/118	32/118		35.4	0.56 (0.34, 0.94)
Total (95% CI)	38/273	90/273		100.0	0.42 (0.31, 0.59)

Test for heterogeneity chi-squared $=4.18$ df$=6$
  $P=0.6528$
Test for overall effect $=-5.13$ $P<0.00001$

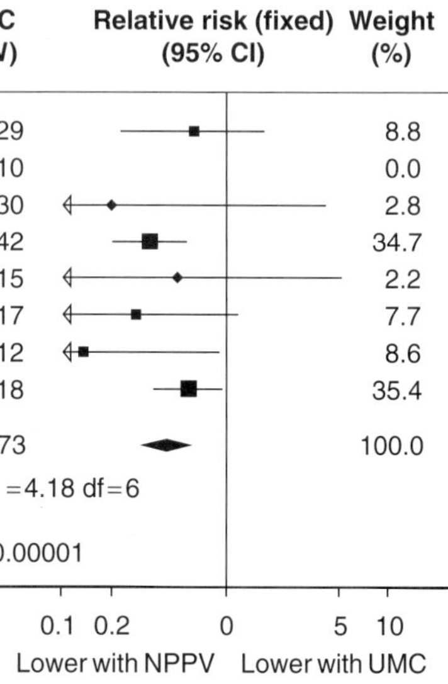

0.1 0.2   0   5 10

Lower with NPPV   Lower with UMC

Figure 3. Acute exacerbations of COPD, NIV and usual medical care versus usual medical care alone; intubation rate. Reproduced with the permission of Ram *et al.*[16]

Review: Non-invasive positive pressure ventilation for treatment of respiratory failure due to exacerbations of chronic obstructive
pulmonary disease

Comparison: 01 NPPV + usual medical care vs usual medical care—Overall

Outcome: 04 Length of hospital stay (days)

Study	N	NPPV [mean (SD)]	N	UMC [mean (SD)]	WMD (fixed) (95% CI)	Weight (%)	WMD (fixed) (95% CI)
Avdeev (1998)	29	26.00 (7.00)	29	34.00 (10.00)		7.1	−8.000 (−12.443, −3.557)
Barbe (1996)	10	10.60 (3.24)	10	11.30 (3.90)		14.1	−0.700 (−3.843, 2.443)
Bott (1993)	30	10.50 (5.30)	30	11.90 (8.80)		10.3	−1.400 (−5.076, 2.276)
Brochard (1995)	43	23.00 (17.00)	42	35.00 (33.00)		1.1	−12.000 (−23.199, −0.801)
Celikel (1998)	15	11.70 (3.50)	15	14.60 (4.70)		15.8	−2.900 (−5.866, 0.066)
Dikensoy (2002)	17	8.00 (2.10)	17	12.30 (3.30)		40.3	−4.300 (−6.159, −2.441)
Kramer (1995)	11	14.90 (10.44)	12	17.30 (9.95)		2.0	−2.400 (−10.752, 5.952)
Plant (2000)	118	13.82 (13.92)	118	14.44 (16.26)		9.3	−0.620 (−4.482, 3.242)
Total (95% CI)	273		273			100.0	−3.237 (−4.417, −2.057)

Test for heterogeneity chi-squared $=13.34$ df$=7$ $P=0.0643$
Test for overall effect z$=-5.38$ $P=0.00$

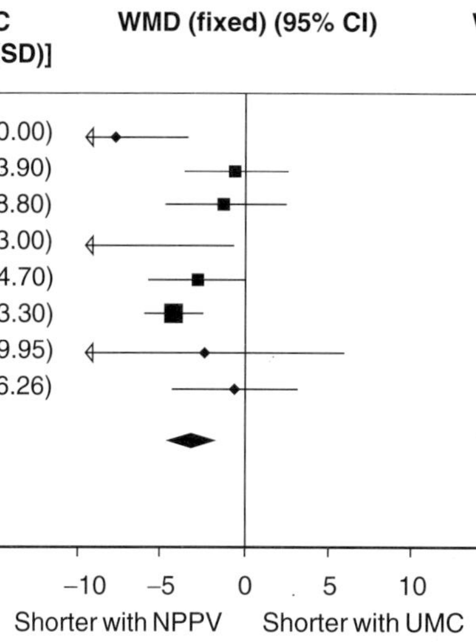

−10 −5   0 . 5   10

Shorter with NPPV   Shorter with UMC

Figure 4. Acute exacerbations of COPD, NIV and usual medical care versus usual medical care alone; length of hospital stay. Reproduced with the permission of Ram *et al.*[16]

initial disease severity or the location of treatment (Table 3). However, length of stay was not different for those with milder ARF (pH 7.35–7.30).

Concerns remain that NIV may adversely affect outcomes by delaying intubation, although this has not been demonstrated in the trials in COPD. NIV did demonstrate a signifi-cant improvement in arterial blood gas pH within 1 hour of commencement in 408 patients: WMD 0.03 (95% CI 0.02–0.04).

An economic analysis of the effect of NIV in acute exacerbations of COPD was carried out on the subjects reported by Plant *et al.*[17] This demonstrated that a ward-based NIV pro-

Table 3. Effects of non-invasive ventilation (NIV) positive pressure ventilation as an adjunct to usual medical care, compared with usual care alone in subjects with COPD: comparison of outcomes by severity of acute respiratory acidosis and site of treatment with NIV.

Outcome	Initial pH < 7.30 (95% CI)	Initial pH 7.35–7.30 (95% CI)	ICU-based treatment (95% CI)	Ward-based treatment (95% CI)
Treatment failure (RR)	0.40 (0.27–0.59)	0.63 (0.43–0.95)	0.33 (0.2–0.54)	0.61 (0.44–0.86)
Mortality (RR)	0.34 (0.17–0.71)	0.45 (0.26–0.80)	0.33 (0.12–0.88)	0.43 (0.26–0.71)
Intubation (RR)	0.36 (0.23–0.55)	0.54 (0.32–0.89)	0.31 (0.19–0.53)	0.56 (0.34–0.79)
Length of stay (WMD)	−4.43 (−5.88 to −2.98)	−0.89 (−2.92 to 1.14)	−3.38 (−6.09 to −0.67)	−3.20 (−4.51 to −1.89)

RR, relative risk; 95% CI, 95% confidence intervals; WMD, weighted mean difference.

gramme led to a substantial reduction in costs (£49 362 or US$78 741), largely accounted for by the reduced use of ICU beds and, to a lesser extent, reduced mortality.

One prospective RCT compared NIV with treatment with the chemical respiratory stimulant doxapram.[18] NIV was found to be more effective and led to a sustained improvement in blood gases that was not seen with doxapram beyond the first 2 hours.

There are no prospective RCTs of CPAP in the treatment of ARF in COPD. Case series reported physiological improvement,[19] but treatment failure and intubation rates remained high.[20]

The evidence is strongly in favour of NIV to treat ARF in COPD. It reduces length of stay, ICU admission and mortality. Treatment has been initiated successfully both in the ICU and in a dedicated ward-based setting. A dedicated NIV treatment area outside the ICU appears to offer the best prospects for reducing costs.

ARF and pneumonia

One multicentre prospective RCT has been performed in 56 adults with confirmed severe pneumonia.[21] All subjects had radiographic evidence of severe CAP and evidence of either type I or type II respiratory failure and were treated with bilevel PSV or standard medical treatment and oxygen in an ICU setting. There were 23 subjects with COPD. Subjects were excluded if they required immediate intubation, were haemodynamically unstable, had severe neurological impairment, were on long-term oxygen or ventilatory support, unable to expectorate or had a pre-existing terminal disease. The use of NIV was associated with a reduced need for intubation (21% versus 50%, $P = 0.03$) and a significant reduction in length of stay in the ICU (1.8 ± 0.7 days versus 6 ± 1.8 days, $P = 0.04$). There were no differences in hospital mortality. A post hoc analysis dividing the subjects by diagnosis of COPD demonstrated that those with COPD appeared to benefit most from NIV: they were less likely to meet intubation criteria (0 versus 6, $P < 0.01$) and had shorter ICU stays (0.25 ± 2.1 days versus 7.6 ± 2.2 days, $P = 0.02$). However, a significant benefit was not seen in those without COPD treated with NIV.

Two further RCTs were performed in the ICU comparing NIV with conventional mechanical ventilation in patients with respiratory failure in whom the aetiology for ARF was a mixture of pneumonia or cardiac failure.[22,23] In the study by Wysocki et al.,[22] 41 patients were randomized to NIV or invasive ventilation, and they found no difference in intubation rates or length of stay, with the only benefit being seen in those who had type II respiratory failure. Antonelli et al.[23] randomized 64 patients with acute hypoxaemic respiratory failure. The NIV arm had fewer complications overall, particularly less risk of nosocomial pneumonia or sinusitis compared with the invasively ventilated arm (31% compared with 3%, $P < 0.01$), but there was no difference in survival.

Treatment of type I (hypoxic) respiratory failure secondary to pneumonia with CPAP has only been assessed in case series[24] and one prospective RCT.[25] In the study by Delclaux et al.,[25] 123 adults with acute non-hypercapnoeic respiratory failure were recruited; subjects with cardiac failure were included, but COPD was an exclusion factor. Of these subjects, 21 were thought to have pulmonary oedema, and the remainder had acute lung injury with no previous cardiac disease. Of these, 52 subjects had CAP, three had aspiration pneumonia, eight near drowning and five systemic inflammatory response syndrome. Overall, CPAP led to an initial improvement in hypoxaemia, and there was no difference in numbers intubated (21 versus 24, $P = 0.5$), hospital mortality (19 versus 18, $P = 0.5$) and length of ICU stay (6.5 versus 6.0 days, $P = 0.4$). A treatment effect could not be seen in those without cardiac failure. There were more adverse events in the CPAP group with four cardiac arrests, possibly reflecting a delay in intubation.

Outside the context of COPD, there is no good evidence to support the use of NIV or CPAP in ARF secondary to pneumonia, even though the trials have occurred within ICU settings. This may reflect important differences in the clinical condition of patients with severe pneumonia compared with acute exacerbations of COPD. Patients with pneumonia are more likely to have multiorgan dysfunction, hypoxaemia due to worsening ventilation–perfusion mismatch from consolidation, which is not quickly reversed, as is the physiological abnormality in an exacerbation of COPD, and there are limitations of the PSV used for NIV to delivery an adequate Fio_2.

The evidence so far does not support the use of either NIV or CPAP in the routine treatment of severe CAP, and this should only be undertaken where there is rapid access to invasive ventilation and an ICU.

ARF in the immunosuppressed

There are two RCTs demonstrating effectiveness of NIV in immunosuppressed patients with ARF. Hilbert et al.[26] randomized 52 patients with pre-existing immunosuppression (15 had haematological malignancy and neutropenia) and ARF, pulmonary infiltrates and fever to intermittent NIV (45 min to 3 hours' duration at a time) or oxygen alone. The NIV arm was less likely to require intubation (12 versus 20, $P = 0.03$), had fewer complications (13 versus 21, $P = 0.02$) and was less likely to die in hospital (13 versus 21, $P = 0.02$).

A group of 238 patients who underwent solid organ transplantation was followed, and 40 were randomized to treatment with NIV or treatment with oxygen when they developed acute respiratory distress and hypoxaemia.[27] All patients were treated in an ICU, and NIV was given using ICU standard ventilators. There were preset criteria for intubation. Causes of ARF were acute respiratory distress syndrome (ARDS) (15 patients), pneumonia (4), cardiogenic pulmonary oedema (9), atelectasis (10) and pulmonary embolus (2). A sustained improvement in oxygenation was seen in the NIV group by 12 hours compared with the oxygen arm (12 versus 5, $P = 0.03$). The NIV arm had a significant reduction in rate of intubation (20% versus 50%, $P = 0.002$) and a shorter length of ICU stay (mean 5.5 days compared with 9 days, $P = 0.03$). There was a trend to improved ICU mortality, but overall hospital mortality was not different.

CPAP has become widely used in the treatment of pneumonia in the immunosuppressed, particularly the treatment of ARF secondary to *Pneumocystis carinii* associated with human immunodeficiency virus (HIV) infection, and is now established treatment. Despite this, the evidence for effectiveness is confined to uncontrolled studies[28,29] where the addition of CPAP improved mortality, reduced the risk of intubation and the rate of nosocomial pneumonia compared with historical controls.

In the immunosuppressed patient with ARF, even with evidence of severe respiratory compromise and ARDS, NIV improves outcomes and reduces the need for intubation. The improvement in outcomes is, at least in part, due to the avoidance of intubation and invasive ventilation where the risk of nosocomial infection (especially pneumonia) and its mortality is very high. This makes NIV a reasonable first choice in ARF; however, these trials were performed in an ICU setting with advanced ventilators, and it is not clear whether success rates will be affected by treatment in a ward setting or with PS NIV that deliver variable oxygen flow rates.

ARF and asthma

There are no prospective RCTs of the use of NIV in ARF and asthma. There is one case series of 17 adults admitted to an ICU with persistent ARF despite treatment of acute asthma.[30] All were given NIV using ICU ventilators: two subjects required invasive mechanical ventilation, and the remainder demonstrated a significant improvement in arterial blood gases within 2–6 hours.

Several uncontrolled trials have applied NIV to treat acute asthma. CPAP is reported to enhance bronchodilatation,[31] improve gas exchange[32] and reduce the work of breathing.[33] In a single-blinded RCT of NIV in acute asthma, 30 subjects with acute asthma presenting to the emergency room were treated with NIV for 3 hours [bilevel positive airway pressure (BiPAP) ST] using a fixed protocol to adjust pressures.[34] Subjects had severe airflow obstruction [forced expiratory volume in 1 second (FEV_1) less than 60% predicted], but derangements in gas exchange were not severe with mean $Paco_2$ and Pao_2 not being in the range of ARF. It is unclear how many, if any, of the subjects had ARF at presentation. The use of NIV significantly improved lung function at 4 hours with a mean percentage improvement in FEV_1 with treatment of 53.5%, compared with 28.5% with placebo ($P = 0.006$). A similar improvement was seen with respiratory rate. Fewer subjects treated with NIV required hospitalization, 17.6% compared with 62.5% ($P = 0.01$). However, no subjects were reported to deteriorate and develop worsening respiratory failure or require ICU admission.

Pilot studies suggest that NIV may be beneficial in acute asthma, improving lung function and reducing the work of breathing. It appears to be well tolerated and does not seem to compromise patients. However, data for its use in ARF are limited, and it is difficult to draw conclusions as to its efficacy over usual medical practice given the overall good response of asthmatic subjects to pharmacological treatment.

ARF and chest trauma

There is one prospective RCT of CPAP in 69 adults.[35] All subjects had been admitted following chest trauma with at least two rib fractures and hypoxaemia. They were randomized to treatment with CPAP and regional anaesthesia or invasive mechanical ventilation. The most severely affected subjects with a $Pao_2 < 56$ mmHg (8.0 kPa) were excluded. Subjects treated with invasive mechanical ventilation had higher injury scores. Those treated with CPAP had a reduced length of stay in ICU, 5.3 ± 2.9 days compared with 9.5 ± 4.4 days ($P < 0.001$), and an overall reduced length of stay in hospital, 8.4 ± 7.1 days compared with 14.6 ± 8.6 days ($P < 0.01$). The CPAP group also had fewer complications, the majority of which were nosocomial pneumonias, 28% compared with 73% ($P < 0.05$).

These results demonstrate that CPAP is a safe, well-tolerated treatment for ARF secondary to chest trauma, although this was demonstrated in an ICU setting, and the results may have been exaggerated due to more severe disease in the invasive ventilation arm. Issues that are uncertain are the use of CPAP in more severe respiratory failure, the role of PS

NIV particularly in hypercapnoeic respiratory failure or COPD and chest trauma.

ARF and cystic fibrosis or bronchiectasis

There are no prospective RCTs of NIV for ARF in either of these conditions. While in both cases patients often have severe fixed airflow obstruction as in COPD, excessive purulent secretions complicate the clinical situation, and excess secretions may reduce the effectiveness of NIV.[36] In bronchiectasis, it is unclear whether NIV helps or hinders sputum clearance acutely. The use of NIV in chronic respiratory failure in CF has been the subject of a systematic review.[37] This found that, in CF patients with chronic nocturnal hypercapnoea, NIV during sleep demonstrated improvements in gas exchange and sleep architecture in two RCTs.[37] In the study by Milross et al.,[38] NIV was compared with low-flow oxygen with improvements in sleep architecture and hypercapnoea only occurring in the NIV arm. Similarly, case reports describe the use of NIV as a bridge to transplantation in CF in patients with worsening respiratory failure.[39] These results suggest that, at least in chronic respiratory failure, NIV can correct hypercapnoea. Given the poor prognosis of ARF and invasive mechanical ventilation in CF, it is reasonable to treat these patients initially with NIV and decide at this time whether further treatment with invasive ventilation should be employed.

ARF associated with thoracic cage deformity or neuromuscular weakness

There are no prospective RCTs of NIV in ARF associated with restrictive thoracic cage deformities or in type II respiratory failure due to neuromuscular disease. However, NIV has become the treatment of choice for chronic hypercapnoeic respiratory failure in these patients, with retrospective series suggesting dramatic improvements in quality of life and mortality compared with historic controls.[40] This does not translate directly to success in ARF, especially when many of these patients will be suffering acutely from sputum retention, pneumonia or recurrent aspiration, all of which will potentially reduce the efficacy of NIV. Nonetheless, an acute trial of NIV would be reasonable, given the potential complications of invasive mechanical ventilation in these people. Of particular future interest would be the use of NIV in acute neurological diseases with respiratory impairment, as is seen with Guillain–Barre syndrome or strokes. In both cases, bulbar dysfunction may compromise the airway acutely making NIV impractical, while in the case of Guillain–Barre syndrome, the profound respiratory weakness that can occur along with the prolonged course of illness may at best only delay the need for intubation and ventilation.

ARF following extubation

Given the success of NIV as a primary treatment in ARF, it has been proposed that it may prevent respiratory decompensa-tion and failure occurring in patients following extubation. The success of NIV has varied for this purpose however.

NIV was tested in 50 patients admitted to one ICU with an exacerbation of COPD and acute hypercapnoeic respiratory failure who had woken after 48 hours of mechanical ventilation, but who had failed a 2-hour T-piece weaning trial. They were then either randomized to NIV or continued with invasive mechanical ventilation.[41] The arm randomized to NIV had a reduction in the overall duration of ventilatory support (10.2 ± 6.8 days versus 16.6 ± 11.8 days, $P=0.02$) and a reduced length of stay in ICU (15.1 ± 5.4 days versus 24 ± 13.7 days, $P < 0.001$). They also had better overall survival at 60 days (92% versus 72%, $P < 0.01$) with less nosocomial pneumonia (no cases versus seven cases, $P < 0.05$).

In a similarly designed trial, Girault et al.[42] randomized 33 general ICU patients (17 of whom had COPD) who had been invasively ventilated and who met weaning criteria but had failed a 2-hour T-piece trial to extubation on to NIV or continuing intubation and ventilation. The NIV arm demonstrated a shorter duration of mechanical ventilatory support (4.56 ± 1.85 days versus 7.69 ± 3.79 days, $P < 0.001$), but no differences were seen in terms of length of stay in ICU or mortality at 3 months.

In an important variation from the above studies, Keenan et al.[43] randomized 81 ICU patients who were within 48 hours of extubation, with a history of cardiac or respiratory disease or who had been intubated and ventilated for more than 2 days and who then developed respiratory distress, to NIV or usual medical treatment and oxygen. They did not find any differences between NIV and usual treatment, in any of the outcomes, including reintubation rates (RR 1.04 95% CI 0.78–1.38), hospital mortality (RR 0.99 95% CI 0.52–1.91) or overall length of stay (32.2 ± 25.4 days versus 29.8 ± 28.4 days, $P=0.7$).

The evidence supports the use of extubation on to ventilatory support with NIV to prevent reintubation in patients with COPD who have failed a T-piece weaning trial. However, the effect of delaying initiation of NIV and applying it to those extubated COPD patients who develop respiratory distress has not been determined. In a mixed group of patients, the efficacy of NIV is less clear. In this group, maximal benefit may only be gained if NIV allows earlier extubation, and its effect may be lost by applying it only after respiratory distress has developed. Further work to define whether other early factors may predict an increased risk of reintubation and earlier application of NIV would be of value. Whether other subgroups, such as people with respiratory muscle weakness and other forms of chronic respiratory disease such as CF or the immunosuppressed, may benefit from NIV post extubation, given success in ARF, remains uncertain and requires investigation to establish efficacy.

Predicting a successful outcome for NIV in ARF

In both the early RCTs of NIV to treat patients with COPD and acute hypercapnoeic respiratory failure, an improvement in pH and respiratory rate was seen within 2 hours in those who were treated successfully. Those who failed to respond by this time were at a higher risk of treatment failure, inferring that early response and tolerance of treatment were predictors of a favourable outcome.[44,45] In the systematic review of NIV in exacerbations of COPD, significant changes in respiratory acidosis, $Paco_2$ and respiratory rate but not Pao_2 had occurred within this time frame, supporting the conclusion that an early improvement in respiratory acidosis and a reduction in the work of breathing are predictors of treatment success.[16] Severity of initial ARF (pH < 7.25) was found by Plant et al.[46] in their ward-based study to be associated with a higher rate of treatment failure. This was also seen in the study by Ambrosino et al.,[47] in which more severe respiratory acidosis at baseline was associated with treatment failure. In addition, the presence of radiographic pneumonia in COPD was also associated with reduced success. In the uncontrolled trial by Soo Hoo et al.[36] in patients with COPD, treatment failure was associated with more severe overall clinical disease (expressed by APACHE II score), excess secretions, pneumonia and, again, more severe acute hypercapnoeic respiratory failure. Those subjects who were able to tolerate the nasal mask and adapted to breathing on the machine more quickly also had a better outcome. A factor associated in this group with failure was pursed lip breathing and intolerance of the nasal mask due to mouth breathing. This reinforces the importance of the interface between the patient and the ventilator in maximizing success, which means tailoring the mask to suit the individual and adjusting ventilator parameters to relieve respiratory distress in the crucial first hour of treatment.

In summary, the likelihood of success with NIV is reduced in people with very severe ARF and additional problems such as pneumonia. Not surprisingly, difficulty in tolerating NIV makes success with NIV unlikely. Finally, improvement within 2 hours in ARF parameters, such as pH, $Paco_2$ and respiratory rate, indicate a successful outcome.

Conclusions

In recent years, there has been a dramatic increase in the use of NIV to treat patients with ARF. The evidence for a successful outcome with NIV is strongest in the context of acute type II respiratory failure during exacerbations of COPD. Treatment has been shown to reduce mortality, the need for intubation and the length of stay in ICU. As a consequence, there is a substantial cost reduction. Taking into consideration that COPD is a common disease with increasing prevalence and its exacerbations cause high morbidity, mortality and cost especially associated with ventilation and ICU admission, the use of NIV is one of the most important advances in COPD treatment in decades. To a lesser extent, NIV benefits COPD patients with pneumonia and

acts as an aid to extubation, again largely by avoiding the complications of prolonged ICU stay. Despite these successes, further work is needed to see whether more can be done to enhance patient compliance and improve success in avoiding intubation, particularly in those with more severe initial ARF. More information is needed on how long support with NIV is needed and how to wean this effectively. In the cases of ARF in other chronic respiratory diseases, the evidence is less clear. In diseases such as CF, neuromuscular disease or restrictive thoracic disorders, RCTs of NIV in ARF will remain difficult to perform and be small in size. All these conditions share a poor outcome for ARF even with invasive mechanical ventilation in the ICU, and this will make it difficult to withhold treatment by using NIV and to conduct placebo-controlled trials. Outside of subjects with chronic lung disease, the benefits for NIV are not clear, and the benefits are unlikely to be as great. Support with CPAP in chest trauma is effective, safe and well tolerated. However, in the case of pneumonia, the benefits of NIV over treatment with invasive mechanical ventilation are not established. Overall, prognosis for these patients is not adversely affected by mechanical ventilation except in the most severe cases where NIV is unlikely to influence outcomes. In this situation, there is a greater risk of delaying appropriate support and treating these individuals in under-resourced areas. A role may still exist for NIV in this context, but more work needs to be done cautiously, establishing clear efficacy, appropriate patient selection, place of treatment and the ventilator best suited to provide support.

References

1 National Centre for Health Statistics, Centres for Disease Control and Prevention. *Advance Report of Final Mortality Statistics 1992.* Hyattsville, MD, US Department of Health and Human Services, 1992.

2 Marston BJ, Plouffe JF, File TM Jr et al. Incidence of community acquired pneumonia requiring hospitalization: results of a population-based active surveillance study in Ohio. *Arch Intern Med* 1997; **157**:1709–18.

3 Restrepo MI, Jorgensen JH, Mortensen EM, Anzueto A. Severe community-acquired pneumonia: current outcomes, epidemiology, etiology and therapy. *Curr Opin Infect Dis* 2001; **14**:703–9.

4 Fuso L, Incalzi RA, Pistrelli R et al. Predicting mortality of patients hospitalised for acutely exacerbated chronic obstructive pulmonary disease. *Am J Med* 1995; **98**:272–7.

5 Plant PK, Owen J, Elliot MW. One year period prevalence study of respiratory acidosis in acute exacerbations of COPD: implications for the provision of non-invasive ventilation and oxygen administration. *Thorax* 2000; **55**:550–4.

6 Jeffrey AA, Warren PM, Flenley DC. Acute hypercapnoeic respiratory failure in patients with chronic obstructive lung disease: risk factors and use of guidelines for management. *Thorax* 1992; **47**:34–40.

7 Breen D, Churches T, Hawker F, Torzillo PJ. Acute respiratory failure secondary to chronic obstructive pulmonary disease treated in the intensive care unit: a long term follow up study. *Thorax* 2002; **57**:29–33.

8 Chien JW, Ciufo R, Novak R et al. Uncontrolled oxygen administration and respiratory failure in acute asthma. *Chest* 2000; **117**: 728–33.

9 Mountain RD, Sahn SA. Clinical features and outcome in patients with acute asthma presenting with hypercapnia. *Am Rev Respir Dis* 1988; **138**:535–9.

10 Berlinski A, Leland LF, Kozinetz CA, Oermann CM. Invasive mechanical ventilation for acute respiratory failure in children with cystic fibrosis. *Pediatr Pulmonol* 2002; **34**:297–303.

11 Sulica R, Teirstein A, Padilla ML. Lung transplantation in interstitial lung disease. *Curr Opin Pulm Med* 2001; **7**:314–22.

12 Laghi F, Tobin MJ. Disorders of the respiratory muscles. *Am J Respir Crit Care Med* 2003; **168**:10–48.

13 Baudoin S, Blumenthal S, Cooper B *et al.* Non-invasive ventilation in acute respiratory failure. *Thorax* 2002; **57**:192–211.

14 Elliot MW, Simonds AK. Nocturnal assisted ventilation using bilevel airway pressure: the effect of expiratory airway pressure. *Eur Respir J* 1995; **8**:436–40.

15 Lightowler JV, Wedzicha JA, Elliot MW, M. Ram FS. Non-invasive positive pressure ventilation to treat respiratory failure resulting from exacerbations of chronic obstructive pulmonary disease: Cochrane systematic review and meta-analysis. *BMJ* 2003; **326**:1–5.

16 Ram FSM, Lightowler JV, Wedzicha JA. Non-invasive positive pressure ventilation to treat respiratory failure resulting from exacerbations of chronic obstructive pulmonary disease (Cochrane review). In: *The Cochrane Library*, Issue 3. Oxford, Update Software, 2003.

17 Plant PK, Owen J, Parrott S, Elliot MW. Cost effectiveness of ward based non-invasive ventilation for acute exacerbations of chronic obstructive pulmonary disease: economic analysis of randomised controlled trial. *BMJ* 2003; **326**:1–5.

18 Angus RM, Ahmed AA, Fenwick IJ *et al.* Comparison of the acute effects on gas exchange of nasal ventilation and doxapram in exacerbations of chronic obstructive pulmonary disease. *Thorax* 1997; **51**:1048–50.

19 Appendini I, Patessio A, Zannobonni S *et al.* Physiological effects of positive end-expiratory pressure and mask pressure support during exacerbations of chronic obstructive pulmonary disease. *Am J Respir Crit Care Med* 1994; **149**:1069–76.

20 Lim TK. Treatment of severe exacerbations of chronic obstructive pulmonary disease with mask applied continuous positive airway pressure. *Respirology* 1996; **1**:189–93.

21 Confalonieri M, Potena A, Carbone G, Della Porta R, Tolley E, Meduri GU. Acute respiratory failure in patients with severe community acquired pneumonia. *Am J Respir Crit Care Med* 1999; **160**:1585–91.

22 Wysocki M, Tric L, Wolff MA *et al.* Non-invasive pressure support ventilation in patients with acute respiratory failure. A randomised comparison with conventional therapy. *Chest* 1995; **107**:761–8.

23 Antonelli M, Conti G, Rocco M *et al.* A comparison of non-invasive positive-pressure support ventilation and conventional mechanical ventilation in acute respiratory failure. *N Engl J Med* 1998; **339**:429–34.

24 Brett A, Sinclair DG. Use of continuous positive airway pressure in the management of community acquired pneumonia. *Thorax* 1993; **48**:1280–1.

25 Delclaux C, L'Her E, Alberti C *et al.* Treatment of acute hypoxaemic non-hypercapnic respiratory insufficiency with continuous positive airway pressure delivered by a face mask. *JAMA* 2000; **284**: 2352–60.

26 Hilbert G, Gruson D, Vargas F *et al.* Noninvasive ventilation in immunosuppressed patients with pulmonary infiltrates, fever and acute respiratory failure. *N Engl J Med* 1999; **344**:481–7.

27 Antonelli M, Conti G, Bufi M *et al.* Noninvasive ventilation for treatment of acute respiratory failure in patients undergoing solid organ transplantation. *JAMA* 2000; **283**:235–41.

28 Prevedoros HP, Lee RP, Marriott D. CPAP, effective respiratory support in patients with AIDS related *Pneumocystis carinii* pneumonia. *Anaesth Intens Care* 1991; **19**:561–6.

29 Kesten S, Rebuck AS. Nasal continuous positive airway pressure in *Pneumocystis carinii* pneumonia. *Lancet* 1988; **ii**:1414–15.

30 Meduri GU, Cook TR, Turner RE *et al.* Noninvasive positive pressure ventilation in status asthmaticus. *Chest* 1996; **110**:767–74.

31 Wang CH, Lin HC, Huang TJ *et al.* Differential effects of nasal continuous positive airway pressure on reversible or fixed upper and lower airway obstruction. *Eur Respir J* 1996; **9**:952–9.

32 Shivraam U, Donath J, Khan FA *et al.* Effects of continuous positive airway pressure in acute asthma. *Respiration* 1987; **52**:157–62.

33 Martin JG, Shore S, Engel LA. Effect of nasal continuous positive airway pressure on respiratory mechanics and pattern of breathing in acute asthma. *Am Rev Respir Dis* 1982; **126**:812–17.

34 Soroksky A, Stav D, Shpirer I. A pilot prospective, randomized, placebo-controlled trial of bilevel positive airway pressure in acute asthmatic attack. *Chest* 2003; **123**:1018–25.

35 Bolliger CT, Van Eeden SF. Treatment of multiple rib fractures. Randomised controlled trial comparing ventilatory with nonventilatory management. *Chest* 1990; **97**:943–8.

36 Soo Hoo GW, Santiago S, Williams AJ. Nasal mechanical ventilation for hypercapnoeic respiratory failure in chronic obstructive pulmonary disease: determinants of success and failure. *Crit Care Med* 1994; **22**:1253–61.

37 Moran F, Bradley J. Non-invasive ventilation for cystic fibrosis. In: *The Cochrane Library*, Issue 3. Oxford, Update Software, 2003.

38 Milross MA, Piper AJ, Norman M *et al.* Low flow oxygen and bilevel ventilatory support. *Am J Respir Crit Care Med* 2001; **163**:129–34.

39 Hodson ME, Madden BP, Steven MH *et al.* Non-invasive mechanical ventilation for cystic fibrosis patients — a potential bridge to transplantation. *Eur Respir J* 1991; **4**:524–7.

40 Simonds AK, Elliot MW. Outcome of domiciliary nasal intermittent positive pressure ventilation in restrictive and obstructive disorders. *Thorax* 1995; **50**:604–9.

41 Nava S, Ambrosino N, Clini E *et al.* Noninvasive mechanical ventilation in the weaning of patients with respiratory failure due to chronic obstructive pulmonary disease. A randomised controlled trial. *N Engl J Med* 1998; **128**:721–8.

42 Girault C, Daudenthun I, Chevron V, Tamion F, Leroy J, Bonmarchand G. Noninvasive ventilation as a systemic extubation and weaning technique in acute or chronic respiratory failure. *Am J Respir Crit Care Med* 1999; **160**:86–92.

43 Keenan SP, Powers C, McCormack DG, Block G. Noninvasive positive pressure ventilation for post extubation respiratory distress. *JAMA* 2002; **287**:3238–44.

44 Bott J, Carroll MP, Conway JH *et al.* Randomised controlled trial of nasal ventilation in acute ventilatory failure due to chronic obstructive airways disease. *Lancet* 1993; **341**:1555–7.

45 Brochard L, Mancebo J, Wysocki M *et al.* Noninvasive ventilation for acute exacerbation of chronic obstructive pulmonary disease. *N Engl J Med* 1995; **333**:817–22.

46 Plant PK, Owen J, Elliot MW. Early use of non-invasive ventilation for acute exacerbations of chronic obstructive pulmonary disease on general respiratory wards. *Lancet* 2000; **355**:1931–5.

47 Ambrosino N, Foglio K, Rubini F *et al.* Non-invasive mechanical ventilation in acute respiratory failure due to chronic obstructive airways disease: correlates for success. *Thorax* 1995; **50**:755–7.

48 Celikel T, Sungur M, Ceyhan B, Karakurt S. Comparison of non-invasive positive pressure ventilation with standard medical therapy in hypercapnoeic acute respiratory failure. *Chest* 1998; **114**:1636–42.

49 Kramer N, Meyer TJ, Meharg J, Cece RD, Hill NS. Randomized prospective trial of non-invasive positive pressure ventilation in

acute respiratory failure. *Am J Respir Crit Care Med* 1995; **151**:1799–806.

50 Avdeev SN, Tretyakov AV, Grigoryants RA, Kutsenko MA, Chuchalin AG. Non-invasive positive airway pressure ventilation: role in treating acute respiratory failure caused by chronic obstructive pulmonary disease. *J Anestiziol Reanimatol* 1998; **May**:45–51.

51 Dikensoy O, Ikidag B, Filiiz A, Bayram N. Comparison of non-invasive ventilation and standard medical therapy in acute hypercapnoeic respiratory failure: a randomized controlled trial at a tertiary health centre in SE Turkey. *Int J Clin Pract* 2002; **56**:85–8.

52 Barbe R, Togores B, Rubi M, Pons S, Maimo A, Agusti AGN. Non-invasive ventilatory support does not facilitate recovery from acute respiratory failure in chronic obstructive pulmonary disease. *Eur Respir J* 1996; **9**:1240–5.

CHAPTER 5.3

Non-invasive positive pressure ventilation in stable patients with chronic obstructive pulmonary disease. What is the evidence?

Peter J Wijkstra

Description of problem

Chronic obstructive pulmonary disease (COPD) is an important cause of morbidity and mortality worldwide. While a wide range of therapeutic approaches exists to assist patients with this condition, only long-term oxygen therapy for patients with resting awake hypoxaemia has been shown to prolong life.[1,2] Other treatments are largely symptomatic, such as bronchodilators to improve airflow and relieve dyspnoea. Even with optimal use of medication, patients with COPD often suffer from dyspnoea that limits their exercise tolerance and health-related quality of life. Randomized trials have demonstrated that respiratory rehabilitation improved dyspnoea, exercise tolerance and health-related quality of life.[3–6] As a result, rehabilitation has now become part of the standard of care for the more severely affected patients. Newer approaches to the management of COPD, such as lung volume reduction surgery (LVRS), are likely to benefit only a small number of highly selected individuals.[7]

In case of acute respiratory failure, non-invasive positive pressure ventilation (NIPPV) provides a safe, effective way of stabilizing the arterial blood gases while avoiding the risks and inconvenience of intubation.[8,9] Short-term NIPPV has therefore become an accepted management approach for patients with acute hypercapnia. However, it remains unclear as to whether NIPPV can also play a useful role in improving either arterial blood gases or functional ability among stable patients with chronic respiratory failure.

In this chapter, we will start to discuss the rationale of NIPPV and how it can be administered. Secondly, all randomized controlled trials (RCTs) will be discussed, both short term and long term, that have been published investigating the effects of NIPPV in stable patients with COPD. Finally, we will elaborate on different issues that might be important in making NIPPV effective.

Description of treatment

While negative pressure ventilation was started decades ago in patients with thoracic cage abnormalities or in patients with neuromuscular disease, NIPPV is nowadays the most frequently used mode of ventilatory support in patients with chronic respiratory failure. During NIPPV, the patients are ventilated through a nose mask or full-face mask, while oral masks are on the market as well. Although most patients are ventilated for a considerable number of hours during the night, daytime NIPPV has been shown to be effective as well.[10,11] One of the most crucial elements in obtaining effective NIPPV is the compliance of the patient. An appropriate mask to ensure comfort and optimal fit are the first steps in this respect. Patients will only sleep with the mask for a considerable number of hours if it is comfortable. Next to mask fitting, effective ventilation is an important issue. While in recent years bilevel ventilation has been used more frequently, volume-limited ventilators have been used in the past as well. Studies investigating these ventilator modes in patients with acute exacerbations suggested that pressure ventilation was tolerated better by the patients.[12,13] Finally, correct ventilator settings are necessary to provide effective ventilation on the one hand, while on the other hand patients must tolerate these pressures or volumes. The best way to deal with all these issues is to admit patients to the hospital for a number of days. Although there is no evidence that the setting of initiating NIPPV is of influence towards effective ventilation, one might expect that, if patients are admitted to the hospital, they get more time to adjust to the ventilator. At the end of this chapter, these issues will be discussed in detail.

Rationale of NIPPV

There are some theoretical reasons why NIPPV might be effective: (a) resetting of the respiratory centre to improve daytime gases; (b) resting dysfunctional respiratory muscles, thereby increasing their daytime strength and endurance; (c) improving peripheral muscle function from a better milieu (pH, Pa_{O_2}, Pa_{CO_2}); and (d) preventing repeated nocturnal arousals, thereby improving the quality of sleep. We all know that the respiratory muscles are in an unfavourable position in patients with severe COPD due to hyperinflation. Bellemare and Grassino showed that, in patients with COPD, the diaphragm is susceptible to fatigue.[14] They introduced the so-called time tension index (TTI) containing two elements: respiratory load and respiratory duty cycle. The respiratory load is represented by the pressure generated by the diaphragm (Pdi) as a proportion of the maximal inspiratory pressure (Pdimax). The duty cycle is represented by the inspiratory time (Ti) as a proportion of the duration of the total respiration (Ttot). As a formula: $TTI = Pdi/Pdimax \times Ti/Ttot$. If this product exceeds 0.15, one might expect that fatigue of the diaphragm will occur. The hypothesis is that NIPVV might increase Pdimax, which decreases the TTI and thereby postpones fatigue. Resting inspiratory muscles was the hypothesis behind a major trial of negative pressure ventilation (NPV). Shapiro et al.[15] randomized 184 patients with severe COPD to active or sham ventilation with a poncho wrap negative pressure ventilator. There were no significant changes in respiratory muscle strength; however, although patients were encouraged to use the ventilator for at least 5 hours each day, the average duration of use was closer to 3 hours, and the intensity of the treatment intervention was quite variable. Celli et al.[16] and Zibrak et al.[17] also failed to identify improvements in arterial blood gases or respiratory muscle strength with NPV. In contrast, studies that included patients with higher Pa_{CO_2} levels showed improvements in respiratory muscle function after NPV.[18] One uncontrolled study showed that NIPPV had induced a significant decrease in Pa_{CO_2} in association with a decrease in the pressure time product of the diaphragm. A subgroup of responders had a significantly increased trans-diaphragmatic pressure and were better able to clear CO_2 by their ventilatory pump.[19] In addition, Belman et al.[20] showed that positive pressure ventilation (PPV) was more effective in unloading the diaphragm than NPV. Another consequence of flow limitation in COPD is the incomplete alveolar emptying at the end of the inspiration, leading to the so-called auto positive end-expiratory pressure (PEEP) or intrinsic PEEP. A recent randomized controlled study by Diaz et al.[11] showed that NIPPV could lower the Pa_{CO_2} by lowering the level of hyperinflation and PEEPi. So, while there is some evidence that NIPPV can be effective in unloading the respiratory muscles, there is currently no RCT that found a significant improvement in respiratory muscle function.

Another theoretical explanation for the effects of NIPPV is improved sleep efficiency. Meecham Jones, who achieved effective ventilation in clearly hypercapnic patients, showed improved sleep efficiency.[21] In an uncontrolled very short-term trial (3 days), Criner et al.[22] investigated gas exchange and sleep efficiency in patients with COPD. They compared low-level continuous positive airway pressure (CPAP) with bilevel positive airway pressure (BiPAP) on two consecutive nights in patients with a mean Pa_{CO_2} of 58($\pm$4) mmHg. No significant changes were found in Pa_{CO_2}, while there was a significant improvement in sleep efficiency and total sleep time.

In conclusion, currently, there are no studies on NPV or NIPPV that have provided evidence whether the benefits they found in respiratory muscle function or sleep efficiency were related to improvements in gas exchange.

Randomized controlled trials

Literature search

RCTs were identified from several sources, such as MEDLINE, EMBASE and CINAHL (Cumulated Index to Nursing and Allied Health). In addition, records were identified through hand searching of abstracts from meetings of the American Thoracic Society, the American College of Chest Physicians and the European Respiratory Society. We included in this chapter both nocturnal NIPPV as well as daytime NIPPV if they have been published as a full paper. Patients in the group treated by NIPPV continued to receive their usual management for COPD. The control group received the same management as the study group with the exception of their not receiving NIPPV.

Short-term NIPPV

Until now, six RCTs with a maximum duration of 3 months have been published as a full paper.[10,11,21,23–25] Details of the studies are presented in Table 1. The first study was published by Strumpf et al.[25] in 1991 and, except for neuropsychological function, no significant changes were detected. The reason for this negative study might be the fact that only seven out of the 19 patients completed it, which underpowers the study. Secondly, the patients were not clearly hypercapnic, while some patients were even normocapnic. Gay et al.[24] assessed the effects of NIPPV in hypercapnic patients and did not find improvements in clinical parameters. In this study also, only a small number of patients completed it. In contrast to the previous studies, Lin[23] investigated the effects of 2 weeks of NIPPV and found only a positive effect for the combination of NIPPV and oxygen on night-time oxygenation. A probable reason for this negative result is that some patients need more than 2 weeks of acclimatization before they are comfortable and feel confident with the ventilator during the night. Meecham Jones[21] produced the only study showing clear evidence of clinical benefits for nocturnal NIPPV in patients with COPD. After 3 months, the combination of NIPPV and oxygen was better than oxygen alone for gas exchange, sleep efficiency and health status.

In contrast to the previous studies, Renston et al.[10] investigated the effects of daytime NIPPV (2 hours a day for five consecutive days). Despite the fact that no significant changes were found in gas exchange, patients in the BiPAP group

Table 1. Randomized controlled trials of short-term NIPPV.

Trial	No. of patients (treatment/ controls)	FEV$_1$ mean (range) or ($\pm$ SD)	Paco$_2$ mean (range) or ($\pm$ SD)	Length	IPAP/ EPAP	Outcome measures	Effects
Strumpf et al.[25]	Crossover trial Enrolled: 19 Completed: 7	0.54 (0.46–0.88)	49 (35–67)	3 months	15/2	ABG, RM, walking test, dyspnoea, PFT, sleep study, NP function	Significant effects for NP function
Gay et al.[24]	Parallel group trial Randomized: 7/6 Completed: 4/6	0.68 (0.5–1.1)	55 (45–89)	3 months	10/2	ABG, 6MWD, dyspnoea, PFT, sleep study	No significant effects
Meecham Jones et al.[21]	Crossover trial Enrolled: 18 Completed: 14	0.86 (0.33–1.7)	56 (52–65)	3 months	18/2	ABG, 6MWT, HRQL, PFT, sleep study	Significant effects for ABG, sleep efficiency, HRQL
Lin[23]	Crossover trial Enrolled: 12	33% pred.	51 ($\pm$ 4)	2 weeks	12/2	ABG, PFT, RVEL, LVEF, sleep study	Significant effects of NIPPV and O$_2$ on nocturnal oxygenation
Renston et al.[10]	Completed: 12	0.75 (0.45–1.05)	–	5 days for 2 h	15–20/2	ABG, EMG, RM, 6MWD, dyspnoea	Significant effects for dyspnoea and 6MWD
Diaz et al.[11]	Parallel group trial Randomized: 9/8 Completed: 9/8 Parallel group trial Randomized: 18/18 Completed: 18/18	0.75 ($\pm$ 0.2)	56 ($\pm$ 5)	3 h/day 5 days/week 3 weeks	18/2	ABG, RM, PFT, respiratory mechanics	Significant effects for ABG, lung volumes, respiratory mechanics, PEEPi

ABG, arterial blood gases; RM, respiratory muscles; PFT, pulmonary function tests; NP, neuropsychological; HRQL, health-related quality of life; RVEL, right ventricular ejection fraction; LVEF, left ventricular ejection fraction; EMG, electromyography.

showed both a significant decrease in level of dyspnoea and an improvement in 6-min walking distance (6MWD). However, it is not clear from the paper whether BiPAP is significantly better than sham treatment. Recently, Diaz et al.[11] showed benefits by daytime NIPPV for 3 hours per day during 5 days a week for 3 weeks. Significant improvements were found in blood gases, lung volumes and respiratory mechanics. In addition, the changes in Paco$_2$ were significantly related to changes in dynamic intrinsic PEEP, inspiratory lung impedance, tidal volume and functional residual capacity (FRC) (Fig. 1).

Recently, a meta-analysis of individual data from RCTs compared NIPPV with conventional management in patients with COPD and stable respiratory failure.[26] RCTs were identified from several sources. Only studies investigating nocturnal NIPPV applied via a nasal or face mask for at least 5 hours each day for at least 3 weeks were included. Patients in the actively treated group continued to receive their usual management for COPD next to NIPPV. The control group received the same management as the study group with the exception of their

not receiving NIPPV. Only four RCTs fulfilled the above-mentioned criteria (Table 2).[21,24,25,27] Three months of data from the study by Casanova et al.[27] were included as well. The study by Lin[23] was excluded because the intervention period was only 2 weeks, whereas the studies by Renston et al.[10] and Diaz et al.[11] were excluded because they applied daytime ventilation. The long-term study by Clini et al.[28] was not included as it was not published as a full paper at the time that we did our analysis. Our analysis showed that 3 months of NIPPV in patients with stable COPD did not improve lung function, gas exchange or sleep efficiency. The high upper limit of the confidence interval for the 6MWD suggests that some people do improve their walking distance. Still, the limited number of patients included in this meta-analysis precluded a clear clinical direction regarding the effects of NIPPV in COPD.

Long-term NIPPV
Casanova et al.[27] were the first to investigate the long-term effects of NIPPV with a duration of 1 year. Fifty-two patients

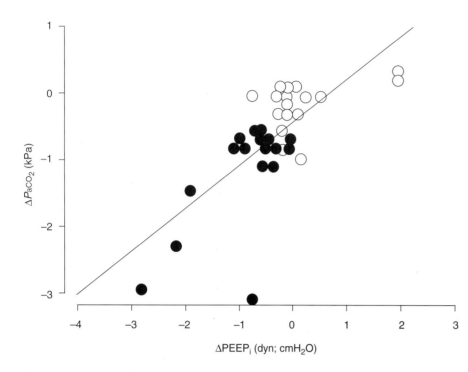

Figure 1. Relationship between changes (Δ) in the carbon dioxide tension in arterial blood (Pa_{CO_2}) and dynamic intrinsic positive end-expiratory pressure (PEEPi, dyn). Closed circles, non-invasive mechanically ventilated patients; open circles, control subjects ($r^2 = 0.52$; $P < 0.0001$).

Table 2. Primary results of a meta-analysis on nocturnal NIPPV.

Outcomes	Contributing trials (references*)	Sample size (NIPPV/control)	Treatment effect Mean	95% CI
FEV_1	21,24,25,27	33/33	0.02 L	−0.04 to 0.09
FVC	21,24,25,27	33/33	−0.01 L	−0.14 to 0.13
Pimax	24,25,27	24/24	6.2 cm H_2O	0.2–12.2
Pemax	24,25,27	24/24	18.4 cm H_2O	−11.8 to 48.6
Pa_{O_2}	21,24,25,27	33/33	0.0 mmHg	−3.8 to 3.9
Pa_{CO_2}	21,24,25,27	34/33	−1.5 mmHg	−4.5 to 1.5
6-min walk test	21,24	12/11	27.5 m	−26.8 to 81.8
Sleep efficiency	21,24,25	13/11	−4.0%	−14.7 to 6.7

*Contributing trials.[21,24,25,27]

were randomized to either NIPPV plus standard care or standard care alone. The level of BiPAP was modest [inspiratory positive airway pressure (IPAP) 12–14 cm H_2O], and its effect was not controlled during the night. Although the number of hospital admissions was less in the NIPPV group after 3 months (5% versus 15%), this was not the case after 6 months. After 12 months, there were only modest improvements in both dyspnoea and neuropsychological function. Recently, Clini et al.[28] reported a prospective RCT comparing the combination of NIPPV and long-term oxygen therapy (LTOT) with LTOT alone for a period of 2 years. COPD patients with a $Pa_{CO_2} > 6.6$ kPa were included. While 120 patients were considered, 90 were randomized and only 47 completed the study. The level of NIPPV was modest again (IPAP of 14 ± 3 cm H_2O), while the ventilator was used for a considerable number of hours (9 ± 2 h). Compared with the period before the study, total hospital admissions decreased by 45% in the NIPPV group, but increased by 27% in the LTOT group. Intensive care unit (ICU) admissions decreased in the NIPPV group by 75%, but in the LTOT group by 20%. However, both outcomes were not significantly different between both groups. After 2 years, dyspnoea decreased, and health-related quality of life improved significantly in the NIPPV group compared with the LTOT group. The study by Clini et al.[28] suggests that NIPPV might lead to beneficial effects in some patients with COPD. However, it does not advocate the widespread use of NIPPV in these patients as only minor improvements were found. The long-term trial by Muir et al.[29] was not included in this systematic overview as no full paper had been published.

Uncontrolled trials

In contrast to the aforementioned RCTs, most uncontrolled

trials of NIPPV did show positive results. Elliot *et al.*,[30,31] in two studies, showed positive effects of NIPPV. In one study, they included eight patients with severe COPD [mean forced expiratory volume in 1 second (FEV_1) 0.53 L] and hypercapnia (mean Pa_{CO_2} 8.0 kPa), showing that NIPPV could lead to a significant decrease in Pa_{CO_2} that was significantly correlated with a decrease in both residual volume (RV) and gas trapping.[30] They could not detect a relationship between improved gas exchange and relief of muscle fatigue. In the other study from this group, after 12 months of NIPPV, they found a significant decrease in Pa_{CO_2} and improved sleep efficiency, while the quality of life was unchanged.[31] In contrast, Perrin *et al.*[32] showed that quality of life improved significantly after 6 months of NIPPV. In this study, 14 patients were included with a mean Pa_{CO_2} of 7.8 kPa, and they received volume ventilation during the night. Next to an improved quality of life, they also found significantly improved gas exchange. The same positive results were seen in the study by Sivasothy *et al.*[33] Twenty-six patients with severe COPD (mean FEV_1 0.7 L) and hypercapnia (Pa_{CO_2} 8.6 kPa) were ventilated by a volume ventilator during the night. After 18 months (range 4–74 months), both gas exchange and quality of life improved significantly. Finally, a long-term study by Jones *et al.*[34] showed significant improvements in gas exchange and reduction in hospital admissions and general practitioner visits after 24 months of pressure ventilation. In summary, these uncontrolled studies showed that, in patients with severe hypercapnia, NIPPV can improve gas exchange. However, this does not lead to a concomitant decrease in pulmonary artery pressure, as shown recently.[35]

Discussion

From the available studies, we do not get a clear picture of whether NIPPV leads to clear benefits in patients with COPD. In the next section, we will elaborate about the various issues that might explain the differences in outcome between all studies.

Selection of patients

It seems that patients who are more hypercapnic at entry to the study have more benefits from NIPPV. In contrast to other RCTs, Meecham Jones *et al.*[21] and Clini *et al.*[28] included only patients with a Pa_{CO_2} above 6.6 kPa, and both showed significant benefits in different outcome parameters. In addition, Meecham Jones *et al.*[21] showed that the patients who had an increase in Pa_{CO_2} during the night before they were on NIPPV had the most benefit in decreasing daytime Pa_{CO_2} after starting NIPPV (Fig. 2). The other RCTs included normocapnic patients[25,27] or patients who were just hypercapnic.[23,24] The uncontrolled studies in which only hypercapnic patients (lowest value of 6.3 kPa) were included also had only positive outcomes. In our meta-analysis, we expected heterogeneity between the four studies based on different levels of Pa_{CO_2} at inclusion. However, probably because of the low number of patients included in our analysis, we could not detect such a difference. Nevertheless, all available studies suggest that patients who are clearly hypercapnic are the best candidates for NIPPV.

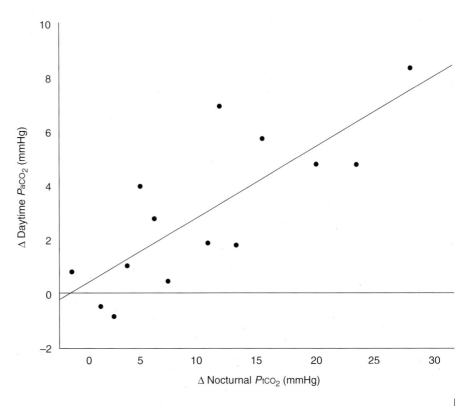

Figure 2. Correlation between change in daytime arterial Pa_{CO_2} and change in mean overnight transcutaneous Pa_{CO_2} for individual patients ($r^2 = 0.69$; $P = 0.01$).

Adequacy of ventilation

At this moment, there is no evidence that pressure-cycled ventilation is better or worse than volume-cycled ventilation. While all RCTs using BiPAP showed different outcomes, the uncontrolled studies used mainly volume-cycled ventilation. Assisted control ventilation is frequently selected as the mode of choice to enhance synchrony between patient and ventilator. One study did use time-cycled ventilation to reduce the level of inspiratory muscle effort; however, asynchrony between patient and machine was present in 20%.[25] Another important aspect is the lack of control in most studies whether the ventilation was effective or not. The study by Meecham Jones et al.[21] was the only one that controlled for the level of ventilation by transcutaneous CO_2, while Strumpf et al.[25] controlled it discontinuously by end-tidal CO_2. The latter might easily miss hypoventilation, leading to ineffective ventilation. In all other studies,[10,11,23,24,27,28] the effectiveness of ventilation was not controlled. So, as most studies did not control for effective ventilation, we cannot draw strong conclusions about the possible effect of NIPVV. It means that we do not know whether the IPAP used in the so-called negative studies was high enough. In the study by Meecham Jones et al.,[21] mean inspiratory pressures of 18 were used, showing positive effects on most outcomes, including gas exchange. Probably, they needed these higher levels to achieve effective ventilation. Finally, as it takes time to get used to the mask and to find the appropriate settings of the ventilator, it seems better to admit patients to hospital. In this way, effective ventilation can be achieved as shown in the study by Meecham Jones et al.[21]

Number of hours on NIPPV

Currently, it is not known what the optimal duration of ventilatory support is, so different approaches have been used. There are two RCTs[10,11] treating patients with COPD for a short period with ventilatory support during the day. In one study, patients received BiPAP for 2 hours daily for 5 days a week, while in the other study, BiPAP was given for 3 hours daily, 5 days a week for three consecutive weeks. These short periods produced significant benefits in clinical parameters. In addition, the study by Diaz et al.[11] showed that the decrease in Pa_{CO_2} was significantly related to a reduction in PEEPi. A possible explanation for the positive effects of short daytime NIPPV might be that, during ventilatory support in the daytime, there is no leakage as the patients are awake. In this way, it might be more effective than at night-time as leakage occurs frequently if the patient starts to sleep. On the other hand, night-time NIPPV can be positive if patients receive ventilatory support for a considerable number of hours. In the long-term trial by Clini et al.,[28] the mean number of hours on BiPAP was 9 ± 2 hours. In addition, in the study by Meecham Jones et al.,[21] the median number of hours was 6.9 hours (range 4.2–10.8 hours). Until now, there has been no study showing that more hours on ventilatory support are better in reducing the work of breathing, in resting the respiratory muscles or in improving sleep quality. Because it is more practical, NIPPV is still being advocated for use during the night for as many hours as possible.

Length of ventilation

The length of ventilatory support can also influence the outcomes. Most studies were of relatively short duration (3 months), and some of them could detect significant clinical benefits after such a short period. Two European studies followed the patients for the longest period.[28,29] Clini et al.[28] showed an improved quality of life after 2 years and improved dyspnoea even after 1 year. In addition, they showed a reduction in both hospital admissions and ICU admissions. Cumulative days spent in hospital due to respiratory exacerbations showed a trend in favour of those receiving NIPPV (12.6 ± 7.9

Table 3. Randomized controlled trials of long-term nocturnal NIPPV.

Trial	Type of trial Number of patients (treatment/controls)	FEV$_1$ mean (range)	Pa$_{CO_2}$ mean (range)	Length (months)	IPAP/ EPAP	Outcome measures	Effects
Casanova et al.[27]	Parallel group trial Randomized: 26/26 Completed: 17/19	0.85 (0.44–1.28)	51 (37–66)	12	12–14/4	ABG, RM, dyspnoea, PFT	Significant effect for dyspnoea and NP function
Clini et al.[28]	Parallel group trial Randomized: 43/47 Completed: 23/24	0.70 (0.30–1.35)	55 (50–75)	24	14/2	ABG, RM, dyspnoea, sleep study, HRQL, hospitalizations	Significant long-term effects for dyspnoea and HRQL Positive trends for hospital admissions and ICU stay

IPAP, inspiratory positive airway pressure; EPAP, expiratory positive airway pressure; ABG, arterial blood gases; RM, respiratory muscles: PFT, pulmonary function tests; NP, neuropsychological; HQRL, health-related quality of life; ICU, intensive care unit.

versus 16.9 ± 10.3 respectively). Muir et al.[29] compared 60 patients with severe COPD who received LTOT and NIPPV with 62 patients who received LTOT alone. After a median follow-up of 4.7 years, there were no significant differences in survival between the groups, with the exception of patients older than 65 years in whom survival was better in the NIPPV + LTOT group. In contrast to these long-term studies, patients in the study by Meecham Jones et al.[21] needed only 3 months to get significant clinical benefits.

Summary

In conclusion, until now, there has been no conclusive evidence that NIPPV should be provided routinely to stable patients with COPD. However, a small group of patients might have clinical benefits from it. Good candidates are probably patients who are clearly hypercapnic, who receive adequately controlled ventilation and who get enough time to adjust to the ventilator. In this selected group of patients, a trial with ventilatory support can be considered.

References

1 Kvale PA, Cugell DW, Anthonisen NR, Timms RM, Petty TL, Boylen CT. Continuous or nocturnal oxygen therapy in hypoxemic chronic obstructive lung disease. *Ann Intern Med* 1980; **93**:391–8.

2 Report of the Medical Research Council Working Party. Long term domiciliary oxygen therapy in chronic hypoxic cor pulmonale complicating chronic bronchitis and emphysema. *Lancet* 1981; **1**: 681–6.

3 Lacasse Y, Wong E, Guyatt GH, King D, Cook DJ, Goldstein RS. Meta-analysis of respiratory rehabilitation in chronic obstructive pulmonary disease. *Lancet* 1996; **348**:1115–19.

4 Goldstein RS, Gort EH, Stubbing D, Avendano MA, Guyatt GH. Randomised controlled trial of respiratory rehabilitation. *Lancet* 1994; **344**:1394–7.

5 Griffiths TL, Burr ML, Campbell IA et al. Results at 1 year of outpatient multidisciplinary pulmonary rehabilitation: a randomised controlled trial. *Lancet* 2000; **355**:362–8.

6 Wijkstra PJ, van Altena R, Kraan J, Otten V, Postma DS, Koeter GH. Quality of life in patients with chronic obstructive pulmonary disease improves after rehabilitation at home. *Eur Respir J* 1994; **7**:269–73.

7 National Emphysema Treatment Trial Research Group. A randomized trial comparing lung-volume-reduction surgery with medical therapy for severe emphysema. *N Engl J Med* 2003; **348**:2059–73.

8 Brochard L, Mancebo J, Wysocki M et al. Noninvasive ventilation for acute exacerbations of chronic obstructive pulmonary disease. *N Engl J Med* 1995; **333**:817–22.

9 Kramer N, Meyer TJ, Meharg J et al. Randomized, prospective trial of noninvasive positive pressure ventilation in acute respiratory failure. *Am J Respir Crit Care Med* 1995; **151**:1799–806.

10 Renston JP, DiMarco AF, Supinski GS. Respiratory muscle rest using nasal BiPAP ventilation in patients with stable severe COPD. *Chest* 1994; **105**:1053–60.

11 Diaz O, Begin P, Torrealba B, Jover E, Lisboa C. Effects of noninvasive ventilation on lung hyperinflation in stable hypercapnic COPD. *Eur Respir J* 2002; **20**:1490–8.

12 Girault C, Richard JC, Chevron V et al. Comparative physiological effects of non invasive assist control and pressure support ventilation in acute hypercapnic respiratory failure. *Chest* 1997; **111**:1639–48.

13 Vitacca M, Rubini, Foglio K et al. Non invasive modalities of positive pressure ventilation improved the outcomes of acute exacerbations in COPD patients. *Intens Care Med* 1993; **19**:450–5.

14 Bellamare F, Grassino A. Effect of pressure and timing of contraction on human diaphragm fatigue. *J Appl Physiol* 1982; **53**:1190–5.

15 Shapiro SH, Ernst P, Gray-McDonald K. Effect of negative pressure ventilation in severe chronic obstructive pulmonary disease. *Lancet* 1992; **340**:1425–9.

16 Celli B, Lee H, Criner G et al. Controlled trial of external negative pressure ventilation in patients with severe chronic airflow obstruction. *Am Rev Respir Dis* 1989; **140**:1251–6.

17 Zibrak JD, Hill NS, Federman EC, Kwa SL, O'Donnell C. Evaluation of intermittent long-term negative-pressure ventilation in patients with severe chronic obstructive pulmonary disease. *Am Rev Respir Dis* 1988; **138**:1515–18.

18 Clinical indications for noninvasive positive pressure ventilation in chronic respiratory failure due to restrictive lung disease, COPD, and nocturnal hypoventilation – a consensus conference report. *Chest* 1999; **116**:521–34.

19 Nava S, Fanfulla F, Frigerio P, Navalesi P. Physiologic evaluation of 4 weeks of nocturnal nasal positive pressure ventilation in stable hypercapnic patients with chronic obstructive pulmonary disease. *Respiration* 2001; **68**:573–83.

20 Belman MJ, Soo Hoo GW, Kuei JH, Shadmehr R. Efficacy of positive vs negative pressure ventilation in unloading the respiratory muscles. *Chest* 1990; **98**:850–6.

21 Meecham Jones DJ, Paul EA, Jones PW, Wedzicha JA. Nasal pressure support ventilation plus oxygen compared with oxygen therapy alone in hypercapnic COPD. *Am J Respir Crit Care Med* 1995; **152**:538–44.

22 Criner GJ, Brennan K, Travaline JM, Kreimer D. Efficacy and compliance with noninvasive positive pressure ventilation in patients with chronic respiratory failure. *Chest* 1999; **116**:667–75.

23 Lin CC. Comparison between nocturnal nasal positive pressure ventilation combined with oxygen therapy and oxygen monotherapy in patients with severe COPD. *Am J Respir Crit Care Med* 1996; **154**(2 Pt 1):353–8.

24 Gay PC, Hubmayr RD, Stroetz RW. Efficacy of nocturnal nasal ventilation in stable, severe chronic obstructive pulmonary disease during a 3-month controlled trial. *Mayo Clin Proc* 1996; **71**:533–42.

25 Strumpf DA, Millman RP, Carlisle CC et al. Nocturnal positive-pressure ventilation via nasal mask in patients with severe chronic obstructive pulmonary disease. *Am Rev Respir Dis* 1991; **144**:1234–9.

26 Wijkstra PJ, Lacasse Y, Guyatt GH et al. A meta-analayis of nocturnal non-invasive positive pressure ventilation in patients with stable COPD. *Chest* 2003; **124**:337–43.

27 Casanova C, Celli BR, Tost L et al. Long-term controlled trial of nocturnal nasal positive pressure ventilation in patients with severe COPD. *Chest* 2000; **118**:1582–90.

28 Clini E, Sturani C, Rossi A et al. The Italian multicentre study on non-invasive ventilation in chronic obstructive pulmonary disease patients. *Eur Respir J* 2002; **20**:529–38.

29 Muir JF, de la Salmoniere P, Cuvelier A. Survival of severe hypercapnic COPD under long-term home mechanical ventilation with NIPPV + oxygen versus oxygen therapy alone. Preliminary results of a European multicentre study. *Am J Respir Crit Care Med* 1999; **159**:A295.

30 Elliott MW, Mulvey DA, Moxham J, Green M, Branthwaite MA. Domiciliary nocturnal nasal intermittent positive pressure ventilation in COPD: mechanisms underlying changes in arterial blood gas tensions. *Eur Respir J* 1991; **4**:1044–52.

31 Elliott MW, Simonds AK, Carroll MP, Wedzicha JA, Branthwaite MA. Domiciliary nocturnal nasal intermittent positive pressure ventilation in hypercapnic respiratory failure due to chronic obstructive lung disease: effects on sleep and quality of life. *Thorax* 1992; **47**:342–8.

32 Perrin C, El Far Y, Vandenbos F *et al*. Domiciliary nasal intermittent positive pressure ventilation in severe COPD: effects on lung function and quality of life. *Eur Respir J* 1997; **10**:2835–9.

33 Sivasothy P, Smith IE, Shneerson JM. Mask intermittent positive pressure ventilation in chronic hypercapnic respiratory failure due to chronic obstructive pulmonary disease. *Eur Respir J* 1998; **11**:34–40.

34 Jones SE, Packham S, Hebden M, Smith AP. Domiciliary nocturnal intermittent positive pressure ventilation in patients with respiratory failure due to severe COPD: long-term follow up and effect on survival. *Thorax* 1998; **53**:495–8.

35 Schonhofer B, Barchfeld T, Wenzel M, Kohler D. Long term effects of non-invasive mechanical ventilation on pulmonary haemodynamics in patients with chronic respiratory failure. *Thorax* 2001; **56**:524–8.

CHAPTER 5.4

The treatment of the obstructive sleep apnoea–hypopnoea syndrome

Michael J Hensley and Cheryl D Ray

Summary

Nasal continuous positive airway pressure (CPAP) in severe obstructive sleep apnoea–hypopnoea syndrome (OSAHS). Systematic reviews have found that nasal CPAP reduces daytime sleepiness, improves health status, reduces depression and possibly improves blood pressure and driving performance compared with placebo, no treatment, sham or subtherapeutic nasal CPAP or conservative treatment in people with severe OSAHS.

Nasal CPAP in non-severe OSAHS. Systematic reviews found that CPAP treatment of patients with non-severe OSAHS did not improve daytime sleepiness when compared with conservative treatment, sham or subtherapeutic CPAP or placebo tablets, but found significant improvement in some measures of cognitive performance and functional outcomes.

Oral appliance in severe OSAHS. Randomized controlled trials (RCTs) have found that oral appliances that produce anterior advancement of the mandible improve sleep-disordered breathing (SDB) and may improve daytime sleepiness in patients with severe OSAHS compared with no treatment or control oral appliances, but are less effective than CPAP treatment.

Oral appliance in non-severe OSAHS. A systematic review and RCTs found oral appliances that produce mandibular advancement reduced SDB, snoring and daytime sleepiness and improved general health status and quality of life when compared with no treatment or control oral appliance, but was less effective than CPAP treatment in people with non-severe OSAHS. Oral appliances reduced SDB more than uvulopalatopharyngoplasty, but both treatments improved daytime sleepiness and quality of life similarly.

Weight loss in OSAHS. Level 1 evidence for the effects of weight loss in people with severe OSAHS and non-severe OSAHS was not identified. No RCTs were found on the effects of weight loss in people with OSAHS.

Lifestyle modifications in OSAHS. A systematic review found insufficient evidence to support the use of lifestyle changes as a treatment for OSAHS.

Drug treatments in OSAHS. A systematic review found insufficient evidence to support the use of drugs as a treatment for OSAHS.

Surgery in OSAHS. A systematic review found insufficient evidence to support the use of surgery as a permanent cure for OSAHS.

Introduction

Obstructive sleep apnoea (OSA) is a recently recognized disorder of sleep in which there is periodic partial or complete cessation of breathing caused by upper airway obstruction. OSA is one form of sleep-disordered breathing (SDB) that causes recurrent arousals, sleep fragmentation and nocturnal hypoxaemia. These in turn lead to daytime sleepiness, impaired vigilance and cognitive functioning, reduced quality of life, increased risk of hypertension and difficulty with its control, together with the possibility of other cardiovascular disorders such as cardiac failure and stroke. OSA has been recognized clinically for more than 30 years.[1,2] The obstructive sleep apnoea–hypopnoea syndrome (OSAHS) is OSA together with its health impact, especially excessive daytime sleepiness. The terms associated with OSA, SDB and OSAHS are summarized in Table 1.

This chapter reviews the evidence for current treatments for OSAHS. Tracheostomy was the first effective treatment for OSAHS[3] and was used for very severe disease before less invasive alternatives became available. Currently, the most common treatment is nasal CPAP, which was first described for OSA about 25 years ago.[4] Other treatments include oral appliances, surgery, drugs and conservative treatments such as weight loss and lifestyle changes. The major objective of treatment is to reduce the symptoms of daytime sleepiness and improve vigilance and quality of life. Associated benefits would be reducing the increased risk of motor vehicle accidents and cardiovascular events. As with all other effective treatments, the aim is to achieve good compliance and have minimal adverse effects. This chapter concerns SDB caused by upper airway obstruction. Central sleep apnoea and sleep-associated hypoventilation syndromes are not considered. This chapter draws on much of the material published by the authors in *Clinical Evidence*.[5]

Diagnosis and severity of OSAHS

Criteria for the diagnosis of significant OSA have been set by consensus and convention.[6,7] An apnoea/hypopnoea index (AHI) of less than 5/hour is considered normal. Diagnostic

Table 1. Glossary of terms.

Term (abbreviation)	Definition
Apnoea (A)	Absence of airflow at the nose and mouth for at least 10 seconds. Sometimes defined indirectly in terms of oxygen desaturation index (impact on pulse oximetry saturation is measured as the number of occasions an hour when oxygen saturation falls by ≥4%). Apnoeas may be 'central', in which there is cessation of inspiratory effort, or 'obstructive', in which inspiratory efforts continue but are ineffective because of upper airway obstruction.
Apnoea/hypopnoea index (AHI)	The sum of apnoeas and hypopnoeas per hour of sleep determined by polysomnography, which measures sleep time and respiratory events. Although the generally accepted cut-off level for 'normal' is an AHI of <5 per hour, there are several definitions of 'normal', of which at least four are applicable to sleep-disordered breathing: levels that are inside the range in a 'normal' (i.e. healthy) population; levels that are well removed from those found in a target disorder such as OSAHS; levels that are not associated with a significant risk of disease/disability; levels for which there is no evidence of a significant benefit of treatment.[7]
Continuous positive airway pressure (CPAP)	Involves applying positive pressure from a blower motor to the upper airway through tubing and a soft nasal mask or a facemask. It provides a 'pneumatic splint' to the upper airway. Because nasal delivery is the most common in the published literature, we refer to 'nasal CPAP'.
Excessive daytime sleepiness (EDS)	Is a condition in which an individual has an overwhelming urge to fall asleep. People with EDS feel drowsy and tired and often nod or doze easily in relaxed or sedentary situations or fall asleep in situations where they need to be or want to be fully awake and alert. It can interfere with a person's ability to concentrate and perform daily tasks and routines. It can be measured objectively in a sleep laboratory with a Multiple Sleep Latency Test (MSLT) or a Maintenance of Wakefulness Test (MWT) or, subjectively, with questionnaires such as the Epworth Sleepiness Scale (ESS) or Stanford Sleepiness Scale.
Hypopnoea (H)	A major reduction (>50%) in airflow at the nose and mouth for at least 10 seconds. A smaller reduction in airflow may be accepted as hypopnoea if it is associated with either an arousal or a reduction in oxygen saturation of 4% or more.
Laser-assisted uvulopalatopharyngoplasty (LAUP)	Developed as an alternative procedure to UPPP that can be performed under a local anaesthetic. Vertical through-and-through troughs are created in the soft palate and the uvula is shortened.
Obstructive sleep apnoea–hypopnoea syndrome (OSAHS)	Is characterized by sleep-disordered breathing with an AHI ≥ 5 plus abnormal daytime function, especially excessive daytime sleepiness. In some instances, the 'syndrome' may include other outcomes such as poorly controlled cardiac failure or hypertension.
Oral appliance	The term 'oral appliance' is generic for devices that are placed in the mouth in order to change the position of the mandible, tongue and other structures in the upper airway to reduce the upper airway obstruction of OSAHS and snoring. Specific types are referred to as mandibular advancement devices or splints (MAD or MAS).
Respiratory disturbance index (RDI)	Often interchanged with AHI. However, RDI is a more general term that covers a range of methods used to measure sleep-disordered breathing, that is the rate of abnormal breathing events. The respiratory events include apnoeas and hypopnoeas but, in some cases, RERA. The events may be measured by non-supervised portable monitoring, oximetry or full polysomnography. Determinations of sleep time will vary between very accurate with polysomnography and an estimate (time in bed) with portable devices.
Respiratory effort-related arousal event (RERA)	Does not fit the criteria of an apnoea or a hypopnoea, but is a sequence of breaths requiring increasing respiratory effort, lasting at least 10 seconds, resulting in an arousal from sleep.
Sham/subtherapeutic nasal CPAP (sham CPAP)	This involves the use of the nasal mask and CPAP machine, but the pressure delivered to the upper airway is inadequate to overcome upper airway obstruction during sleep.

Continued

Term (abbreviation)	Definition
Sleep-disordered breathing (SDB)	Incorporates all abnormalities of breathing during sleep including obstructive and central apnoeas, REM-related hypoventilation and progressive hypoventilation. Other features of sleep-disordered breathing include snoring, witnessed episodes of absent breathing (apnoeas), abnormal breathing during sleep, nocturnal hypoxaemia and abnormal sleep architecture.
Upper airway resistance syndrome (UARS)	Measurement of inspiratory effort by oesophageal pressure shows recurrent episodes of increased inspiratory effort that maintain stable ventilation but are associated with arousals and sleep fragmentation. These episodes are also referred to as RERA events.[11] More recent techniques of measuring nasal airflow can show changes consistent with upper airway resistance syndrome without the need for an oesophageal pressure catheter.[73]
Uvulopalatopharyngoplasty (UPPP)	Surgical removal of the posterior portion of the uvula and palate and tonsillectomy under general anaesthetic.

criteria for the severity of OSA vary. For example, an AHI of 5–20 episodes/hour is often used to define borderline to mild OSA, 20–35 to define moderate and more than 35 severe OSA[8] (Table 2). However, people with upper airway resistance syndrome (UARS) (Table 1) have an index below five episodes/hour,[9] and many healthy elderly people have an index greater than five episodes/hour.[10]

The severity of OSAHS should be classified by reference to its major components: OSA and impaired daytime function, usually excessive daytime sleepiness. In an effort to obtain an international consensus, new criteria have been proposed and are becoming more widely used[11] (Tables 2 and 3).

Severe OSAHS is defined as severe OSA [respiratory disturbance index (RDI) > 35] plus symptoms of excessive daytime sleepiness (EDS). Measures of daytime function other than Table 3 may be used: for instance, an Epworth Sleepiness Scale (ESS) score of > 10 or a Multiple Sleep Latency Test (MSLT) of < 7 min. A very pragmatic test for clinically significant OSAHS is to show significant clinical improvement in daytime symptoms after treatment for OSA. This must allow for a placebo effect that has been shown with sham CPAP.

Incidence/prevalence

Epidemiological studies have demonstrated a range of prevalence of OSAHS in different populations (Tables 4 and 5). The Wisconsin Sleep Cohort Study of over 1000 people (mean age 47 years) in North America found a prevalence of AHI greater than five episodes/hour in 24% of men and 9% of women, and of OSAHS (AHI > 5 plus excessive sleepiness) in 4% of men and 2% of women.[12] There are international differences in the occurrence of OSAHS, for which obesity is considered to be an important determinant.[13] Ethnic differences in prevalence have also been found after adjustment for other risk factors.[10,13] Little is known about the burden of illness in developing countries.

Table 2. Classification of the severity of OSA.[11]

Severity of OSA	AHI or RDI
Mild	5–20
Moderate	20–35
Severe	>35

Aetiology/risk factors

The site of the upper airway obstruction in OSAHS is around the level of the tongue, soft palate or epiglottis. Disorders that predispose to either narrowing of the upper airway or reduction in its stability (e.g. obesity, certain craniofacial abnormalities, vocal cord abnormalities and enlarged tonsils) have been associated with an increased risk of OSAHS. Other strong associations include increasing age and sex (male to female ratio is 2 : 1). Weaker associations include menopause, family history, smoking and night-time nasal congestion.[13]

Prognosis

The long-term prognosis of people with untreated severe OSAHS is poor with respect to quality of life, likelihood of motor vehicle accidents, hypertension and, possibly, cardiovascular disease and premature mortality.[14] Unfortunately, the prognosis of both treated and untreated OSAHS is unclear.[10] A study of an historical cohort of patients with OSAHS demonstrated an increased mortality rate of patients not treated for OSAHS. Patients treated for OSAHS with diet, nasal CPAP or surgery had a similar mortality rate to the general population.[15] The limitations in the evidence include bias in the selection of participants, short duration of follow-up and variation in the measurement of potential confounders (e.g. smoking, alcohol use and other cardiovascular risk factors). As treatment is now widespread, it is very difficult to find

Table 3. Severity of impairment of daytime function.[11]

Severity of daytime sleepiness	Activities where unwanted sleepiness or involuntary sleep episodes occur	Effect of symptoms
Mild	Activities that require little attention, e.g. watching TV, reading	Only minor impairment of social or occupational function
Moderate	Activities that require some attention, e.g. attending concerts, meetings or presentations	Moderate impairment of social or occupational function
Severe	Activities that require more active attention, e.g. eating, during conversation, walking, driving	Marked impairment in social or occupational function

Table 4. Summary of epidemiological studies on the prevalence of OSAHS.

	N	Age (years)	Men	Women	Diagnosis of OSAHS
Wisconsin, USA[12]	1201	36–60	4%	2%	AHI > 5, EDS
San Diego, USA[74]	355	40–64	9%	5%	AHI > 15, O$_2$ sat 4%
Pennsylvania, USA[75]	1741	≥20	3.9%	1.2%	AHI ≥ 10, EDS
Vitoria-Gasteiz, Spain[76]	555	30–70	3.4%	3%	AHI ≥ 10, EDS

Table 5. Summary of epidemiological studies on the prevalence of OSA.

	N	Age (years)	Men	Women	OSA
Busselton, Australia[77]	400	40–85	10%	7%	RDI ≥ 10
Wisconsin, USA[12]	1201	36–60	9%	4%	AHI ≥ 15
Pennsylvania, USA[75]	1741	≥20	7%	2%	AHI ≥ 15
Newcastle, Australia[78]	2202	35–69	5%	1.2%	RDI ≥ 15

evidence on the prognosis of people with untreated OSAHS. Observational studies support a causal association between OSAHS and systemic hypertension, which increases with the severity of OSAHS [odds ratio (OR) 1.21 for mild OSAHS to 3.07 for severe OSAHS].[14] OSAHS increases the risk of motor vehicle accidents three- to sevenfold[14,16] and is associated with increased risk of premature mortality, cardiovascular disease and impaired neurocognitive functioning.[14]

Aims of intervention

Treatments for OSAHS evaluated in this chapter include CPAP, oral appliances, weight loss and lifestyle modifications, medications and surgery in people with severe and non-severe OSAHS. Successful therapy aims to minimize or eliminate symptoms of daytime sleepiness, to improve vigilance and quality of life, to reduce or abolish the increased risk of motor vehicle accidents and cardiovascular events, to enhance compliance with treatment and to minimize adverse effects of treatment.

In order to assess these aims, the effects of treatment were examined on the following outcomes: daytime sleepiness,

quality of life, psychological assessment, cognitive performance measures, mortality and morbidity and intermediate outcomes.

For daytime sleepiness, both subjective and objective measures were examined: for instance, the Epworth Sleepiness Scale, Multiple Sleep Latency Test (MSLT) and Maintenance of Wakefulness Test (MWT). General quality of life measures included the Medical Outcomes Study 36-item Short Form Health Survey and the General Health Questionnaire (GHQ). More specific measures included measurements of mood with the Hospital Anxiety and Depression Scale (HADS), the Beck Depression Inventory and the Profile of Mood States and measures of energy and vitality such as the 36-item Short Form energy scale, the UWIST Mood Adjective Checklist and the energy and vitality scale of the Nottingham Health Profile (NHP). Disease-specific quality of life measures included the Functional Outcomes of Sleep Questionnaire (FOSQ). Examples of cognitive performance tests are the Steer Clear, Trail-making Test B, Digit Symbol Substitution and Paced Auditory Serial Addition–2 Second Timing. Mortality and morbidity can be measured by road traffic accidents, hypertension, stroke, cardiac failure and ischaemic heart disease. Intermedi-

Table 6. Validated outcome measures.

Outcome measure (abbreviation)	Description	Scoring
Daytime sleepiness Epworth sleepiness scale (ESS)	Questionnaire developed to measure the general level of sleepiness, the likelihood of falling asleep in eight common situations. A lower score indicates less daytime sleepiness in the last week.	The score for each question ranges from 0 (no likelihood of falling asleep) to 3 (highly likely to fall asleep). Maximum score = 24. <10 is normal. >12 is pathological.
Multiple Sleep Latency Test (MSLT)	A daytime sleep laboratory-based test in which the subject is asked to try and fall asleep when placed in a quiet, dark room for 20 min at 2-hourly intervals. They are monitored electroencephalographically. The time between lights out and sleep onset (sleep latency) is measured in minutes. The mean value of 4–5 test sleeps in the day is calculated. The mean sleep latency is considered an 'objective' sleep measure of daytime sleepiness. A reduced score indicates a reduction in daytime sleepiness.	By convention: mean adult sleep latency of <5 min is indicative of pathological sleepiness. Mild 5–7 min. Borderline 8–9 min. Normal ≥10 min. However, MSLT does not discriminate well between clinical and control populations with 95% of values for control populations falling between 1.8 and 19 min.[79]
Maintenance of Wakefulness Test (MWT)	Similar to the MSLT, but the subject is asked to stay awake during the four trials of 40 minutes in the dark room.	By convention: sleep latencies of <20 min are indicative of pathological sleepiness but 95% of values for control populations fall between 8 and 40 min.[79]
Quality of life Medical Outcomes Survey Short form 36 (SF-36)	A short-form health survey that measures generic health-related quality of life. The instrument is used widely to evaluate health-related quality of life across various populations. It is a 36-item questionnaire encompassing eight health concepts which include: physical functioning; role limitations due to physical health problems; bodily pain; social functioning; general mental health; role limitations due to emotional problems; vitality, energy or fatigue; general health perceptions.	Variable scaling for different questions including: excellent, very good, good, fair, poor; limited a lot, limited a little, not limited at all; yes/no; not at all, slightly, moderately, quite a bit, extremely; none, very mild, mild, moderate, severe, very severe; all of the time, most of the time, a good bit of the time, some of the time, a little of the time, none of the time; and others. 36 items, most scored on a three- to six-point Likert scale with a higher score indicating better health-related quality of life.
General Health Questionnaire-28 (GHQ-28)	A self-administered screening test, designed to identify short-term changes in mental health. The most popular of the GHQ, it has 28 questions, seven in each subscale of depression, anxiety, social dysfunction and somatic symptoms.	Four subscores as well as a total score are obtained. The higher the score, the more severe the condition. A four-point scoring system ranges from a 'better/healthier than normal' option, through a 'same as usual' and a 'worse/more than usual' to a 'much worse/more than usual' option.
Nottingham Health Profile (NHP)	Generic health-related quality of life measure made up of 38 items that can be used to produce scores for six domains of health including: physical mobility (eight items), pain (eight items), social isolation (five items), emotional reactions (nine items), energy (three items), sleep (five items).	Each item is weighted; weights were derived from patients and non-patients. Dimension scores range from 0 to 100, the higher the score the greater the health problem. Scores are presented as a profile rather than an overall score. Mean score is calculated across all items within each domain. Overall score is the mean across all items.

Continued

Outcome measure (abbreviation)	Description	Scoring
Functional Outcomes of Sleep Questionnaire (FOSQ)	A sleep-specific functional measure designed to evaluate the impact of sleep disorders and excessive sleepiness on physical, mental and social functioning in everyday activities. Thirty items represent five subscales: activity level; vigilance; intimacy and sexual relationships; general productivity; and social outcome.	Mean-weighted item score for each subscale; subscale scores are totalled to produce a global score. The lower the score, the greater dysfunction as a result of sleepiness. Four levels of response are possible: no difficulty; a little; moderate; or extreme plus non-participation.
Psychological assessment Hospital Anxiety and Depression scale (HAD)	A 14-item questionnaire designed to identify clinical depression and anxiety. Seven items conceptually assess depression and seven items were derived from psychic manifestations of anxiety neurosis.	Overall level of severity of each mood on a four-point scale (0–3). A score of 8 is significant, a score of 11 or more highly significant
Beck Depression Inventory (BDI)	A measurement of clinical depression with 21 statements regarding a symptom associated with depression (e.g. appetite, mood, sense of failure).	Scores range from 0, indicating the absence of the particular symptom, to 3 for most severe.
Profile of Mood States (POMS)	A self-report designed to measure six dimensions of mood which include: tension–anxiety; depression–dejection; anger–hostility; vigour–activity; fatigue–inertia; and confusion–bewilderment. It consists of 65 short phrases describing feeling and mood with respondents asked to indicate mood reactions for the 'past week including today' or for shorter periods such as 'right now'.	A five-point Likert-type scale ranging from 0 for not at all to 4 indicating extremely.
University of Wales Institute of Science and Technology (UWIST) Mood Adaptive Checklist (UMACL)	A measurement of mood with four subscales: hedonic tone; anger; tense arousal; and energetic arousal. Except for anger, which only has positively loaded items, each one is made up of a combination of positively loaded and negatively loaded items.	The final score is the result of adding the positively loaded answers and subtracting the negatively loaded answers.
Cognitive performance measures SteerClear (SC)	A computer-based program designed to simulate a long, mundane highway drive and to characterize the decrements in driving ability. The subject is required to avoid obstacles that appear randomly on a two-lane highway by pressing a single computer key. Performance on this 30-min task is reflected by the number of obstacles passed and the number hit.	Reducing the number of obstacles hit reflects improved vigilance.
Trailmaking B tests (TTB)	A test for broad cognitive performance that utilizes the connect-a-dot concept requiring the subject to draw lines from circle to circle to link numbers and letters (TTB) consecutively in the quickest time possible.	Better cognitive performance is indicated by a reduction in score, which reflects the time taken to complete the task.
Digit Symbol Substitution (DSS)	Cognitive speed is tested by the subject matching individually presented symbols to their numbers using a reference key.	Improved speed of performance is reflected by an increased score.
Paced Auditory Serial Addition Task – 2-second timing (PASAT-2)	A test of auditory attention and concentration by evaluating how rapidly consecutive numbers presented every 2 seconds can be added.	An increase in the score indicates improved ability to maintain concentration under distraction.

ate outcomes include measures of the degree of sleep-disordered breathing and breathing-disordered sleep, such as the AHI, the frequency of arousals and the degree of sleep fragmentation. Some details of validated outcome measures for daytime sleepiness, quality of life, psychological and cognitive performance are listed in Table 6.[17–29]

Relevant studies were identified by a search of electronic databases (August 2003) and ongoing additional hand searches by the author. The majority of references were identified as part of the search process of *Clinical Evidence*.[5] An important issue is the heterogeneity of studies, including different definitions of OSAHS. An attempt has been made to provide some details of the definitions used.

Treatment of OSAHS

Question: What is the effect of nasal CPAP in severe and non-severe OSAHS?

With the increasing interest in the treatment of OSAHS over the past few years, many studies have been published that investigate the effect of nasal CPAP on OSAHS. The information has been consolidated in a number of systematic reviews[8,30–32] (Table 7). Each of these systematic reviews has included at least 11 studies with four studies being included in all four reviews. One review[30] of 26 studies was a qualitative review. The studies included in the systematic reviews used various controls for comparison with CPAP including: no treatment; sham/subtherapeutic CPAP; oral appliances; oral placebo tablets; and

conservative treatment or lifestyle changes including sleep hygiene and weight loss. Sham CPAP is the only comparison where the patients may be blinded to the treatment they are receiving.

In patients with severe OSAHS, nasal CPAP has a beneficial effect on both subjective and objective measures of daytime sleepiness. Two reviews separated the studies with respect to the severity of the OSAHS,[8,31] one with two studies[33,34] and the other with six studies.[34–39] They found that CPAP treatment reduced ESS score in patients with severe OSAHS. However, no significant improvement in daytime sleepiness was observed in patients with non-severe OSAHS (Fig. 1). Similarly, using objective measures of daytime sleepiness, MSLT and MWT, CPAP significantly improved daytime sleepiness in patients with severe OSAHS, but not in patients with non-severe OSAHS (Fig. 2).

Small significant improvements were found in the quality of life outcomes and mood indicators (NHP part 2, GHQ-28),[40–42] whereas there were large improvements in health status when considering SF-36[36,42] domains of vitality, physical role, bodily pain and mental health (Fig. 3).

The final systematic review[30] (search date June 1999) is a qualitative systematic review of 26 prospective studies. Analysis of the seven randomized controlled trials (RCTs)[34–36,40–43] found that CPAP has a significant beneficial effect on subjective sleepiness and depression. When all studies were considered, fatigue, generic health-related quality of life, vigilance and driving performance are all improved by CPAP treatment. These improvements may be sensitive to the duration of treatment and compliance.

The RCTs have problems with their methods and with

Table 7. Summary of systematic reviews.

Systematic review	Dates for search	Number of studies	Comparison and conditions	Outcomes
NHMRC of Australia[8]	Up to 1999	11 (all RCTs)	CPAP treatment for >4 weeks versus minimal or no CPAP RCTs	Patient preference Daytime sleepiness Cognitive performance Quality of life Symptoms
McMahon[30]	Up to June 1999	26 (7 RCTs)	CPAP treatment Prospective studies	Neurobehavioural outcomes Quality of life Daytime sleepiness
Patel[31]	Jan 1966 to October 2001	12 (all RCTs)	CPAP treatment and daytime sleepiness measures	Daytime sleepiness
White[32]	1966 to December 2000	12 (all RCTs)	CPAP treatment versus placebo or other treatments	Daytime sleepiness Quality of life Cognitive performance

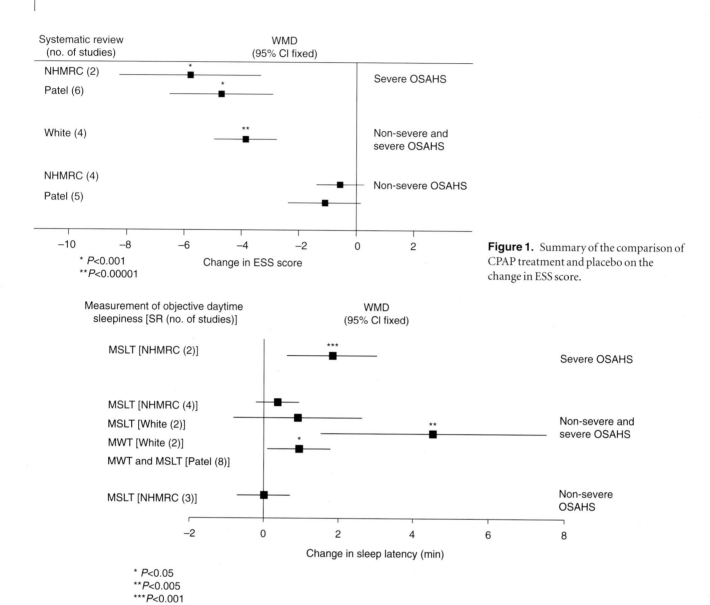

Figure 1. Summary of the comparison of CPAP treatment and placebo on the change in ESS score.

Figure 2. Summary of the comparison of CPAP and placebo on the change in sleep latency (min).

applicability of results. First, severity of OSA (using AHI, etc.) is not a good guide to severity of daytime sleepiness, which is a major symptom. For instance, one RCT[44] demonstrated no benefit of CPAP treatment in patients with severe OSA but with no daytime sleepiness. Secondly, it is not clear whether the sham or subtherapeutic CPAP used in some 'placebo' groups is a truly inactive treatment. Thirdly, RCT evidence reports short-term symptomatic outcomes only, rather than longer term complications, such as mortality, motor vehicle accident rate, hypertension, stroke and ischaemic heart disease. Finally, there is repeated evidence of a significant placebo effect in the treatment of OSAHS for both OSA and daytime sleepiness outcomes.[45]

More recent clinical trials support the evidence from the systematic reviews about the effectiveness of CPAP using a range of outcome measures (Table 8).

Simulated driving performance measures have been shown to be improved significantly after 1 month of CPAP treatment.[46] These improvements in vigilance in patients with severe OSAHS support the hypothesis that untreated OSAHS may increase the rate of motor vehicle accidents.

CPAP therapy has also been found to be more effective when compared with a conservative lifestyle strategy in OSAHS.[47] Lifestyle intervention included educating the patient on strategies for sleep hygiene, quitting smoking, reducing alcohol consumption and controlling stress in addition to advice on achieving an ideal body weight with exercise and diet. The study (71 patients, AHI 49 ± 28) showed that, after 3 months of CPAP therapy, AHI and ESS were reduced more compared with lifestyle changes. CPAP treatment reduced AHI from 55 ± 28.7 to 8 ± 28 ($P < 0.001$) and ESS from 16 ± 5.6 to 8 ± 6.4 ($P < 0.001$), whereas AHI was unchanged (35 ± 19.1

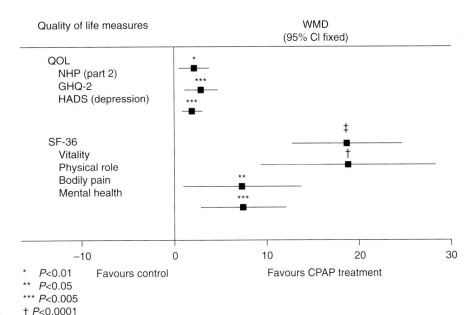

Figure 3. The effect of CPAP treatment on quality of life measures in patients with severe OSAHS.

* $P<0.01$
** $P<0.05$
*** $P<0.005$
† $P<0.0001$
‡ $P<0.00001$

Table 8. Clinical trials examining the effectiveness of nasal CPAP on a range of outcome measures.

Study	N	ESS	AHI	Control	Outcomes	
Hack[46]	59 men	>10		Sham nasal CPAP	Daytime sleepiness Simulated driving performance	Improved driving performance
Chakravorty[47]				Conservative therapy	Quality of life AHI ESS	Improved quality of life
Kaneko[48]	32			Medical therapy	Heart failure Blood pressure	Improved left ventricular function

to 34 ± 21, NS) and ESS reduced from 14 ± 4.2 to 11 ± 5 ($P < 0.05$) after changes in lifestyle. There was a 23% improvement in general health status of patients receiving CPAP compared with a 4% improvement with lifestyle changes. The study estimated that there was an increase of 8.2 quality of life years (QALYs) with CPAP therapy compared with 4.7 QALYs with lifestyle changes.

Kaneko and co-workers[48] examined the effects of CPAP on patients with mild to moderate symptoms of heart failure and OSAHS. The control group of patients received only medical therapy, while the experimental group received CPAP treatment for 1 month as well as medical therapy. Twenty-four patients with a depressed left ventricular ejection fraction (45% or less) were studied with 12 patients in each group. Medical treatment alone did not significantly change the severity of OSAHS, daytime blood pressure, heart rate, left ventricular end-systolic dimension or left ventricular ejection fraction. With the addition of CPAP treatment, AHI was reduced from 37.1 ± 6.4 to 8.3 ± 2.8 ($P < 0.001$). The changes in left ventricular ejection fraction (8.8 ± 1.6% versus 1.5 ± 2.3%, $P = 0.009$) and left ventricular end-systolic dimension (–2.8 ± 1.1 versus 0.7 ± 0.8mm, $P = 0.02$) were significantly greater in the group having CPAP treatment. In association with these improvements in systolic function were a decrease in systolic pressure (126 ± 6 to 116 ± 5, $P = 0.008$ between groups) and a decrease in heart rate (68 ± 3 to 64 ± 3, $P = 0.09$ between groups). Kaneko et al.[48] suggested that the cardiovascular effects are primarily due to the alleviation of OSA.

Although there appears to be little improvement in objective or subjective daytime sleepiness (Figs 1 and 2), significant improvement in two other measures of cognitive performance [Trailmaking Test B[41,42,49] $P = 0.003$ and Paced Auditory Serial Addition–2 Second Timing[41,42] $P < 0.0001$; confidence interval (CI) not reported] have been reported. In addition, no significant difference between nasal CPAP and oral placebo tablets for quality of life (SF-36 general perception[42,49]) and anxiety measures (HADS[41,42]) have been demonstrated, but there is significant improvement in depression (HADS,[41,42] Beck Depression Inventory[43]) and energy and vitality (SF-36 vitality,[42,49] UWIST Mood Adjective Checklist Energetic Arousal Score;[41] combined $P = 0.13$, energy/fatigue subscore of MOD[43] $P < 0.05$). The three RCTs that reported a symptom score (in-house questionnaires using an analogue scale) showed significant benefit of CPAP over placebo (combined $P = 0.006$).[41,42,49] However, these were all crossover trials and need to be considered with care.

People with non-severe OSAHS find nasal CPAP less acceptable. For instance, people with an AHI below 15/hour have been found to have half the long-term use of nasal CPAP compared with people with an AHI greater than 15/hour.[50] One RCT showed that adherence by people with mild OSAHS was moderately high (4.8 hours/day),[51] and treatment acceptance was also good to reasonable (62% of people who finished the trial chose to continue CPAP).

Adverse effects

The systematic reviews did not summarize any harmful effects found in the RCTs that were reviewed.[8,30–32] One systematic review reported a high prevalence of minor adverse effects from nasal CPAP treatment, the most common being dry mouth, nose and throat (40%).[8] We found one case series (52 consecutive people with severe OSAHS, mean oxygen desaturation index 43/hour), in which the occurrence of nasopharyngeal symptoms was studied systematically before and after nasal CPAP.[52] It found that nasopharyngeal symptoms were common before nasal CPAP in OSAHS (nasal dryness 74%, sneezing 51%, blocked nose 43% and rhinorrhoea 37%) with greater discomfort in winter. Other adverse effects of nasal CPAP include local effects of the mask on the nasal bridge, mask discomfort, nasal congestion, rhinitis, sore eyes, headache, chest discomfort and noise disturbance. Adoption of and adherence to CPAP treatment is a widely acknowledged problem but less so in patients with more severe OSAHS. One RCT in non-severe OSAHS[53] found that 95% of the patients undergoing CPAP treatment had at least one side-effect, but none was serious. The side-effects were divided into five categories: (a) nasal, which included dryness, congestion, bleeding and/or sinusitis; (b) sleep including delayed sleep and/or subjective sleep fragmentation; (c) inconvenience including noise and/or spouse objection; (d) air mechanics including aerophagia, chest wall discomfort and/or mouth breathing; and (e) skin and eye problems.

Summary

In people with severe OSAHS, CPAP reduces daytime sleepiness, improves health status, reduces depression and possibly improves blood pressure and driving performance compared with placebo, no treatment, sham or subtherapeutic nasal CPAP or conservative treatment.

In people with non-severe OSAHS, CPAP treatment does not improve daytime sleepiness when compared with conservative treatment, sham or subtherapeutic CPAP or placebo tablets, but there do appear to be some benefits on some measures of cognitive performance, functional outcomes, symptoms, energy and vitality and depression.

Question: What is the effect of oral appliances in severe and non-severe OSAHS?

Although CPAP treatment is the 'gold standard' treatment for the relief of the upper airway obstruction of OSA, many patients are not willing to or cannot tolerate the treatment. A more acceptable alternative treatment is the oral appliance. There are a variety of oral appliances with a similar basic function to advance the mandible or tongue, thereby increasing the oropharyngeal space and improving airflow. They are often referred to as mandibular advancement devices (MAD) or splints (MAS). Two recent systematic reviews have examined the effectiveness of MADs[32,54] (Table 9). Many of the studies examined in these reviews did not stratify the patients for severity of OSAHS. However, White et al.[32] examined studies in which the effect of MADs was compared with CPAP treatment in patients with non-severe OSAHS. Despite CPAP being more effective than oral appliances in the management of OSAHS, overall, the review found that people preferred an oral appliance over nasal CPAP [odds ratio (OR) 9.5, 95% CI

Table 9 . Systematic reviews examining the effectiveness of mandibular advancement devices.

Systematic review	Dates for search	Number of RCTs	Comparison	Outcome
White[32]	1966 to December 2000	3	CPAP versus MAD	Daytime sleepiness
Lim[54]	1966 to July 2003	12	Inactive MAD (4 RCTs) CPAP (7 RCTs) Surgery (1 RCT)	Daytime sleepiness Symptoms Quality of life Cognitive performance

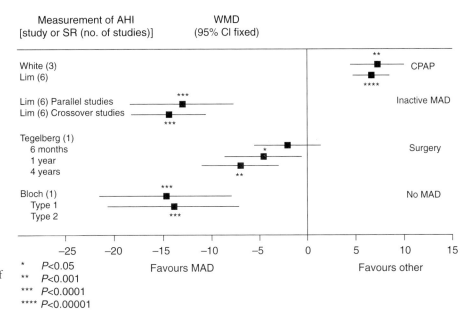

Figure 4. Summary of the comparison of the effect of MAD and other treatments on AHI.

* $P<0.05$
** $P<0.001$
*** $P<0.0001$
**** $P<0.00001$

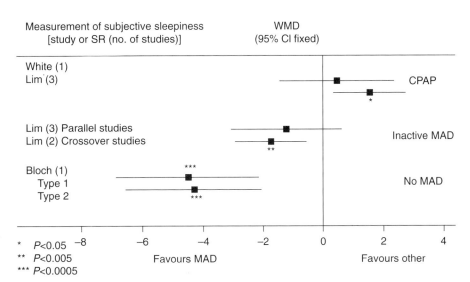

Figure 5. Summary of the comparison of the effect of MAD and other treatments on daytime sleepiness.

* $P<0.05$
** $P<0.005$
*** $P<0.0005$

4.3–21.1]. The one study that measured subjective sleepiness[55] found that both treatments improved ESS equally. The effect of MAD on AHI when compared with CPAP treatment, surgery, an inactive MAD or no appliance is summarized in Figure 4.

When compared with an inactive MAD, surgery or no MAD, MAD reduced AHI significantly. While MAD and surgery have a similar effect on AHI in the first 6 months after surgery, after 12 months, MAD significantly improved the AHI compared with uvulopalatopharyngoplasty (78% improved with oral appliance versus 51% improved with uvulopalatopharyngoplasty; $P < 0.05$). This difference in effectiveness was maintained 4 years after surgery.[56] Associated with these changes in AHI by MAD are improvements in daytime sleepiness when compared with inactive or no MAD. MAD and uvulopalatopharyngoplasty significantly improved qual-

ity of life dimensions of vitality and sleep similarly, but the uvulopalatopharyngoplasty group had a better contentment score (Fig. 5).

In addition, MAD significantly reduced interference with daily tasks, snoring frequency and loudness, and improved performance ability and energy level compared with no treatment.[57]

Adverse effects

One small series (22 people involved in the RCT) investigated adverse effects of oral appliances over 12–30 months.[58] It found that adverse effects were common (mucosal dryness 86%, tooth discomfort 59% and hypersalivation 55%) but did not require discontinuation of treatment. Johnston *et al.*[59] found that the most commonly reported complication was excessive salivation.

The RCTs on oral appliances have generally been too brief to evaluate clinically important adverse effects.

Comment

Oral appliances are commonly used for snoring with or without mild sleep apnoea. We found one systematic review that used all studies[60] (search date 1994, 304 people with mean AHI in the severe range, 21 publications, 19 case series), which found that about 70% of people had a 50% or greater reduction in AHI. There is insufficient evidence about long-term effectiveness and adverse effects. One RCT (24 people, crossover design), which compared an oral appliance with a small bite opening (4 mm) versus one with a larger opening (14 mm), found no significant difference in OSA or ESS.[61]

Summary

Oral appliances that produce mandibular advancement reduce OSA and daytime sleepiness in some patients with OSAHS but are less effective than CPAP treatment. The beneficial effects have been seen in non-severe OSAHS. In people with non-severe OSAHS, there may also be improvements in general health status and quality of life. Oral appliances reduced OSA more than uvulopalatopharyngoplasty, but both treatments improved daytime sleepiness and quality of life similarly.

Question: What is the effect of weight loss in OSAHS?

An increased risk of OSAHS has been associated with disorders that predispose to either narrowing of the upper airway or reduction in its stability, of which obesity is a prime example. Young and Peppard[13] estimated that a 30% increase (95% CI 13–50%) in the relative risk of developing abnormal sleep-disordered breathing (AHI $\geq$ 5/hour) over a period of 4 years could be triggered by a $1\,kg/m^2$ increase in body mass index (3.2 kg for a person 1.8 m tall). However, a systematic review (search date 2000) identified no RCTs on the effect of weight loss in people with OSAHS.[62]

One large population-based cohort study (690 people with OSA, including those who did not qualify for diagnosis of OSAHS) that evaluated OSA at 4-year intervals over 10 years[63] found an association between changes in weight and AHI. A weight gain of 10% was associated with an increase in AHI of 32% (95% CI 20–45%), and a weight loss of 10% was associated with a decrease in AHI of 26% (95% CI 18–34%).

One review reported a case series in which weight loss, especially that achieved by surgery, was associated with improvement, mainly in people with severe OSAHS.[64] Large relative improvements in AHI (−72% to −98%) were found after a weight loss of 30–70% of initial weight. It seems that weight loss has the potential to benefit obese persons with OSAHS. There is consensus that advice about weight reduction is an important component of management. However, weight loss is difficult, and advice may need to be combined with nasal CPAP in people with severe OSAHS.

Summary

We found no RCTs on the effect of weight loss in people with OSAHS.

Question: What is the effect of other lifestyle modifications in OSAHS?

Besides weight loss, other lifestyle modifications, such as exercise and sleep hygiene, are often recommended to patients with OSAHS. Exercise has been recommended to lose weight, but may also change sleep structure. Sleep hygiene includes measures to improve the sleep environment such as having a warm comfortable bed, with the bedroom dark and quiet, avoiding caffeine and other stimulants in the evenings as well as improving the sleep/wake patterns by not having naps during the day. From a recent review on the effect of lifestyle modification on OSA, there appears to be no evidence to substantiate the concept that the strategies for improving sleep hygiene or exercise can prevent or reduce the symptoms of OSA.[62]

Summary

We found no RCTs on the effect of lifestyle modifications in people with OSAHS.

Question: What is the effect of medications in OSAHS?

Another treatment suggested for OSAHS is drug therapy. A recent review did not find any evidence to support the use of drugs as a therapy for OSA.[65] Drugs that have been tested include acetazolamide, protryptyline, medroxyprogesterone, clonidine, busipirone, aminophylline, theophylline and sabeluzole. Only acetazolamide reduced AHI, but was poorly tolerated and did not reduce symptoms. In contrast, protryptyline improved symptoms but had no effect on AHI. The authors of the review considered that, even though many of the studies were small and had methodological limitations, there was little justification in undergoing further trials of these particular drugs. A recent study demonstrated that physostigmine reduced AHI during both rapid eye movement (REM) and non-REM sleep as well as increasing the minimum oxygen saturation. However, as the administration of physostigmine was by continuous overnight infusion, its clinical relevance is questionable.[66]

Summary

We found no evidence to support the use of drugs for the treatment of OSAHS.

Question: What is the effect of surgery in OSAHS?

A major reason for the enthusiasm for surgery is the possibility of a cure: the daily use of a CPAP or a MAD is a major burden for patients and their families. The principal surgical procedures that have been used in OSAHS include tracheostomy, uvulopalatopharyngoplasty (UPPP), laser-assisted uvulopalatoplasty (LAUP), a modified version of UPPP, temperature-controlled radiofrequency tissue ablation (TCRFTA), often referred to by its trade name of Somnoplasty, and maxillofacial surgery. The two most common surgical procedures are UPPP and LAUP, with TCRFTA, a recent innovation in surgery, becoming more widely used.

UPPP is a procedure used to remove excess tissue at the back of the throat including the tonsils, uvula and parts of the soft palate under a general anaesthetic. The width of the airway at the throat opening is increased, but obstructions at the base of the tongue are not addressed. Its effectiveness as a cure for OSAHS lacks good trial-based evidence.[67] Adverse effects include pain, bleeding, risk of infection, changes in voice frequency and decreased efficacy of CPAP after UPPP.

Kamami[68] developed LAUP as a modification of UPPP, replacing the scalpel with a CO_2 laser. It is a simpler surgical procedure, which is performed under local anaesthetic reducing far less palatal tissue and does not alter the tonsils or the pharyngeal pillars. No wound closure or postoperative stay are required. Although surgery has been widely used for snoring and OSAHS, only recently has there been a controlled study of the effectiveness of LAUP[69] in patients with non-severe OSAHS. This study found that side-effects were common within the first week of treatment and included sore throat, difficulty swallowing, bleeding, change in vocal quality, nasal regurgitation and infection. Less than 25% of the patients were considered to be treated successfully with surgery that achieved an AHI of less than 10/hour. More success was achieved with the improvement in snoring; however, this was still less than 50% of the patients. Their conclusion was that LAUP may be effective in some patients with non-severe OSA for the treatment of snoring, but there was minimal improvement in the reduction of AHI and symptoms. This confirms the summary findings of the American Academy of Sleep Medicine, who reviewed the literature in 2000 and concluded that LAUP should not be recommended as a substitute for UPPP or as a treatment of OSAHS; it is comparable to UPPP in relieving subjective snoring.[70] It has been suggested that LAUP may even lead to a worsening of OSA.[71]

Another relatively new surgical procedure for OSA is TCRFTA. It is also one typically done in the doctor's office. It is used to shrink the size of the tongue and/or palate with radiofrequency energy. As with LAUP, multiple treatments are often necessary. Preliminary results from a study comparing LAUP with TCRFTA found that the latter produced less pain for a shorter period.[72] A recent study[53] (90 patients, AHI 10–30, age 18–65 years) compared the effectiveness of this surgery with CPAP and a placebo of sham surgery on patients with non-severe OSAHS (AHI 5–40). Both CPAP treatment and TCFRTA improved FOSQ (1.5 ± 2.1, $P < 0.02$ and 1.2 ± 1.6, $P < 0.005$), Symptoms of Nocturnal Obstruction and Related Events Questionnaire (–3.0 ± 0.52, $P < 0.005$ and –0.43 ± 0.56, $P < 0.001$) and ESS (–2.3 ± 5.2, $P < 0.02$ and –2.1 ± 3.9, $P < 0.005$). However, TCRFTA also reduced reaction times using the Psychomotor Vigilance Task; the reciprocal of slowest reaction time (0.32 ± 0.57, $P < 0.006$), reaction time (–10.0 ± 19.5, $P < 0.03$) and fastest reaction time (–10.2 ± 21.9, $P < 0.02$). Outcomes were comparable between TCRFTA and CPAP groups with no significant differences between treatments. When compared with sham surgery, only the effect on FOSQ was significantly increased (1.2, 5% CI 0.1–2.3, $P < 0.02$) by CPAP treatment. Only 38% of patients on CPAP treatment were considered to be using it adequately. Pain and swallowing difficulty were evident in patients undergoing surgery and sham surgery at 1 week after the procedures; however, both returned to normal 3 weeks after surgery. These authors suggest that TCRFTA may have an important role as an alternative treatment of OSAHS in patients who cannot tolerate CPAP. However, long-term effectiveness was not determined as only an 8-week follow-up was undertaken.

Summary

No evidence was found to support the use of surgery as a permanent cure for OSAHS.

Conflict of interest statement

MJH is chief investigator of a multicentre research study funded by the NHMRC of Australia that has an untied research grant from ResMed consisting of the loan of equipment valued at $A40 000 and direct costs of $A50 000. Masimo has loaned oximetry equipment for the same study valued at $A60 000.

References

1 Gastaut H, Tassinari CA, Duron B. Polygraphic study of the episodic diurnal and nocturnal (hypnic and respiratory) manifestations of the Pickwick syndrome. *Brain Res* 1966; **1**:167–86.
2 Bassari AG, Guilleminault C. Clinical features and evaluation of obstructive sleep apnea hypopnea syndrome. In: Kryger MH,

Roth T, Dement WC, eds. *Principles and Practice of Sleep Medicine.* Philadelphia, PA, WB Saunders, 2000:869–78.

3 He J, Kryger MH, Zorick FJ, Conway W, Roth T. Mortality and apnea index in obstructive sleep apnea. Experience in 385 male patients. *Chest* 1988; **94**:9–14.

4 Sullivan CE, Issa FG, Berthon-Jones M, Eves L. Reversal of obstructive sleep apnoea by continuous positive airway pressure applied through the nares. *Lancet* 1981; **1**:862–5.

5 Hensley M, Ray C. Sleep apnoea. *Clin Evid* 2003; **10**:1958–74.

6 Ross SD, Sheinhait IA, Harrison KJ *et al.* Systematic review and meta-analysis of the literature regarding the diagnosis of sleep apnea. *Sleep* 2000; **23**:519–32.

7 Strauss SE, Richardson WS, Glasziou P, Haynes RB. *Evidence Based Medicine: How to Practice and Teach EBM*, 3rd edn. Edinburgh, Churchill Livingstone, 2005:69–70.

8 National Health and Medical Research Council of Australia. *Effectiveness of Nasal Continuous Positive Airway Pressure (nCPAP) in Obstructive Sleep Apnoea in Adults.* Canberra, Australia, NHMRC, 2000.

9 Guilleminault C, Stoohs R, Clerk A, Cetel M, Maistros P. A cause of excessive daytime sleepiness. The upper airway resistance syndrome. *Chest* 1993; **104**:781–7.

10 Lindberg E, Gislason T. Clinical review article: epidemiology of sleep-related obstructive breathing. *Sleep Med Rev* 2000; **4**:411–33.

11 American Academy of Sleep Medicine Task Force. Sleep-related breathing disorders in adults: recommendations for syndrome definition and measurement techniques in clinical research. The Report of an American Academy of Sleep Medicine Task Force. *Sleep* 1999; **22**:667–89.

12 Young T, Palta M, Dempsey J, Skatrud J, Weber S, Badr S. The occurrence of sleep-disordered breathing among middle-aged adults. *N Engl J Med* 1993; **328**:1230–5.

13 Young TB, Peppard P. Epidemiology of obstructive sleep apnea. In: McNicholas WT, Phillipson EA, eds. *Breathing Disorders in Sleep.* London, WB Saunders, 2002:31–43.

14 Redline S. Morbidity, mortality and public health burden of sleep apnea. In: McNicholas WT, Phillipson EA, eds. *Breathing Disorders in Sleep.* London, WB Saunders, 2002:222–35.

15 Marti S, Sampol G, Munoz X *et al.* Mortality in severe sleep apnoea/hypopnoea syndrome patients: impact of treatment. *Eur Respir J* 2002; **20**:1511–18.

16 George CF. Reduction in motor vehicle collisions following treatment of sleep apnoea with nasal CPAP. *Thorax* 2001; **56**: 508–12.

17 Quality of Life Resource. American Thoracic Society: www.atsqol.org.

18 Beck AT, Ward CH, Mendelson M *et al.* An inventory for measuring depression. *Arch Gen Psychiatr* 1961; **4**:561–71.

19 McNair D, Lorr M, Droppleman L. *EITS Manual for the Profile of Mood States.* San Diego, Educational and Industrial Test Services, 1971.

20 Zigmond AS, Snaith RP. The hospital anxiety and depression scale. *Acta Psychiatr Scand* 1983; **67**:361–70.

21 Hunt SM, McEwen J, McKenna SP. Measuring health status: a new tool for clinicians and epidemiologists. *J Roy Coll Gen Pract* 1985; **35**:185–8.

22 Carskadon MA, Dement WC, Mitler MM, Roth T, Westbrook PR, Keenan S. Guidelines for the Multiple Sleep Latency Test (MSLT): a standard measure of sleepiness. *Sleep* 1986; **9**:519–24.

23 Findley LJ, Fabrizio MJ, Knight H, Norcross BB, LaForte AJ, Suratt PM. Driving simulator performance in patients with sleep apnea. *Am Rev Respir Dis* 1989; **140**:529–30.

24 Matthews G, Jones DM, Chamberlain AG. Refining the measurement of mood: the UWIST Mood Adjective Checklist. *Br J Psychol* 1990; **81**:17.

25 Johns MW. A new method for measuring daytime sleepiness: the Epworth sleepiness scale. *Sleep* 1991; **14**:540–5.

26 Poceta JS, Timms RM, Jeong DU, Ho SL, Erman MK, Mitler MM. Maintenance of wakefulness test in obstructive sleep apnea syndrome. *Chest* 1992; **101**:893–7.

27 Ware JE Jr, Sherbourne CD. The MOS 36-item short-form health survey (SF-36). I. Conceptual framework and item selection. *Med Care* 1992; **30**:473–83.

28 Weaver TE, Laizner AM, Evans LK *et al.* An instrument to measure functional status outcomes for disorders of excessive sleepiness. *Sleep* 1997; **20**:835–43.

29 Weaver TE. Outcome measurement in sleep medicine practice and research. Part 2: assessment of neurobehavioral performance and mood. *Sleep Med Rev* 2001; **5**:223–36.

30 McMahon JP, Foresman BH, Chisholm RC. The influence of CPAP on the neurobehavioral performance of patients with obstructive sleep apnea hypopnea syndrome: a systematic review. *Wisconsin Med J* 2003; **102**:36–43.

31 Patel SR, White DP, Malhotra A, Stanchina ML, Ayas NT. Continuous positive airway pressure therapy for treating sleepiness in a diverse population with obstructive sleep apnea: results of a meta-analysis. *Arch Intern Med* 2003; **163**:565–71.

32 White J, Cates C, Wright J. Continuous positive airways pressure for obstructive sleep apnoea (Cochrane Review). In: *The Cochrane Library.* Chichester, John Wiley & Sons, 2003.

33 Douglas NJ. Systematic review of the efficacy of nasal CPAP (comment). *Thorax* 1998; **53**:414–15.

34 Ballester E, Badia JR, Hernandez L *et al.* Evidence of the effectiveness of continuous positive airway pressure in the treatment of sleep apnea/hypopnea syndrome (erratum appears in *Am J Respir Crit Care Med* 1999; **159**(5 Pt 1):1688). *Am J Respir Crit Care Med* 1999; **159**:495–501.

35 Engleman HM, Martin SE, Kingshott RN, Mackay TW, Deary IJ, Douglas NJ. Randomised placebo controlled trial of daytime function after continuous positive airway pressure (CPAP) therapy for the sleep apnoea/hypopnoea syndrome. *Thorax* 1998; **53**:341–5.

36 Jenkinson C, Davies RJ, Mullins R, Stradling JR. Comparison of therapeutic and subtherapeutic nasal continuous positive airway pressure for obstructive sleep apnoea: a randomised prospective parallel trial. *Lancet* 1999; **353**:2100–5.

37 Faccenda JF, Mackay TW, Boon NA, Douglas NJ. Randomized placebo-controlled trial of continuous positive airway pressure on blood pressure in the sleep apnea–hypopnea syndrome. *Am J Respir Crit Care Med* 2001; **163**:344–8.

38 Henke KG, Grady JJ, Kuna ST. Effect of nasal continuous positive airway pressure on neuropsychological function in sleep apnea–hypopnea syndrome. A randomized, placebo-controlled trial. *Am J Respir Crit Care Med* 2001; **163**:911–17.

39 Montserrat JM, Ferrer M, Hernandez L *et al.* Effectiveness of CPAP treatment in daytime function in sleep apnea syndrome: a randomized controlled study with an optimized placebo. *Am J Respir Crit Care Med* 2001; **164**:608–13.

40 Engleman HM, Martin SE, Deary IJ, Douglas NJ. Effect of continuous positive airway pressure treatment on daytime function in sleep apnoea/hypopnoea syndrome. *Lancet* 1994; **343**:572–5.

41 Engleman HM, Martin SE, Deary IJ, Douglas NJ. Effect of CPAP therapy on daytime function in patients with mild sleep apnoea/hypopnoea syndrome. *Thorax* 1997; **52**:114–19.

42 Engleman HM, Kingshott RN, Wraith PK, Mackay TW, Deary IJ, Douglas NJ. Randomized placebo-controlled crossover trial of continuous positive airway pressure for mild sleep apnea/hypopnea syndrome. *Am J Respir Crit Care Med* 1999; **159**:461–7.

43 Redline S, Adams N, Strauss ME, Roebuck T, Winters M, Rosenberg C. Improvement of mild sleep-disordered breathing with CPAP

compared with conservative therapy. *Am J Respir Crit Care Med* 1998; **157**(3 Pt 1):858–65.

44 Barbe F, Mayoralas LR, Duran J *et al.* Treatment with continuous positive airway pressure is not effective in patients with sleep apnea but no daytime sleepiness. a randomized, controlled trial. *Ann Intern Med* 2001; **134**:1015–23.

45 Profant J, Ancoli-Israel S, Dimsdale JE. A randomized, controlled trial of 1 week of continuous positive airway pressure treatment on quality of life. *Heart Lung: J Acute Crit Care* 2003; **32**:52–8.

46 Hack M, Davies RJ, Mullins R *et al.* Randomised prospective parallel trial of therapeutic versus subtherapeutic nasal continuous positive airway pressure on simulated steering performance in patients with obstructive sleep apnoea. *Thorax* 2000; **55**:224–31.

47 Chakravorty I, Cayton RM, Szczepura A. Health utilities in evaluating intervention in the sleep apnoea/hypopnoea syndrome. *Eur Respir J* 2002; **20**:1233–8.

48 Kaneko Y, Floras JS, Usui K *et al.* Cardiovascular effects of continuous positive airway pressure in patients with heart failure and obstructive sleep apnea. *N Engl J Med* 2003; **348**:1233–41.

49 Barnes M, Houston D, Worsnop CJ *et al.* A randomized controlled trial of continuous positive airway pressure in mild obstructive sleep apnea. *Am J Respir Crit Care Med* 2002; **165**:773–80.

50 McArdle N, Kingshott R, Engleman HM, Mackay TW, Douglas NJ. Partners of patients with sleep apnoea/hypopnoea syndrome: effect of CPAP treatment on sleep quality and quality of life. *Thorax* 2001; **56**:513–18.

51 Monasterio C, Vidal S, Duran J *et al.* Effectiveness of continuous positive airway pressure in mild sleep apnea–hypopnea syndrome. *Am J Respir Crit Care Med* 2001; **164**:939–43.

52 Brander PE, Soirinsuo M, Lohela P. Nasopharyngeal symptoms in patients with obstructive sleep apnea syndrome. Effect of nasal CPAP treatment. *Respiration* 1999; **66**:128–35.

53 Woodson BT, Steward DL, Weaver EM, Javaheri S. A randomized trial of temperature-controlled radiofrequency tissue ablation, continuous positive airway pressure, and placebo for obstructive sleep apnea syndrome. *Otolaryngol – Head Neck Surg* 2003; **128**:848–61.

54 Lim J, Lasserson TJ, Fleetham J, Wright J. Oral appliances for obstructive sleep apnoea (Cochrane Review). In: *The Cochrane Library*. Chichester, John Wiley & Sons, 2003.

55 Ferguson KA, Ono T, Lowe AA, al-Majed S, Love LL, Fleetham JA. A short-term controlled trial of an adjustable oral appliance for the treatment of mild to moderate obstructive sleep apnoea. *Thorax* 1997; **52**:362–8.

56 Tegelberg A, Wilhelmsson B, Walker-Engstrom ML *et al.* Effects and adverse events of a dental appliance for treatment of obstructive sleep apnoea. *Swed Dent J* 1999; **23**:117–26.

57 Bloch KE, Iseli A, Zhang JN *et al.* A randomized, controlled crossover trial of two oral appliances for sleep apnea treatment. *Am J Respir Crit Care Med* 2000; **162**:246–51.

58 Fritsch KM, Iseli A, Russi EW, Bloch KE. Side effects of mandibular advancement devices for sleep apnea treatment. *Am J Respir Crit Care Med* 2001; **164**:813–18.

59 Johnston CD, Gleadhill IC, Cinnamond MJ, Gabbey J, Burden DJ. Mandibular advancement appliances and obstructive sleep apnoea: a randomized clinical trial. *Eur J Orthodont* 2002; **24**:251–62.

60 Schmidt-Nowara W, Lowe A, Wiegand L, Cartwright R, Perez-Guerra F, Menn S. Oral appliances for the treatment of snoring and obstructive sleep apnea: a review. *Sleep* 1995; **18**:501–10.

61 Pitsis AJ, Darendeliler MA, Gotsopoulos H, Petocz P, Cistulli PA. Effect of vertical dimension on efficacy of oral appliance therapy in obstructive sleep apnea. *Am J Respir Crit Care Med* 2002; **166**:860–4.

62 Shneerson J, Wright J. Lifestyle modification for obstructive sleep apnoea. *Cochrane Database Syst Rev* 2001; **1**:CD002875.

63 Peppard PE, Young T, Palta M, Dempsey J, Skatrud J. Longitudinal study of moderate weight change and sleep-disordered breathing. *JAMA* 2000; **284**:3015–21.

64 Barvaux VA, Aubert G, Rodenstein DO. Clinical review article: weight loss as a treatment for obstructive sleep apnoea. *Sleep Med Rev* 2000; **4**:435–52.

65 Smith I, Lasserson TJ, Wright J. Drug treatments for obstructive sleep apnea (Cochrane Review). In: *The Cochrane Library*. Chichester, John Wiley & Sons, 2004.

66 Hedner J, Kraiczi H, Peker Y, Murphy P. Reduction of sleep-disordered breathing after physostigmine. *Am J Respir Crit Care Med* 2003; **168**:1246–51.

67 Bridgman SA, Dunn KM. Surgery for obstructive sleep apnoea. In: *The Cochrane Library*. Chichester, John Wiley & Sons, 2004.

68 Kamami YV. Outpatient treatment of sleep apnea syndrome with CO_2 laser: laser-assisted UPPP. *J Otolaryngol* 1994; **23**:395–8.

69 Ferguson KA, Heighway K, Ruby RR. A randomized trial of laser-assisted uvulopalatoplasty in the treatment of mild obstructive sleep apnea. *Am J Respir Crit Care Med* 2003; **167**:15–19.

70 Littner M, Kushida CA, Hartse K *et al.* Practice parameters for the use of laser-assisted uvulopalatoplasty: an update for 2000. *Sleep* 2001; **24**:603–19.

71 Finkelstein Y, Stein G, Ophir D, Berger R, Berger G. Laser-assisted uvulopalatoplasty for the management of obstructive sleep apnea. *Arch Otolaryngol Head Neck Surg* 2002; **128**:429–34.

72 Terris DJ, Coker JF, Thomas AJ, Chavoya M. Preliminary findings from a prospective, randomized trial of two palatal operations for sleep-disordered breathing. *Otolaryngol – Head Neck Surg* 2002; **127**:315–23.

73 Ayappa I, Norman RG, Krieger AC, Rosen A, O'Malley RL, Rapoport DM. Non-invasive detection of respiratory effort-related arousals (RERAs) by a nasal cannula/pressure transducer system. *Sleep* 2000; **23**:763–71.

74 Kripke DF, Ancoli-Israel S, Klauber MR, Wingard DL, Mason WJ, Mullaney DJ. Prevalence of sleep-disordered breathing in ages 40–64 years: a population-based survey. *Sleep* 1997; **20**:65–76.

75 Bixler EO, Vgontzas AN, Lin HM *et al.* Prevalence of sleep-disordered breathing in women: effects of gender. *Am J Respir Crit Care Med* 2001; **163**(3 Pt 1):608–13.

76 Duran J, Esnaola S, Rubio R, Iztueta A. Obstructive sleep apnea–hypopnea and related clinical features in a population-based sample of subjects aged 30 to 70 yr. *Am J Respir Crit Care Med* 2001; **163**:685–9.

77 Bearpark H, Elliott L, Grunstein R *et al.* Occurrence and correlates of sleep disordered breathing in the Australian town of Busselton: a preliminary analysis. *Sleep* 1993; **16**(8 Suppl):S3–5.

78 Olson LG, King MT, Hensley MJ, Saunders NA. A community study of snoring and sleep-disordered breathing. Prevalence. *Am J Respir Crit Care Med* 1995; **152**:711–16.

79 American Academy of Sleep Medicine. Standards of Practice Committee. Practice parameters for clinical use of the Multiple Sleep Latency Test and the Maintenance of Wakefulness Test. *Sleep* 2005; **28**:113–21.

CHAPTER 5.5

Long-term oxygen therapy for chronic respiratory failure in chronic obstructive pulmonary disease

Peter G Gibson

Introduction

The use of domiciliary oxygen for chronic obstructive pulmonary disease (COPD) represents an important treatment modality for this chronic and progressive condition. Pivotal studies have demonstrated improved survival in patients with severe COPD treated with supplemental oxygen.[1,2] Consequently, long-term oxygen therapy now plays a key role in the management of respiratory failure associated with COPD. Supplemental oxygen may also improve other outcomes in chronic respiratory illness, such as exercise tolerance and quality of life. However, the evidence is not yet conclusive, and the use of oxygen for these purposes is the subject of further study. This section will examine the evidence base supporting the use of long-term oxygen therapy in COPD.

Rationale for use

Advanced COPD is associated with peripheral airways obstruction, parenchymal destruction and abnormalities of pulmonary vessels.[3] These abnormalities lead to inequality in the ventilation/perfusion ratio, chronic alveolar hypoxia, impaired gas exchange and hypoxaemia. Initially, hypoxaemia is present only during exercise, but eventually occurs at rest. Pulmonary hypertension is a late manifestation of COPD that develops as a result of hypoxic pulmonary vasoconstriction and fixed abnormalities of the pulmonary vasculature, including vascular remodelling and destruction of the vascular bed from emphysema.

Assessment

The presence of hypoxaemia should be assessed in advanced COPD, especially in patients whose forced expiratory volume in 1 second (FEV_1) is below 40% predicted, or if there are signs of cor pulmonale or respiratory failure.[4–7] This is preferably done using arterial blood gas analysis. Arterial oxygen saturation as measured by pulse oximetry (Sao_2) can be used to monitor patients over time. Long-term oxygen therapy is indicated in stage IV disease, i.e. very severe COPD with arterial oxygen tension (Pao_2) < 7.3 kPa (55 mmHg). In hypoxaemic patients with COPD, supplemental long-term oxygen therapy (LTOT) improves survival, exercise, sleep and cognitive performance.[8–10] The therapeutic goal is to maintain $Sao_2 > 90\%$ during rest, sleep and exertion.

Administration

Oxygen can be used as long-term continuous therapy, during exercise and for short-term use to relieve dyspnoea. Available sources of oxygen include gas, liquid oxygen and oxygen via a concentrator. Oxygen delivery methods include nasal continuous flow, pulse demand, reservoir cannulae and transtracheal catheters. The oxygen concentrator is a cost-efficient method of delivering long-term domiciliary oxygen therapy. It uses a compressor and molecular sieve to remove nitrogen from the air. This results in 92–95% oxygen at low flow rates, up to 3 L/min.

Efficacy

The evidence base for the use of domiciliary oxygen therapy for hypoxaemic COPD patients consists of five randomized controlled trials (RCTs; Table 1) that have been examined in a Cochrane systematic review.[11] The trials investigated:

1 Continuous oxygen therapy versus nocturnal oxygen therapy in hypoxaemic chronic obstructive lung disease.[1]

2 Long-term oxygen therapy versus no oxygen therapy in chronic hypoxic cor pulmonale complicating chronic bronchitis and emphysema.[2]

3 Nocturnal oxygen therapy 3 L/min versus room air 3 L/min for patients with COPD and nocturnal sleep desaturation but resting daytime $Pao_2 > 60$ mmHg (8 kPa).[12]

4 Long-term oxygen therapy plus conventional treatment in patients with COPD and moderate hypoxaemia versus conventional treatment alone.[13]

5 Nocturnal oxygen therapy in COPD patients with mild to moderate daytime hypoxaemia and nocturnal sleep desaturation.[14]

Continuous oxygen therapy versus nocturnal oxygen therapy[1]

In this study, 203 patients with hypoxaemic chronic obstructive lung disease were randomly allocated to nocturnal oxygen

Table 1. Characteristics of studies of oxygen therapy in stable COPD.

Study (first author)	Methods	Participants	Interventions	Outcomes
Chaouat (1999)[14]	Randomized, unblinded, controlled study	76 COPD patients were randomized, 41 in the nocturnal oxygen group and 35 in the control group. 46 patients (24 treated and 22 control patients) were available for haemodynamic monitoring at 2 years	Nocturnal oxygen therapy for 8–10 hours a night, at a flow to allow the nocturnal Sao_2 to be constantly >90%	Physiological parameters, pulmonary haemodynamic parameters, survival
Fletcher (1992)[12]	Randomized, double-blind, controlled trial	38 COPD patients with nocturnal desaturation, nine patients were sham treated and seven patients oxygen treated. Daytime $Pao_2 \geq 60$ mmHg	Nocturnal oxygen or room air 3 L/min supplied by home concentrators	Mortality, physiological parameters, FEV_1, FVC, PAP
Gorecka (1997)[13]	Randomized, controlled study	135 patients with COPD and moderate hypoxaemia (Pao_2 56–65 mmHg) referred to nine regional centres in Poland	Conventional treatment consisted of bronchodilators, (theophylline, β_2-agonists and anticholinergic drugs). Antibiotics, diuretics and corticosteroids were prescribed at the discretion of the physician. Long-term oxygen therapy was given at a flow rate adjusted to raise Pao_2 above 65 mmHg	Mortality
MRC (1981)[2]	Randomized controlled trial	87 patients, $FEV_1 < 1.2$ L, Pao_2 between 40 and 60 mmHg breathing air at rest	Long-term domiciliary oxygen therapy versus no oxygen therapy	Mortality, physiological parameters of FEV_1, FVC, Pao_2 and $Paco_2$
NOTT Group (1980)[1]	Randomized controlled trial	203 patients, 101 received continuous oxygen therapy, (77.2% males) and 102 received nocturnal oxygen therapy (80.4% males). Entry criteria: clinical diagnosis of chronic obstructive lung disease, age > 35 years. Hypoxaemia $Pao_2 \leq 55$ mmHg, $Pao_2 \leq 59$ plus one of the following: oedema, haematocrit $\geq 55\%$, cor pulmonale on ECG: 3 mm in leads I, III, AVF. Lung function: FEV_1/FVC < 70% after inhaled bronchodilator. TLC $\geq 80\%$ predicted. Age > 35 years	Continuous oxygen therapy versus 12-hour nocturnal oxygen therapy 1–4 L/min by oxygen concentrators or liquid oxygen systems or compressed gas	Mortality, physiological parameters; quality of life; cardiovascular: right atrial pressure; pulmonary artery pressure; pulmonary wedge pressure; cardiac index; stroke volume index; pulmonary vascular resistance; right ventricular stroke index

therapy ($n = 102$) or continuous oxygen therapy ($n = 101$) at a flow rate of 1–4 L/min. The oxygen source was an oxygen concentrator, liquid oxygen or compressed gas. The population studied was predominantly older men. Although there was a trend for improved survival at 12 months, this was not significant [Peto odds ratio (OR) 0.53; 95% confidence interval (CI) 0.25–1.11]. At 24 months, however, there was a significant reduction in mortality (Peto OR 0.45; 95% CI 0.25–0.81) for the continuous oxygen treatment group. The group treated with continuous oxygen also demonstrated improvement in pulmonary vascular resistance and pulmonary artery pressure.[15]

Oxygen therapy versus no oxygen therapy[2]

This study was a controlled trial of long-term domiciliary oxygen therapy involving 87 patients with COPD and a Pa_{O_2} of between 40 and 60 mmHg (5.3 and 8 kPa) and one or more recorded episodes of right heart failure with ankle oedema. These subjects had very severe COPD, with a mean baseline FEV_1 of between 0.58 and 0.76 L. They were randomized to receive oxygen therapy or no oxygen (control subjects) in an unblinded fashion. Forty-three patients (33 male) received oxygen therapy for at least 15 hours a day at a minimum flow rate of 2 L/min. Oxygen was delivered via liquid oxygen therapy (8), oxygen concentrator or cylinder. Over 5 years, there was a significant reduction in mortality for the group receiving oxygen therapy (Peto OR 0.42, 95% CI 0.18–0.98). This effect appeared to depend on the sex of the patient. There was no difference in mortality for male patients in both treated and control groups up to 500 days from commencement of treatment. However, in female patients, mortality was improved for the oxygen-treated group from the commencement of treatment. Treating five patients with severe hypoxaemic COPD with long-term oxygen therapy saved one life over the 5-year study period: number needed to treat (NNT) = 5.

Long-term oxygen therapy versus no oxygen therapy in moderate hypoxaemia[13]

This unblinded RCT examined oxygen versus no oxygen in patients with COPD and moderate hypoxaemia. A total of 135 patients received oxygen from an oxygen concentrator at a flow rate that raised their resting Pa_{O_2} to >8.7 kPa (65 mmHg). Sixty-seven patients formed the control group, and both treated and control groups received 'usual treatment', which consisted of bronchodilators, antibiotics, corticosteroids and diuretics as required. There was no difference in mortality during the 3-year study period.

Nocturnal oxygen 3 L/min versus room air 3 L/min[12]

This study was a double-blind RCT designed to assess the effect of nocturnal oxygen in 38 patients with COPD and nocturnal sleep desaturation. Oxygen was supplied to the active group through an oxygen concentrator. The control group received gas from an oxygen concentrator rendered ineffective. In the control group of 19 patients, six patients died and four were excluded (two withdrew, one developed daytime hypoxaemia, one was non-compliant). Of the original 19 treated subjects, six developed significant daytime hypoxaemia, one developed worsening of sleep apnoea, and there were five deaths. The remaining 16 subjects were randomized to receive nocturnal oxygen therapy ($n = 7$) or sham treatment ($n = 9$). There was no difference in mortality after 36 months between the oxygen-treated and sham-treated groups. However, the small study size could not exclude the possibility of a type 2 error.

Nocturnal oxygen therapy in patients with mild to moderate hypoxaemia[14]

This study examined a less intensive oxygen treatment regimen using nocturnal oxygen therapy. Oxygen via a concentrator was given for 8–10 hours per night at a flow rate of 2 L/min to 76 patients with COPD and daytime hypoxaemia as well as significant nocturnal desaturation. The control group of 35 patients received no oxygen therapy. Treatment allocation was randomized, and the study was unblinded. There was no difference in mortality between the treated and control groups on an intention-to-treat basis. Twelve patients in the nocturnal oxygen group and 10 control group patients deteriorated and required treatment with conventional long-term oxygen therapy during the follow-up period. Five of these patients subsequently died, two in the treated group and three in the control group. Nocturnal oxygen did not allow delay in the prescription of long-term oxygen therapy.

Meta-analysis

The studies of nocturnal oxygen by Chaouat et al.[14] and Fletcher et al.[12] had similar methodologies, allowing aggregation and meta-analysis.[11] There was no difference in mortality between the treated and control groups. The pooled Peto OR moved closer to unity (0.97; 95% CI 0.41–2.31) than the individual ORs. These data demonstrate that, in COPD with hypoxaemia, nocturnal oxygen therapy does not reproduce the survival benefit that can be achieved by continuous oxygen therapy. The relatively small numbers of patients, the young age of participants and the lack of comorbidities in most of the studies raises concerns about the applicability of the survival outcomes to current clinical situations. Patients with COPD fulfilling prescription guidelines for domiciliary home oxygen therapy appear to be older than the subjects included in these studies. The majority of these COPD patients have multiple comorbidities. The assumption that home oxygen therapy has a beneficial effect in these patients has not been demonstrated.

Implications for practice

Long-term oxygen therapy improved survival in a selected group of COPD patients with severe hypoxaemia. Long-term oxygen therapy did not appear to improve survival in patients with COPD and moderate hypoxaemia, nor in COPD patients with nocturnal desaturation but resting daytime oxygenation above what would qualify for oxygen therapy.

Adverse effects

The main adverse effect reported and directly attributed to oxygen therapy is burns. The simultaneous use of cigarettes and oxygen therapy is most commonly associated with burns.[16] In a retrospective review of 3673 consecutive patients treated at an adult burn centre over a 10-year period, Robb *et al.*[17] identified 27 patients with burns attributable to oxygen therapy. Most patients (*n* = 25) were receiving oxygen for COPD, and 23 were using oxygen at home. Twenty-four patients were smoking while using oxygen, whereas two were lighting pilot lights, and one was lighting his wife's cigarette. These results reinforce the need for complete smoking cessation as part of COPD management.

Cost-effectiveness

Oxygen treatment represents a major cost for ambulatory patients with COPD.[18] The oxygen concentrator is a useful means of delivering supplemental oxygen in COPD because it is reliable, convenient and easy to use. It is probably the most cost-effective of the various oxygen delivery systems from the institutional standpoint.[19] Initiation of domiciliary oxygen therapy requires careful assessment. Dedicated oxygen assessment clinics can assist with cost minimization by avoiding unnecessary use.[20,21]

Use of oxygen during exercise/rehabilitation

Exercise rehabilitation is an effective therapy for COPD. Oxygen can be added during exercise to enhance performance;[22] however, controversy surrounds the use of supplemental oxygen to enhance further the effectiveness of exercise and respiratory rehabilitation in patients with COPD. Many investigators have assessed the short-term effect of increased oxygen availability during exercise,[23] predominantly in laboratory-based studies. The rationale for the use of oxygen in this setting is that it allows patients to tolerate higher exercise intensities or longer exercise times, which leads to larger training effects.[24,25] Other researchers, however, argue that peripheral muscles require an adequate hypoxaemic stimulus to improve exercise capacity, and that supplemental oxygen prevents this. Two systematic reviews have examined the effect of supplemental oxygen during exercise in COPD.[26,27]

Puhan *et al.*[26] identified five RCTs (Table 2)[28–32] that provided sufficient data for analysis. The methodological quality was low, and sample sizes were too small for most trials to produce meaningful results (median total sample size = 28). Data from five trials showed that supplemental oxygen during exercise did not have clinically meaningful effects on health-related quality of life, while improvements in exercise capacity may be even larger for patients exercising in room air.

The studies are summarized in Figures 1 and 2 and Table 2.

Emtner and co-workers[28] examined the effects of a 7-week high-intensity training programme while breathing air or 30% oxygen in patients with COPD who were normoxic at rest breathing room air. Oxygen supplementation allowed patients to train at higher intensity and for a longer time. As

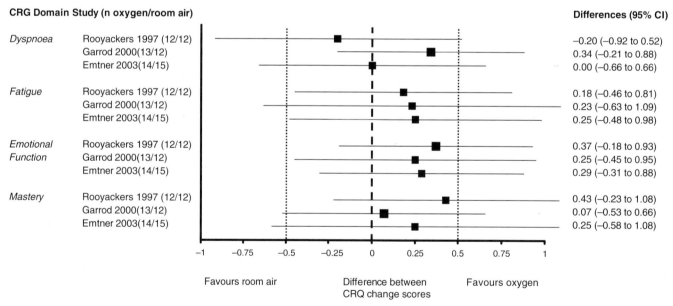

Figure 1. Effect of supplemental oxygen on health-related quality of life. The Forrest plot shows the results from three trials comparing physical exercise with and without oxygen, separately for each domain of the Chronic Respiratory Questionnaire (CRQ). The *x*-axis represents the difference in change scores between study groups with negative values favouring exercise in room air and positive values favouring exercise with supplemental oxygen. A difference of 0 means that both study groups changed to the same amount. Boxes with 95% confidence intervals (CI) represent point estimates for the difference between the CRQ change scores (from baseline to follow-up) of the study groups. Dotted lines represent the minimal important difference of the CRQ (change of 0.5). On the right of the Forrest plot, point estimates for differences between groups and 95% CI are shown. From Puhan *et al.*[26]

Table 2. Characteristics of randomized controlled trials investigating supplemental oxygen and assisted ventilation.

Study (first author)	Total sample size	Mean age (years)	Desaturation during exercise Pa_{O_2} at rest	Mean FEV_1 % predicted	Exercise programme	Exercise session (min) and times/week	Duration exercise programme	Supplemental intervention	Additional interventions in both groups	Outcomes
Emtner (2003)[28]	29 (62% males)	67	Only patients without desaturation ($Sp_{O_2} > 88\%$) $Pa_{O_2} = 9.7\,kPa$	36.6	ET: continuous high-intensity cycling at 80% of Wmax for 35 min (+5 min warming up and cooling down)	45 min 3×/week	7 weeks	3 L oxygen per min	Edu	IET, CWRT, CRQ, SF-36
Fichter (1999)[29]	10 (100% males)	59	Patients ± desaturation $Pa_{O_2} = 9.9\,kPa$	43.2	ET: continuous high-intensity cycling at 80% of Wmax for 45 min	45 min 5×/week	4 weeks	3.5 L oxygen per min	No	IET
Garrod (2000)[30]	25 (72% males)	67	Patients with desaturation during exercise (Sp_{O_2} fall of 4% or ≤90%) $Pa_{O_2} = 8.5\,kPa$	31.6	ET: continuous high-intensity walking at 80% of maximum oxygen consumption in SWT and low-intensity cycling (unloaded) ST: upper and lower extremity	60 min 3×/week	6 weeks	4 L oxygen per min	Edu, BE, Psy, Re	SWT, CRQ, HADS
Rooyackers (1997)[31]	24 (83% males)	61	Patients with desaturation during exercise ($Sp_{O_2} \leq 90\%$) $Pa_{O_2} = 10.4\,kPa$	33.5	ET: interval cycle exercise (2 min exercise/2 min rest) ST: upper and lower extremity	50 min 5×/week	10 weeks	4 L oxygen per min. Patients stopped exercising when $Sp_{O_2} \leq 90\%$	Edu, Psy, Re	IET, CWRT, 6MWT, CRQ
Wadell (2001)[32]	20 (50% males)	67	Only patients with desaturation ($Sp_{O_2} \leq 92\%$) $Pa_{O_2} = 9.4\,kPa$	45.3	ET: interval treadmill exercise (2 min high speed with target dyspnoea of 7/10 on Borg/2 min low speed)	30 min 3×/week	8 weeks	5 L oxygen per min	No	6MWT

Table 2. *Continued.*

Study (first author)	Total sample size	Mean age (years)	Desaturation during exercise Pa$_{O_2}$ at rest	Mean FEV$_1$ % predicted	Exercise programme	Exercise session (min) and times/week	Duration exercise programme	Supplemental intervention	Additional interventions in both groups	Outcomes
Bianchi (2003)[36]	33 (100% males)	64.5	Patients ± desaturation Pa$_{O_2}$ = 10.0	44.2	ET: moderate-intensity cycling at 50–70% of Wmax ST: upper and lower extremity	30 min 3×/week	6 weeks	Proportional assist ventilation during exercise	Edu	6MWT, IET, SGRQ, BDI, TDI
Garrod (2000)[37]	45 (62% males)	65	Patients ± desaturation Pa$_{O_2}$ = 8.7	34.1	ET: walking at 80% of V_{O_2}max of SWT + low-intensity cycling ST: Upper and lower extremity	60 min 2×/week	8 weeks	Overnight non-invasive positive pressure ventilation during training period	Edu, Rel	SWT, CRQ, HADS, LCADL
Hawkins (2002)[38]	19 (89% males)	67	Patients ± desaturation Pa$_{O_2}$ = 8.4	26.9	ET: High-intensity cycling at 70% Wmax	30 min 3×/week	6 weeks	Proportional assist ventilation during exercise	No	IET
Johnson (2002)[39]	32 (68% males)	69	Patients ± desaturation Pa$_{O_2}$ = 9.4	32.1	ET: High-intensity treadmill walking at 50–60% of METmax at baseline	20 min 2×/week	6 weeks	Non-invasive positive pressure ventilation during exercise Heliox 101/min	Edu, BE, Psy, Rel	IET, exercise duration, global ratings

ET, endurance training; ST, strength training; Wmax, maximum exercise capacity; SWT, incremental shuttle walk test; MET, metabolic equivalent; Edu, education; BE, breathing exercises; Psy, psychological support; Rel, relaxation exercises; IET, incremental exercise test; CRQ, Chronic Respiratory Questionnaire; CWRT, constant work rate test; SGRQ, St George's Respiratory Questionnaire; SF-36, Short form survey; HADS, Hospital Anxiety Depression Scale; 6MWT, 6-minute walk test; SGRQ, St George's Respiratory Questionnaire; ESWT, endurance shuttle walk test; BDI and TDI, Baseline and Transitional Dyspnea Index; LCADL, London Chest Activity of Daily Living Scale. From Puhan *et al.* (2004).[26]

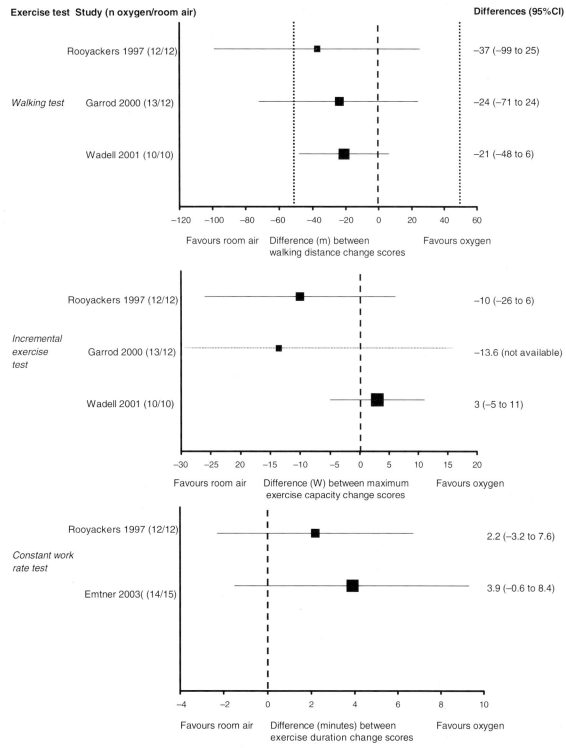

Figure 2. Effect of supplemental oxygen on exercise capacity. The Forrest plot shows the results from five trials comparing respiratory rehabilitation with and without oxygen. Walking tests, incremental and constant work rate exercise tests were used to assess the additional effect of supplemental oxygen during exercise. The x-axis represents the difference in change scores between study groups with negative values favouring exercise in room air and positive values favouring exercise with supplemental oxygen. A difference of 0 means that both study groups changed to the same amount. Boxes with 95% confidence intervals (CI) represent point estimates for the difference between the walking distance and maximum exercise capacity change scores (from baseline to follow-up) of the study groups. Dotted lines represent the minimal important difference of the 6-min walking distance (53 m). On the right of the Forrest plot, point estimates for differences between groups and 95% CI are shown. From Puhan et al.[26]

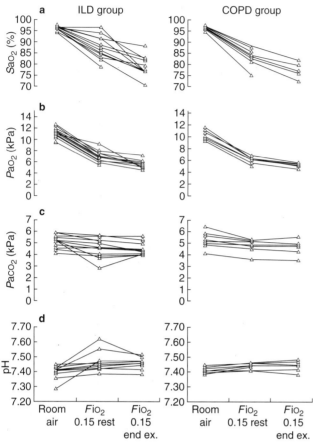

Figure 3. Comparison of arterial blood gas tensions between patients with interstitial lung disease (ILD) and those with chronic obstructive pulmonary disease (COPD) at sea level at rest (room air), on 15% oxygen at rest for 20 min (Fio_2 0.15 rest) and after a walking task on 15% oxygen (Fio_2 0.15 end ex.). Individual and mean values of (a) arterial oxygen saturation (Sao_2), (b) arterial oxygen pressure (Pao_2), (c) arterial carbon dioxide pressure ($Paco_2$) and (d) arterial pH. From Seccombe *et al.*[34] reproduced with permission from the BMJ Publishing Group.

a result, physical performance and health status improved significantly more by training with oxygen than with air. Thus, it appears that patients affected by severe COPD gain additional advantage from rehabilitation programmes if conducted with supplemental oxygen, even if they are not hypoxaemic and do not desaturate during exercise. There was a trend towards larger improvements of health-related quality of life (HRQL) and exercise duration in constant work rate tests in the groups with oxygen, but patients exercising on room air had larger improvements in walking distance. The effects on quality of life were slight but not clinically meaningful (Fig. 1).

In the trial by Rooyackers *et al.*,[31] patients achieved mean exercise intensities corresponding to 124% of maximum exercise capacity in the group with oxygen and 114% of maximum exercise capacity in the group without oxygen ($P = 0.12$).

Given the limited methodological quality of trials, any conclusions are vague. The general use of oxygen is only justified if larger trials of good quality show its benefit on clinically relevant outcomes. The mechanisms of the effects of oxygen during exercise are also still insufficiently understood and more research is required.[23]

Air travel

Air travel represents a period of hypoxia that may be problematic for people with COPD. Commercial aircraft routinely fly at around 38 000 ft and are pressurized to a cabin altitude not exceeding 8000 ft (2438 m). At this altitude, the partial pressure of oxygen is reduced and is equivalent to breathing 15% oxygen. This will cause the arterial oxygen tension (Pao_2) of a healthy person to fall to between 7.0 and 8.5 kPa, and the effects of this usually go unnoticed. However, exposure to this altitude may worsen hypoxaemia in patients with lung disease, especially if the person is already hypoxaemic at sea level.[33] This issue was directly examined by Seccombe *et al.*,[34] who studied 15 subjects with interstitial lung disease (ILD) and 10 subjects with COPD while breathing a hypoxic gas mixture that simulated cabin altitude (15% oxygen), both at rest and during a 50-m walk. The subjects had a resting Pao_2 equal to or above 9.3 kPa. In both groups, Pao_2 fell significantly from that at rest on room air to that breathing 15% oxygen at rest, and again to completion of the walk test. Mean Pao_2 fell to 5.5 kPa after exercise in the ILD group and to 5.3 kPa after exercise in the patients with COPD (Fig. 3).

Preflight assessment can help to determine the oxygen needs of a patient who is intending to fly. Oxygen needs can be estimated using the hypoxia inhalation test or through the use of regression formulae. It is currently recommended that the Pao_2 during air travel should be maintained above 6.7 kPa (50 mmHg).[35] Treatment with 2–3 L/min oxygen by nasal cannula will replace the inspired oxygen partial pressure lost at 2438 m (8000 ft) compared with sea level.[35] For high-risk patients, the goal should be to maintain oxygen pressure during flight at the same level at which the patient is clinically stable at sea level. Most airlines will provide supplemental oxygen on request.[35]

Conclusions

Long-term oxygen therapy improved survival in a selected group of COPD patients with severe hypoxaemia. Long-term oxygen therapy did not appear to improve survival in patients with COPD and moderate hypoxaemia, nor in COPD patients with nocturnal desaturation but resting daytime oxygenation above what would qualify for oxygen therapy.

References

1 Nocturnal Oxygen Therapy Trial Group. Continuous or nocturnal oxygen therapy in hypoxemic chronic obstructive lung disease. *Ann Intern Med* 1980; **93**:391–8.

2 Medical Research Council, Report of the Medical Research Council Working Party. Long-term domiciliary oxygen therapy in chronic hypoxic cor pulmonale complicating chronic bronchitis and emphysema. *Lancet* 1981; **1**:681–5.

3 Global Initiative for Chronic Obstructive Lung Disease. Workshop Report 2004. www.goldcopd.com, 2004.

4 Celli B, MacNee W and ATS/ERS Task Force. Standards for the diagnosis and treatment of patients with COPD: a summary of the ATS/ERS position paper. *Eur Respir J* 2004; **23**:932–46.

5 American Thoracic Society. Standards for the diagnosis and care of patients with chronic obstructive pulmonary disease. *Am J Respir Crit Care Med* 1995; **152**:S77–S121.

6 Siafakas N, Vermiere P, Pride NB *et al*. Optimal assessment and management of chronic obstructive pulmonary disease (COPD). The European Respiratory Society Task Force. *Eur Respir J* 1995; **8**:1398–420.

7 Pauwels R, Buist AS, Calverley PM *et al*. Global strategy for the diagnosis, management, and prevention of chronic obstructive pulmonary disease. NHLBI/WHO Global Initiative for Chronic Obstructive Lung Disease (GOLD) Workshop summary. *Am J Respir Crit Care Med* 2001; **163**:1256–76.

8 Weitzenblum E, Sautegeau A, Ehrhart M *et al*. Long-term oxygen therapy can reverse the progression of pulmonary hypertension in patients with chronic obstructive pulmonary disease. *Am Rev Respir Dis* 1985; **131**:493–8.

9 Oswald-Mammosser M, Weitzenblum E, Quoix E *et al*. Prognostic factors in COPD patients receiving long-term oxygen therapy: importance of pulmonary artery pressure. *Chest* 1995; **107**:1193–8.

10 Zielinski J, Tobiasz M, Hawrylkiewicz I *et al*. Effects of long-term oxygen therapy on pulmonary hemodynamics in COPD patients: a 6-year prospective study. *Chest* 1998; **113**:65–70.

11 Crockett A, Cranstonet J, Moss JR *et al*. Domiciliary oxygen for chronic obstructive pulmonary disease. *Cochrane Database Syst Rev* 2000; **4**:CD001744.

12 Fletcher E, Luckett RA, Goodnight-White SA *et al*. A double-blind trial of nocturnal supplemental oxygen for sleep desaturation in patients with chronic obstructive pulmonary disease and a daytime Pao_2 above 60 mmHg. *Am Rev Respir Dis* 1992; **145**:1070–6.

13 Gorecka D, Gorzelak K, Sliwinski P *et al*. Effect of long-term oxygen therapy on survival in patients with chronic obstructive pulmonary disease with moderate hypoxaemia. *Thorax* 1997; **52**:674–9.

14 Chaouat A, Weitzenblum E, Kessler R *et al*. A randomized trial of nocturnal oxygen therapy in chronic obstructive pulmonary disease patients. *Eur Respir J* 1999; **14**:1002–8.

15 Timms R, Khaja FU, Williams GW. Hemodynamic response to oxygen therapy in chronic obstructive pulmonary disease. *Ann Intern Med* 1985; **102**:29–36.

16 Baruchin O, Yoffe B, Baruchin A. Burns in inpatients by simultaneous use of cigarettes and oxygen therapy. *Burns* 2004; **30**:836–8.

17 Robb B, Hungness ES, Hershko DD *et al*. Home oxygen therapy: adjunct or risk factor? *J Burn Care Rehabil* 2003; **24**:403–6.

18 Pelletier-Fleury N, Lanoe JL, Fleury B *et al*. Cost-effectiveness study of 2 long-term home oxygen therapy management systems. *Rev Epidemiol Sante Publ* 1997; **45**:53–63.

19 Reisfield G, Wilson G. The cost of breathing: an economic analysis of the patient cost of home oxygen therapy. *Am J Hosp Palliat Care* 2004; **21**:348–52.

20 Zinman C, Richards GA, Taylor R *et al*. Long-term domiciliary oxygen therapy—the Johannesburg Hospital experience. *S Afr Med J* 2000; **90**:617–21.

21 McKeon J, Saunders N, Murree-Allen K. Domiciliary oxygen: rationalization of supply in the Hunter region from 1982–1986. *Med J Aust* 1987; **146**:73–8.

22 Cotes J, Gilson J. Effect of oxygen on exercise ability in chronic respiratory insufficiency—use of portable apparatus. *Lancet* 1956; **270**:872–6.

23 Snider G. Enhancement of exercise performance in COPD patients by hyperoxia: a call for research. *Chest* 2002; **122**:1830–6.

24 Casaburi R, Patessio A, Loli F *et al*. Reductions in exercise lactic acidosis and ventilation as a result of exercise training in patients with obstructive lung disease. *Am Rev Respir Dis* 1991; **143**:9–18.

25 Hardman A. Issues of fractionalization of exercise (short vs long bouts). *Med Sci Sports Exer* 2001; **33**:S421–S427.

26 Puhan M, Schuneman HJ, Frey M *et al*. Value of supplemental interventions to enhance the effectiveness of physical exercise during respiratory rehabilitation in COPD patients. A systematic review. *Respir Res* 2004; **5**:25.

27 Ram F, Wedzicha J. Ambulatory oxygen for chronic obstructive pulmonary disease. *Cochrane Database Syst Rev* 2002; **2**:CD000238.

28 Emtner M, Porszasz J, Burns M *et al*. Benefits of supplemental oxygen in exercise training in nonhypoxemic chronic obstructive pulmonary disease patients. *Am J Crit Care Med* 2003; **168**:1034–42.

29 Fichter J, Fleckenstein J, Stahl C *et al*. Effect of oxygen (FiO_2: 0.35) on the aerobic capacity in patients with COPD. *Pneumologie* 1999; **53**:121–6.

30 Garrod R, Paul E, Wedzicha JA. Supplemental oxygen during pulmonary rehabilitation in patients with COPD with exercise hypoxaemia. *Thorax* 2000; **55**:539–43.

31 Rooyackers J, Dekhuijzen PN, van Herwaarden CL *et al*. Training with supplemental oxygen in patients with COPD and hypoxaemia at peak exercise. *Eur Respir J* 1997; **10**:1278–84.

32 Wadell K, Henriksson Larsen K, Lundgren R. Physical training with and without oxygen in patients with chronic obstructive pulmonary disease and exercise-induced hypoxaemia. *J Rehabil Med* 2001; **33**:200–5.

33 Coker R, Partridge M. What happens to patients with respiratory disease when they fly? *Thorax* 2004; **59**:919–20.

34 Seccombe L, Kelly PT, Wong CK *et al*. Effect of simulated commercial flight on oxygenation in patients with interstitial lung disease and chronic obstructive pulmonary disease. *Thorax* 2004; **59**:966–70.

35 BTS Standards of Care Committee. Managing passengers with respiratory disease planning air travel: BTS recommendations. *Thorax* 2002; **57**:289–304.

36 Bianchi L, Foglio R, Baiardi R *et al*. Lack of additional effect of adjunct of assisted ventilation to pulmonary rehabilitation in mild COPD patients. *Respir Med* 2002; **96**:359–67.

37 Garrod R, Mikelsons C, Paul EA *et al*. Randomized controlled trial of domiciliary noninvasive positive pressure ventilation and physical training in severe chronic obstructive pulmonary disease. *Am J Respir Crit Care Med* 2000; **162**(4 Pt 1):1335–41.

38 Hawkins P, Johnson LC, Nikoletou D *et al*. Proportional assist ventilation as an aid to exercise training in severe chronic obstructive pulmonary disease. *Thorax* 2002; **57**:853–9.

39 Johnson J, Gavin D, Dramiga S. Effects of training with heliox and noninvasive positive pressure ventilation on exercise ability in patients with severe COPD. *Chest* 2002; **122**:464–72.

PART 6

Diffuse lung disease/pleural disease/thromboembolism

Diffuse lung disease

CHAPTER 6.1.1

The treatment of cryptogenic fibrosing alveolitis

Barry Plant and Jim Egan

Introduction

The idiopathic interstitial pneumonias are a group of disorders of unknown aetiology. The commonest subgroup is represented by idiopathic pulmonary fibrosis/cryptogenic fibrosing alveolitis, which is synonymous with the histological pattern of usual interstitial pneumonia. This chapter will focus predominantly on this group of patients. A PubMed literature search was performed up to 16 January 2004 and a review of ATS International Annual Conference abstracts from 1996 to 2003. The search terms used are summarized in Table 1. Unfortunately, there is little or no evidence that can support any form of therapy in these conditions. This chapter will briefly summarize the idiopathic pneumonias and overview the treatments that may be considered by clinicians for their patients.

Description of problem

Idiopathic interstitial pneumonias

The idiopathic interstitial pneumonias (IIPs) comprise a number of clinicopathological syndromes, with different histological patterns and clinical courses.[1,2]

Cryptogenic fibrosing alveolitis (CFA) usual interstitial pneumonia (UIP)

Also known as idiopathic pulmonary fibrosis (IPF), this is the commonest subgroup, accounting for 65% of IIP cases.[1] UIP is the histopathological pattern synonymous with the clinical syndrome of CFA. The prevalence is estimated to be between 20 and 30 per 100 000 of the general population.[3]

Men are affected more commonly than women by a ratio of 2 : 1.[4] Most patients are between 40 and 80 years old, with a mean age of 65 years. The clinical diagnosis of CFA is based upon three criteria:[1] (a) exclusion of other causes of interstitial lung disease (ILD); (b) abnormal pulmonary function tests (PFTs), showing a restrictive pattern and/or decreased diffusing lung capacity (D_LCO); (c) a radiological pattern on high-resolution computerized tomography (HRCT) showing peripheral bibasilar reticular abnormalities and minimal 'ground-glass' attenuation.

A clinical and radiological evaluation is usually adequate for diagnostic purposes.[5] In the majority of cases, HRCT caries a specificity of 90% for the diagnosis of CFA. This is im-

portant as a study of 60 UIP patients undergoing surgical lung biopsy demonstrated a mortality of 17% within 30 days of the procedure.[6] However, if there are atypical features on HRCT, including nodules or predominant ground-glass attenuation or consolidation, particularly in a younger patient, careful consideration should be given to surgical biopsy.

The histological features of UIP show fibrotic areas of varying age and activity.[4] Typically, honeycombing is interspersed with areas of relatively normal lung tissue. Interstitial inflammation is mild, and fibroblastic foci are a major characteristic feature.[4]

Clinical course in CFA

Unfortunately, many reported cases of CFA present with advanced disease.[7] The median survival is 2.9 years from diagnosis.[2] Respiratory failure is the most frequent cause of death, accounting for 40% of deaths. Other causes include heart failure, ischaemic heart disease, infection and pulmonary emboli.[8] Bronchogenic carcinoma is seen in 10–15% of advanced cases. Surrogate markers for longer survival include:[9] younger age (<50 years); female sex; shorter symptomatic period (<1 year); increased proportion of lymphocytes (20–25%) in bronchoalveolar lavage (BAL) fluid; and a beneficial response 3–6 months after corticosteroid therapy. Surrogate markers for limited survival include: older age (>65 years); male; honeycombing and traction bronchiectasis on HRCT; excess neutrophils (>5%) and/or eosinophils (>5%) in the BAL fluid.

Non-specific interstitial pneumonia (NSIP)

The clinical presentation of NSIP is similar to UIP, but affects younger patients, mean age 57 years.[10] NSIP is likely to have been described formerly as 'cellular' CFA.[11] HRCT shows bilateral symmetric ground-glass opacities or mixed bilateral air space consolidation and interstitial thickening, but the specificity of HRCT-based diagnosis of NSIP is unknown.[10] NSIP patients have a limited prognosis but, relative to UIP, it is better with a median survival of greater than 10 years.[12] Many show improvement after treatment with corticosteroids.

The histopathological pattern reveals a chronic interstitial pneumonia that lacks the characteristic variegated pattern of UIP. The changes are uniform with a cellular interstitial infiltrate of mononuclear inflammatory cells associated with varying degrees of interstitial fibrosis.[13] NSIP is the

Table 1. Search terms used for preparation of text.

Idiopathic interstitial pneumonias (IIPs)
Idiopathic pulmonary fibrosis (IPF)
Cryptogenic fibrosing alveolitis (CFA)
Usual interstitial pneumonia (UIP)
Non-specific interstitial pneumonia (NSIP)
Desquamative interstitial pneumonia (DIP)
Respiratory bronchiolitis-associated interstitial lung disease (RBILD)
Acute interstitial pneumonia (AIP)
Hamman-Rich syndrome
Fibrosing alveolitis associated with systemic sclerosis (FASSc)
Interstitial lung disease in rheumatoid arthritis
Interstitial lung disease in connective tissue disorders
Corticosteroids
Azathioprine
Cyclophosphamide
Cyclosporin
Methotrexate
Penicillamine
Antioxidants in IPF
N-acetylcysteine
Colchicine
Pirfenidone
Interferon gamma
Reflux in IPF
Lignocaine and cough
Hypoxaemia and CFA
Pulmonary hypertension primary and secondary to lung fibrosis
Iloprost
Phosphodiesterase inhibitors
Nitric oxide
Lung transplantation and IPF
Palliation in IPF

commonest histological pattern of IIP associated with systemic sclerosis.[14]

Desquamative interstitial pneumonia (DIP)

DIP typically affects cigarette smokers in their fourth or fifth decade of life with a subacute (weeks to months) illness characterized by dyspnoea and cough. It is rare, with an incidence <3% of all interstitial lung disease (ILDs). HRCT shows ground-glass attenuation. Clinical recognition of DIP is important because the prognosis is excellent, and it responds to corticosteroid treatment. It rarely progresses to advanced pulmonary fibrosis and has an overall survival of about 70% after 10 years.[2] Lung biopsy reveals uniform, diffuse, intra-alveolar macrophage accumulation.[1] As a consequence, it has been suggested that DIP should be renamed 'acute macrophage pneumonia'.

Respiratory bronchiolitis-associated interstitial lung disease (RBILD)

RBILD typically affects current or former cigarette smokers during the fourth or fifth decades of life.[15] It is a rare condition presenting with cough, breathlessness and sparse crackles on auscultation. HRCT scanning shows mild, diffuse, fine, reticulonodular opacities in a bibasilar distribution. RBILD appears to be a relatively benign and self-limited condition.[16] Smoking cessation is critical.[9]

Histologically, RBILD is defined by the presence of pigmented intraluminal macrophages within first- and second-order respiratory bronchioles. The changes are patchy at low magnification and have a bronchiolocentric distribution, accompanied by a patchy submucosal and peribronchiolar infiltrate of lymphocytes and histiocytes.[16]

Acute interstitial pneumonia (AIP)

AIP (also known as Hamman-Rich syndrome) is a rare, acute, fulminant form of lung injury, usually in a previously healthy individual.[17] Symptoms are primarily confined to the respiratory tract, with the majority reporting cough (≥80%), dyspnoea (≥90%) and a significant minority fever. While the absolute mean symptom duration to presentation is variable, the fact that most present within 60 days of onset of symptoms helps to differentiate it from IPF.[18] Diffuse, bilateral, air space opacification is seen on chest radiograph, and HRCT scans shows mixed areas of ground-glass attenuation and consolidation. AIP is distinguished from acute respiratory distress syndrome (ARDS) clinically by the absence of a known cause and the lack of systemic involvement such as multiorgan failure.[18]

In AIP, the histological pattern is typical of diffuse alveolar damage (DAD), including oedema, hyaline membranes and interstitial acute inflammation.[18] Loose organizing fibrosis is mostly seen within alveolar septa, but it may also be observed within air spaces. The latter pattern may be a prominent feature in more than one-third of cases. Of note, a number of studies have found no correlation between the degree of lung involvement on biopsy, including fibroblastic proliferation and degree of fibrosis, and long-term prognosis.[17,18]

Ventilatory support is invariably required. The recommended treatment is high-dose intravenous corticosteroids, although the benefits of this therapy remain unproven.[17,18] AIP has a poor prognosis. In a recent meta-analysis of data on 82 patients with AIP, there was 74% mortality. If the patient survives, complete recovery is possible, with one study showing that five out of six survivors had normal or improving lung spirometry at 12–24 months.[17] Approximately 25% of cases can recur, progressing to chronic interstitial fibrosis potentially requiring lung transplantation.[17]

In contrast, a recent study on 13 AIP cases reported a much higher survival rate (67%). However, secondary chronic progressive interstitial lung disease was more common than in previous studies.[18] This pattern may be explained by a survivor selection bias, as the centre was referred a number of patients who had already survived initial hospitalization elsewhere.

Fibrosing alveolitis associated with systemic sclerosis (FASSc)

Pulmonary disease occurs more frequently in systemic sclerosis than in any other connective tissue diseases.[19] The most common type of pulmonary manifestation is fibrosing alveolitis, which occurs in approximately 80% of cases.[20] FASSc has a better prognosis than lone CFA.[21] In patients with diffuse, cutaneous, systemic sclerosis and pulmonary disease, the median survival is 78 months.[22] This may be explained by the fact that > 75% of patients with FASSC have a histological diagnosis of NSIP.[23] ILD is seen in both diffuse and limited cutaneous scleroderma, although it usually occurs at an earlier stage and may progress more rapidly in diffuse sclerosis. The most common symptoms of ILD are fatigue, breathlessness on exertion and a dry cough. A pronounced reduction in D_LCO is usually associated with a restrictive pattern on pulmonary function testing.[24] In a study of 64 patients with FASSc, the percentage predicted D_LCO best reflects the extent of disease on CT and should therefore be measured in routine evaluations.[24] In a recent study of 80 biopsy-proven patients with FASSc, mortality increased with decreasing initial forced vital capacity (FVC) and D_LCO levels. Mortality was not influenced by age, sex, smoking status or BAL findings.[23]

Interstitial lung disease in rheumatoid arthritis (RA)

ILD associated with RA is most common in men (M : F = 3 : 1) between 50 and 60 years of age and is most frequently associated with seropositive and erosive joint disease.[25] A study of 36 patients with recent onset rheumatoid disease (joint symptoms <2 years) demonstrated clinically apparent pulmonary involvement in 14% of patients; however, 58% of patients had evidence of ILD on chest X-ray (CXR), HRCT, bronchial lavage or lung physiology.[26] The onset of pulmonary symptoms usually postdates the onset of joint symptoms by up to 5 years. Smoking is an important risk factor for ILD in RA. In a study of 336 RA patients, it was observed that those with a >25 pack–year smoking history were significantly associated with radiographic evidence of ILD.[27] The prognosis and natural history of IIP associated with RA is not precisely defined but, in general, it appears to be better than IPF. However, when hospital admission for pulmonary disease is required, the median survival is limited. In a study of 49 RA patients who required hospitalization for ILD, the median survival was only 3.5 years.[28]

In a HRCT surveillance study of 84 RA patients, heterogeneous changes were identified. Bronchiectasis in the absence of fibrosis occurred in 30% of patients, pulmonary nodules in 22%, subpleural micronodules in 17%, ground-glass attenuation in 14%, non-septal linear attenuation in 18% and honeycombing in 10%.[29] In another HRCT study, bullous emphysema was an additional common finding, occurring in 66% of patients.[30] Histopathologically, a spectrum of findings may be present, including inflammatory disease, a mixed pattern or, more commonly, UIP.[31]

Description of treatment

Management regimens can be considered as follows: disease-modifying therapy, symptomatic control, lung transplantation and palliation.

Disease-modifying therapy

When discussing the treatment of CFA, it is important to acknowledge that no pharmacological therapy to date has been proven to alter or reverse the clinical course of CFA.[9,32] Indeed, the joint statement of the ATS/ERS on CFA believes that therapy is not indicated in all patients. Given the limited success of current therapies, the potential benefits of any treatment may be outweighed by the risk of treatment-related complications. Special consideration should be given before commencing therapy in patients older than 70 years or with comorbidities including extreme obesity, cardiac disease, diabetes mellitus, osteoporosis or very advanced disease.[9]

Anti-inflammatory therapy has been utilized for CFA based around the concept that untreated 'alveolitis' (inflammation of the lower respiratory tract) progresses to pulmonary fibrosis. Treatment regimens traditionally include corticosteroids and cytotoxic agents, alone and in combination. The joint statement of the ATS/ERS advises oral corticosteroids in combination with either oral azathioprine or cyclophosphamide.[9] If therapy is offered to patients, it should be started early, at the first identification of clinical deterioration. Treatment should be continued for at least 6 months, at which time repeat studies should be performed to determine response to therapy. Therapy should be continued at the same doses if the patient has improved or remained stable. If the patient deteriorates, therapy should be altered and consideration given to lung transplantation.[9]

The importance of inflammation in the pathogenesis of CFA has been challenged, and it has been alternatively proposed that the burden of fibroblasts and the presence of viral infection influence disease progression.[33,34] This has led some authors to argue that current anti-inflammatory therapy for CFA provides no benefit and may even be detrimental.[35,36] Consequently, acknowledging the importance of fibroblast activity, antifibrotic therapy is receiving greater attention. For a treatment summary of standard immunosuppressive agents in CFA, see Table 2.

Corticosteroids

There are no randomized controlled trials (RCTs) on the use of corticosteroids in CFA.[32,37] What constitutes the most effective dose and period of treatment is also unknown. Despite this, a dose of 0.5 mg/kg/day for 4 weeks followed by dose reduction to 0.25 mg/kg/day has been recommended as therapy for CFA.[9] The application of corticosteroids is based on a variety of historical reports. In a retrospective analysis of 127 patients who received oral corticosteroid therapy with a follow-up of 4 years, 17% of patients demonstrated an objec-

Table 2. A treatment summary of standard immunosuppressive agents in CFA.

Drug	Dosage	Evidence	Comment	Important side-effects
Corticosteroids (oral)	0.5 mg/kg/day for 4 weeks then 0.25 mg/kg/day[9]	B	A retrospective study[38] and a prospective study[39] showed a response to therapy in 17% and 11% respectively. A trial, particularly in younger patients (<65 years), is recommended	76% insomnia, 73% cushingoid, 61% visual blurring[9]
Azathioprine (oral)	2–3 mg/kg/day to max. 150 mg/day[9,32] in combination with oral corticosteroids	A	A prospective, double-blind, randomized, placebo-controlled study showed a survival benefit at 4 years[41] with combination therapy over corticosteroids, but high mortality within the first year (27%) and female weighting (63%)	Non-specific gastrointestinal. ↑ Bone marrow suppression in thiopurine methytransferase deficiency
Cyclophosphamide (oral)	2 mg/kg/day to max. 150 mg/day[9] in combination with oral corticosteroids	B	A randomized study showed a marginal benefit for oral cyclophosphamide 100 plus low-dose corticosteroids over corticosteroids alone.[42] However, the group on cyclophosphamide had better lung function.	Alopecia, infertility, haemorrhagic cystitis, bone marrow suppression. ↑ risk of malignancy[45]
(intravenous)	500–1800 mg[9] every 2–4 weeks	No evidence	No randomized studies involving IV cyclophosphamide	
Cyclosporin A (oral)	1–7 mg/kg/day pending study[49–52]	C	Has a role as a steroid sparing agent.[49] Two open, non-randomized, small studies (n = 10) suggested a survival benefit,[50,51] and one retrospective study highlighted a possible role in the prevention of exacerbations of CFA[52]	Dose-dependent nephrotoxicity, gingival hypertrophy, hypertension. ↑ risk of malignancy and lymphoproliferative disorders
Methotrexate	No role	No evidence	No published data on therapeutic role[9,32]	Pulmonary toxicity[9,32]
Penicillamine (oral)	125–150 mg/day, gradual ↑ to 500 mg/day	C	Open-label, non-randomized, controlled trials demonstrate little benefit[55,56]	Loss of taste, nephrotoxicity[9]

tive response to treatment.[38] Of note, this study identified a subgroup with an improved survival who were younger patients with a more cellular lung biopsy. In retrospect, these patients may be reclassified as suffering from NSIP. An additional study describes the clinical outcome of patients with DIP and UIP exposed to corticosteroids. Of 40 DIP patients and 53 UIP patients, 66% of the DIP patients responded to corticosteroid therapy compared with only 11% of UIP patients.[39]

Therefore, a trial of corticosteroids may have a role in selecting patients with suspected treatment-responsive disease (DIP, NSIP), particularly younger patients less than 65 years of age.[38] By implication, the majority of patients not responding to corticosteroid therapy may have UIP. These patients are commonly elderly (mean age 65 years), male, have a BAL characterized by an excess of neutrophils and a HRCT with honeycombing, traction bronchiectasis and no ground-glass attenuation.

Side-effects In UIP patients exposed to corticosteroid therapy in line with international guidelines, 76% of these patients complained of insomnia, 73% became cushingoid, while 61% of patients suffered with irritability and blurred vision.[40] Other side-effects include peptic ulcer disease, posterior capsular cataracts, hypertension, hyperglycaemia, hypokalaemia, metabolic alkalosis, secondary adrenal insufficiency, osteoporosis, vertebral compression fractures, aseptic necrosis of femoral/humeral heads and mood disturbances.[9] In view of the significant side-effect profile of corticosteroids, and the lack of documented efficacy in UIP, CFA patients should only be exposed to corticosteroids after careful consideration.

Immunosuppression

Immunosuppressive drugs, alone but largely with corticosteroids, have been employed in the treatment of CFA. These agents include azathioprine, cyclophosphamide, methotrexate and cyclosporin. Most treatments are intended to suppress inflammation, but none has been proven to alter disease progression. There is little good-quality information regarding the efficacy of non-corticosteroid agents in CFA.

Azathioprine ATS and BTS guidelines recommend a dose of 2–3 mg/kg/day to a maximum dose of 150 mg/day.[9,32] The ATS recommends the use of azathioprine in combination with corticosteroids.[9] In a double-blind, randomized, placebo-controlled study, the combination of corticosteroids and azathioprine at 3 mg/kg/day conferred a survival advantage in comparison with those patients receiving oral corticosteroids 20 mg/day[41] in one study. When the survival analysis was adjusted for age, there was a significantly better survival in those patients receiving azathioprine. However, 27% of patients died in the first year, and a difference in survival only became apparent after 4 years of follow-up. We now recognize that survival beyond 3 years is unusual in patients with UIP, and therefore, inadvertently, the prolonged survival associated with azathioprine may reflect the fact that 63% of the azathioprine patients were female. Nevertheless, the trend towards improved survival from a prospective randomized study has resulted in azathioprine and corticosteroids being a recommended form of therapy.

Side-effects The most common side-effects of azathioprine are gastrointestinal (GI) side-effects, including nausea, vomiting and diarrhoea. There is an increased risk of bone marrow suppression in patients who are deficient in thiopurine methyltransferase. Mild thiopurine methyltransferase deficiency occurs in 11% of the general population.

Cyclophosphamide If clinicians consider cyclophosphamide for therapy, current ATS guidelines recommend cyclophosphamide 2 mg/kg/day, maximum of 150 mg/day in combination with corticosteroids.[9] However, no convincing data exist to show a superiority of cyclophosphamide over corticosteroids in treating CFA.[32] No studies have directly compared cyclophosphamide with other immunosuppressive or cytotoxic agents.[42] A randomized study showed a marginal benefit for cyclophosphamide 100 mg daily plus prednisolone 20 mg on alternate days over prednisone 60 mg/day tapering to 20 mg on alternate days alone.[42] These data were widely interpreted as suggesting that cyclophosphamide conferred a significant survival advantage. However, the data were biased in favour of cyclophosphamide. More than 50% of patients receiving cyclosphosphamide had a total lung capacity of >80%

predicted, in contrast to > 50% of patients receiving prednisolone alone having a total lung capacity below 60% of predicted. Fundamentally, there was still no significant difference in survival between the two groups.

Intravenous (IV) 'pulse' cyclophosphamide (dose range 500–1800 mg every 2–4 weeks)[9] is an alternative to oral cyclophosphamide. Results are generally unimpressive. There are no randomized studies involving the use of IV cyclophosphamide. An open non-controlled study[43] reported on 33 patients, 30% of whom died in the first 6 months of the study period. This study demonstrated that IV cyclophosphamide had little impact in patients with progressive disease but facilitated steroid tapering in patients who selected themselves out as having non-progressive disease. In a further retrospective study of 18 patients with progressive CFA treated with intermittent IV cyclophosphamide and oral prednisolone for 1 year, 11 patients were defined as responding to treatment.[44] It should be noted that the vital capacity (VC) was higher at the initiation of therapy in those patients who responded.

Side-effects Cyclophosphamide has a significant side-effects profile. Nausea, alopecia, infertility, haemorrhagic cystitis and bone marrow suppression are common side-effects. The increased risk of malignancy in patients receiving cyclophosphamide[45] is important, especially when CFA patients are inherently at greater risk of the development of lung cancer[46] and are recognized as having increased p53 oncogene expression in pulmonary tissues.[47] Late after lung transplantation, malignant disorders are the second commonest cause of death (15%) in CFA patients.[48] This may reflect the use of cyclophosphamide in CFA patients prior to transplantation.

Cyclosporin Cyclosporin A has occasionally been used in the treatment of CFA.[9,32] However, further studies are required prior to cyclosporin being a recommended form of therapy. Cyclosporin has been advocated as an effective means of facilitating steroid withdrawal or reduction.[49] In a study of 10 patients awaiting lung transplantation receiving high-dose prednisolone (>50 mg/day), giving cyclosporin (4–7 mg/kg/day) achieved cyclosporin levels of 300–400 ng/ml, with a reduction in dose of steroids and a mild improvement in 6-min walk test in five out of 10 patients.[49] Two other open non-randomized studies have reported on the application of cyclosporin in CFA. In a study of 10 patients (five UIP and five NSIP) receiving cyclosporin 3 mg/kg/day for 9 months, all five patients with NSIP and three patients with UIP experienced an improvement in exercise capacity and VC.[50] In once-daily cyclosporin at a dose of 5 mg/kg/day in 10 patients in whom cyclophosphamide therapy failed, there was an improvement in survival of 2.5–5 months in comparison with a matched historical control group of seven patients receiving cyclosporin.[51]

An emerging novel role for cyclosporin in CFA may be the prevention of re-exacerbations and improvement of the patients' chances of long-term survival.[52] A recent study of 13 patients with an acute exacerbation of CFA was analysed retrospectively. All 13 patients received pulse therapy with methylprednisolone (1000 mg/day for 3 days), followed by oral prednisolone (40–60 mg/day). Seven were given cyclosporin (1.0–2.0 mg/kg/day) after the treatment with corticosteroids. Of this group, four patients survived 60, 120, 276 and 208 weeks respectively. All six patients treated without cyclosporin died within 66 weeks of the acute exacerbation, despite the fact that four initially responded to methylprednisolone.

Side-effects Classically, cyclosporin causes a dose-dependent increase in serum creatinine and urea. Common problems include gingival hypertrophy, hypertrichosis, GI disturbances and hypertension and increased incidence of malignancies and lymphoproliferative disorders.

Methotrexate At present, there is no evidence to support its application in CFA. Probably because of its known pulmonary toxicity, published data evaluating methotrexate as a therapy for CFA are lacking.[9,32]

Penicillamine D-penicillamine appears to inhibit collagen deposition by interfering with the intramolecular cross-linking of mature collagen,[53] and may inhibit collagen accumulation in rats following intratracheal bleomycin.[54] Responses to penicillamine have been noted in idiopathic or connective tissue disease-associated pulmonary fibrosis. There are a number of open-label, non-randomized, uncontrolled trials[55,56] and one case series in the literature[57] demonstrating that penicillamine has little or no benefit in CFA, and side-effects appear to be frequent. If initiated, the dose is 125 or 250 mg given orally as a single daily dose, with gradual increments to a final dose of 500 mg/day.

Side-effects Loss of taste, vomiting, stomatitis, nephrotoxicity.[9]

Antioxidant therapy

An increased oxidant burden contributes to tissue remodelling and fibroblast activation in CFA and related pulmonary fibrotic conditions.[58] Consequently, there is interest in the impact of antioxidant therapy in CFA. For a treatment summary of novel/new agents in CFA, see Table 3.

Glutathione (GSH) GSH is a tripeptide that plays a pivotal role in metabolic and cell cycle-related functions in virtually all cells. It directly scavenges free radicals and acts as a co-substrate in GSH peroxidase-catalysed reduction in H_2O_2 and lipid hydroperoxides making it central to the defence against intra- and extracellular oxidative stress.[59] The antioxidant substance glutathione is deficient in the alveolar lining fluid of CFA patients. Recent studies reported a fourfold deficiency of GSH in BAL[58] and induced sputum[60] in CFA. *N*-acetylcysteine (NAC) is a known precursor for glutathione synthesis. A sin-

Table 3. A treatment summary of novel/new agents in CFA.

Drug and dosage	Proposed mechanism	Comment	Important side-effects
N-acetylcysteine (NAC) 600 mg tds[61]	There is a fourfold deficiency in glutathione in CFA.[58,59] NAC a known precursor	A single open-label study was associated with an improvement in lung function[61]	Diarrhoea
Colchicine 0.6 mg od/bd[9,32]	Colchicine *in vitro* inhibits fibroblastic proliferation[64] and collagen formation[62,64]	A small prospective randomized study showed similar efficacy but fewer side-effects with colchicine compared with corticosteroids[66]	57% diarrhoea, 14% muscle cramps[66]
Pirfenidone 40 mg/kg/day[70,71] to a max. dose of 3600 mg/day[70]	Pirfenidone *in vitro* inhibits TGF-β collagen synthesis and fibroblast proliferation[70]	Two open-label studies outline its potential role.[70,71] Data suggest a stabilization of lung function with treatment[70]	64% gastrointestinal, 37% dermatological, 42% fatigue[70]
Interferon gamma (IFN-γ)-1b 200 μg three times weekly[74,76]	IFN-γ inhibits TGF-β gene.[73] CFA patients have reduced levels of IFN-γ in BAL[72]	An open randomized pilot study over 1 year showed a statistically significant 9% improvement in lung capacity.[75] A subsequent large, randomized, double-blind, placebo-controlled study had no effect on pulmonary function, gas exchange or quality of life.[77] IFN-γ may confer a survival advantage in patients with limited disease.[77] However, it may hasten disease progression in advanced CFA[77–79]	Fever, chills, influenza-like illness[77]

gle, 12-week, open-label study of oral NAC 600 mg three times a day in a group of 18 patients with pulmonary fibrosis was associated with a significant improvement in lung function and a subjective improvement in dyspnoea reported by 50% of the patients.[61] Interestingly, the positive effects of NAC treatment were restricted to patients on maintenance immunosuppressive therapy, suggesting that it may have a role as adjunctive therapy. A randomized study has been undertaken using antioxidant therapy, and its results are awaited.

Side-effects NAC is very well tolerated. In the above study, one patient had persistent diarrhoea, three experienced a single episode of diarrhoea and four complained of temporary nausea.[61]

Antifibrotic agents

Colchicine Colchicine, an antimicrotubular agent, inhibits collagen formation[62] and increases collagen degradation[63] by fibroblasts *in vitro*. *In vitro* studies have demonstrated that colchicine is an inhibitor of fibroblast function, particularly fibroblast proliferation.[64] It also suppresses the release of fibronectin from alveolar macrophages isolated from CFA patients.[64] Oral colchicine, 0.6 mg once or twice daily, may be considered as a first-line therapy or for patients refractory to corticosteroids, either alone or in combination with immunosuppressive/cytotoxic agents.[9,32] A study in which colchicine 600 μg/day was administered to 23 patients who had received previous corticosteroid therapy showed that 30% of patients improved, 30% remained stable and 40% of patients worsened.[65] Subsequently, a prospective, randomized study compared 12 subjects treated with prednisolone and 14 patients treated with colchicine. There was no difference in the impact on lung function, but fewer side-effects were identified in the colchicine group.[66]

Side-effects At the proposed dosage regimen, 57% of patients had diarrhoea, 21% nausea and proteinuria and 14% muscle cramps.[66]

Pirfenidone Pirfenidone is a pyridone molecule that inhibits transforming growth factor β (TGF-β)-stimulated collagen synthesis, decreases the extracellular matrix and blocks fibroblast proliferation *in vitro*.[67] Animal model studies have shown that pirfenidone ameliorates bleomycin-induced[68] and amiodarone-induced pulmonary fibrosis.[69] Two open-label studies have highlighted its potential role in advanced CFA.[70,71] A study in 54 patients with CFA administered oral pirfenidone from 40 mg/kg/day starting dose to a maximum dose of 3600 mg/day over 15 days of follow-up suggests that it may facilitate the stabilization of lung function.[70] Patients whose lung function had deteriorated prior to enrolment appeared to stabilize after beginning treatment. Conventional therapy was discontinued in 38 out of 46 patients: the other

eight were able to decrease their prednisolone dosage. Eight had no previous therapy. One- and 2-year survival was 78% and 63% respectively.[70] Further studies are required of this potentially important compound.

Side-effects The drug was reasonably well tolerated. Gastrointestinal side-effects are the most common at 64% (nausea 44%, anorexia 13%, abdominal bloating 11%), and dermatological problems are also prevalent 37% (photosensitivity 24%, itch 9%). Fatigue was seen in 42%.[70]

Interferon gamma-1b Interferon gamma (IFN-γ)-1b is a potential therapeutic compound for the treatment of CFA. CFA patients have reduced levels of IFN-γ in BAL compared with control subjects.[72] It is believed that an imbalance between IFN-γ and TGF-β in IPF may contribute to the disease process. IFN-γ inhibits transcription of the TGF-β gene and inhibits TGF-β-induced gene expression through the induction of Smad7, an intracellular signalling molecule.[73] Activation of Smad7 may be a crucial mediator of IFN-γ antifibrotic activity as transient overexpression of Smad7 *in vivo* attenuates bleomycin-induced fibrosis.[74] In an open randomized pilot study, patients receiving IFN-γ demonstrated a statistically significant 9% improvement in total lung capacity over 1 year and a reduction in TGF-β expression in tissue obtained by serial transbronchial biopsy.[75] In this study, nine IPF patients received subcutaneous IFN-γ 200 μg three times a week with 7.5 mg of oral corticosteroids per day, and nine patients received a symptom-driven schedule of oral corticosteroids. The CFA patients were carefully selected on the basis of two criteria: first, a failure to respond to steroids over 1 year and, secondly, histological evidence of UIP acquired by open lung biopsy. When interpreting the data, important factors need to be considered. The steroid-only group, who clearly had steroid-unresponsive disease, were exposed to ongoing oral corticosteroids, potentially worsening lung function by increasing body mass or possibly promoting Epstein–Barr virus replication.[76] It is unclear how representative the cohort was of CFA in general. Also, a subsequent independent review suggested that two of the interferon group did not suffer from CFA. Furthermore, patients with a total lung capacity of <45% of the predicted normal value were excluded. The group consisted of non-smokers. While 15 of the 18 patients had surgical biopsies with findings consistent with UIP, the remaining three had transbronchial biopsies, which are inadequate for the diagnosis of most diffuse lung diseases, especially for distinguishing UIP from NSIP. Also, all patients in both groups were alive 3 years after the study began, which is unusual for CFA.

New data from a large, randomized, multinational, double-blind, placebo-controlled trial of IFN-γ 1b in 330 IPF patients followed up for a median of 58 weeks have been reported.[77] A total of 162 CFA patients were treated with IFN-γ 100 μg subcutaneously three times weekly for the first 2 weeks, increased to IFN-γ 200 µg subcutaneously three times weekly, and 168 with placebo. There was no statistically significant advantage to the IFN-γ group as determined by the primary endpoints of death or disease progression (≥10% fall in %predicted FVC or ≥ 5 mmHg increase in alveolar to arterial (A–a) oxygen gradient from baseline) and the secondary endpoint including lung function, gas exchange or quality of life.[77] Post hoc subgroup analysis showed a statistically significant benefit in the group with limited disease (baseline FVC > 62% of the predicted value) with death occurring in 4% of the IFN-γ group compared with 12% of the placebo group. This suggests that therapy with IFN-γ in patients with limited disease may confer a survival advantage.[77] In contrast, if IFN-γ is administered to patients with advanced disease, there is a suggestion that treatment may hasten disease progression. This has been suggested by two small cohort studies in which adverse outcomes were associated with the administration of IFN-γ.[78,79]

Side-effects Fever, chills, headache and influenza-like illness are common but usually subside within the first 4 weeks. Paracetamol and ibuprofen can control these side-effects.[77]

Symptom control

The treatment of CFA includes the management of the concurrent pulmonary problems associated with advanced CFA. These include reflux oesophagitis, cough, hypoxaemia and pulmonary hypertension. The following outlines the management of these conditions, summarized in Table 4.

Reflux oesophagitis

CFA patients have a significantly increased incidence of acid reflux in comparison with control subjects. In a study of 17 CFA patients, 16 had acid reflux. Very importantly, only 25%

of these were symptomatic.[80] Interim data from an ongoing prospective study of 65 CFA patients indicate a prevalence of 95% (*P* = 0.01), with only 40% of patients reporting symptoms.[81] No significant difference in pulmonary function tests was found between patients with and without gastro-oesophageal reflux (GOR). Some centres are recommending 24-hour oesophageal monitoring as part of the basic workup for patients with CFA, and those patients positive for GOR are treated for 6 weeks with a proton pump inhibitor and re-evaluated.

Cough

Cough is a major problem in CFA patients. There are no data in the literature as to what is the best management strategy for this problem. Inhaled beclomethasone, which is administered using the hydrofluoroalkane (HFA) propellant in order to achieve small airway distribution, may offer relief to some individuals. In the context of cough, treatment of reflux oesophagitis with proton pump inhibitors is vital. Nebulized lignocaine and nebulized narcotic therapy do not substantially ameliorate the symptoms.[82]

Hypoxaemia

Formerly, it had been hypothesized that oxygen might facilitate disease progression by promoting oxygen free radical lung tissue damage. This was refuted in a multivariate analysis demonstrating that oxygen therapy was not associated with a decline in clinical status in CFA.[83] Indeed, oxygen therapy is beneficial for patients with pulmonary hypertension secondary to pulmonary fibrosis. An acute oxygen challenge significantly reduces the mean pulmonary artery pressure. Patients with nocturnal hypoxemia have impaired daytime quality of life scores. Nocturnal oxygen therapy attenuates the daytime

Table 4. A symptom control treatment summary in CFA.

Symptom	Treatment	Evidence	Comment
Reflux	Proton pump inhibitor	B	A 95% prevalence in an ongoing prospective study of CFA[81]
Cough	Inhaled beclamethasone	C	A recent Cochrane report showed that nebulized lignocaine and narcotic therapy does not substantially reduce symptoms[82]
Hypoxaemia	Titrated O_2	B	In a retrospective study, O_2 was not associated with a better or worse outcome.[83] Nocturnal O_2 attenuates daytime symptoms and improves QoL scores in nocturnal hypoxaemia[84]
Pulmonary hypertension	Iloprost	B	In an acute challenge, nebulized iloprost significantly reduced pulmonary artery pressure in eight patients with CFA[86]
	Sildenafil	B	Adjunctive sildenafil in 14 patients unresponsive to inhaled iloprost reversed clinical deterioration and increased 6-min walking test[91]
	Nitric oxide (NO)	C	Isolated case reports exist of inhaled NO in CFA. However, it is limited by the lack of suitable delivery systems[93,95]

symptoms and improves quality of life.[84] In prescribing oxygen therapy, both the concentration and the flow should be considered. It is reasonable to titrate the oxygen therapy according to resting oxygen saturations, but it must be remembered that additional oxygen is required immediately following exercise and coughing in order to correct for deficits. For instance, an additional cylinder delivering a higher flow of oxygen should be available at the top of the stairs.

Side-effects Predominantly local irritation and epistaxis caused by cold, dry oxygen. To overcome this problem, an alternative method for oxygen delivery is the transtracheal route, although this method is not widely applied. Complications include mucous plugging, local infection and potentiating the patient's existing cough.

Pulmonary hypertension
Pulmonary hypertension is an important but late complication of CFA. Aetiology is multifactorial including: hypoxaemia (see oxygen therapy section), architectural disruption of the arterial bed by fibrosis (see immunomodulatory therapy section), imbalance of vasomotor tone and *in situ* arteriolar thrombosis.

Iloprost Iloprost is a stable analogue of prostacyclin that is associated with a prolonged duration of vasodilation,[85] its effects lasting for 30–90 min. In an acute challenge study of eight patients with pulmonary hypertension secondary to lung fibrosis, nebulized iloprost (total nebulized dose 54–68 μg) significantly reduced pulmonary artery pressures without augmenting the pulmonary shunt.[86]

While this study primarily addressed the acute benefits of nebulized iloprost, long-term therapy in one patient with a total daily dose of 135 μg of iloprost showed an improvement in clinical state over the subsequent 18 months.[86] Exercise tolerance increased and, after 12 months, a 6-min walk test improved from 240 m before to 314 m just after inhalation of iloprost.

Side-effects Flushing (26.7%) and jaw pain (11.9%) are documented, but these were mild and mostly transient. Syncope has been documented as a serious adverse event in one study, occurring in 5% of patients; however, it occurred with similar frequencies in both iloprost and placebo groups and of note was not associated with a clinical deterioration.[85] Overshooting 'rebound' pulmonary hypertension does not occur.[87] Compliance may be a problem as daily inhalations of iloprost need to be nebulized every 3 hours, and a specific ultrasonic nebulizer, which achieves particles of less than 3 μg, is recommended.[88]

Oral phosphodiesterase (PDE) inhibitors Recent reports have described a role for PDE inhibitors in the treatment of second-ary pulmonary hypertension. Phosphodiesterases in lung tissue inhibit second-line messengers of prostacyclin and nitric oxide (cyclic adenosine monophosphate and cyclic guanosine monophosphate).[89]

In a study of 16 individuals with pulmonary hypertension specifically secondary to lung fibrosis, oral sildenafil (50 mg) reduced the pulmonary vascular resistance index [–32.5%, 95% confidence interval (CI) –10.2 to 54.1] and maintained V/Q matching (3.3%, 95% CI 0.0–11.3; 0.0%, 95% CI 0.0–12.4), with raised arterial partial pressure of oxygen (14.3 mmHg, 95% CI –1.7 to 31.3).[90]

The benefits of long-term adjunct oral sildenafil therapy in pulmonary hypertension have been shown in two recent studies on patient cohorts with both primary and secondary pulmonary hypertension.[91,92] In 14 patients unresponsive to long-term inhaled iloprost therapy, the commencement of adjunctive sildenafil significantly reversed clinical deterioration and increased 6-min walk test from 256 ± 30 m to 346 ± 26 m at 3 months, with a sustained efficacy up to 12 months.[91]

Nitric oxide (NO) Inhalation of NO in CFA patients with secondary pulmonary hypertension leads to a significant fall in pulmonary artery pressure.[93] NO is strictly pulmonary vessel selective owing to its immediate inactivation by binding haemoglobin on entering the intravascular space. The therapeutic application of NO is potentially limited by the lack of availability of suitable continuous delivery systems for outpatients given its very short half-life, and owing to possible rebound pulmonary hypertensive crisis[94] on abrupt cessation of the gas flow. A recent report described the chronic application of NO to a CFA patient as a bridge to lung transplantation.[95]

Lung transplantation
Lung transplantation should be considered for those who experience progressive disease.[9,32] Lung transplantation for CFA has been shown to confer an improved survival compared with patients remaining on the waiting list.[48] Recent data on 46 CFA patients accepted for lung transplantation during a 12-year period showed that lung transplantation reduced the risk of death by 75%.[96] The survival after lung transplantation was 80% at 1 year and 60% at 5 years.

Currently, international recommendations suggest that lung transplantation should be restricted to patients less than 60 years of age. This potentially limits access to transplantation to patients suffering with CFA. Increasingly, programmes are considering CFA patients up to the age of 70 years. However, such patients should have no other relative contraindications to transplantation.

A limited window for transplantation of just 22 months exists, reflected by the fact that CFA patients still have the highest death rate while awaiting lung transplantation.[48] Of note, in a study of 46 CFA patients awaiting lung transplantation, 16 died on the waiting list.[96] The expected median survival is

34 months after the diagnosis of CFA, and the mean waiting list for transplantation is 12 months in the UK.

International guidelines from 1998 recommend that symptomatic patients with CFA younger than 65 years of age should be discussed with the transplant centre after a failed trial of corticosteroid therapy and referred in any of the following circumstances: $D_LCO < 50–60\%$; FVC < 60–70%; resting hypoxia or pulmonary hypertension.[97] A recent study has shown that 2-year survival can be best estimated in CFA patients utilizing D_LCO percentage predicted and HRCT fibrosis score. In a study of 115 CFA patients less than 65 years of age, a D_LCO of less than 40% of predicted combined with a HRCT fibrosis score of greater than 2 has a sensitivity and specificity of 80% in predicting 2-year survival.[98] Essentially, early referral for transplantation is critical and is recommended in patients whose D_LCO is < 40% predicted.

Palliation

Palliation involves avoiding unnecessary immunosuppression, dose reduction or drug withdrawal. It has particular application in patients who have failed to show a response to medical therapy.[36] Such patients are commonly elderly, males, with an excess of neutrophils in the BAL and a HRCT with honeycombing, traction bronchiectasis and no ground-glass attenuation. Indeed, much of the data support a strategy of drug withdrawal or dose reduction. One study showed that low-dose corticosteroid therapy was as effective as high-dose steroid therapy, and the addition of cyclophosphamide failed to improve survival.[42] Colchicine may be a less hazardous alternative to prednisolone in the treatment of patients with UIP.[99] There is no indication for mechanical ventilation in CFA patients. The outcome of CFA patients receiving mechanical ventilation is dismal.[100,101] Significant ventilatory pressure support is required for oxygenation, and barotrauma manifesting in pneumothorax is inevitable. Furthermore, the need for pressure support inevitably results in impaired cardiac output and multiorgan failure.

Clinical surveillance to predict prognosis and anticipate the need for palliation is vitally important. The symptoms of distressing breathlessness, cough and pain also result in fear and anxiety. Addressing each symptom and explaining the type of therapy available for alleviating each individual symptom is very important. Emphasizing that the patient's wishes are the key factor in determining what form of therapy can be offered is important.

Adequate flows of oxygen are important when dealing with breathlessness. Opiates are indicated for distressing breathlessness and should be administered according to local policies and guidelines. Attention should be given to opiate-induced side-effects, in particular nausea and constipation. Anxiolytic therapy including midazolam should be combined with the opiates in order to prevent disinhibition or euphoria. Occasionally, a patient may wish to die at home, in which case every effort should be made to accommodate this wish.

Gentle, compassionate and transparent discussion regarding death is essential. Clearly, individual patients approach their illness in a unique fashion, and this must be respected when introducing discussion regarding death. It is very important that clear and open discussion occurs among the multidisciplinary team caring for the patient. This must be undertaken regularly so that the patient and their family do not perceive that there is any confusion regarding the terminal care. In particular, resuscitation orders should be clearly documented with the knowledge of the patient and relatives.

Summary for clinicians

CFA is the commonest subgroup of the IIPs, accounting for 65% of all cases and synonymous with the histopathological pattern of UIP.

The prevalence is 20–30 per 100 000, with men twice as likely to be affected. A clinical and radiological evaluation is usually diagnostic.

At diagnosis, the mean age is 65 years and median survival 2.9 years. Older age (> 65 years), male sex, honeycombing and traction bronchiectasis on HRCT, neutrophils or eosinophils > 5% on BAL are markers of limited survival.

No pharmacological therapy to date has been proven to alter or reverse the clinical course of CFA. Treatment is not offered to all patients. It may be outweighed by treatment-associated complications. Careful consideration should be given to patients over 70 years old or with comorbidities. When offered, treatment should be given early at the first sign of lung impairment or deterioration.

First-line therapy should be oral corticosteroids in combination with either oral azathioprine or cyclophosphamide, continued for at least 6 months. If the patient improves or stabilizes, continue therapy at the same doses. Lung transplantation should be considered for those with progressive disease.

Treat concurrent problems including reflux, cough, hypoxaemia and pulmonary hypertension as appropriate.

Anticipate the need for palliation. Avoid unnecessary immunosuppression. Treat any distressing symptoms. Compassionate and transparent discussion is essential regarding death. Mechanical ventilation is not indicated in CFA.

References

1 American Thoracic Society/European Respiratory Society. International multidisciplinary consensus classification of the idiopathic interstitial pneumonias. *Am J Respir Crit Care Med* 2002; **165**:277–304.

2 Bjoraker JA, Ryu J, Edwin MK *et al*. Prognostic significance of histologic subsets in idiopathic pulmonary fibrosis. *Am J Respir Crit Care Med* 1998; **157**:199–203.

3 Katzenstein AA, Myers JL. Idiopathic pulmonary fibrosis, clinical relevance of pathologic classification. *Am J Respir Crit Care Med* 1998; **157**:1301–15.

4 Coultas DB, Zumwalt ZE, Black WC, Sobonya RE. The epidemiology of interstitial lung diseases. *Am J Respir Crit Care Med* 1994; **150**:967–72.

5 Raghu G, Mageto YN, Lockhart D, Schmidt RA, Wood DE, Godwin JD. The accuracy of the clinical diagnosis of new-onset idiopathic pulmonary fibrosis and other interstitial lung disease: a prospective study. *Chest* 1999; **116**:1168–74.

6 Utz JP, Ryu JH, Douglas WW *et al*. High short-term mortality following lung biopsy for usual interstitial pneumonia. *Eur Respir J* 2001; **17**:175–9.

7 Schwartz DA, Helmers RA, Galvin JR *et al*. Determinants of survival in idiopathic pulmonary fibrosis. *Am J Respir Crit Care Med* 1994; **149**:450–4.

8 Panos RJ, Mortenson RL, Niccoli SA, King TE Jr. Clinical deterioration in patients with idiopathic pulmonary fibrosis: causes and assessment. *Am J Med* 1990; **88**:396–404.

9 American Thoracic Society. Idiopathic pulmonary fibrosis: diagnosis and treatment. International consensus statement. American Thoracic Society (ATS), and the European Respiratory Society (ERS). *Am J Respir Crit Care Med* 2000; **161**:646–64.

10 Park JS, Lee KS, Kim JS *et al*. Nonspecific interstitial pneumonia with fibrosis: radiographic and CT findings in seven patients. *Radiology* 1995; **195**:645–8.

11 Scadding JG, Hinson KFW. Diffuse fibrosing alveolitis (diffuse interstitial fibrosis of the lungs): correlation with histology of biopsy with prognosis. *Thorax* 1967; **22**:291–304.

12 Daniil ZD, Gilchrist FC, Nicholson AG *et al*. A histologic pattern of nonspecific interstitial pneumonia is associated with a better prognosis than usual interstitial pneumonia in patients with cryptogenic fibrosing alveolitis. *Am J Respir Crit Care Med* 1999; **160**:899–905.

13 Katzenstein AL, Fiorelli RF. Nonspecific interstitial pneumonia/fibrosis: histologic features and clinical significance. *Am J Surg Pathol* 1994; **18**:136–47.

14 Fugita J, Yoshinouchi T, Ohtsuki Y *et al*. Non-specific interstitial pneumonia as pulmonary involvement of systemic sclerosis. *Ann Rheum Dis* 2001; **60**:281–3.

15 Myers JL. Respiratory bronchiolitis associated interstitial lung disease. In: Epler GR, ed. *Diseases of the Bronchioles*. New York, Raven Press, 1994.

16 Nicholson AG, Colby TV, du Bois RM, Hansell DM, Wells AU. The prognostic significance of the histologic pattern of interstitial pneumonia in patients presenting with the clinical entity of cryptogenic fibrosing alveolitis. *Am J Respir Crit Care Med* 2000; **162**:2213–17.

17 Olsen J, Colby T, Elliott C. Hamman-Rich syndrome revisited. *Mayo Clin Proc* 1990; **65**:1538–48.

18 Vourlekis JS, Brown KK, Cool CD *et al*. Acute interstitial pneumonitis. Case series and review of the literature. *Medicine* 2000; **79**: 369–78.

19 Minai OA, Dweik RA, Arroliga AC. Manifestations of scleroderma pulmonary disease. *Clin Chest Med* 1998; **19**:713–31.

20 Arroliga AC, Podel DN, Mathay RA. Pulmonary manifestations of scleroderma. *J Thorac Imaging* 1992; **7**:30–45.

21 Wells Au, Hansell DM, Rubens MB, Cailes JB, Black CM, du Bois RM. Functional impairment in lone cryptogenic fibrosing alveolitis and fibrosing alveolitis associated with systemic sclerosis: a comparison. *Am J Respir Crit Care Med* 1997; **155**:1657–64.

22 Altman RD, Medsger TA Jr, Bloch DA, Michel BA. Predictors of survival in systemic sclerosis (scleroderma). *Arthritis Rheum* 1991; **34**:403–13.

23 Bouros D, Wells AU, Nicholson AG *et al*. Histopathologic subsets of fibrosing alveolitis in patients with systemic sclerosis and their relationship to outcome. *Am J Respir Crit Care Med* 2002; **165**:1581–6.

24 Wells AU, Hansell DM, Rubens MB *et al*. Fibrosing alveolitis in systemic sclerosis. Indices of lung function in relation to extent of disease on computed tomography. *Arthritis Rheum* 1997; **40**:1229–36.

25 Hunninghake GW, Fauci AS. Pulmonary involvement in collagen vascular diseases. *Am Rev Respir Dis* 1979; **119**:471–503.

26 Gabbay E, Tarala R, Will R *et al*. Interstitial lung disease in recent onset rheumatoid arthritis. *Am J Respir Crit Care Med* 1997; **156**:528–35.

27 Saag KG, Kolluri S, Koehnke RK *et al*. Rheumatoid arthritis lung disease: determinants of radiographic and physiologic abnormalities. *Arthritis Rheum* 1996; **39**:1711–19.

28 Hakala M. Poor prognosis in patients with rheumatoid arthritis hospitalized for interstitial lung fibrosis. *Chest* 1988; **93**:114–18.

29 Remy-Jardin M, Remy J, Cortet B, Mauri F, Delcambre B. Lung changes in rheumatoid arthritis: CT findings. *Radiology* 1994; **193**:375–82.

30 Dawson JK, Fewins HE, Desmond J, Lynch MP, Graham DR. Fibrosing alveolitis in patients with rheumatoid arthritis as assessed by high resolution computed tomography, chest radiography, and pulmonary function tests. *Thorax* 2001; **56**:622–7.

31 Yousem SA, Colby TV, Carrington CB. Lung biopsy in rheumatoid arthritis. *Am Rev Respir Dis* 1985; **131**:770–7.

32 The Diffuse Parenchymal Lung Disease Group of the British Thoracic Society. The diagnosis, assessment and treatment of diffuse parenchymal lung disease in adults. *Thorax* 1999: **54**(Suppl 1).

33 King TE Jr, Schwarz MI, Brown K *et al*. Idiopathic pulmonary fibrosis: relationship between histopathologic features and mortality. *Am J Respir Crit Care Med* 2001; **164**:1025–32.

34 Selman M, King TE, Pardo A. Idiopathic pulmonary fibrosis: prevailing and evolving hypotheses about its pathogenesis and implications for therapy. *Ann Intern Med* 2001; **134**:136–51.

35 Gross TJ, Hunninghake GW. Idiopathic pulmonary fibrosis. *N Engl J Med* 2001; **345**: 517–25.

36 Egan JJ. Pharmacologic therapy of idiopathic pulmonary fibrosis. *J Heart Lung Transplant* 1998; **17**:1039–44.

37 Richeldi L, Davies HR, Ferrara G, Franco F. Corticosteroids for idiopathic pulmonary fibrosis (Cochrane Review). In: *The Cochrane Library*, Issue 3, 2003.

38 Turner-Warwick M, Burrows B, Johnson A. Cryptogenic fibrosing alveolitis: response to corticosteroid treatment and its effect on survival. *Thorax* 1980; **35**:593–9.

39 Carrington CB, Gaensler EA, Coutu RE, FitzGerald MX, Gupta RG. Natural history and treated course of usual and desquamative interstitial pneumonia. *N Engl J Med* 1978; **298**:801–9.

40 Flaherty KR, Toews GB, Lynch JP *et al*. Steroids in idiopathic pulmonary fibrosis: a prospective assessment of adverse reactions, response to therapy, and survival. *Am J Med* 2001; **110**:278–82.

41 Raghu G, Depaso WJ, Cain K *et al*. Azathioprine combined with prednisolone in the treatment of idiopathic pulmonary fibrosis: a prospective, double-blind randomised, placebo-controlled clinical trial. *Am Rev Respir Dis* 1991; **144**:291–6.

42 Johnson MA, Kwan S, Snell NJC, Nunn AJ, Darbyshire JH, Turner-Warwick M. Randomised controlled trial comparing prednisolone alone with cyclophosphamide and low dose prednisolone in combination in cryptogenic fibrosing alveolitis. *Thorax* 1989; **44**:280–8.

43 Baughman RP, Lower EE. Use of intermittent, intravenous cyclophosphamide for idiopathic pulmonary fibrosis. *Chest* 1992; **102**:1090–4.

44 Kolb M, Kirschner J, Riedel W, Wirtz H, Schmidt M. Cyclophosphamide pulse therapy in idiopathic pulmonary fibrosis. *Eur Respir J* 1998; **12**:1409–14.

45 Hoffman GS, Kerr GS, Leavitt RY *et al*. Wegeners granulomatosis: an analysis of 158 patients. *Ann Intern Med* 1992; **116**:488–98.

46 Turner-Warwick M, Lebowit M, Burrows B, Johnson A. Cryptogenic fibrosing alveolitis and lung cancer. *Thorax* 1980; **35**:496–9.

47 Kuwano K, Kunitake R, Kawasaki M *et al*. P21 WAFI/CIPI/SD11 and p53 expression in association with DNA strand breaks in idiopathic pulmonary fibrosis. *Am J Respir Crit Care Med* 1996; **154**:477–83.

48 Hosenpud JD, Bennett LE, Keck BM, Edwards EB, Novick RJ. Effect

of diagnosis on survival benefit of lung transplantation for end-stage lung disease. *Lancet* 1998; **351**:24–7.

49 Venuta F, Rendina EA, Ciriaco P *et al.* Efficacy of cyclosporine to reduce steroids in patients with idiopathic pulmonary fibrosis before lung transplantation. *J Heart Lung Transplant* 1993; **12**:909–14.

50 Moolman JA, Bardin PG, Roussouw DJ, Joubert JR. Cyclosporin as a treatment for interstitial lung disease of unknown etiology. *Thorax* 1991; **46**:592–5.

51 Alton EWF, Johnson M, Turner-Warwick M. Advanced cryptogenic fibrosing alveolitis: preliminary report on treatment with cyclosporine A. *Respir Med* 1989; **83**:277–9.

52 Inase N, Sawada M, Ohtani Y *et al.* Cyclosporin A followed by the treatment of acute exacerbation of idiopathic pulmonary fibrosis with corticosteroid. *Intern Med* 2003; **42**:565–70.

53 Herbert CM, Lindberg KA, Jayson MI *et al.* Biosynthesis and maturation of skin collagen in scleroderma, and effect of D-penicillamine. *Lancet* 1974; **1**:187–92.

54 Geismar LS, Hennessey S, Reiser KM *et al.* D-penicillamine prevents collagen accumulation in lungs of rats given bleomycin. *Chest* 1986; **89**:153S–154S.

55 Chapela R, Zuniga G, Selman M. D-penicillamine in the therapy of fibrotic lung diseases. *Int J Clin Pharmacol Ther Toxicol* 1986; **24**:16–17.

56 Selman M, Carrillo G, Salas J *et al.* Colchicine, D-penicillamine and prednisolone in the treatment of idiopathic pulmonary fibrosis. *Chest* 1998; **114**:507–12.

57 Liebetrau G, Pielesch W, Ganguin HG, Jung A, Jung H. Die therapie der lungenfibrosen mit D-penizillamin. *Z Ges Inn Med* 1982; **37**: 263–6.

58 Cantin AM, Hubbard RC, Crystal RG. Glutathione deficiency in the epithelial lining fluid of the lower respiratory tract in idiopathic pulmonary fibrosis. *Am Rev Respir Dis* 1989; **139**:370–2.

59 Davis WB, Pacht ER. Extracellular antioxidant defenses. In: Crystal RG, West JB, eds. *The Lung. Scientific Foundations*. New York, Raven Press, 1991.

60 Beeh KM, Beier J, Haas IC, Kornmann O, Mocke P, Buhl R. Glutathione deficiency of lower respiratory in patients with idiopathic pulmonary fibrosis. *Eur Respir J* 2002; **19**:1119–23.

61 Behr J, Maier K, Degenkolb B, Krombach F, Vogelmeier C. Antioxidative and clinical effects of high-dose N-acetylcysteine in fibrosing alveolitis. Adjunctive therapy to maintenance immunosuppression. *Am J Respir Crit Care Med* 1997; **156**:1897–901.

62 Mansour MM, Dunn MA, Salah LA. Effect of colchicine on collagen synthesis by liver fibroblasts in murine schistosomiasis. *Clin Chim Acta* 1988; **177**:11–20.

63 Bauer EA, Valle KJ. Colchicine-induced modulation of collagenase in human skin fibroblast cultures. I. Stimulation of enzyme synthesis in normal cells. *J Invest Dermatol* 1982; **79**:398–402.

64 Rennard SI, Bitterman PB, Ozaki T, Rom WN, Crystal RG. Colchicine suppresses the release of fibroblast growth factors from alveolar macrophages *in vitro*. *Am Rev Respir Dis* 1988; **137**:181–5.

65 Peters SG, McDougall JC, Douglas WW, Coles DT, DeRemee RA. Colchicine in the treatment of pulmonary fibrosis. *Chest* 1993; **103**:101–4.

66 Douglas WW, Ryu JH, Swensen SJ *et al.* Colchicine versus prednisolone in the treatment of idiopathic pulmonary fibrosis. *Am J Respir Crit Care Med* 1998; **158**:220–5.

67 Lurton JM, Trejo T, Narayanan AS, Raghu G. Pirfenidone inhibits the stimulatory effects of profibrotic cytokines on human lung fibroblasts *in vitro* (abstract). *Am J Respir Crit Care Med* 1996; **153**:A403.

68 Iyer SN, Wild JS, Schiedt MJ, Hyde DM, Margolin SB, Giri SN. Dietary intake of pirfenidone ameliorates bleomycin-induced fibrosis in hamsters. *J Lab Clin Med* 1995; **125**:779–85.

69 Card JW, Racz WJ, Brien JF, Margolin SB, Massey TE. Differential effects of pirfenidone on acute pulmonary injury and ensuing fibrosis in the hamster model of amiodarone-induced pulmonary toxicity. *Toxicol Sci* 2003; **75**:169–80.

70 Raghu G, Johnson WC, Lockhart D, Mageto Y. Treatment of idiopathic pulmonary fibrosis with a new antifibrotic agent, perfenidone. *Am J Respir Crit Care Med* 1999; **159**:1061–9.

71 Nagai S, Hamada K, Shigematsu M, Taniyama M, Yamauchi S, Izumi T. Open-label compassionate use one year-treatment with pirfenidone to patients with chronic pulmonary fibrosis. *Intern Med* 2002; **41**:1118–23.

72 Prior C, Haslam CM. *In vivo* levels and *in vitro* production of interferon-gamma in fibrosing interstitial lung diseases. *Clin Exp Immunol* 1992; **88**:280–7.

73 Ulloa L, Doody J, Massague J. Inhibition of transforming growth factor-β/SMAD signalling by the interferon-gamma/STAT pathway. *Nature* 1999; **397**:710–13.

74 Nakao A, Fujii M, Matsumura R *et al.* Transient gene transfer and expression of Smad7 prevents bleomycin-induced lung fibrosis in mice. *J Clin Invest* 1999; **104**:5–11.

75 Ziesche R, Hofbauer E, Wittmann K, Petkov V, Block LH. A preliminary study of long-term treatment with interferon-gamma-1b and low dose prednisolone in patients with idiopathic pulmonary fibrosis. *N Engl J Med* 1999; **341**:1246–9.

76 Stewart JP, Egan JJ, Haselton PS, Lok S, Nash AA, Woodcock AA. The detection of EBV DNA in lung biopsy specimens from patients with idiopathic pulmonary fibrosis. *Am J Respir Crit Care Med* 1999; **159**:1336–41.

77 Raghu G, Brown K, Bradford W *et al.* Idiopathic Pulmonary Fibrosis Study Group. A placebo-controlled trial of interferon gamma-1b in patients with idiopathic pulmonary fibrosis. *N Engl J Med* 2004; **350**:125–33.

78 Honore I, Nunes H, Groussard O *et al.* Acute respiratory failure after interferon-gamma therapy of end-stage pulmonary fibrosis. *Am J Respir Crit Care Med* 2003; **167**:953–7.

79 Prasse A, Müller K-M, Kurz C, Hamm H, Virchow JC Jr. Does interferon-γ improve pulmonary function in idiopathic pulmonary fibrosis? *Eur Resp J* 2003; **22**: 906–11.

80 Tobin RW, Pope CE, Pellefrini CA, Emond MJ, Sillery J, Raghu G. Increased prevalence of gastroesophageal reflux in patients with idiopathic pulmonary fibrosis. *Am J Respir Crit Care Med* 1998; **158**:1804–8.

81 Raghu G. The role of gastroesophageal reflux in idiopathic pulmonary fibrosis. *Am J Med* 2003; **115**(Suppl 3A):60S–64S.

82 Polosa R, Simidchiev A, Walters EH. Nebulised morphine for severe interstitial lung disease (Cochrane Review). In: *The Cochrane Library*, Issue 3, 2003.

83 Douglas WW, Ryu JH, Schroeder DR. Idiopathic pulmonary fibrosis: impact of oxygen and colchicine, prednisolone or no therapy on survival. *Am J Respir Crit Care Med* 2000; **161**:1172–8.

84 Clark M, Cooper B, Singh S, Cooper M, Carr N, Hubbard R. A survey of nocturnal hypoxaemia and health related quality of life in patients with cryptogenic fibrosing alveolitis. *Thorax* 2001; **56**:482–6.

85 Olschewski H, Simonneau G, Galie N *et al.* Aerosolized Iloprost Randomized Study Group. Inhaled iloprost for severe pulmonary hypertension. *N Engl J Med* 2002; **347**:322–9.

86 Olschewski H, Ghofrani HA, Walmrath D *et al.* Inhaled prostacyclin and ilioprost in severe pulmonary hypertension secondary to lung fibrosis. *Am J Respir Crit Care Med* 1999; **160**:600–7.

87 Olschewski H, Walmrath D, Schermuly R, Ghofrani HA, Grimminger F, Seeger W. Aerosolized prostacyclin and iloprost in severe pulmonary hypertension. *Ann Intern Med* 1996; **125**:820–4.

88 Gessler T, Schmehl T, Hoeper M *et al.* Ultrasonic versus jet nebuliza-

tion of iloprost in severe pulmonary hypertension. *Eur Resp J* 2001; **17**:14–19.

89 Beavo JA. Cyclic nucleotide phophodiesterases: functional implications of multiple isoforms. *Physiol Rev* 1995; **75**:725–48.

90 Ghofrani HA, Wiedemann R, Rose F *et al.* Sildenafil for treatment of lung fibrosis and pulmonary hypertension: a randomised controlled trial. *Lancet* 2002; **360**:895–900.

91 Ghofrani HA, Rose F, Schermuly RT *et al.* Oral sildenafil as long-term adjunct therapy to inhaled iloprost in severe pulmonary arterial hypertension. *J Am Coll Cardiol* 2003; **42**:158–64.

92 Stiebellehner L, Petkov V, Vonbank K *et al.* Long-term treatment with oral sildenafil in addition to continuous IV epoprostenol in patients with pulmonary arterial hypertension. *Chest* 2003; **123**:1293–5.

93 Channick RN, Hoch RC, Newhart JW, Johnson FW, Smith CM. Improvement in pulmonary hypertension and hypoxemia during nitric oxide inhalation in a patient with end-stage pulmonary fibrosis. *Am J Respir Crit Care Med* 1994; **149**:811–14.

94 Higenbottam T, Stenmark K, Simmoneau G. Treatments for severe pulmonary hypertension. *Lancet* 1999; **353**:338–40.

95 Yung GL, Kriett JM, Jamieson SW *et al.* Outpatient inhaled nitric oxide in a patient with idiopathic pulmonary fibrosis: a bridge to lung transplantation. *J Heart Lung Transplant* 2001; **20**:1224–7.

96 Thabut G, Mal H, Castier Y *et al.* Survival benefit of lung transplantation for patients with idiopathic pulmonary fibrosis. *J Thorac Cardiovasc Surg* 2003; **126**:469–75.

97 Maurer J, Frost A, Estenne M, Higenbottam T, Glanville AR. Intertonal guidelines for the selection of lung transplant candidates. *Am J Respir Crit Care Med* 1998; **158**:335–9.

98 Mogulkoc N, Brutsche MH, Bishop PW, Greaves MS, Horrocks AW, Egan JJ. Pulmonary function in idiopathic pulmonary fibrosis and referral for lung transplantation. *Am J Respir Crit Care Med* 2001; **164**:103–8.

99 Douglas WW, Ryu JH, Bjoraker JA *et al.* Colchicine versus prednisolone as treatment of usual interstitial pneumonia. *Mayo Clin Proc* 1997; **72**:201–9.

100 Stern JB, Mal H, Groussard O *et al.* Prognosis of patients with advanced idiopathic pulmonary fibrosis requiring mechanical ventilation for acute respiratory failure. *Chest* 2001; **120**:213–19.

101 Blivet S, Philit F, Sab JM *et al.* Outcome of patients with idiopathic pulmonary fibrosis admitted to the ICU for respiratory failure. *Chest* 2001; **120**:209–12.

CHAPTER 6.1.2

Evidence-based approach to the treatment of sarcoidosis

Robert P Baughman and Olof Selroos

The aetiology of sarcoidosis remains unknown. Therapy for sarcoidosis has been directed towards patients' symptoms. Since the first reports of the dramatic effects of corticosteroids for some cases of sarcoidosis,[1] corticosteroids have been widely used, particularly in some patients with symptomatic, progressive pulmonary sarcoidosis and in many types of extrapulmonary disease.

As in many diseases where corticosteroids are used for treatment, alternatives have been sought to reduce toxicity. In addition, there are cases in which corticosteroids are not effective. Table 1 lists the various drugs reported as useful for some patients with sarcoidosis.

For this chapter, we have chosen to study those agents in which there is some evidence to support their use in sarcoidosis. We have divided the chapter into two sections: corticosteroids and non-corticosteroid agents. This division has been used by others when performing evidence-based reviews of the benefits of these agents.[2,3]

Literature search

For this analysis, we searched MEDLINE for all clinical trials regarding specific agents used for sarcoidosis. Individual articles were reviewed for additional citations not retrieved by the original PubMed search. In addition, we reviewed all available abstracts from international meetings (World Association of Sarcoidosis and Other Granulomatous Disease, American Thoracic Society, American College of Chest Physicians). We also reviewed our own files on these areas.

For the non-steroidal section, a trial was included in the initial analysis if the report was of more than one patient. In addition, therapy had to be specified in the report. Additional information regarding response to therapy, steroid sparing and toxicity was noted when reported. If the authors provided sufficient information, the response was divided into complete response, partial response or stable using their criteria.

Level of evidence to support a recommendation

We have chosen to grade the evidence based on the available information from published manuscripts and abstracts. Table 2 summarizes the grade of evidence (A to D, and U) to support a particular recommendation.

The quality of individual studies was scored by study design into level I, double blind, randomized; level II, open, random-ized or cohort studies; level III, retrospective case series with specified protocols and outcome stated; and level IV, other studies with no comments on protocols or toxicity. A cohort study required that the authors indicate how the patients were identified, the total number of patients treated and the outcome of all patients, especially those who discontinued the drug. The quality of the individual studies was also graded. The quality of the individual studies is also summarized in Table 2.

Corticosteroid therapy

Tables 3 and 4 summarize the trials of oral and inhaled corticosteroids for sarcoidosis.

Patients with erythema nodosum and bilateral hilar adenopathy frequently achieve a spontaneous remission, and they have normally been excluded from clinical trials. No controlled studies have been performed. Most patients included in controlled clinical trials have had radiographic stage II or III. Some studies, but not all, have applied at least a 6-month run-in period without treatment with the aim of excluding patients undergoing spontaneous remission.

There are no controlled trials in patients with extrapulmonary sarcoidosis of any type as a study inclusion criterion.

Pulmonary sarcoidosis

Oral corticosteroids

Only three double-blind, randomized, placebo-controlled trials (level I) have been reported.[4-6] Two of these studies were of only 6 months' duration, with no follow-up in one of them.[4] No single-blind studies have been reported. The majority of the studies have been open but randomized. Five studies have been placebo controlled.

Most of the studies have demonstrated an early benefit from oral corticosteroids in terms of symptomatic, lung functional and chest radiographic improvements. After cessation of treatment, after various periods of time, the differences between steroid-treated and placebo-treated or untreated, randomized or matched controls have been less clear or non-existing. The required duration of treatment is therefore an open question.

The largest study, although not blinded, is the British Thoracic Society trial[7] evaluating four groups of patients.

Table 1. Treatments for sarcoidosis.

Classification	Drugs
Anti-inflammatory/immunomodulators	Corticosteroids
	Cyclosporin
	Phenoxybutazone
Cytotoxic agents	Methotrexate
	Azathioprine
	Cyclophosphamide
	Chlorambucil
	Leflunomide
Antimicrobial agents	Chloroquine
	Hydroxychloroquine
	Minocycline
	Doxycycline
Cytokine modulators	Thalidomide
	Infliximab
	Etanercept
Miscellaneous	Fumaric acid esters
	Radiation

Table 2. Grading of recommendations.

Grade of recommendation	Definition
A	Supported by at least two double-blind, randomized, control trials
B	Supported by prospective cohort studies
C	Supported primarily by two or more retrospective studies
D	Only one retrospective study or based on experience in other diseases
U	No support

Quality of study Level:

I	Double-blind, placebo-controlled trial
II	Randomized trial or cohort study with outcome of all patients specifically stated
III	Case series with outcome of all patients stated. The treatment protocol is specified and frequency of toxicity and modifications of regimen noted
IV	Case series with no comment on toxicity

Patients requiring immediate treatment formed one group. The other patients were observed without treatment for 6 months. At that time point, patients demonstrating spontaneous improvements were included in an untreated observation group. Patients who did not improve spontaneously were randomized, partly blinded, into a selective group (treatment for 6–9 months) or a long-term treatment group (18 months of treatment). The long-term treatment group showed clear benefits compared with the selective, short-term treatment group in terms of symptomatic, lung functional and chest radiographic improvements.

No dose–response studies have been reported. It appears to be most appropriate to start treatment with 30–40 mg of prednisolone or equivalents per day and reduce the dose by 5–10 mg every month until a maintenance dose of 5–10 mg/day is achieved. Compared with prednisone/prednisolone, methylprednisolone has a more favourable lung pharmacokinetic profile.

Inhaled corticosteroids

The studies with inhaled corticosteroids have focused on pulmonary sarcoidosis and disease activity measured with serum and bronchoalveolar lavage (BAL) variables.

The quality of the studies performed with inhaled corticosteroids is generally better than the studies with oral corticosteroids. A total of seven double-blind, randomized, placebo-controlled studies were identified,[8–14] and an eighth was reported as an abstract.[15] Three studies have used follow-up periods without treatment in order to document persisting effects.[10–12]

Regarding patient populations, the studies fall into three categories: (a) patients with newly detected pulmonary disease;[12] (b) patients with stage I–III pulmonary sarcoidosis and impaired lung function, not previously treated;[8–11] (c) patients with chronic sarcoidosis using systemic corticosteroids.[13,14] The patient population in the Niven study was not specifically reported.[15]

In two short-term studies (8–10 and 16 weeks respectively), treatment with budesonide resulted in statistically significant changes in BAL cell populations compared with placebo, indicating that treatment with budesonide may modulate the immunopathogenesis of sarcoidosis in a favourable direction.[8,16]

In patients with newly detected pulmonary stage I–II disease, treatment with budesonide resulted in statistically significant changes in lung function [diffusing lung capacity $(D_L CO)$] and markers of disease activity in stage II patients compared with placebo.[12] Differences remained statistically significant during a 5-year follow-up period.[17] In patients with stage I disease, no differences were found between budesonide- and placebo-treated groups. This suggests that patients with radiographic stage I lesions (bilateral lymphadenopathy without radiographic parenchymal lesions) do not need (or do not benefit from) treatment for their lung disease.

No clinically important changes in lung function compared with placebo were seen when untreated patients received

Table 3. Clinical studies with oral corticosteroids.

Reference (first author)	Design	No. of pts Duration	X-ray stage	Treatment Active	Control	Results	Follow-up	Level of quality I–IV
James[4]	DB, R, P	75 6 months	I (n = 39) II (n = 25) III (n = 11)	Prednisolone 20 mg × 1 or oxyphenbutazone one	Placebo	Pred and Ox > P for chest X-ray. Best efficacy in early cases	None	I
Hapke[125]	O, R	32 (16 pairs) 6 months	I–II	Prednisolone, 15 mg × 1	Matched untreated controls (age, sex, duration of disease, lung function)	9 months: chest X-ray Predn > controls. Lung function Predn = controls	4 years, 11 pairs chest X-ray Predn = P	IV
Israel[126]	O, R, P	83 3 months	I (n = 37) II–III (n = 46)	Predn 15 mg × 1	Placebo	Chest X-ray Stage II Predn > P. Stage I predn = P	5.3 years Chest X-ray Predn = P	III
Mikami[5]	DB, R	101 6 months	I (n = 51) II (n = 50)	Prednisolone 30 mg 4 weeks, 20 mg 4 weeks, 10 mg 4 weeks, 5 mg 12 weeks	Placebo	Chest X-ray: Predn > P up to 12 weeks, thereafter predn = P	1 year Chest X-ray Predn = P	I
Selroos[127]	O, R	37 7 months	II without spontaneous improvement	Methylpred 32–4 mg × 1 or alt days	Untreated controls	Chest X-ray, VC, D$_L$CO Methylpred > controls	2 years Methylpred = controls	IV
Yamamoto[128]	O, R	74 (37 matched pairs)	I (n = 32) II (n = 42)	Alternate-day prednisolone	Matched untreated controls selected	No difference in chest X-ray resolution rates	3 years No difference in	IV

Table 3. *Continued.*

Reference (first author)	Design	No. of pts Duration	X-ray stage	Treatment Active	Control	Results	Follow-up	Level of quality I–IV
		18 months		60 mg to 5 mg, selected from 47 treated cases	from 106 untreated cases		chest X-ray resolution rates	
Harkleroad[129]	O, R	25 6 months	$D_LCO < 80\%$ pred or $Pao_2 < 80$ mmHg	Prednisone 60 mg 1 month, 20 mg at least 5 months	Placebo	Chest X-ray and lung function: Predn = P	15 years Chest X-ray and lung function: Predn = P	III
Zaki[6]	R, DB, P	159 2 years	0 ($n = 17$) I ($n = 64$) II ($n = 59$) III ($n = 19$)	Pred 40 mg × 1 3 months 20 mg × 1 ad 2 years	Placebo	Chest X-ray and lung function: Predn = P	> 3 years Chest X-ray and lung function: Predn = P	I
Gibson[7]	O, Controlled. Partly blinded and randomized	149 7–10 months	II–III	'Selective therapy' (S, $n = 31$) after 6 months' observation without treatment: Predn 30 mg × 11 mo, gradual tapering to 0 over 6–9 mo	(a) Observation group without treatment (O, $n = 58$); (b) Long-term group (L, $n = 27$), predn for 18 mo after 6 mo observation without treatment; (c) Immediate predn group (P, $n = 33$)	L > S for improvements in chest X-ray, symptoms and lung function	5 years Advantage of long-term treatment in terms of chest X-ray, lung function and symptoms	IV

R, randomized; DB, double blind; O, open; P, placebo controlled; Predn, prednisone/prednisolone; Ox, oxyphenbutazone; VC, vital capacity; D_LCO, diffusion capacity for carbon monoxide.

Table 4. Clinical studies with inhaled corticosteroids.

Reference (first author)	Design	No. of pts Duration	Disease	Treatment Active control		Result	Follow-up	Level of quality I–IV
Selroos[21]	O	12 6–27 months	Relapsing stage II–III after previous treatment with oral steroids*	BUD 1.2–2.4 mg/day	None	Significant improvements in chest X-ray, lung function and biochemical markers in 8/12 patients	None	IV
Erkkilä[8]	DB, R, P	19 8–10 weeks	Stage II–III	BUD 1.6 mg/day	Placebo	BUD > P (S-ACE, S-β_2-M, BAL hyaluronan, T-ly CD4+/CD8+ ratio)	None	I
Selroos[19]	O	10 + 10 age-, sex- and stage-matched control subjects 18 months	Stage II $D_LCO < 70\%$ PN, VC <75% PN	Methylpredn 32–8 mg/day for 8–12 weeks followed by BUD 1.6 mg/day	Oral steroids in indiv. adjusted doses	Oral therapy followed by inhaled = oral therapy	None	IV
Spiteri[16]	O, R, P	15 16 weeks	Stage III	BUD 1.6 mg/day	Placebo	BUD > P Symptoms (cough, dyspnoea) BAL lymph, BAL antigen-presenting cells	None	III
Zych[9]	DB, R	40 1 year	Stage II–III	Pred 40–30–20 mg/day 6 months, Thereafter BUD 1.6 mg	Prednisolone 40–10 mg/day for 1 year	BUD = Predn as maintenance treatment (chest X-ray, lung function, S-ACE)	None	IV
Milman[10]	DB, R, P	21 (1 + 2) 8 (3) 1 year	(a) I, normal lung function; (b) II–III; (c) oral pred	BUD 1.2 or 2.0 mg/day	Placebo	BUD = P Chest X-ray, lung function, S-ACE	6 months F-U data not presented	I

Table 4. *Continued.*

Reference (first author)	Design	No. of pts Duration	Disease	Treatment Active control	Result	Follow-up	Level of quality I–IV
Selroos[18]	O	47 18 months	Stage II not spontaneously improving in 6–12 months	Methylpredn 48–4 mg/day over 8 weeks. Thereafter BUD 1.6mg/day	Clinically significant response in 31/38 with BUD alone. Nine pts required combined treatment	3 years	IV
Alberts[11]	DB, R, P	47 6 months	I–III	BUD 1.2 mg/day	BUD > P GCI, IVC	6 months BUD > P IVC	I
Niven[15]	DB, R, P	11 24 weeks	Not mentioned	Triamcinolone 1800 g/day	TA = P	None	I
Pietinalho[12,17]	DB, R, P	189 18 months	I–II Newly detected	Predn 20–10 mg/day 3 mo, then BUD 1.6 mg for 15 months	BUD > P for stage II, D_LCO, S-ACE	5 years BUD > P, FVC, D_LCO, more P-treated patients required oral steroids	I
Du Bois[13]	DB, R, P	44 6 months	II–III	Fluticasone, 2 mg/day	FP = P (FP > P for SF-36)	None	I
Baughman[130]	DB, R, P	22 48 weeks	Requiring oral steroids, at least 20 mg × 1	Fluticasone, 0.88 g × 2 (2.0 g/day metered dose)	FP = P	None	I

DB, double blind; R, randomized; P, placebo controlled; O, open trial; BUD, budesonide; FP, fluticasone propionate; TA, triamcinolone acetonide; S-ACE, serum angiotensin-converting enzyme; S-β_2-M, serum β_2-microglobulin; BAL, bronchoalveolar lavage; GCI, patient's global clinical impression; IVC, inspiratory vital capacity; D_LCO, diffusion capacity for carbon monoxide; FVC, forced vital capacity; SF-36, general health perception questionnaire, short form 36.

*Patients relapsing after treatment with oral corticosteroids rarely improve spontaneously. The results of this open study indicate that inhaled treatment with BUD was clinically effective.

budesonide as initial treatment.[10,11,15] Symptomatic improvement was documented.[10,11]

Patients treated with oral prednisolone for 6 months followed by low-dose prednisolone or budesonide showed no difference between the two types of maintenance treatments but with a lower incidence of side-effects in the budesonide-treated group.[9] These findings are in agreement with the results of open studies.[18,19]

Chronic pulmonary sarcoidosis on treatment with systemic corticosteroids

Two studies with fluticasone propionate (FP) have failed to demonstrate an oral steroid sparing capacity compared with placebo,[13,14] which was seen with budesonide in early uncontrolled pilot studies.[20] In one FP study, an improvement in patients' perception of disease was seen measured with the SF-36 questionnaire.[14]

In an open study, patients relapsing after treatment with oral corticosteroids achieved normal chest X-rays and improved lung function on inhaled budesonide alone.[21] As spontaneous improvements are almost never seen in this clinical situation, the findings indicate the efficacy of inhaled budesonide.

The pulmonary pharmacokinetics of inhaled corticosteroids differ to a large extent. While FP is a highly lipophilic corticosteroid, which after inhalation is retained in fatty tissues in the body, budesonide forms inactive, reversible, intracellular lipid esters, which form an inner depot from which active budesonide is continuously released.[22] This kinetic mechanism may result in higher tissue concentrations of active budesonide. The concentration of budesonide in lung biopsies obtained during surgery, when patients have inhaled the drug immediately before intubation, has also been sufficiently high to give an anti-inflammatory effect in the lung parenchyma.[23] As budesonide is the only inhaled corticosteroid that can form these corticosteroid esters, it is therefore possible that effects described with budesonide cannot be considered class effects but specific for budesonide.

Extrapulmonary sarcoidosis

No controlled clinical studies have been performed in patients with extrapulmonary sarcoidosis. All knowledge is based on case reports and small series of patients.

There appears to be agreement that patients with myocardial and neurological sarcoidosis and disease affecting endocrine organs should be treated with systemic corticosteroids (level IV).[24–26] The daily doses required initially may be higher (40–80 mg of methylprednisolone) than for treatment of pulmonary sarcoidosis.[27] Eye lesions can be treated with topical application of corticosteroids (level IV).[28] Greatly enlarged lymph nodes and parotid glands respond well to corticosteroid treatment (level IV).[29] Hypercalcaemia should be treated with corticosteroids, and the response is usually good

(level IV).[30] Sarcoidosis-induced nephrocalcinosis is reversible with corticosteroids (level III).[31,32]

Alternatives to corticosteroids

Although there is a long list of drugs that have been used for treating sarcoidosis, only a few have been well studied. Limitations have been noted for almost all the previously reported studies.[3] Table 1 lists all the various agents and those studies in which at least two patients have been studied.

Study design

Table 5 includes the type of study. The majority of studies were retrospective series. Results from these studies can only really lead to grade C evidence to support the use of these drugs. There were only a few randomized trials. These included only three studies in which a placebo was employed.[4,33,34] Two other studies randomized the patients in a non-blinded manner. One study treated all patients with high-dose chloroquine, then randomized patients to either continue on drug or go on placebo.[35] The other study treated all patients with high doses of prednisone and added an open-label randomization of cyclosporin.[36] One study was specifically designed as a dose escalation trial.[37]

Outcome measurement

The measurement of outcome is poorly defined in many sarcoidosis studies. For lung involvement, some authors report improvement in pulmonary function or chest roentgenogram. However, different patients may have different parameters improving during the course of therapy.[38] If one parameter was used, the vital capacity was the most common value followed. The amount of improvement also varied between studies and often was not specified. In one study of prolonged methotrexate, Lower and Baughman[39] found that 22 out of 40 patients with pulmonary disease had a 10% or greater improvement in their vital capacity, while only 17 had a >15% improvement in their vital capacity. Most studies used a combination of pulmonary function studies and chest roentgenogram in determining patient improvement. Attempts to incorporate changes in chest roentgenogram, pulmonary function studies and dyspnoea score have been used to assess the value of serial angiotensin-converting enzyme level,[40] but not systematically in clinical trials.

Moreover, sarcoidosis is a multiorgan disease, and improvement may be more important in one organ than another. Most authors would report that the patient improved if one or more organ improved. In one study, the authors refer to the organ that led to therapy as the 'index organ'.[41] In other cases, the specialty of the treating physician (dermatologist, ophthalmologist, pulmonologist) led to focus on one organ. When stated in the study, they are included in Table 5. Only one study provided a specific score that tried to incorporate the multiorgan nature of the disease.[42]

One potential difficulty is that an agent may work more ef-

Table 5. Alternatives to corticosteroids: antimalarial agents.

Reference (first author)	Drug	Study design	Indication	Number on Drug Pred Pla	Outcome	Quality of study
Br TB Assoc[44]	Chlor	DB, R, P	Pulm	29 Clron 28 Plac	Improve with Chlor	I
Adams[48]	Chlor	Retrospect	Hypercalcaemia	2	2 responded	III
Baltzan[35]	Chlor	R	Chronic pulm	23 treated with drug, then randomize 18: 10 drug 8 observation	Slowed worsening of disease in observation group 3/23 had severe AE	II
Baughman[51]	H-C	Retrospect	Refract sarc	41	11 CR 3 stable	III
Davies[131]	Chlor	Retrospect	Pulm	5	2 respond	III
Hirsch[132]	Chlor	Retrospect	Pulm and cutaneous	8 total 7 skin 7 pulm	7/7 skin respond, 2/7 pulm respond	III
Jones[47]	Chlor	Retrospect	Cutaneous	17	12 CR 3 PR 2 stable	III
Morse[45]	Chlor	Cohort	Cutaneous	7	7 respond	II
O'Leary[49]	Chlor	Retrospect	Hypercalcaemia	2	2/2 respond	III
Sharma[50]	Chlor/H-C	Retrospect	CNS	12	10/12 respond	IV
Siltzbach[46]	Chlor	Cohort	Cutaneous and pulm	43 total 43 pulm 14 skin	31/43 pulm respond 14/14/ skin respond	II

Chlor, chloroquine; H-C, hydroxychloroquine; DB, double blind; P, placebo; R, randomized; AE, adverse event; CR, complete response; PR, partial response; Pulm, pulmonary; VC, vital capacity; SS, steroid sparing; CNS, central nervous system.

fectively for one indication than another. For example, agents often have a higher response rate for skin lesions than elsewhere. However, this differential effect on organ involvement is usually not commented upon. Veien and Brodthagen[43] noted a similar percentage response to methotrexate. Lower and Baughman[39] found that the rate of response for skin, lung, neurological and eye involvement was similar. On the other hand, thalidomide appears to be more effective for one organ than another. In one study, all patients had improvement of their skin lesions, most had improved sinus symptoms, but none had objective improvement of their lung disease.[37]

Several of the drugs listed in Table 1 were used to avoid the toxicity of corticosteroids. The steroid sparing property of several of these drugs was specified by authors in their studies, and these are included in Table 1. However, the rate of reduc-

tion of prednisone was not usually followed in any standard protocol. Only one study of a steroid alternative, methotrexate, specified that the two treating physicians used the same criteria for tapering prednisone, but the criteria were not specified.[34] A study of inhaled fluticasone did provide specific criteria for tapering prednisone. It demonstrated that at only 80% of the visits was the corticosteroid dose adjusted on the basis of the specified protocol.[14]

Specific agents

Antimalarial agents (Table 5)

The longest experience with an alternative to corticosteroids for sarcoidosis has been the antimalarial agents. Chloroquine and its derivative hydroxychloroquine have been studied and found to be effective for sarcoidosis.[44–46] It has been employed most effectively for cutaneous disease. In open-label series, the drug has been effective for skin lesions in more than 50% of cases.[44,46,47] In small series, it also appears to be effective in controlling hypercalcaemia to some extent.[48,49] One open-label study found that 10 out of 12 selected patients with neurosarcoidosis had a response to either chloroquine or hydroxychloroquine.[50]

The use of these agents for pulmonary disease is not so clear. The response rate in open-label studies has been as low as 20–30%.[38,51] In one randomized trial, all patients were given high-dose chloroquine, then randomized to maintenance low-dose chloroquine or observation. Those patients on chloroquine had a slower decline in lung function and were less likely to have a clinical relapse of their disease.[35]

Toxicity of these drugs is dose related.[35] The major limitation is gastrointestinal. An additional concern is ocular toxicity.[52] Hydroxychloroquine appears to be much less likely to cause ocular toxicity. However, patients on either antimalarial agent need to undergo routine ophthalmological evaluation.[53,54]

Methotrexate (Table 6)

This cytotoxic agent was first reported to be useful for sarcoidosis by Lacher.[55] It has been a well-established agent in rheumatoid arthritis, based on double-blind, randomized, clinical trials.[56,57] For sarcoidosis, there are several series demonstrating effectiveness of the drug for many forms of the disease. These include large series followed for more than 2 years.[51,58] These are included in Table 6. Response rates of 50–100% have been reported for pulmonary,[39] ocular,[43,59–62] cutaneous,[39,43,63,64] cardiac[65] and neurological[24,60] disease.

There has been one double-blind, randomized trial of methotrexate.[34] The study was designed to determine the steroid sparing effect of the drug. All patients were treated with prednisone at 40 mg/day at the time of starting the study. The dose was tapered as clinically indicated by one of two treating physicians, using standard guidelines that they use in their clinic. The criteria for changing dose were not specified. Those patients on placebo received significantly more prednisone than the methotrexate group during the second 6 months of the study. In addition, there were patients on placebo who relapsed and had to have their prednisone dose increased.

Methotrexate causes bone marrow suppression in a dose-dependent manner. The drug is cleared by the kidney. Routine monitoring should include a complete blood count as well as a serum creatinine. Methotrexate toxicity includes gastrointestinal symptoms, which can be minimized by folic acid supplementation.[66] Pulmonary toxicity has also been reported with methotrexate use for malignancy and rheumatoid arthritis.[67] Six out of 209 sarcoidosis patients treated with methotrexate developed cough attributed to the methotrexate.[51] There appears to be limited risk of malignancy associated with methotrexate.[68,69]

A major concern with the use of methotrexate in sarcoidosis is hepatotoxicity. Although irreversible cirrhosis has not been reported with use, changes on liver biopsy have been seen in patients undergoing surveillance biopsies.[39] In a series of 100 consecutive biopsies done on 68 patients at one institution, 14 patients were felt to have changes that suggested methotrexate toxicity and had the drug discontinued.[70] The finding of these changes was not associated with the duration of therapy, cumulative dose or liver function studies. The authors recommended that liver biopsies be performed for patients who are receiving prolonged therapy with methotrexate.

Azathioprine (Table 7)

Azathioprine has been widely used as a treatment for solid organ transplant. It has also been employed as a treatment for idiopathic pulmonary fibrosis.[71] Some centres are more familiar with this drug than with methotrexate. Table 7 lists open-label studies that have reported a response rate from 30%[38,72] and studies reporting that all patients had some response for pulmonary[73,74] or optic neuritis.[75] There have been no randomized trials of the drug for sarcoidosis.

The toxicity of azathioprine includes haematological and gastrointestinal effects. As the drug is metabolized by methyltransferase,[76,77] care must be taken to monitor for toxicity even at relatively low doses. Nausea is a problem for some patients. In a study comparing various cytotoxic drugs for rheumatoid arthritis, methotrexate was better tolerated than azathioprine.[78,79] The risk of malignancy with azathioprine in non-transplant patients has been estimated to be low, but not zero.[80,81]

Other cytotoxic agents (Table 8)

Leflunomide was developed as an alternative to methotrexate. It has been useful for the treatment of rheumatoid arthritis as a single agent[82,83] or in combination with methotrexate.[84] A recent open-label report has found leflunomide to be useful for both pulmonary and ocular sarcoidosis,[85] with over 50% of patients in both groups responding. The drug was more effective when given with methotrexate. The toxicity was similar to methotrexate, with the exception that pulmonary toxicity was not encountered. In 17 patients treated with leflunomide because of methotrexate toxicity, nine out of 12 did not have the nausea they had with methotrexate. All five cases who stopped methotrexate because of pulmonary symptoms tolerated leflunomide.

Chlorambucil is another cytotoxic agent associated with response in over 80% of patients reported in two studies.[86,87] The drug is associated with an increased risk of malignancy, including leukaemia,[88] and has been used fairly infrequently as safer alternatives are available.

Cyclophosphamide is another cytotoxic agent useful in conditions such as Wegener's granulomatosis, in which corticosteroids are not effective.[89] Cyclophosphamide has been reported as useful in neurosarcoidosis, refractory to

Table 6. Alternatives to corticosteroids: methotrexate.

Reference (first author)	Drug	Study design	Indication	Number on drug	Outcome	Quality of study
Baughman[34]	MTX	DB, R, P	Acute pulm	16 MTX 9 placebo All on pred	Less steroids for MTX group in second 6 mo No difference in change in VC	I
Baughman[51]	MTX	Retrospect	Refractory	209	108 responded 33 stable	III
Dev[59]	MTX	Retrospect	Uveitis	11	4 CR 3 PR 4 stable 9/9 SS	III
Gedalia[42]	MTX	Cohort	Juvenile	7	5 CR 1 PR	II
Kaye[133]	MTX	Retrospect	Musculoskeletal	5	4 improved, SS	III
Lower[24]	MTX	Cohort	CNS	28	17 responded	II
Lower[39]	MTX	Cohort	Refractory	50	33 responded 25/30 SS	II
Maust[60]	MTX	Retrospect	Optic neuritis	3	3 responded	III
Morishita[65]	MTX	Retrospect	Cardiac	9	5 responded	IV
Rajendran[63]	MTX	Retrospect	Cutaneous	12	7 CR 4 PR	III
Samson[61]	MTX	Retrospect	Ocular	10	10 responded	IV
Shetty[62]	MTX	Retrospect	Iritis	2	Improved	III
Veien[43]	MTX	Retrospect	Cutaneous, uveitis	16	12/16 skin responded 3 of 4 uveitis responded	III
Vucinic[58]	MTX	Retrospect	Chronic	91	80% responded 49/49 SS	III
Webster[64]	MTX	Retrospect	Cutaneous	3	3 CR	III

DB, double blind; P, placebo; R, randomized; MTX, methotrexate; AE, adverse event; CR, complete response; PR, partial response; Pulm, pulmonary; VC, vital capacity; SS, steroid sparing; CNS, central nervous system.

conventional doses of corticosteroids.[24,90] In one series, the drug was effective in patients who had also failed methotrexate treatment.[24] The toxicity of cyclophosphamide includes significant bone marrow suppression and nausea. We use a regimen of intermittent intravenous therapy to moderate this toxicity.[91] Bladder toxicity can also be seen with the drug, especially when used as a daily oral medication. In one study of prolonged oral use, bladder cancer was encountered.[92]

Biological agents blocking tumour necrosis factor (TNF) (Table 9)

Three different agents have been approved that specifically block TNF. Etanercept is a soluble TNF receptor antagonist, while infliximab and adalimumab are monoclonal antibodies directed against TNF. Infliximab and etanercept have both been studied in sarcoidosis. Both drugs have been found to be effective for rheumatoid arthritis,[93–95] but only infliximab has

Table 7. Alternatives to corticosteroids: azathioprine.

Author	Drug	Study design	Indication	Number on drug	Outcome	Quality of study
Baughman[51]	AZA	Retrospect	Refract sarc	35	6 respond 13 stable 3 tox	III
Diab[74]	AZA	Retrospect	Refractory	7	7 respond	IV
Gelwan[75]	AZA	Retrospect	Optic nerve	2	2 respond 2/2 SS	III
Lewis[72]	AZA	Cohort	Refract pulm	10	2 respond 2 PR 5 NR 1 NE	II
Muller-Quernheim[73]	AZA	Cohort	Pulm	11	8 CR 3 PR	II
Pacheo[134]	AZA	Retrospect	Refractory	10	8 respond	III
Sharma[38]	AZA	Retrospect	Refractory	10	3 respond	III

DB, double blind; P, placebo; R, randomized; AZA, azathioprine; AE, adverse event; CR, complete response; PR, partial response; Pulm, pulmonary; VC, vital capacity; SS, steroid sparing; CNS, central nervous system.

Table 8. Alternatives to corticosteroids: other cytotoxic agents.

Reference (first author)	Drug	Study design	Indication	Number on drug	Outcome	Quality of study
Chlorambucil Israel[86]	Chloram	Retrospect	Refractory	31	15 CR 13 PR	III
Kataria[87]	Chloram	Cohort	Refractory	10	3 CR 5 PR	II
Cyclophosphamide Doty[90]	CTX	Cohort	CNS	7	7 respond 7 SS	II
Lower[24]	CTX	Cohort	CNS	10	8 CR 1 NR 1 Tox	II
Leflunamide Baguhman[85]	Lefl	Retrospect	Refract sarc	33 total 28 ocular 16 pulmonary	13 CR 9 PR 3 Tox Ocular 23/28 respond Pulm 12/16 respond	III

DB, double blind; P, placebo; R, randomized; LEF, leflunomide; Chloram, chlorambucil; Cyc, cyclophosphamide; TCN, tetracyclines; AE, adverse event; CR, complete response; PR, partial response; Pulm, pulmonary; VC, vital capacity; SS, steroid sparing; CNS, central nervous system.

Table 9. Alternatives to corticosteroids: tumour necrosis factor inhibitors.

Reference (first author)	Drug	Study design	Indication	Number on drug	Outcome	Quality of study
Infliximab						
Baughman[98]	Inflix	Retrospect	Ocular	7	7 CR	III
Baughman[41]	Inflix	Retrospect	Refractory	3	3 respond	III
Etanercept						
Baughman[33]	Etaner	DB, R, P	Refract uveitis	10	3/10 respond, 3/10 respond to placebo	I
Utz[97]	Etaner	Cohort	Pulm	17	5 responded 11 failed therapy	II

DB, double blind; P, placebo; R, randomized; CR, complete response; Pulm, pulmonary; VC, vital capacity.

been shown to be effective for Crohn's disease.[96] Both drugs have been reported to be useful in sarcoidosis, but to varying degrees of efficacy. Utz *et al.*[97] reported that only five out of 17 patients with pulmonary sarcoidosis responded to etanercept. In the original case report of sarcoidosis patients treated with infliximab, all three cases had refractory disease despite treatment with corticosteroids and at least one other agent. All three cases had improvement with therapy.[41] In a follow-up report from that centre, 10 out of 11 patients responded to infliximab.[98] There have been several other case reports of the utility of infliximab for sarcoidosis.[99–103]

There is one double-blind, placebo, randomized trial of etanercept for ocular sarcoidosis.[33] That study included only patients who had persistent ocular disease despite at least 6 months of methotrexate. Patients were continued on methotrexate. There was no significant difference in changes in steroid usage or ocular inflammation between the etanercept versus the placebo group after 6 months of therapy. This lack of efficacy for etanercept for ocular disease was also noted in another placebo-controlled trial of chronic uveitis due to many causes (none with sarcoidosis).[104]

The major toxicities reported with infliximab and etanercept have been allergic reactions. For the intravenously administered infliximab, these can be severe systemic effects leading to drug discontinuation. Infliximab should be administered in a closely observed area by a team prepared to treat any reactions that occur. While both agents are associated with increased risk of infection, infliximab in particular has also been associated with an increased risk of tuberculosis.[105] Both drugs have been found to have increased risk of worsening severe heart failure.[106,107]

Miscellaneous agents (Table 10)

Thalidomide
The drug, originally marketed as a hypnotic but withdrawn from the market when it became clear that it was severely teratogenic, has been reintroduced over the past few years for several indications. One property of thalidomide is its anti-inflammatory properties, including activity suppressing TNF and interleukin (IL)-12.[108,109] It has also been used as an adjuvant therapy in tuberculosis.[110] Its use in sarcoidosis has mostly been limited to cutaneous manifestations, where the drug seems to work in over 80% of cases.[37,111,112] One dose escalation study demonstrated that skin lesions responded in 12 out of 14 cases at 100 mg.[37] The toxicity of sleepiness, constipation and peripheral neuropathy are all dose dependent. Patients receiving the drug have to be carefully monitored for pregnancy. This included male patients, who are required to use barrier precautions when taking the agent.

Pentoxifylline
The phosphodiesterase inhibitor pentoxifylline has been shown to suppress TNF release by alveolar macrophages.[113] One study did demonstrate benefit from the drug in treating patients with acute disease.[114] Confirmation of this initial study is still lacking. Many clinicians have been disappointed with the efficacy of this drug. It is associated with gastrointestinal toxicity, which may be why it appears to be of limited use in sarcoidosis.

Cyclosporin
The use of cyclosporin seemed an ideal drug for sarcoidosis. It has been shown that cyclosporin successfully downregulated T-cell activation, one of the hallmarks of active disease.[115] However, patients in this study showed no improvement in their pulmonary status. Others have reported in open-label studies that the drug was useful in some cases of pulmonary[116] or neurological[117,118] disease.

In a randomized trial of pulmonary sarcoidosis patients treated with corticosteroids, patients were randomized to receive either cyclosporin or placebo.[36] The groups responded

Table 10. Alternatives to corticosteroids: miscellaneous.

Author	Drug	Study design	Indication	Number on drug	Outcome	Quality of study
Thalidomide Baughman[37]	Thal	Cohort	Lupus pernio	14	14 responded	II
Carlesimo[111]	Thal	Retrospect	Cutaneous and pulm	2	2 responded	III
Oliver[112]	Thal	Cohort	Cutaneous	8	8 responded	II
Pentoxifylline Zabel[114]	Pentoxy	Retrospect	Pulm	17	11 responded	III
Cyclosporin Bielory[117]	Cyclo	Retrospect	Optic neuro	3	3 responded	III
Martinet[115]	Cyclo	Cohort	Pulm	8	8 NR	II
Pia[135]	Cyclo/MTX / Ster oids	Retrospect	Refract	11	11	III
Rebuck[116]	Cyclo	Retrospect	Pulm	3	1 CR 2 PR (1 died)	III
Stern[118]	Cyclo	Retrospect	CNS	6	2 responded 4 relapses with 1 death	III
Wyser[36]	Cyclo	R	Pulm	All pts on pred Pred alone 18 Pred + Cyclo 19	Groups responded equally, Not steroid sparing Higher rate of relapse with Cyclo	II
Tetracyclines Bachelez[119]	TCN	Retrospect	Cutaneous	12	8 CR 2 PR	III
Radiation Kang[124]	Rads	Retrospect	CNS	3	2 CR	III
Fumaric acids Nowack[136]	Fum acids	Open cons	Cutaneous	3	3 responded	
Oxyphenbutazone James[4]	Oxyphen	DB, R, P	Pulm	24 Oxyphen 27 Prednisolone 24 Placebo	Oxyphen: 13 improved, 7 stable; Pred: 16 improved 8 stable Placebo 4 improved 13 stable	I

DB, double blind; P, placebo, R; randomized; MTX, methotrexate; Cyc, cyclophosphamide; TCN, tetracyclines; AE, adverse event; CR, complete response; PR, partial response; Pulm, pulmonary; VC, vital capacity; SS, steroid sparing; CNS, central nervous system.

equally: there was no difference in the amount of corticosteroids used in the two groups. There was a significantly higher rate of relapse for the patients treated with cyclosporin compared with the placebo group.

Cyclosporin is associated with renal toxicity, hypertension and increased risk of infection. In addition, there is an increased risk of malignancy.

Tetracyclines

Bachelez et al.[119] reported successful treatment of cutaneous sarcoidosis with either minocycline or doxycycline. The study is intriguing, as it seems to support the hypothesis that *Propiniobacter acnes* may be a causative agent of sarcoidosis.[120] However, minocycline has immunoregulatory activity independent of its antibacterial properties.[121,122] Although generally safe, there is some toxicity, such as nausea and rash, associated with the use of these agents, with minocycline seeming to be the more toxic.[123]

Radiation

The use of radiation for refractory sarcoidosis has usually been limited to case reports. Kang and Suh[124] presented a series of three cases at their institution, all with neurological disease, of whom two had response. Radiation is associated with damage to local, healthy tissue. Its major limitation in sarcoidosis is that it is most useful for small, specific lesions. As sarcoidosis is a systemic disease, radiation is most often employed when there is a small, well-specified and persistent lesion.

Fumaric acid esters

These have been reported in a series of three cases of cutaneous sarcoidosis, with all three responding. Gastrointestinal toxicity was the major limitation.

Oxyphenbutazone

This is one of the early non-steroidal anti-inflammatory agents. In a double-blind, randomized trial by James et al.,[4] the drug was as effective as prednisone and was significantly better than placebo in controlling disease. This drug has been removed from the market because of toxicity. The use of other non-steroidal agents does not seem to influence the outcome of sarcoidosis. However, this has not been studied in a systematic way.

Conclusions

Patients with pulmonary radiographic stage I disease, with or without erythema nodosum, no dyspnoea and with normal lung function (VC, D_LCO) do not require treatment with corticosteroids (grade A).

Symptomatic patients with stage II–III pulmonary lesions and impaired lung function respond to treatment with oral corticosteroids (grade A). Patients with newly detected disease respond better than patients who have had sarcoidosis for more than 2 years (grade A). It is unknown for how long treatment has to be continued and what markers should be used in the decision making for tapering the dose during treatment, and when to stop treatment.

No dose–response studies have been performed. It appears that a starting dose of 30–40 mg of prednisolone per day or its equivalents is sufficient (grade U).

Inhaled corticosteroids (all) can be used for treatment of bronchial sarcoidosis causing symptoms such as cough and in patients with airway obstruction and bronchial hyper-responsiveness (grade D).

After induction with oral corticosteroids, inhaled budesonide can be used as an alternative to oral cortiocosteroids for long-term maintenance treatment (grade B). Budesonide can be recommended for patients at risk of systemic side-effects with oral corticosteroids, and in combination with lower doses of oral corticosteroids as an oral corticosteroid sparing treatment. These effects have been demonstrated only with budesonide.

Extrapulmonary sarcoidosis affecting vital organs with risk of organ failure development should be treated with corticosteroids on an individual patient basis (grade D).

The use of the antimalarial agent chloroquine is effective for some forms of sarcoidosis (grade B). Hydroxychloroquine, which is less toxic, may also be effective (grade C). Patients need to have routine eye examinations while on therapy (grade D).

Methotrexate is steroid sparing for patients with pulmonary disease (grade B). It is effective for pulmonary, ocular, cutaneous and neurological disease (grade C). Patients on drug should undergo routine renal and haematological monitoring (grade D). Folic acid may reduce gastrointestinal toxicity (grade B). Liver biopsy should be considered if the patient has received prolonged treatment to a cumulative dose of >1–2 g (grade B).

Azathioprine appears to be effective as a steroid sparing agent in sarcoidosis in some cases (grade B). Leflunomide alone or in combination with methotrexate is effective for ocular or pulmonary sarcoidosis (grade D). Chlorambucil is as effective as other cytotoxic drugs for sarcoidosis, but is more toxic without any apparent increased efficacy compared with methotrexate or azathioprine (grade C). Cyclophosphamide appears to be useful for refractory neurosarcoidosis (grade B). Use of these cytotoxic drugs requires close monitoring for haematological toxicity. Cyclophosphamide is associated with bladder toxicity, and urine should be monitored at least once a month (grade B).

Thalidomide is effective for cutaneous sarcoidosis (grade B). Patients need to be monitored for risk of pregnancy while taking the agent (grade C).

Infliximab is effective for chronic sarcoidosis (grade C). Patients receiving drug must be carefully monitored during infusion. Etanercept is not effective for most patients with sarcoidosis (grade C). The drug should be given with caution in patients with a history of heart failure or exposure to tuberculosis (grade C).

Tetracyclines benefit some forms of cutaneous sarcoidosis (grade D). Cyclosporin has no apparent benefit for pulmonary sarcoidosis (grade B) but may help some neurosarcoidosis (grade D). Radiation may be useful for small, refractory sarcoidosis lesions (grade D). There is incomplete evidence and experience to comment on the role of pentoxifylline or formic acid esters for sarcoidosis.

References

1 Siltzbach LE. Effects of cortisone in sarcoidosis: a study of thirteen patients. *Am J Med* 1952; **12**:139–60.

2 Paramothayan S, Jones PW. Corticosteroid therapy in pulmonary sarcoidosis: a systematic review. *JAMA* 2002; **287**:1301–7.

3 Paramothayan S, Lasserson T, Walters EH. Immunosuppressive and cytotoxic therapy for pulmonary sarcoidosis. *Cochrane Database Syst Rev* 2003;CD003536.

4 James DG, Carstairs LS, Trowell J, Sharma OP. Treatment of sarcoidosis: report of a controlled therapeutic trial. *Lancet* 1967; **2**:526–8.

5 Mikami R, Hiraga Y, Iwai K *et al.* A double-blind controlled trial on the effect of corticosteroid therapy in sarcoidosis. In: Iwai K, Hosoda Y, eds. *Proceedings of the VI International Conference on Sarcoidosis.* Tokyo, University of Tokyo Press, 1974:533–8.

6 Zaki MH, Lyons HA, Leilop L, Huang CT. Corticosteroid therapy in sarcoidosis: a five year controlled follow-up. *NY State J Med* 1987; **87**:496–9.

7 Gibson GJ, Prescott RJ, Muers MF *et al.* British Thoracic Society Sarcoidosis study: effects of long term corticosteroid treatment. *Thorax* 1996; **51**:238–47.

8 Erkkila S, Froseth B, Hellstrom PE *et al.* Inhaled budesonide influences cellular and biochemical abnormalities in pulmonary sarcoidosis. *Sarcoidosis* 1988; **5**:106–10.

9 Zych D, Pawlicka L, Zielinski J. Inhaled budesonide vs prednisone in the maintenance treatment of pulmonary sarcoidosis. *Sarcoidosis* 1993; **10**:56–61.

10 Milman N, Graudal N, Grode G, Munch E. No effect of high-dose inhaled steroids in pulmonary sarcoidosis: a double-blind, placebo-controlled study. *J Intern.Med* 1994; **236**:285–90.

11 Alberts C, van der Mark TW, Jansen HM. Inhaled budesonide in pulmonary sarcoidosis: a double-blind, placebo-controlled study. Dutch Study Group on Pulmonary Sarcoidosis. *Eur Respir J* 1995; **8**:682–8.

12 Pietinalho A, Lindholm A, Haahtela T, Tukiainen P, Selroos O. Inhaled budesonide for treatment of pulmonary sarcoidosis. Results of a double-blind, placebo-controlled, multicentre study. *Eur Respir J* 1996; **9**(Suppl 23): 406s.

13 du Bois RM, Greenhalgh PM, Southcott AM, Johnson NM, Harris TA. Randomized trial of inhaled fluticasone propionate in chronic stable pulmonary sarcoidosis: a pilot study. *Eur Respir J* 1999; **13**:1345–50.

14 Baughman RP, Iannuzzi MC, Lower EE *et al.* The use of fluticasone for acute symptomatic pulmonary sarcoidosis. *Sarcoidosis Vasc Diffuse Lung Dis* 2002; **19**:198–204.

15 Niven AS, Poropatich RK, Phillips YY, Parker JM, Torrington KG. High dose triamcinolone acetonide (TA) as induction therapy for pulmonary sarcoidosis. *Am J Respir Crit Care Med* 1997; **155**:A944.

16 Spiteri MA, Newman SP, Clarke SW, Poulter LW. Inhaled corticosteroids can modulate the immunopathogenesis of pulmonary sarcoidosis. *Eur Respir J* 1989; **2**:218–24.

17 Pietinalho A, Tukiainen P, Haahtela T, Persson T, Selroos O and the Finnish Pulmonary Sarcoidosis Study Group. Early treatment of

18 Selroos O, Lofroos AB, Pietinalho A, Niemisto M, Riska H. Inhaled budesonide for maintenance treatment of pulmonary sarcoidosis. *Sarcoidosis* 1994; **11**:126–31.

19 Selroos O. Further experience with inhaled budesonide in the treatment of pulmonary sarcoidosis. In: Grassi C, Rizzato G, Pozzi E, eds. *Sarcoidosis and other Granulomatous Disorders.* Amsterdam. Elsevier, 1988:637–40.

20 Morgan AD, Johnson MA, Kerr I, Turner-Warwick M. The action of an inhaled corticosteroid as a steroid sparing agent in chronic pulmonary sarcoidosis. *Am Rev Respir Dis* 1987; **135**:A349.

21 Selroos O. Use of budesonide in the treatment of pulmonary sarcoidosis. In: Ellul-Micallef R, Lam WK, Toogood JH, eds. *Advances in the Use of Inhaled Corticosteroids.* Hong Kong, Exerpta Medica, 1987:188–97.

22 Edsbacker S, Brattsand R. Budesonide fatty-acid esterification: a novel mechanism prolonging binding to airway tissue. Review of available data. *Ann Allergy Asthma Immunol* 2002; **88**:609–16.

23 van den Bosch JMM, Westermann CJJ, Aumann J, Edsbacker S, Tonnesson M, Selroos O. Relationship between lung disposition and blood plasma concentrations of inhaled budesonide. *Biopharm Drug Dispos* 1993; **14**:455–9.

24 Lower EE, Broderick JP, Brott TG, Baughman RP. Diagnosis and management of neurologic sarcoidosis. *Arch Intern Med* 1997; **157**:1864–8.

25 Yazaki Y, Isobe M, Hiroe M *et al.* Prognostic determinants of long-term survival in Japanese patients with cardiac sarcoidosis treated with prednisone. *Am J Cardiol* 2001; **88**:1006–10.

26 Roberts WC, McAllister HA Jr, Ferrans VJ. Sarcoidosis of the heart. A clinicopathologic study of 35 necropsy patients (group 1) and review of 78 previously described necropsy patients (group 11). *Am J Med* 1977; **63**:86–108.

27 Oksanen V. Neurosarcoidosis: clinical presentations and course in 50 patients. *Acta Neurol Scand* 1986; **73**:283–90.

28 Jabs DA, Johns CA. Ocular involvement in chronic sarcoidosis. *Am J Ophthalmol* 1986; **102**:297–301.

29 James DG, Sharma OP. Parotid gland sarcoidosis. *Sarcoidosis Vasc Diffuse Lung Dis* 2000; **17**:27–32.

30 Adams JS. Hypercalcemia and hypercalcuria. *Semin Respir Med* 1992; **13**:402–10.

31 Rizzato G, Colombo P. Nephrolithiasis as a presenting feature of chronic sarcoidosis: a prospective study. *Sarcoidosis* 1996; **13**:167–72.

32 Rizzato G, Fraioli P, Montemurro L. Nephrolithiasis as a presenting feature of chronic sarcoidosis. *Thorax* 1995; **50**:555–9.

33 Baughman RP, Bradley DA, Raymond LA *et al.* Double blind randomized trial of a tumor necrosis factor receptor antagonist (etanercept) for treatment of chronic ocular sarcoidosis. *Am J Respir Crit Care Med* 2002; **165**:A495.

34 Baughman RP, Winget DB, Lower EE. Methotrexate is steroid sparing in acute sarcoidosis: results of a double blind, randomized trial. *Sarcoidosis* 2000; **17**:60–6.

35 Baltzan M, Mehta S, Kirkham TH, Cosio MG. Randomized trial of prolonged chloroquine therapy in advanced pulmonary sarcoidosis. *Am J Respir Crit Care Med* 1999; **160**:192–7.

36 Wyser CP, van Schalkwyk EM, Alheit B, Bardin PG, Joubert JR. Treatment of progressive pulmonary sarcoidosis with cyclosporin A: a randomized controlled trial. *Am J Respir Crit Care Med* 1997; **156**:1571–6.

37 Baughman RP, Judson MA, Teirstein AS, Moller DR, Lower EE. Thalidomide for chronic sarcoidosis. *Chest* 2002; **122**:227–32.

38 Sharma OP, Hughes DTD, James DG, Naish P. Immunosuppressive therapy with azathioprine in sarcoidosis. In: Levinsky L, Macholoa F,

stage II sarcoidosis improves 5-year pulmonary function. *Chest* 2002; **121**:24–31.

eds. *Fifth International Conference on Sarcoidosis and other Granulomatous Disorders*. Prague, Universita Karlova, 1971:635–7.

39 Lower EE, Baughman RP. Prolonged use of methotrexate for sarcoidosis. *Arch Intern Med* 1995; **155**:846–51.

40 DeRemee RA, Rohrbach MS. Serum angiotensin-converting enzyme in evaluating the clinical course of sarcoidosis. *Ann Intern Med* 1980; **92**:361–5.

41 Baughman RP, Lower EE. Infliximab for refractory sarcoidosis. *Sarcoidosis Vasc Diffuse Lung Dis* 2001; **18**:70–4.

42 Gedalia A, Molina JF, Ellis GS, Galen W, Moore C, Espinoza LR. Low-dose methotrexate therapy for childhood sarcoidosis. *J Pediatr* 1997; **130**:25–9.

43 Veien NK, Brodthagen H. Cutaneous sarcoidosis treated with methotrexate. *Br J Dermatol* 1977; **97**:213–16.

44 British Tuberculosis Association. Chloroquine in the treatment of sarcoidosis. *Tubercle* 1967; **48**:257–72.

45 Morse SI, Cohn ZA, Hirsch JG, Shaedler RW. The treatment of sarcoidosis with chloroquine. *Am J Med* 1961; **30**:779–84.

46 Siltzbach LE, Teirstein AS. Chloroquine therapy in 43 patients with intrathoracic and cutaneous sarcoidosis. *Acta Med Scand* 1964; **425**:302S–8S.

47 Jones E, Callen JP. Hydroxychloroquine is effective therapy for control of cutaneous sarcoidal granulomas. *J Am Acad Dermatol* 1990; **23**:487–9.

48 Adams JS, Diz MM, Sharma OP. Effective reduction in the serum 1,25-dihydroxyvitamin D and calcium concentration in sarcoidosis-associated hypercalcemia with short-course chloroquine therapy. *Ann Intern Med* 1989; **111**:437–8.

49 O'Leary TJ, Jones G, Yip A, Lohnes D, Cohanim M, Yendt ER. The effects of chloroquine on serum 1,25-dihydroxyvitamin D and calcium metabolism in sarcoidosis. *N Engl J Med* 1986; **315**:727–30.

50 Sharma OP. Effectiveness of chloroquine and hydroxychloroquine in treating selected patients with sarcoidosis with neurologic involvement. *Arch Neurol* 1998; **55**:1248–54.

51 Baughman RP, Lower EE. Alternatives to corticosteroids in the treatment of sarcoidosis. *Sarcoidosis* 1997; **14**:121–30.

52 Bartel PR, Roux P, Robinson E, Anderson IF. Visual function and long-term chloroquine treatment. *South Afr Med J* 1994; **84**:32–4.

53 Jones SK. Ocular toxicity and hydroxychloroquine: guidelines for screening. *Br J Dermatol* 1999; **140**:3–7.

54 Mazzuca SA, Yung R, Brandt KD, Yee RD, Katz BP. Current practices for monitoring ocular toxicity related to hydroxychloroquine (Plaquenil) therapy. *J Rheumatol* 1994; **21**:59–63.

55 Lacher MJ. Spontaneous remission response to methotrexate in sarcoidosis. *Ann Intern Med* 1968; **69**:1247–8.

56 Anderson PA, West SG, O'Dell JR, Via CS, Claypool RG, Kotzin BL. Weekly pulse methotrexate in rheumatoid arthritis. *Ann Intern Med* 1985; **103**:489–96.

57 Kremer JM, Lee JK. The safety and efficacy of the use of methotrexate in long-term therapy for rheumatoid arthritis. *Arthritis Rheum* 1986; **29**:822–31.

58 Vucinic VM. What is the future of methotrexate in sarcoidosis? A study and review. *Curr Opin Pulm Med* 2002; **8**:470–6.

59 Dev S, McCallum RM, Jaffe GJ. Methotrexate for sarcoid-associated panuveitis. *Ophthalmology* 1999; **106**:111–18.

60 Maust HA, Foroozan R, Sergott RC, Niazi S, Weibel S, Savino PJ. Use of methotrexate in sarcoid-associated optic neuropathy. *Ophthalmology* 2003; **110**:559–63.

61 Samson CM, Waheed N, Baltatzis S, Foster CS. Methotrexate therapy for chronic noninfectious uveitis: analysis of a case series of 160 patients. *Ophthalmology* 2001; **108**:1134–9.

62 Shetty AK, Zganjar BE, Ellis GS Jr, Ludwig IH, Gedalia A. Low-dose methotrexate in the treatment of severe juvenile rheumatoid arthritis and sarcoid iritis. *J Pediatr Ophthalmol Strabismus* 1999; **36**:125–8.

63 Rajendran R, Theertham M, Salgia R, Muthuswamy P. Methotrexate in the treatment of cutaneous sarcoidosis. *Sarcoidosis* 1994; **11**: S335–S338.

64 Webster GF, Razsi LK, Sanchez M, Shupack JL. Weekly low-dose methotrexate therapy for cutaneous sarcoidosis. *J Am Acad Dermatol* 1991; **24**:451–4.

65 Morishita M, Matsuda R, Satoh S et al. Prolonged low dose methotrexate for cardiac sarcoidosis. *Am J Respir Crit Care Med* 1998; **157**:A809.

66 Morgan SL, Baggott JE, Vaughn WH et al. Supplementation with folic acid during methotrexate therapy for rheumatoid arthritis. *Ann Intern Med* 1994; **121**:833–41.

67 Zisman DA, McCune WJ, Tino G, Lynch JP III. Drug-induced pneumonitis: the role of methotrexate. *Sarcoidosis Vasc Diffuse Lung Dis* 2001; **18**:243–52.

68 Balin PL, Tindall JP, Roenigk HH, Hogan MD. Is methotrexate therapy for psoriasis carcinogenic? A modified retrospective–prospective analysis. *JAMA* 1975; **232**:359–62.

69 Nyfors A, Jensen H. Frequency of malignant neoplasms in 248 long-term methotrexate treated psoriatics. *Dermatologica* 1983; **167**:260–1.

70 Baughman RP, Koehler A, Bejarano PA, Lower EE, Weber FL Jr. Role of liver function tests in detecting methotrexate-induced liver damage in sarcoidosis. *Arch Intern Med* 2003; **163**:615–20.

71 Raghu G, Depaso WJ, Cain K et al. Azathioprine combined with prednisone in the treatment of idiopathic pulmonary fibrosis: a prospective double-blind, randomized, placebo-controlled clinical trial. *Am Rev Respir Dis* 1991; **144**:291–6.

72 Lewis SJ, Ainslie GM, Bateman ED. Efficacy of azathioprine as second-line treatment in pulmonary sarcoidosis. *Sarcoidosis Vasc Diffuse Lung Dis* 1999; **16**:87–92.

73 Muller-Quernheim J, Kienast K, Held M, Pfeifer S, Costabel U. Treatment of chronic sarcoidosis with an azathioprine/prednisolone regimen. *Eur Respir J* 1999; **14**:1117–22.

74 Diab SM, Karnik AM, Ouda BA, Denath FM, Fettich J, Francis IM. Sarcoidosis in Arabs: the clinical profile of 20 patients and review of the literature. *Sarcoidosis* 1991; **8**:56–62.

75 Gelwan MJ, Kellen RI, Burde RM, Kupersmith MJ. Sarcoidosis of the anterior visual pathway: successes and failures. *J Neurol Neurosurg Psychiatr* 1988; **51**:1473–80.

76 Ben Ari Z, Mehta A, Lennard L, Burroughs AK. Azathioprine-induced myelosuppression due to methyltransferase defiency in a patient with autoimmune hepatitis. *J Hepatol* 1995; **23**:351–4.

77 Escousse A, Mousson C, Santona L et al. Azathioprine-induced pancytopenia in homogeneous thioprine methyltransferase-deficient renal transplant recipients: a family study. *Transplant Proc* 1995; **27**:1739–42.

78 McKendry RJR, Cyr M. Toxicity of methotrexate compared with azathioprine in the treatment of rheumatoid arthritis: a case–control study of 131 patients. *Arch Intern Med* 1989; **149**:685–9.

79 Wilkens RF, Urowitz MB, Stablein DM et al. Comparison of azathioprine, methotrexate, and the combination of both in the treatment of rheumatoid arthritis. A controlled clinical trial. *Arthritis Rheum* 1992; **35**:849–56.

80 Confavreux C, Saddier P, Grimaud J, Moreau T, Adeleine P, Aimard G. Risk of cancer from azathioprine therapy in multiple sclerosis: a case–control study. *Neurology* 1996; **46**:1607–12.

81 Lamers CB, Griffioen G, Van HR, Veenendaal RA. Azathioprine: an update on clinical efficacy and safety in inflammatory bowel disease. *Scand J Gastroenterol* 1999; **230**:111–15.

82 Emery P, Breedveld FC, Lemmel EM et al. A comparison of the efficacy and safety of leflunomide and methotrexate for the

treatment of rheumatoid arthritis. *Rheumatology (Oxford)* 2000; **39**:655–65.

83 Scott DL, Smolen JS, Kalden JR *et al.* Treatment of active rheumatoid arthritis with leflunomide: two year follow up of a double blind, placebo controlled trial versus sulfasalazine. *Ann Rheum Dis* 2001; **60**:913–23.

84 Kremer JM, Caldwell JR, Cannon GW *et al.* The combination of leflunomide and methotrexate in patients with active rheumatoid arthritis who are failing on methotrexate treatment alone: a double-blind placebo controlled study. *Arthritis Rheum* 2000; **43**:S224.

85 Baughman RP, Lower EE. Leflunomide for chronic sarcoidosis. *Sarcoidosis Vasc Diffuse Lung Dis* 2004; **21**:43–8.

86 Israel HL, McComb BL. Chlorambucil treatment of sarcoidosis. *Sarcoidosis* 1991; **8**:35–41.

87 Kataria YP. Chlorambucil in sarcoidosis. *Chest* 1980; **78**:36–42.

88 Lerner HJ. Acute myelogenous leukemia in patients receiving chlorambucil as long-term adjuvant chemotherapy for stage II breast cancer. *Cancer Treat Rep* 1978; **62**:1135–8.

89 Hoffman GS, Kerr GS, Leavitt RY *et al.* Wegener granulomatosis: an analysis of 158 patients. *Ann Intern Med* 1992; **116**:488–98.

90 Doty JD, Mazur JE, Judson MA. Treatment of corticosteroid-resistant neurosarcoidosis with a short-course cyclophosphamide regimen. *Chest* 2003; **124**:2023–6.

91 Baughman RP, Lower EE. Use of intermittent, intravenous cyclophosphamide for idiopathic pulmonary fibrosis. *Chest* 1992; **102**:1090–4.

92 Talar-Williams C, Hijazi YM, Walther MM *et al.* Cyclophosphamide-induced cystitis and bladder cancer in patients with Wegener granulomatosis. *Ann Intern Med* 1996; **124**:477–84.

93 Jack D. 54-week results on infliximab attract attention at EULAR. European League against Rheumatism [news]. *Lancet* 1999; **353**: 2132.

94 Lovell DJ, Giannini EH, Reiff A *et al.* Etanercept in children with polyarticular juvenile rheumatoid arthritis. Pediatric Rheumatology Collaborative Study Group. *N Engl J Med* 2000; **342**:763–9.

95 Maini R, St CE, Breedveld F *et al.* Infliximab (chimeric anti-tumour necrosis factor α monoclonal antibody) versus placebo in rheumatoid arthritis patients receiving concomitant methotrexate: a randomised phase III trial. ATTRACT Study Group. *Lancet* 1999; **354**:1932–9.

96 Rutgeerts P, D'Haens G, Targan S *et al.* Efficacy and safety of retreatment with anti-tumor necrosis factor antibody (infliximab) to maintain remission in Crohn's disease. *Gastroenterology* 1999; **117**:761–9.

97 Utz JP, Limper AH, Kalra S *et al.* Etanercept for the treatment of stage II and III progressive pulmonary sarcoidosis. *Chest* 2003; **124**: 177–85.

98 Baughman RP, Bradley DA, Lower EE. Infliximab for chronic ocular inflammation. *Int J Clin Pharmacol Ther* 2005; **43**:7–11.

99 Mallbris L, Ljungberg A, Hedblad MA, Larsson P, Stahle-Backdahl M. Progressive cutaneous sarcoidosis responding to anti-tumor necrosis factor-α therapy. *J Am Acad Dermatol* 2003; **48**:290–3.

100 Meyerle JH, Shorr A. The use of infliximab in cutaneous sarcoidosis. *J Drugs Dermatol* 2003; **2**:413–14.

101 Pettersen JA, Zochodne DW, Bell RB, Martin L, Hill MD. Refractory neurosarcoidosis responding to infliximab. *Neurology* 2002; **59**: 1660–1.

102 Roberts SD, Wilkes DS, Burgett RA, Knox KS. Refractory sarcoidosis responding to infliximab. *Chest* 2003; **124**:2028–31.

103 Yee AMF, Pochapin MB. Treatment of complicated sarcoidosis with infliximab anti-tumor necrosis-α therapy. *Ann Intern Med* 2001; **135**:27–31.

104 Foster CS, Tufail F, Waheed NK *et al.* Efficacy of etanercept in preventing relapse of uveitis controlled by methotrexate. *Arch Ophthalmol* 2003; **121**:437–40.

105 Keane J, Gershon S, Wise RP *et al.* Tuberculosis associated with infliximab, a tumor necrosis factor-α neutralizing agent. *N Engl J Med* 2001; **345**:1098–104.

106 Anker SD, Coats AJ. How to recover from renaissance? The significance of the results of recover, renaissance, renewal and attach. *Int J Cardiol* 2002; **86**:123–30.

107 Chung ES, Packer M, Lo KH, Fasanmade AA, Willerson JT. Randomized, double-blind, placebo-controlled, pilot trial of infliximab, a chimeric monoclonal antibody to tumor necrosis factor-α, in patients with moderate-to-severe heart failure: results of the anti-TNF Therapy Against Congestive Heart Failure (ATTACH) trial. *Circulation* 2003; **107**:3133–40.

108 Moller DR, Wysocka M, Greenlee BM *et al.* Inhibition of IL-12 production by thalidomide. *J Immunol* 1997; **159**:5157–61.

109 Tavares JL, Wangoo A, Dilworth P, Marshall B, Kotecha S, Shaw RJ. Thalidomide reduces tumour necrosis factor-α production by human alveolar macrophages. *Respir Med* 1997; **91**:31–9.

110 Tramontana JM, Utaipat U, Molloy A *et al.* Thalidomide treatment reduces tumor necrosis factor α production and enhances weight gain in patients with pulmonary tuberculosis. *Mol Med* 1995; **1**:384–97.

111 Carlesimo M, Giustini S, Rossi A, Bonaccorsi P, Calvieri S. Treatment of cutaneous and pulmonary sarcoidosis with thalidomide. *J Am Acad Dermatol* 1995; **32**:866–9.

112 Oliver SJ, Kikuchi T, Krueger JG, Kaplan G. Thalidomide induces granuloma differentiation in sarcoid skin lesions associated with disease improvement. *Clin Immunol* 2002; **102**:225–36.

113 Marques LJ, Zheng L, Poulakis N, Guzman J, Costabel U. Pentoxifylline inhibits TNF-α production from human alveolar macrophages. *Am J Respir Crit Care Med* 1999; **159**:508–11.

114 Zabel P, Entzian P, Dalhoff K, Schlaak M. Pentoxifylline in treatment of sarcoidosis. *Am J Respir Crit Care Med* 1997; **155**:1665–9.

115 Martinet Y, Pinkston P, Saltini C, Spurzem J, Muller-Quernheim J, Crystal RG. Evaluation of the *in vitro* and *in vivo* effects of cyclosporine on the lung T-lymphocyte alveolitis of active pulmonary sarcoidosis. *Am Rev Respir Dis* 1996; **138**:1242–8.

116 Rebuck AS, Stiller CR, Braude AC, Laupacis A, Cohen RD, Chapman KR. Cyclosporin for pulmonary sarcoidosis. *Lancet* 1984; **1**:1174.

117 Bielory L, Frohman LP. Low-dose cyclosporine therapy of granulomatous optic neuropathy and orbitopathy. *Ophthalmology* 1991; **98**:1732–6.

118 Stern BJ, Schonfeld SA, Sewell C, Krumholz A, Scott P, Belendiuk G. The treatment of neurosarcoidosis with cyclosporine. *Arch Neurol* 1992; **49**:1065–72.

119 Bachelez H, Senet P, Cadranel J, Kaoukhov A, Dubertret L. The use of tetracyclines for the treatment of sarcoidosis. *Arch Dermatol* 2001; **137**:69–73.

120 Eishi Y, Suga M, Ishige I *et al.* Quantitative analysis of mycobacterial and propionibacterial DNA in lymph nodes of Japanese and European patients with sarcoidosis. *J Clin Microbiol* 2002; **40**:198–204.

121 Kloppenburg M, Verweij CL, Miltenburg AM *et al.* The influence of tetracyclines on T cell activation. *Clin Exp Immunol* 1995; **102**: 635–41.

122 Le CH, Morales A, Trentham DE. Minocycline in early diffuse scleroderma. *Lancet* 1998; **352**:1755–6.

123 Shapiro LE, Knowles SR, Shear NH. Comparative safety of tetracycline, minocycline, and doxycycline. *Arch Dermatol* 1997; **133**:1224–30.

124 Kang S, Suh JH. Radiation therapy for neurosarcoidosis: report of three cases from a single institution. *Radiat Oncol Invest* 1999; **7**:309–12.

125 Hapke EJ, Meek JC. Steroid treatment in pulmonary sarcoidosis. In: Levinsky L, Macholoa F, eds. *Fifth International Conference on Sarcoidosis*. Praha, Univ. Karlova, 1971:621–5.

126 Israel HL, Fouts DW, Beggs RA. A controlled trial of prednisone treatment of sarcoidosis. *Am Rev Respir Dis* 1973; **107**:609–14.

127 Selroos O, Sellergren TL. Corticosteroid therapy of pulmonary sarcoidosis. *Scand J Resp Dis* 1979; **60**:215–21.

128 Yamamoto M, Saito N, Tachibabana T *et al*. Effects of 18-month corticosteroid therapy on stage I and stage II sarcoidosis patients (a control trial). In: Chretien J, Marsac J, Saltiel JC, eds. *Sarcoidosis and other Granulomatous Disorders: Ninth International Conference*. Paris, Pergamon Press, 1981:470–4.

129 Harkleroad LE, Young RL, Savage PJ, Jenkins DW, Lorden RE. Pulmonary sarcoidosis. Long-term follow-up of the effects of steroid therapy. *Chest* 1982; **82**:84–7.

130 Baughman RP, Iannuzzi MC, Lower EE *et al*. Use of fluticasone in acute symptomatic pulmonary sarcoidosis. *Sarcoidosis Vasc Diffuse Lung Dis* 2002; **19**:198–204.

131 Davies D. Sarcoidosis treated with chloroquine. *Br J Dis Chest* 1963; **57**:30–6.

132 Hirsch JG. Experimental treatment with chloroquine. *Am Rev Respir Dis* 1961; **84**:52–8.

133 Kaye O, Palazzo E, Grossin M, Bourgeois P, Kahn MF, Malaise MG. Low-dose methotrexate: an effective corticosteroid-sparing agent in the musculoskeletal manifestations of sarcoidosis. *Br J Rheumatol* 1995; **34**:642–4.

134 Pacheo Y, Marechal C, Marechal F, Biot N, Perrin-Fayolle M. Azathioprine treatment of chronic pulmonary sarcoidosis. *Sarcoidosis* 1985; **2**:107–13.

135 Pia G, Pascalis L, Aresu G, Rosetti L, Ledda MA. Evaluation of the efficacy and toxicity of the cyclosporine A–flucortolone–methotrexate combination in the treatment of sarcoidosis. *Sarcoidosis Vasc Diffuse Lung Dis* 1996; **13**:146–52.

136 Nowack U, Gambichler T, Hanefeld C, Kastner U, Altmeyer P. Successful treatment of recalcitrant cutaneous sarcoidosis with fumaric acid esters. *BMC Dermatol* 2002; **2**:15.

CHAPTER 6.1.3

Hypersensitivity pneumonitis

Yves Lacasse and Yvon Cormier

Definition of problem

Hypersensitivity pneumonitis (HP) is a pulmonary disease with symptoms of dyspnoea and cough resulting from the inhalation of an allergen to which the subject has been previously sensitized. Acute and subacute HP represent the most active forms of the disease, which may become chronic while remaining progressive. HP may also evolve to end-stage lung disease.[1] The diagnosis of HP has most often relied on an array of non-specific clinical symptoms and signs developed in an appropriate setting,[2] with the demonstration of interstitial markings on chest radiographs, serum precipitating antibodies against offending antigens, a lymphocytic alveolitis on bronchoalveolar lavage (BAL) and/or a granulomatous reaction on lung biopsies.

A wide spectrum of antigens may trigger the disease. These antigens have often led to a graphic and most descriptive nomenclature detailed in several case reports. A complete review of these antigens is beyond the scope of this chapter. The offending antigens can be classified in five broad categories represented by disease prototypes (Table 1).

Literature search

HP is an orphan disease. We nevertheless conducted three broad MEDLINE searches using 'alveolitis, extrinsic allergic' as the unique medical subject heading (MeSH) term. We restricted the searches to the following subheadings, diagnosis, therapy and prevention and control, and limited our review to the English and French literature. These searches covered the period 1980–2003. The following discussion focuses on the best available evidence. In the case of articles on diagnostic strategies, priority was given to studies reporting on the sensitivity and/or specificity of diagnostic strategies. In the case of articles on therapy, priority was given to controlled trials.

Diagnostic criteria

A number of diagnostic criteria recommendations for HP have been published[3–6] (Table 2). The most widely used are those from Richerson and colleagues.[4] None of these sets of criteria has been validated. Their diagnostic accuracy is therefore unknown. They correspond in effect to definitions of the disease.

Others have developed prediction rules (i.e. clinical tools that quantify the contribution of various components of the history, physical examination and basic laboratory results in the diagnosis of an individual patient[7]) for periodic surveillance in high-risk workers or case finding in outbreaks of HP.[8–10] Although these rules are meant to be sensitive (i.e. able to detect most cases of work-related HP), it is likely that their specificity is limited in work environments with a high prevalence of other respiratory diseases. Little information is provided for their accuracy.

The HP study

We recently addressed the issue of the clinical diagnostic criteria of HP in a prospective multicentre cohort study.[11] Its objective was to develop a clinical prediction rule for the diagnosis of active HP. Such a rule aims at helping clinicians to arrive at a more accurate estimate of probability of HP and decide whether further investigation is needed to either rule in or rule out HP.

Consecutive adult patients presenting with a pulmonary syndrome for which active HP was considered in the differential diagnosis were included in this study. This cohort thus included a wide range of patients presenting for the investigation of a suspected interstitial lung disease, including patients with HP (the 'cases') and patients without HP (the 'controls'). The criteria under study included data usually collected during the initial investigation of the patients with suspected HP (clinical history, physical examination, pulmonary function testing, blood gases, blood count, serum precipitating antibodies).

The investigators had to classify each patient as HP or non-HP. In the absence of a unique gold standard defining the presence or absence of HP, the final diagnosis relied on findings of BAL, high-resolution computerized tomography (HRCT) and, if needed, other diagnostic procedures. BAL lymphocytosis (≥30% for non- and ex-smokers and ≥20% for current smokers[12]) and bilateral ground-glass or poorly defined centrilobular nodular opacities on HRCT[13] were required for the diagnosis of HP to be accepted without resorting to additional diagnostic procedures. When the association of HRCT and BAL did not allow the investigators to make a final diagnosis of HP or non-HP with confidence, the decision regarding additional procedures (including for instance BAL fluid cytology or culture, transbronchial or endobronchial biopsy or medi-

Table 1. Prototypes of hypersensitivity pneumonitis according to major classes of antigens.

Class of antigens	Specific antigen	Disease
Bacteria	*Saccharopolyspora rectivirgula*	Farmer's lung
Fungus	*Trichosporon cutaneum*	Summer-type HP
Mycobacteria	*Mycobacterium avium-intracellulare*	Hot-tub lung
Proteins	Altered pigeon serum (probably IgA)	Pigeon-breeder's disease
Chemical products	Diphenylmethane diisocyanate (MDI)	MDI HP

Table 2. Proposed diagnostic criteria for hypersensitivity pneumonitis for clinical purposes.

Study (first author)	Major criteria	Minor criteria
Terho[3]	Exposure to offending antigens (revealed by history of aerobiological or microbiological investigations of the environment or measurements of antigen-specific IgG antibodies) Symptoms compatible with HP present and appearing or worsening some hours after antigen exposure Lung infiltrations compatible with HP visible on chest X-ray	Basal crepitant rales Impairment of the diffusing capacity Oxygen tension (or saturation) of the arterial blood either decreased at rest or normal at rest but decreased during exercise Restrictive ventilation defect in the spirometry Histological changes compatible with HP Positive provocation test whether by work exposure or controlled inhalation challenge
Richerson[4]	The history and physical findings and pulmonary function tests indicate an interstitial lung disease The X-ray film is consistent There is exposure to a recognized cause There is antibody to that antigen	
Cormier[5]	Appropriate exposure Inspiratory crackles Lymphocytic alveolitis (if BAL is done) Dyspnoea Infiltrates on chest radiographs (or HRCT)	Recurrent febrile episodes Decreased $D_L CO$ Precipitating antibodies to HP antigens Granulomas on lung biopsy (usually not required) Improvement with contact avoidance or appropriate treatment
Schuyler[6]	Symptoms compatible with HP Evidence of exposure to appropriate antigen by history or detection in serum and/or BAL fluid antibody Findings compatible with HP on chest radiograph or HRCT BAL fluid lymphocytosis Pulmonary histological changes compatible with HP Positive 'natural challenge'	Bibasilar rales Decreased $D_L CO$ Arterial hypoxaemia, either at rest or during exercise

astinoscopy) was not protocol based but left to the investigators, according to clinical circumstances and their usual practice. Patients underwent surgical lung biopsy when the HRCT, the BAL and other diagnostic procedures failed to confirm a diagnosis.

Regression analyses identified six significant predictors of active HP (Table 3). The clinical prediction model produced an equation expressing the probability of HP as a function of the statistically significant variables. From this equation, we constructed a table of probability for combinations of predictors (Table 4). In clinical practice, the best diagnostic strategy will then depend on the probability of HP determined from Table 4. For instance, in a farmer presenting with recurrent episodes of respiratory symptoms, inspiratory crackles and testing positive for the corresponding precipitating antibodies, the probability of HP would be 81% (Table 4).

Another patient presenting with progressive dyspnoea and inspiratory crackles as the unique criteria of HP would have a probability of HP of <1%. Further investigation would be mandated only in the former. Typical findings of an alveolar lymphocytosis and/or bilateral ground-glass opacities on HRCT in the former patient would secure the diagnosis of HP, without resorting to surgical lung biopsy. HP would be confidently ruled out in the latter and the investigation oriented towards another diagnosis. We submit that a probability ≥90% or "10% should be sufficient in most cases to rule in or rule out HP, respectively, especially in areas of high or low prevalence

of HP respectively. However, the 'test threshold' (that is the probability below which a clinician would dismiss the diagnosis and order no further test) and the 'treatment threshold' (that is the probability above which a clinician could consider the diagnosis confirmed and would stop testing) are likely to differ according to the clinical implications of the diagnosis.[14] A clinician and his/her patient will be more likely to accept the diagnosis of bird-fancier's disease when the offending antigen is a pet, even if the probability of HP is 75%. In such a case, antigen avoidance would be appropriate. Further investigation would be required only if the clinical course is unusual. On the other hand, a clinician and his/her patient will want to secure the diagnosis of farmer's lung even if the probability of HP is around 90%, given that more than 50% will quit farming within 6 years of a diagnosis of farmer's lung.[15]

Ancillary tests

Chest radiology

Chest X-ray

Chest radiography is often the initial step in the investigation of a patient presenting with a pulmonary syndrome suggesting HP. The first objective of chest X-rays is not to rule in HP but rather to rule out other diseases for the patient's illness. In acute HP, one expects to find ground-glass infiltrates, nodular and/or striated patchy opacities.[16,17] The distribution of these

Table 3. Significant predictors of hypersensitivity pneumonitis.

Variables	Odds ratio	Confidence interval (95%)
Exposure to a known offending antigen	38.8	11.6–129.6
Positive precipitating antibodies	5.3	2.7–10.4
Recurrent episodes of symptoms	3.3	1.5–7.5
Inspiratory crackles	4.5	1.8–11.7
Symptoms 4–8 hours after exposure	7.2	1.8–28.6
Weight loss	2.0	1.0–3.9

From Lacasse *et al.*,[11] reproduced with permission of the American Thoracic Society.

Table 4. Probability (%) of having hypersensitivity pneumonitis*.

Exposure to a known offending antigen	Recurrent episodes of symptoms	Symptoms 4–8 hours after exposure	Weight loss	Crackles + Serum precipitins +	Crackles + Serum precipitins −	Crackles − Serum precipitins +	Crackles − Serum precipitins −
+	+	+	+	98%	92%	93%	72%
+	+	+	−	97%	85%	87%	56%
+	+	−	+	90%	62%	66%	27%
+	+	−	−	81%	45%	49%	15%
+	−	+	+	95%	78%	81%	44%
+	−	+	−	90%	64%	68%	28%
+	−	−	+	73%	33%	37%	10%
+	−	−	−	57%	20%	22%	5%
−	+	+	+	62%	23%	26%	6%
−	+	+	−	45%	13%	15%	3%
−	+	−	+	18%	4%	5%	1%
−	+	−	−	10%	2%	2%	0%
−	−	+	+	33%	8%	10%	2%
−	−	+	−	20%	4%	5%	1%
−	−	−	+	6%	1%	1%	0%
−	−	−	−	3%	1%	1%	0%

*All the predictors are dichotomous variables. − indicates absent; + , present; from Lacasse *et al.*,[11] reproduced with permission of the American Thoracic Society.

infiltrates is reported as diffuse but often sparing the bases in the subacute form.[18] A variety of different distributions have been described.[19,20] None of these findings is specific for HP. The number of patients studied to support these frequently quoted characteristics is small. A systematic review of the 31 available references (including 13 reports of acute HP and 12 reports of chronic HP) suggested that up to 20% of individuals with acute HP have normal chest X-rays (i.e. sensitivity 80%).[21] Chest X-ray abnormalities were more likely to be present if the radiographs were done at the time of symptoms ('concurrent with disease') than if they were done after symptoms had resolved. In addition, when reports were based on a series of cases rather than actual population-based studies, the proportion of abnormal chest X-rays was significantly higher. This notion is consistent with the results of the HP study, in which 22 of the 199 patients with active HP [11%; 95% confidence interval (CI) 7–16%] had their initial chest X-rays interpreted as normal.[11]

CT scanning

Our ability to define the value of HRCT in HP is limited by the small number of cases studied. Table 5 summarizes selected reports of HRCT findings according to the phase of disease.[22–29] A noteworthy pictorial essay was published recently by Matar and collaborators.[13] The patterns described are not specific. For instance, ground-glass opacities can be

seen in a variety of other diseases including desquamative interstitial pneumonitis, *Pneumocystis carinii* pneumonia, bronchiolitis obliterans with organizing pneumonia, bronchoalveolar carcinoma, alveolar proteinosis and alveolar haemorrhage.

All but one report showed that HRCT was always abnormal in HP.[30] In that study, Lynch *et al.* specifically addressed the issue of sensitivity of HRCT in active HP during an outbreak of HP that had occurred among employees at a local swimming pool. Thirty-one symptomatic employees were referred for examination for possible HP. For the purposes of the study, the diagnostic criteria of HP consisted of the combination of (a) ≥ two work-related signs or symptoms (including cough, chest tightness, dyspnoea and fever); (b) >33% lymphocytes in BAL fluid; and (c) transbronchial biopsies showing noncaseating granulomas, bronchiolitis, peribronchial or perivascular mononuclear cell aggregate or interstitial fibrosis. Based on these criteria, HP was diagnosed in 11 of the 31 symptomatic employees. HRCT findings were abnormal in five subjects (sensitivity of HRCT = 45%). The authors did not compute any confidence interval around this result. Doing so, we calculated that the 95% CI around this sensitivity is actually 17–77%, indicating lack of precision in this estimate of sensitivity. The authors commented on potential explanations of their finding, including a higher index of suspicion for the disease, which led to earlier diagnosis. It is nevertheless our

Table 5. High-resolution computerized tomography findings in hypersensitivity pneumonitis.

Stage of disease	References (first author)	Sample size	Findings*
Acute	Cormier[29]	n = 20 (farmer's lung)	Ground-glass opacities Micronodules Mosaic perfusion Emphysema Honeycombing Mediastinal lymphadenopathies
Subacute	Hansell[23]	n = 17 (including nine with pigeon-breeder's disease and four with farmer's lung)	Generalized increase in attenuation of the lung Nodular pattern Reticular pattern Patchy air space opacification
	Remy-Jardin[27]	n = 21 (pigeon-breeder's disease)	Micronodular pattern (<5 mm in diameter) Ground-glass attenuation Emphysematous changes Honeycombing
Chronic	Adler[24]	n = 16 (antigen = ?)	Fibrosis Ground-glass attenuation Nodules
	Remy-Jardin[27]	n = 24 (pigeon-breeder's disease)	Honeycombing Ground-glass attenuation Micronodules Emphysema

*The findings are ranked according to their decreasing order of prevalence in the study population.

opinion that a normal HRCT is a strong argument against the diagnosis of HP. A normal HRCT in HP should be the exception rather than the rule. As discussed by Lynch et al.,[30] the time interval between the removal from the offending antigen and HRCT may be an explanation for a normal HRCT in HP, although the short-term 'kinetics' of HP-associated ground-glass opacities have not been well described. In the HP study, among the 199 patients with HP who contributed to the analysis, eight patients (4%) had neither bilateral ground-glass nor poorly defined centrilobular nodular opacities on their CT scan.[11] All were submitted to additional diagnostic procedures.

Can HRCT alone be used to make the diagnosis of HP? This question was addressed by Lynch and collaborators who looked at whether HRCT can distinguish HP from idiopathic pulmonary fibrosis (IPF).[31] In a blind comparison of HRCT from biopsy-proven cases of IPF ($n = 36$) and HP ($n = 27$), two radiologists could make a CT diagnosis with confidence in 39 patients (62%). Desquamative interstitial pneumonia could not be reliably distinguished from acute or subacute HP, whereas chronic HP had images identical to those of usual interstitial pneumonia. Of note, only cases of HP and IPF were included in this study. Had other diseases been included, it is very likely that the capacity to distinguish HP would have been even lower. We therefore conclude that HRCT alone cannot adequately diagnose HP.

Pulmonary function tests (PFTs)

The typical physiological profile of acute HP is a restrictive pattern with low $D_L CO$.[32] In chronic disease, the pattern can be restrictive but, at least in farmer's lung, the most frequent profile is an obstructive defect resulting from emphysema.[33] In the HP study, we observed different physiological patterns depending on the offending antigens (Table 6). On average, compared with HP from bacterial or fungal antigen exposure, avian-related HP seldom presented with acute symptoms (chills, tightness of chest, body aches), but typically with manifestations of fibrosis (clubbing, restrictive pattern on PFTs, fibrosis on HRCT).[34] A currently held belief is that a decreased $D_L CO$ is always present in HP.[35] Nevertheless, in the HP study, 39 of the 177 patients in whom $D_L CO$ could be measured

(22%, 95% CI 16–29%) had normal results (defined as a $D_L CO \geq 80\%$ predicted) at the time of diagnosis (HP Study Group, unpublished data).

Hence, the utility of PFTs is primarily to describe the physiological abnormalities and the associated impairment. The results of PFTs may also guide therapy by helping the clinician in selecting those for whom a treatment with corticosteroids may be justified. Pulmonary function tests have no discriminative properties in differentiating HP from other interstitial lung diseases.[11]

Specific antibodies

Most reports on the sensitivity and specificity of serum-specific antibodies are limited by the inclusion of inappropriate controls, who are often represented by healthy subjects. A diagnostic test is really useful only to the extent that it distinguishes between target disorders or states that might otherwise be confused.[36] Almost any test can distinguish the healthy from the affected. This ability tells nothing about the clinical utility of the test. The true, pragmatic value of a test is therefore established only in a study that closely resembles clinical practice. Also, consecutive patients are important for the test to be evaluated in a sample of patients that includes an appropriate spectrum of mild and severe diseases with different but commonly confused disorders (e.g. HP versus sarcoidosis versus idiopathic pulmonary fibrosis).

A critical appraisal based on published methodological criteria[37,38] of the best available study of the accuracy of specific antibodies in HP[39] is provided in Table 7. Regardless of the limitations of the available reports, a general conclusion is that there are important problems with false-positive and false-negative results. HP cannot be ruled in solely on the basis of positive antibodies or ruled out on the basis of negative antibodies. Many asymptomatic farmers (10%) and pigeon breeders (40%) have positive results,[40–42] and many cases of HP have negative specific antibodies.[43] In addition, a study showed fluctuations over 4 years in the precipitin status of dairy farmers who had repeated measurements of serum antibodies against *Saccharopolyspora rectivirgula*, *Thermoactinomyces vulgaris* and *Aspergillus fumigatus*.[44] It is currently

Table 6. Results of pulmonary function testing in the HP study.

	Total cohort ($n = 199$)	Pigeon-breeder's/ bird-fancier's disease ($n = 132$)	Farmer's lung ($n = 38$)	Exposure to various fungi ($n = 26$)	P-value
Normal pattern	34%	23%	68%	42%	
Obstructive pattern*	1%	0%	3%	0%	
Restrictive pattern*	64%	77%	26%	54%	
Mixed pattern (both obstructive and restrictive)	1%	0%	3%	4%	<0.0001

*Obstructive pattern: $FEV_1 < 80\%$ predicted and $FEV_1/FVC < 0.7$. Restrictive pattern: total lung capacity $< 85\%$ predicted.

Table 7. Critical appraisal of a study looking at the accuracy of specific antibodies in bird-breeder's disease*.

Guide	Comments
Are the results of the study valid?	
Was there an independent 'blind' comparison with a reference standard?	The gold standard used in this study for positive diagnosis of bird-breeder's disease was the physician's final diagnosis based on criteria that were not reported. The definitive diagnosis was obtained within 9 months after precipitin determination, indicating that the 'incorporation bias' (the situation occurring when the result of a test is actually incorporated into the evidence used to diagnose the disease) might have operated
Did the patient sample include an appropriate spectrum of patients to whom the test will be applied in clinical practice?	128 sera were received for determination of serum precipitins against avian antigens. Accurate clinical and biological information was obtained for 99 patients. Nine cases were excluded because of uncertainty regarding diagnosis, leaving 90 patients (70% of the initial cohort) in the study (14 HP, 76 control subjects with a variety of pulmonary diseases)
Did the result of the test being evaluated influence the decision to perform the reference standard?	Cannot tell
Were the methods of the test described in sufficient detail to permit replication?	A brief description of the method used (immunoelectrophoresis) is provided
What are the results?	
What were the likelihood ratios?	Reported sensitivity: 12/14 (86%); reported specificity: 71/76 (93%). The sample size (especially the number of HP) is small; the 95% confidence intervals must be wide Calculated likelihood ratio: 12
Will the results improve my patient care?	
Will the reproducibility of the test result and its interpretation be satisfactory in my setting?	No data on the reproducibility of the test are reported. A guide for interpretation is provided however
Are the results applicable to my patient?	The antigens tested were from six bird species most frequently involved in bird-breeder's disease in Switzerland. The sensitivity and specificity of serum precipitins may vary according to the offending antigen
Will the result change my management?	More data are needed to tell
Will patients be better off as a result of the test?	More data are needed to tell

*The criteria used are those of the Evidence-Based Medicine Working Group;[37,38] the article that is appraised is from Reynaud *et al.*[39]

unclear whether the false negatives result from inappropriate antigens tested or if HP can occur in the absence of specific antibodies to the responsible allergen.

Despite the pitfalls discussed above, specific antibodies analysis can be useful as supportive evidence. The results of the HP study demonstrate that positive serum antibodies are a significant predictor of HP [odds ratio (OR) 5.3; 95% CI 2.7–10.4].[11] Antigens available for testing in most centres include pigeon and parakeet sera, dove feather antigen, *Aspergillus sp.*, *Penicillium*, *S. rectivirgula* and *Thermoactinomyces viridans*. These antigens cover most cases of HP including pigeon-breeder's disease, bird-fancier's lung,

farmer's lung and humidifier lung. The antigen *Trichosporon cutaneum* is also available in Japan for cases of summer-type HP.[45] The selection of antigens to be tested often needs to be determined locally according to the prevalent antigens.[11,46]

Several methods for the determination of precipitins or total immunoglobulin (Ig)G antibodies [immunodiffusion, immunoelectrophoresis, enzyme-linked immunosorbent assays (ELISA)] and different antigen preparations have been described.[39] A brief review of these techniques and their limitations was provided recently by Reboux and Dalphin.[47] ELISA is usually the preferred method. In the HP study, six of the seven clinical sites that participated in the study currently use this technique.[11] When sera with optical density readings above 3 standard deviations of the control were considered positive, ELISA was more sensitive than immunodiffusion in the detection of abnormal antibodies in pigeon-breeder's disease.[48] Unfortunately, even the ELISA technique lacks standardization.[49] The importance of the proper determination of reference values for serum antibodies against pigeon serum antigen has also been emphasized.[50]

Inhalation challenge

Inhalation challenges to suspected environments, usually at the workplace, as well as specific provocation tests in controlled conditions have been described.[51] These tests lack standardization in both the inhalation protocols and the criteria defining a positive response. Two selected and recent examples are provided in Table 8.[52,53] The small number of patients studied limits the interpretation of these investigations. Further studies are needed before recommending inhalation challenges in the diagnosis of HP.

Bronchoalveolar lavage (BAL)

BAL plays an important role in the investigation of patients suspected of having HP.[54] BAL can provide useful, supportive elements in the diagnosis of HP. A normal number of lymphocytes rules out all but residual disease.[55] However, the presence of an alveolar lymphocytosis does not, by any means, establish the diagnosis because asymptomatic, exposed individuals can also have increased numbers of lymphocytes in their BAL,[56] and many other diseases (including sarcoidosis, interstitial pneumonia associated with collagen vascular disease, silicosis,

bronchiolitis obliterans with organizing pneumonia, HIV-associated pneumonitis and drug-induced pneumonitis) are also characterized by an alveolar lymphocytosis.[54] Positive BAL findings (especially if the observed lymphocytosis is marked;[57,58] Table 9) in a patient with interstitial lung disease of unknown origin should direct the clinician towards the possible diagnosis of HP.[54]

As in the case of serum precipitins and inhalation challenge, the BAL technique lacks standardization. Data on proportions of BAL cells reported by various groups performing lavage with different amounts of saline suggested that, at least in normal subjects, the information about cell types obtained in volumes of 100–250 mL are comparable.[59] Also, the usual threshold values used to define BAL lymphocytosis ($\geq$30% for non- and ex-smokers and $\geq$20% for current smokers) are from the BAL Cooperative Group report.[12] They represent the 95th percentile of expected % lymphocytes in healthy individuals (healthy never smokers, 34.3%; healthy ex-smokers, 29.3%; healthy current smokers, 18.6%). We are not aware of any data documenting the specificity of 30% BAL lymphocytes in smokers or 20% BAL lymphocytes in non-smokers for identifying HP.

Lymphocyte subsets, especially the CD4/CD8 ratio and activation, were previously thought to be helpful in differentiating HP from sarcoidosis. This is now challenged as the CD4/CD8 ratio can be increased in HP to levels as high as those seen in sarcoidosis.[60–62]

Lung biopsy

The histopathology of HP has been well described.[63–65] Its description is beyond the scope of this chapter. In the acute

Table 8. Selected examples of inhalation challenge for HP.

Reference (first author)	Antigen	Inhalation protocol	Criteria defining a positive response	Accuracy
Ramirez-Venegas[52]	Pigeon serum	20-min inhalation through a nebulizer	Within 24 hours following challenge, either: (1) increase in body temperature by $\geq$0.5°C; (2) decrease in FVC by $\geq$16%; (3) decrease in oxygen saturation by $\geq$3%; (4) decrease in oxygen arterial pressure by $\geq$3 mmHg	Sensitivity: from 17/17 (100% criteria 1) to 13/17 (76% criteria 2) Specificity: from 18/22 (81% criteria 2) to 19/22 (86% criteria 4)
Ohtani[53]	Pigeon or budgerigar dropping extracts	10-min inhalation through a hand nebulizer	$\geq$3 of the following 24 hours after challenge: (1) increased radiological abnormalities; (2) increase in alveolo-arterial oxygen pressure difference by >10 mmHg or decrease in D_LCO by >20%; (3) decrease in FVC by >15%; (4) increase in peripheral leucocyte count by >30%; (5) increase in C-reactive protein by >1.0 mg/dL; (6) increase in body temperature by >1.0°C and/or chills/general fatigue; (7) development of cough/dyspnoea	Sensitivity: 8/11 (72.7%) Specificity: 6/6 (100%)

Table 9. General characteristics of BAL fluid from control subjects and patients with sarcoidosis and HP.

Subset of patients	Recovery of infused lavage fluid (%)	Total cells recovered ($\times 10^6$)	Cell viability (%)	Macrophages		Lymphocytes	
				Total cells ($\times 10^6$)	%	Total cells ($\times 10^6$)	%
Smokers (with chronic bronchitis)	57.4 ± 8.1	60.5 ± 3.2	81.2 ± 2.0	56.7 ± 0.3	85.2 ± 3.4	2.9 ± 0.01	5.3 ± 2.1
Non-smokers	56.2 ± 7.3	27.4 ± 4.1	87.4 ± 3.4	20.7 ± 0.2	54.9 ± 2.2	6.2 ± 0.08	18.6 ± 1.3
Sarcoidosis	62.5 ± 3.3	24.3 ± 3.5	84.4 ± 1.5	10.7 ± 1.8	42.1 ± 3.3	9.3 ± 1.6	43.0 ± 5.1
Hypersensitivity pneumonitis	64.2 ± 8.4	168.5 ± 5.1	87.4 ± 2.8	30.2 ± 1.3	19.8 ± 3.9	101.0 ± 7.2	68.9 ± 4.8

*Results are expressed as mean ± SEM. Godard P, Clot J, Jonquet O, Bousquet J, Michel FB. Lymphocyte subpopulations in bronchoalveolar lavages of patients with sarcoidosis and hypersensitivity pneumonitis. *Chest* 1981; **80**:447–52 with permission.

stages, reports on open lung biopsies revealed features of interstitial lymphocyte infiltrates and fibrosis, oedema, non-caseating granulomas and bronchiolitis obliterans. Macrophages with foamy cytoplasm are also found within the alveolar space. In chronic stages, widespread fibrotic reaction is a prominent feature, often without predominant involvement of upper lobes with contraction. Even if emphysema was found at necropsy in chronic HP, it is only recently that emphysema has been recognized as a long-term complication of HP.[33] A report of six cases meeting Richerson's criteria for HP emphasized that non-specific interstitial pneumonitis may be the sole histological expression of the disease.[66]

Transbronchial biopsy

We reported in 1997 a study that evaluated whether transbronchial biopsy is useful for the diagnosis of acute farmer's lung (FL).[67] Two independent pathologists conducted a retrospective and blinded analysis of 105 transbronchial biopsies with adequate material from patients with parenchymal diseases (55 cases of farmer's lung matched with 50 controls). The pathologists were asked to classify each patient in four diagnostic categories: (a) probable FL; (b) possible FL; (c) non-specific; (d) alternative diagnosis. Interobserver agreement was fair. Almost half the transbronchial biopsies were read as non-specific. The best likelihood ratio of the four diagnostic categories was: (a) probable FL, 2.6 ; (b) possible FL, 2.2; (c) non specific, 0.6; (d) alternative diagnosis, 0.0. We concluded that haematoxylin–eosin-stained transbronchial biopsy is of limited usefulness for the diagnosis of FL.

Surgical lung biopsy

The utility of surgical lung biopsy has been reported most often in terms of 'diagnostic yield', i.e. the proportion of specific diagnoses obtained from the procedure. In addition, whether the procedure alters the clinical management represents an important outcome. Several retrospective studies addressing these issues in series of patients with a variety of diffuse parenchymal diseases are available.[68–79] In selected reports, the results have been very heterogeneous: the diagnostic yield ranged from 34% to 100%; therapy was altered in 46–75% of the cases. This heterogeneity may stem from several factors, including the selection of candidates for open lung biopsy, the timing of the procedure along the course of the disease as well as the expertise of the attending pathologist. The decision to submit a patient to open lung biopsy must be balanced against the associated morbidity. If HP is suspected, it has been our recommendation to reserve surgical lung biopsy for rare cases with puzzling clinical presentation or to verify the clinical diagnosis when the clinical course or response to therapy is unusual.[5] This recommendation is not based on evidence but emphasizes the limitations of surgical lung biopsy and the necessity of a thorough clinical investigation that comprises a high index of suspicion and a careful exposure history.

Therapy

Active HP

HP being an allergic reaction of the lung, the most obvious treatment is avoidance of contact with the allergen. Systemic corticosteroids represent the only reliable pharmacological treatment of HP. The best available evidence comes from a unique, randomized, placebo-controlled trial.[80] In this trial, 36 patients with acute farmer's lung were randomized to receive either 40 mg of prednisolone tapering over 8 weeks or placebo. All patients were instructed to avoid contact with the farm during the drug trial. After 1 month of treatment, there was no difference in forced expiratory volume in 1 second (FEV_1), forced vital capacity (FVC) and Pao_2 between the two groups (Fig. 1). However, a small but significant difference in D_LCO was observed. Corticosteroids had no beneficial effect on the long-term (5-year) prognosis however. The results of this trial confirmed other observations from controlled but non-randomized trials[81,82] and case series: corticosteroids hasten the recovery from the acute stage of HP, but have no beneficial effect on long-term prognosis.

If so, who should be given corticosteroids? The decision to treat with corticosteroids may be guided by the severity of

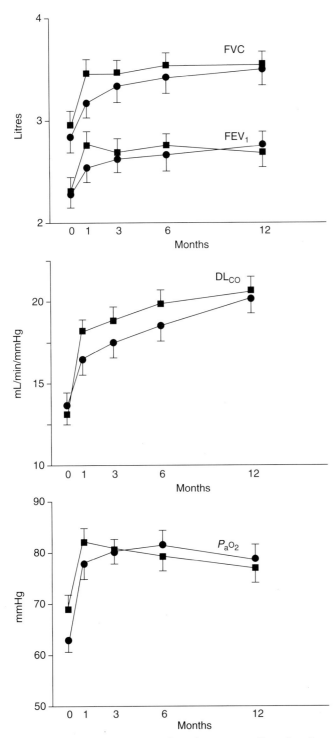

Figure 1. Effect of corticosteroids on the recovery of lung function in farmer's lung. FEV_1, FVC, D_LCO and Pao_2 during the first years of follow-up in the corticosteroid (squares) and placebo (circles) groups. The only significant difference between the two groups at 1-month follow-up was in D_LCO ($P = 0.03$). Reproduced from Kokkarinen *et al.*,[80] reproduced with permission of the American Lung Association.

symptoms and physiological abnormalities. In a prospective study of 101 patients followed from initial diagnosis, 70 received corticosteroid treatment at the time of diagnosis based on severity of symptoms and physiological abnormalities.[83] Eighty-three were still available at 58-month follow-up. Recovery of pulmonary function in patients who did not receive corticosteroid was slower during the first months of follow-up; still, the maximum values for FVC and D_LCO were achieved at the same time as in the overall study group. Corticosteroid therapy should not be prolonged: in Monkare's study, 12 weeks of steroids was no better than 4 weeks.[82] In some circumstances, total contact avoidance is impossible. In such circumstances, small-dose corticosteroid treatment is a valid alternative.[81] The use of inhaled steroids is anecdotal.[84]

Residual HP
The treatment of chronic or residual disease is supportive.

Prevention of HP

Primary prevention
In a high-risk environment (such as farming activities), education may prevent respiratory problems.[85] Ideally, all farmers should be informed of the hazards of exposure to barn dust and encouraged to use adequate preventive measures. For practical purposes, however, major preventive measures (such as mask wearing, increasing barn ventilation, avoiding the barn when the animals are feeding) cannot be recommended for primary prevention and are usually reserved for individuals with a past history of HP.[86]

Secondary prevention
The elimination of the offending antigen is the cornerstone of disease prevention.[87,88] In addition, several interventions have been proposed in order to avoid recurrence of the disease if contacts with the offending antigen cannot be avoided, especially in work-related cases. Although more than 50% of patients with farmer's lung will quit farming within 6 years after the diagnosis,[15] there is some evidence from uncontrolled studies that most agricultural workers who develop HP may be able to continue their occupation if appropriate measures are taken.[89,90] These interventions include appropriate measures of hay-making and storage,[91] use of additives to hay or silage to prevent the development of mould,[92] barn ventilation and use of masks or respirators at work.[93–96] Their description is beyond the scope of this chapter; relevant references are available however.[86]

Summary for clinicians

The diagnosis of HP can often be made or rejected with confidence, especially in areas of high or low prevalence, respectively, using simple diagnostic criteria.

Chest X-rays may be normal in active HP; HRCT is sensitive but not specific for the diagnosis of HP.

The utility of pulmonary function tests is to describe the physiological abnormalities and the associated impairment.

Despite the pitfalls of false-positive and false-negative results, precipitin analysis can be useful as supportive evidence for HP.

Further studies are needed before recommending inhalation challenges for the diagnosis of HP.

Bronchoalveolar lavage plays an important role in the investigation of patients suspected of having HP. A normal number of lymphocytes rules out all but residual disease.

Haematoxylin–eosin-stained transbronchial biopsy is of limited usefulness for the diagnosis of FL; surgical lung biopsy should be reserved for rare cases with puzzling clinical presentation or to verify the clinical diagnosis when the clinical course or response to therapy is unusual.

HP being an allergic reaction of the lung, the most obvious treatment is avoidance of contact with the allergen. Systemic corticosteroids represent the only reliable pharmacological treatment of HP but do not alter long-term outcome.

References

1 Selman M. Hypersensitivity pneumonitis. In: Schwarz MI, King TE Jr, eds. *Interstitial Lung Disease*, 3rd edn. Hamilton, BC Decker, 1998:393–422.

2 Schwartz M, Patterson R. Hypersensitivity pneumonitis—general considerations. *Clin Rev Allergy* 1983; 1:451–67.

3 Terho EO. Diagnostic criteria for farmer's lung disease. *Am J Ind Med* 1986; 10:329.

4 Richerson HB, Bernstein IL, Fink JN *et al.* Guidelines for the clinical evaluation of hypersensitivity pneumonitis. *J Allergy Clin Immunol* 1989; 84:839–44.

5 Cormier Y, Lacasse Y. Keys to the diagnosis of hypersensitivity pneumonitis: the role of serum precipitins, lung biopsy, and high-resolution computed tomography. *Clin Pulm Med* 1996; 3:72–7.

6 Schuyler M, Cormier Y. The diagnosis of hypersensitivity pneumonitis. *Chest* 1997; 111:534–6.

7 Laupacis A, Sekar N, Stiell IG. Clinical prediction rules: a review and suggested modifications of methodological standards. *JAMA* 1997; 277:488–94.

8 Sullivan PA, Odencrantz JR, Petsonk EL *et al.* Development and validation of a hypersensitivity pneumonitis surveillance questionnaire (abstract). *Am J Respir Crit Care Med* 1997; 155:A946.

9 Fox J, Anderson H, Moen T, Gruetzmacher G, Hanrahan L, Fink J. Metalworking fluid associated with hypersensitivity pneumonitis: an outbreak investigation and case control study. *Am J Ind Med* 1999; 35:58–67.

10 Dangman KH, Cole SR, Hodgson MJ *et al.* The Hypersensitivity Pneumonitis Diagnostic Index: use of non-invasive testing to diagnose hypersensitivity pneumonitis in metalworkers. *Am J Ind Med* 2002; 42:150–62.

11 Lacasse Y, Selman M, Costabel U *et al.* for the HP Study Group. Clinical diagnosis of hypersensitivity pneumonitis. *Am J Respir Crit Care Med* 2003; 158:952–8.

12 The BAL Cooperative Group Steering Committee. Bronchoalveolar lavage constituents in healthy individuals, idiopathic pulmonary fibrosis, and selected comparison groups. *Am Rev Respir Dis* 1990; 141:S169–S202.

13 Matar LD, McAdams PH, Sporn TA. Hypersensitivity pneumonitis. *AJR* 2000; 174:1061–6.

14 Pauker SG, Kassirer JP. The threshold approach to clinical decision making. *N Engl J Med* 1980; 302:1109–17.

15 Bouchard S, Morin F, Bedard G, Gauthier J, Paradis J, Cormier Y. Farmer's lung and variables related to the decision to quit farming. *Am J Respir Crit Care Med* 1995; 152:997–1002.

16 Mönkäre S, Ikonen M, Haahtela T. Radiologic findings in farmer's lung: prognosis and correlation to lung function. *Chest* 1985; 87: 460–6.

17 Seal RME, Thomas GO, Griffiths JJ. Farmer's lung. *Proc R Soc Med* 1963; 56:271–3.

18 Cook PG, Wells IP, McGavin CR. The distribution of pulmonary shadowing in farmer's lung. *Clin Radiol* 1988; 39:21–7.

19 Mindell PE. Roentgen findings in farmer's lung. *Radiology* 1970; 97:341–6.

20 Emmanuel DA, Kryda MJ. Farmer's lung disease. *Clin Rev Allergy* 1983; 1:509–32.

21 Hodgson MJ, Parkinson DK, Karpf M. Chest X-rays in hypersensitivity pneumonitis: a meta-analysis of secular trends. *Am J Ind Med* 1989; 16:45–53.

22 Silver SF, Muller NL, Miller RR, Lefcoe MS. Hypersensitivity pneumonitis: evaluation with CT. *Radiology*. 1989; 173:441–5.

23 Hansell DM, Moskovic E. High-resolution computed tomography in extrinsic allergic alveolitis. *Clin Radiol* 1991; 43:8–12.

24 Adler BD, Padley SP, Muller NL, Remy-Jardin M, Remy J. Chronic hypersensitivity pneumonitis: high-resolution CT and radiographic features in 16 patients. *Radiology* 1992; 185:91–5.

25 Akira M, Kita N, Higashihara T, Sakatani M, Kozuka T. Summer-type hypersensitivity pneumonitis: comparison of high-resolution CT and plain radiographic findings. *AJR* 1992; 158: 1223–8.

26 Buschman DL, Gamsu G, Waldron JA Jr, Klein JS, King TE Jr. Chronic hypersensitivity pneumonitis: use of CT in diagnosis. *AJR* 1992; 159:957–60.

27 Remy-Jardin M, Remy J, Wallaert B, Muller NL. Subacute and chronic bird breeder hypersensitivity pneumonitis: sequential evaluation with CT and correlation with lung function tests and bronchoalveolar lavage. *Radiology* 1993; 189:111–18.

28 Small JH, Flower CDR, Traill ZC, Gleeson FV. Air-trapping in extrinsic allergic alveolitis on computed tomography. *Clin Radiol* 1996; 51:684–8.

29 Cormier Y, Brown M, Worthy S, Racine G, Muller NL. High-resolution computed tomographic characteristics in acute farmer's lung and in its follow-up. *Eur Respir J* 2000; 16:56–60.

30 Lynch DA, Rose CS, Way D *et al.* Hypersensitivity pneumonitis: sensitivity of high-resolution CT in a population-based study. *AJR* 1992; 159:469–72.

31 Lynch DA, Newell JD, Logan PM *et al.* Can CT distinguish hypersensitivity pneumonitis from idiopathic pulmonary fibrosis? *AJR* 1995; 165:807–11.

32 Hapke EJ, Seal REM, Thomas GO *et al.* Farmer's lung: a clinical, radiological, functional, and serological correlation of acute and chronic stages. *Thorax* 1968; 23:451–68.

33 Lalancette M, Carrier G, Ferland S *et al.* Long-term outcome and predictive value of bronchoalveolar lavage fibrosing factors in farmer's lung. *Am Rev Respir Dis* 1993; 148:216–21.

34 Lacasse Y, Selman M, Costabel U et al. for the HP Study Group. Clinical manifestations of hypersensitivity pneumonitis from various origins. Am J Respir Crit Care Med 2003; 167;A359.

35 Cormier Y, Bélanger J, Tardif A, Leblanc P, Laviolette M. Relationship between radiographic changes, pulmonary function, and bronchoalveolar lavage fluid in farmer's lung disease. Thorax 1986; 41:28–33.

36 Sackett DL, Haynes RB, Guyatt GH et al. Clinical Epidemiology: a Basic Science for Clinical Medicine, 2nd edn. Boston, Little & Brown, 1991: 51–68.

37 Jaeschke R, Guyatt G, Sackett DL et al. Users' guides to the medical literature. III. How to use an article about a diagnostic test. A. Are the results of the study valid? JAMA 1994; 271:389–91.

38 Jaeschke R, Guyatt G, Sackett DL et al. Users' guides to the medical literature. III. How to use an article about a diagnostic test. B. What are the results and will they help me in caring for my patients? JAMA 1994; 271:703–7.

39 Reynaud C, Slosman DO, Polla BS. Precipitins in bird breeder's disease: how useful are they? Eur Respir J 1990; 3:1155–61.

40 Cormier Y, Bélanger J, Durand P. Factors influencing the development of serum precipitins to farmer's lung antigen in Quebec dairy farmers. Thorax 1985; 40:138–42.

41 Fink JN. Epidemiologic aspects of hypersensitivity pneumonitis. Monogr Allergy 1987; 21:59–69.

42 Dalphin JC, Toson B, Monnet E et al. Farmer's lung precipitins in Doubs (a department of France): prevalence and diagnostic value. Allergy 1994; 49:744–50.

43 Burrel P, Bylander R. A critical review of the role of precipitins in hypersensitivity pneumonitis. Eur J Respir Dis 1981; 62: 332–43.

44 Cormier Y, Bélanger J. The fluctuant nature of precipitating antibodies in dairy farmers. Thorax 1989; 44:469–73.

45 Kawai T, Tamura M, Murao M. Summer-type hypersensitivity pneumonitis: a unique disease in Japan. Chest 1984; 85:311–17.

46 Ojanen T. Class specific antibodies in serodiagnosis of farmer's lung. Br J Ind Med 1992; 49:332–6.

47 Reboux G, Dalphin JC. Hypersensitivity pneumonitis: a technical note on precipitins (in French). Rev Mal Respir 2003; 20:140–3.

48 Simpson C, Shirodaria PV, Evans JP, Simpson DI, Stanford CF. Comparison of immunodiffusion and enzyme linked immunosorbent assay in the detection of abnormal antibodies in pigeon breeder's disease. J Clin Pathol 1992; 45:490–3.

49 Aberer W, Woltsche M, Woltsche-Kahr I, Kranke B. IgG antibodies typical for extrinsic allergic alveolitis – an inter-laboratory quality assessment. Eur J Med Res 2001; 6:498–504.

50 Banales JL, Vazquez L, Mendoza F et al. On the correct determination of reference values for serum antibodies against pigeon serum antigen using a group of healthy blood donors. Arch Med Res 1997; 28:289–91.

51 Edwards JH, Davis BH. Inhalation challenge and skin testing in farmer's lung. J Allergy Clin Immunol 1981; 68:58–64.

52 Ramirez-Venegas A, Sansores RH, Perez-Padilla R, Carillo G, Selman M. Utility of a provocation test for diagnosis of chronic pigeon breeder's disease. Am J Respir Crit Care Med 1998; 158:862–9.

53 Ohtani Y, Kojima K, Sumi Y et al. Inhalation provocation tests in chronic bird fancier's lung. Chest 2000; 118:1382–9.

54 Semenzato G, Bjermer L, Costabel U, Haslam PL, Olivieri D. Clinical guidelines and indications for bronchoalveolar lavage (BAL): report of the European Society of Pneumology Task Group on BAL: extrinsic allergic alveolitis. Eur Respir J 1990; 3:945–6.

55 Cormier Y, Bélanger J, Leblanc P et al. Bronchoalveolar lavage in farmer's lung disease: diagnosis and physiological significance. Br J Ind Med 1986; 43:401–5.

56 Cormier Y, Bélanger J, Laviolette M. Persistent bronchoalveolar lymphocytosis in asymptomatic farmers. Am Rev Respir Dis 1986; 133:843–7.

57 Godard P, Clot J, Jonquet O, Bousquet J, Michel FB. Lymphocyte subpopulations in bronchoalveolar lavages of patients with sarcoidosis and hypersensitivity pneumonitis. Chest 1981; 80:447–52.

58 Valenti S, Scordamaglia A, Crimi P, Mereu C. Bronchoalveolar lavage and transbronchial lung biopsy in sarcoidosis and extrinsic allergic alveolitis. Eur J Respir Dis 1982; 63:564–9.

59 Helmers RA, Dayton CS, Floerchinger C, Hunninghake GW. Bronchoalveolar lavage in interstitial lung disease: effect of volume of fluid infused. J Appl Physiol 1989; 67:1443–6.

60 Soler P, Nioche S, Valeyre D et al. Role of mast cells in the pathogenesis of hypersensitivity pneumonitis. Thorax 1987; 42:565–72.

61 Ando M, Konishi K, Yoneda R, Tamura M. Difference in the phenotypes of bronchoalveolar lavage lymphocytes in patients with summer-type hypersensitivity pneumonitis, farmer's lung, ventilation pneumonitis and bird fancier's lung: report of a nationwide epidemiologic study in Japan. J Allergy Clin Immunol 1991; 87: 1002–9.

62 Wahlstrom J, Berlin M, Lundgren R et al. Lung and blood T cell repertoire in extrinsic allergic alveolitis. Eur Respir J 1997; 10:772–9.

63 Reyes CN, Wenzel FJ, Lawton BR, Emanuel DA. The pulmonary pathology of farmer's lung disease. Chest 1982; 81:142–6.

64 Kawanami O, Basset F, Barrios R, Lacronique JG, Ferrans VJ, Crystal RG. Hypersensitivity pneumonitis in man. Light- and electron-microscopic studies of 18 lung biopsies. Am J Pathol 1983; 110: 275–89.

65 Coleman A, Colby TV. Histologic diagnosis of extrinsic allergic alveolitis. Am J Surg Pathol 1988; 12:514–18.

66 Vourlekis JS, Schwarz MI, Cool CD, Tuder RM, King TE, Brown KK. Nonspecific interstitial pneumonitis as the sole histologic expression of hypersensitivity pneumonitis. Am J Med 2002; 112:490–3.

67 Lacasse Y, Fraser RS, Fournier M, Cormier Y. Diagnostic accuracy of transbronchial biopsy in acute farmer's lung disease. Chest 1997; 112:1459–65.

68 Qureshi RA, Ahmed TA, Grayson AD, Soorae AS, Drakeley MJ, Page RD. Does lung biopsy help patients with interstitial lung disease? Eur J Cardiothorac Surg 2002; 21:621–6.

69 Rena O, Casadio C, Leo F et al. Videothoracoscopic lung biopsy in the diagnosis of interstitial lung disease. Eur J Cardiothorac Surg 1999; 16:624–7.

70 Temes RT, Joste NE, Qualls CR et al. Lung biopsy: is it necessary? J Thorac Cardiovasc Surg 1999; 118:1097–100.

71 Kramer MR, Berkman N, Mintz B, Godfrey S, Saute M, Amir G. The role of open lung biopsy in the management and outcome of patients with diffuse lung disease. Ann Thorac Surg 1998; 65:198–202.

72 Neuhaus SJ, Matar KS. The efficacy of open lung biopsy. Aust NZ J Surg 1997; 67:181–4.

73 Lachapelle KJ, Morin JE. Benefit of open lung biopsy in patients with respiratory failure. Can J Surg 1995; 38:316–21.

74 Bove P, Ranger W, Pursel S, Glover J, Bove K, Bendick P. Evaluation of outcome following open lung biopsy. Am Surg 1994; 60:564–70.

75 Shah SS, Tsang V, Goldstraw P. Open lung biopsy: a safe, reliable and accurate method for diagnosis in diffuse lung disease. Respiration 1992; 59:243–6.

76 Wagner JD, Stahler C, Knox S, Brinton M, Knecht B. Clinical utility of open lung biopsy for undiagnosed pulmonary infiltrates. Am J Surg 1992; 164:104–7.

77 Walker WA, Cole FH Jr, Khandekar A, Mahfood SS, Watson DC. Does open lung biopsy affect treatment in patients with diffuse pulmonary infiltrates? J Thorac Cardiovasc Surg 1989; 97:534–40.

78 Warner DO, Warner MA, Divertie MB. Open lung biopsy in patients with diffuse pulmonary infiltrates and acute respiratory failure. Am Rev Respir Dis 1988; 137:90–4.

79 Venn GE, Kay PH, Midwood CJ, Goldstraw P. Open lung biopsy in patients with diffuse pulmonary shadowing. *Thorax* 1985; **40**: 931–5.

80 Kokkarinen JI, Tukiainen HO, Terho EO. Effect of corticosteroid treatment on the recovery of pulmonary function in farmer's lung. *Am Rev Respir Dis* 1992; **145**:3–5.

81 Cormier Y, Desmeules M. Treatment of hypersensitivity pneumonitis: contact avoidance versus corticosteroid treatment. *Can Respir J* 1994; **1**:223–8.

82 Monkare S. Influence of corticosteroid treatment on the course of farmer's lung. *Eur J Respir Dis* 1983; **64**:283–93.

83 Kokkarinen JI, Tukiainen HO, Terho EO. Recovery of pulmonary function in farmer's lung: a five-year follow-up study. *Am Rev Respir Dis* 1993; **147**:793–6.

84 Carlsen KH, Leegaard J, Lund OD, Skjaervik H. Allergic alveolitis in a 12-year-old boy: treatment with budesonide nebulizing solution. *Pediatr Pulmonol* 1992; **12**:257–9.

85 Hoglund S. Prevention of respiratory problems in agriculture. *Am J Ind Med* 1986; **10**:245–7.

86 American Thoracic Society. Respiratory health hazards in agriculture. *Am J Respir Crit Care Med* 1998; **158**:S1–S76.

87 Yoshida K, Ando M, Sakata T, Araki S. Prevention of summer-type hypersensitivity pneumonitis: effect of elimination of *Trichosporon cutaneum* from the patients' homes. *Arch Environ Health* 1989; **44**:317–22.

88 Jacobs RL, Andrews CP, Jacobs FO. Hypersensitivity pneumonitis treated with an electrostatic dust filter. *Ann Intern Med* 1989; **110**:115–18.

89 Cormier Y, Bélanger J. Long-term physiologic outcome after acute farmer's lung. *Chest* 1985; **87**:796–800.

90 Braun SR, doPico GA, Tsiatis A, Horvarth E, Dickie HA, Rankin J. Farmer's lung disease: a long-term clinical and physiological outcome. *Am Rev Respir Dis* 1979; **119**:185–91.

91 Dalphin JC, Pernet D, Reboux G *et al*. Influence of mode of storage and drying of fodder on thermophilic actinomycete aerocontamination in dairy farms of the Doubs region of France. *Thorax* 1991; **46**:619–23.

92 Baron VS, Greer GG. Comparison of six commercial hay preservatives under simulated storage conditions. *Can J Animal Sci* 1988; **68**:429–37.

93 Nuutinen J, Terho EO, Husman K, Kotimaa M, Harkonen R, Nousiainen H. Protective value of powered dust respirator helmet for farmers with farmer's lung. *Eur J Respir Dis Suppl* 1987; **152**:212–20.

94 Hendrick DJ, Marshall R, Faux JA, Krall JM. Protective value of dust respirators in extrinsic allergic alveolitis: clinical assessment using inhalation provocation tests. *Thorax* 1981; **36**:917–21.

95 Gourley CA, Braidwood GD. The use of dust respirators in the prevention of recurrence of farmer's lung. *Trans Soc Occup Med* 1971; **21**:93–5.

96 Kusaka H, Ogasawara H, Munakata M *et al*. Two-year follow up on the protective value of dust masks against farmer's lung disease. *Intern Med* 1993; **32**:106–11.

CHAPTER 6.2

Pleural disease

Richard Light

Summary

Patients with primary pneumothorax are best initially treated with aspiration and, if this is successful, hospitalization is usually not necessary.

Patients with secondary pneumothorax are best initially hospitalized and treated with tube thoracoscopy.

Thoracoscopy with stapling of blebs and creation of a pleurodesis is more effective at preventing recurrent pneumothorax than is the instillation of a sclerosing agent through a chest tube.

Light's criteria are useful for separating transudative from exudative pleural effusion but, if these criteria are just barely met and the patient clinically should have a transudative effusion, the difference between the serum and the pleural fluid protein should be assessed. If this is >3.1 g/dL, the patient in all probability has a transudative effusion.

Demonstration of a pleural fluid adenosine deaminase level above 40 IU/L is a cost-effective way to diagnose tuberculous pleuritis.

Tumour markers are of limited usefulness in the diagnosis of malignant pleural effusions.

One should consider using an indwelling catheter for the management of symptomatic recurrent malignant pleural effusions.

Approximately 10% of patients post coronary artery bypass graft surgery develop a pleural effusion that occupies more than 25% of the hemithorax.

The great majority of patients with post-coronary artery bypass graft surgery pleural effusions can be managed with one to three therapeutic thoracenteses.

Patients with parapneumonic effusion should undergo a therapeutic thoracentesis as soon as the fluid is recognized.

In patients with parapneumonic effusions, the definitive procedure should be performed within 0–14 days of admission.

The evidence supporting most of the above statements is not strong, and more randomized controlled studies on the diagnosis and treatment of pleural disease are needed.

Literature search

The report was prepared after the following search was performed on Entrez-PubMed: 'pleura or pleural or thoracoscopy or pneumothorax or pleurodesis or empyema or chylothorax or hemothorax'. The titles of all the articles were reviewed, and all articles were retrieved that appeared to be pertinent to the present publication.

Pneumothorax

A pneumothorax occurs when there is air in the pleural space. Pneumothoraces are classified as spontaneous, which occur without preceding trauma or other obvious cause, or traumatic, which occur as a result of trauma to the chest. If the trauma is a diagnostic or therapeutic manoeuvre, the pneumothorax is an iatrogenic pneumothorax. Spontaneous pneumothoraces are subclassified as primary or secondary. A primary spontaneous pneumothorax occurs in an otherwise healthy person without underlying lung disease. A secondary spontaneous pneumothorax complicates an underlying lung disease, most commonly chronic obstructive pulmonary disease (COPD).

Primary pneumothorax

Diagnosis

The diagnosis is usually established by demonstrating a pleural line on the chest radiograph. In the past, it was felt that expiratory films were more sensitive in establishing the diagnosis of pneumothorax than were inspiratory chest films because a larger percentage of the hemithorax is occupied by air on expiration. However, Seow and coworkers[1] compared 85 paired inspiratory and expiratory radiographs with pneumothoraces and 93 pairs without pneumothoraces. The films were randomly arranged and reviewed independently by three radiologists. They found that inspiratory and expiratory films were equally efficient at diagnosing pneumothorax. As radiologists and pulmonologists are more familiar with reading inspiratory chest radiographs, these are recommended for the diagnosis of pneumothorax. The consensus is that chest computerized tomography (CT) scans are not indicated in patients with primary spontaneous pneumothorax.[2,3]

When a patient is seen with a pneumothorax, it is probably important to quantify the size of the pneumothorax. This is most commonly done by expressing the pneumothorax as a percentage of the hemithorax. However, it is not clear how most radiologists arrive at the percentage. Because the volumes of the lung and the hemithorax are roughly proportional to the cube of their diameters, one can estimate the degree of collapse (PNX %) by measuring average diameters of the lung and the hemithorax, cubing these diameters and using the following equation known as the Light index:[4] percentage pneumothorax = $100(1 - \text{lung}^3/\text{hemithorax}^3)$. It has been shown recently that there is an excellent correlation ($r = 0.84$) between the Light index and the amount of air that can be aspirated from a pneumothorax.[5] However, the recent guidelines from the American College of Chest Physicians (ACCP)[3] and those from the British Thoracic Society (BTS)[2] divided pneumothoraces into small and large pneumothoraces. For the ACCP, a small pneumothorax was defined as a pneumothorax where the apex–cupola distance was less than 3 cm,[3] whereas for the BTS, a small pneumothorax was defined as one with a rim of air around the lung of less than 2 cm.[2] The most accurate way to quantify the size of a pneumothorax is with a CT scan.[6] There are no studies that evaluate whether there are advantages to semi-quantifying the percentage of the hemithorax occupied by air or merely separating pneumothoraces into large pneumothoraces and small pneumothoraces.

Treatment

The treatment options for primary pneumothorax include observation, observation with the administration of supplemental oxygen, aspiration, tube thoracostomy with or without the administration of a sclerosing agent, thoracoscopy or thoracotomy. The thoracoscopy can be a medical thoracoscopy or video-assisted thoracic surgery (VATS). Despite these numerous treatment options, there have been very few randomized controlled studies (RCTs) comparing one treatment with another.[3]

As there is a high rate of recurrence after an initial primary spontaneous pneumothorax, consideration should be given to preventing a recurrence when the patient is seen initially. Sadikot and associates[7] followed 153 patients with primary spontaneous pneumothorax for a mean of 54 months and reported that the ipsilateral recurrence rate was 39% and most recurred within the first year. In this same study, 15% of the 153 patients developed a pneumothorax on the contralateral side.[7] Patients who are tall and those who continue to smoke are more likely to have a recurrence.[7] However, there is no relationship between the number of blebs or the size of the blebs on CT[8] or the appearance of the lung at thoracotomy[9] and the risk of recurrence. Once a patient has had one recurrence, the risk of another recurrence increases to more than 50%.[10]

Observation

There is general agreement that asymptomatic patients with small pneumothoraces are best managed with observation.[2,3] The ACCP consensus statement recommends that the patient be observed in the emergency room for 3–6 hours and then discharged if a repeat chest radiograph demonstrates that there is no progression of the pneumothorax. The rate of spontaneous absorption of air from the pleural space with the patient breathing room air is approximately 1.25% of the volume of the hemithorax daily.[11] The rate of air absorption is increased by a factor of four if supplemental oxygen is administered.[12]

Aspiration

The BTS guidelines recommend that simple aspiration be the initial treatment for patients with primary spontaneous pneumothorax who are symptomatic or who have a large pneumothorax.[2] A recent study randomized 60 patients to manual aspiration or tube thoracostomy with 16F or 20F chest tubes.[13] Manual aspiration was successful in 16 of the 27 patients (59%) and 13 of the 16 did not require hospitalization.[13] One might worry that the rate of recurrence would be higher in patients who had a successful aspiration, but the recurrence rates tended to be lower in these patients (19%).[14] The primary advantage of aspiration is that hospitalization is not required in approximately 50% of patients.[14]

Tube thoracostomy

The ACCP consensus statement[3] recommends that all patients with large pneumothoraces be treated with tube thoracostomy, whereas the BTS guidelines[2] recommend that all patients who fail aspiration undergo tube thoracostomy. The ACCP consensus statement[3] recommends that either a small-bore catheter or a 16F to 22F standard chest tube should be used, while the BTS guidelines[2] concluded that smaller (10–14F) tubes can be used unless there is pleural fluid associated with the pneumothorax or the air leak is large. There are no recent randomized studies comparing smaller tubes (10–14F) with larger tubes (16–22F). It should be noted that, in the past, larger (28–32F) tubes were used almost exclusively.[15]

Tube thoracostomy with chemical pleurodesis

Randomized controlled studies have documented that the intrapleural administration of either tetracycline[15,16] or talc slurry[16] through the chest tube reduces the recurrence rates by about 50% to the 20% range. As tetracycline is no longer available, doxycycline 500 mg is presently recommended. Because the administration of talc intrapleurally may be associated with the development of the acute respiratory distress syndrome (ARDS), the author does not recommend its use.[17] However, the rate of recurrence after surgical intervention by either thoracotomy or VATS is far less than after medical pleurodesis.[2] The BTS recommends that chemical pleurodesis be performed only if the patient is either unwilling or unable to undergo surgery. There are no randomized studies comparing the cost-effectiveness of chemical pleurodesis with thoracoscopy in the management of patients with primary spontaneous pneumothorax.

Thoracoscopy

Thoracoscopy, via either VATS or medical thoracoscopy with the insufflation of talc, effectively prevents recurrences of spontaneous pneumothorax. The recurrence rates after thoracoscopy are less than 5%.[4] It is the procedure of choice if the lung remains unexpanded, if there is a persistent air leak for more than 3 days or if the patient has a recurrent pneumothorax. Some have advocated that all patients with their first episode of primary spontaneous pneumothorax be managed with thoracoscopy.[18,19] However, there are no randomized studies comparing the cost-effectiveness of this approach with simple aspiration or tube thoracostomy.

The traditional surgical approach for pneumothorax is to resect any blebs that are apparent and also to do a procedure such as pleurectomy, the instillation of a sclerosing agent or pleural abrasion to create a pleurodesis. Recently, medical thoracoscopy with the insufflation of talc and no treatment for the blebs has been advocated.[20,21] Intuitively, one would hypothesize that treatment strategies that involve resection of the blebs as well as the creation of a pleurodesis would produce the best results. However, there are no RCTs comparing these various techniques. The author, admitting that there is no conclusive evidence, recommends pleural abrasion coupled with endostapling of the blebs.[4] In reality, the procedure that the patient receives is mostly dependent upon the surgeon's preference.

Thoracotomy

The alternative procedure to thoracoscopy in the management of primary spontaneous pneumothorax is thoracotomy. At the time of thoracotomy, the blebs are resected and a procedure is done to create a pleurodesis, as is done with thoracoscopy. The recurrence rates after thoracotomy tend to be less than 1%. In one large series of 362 patients, there were only two documented ipsilateral recurrences with an average follow-up of 4.5 years in 310 patients.[22] In this series, the average postoperative hospitalization was 6 days, and there was only one death.[22] There was one study that randomized 60 patients with pneumothorax to receive VATS (bullectomy and apical pleurectomy) or a posterolateral thoracotomy with the same procedure.[23] In this study, the postoperative pain, hospital stay and pulmonary dysfunction were all less for those undergoing VATS, but the recurrence rates tended to be higher in those patients undergoing VATS.[23]

Secondary pneumothorax

The consequences of a secondary spontaneous pneumothorax are graver than those of a primary spontaneous pneumothorax. The reduction in pulmonary function associated with the pneumothorax in a patient with already reduced pulmonary function may be life-threatening. In addition, the management of the pneumothorax is more difficult because of the underlying lung disease.

The leading cause of secondary spontaneous pneumothorax is COPD, although virtually every pulmonary disease has been associated with a spontaneous pneumothorax. In one recent series of 505 patients with secondary spontaneous pneumothorax, 348 patients had COPD, 92 had tumours, 28 had

sarcoidosis, nine had tuberculosis, 16 had other pulmonary infections and 13 had miscellaneous diseases.[24]

Diagnosis

As with primary spontaneous pneumothorax, the diagnosis is usually made with the chest radiograph. It is important to distinguish a spontaneous pneumothorax from a large, thin-walled, air-containing bulla in patients with COPD. At times, CT examination of the chest is necessary to make this differentiation.[25]

Treatment

The treatment options for secondary spontaneous pneumothorax are the same as those for primary spontaneous pneumothorax. The main difference in the treatment of primary and secondary spontaneous pneumothoraces is that it is more important to prevent recurrences with secondary pneumothoraces because a recurrence of a secondary pneumothorax may be life-threatening. In contrast, the recurrence of a primary pneumothorax is usually not life-threatening. The recurrence rates with secondary spontaneous pneumothorax without treatment are slightly higher than those for primary spontaneous pneumothorax without treatment.[15,26] Although the incidence of secondary spontaneous pneumothorax is comparable to that of primary spontaneous pneumothorax, there have been fewer articles written concerning the treatment of secondary spontaneous pneumothorax and very few randomized studies. The following discussion describes how the treatment for primary and secondary spontaneous pneumothoraces differs.

Observation

The ACCP consensus statement[3] recommends that all patients with secondary spontaneous pneumothorax be hospitalized for observation or tube thoracostomy. The BTS guidelines[2] recommend observation alone only in asymptomatic cases in which the rim of air around the lung is <1 cm.

Aspiration

In general, aspiration is not recommended for secondary spontaneous pneumothorax because it is frequently unsuccessful and does not reduce the recurrence rates.[27,28]

Tube thoracostomy

Virtually all patients with secondary pneumothorax should be treated with tube thoracostomy. In patients with secondary spontaneous pneumothorax, the lung is more difficult to expand and air leaks persist longer than in patients with primary spontaneous pneumothorax. The median time for lung expansion is 5 days in secondary spontaneous pneumothorax resulting from COPD compared with 1 day for primary spontaneous pneumothorax.[29] Approximately 20% of patients will have either an unexpanded lung or a persistent air leak 7 days after tube thoracostomy.[29,30]

Prevention of recurrence

Although there are a limited number of controlled trials, the author believes that all patients with secondary spontaneous pneumothorax should have some treatment to prevent a recurrence.[4] Thoracoscopy or thoracotomy should certainly be performed in patients with a persistent air leak or an unexpanded lung after 72–96 hours. If the lung expands and the air leak ceases within the first 72 hours, an attempt should be made to prevent a recurrence. As outlined above, thoracoscopy and thoracotomy are superior to chemical pleurodesis in preventing recurrences.

Pleural effusion

Diagnostic tests of pleural fluid

Separation of transudates from exudates

When a patient with a pleural effusion is first evaluated, the first question to answer is whether the effusion is transudative or exudative.[31] If the patient has an exudative effusion, more diagnostic tests are indicated to determine the aetiology of the local disease. If the patient has a transudative effusion, the pleura itself can be ignored as the congestive heart failure, cirrhosis or other cause of the effusion is treated. A recent article demonstrated that the pleural fluid must be sampled in order to ascertain whether the effusion is transudative or exudative. Romero-Candeira and coworkers[32] clinically evaluated the history, physical examination and chest radiographs of 249 patients and indicated whether they had transudative or exudative effusions. They reported that 173/185 exudates (94%) were correctly identified clinically, but only 36/64 transudates (56%) were correctly identified.[32] Therefore, biochemical tests on the pleural fluid are necessary to make the differentiation.

For the past several decades, transudates have been differentiated from exudates by measuring the levels of protein and lactate dehydrogenase (LDH) in the pleural fluid and in the serum (Light's criteria).[33] Exudates meet one or more of the following criteria while transudates meet none:

1 A ratio of the pleural fluid protein to the serum protein >0.5.

2 A ratio of the pleural fluid LDH to the serum LDH >0.6.

3 An absolute pleural fluid LDH greater than two-thirds the upper normal limit for serum.

Since these criteria were originally published, several alternative measurements have been proposed for this differentiation. The tests that have been proposed to indicate a pleural exudate have included a pleural fluid cholesterol >60 mg/dL,[34,35] a pleural fluid cholesterol >45 mg/dL,[36] a gradient of <1.2 g/dL for the difference between the serum and the pleural fluid albumin level,[37] a gradient of <3.1 g/dL for the difference between the serum and pleural fluid protein level,[38] a pleural fluid to serum bilirubin ratio above 0.6[39] and a pleural fluid to serum cholinesterase ratio above 0.23.[40]

Two subsequent reports[41,42] have compared Light's criteria with the other proposed tests and have concluded that Light's criteria best separate exudates and transudates. Romero and associates[41] reported that Light's criteria were superior to using cholesterol to make the differentiation in 297 patients, including 44 with transudates and 253 with exudates. In this study, 98% of the exudates and 77% of the transudates were correctly classified with Light's criteria.[41] In another study from South Africa of 393 patients including 123 with transudates and 270 with exudates,[42] Light's criteria were superior to the serum effusion albumin gradient, the effusion cholesterol concentration and the pleura fluid/serum bilirubin ratio.[42] Again, in this study, Light's criteria identified 98% of the exudates correctly, but were less accurate in identifying transudates.[42] Two more recent studies have come to similar conclusions.[43,44] It is unlikely that the pleural fluid cholesterol measurement will provide additional information to the ratio of the pleural fluid to the serum protein as the pleural fluid cholesterol level can be accurately predicted from the serum cholesterol and the ratio of the pleural fluid to the serum protein level.[45]

The number of false positives and false negatives with any test depends upon the cut-off level chosen for the identification of an exudate. If a high cut-off level is chosen, all transudates will be identified correctly, whereas if a low level is chosen, all exudates will be identified correctly. An alternative approach is to choose the cut-off level that identifies the highest percentage of patients correctly. However, when such a cut-off point is chosen, both exudates and transudates will be mislabelled. Heffner and associates[46] analysed the data from eight studies with a total of 1448 patients and concluded that the best cut-off levels for the different pleural fluid tests were as follows: protein ratio 0.5, pleural fluid LDH 0.45 of upper limits of normal, LDH ratio 0.45, cholesterol ratio of 0.3 and albumin gradient of 1.2. Obviously, if these cut-off levels are used in place of the original cut-off levels of Light's criteria, more transudates will be correctly identified, but more exudates will be wrongly classified.

Light's criteria label some patients as having exudative pleural effusions who actually have transudative pleural effusions, but they correctly identify virtually all exudative effusions. This mislabelling occurs most commonly when patients with congestive heart failure are treated with diuretics before thoracentesis is performed. In such patients, the pleural fluid levels of protein and LDH can increase by 50% or more leading to the misclassification of the fluid as an exudate in the majority of cases.[38] Such patients can be identified by measuring the difference (gradient) between the levels of protein in the serum and the pleural fluid. If this difference is greater than 3.1 g/dL, the patient can be said to have a transudative pleural effusion even though Light's exudative criteria are met.[38] The advantage of using the protein gradient rather than an albumin gradient of 1.2, as has been suggested by some,[42] is that the protein gradient is already available from the measurements used to obtain Light's criteria.

In the above discussion, pleural effusions have been dichotomized into transudates or exudates based on a single cut-off point. An alternative approach recommended by Heffner and coworkers is to use likelihood ratios for identifying whether a pleural fluid is a transudate or an exudate.[47,48] The idea behind this approach is that the higher a value, e.g. the pleural fluid LDH, the more likely the effusion is to be an exudate and the lower the value, the less likely the effusion is to be an exudate. Heffner and his coworkers have derived multilevel[47] and continuous[48] likelihood ratios for the usual biochemical tests used to differentiate transudates and exudates. When these likelihood ratios are used in conjunction with pretest probabilities using Bayes' theorem, post-test probabilities can be derived.[48] The difficulty in using this approach is that the pretest probabilities vary significantly from physician to physician. Moreover, most physicians do not understand the mathematics involved. However, this approach does emphasize that it is important to take into consideration the absolute value of the measurements. Very high or very low measurements are almost always indicative of exudates and transudates, respectively, whereas values near the cut-off levels can be associated with either transudates or exudates.

There are no prospective studies that compare the utility of using likelihood ratios with the utility of using dichotomous values.

Other routine laboratory tests on pleural effusions

When a thoracentesis is performed on a patient with an undiagnosed pleural effusion, the following laboratory tests are usually obtained: protein, LDH, glucose, cell count with differential, cultures for bacteria, mycobacteria and fungi, a biochemical test for tuberculosis and pleural fluid cytology for malignancy. If a patient is thought clinically to have a transudative pleural effusion, it is best only to obtain protein and LDH levels on the pleural fluid. If the fluid proves exudative, then other tests can be obtained subsequently. In one older study,[49] the charts of 83 patients with transudative effusions (by Light's criteria) were reviewed. There were 725 additional tests performed on these 83 fluids with nine positive findings. However, the positive findings in at least seven were false-positive findings. Therefore, in addition to the $185/patient for the extra tests, additional costs were incurred in proving that the positive findings were indeed false-positive findings.[49]

There are no controlled studies that address whether it is cost-effective to obtain all the tests outlined in the above paragraph in patients with undiagnosed exudative effusions. It is reasonable to order tests based upon the likelihood of the diagnosis in a given patient. Most patients with an acute febrile illness do not have malignancy, and therefore cytology may be unnecessary in these patients. As most patients with bacterial infections of the pleural space have pleural fluid with predominantly neutrophils, bacterial cultures may not be indicated in patients with lymphocytic predominant pleural effusions.

Several comments can be made about pleural fluid tests. The pleural fluid differential cell count is useful because the presence of neutrophils indicates an acute process, whereas the presence of mononuclear cells indicates a more chronic process. The presence of more than 50% lymphocytes in the pleural effusion is usually associated with pleural tuberculosis, malignant pleural effusion or a pleural effusion post coronary artery bypass graft surgery.[4] When fluid is sent for a cell count and differential, it should be sent in a tube with an anticoagulant because pleural fluid in tubes without anticoagulant may clot and give falsely low counts.[50] Differential cell counts on pleural fluid are inaccurate when they are done with automated cell counters.[50] When bacterial cultures of pleural fluid are obtained, the fluid should be inoculated at the bedside directly into blood culture bottles.[51]

In the past, the author has recommended that amylase determinations be made on pleural fluids from patients with undiagnosed pleural effusion. However, a recent paper[52] has demonstrated that the diagnostic yield with pleural amylase is very low, as the diseases that cause an elevated amylase and the diagnosis of which is suggested by the elevated amylase (pancreatic disease and oesophageal rupture) are very uncommon. Accordingly, pleural fluid amylase measurements are recommended only when there is suspicion of acute pancreatitis, chronic pancreatic disease or oesophageal rupture.[52]

Pleural fluid pH is also frequently ordered on a routine basis. However, with the exception of patients with parapneumonic effusions, it usually has limited independent diagnostic value as the pH tends to be decreased in patients who also have a reduced pleural fluid glucose and a markedly elevated pleural fluid LDH.[4] The pleural fluid pH measurement is accurate only when it is measured with a blood gas machine.[53] Many laboratories do not measure pleural fluid pH with a blood gas machine.[54]

Tests to diagnose pleural tuberculosis

The possibility of tuberculous pleuritis should be considered in every patient with an undiagnosed exudative pleural effusion. In some countries, tuberculosis is the most common cause of pleural effusion, even though only a small percentage of such effusions are due to tuberculosis in the United States. For the past 40 years, the most common way to establish the diagnosis of tuberculous pleuritis has been with needle biopsy of the pleura. However, in recent years, three pleural fluid tests have been developed that may be useful in establishing or excluding the diagnosis of tuberculous pleuritis:[4] (a) the level of adenosine deaminase (ADA) in the pleural fluid; (b) the level of interferon gamma in the pleural fluid; and (c) the polymerase chain reaction (PCR) for mycobacterial DNA. One disadvantage of these tests is that they do not provide bacteria for antibiotic sensitivity testing.

Adenosine deaminase is an enzyme that catalyses the conversion of adenosine to inosine. It has two isoenzymes, ADA1 and ADA2.[55] ADA1 is ubiquitous in all cells, including lymphocytes and monocytes, whereas ADA2 is found only in monocytes.[55] ADA2 is the isoenzyme elevated with tuberculous pleuritis.[55] The pleural fluid ADA is relatively sensitive and specific for the diagnosis of tuberculous pleuritis. The pleural fluid ADA was above 47 U/L in 383 of 397 patients (96.5%) with tuberculosis when two studies were combined.[56,57] Pleural fluid ADA levels are elevated to a comparable degree in human immunodeficiency virus-positive and -negative patients with tuberculous pleuritis.[58] Patients with empyema and rheumatoid pleuritis also have elevated pleural fluid ADA levels, but these conditions should be relatively easy to distinguish from tuberculous pleuritis clinically. The specificity of the pleural fluid ADA level for tuberculosis can be increased it if is combined with a pleural fluid lymphocyte/neutrophil ratio of >0.75.[57] The ADA can also be used to exclude the diagnosis of tuberculosis. In one study, none of 19 patients with a positive tuberculin skin test result, an ADA below 45 IU/L and an exudative pleural effusion followed for a mean of 62 months without treatment for tuberculosis developed tuberculosis.[59] With the exception of Q fever[60] and brucellosis,[61] the pleural fluid level of ADA is not elevated in patients with lymphocytic pleural effusions of other aetiologies.[62,63]

Measurement of the interferon gamma (IFN-γ) levels is also useful in the diagnosis of tuberculous pleuritis. IFN-γ is a lymphokine produced by T lymphocytes in response to antigen stimulation. In one recent study of 595 patients with pleural effusion including 82 patients with tuberculosis, a cut-off level of 3.7 IU/mL yielded only two false negatives (2%) and 12 false positives (2%).[64] In general, measurement of pleural fluid ADA levels and IFN-γ levels is comparable in its diagnostic capability for pleural tuberculosis.[65] The primary advantage of ADA over IFN-γ is the lower cost of the ADA measurement. However, it is difficult to find commercial laboratories that measure ADA in the United States.

A PCR test for tuberculous DNA on pleural fluid may also be useful in the diagnosis of tuberculous pleuritis. In one study,[66] the sensitivity and specificity of PCR were similar to those of ADA but, in another study,[67] the sensitivity for PCR was only 42%. It is likely that the results with PCR will improve as its technology is refined. In a recent study in which PCR was compared with ADA and IFN-γ, PCR was inferior to the other two tests.[65] Accordingly, it is not recommended presently.

Tests to diagnose malignant pleural effusions

Malignancy is the most common cause of a chronic pleural effusion in older patients. Tests on the fluid that have been used to diagnose malignancy include cytology, measurement of tumour markers and flow cytometry.

Cytological examination of the pleural fluid is a fast, efficient and minimally invasive means by which to establish the diagnosis. The percentage of malignant pleural effusions diagnosed with cytology has been reported to be anywhere between 40% and 87%.[4] The diagnostic yield with cytology is influenced by several factors. Almost all adenocarcinomas will be diagnosed with cytology, but the yield is less with squamous cell carcinoma, lymphomas including Hodgkin's disease and mesothelioma.[4] Obviously, the yield is also dependent upon the skill of the cytologist. Overall, if three separate pleural fluid specimens are submitted to an experienced cytologist, a positive diagnosis should be expected in 70–80% of patients.

Flow cytometry on pleural fluid is useful in establishing the diagnosis of lymphoma. If the cells in the pleural fluid are demonstrated to be homogeneous, the diagnosis of lymphoma is established.[68] Flow cytometry can also provide the rapid quantification of nuclear DNA. However, as some benign effusions have abnormal DNA levels and some malignancies have normal DNA levels, the diagnosis of malignancy cannot be confirmed or rejected with this test.[69] Therefore, it is not recommended in this situation.

Many articles have been written regarding the utility of tumour markers such as carcinoembryonic antigen (CEA), carbohydrate antigens CA 15-3, CA 19-9, CA 72-4, cytokeratin 19 fragments, sialyl stage-specific antigen, neuron-specific enolase and squamous cell carcinoma antigen.[4] The problem with the use of tumour markers in the diagnosis of malignancy is that, if a high enough cut-off level is set so that there are no false positives, then they are relatively insensitive.[4] Although the author will use pleural fluid ADA levels to establish the diagnosis of pleural tuberculosis, the author does not use pleural fluid tumour markers to establish the diagnosis of pleural malignancy. The life expectancy of a patient with pleural malignancy is only about 90 days so one does not want to make this diagnosis in error. One possible use of the levels of tumour markers in the pleural fluid is to screen patients for additional invasive procedures. If the tumour marker level is in the range associated with malignancy, this might, for example, lead one to proceed with thoracoscopy.

Immunohistochemistry is used extensively in the diagnosis of pleural malignancy.[70] The primary use of immunohistochemistry in the diagnosis of pleural disease is the differentiation of adenocarcinoma from mesothelioma. A panel of monoclonal antibodies should be used when making this differentiation. The best antibodies for identifying adenocarcinoma are CEA and MOC-31 while the best antibodies for identifying mesothelioma are calretinin and cytokeratin 5/6.[71] Immunohistochemistry cannot distinguish malignant mesothelioma cells from benign mesothelial cells. The basis for immunohistochemical tests is that monoclonal antibodies are developed that are thought to be specific for adenocarcinoma or mesothelioma. When cells from pleural fluid or pleural tissue are counterstained after incubation with the monoclonal antibody, adenocarcinoma or mesothelioma can be identified.[70,71]

Approach to patient with no diagnosis after initial thoracentesis

Approximately 25% of patients have no definitive diagnosis established after the initial diagnostic thoracentesis, which usually includes cytology and a marker for pleural tuberculosis such as ADA. At this time, there are basically six different options available, namely computerized tomography (CT), observation, needle biopsy of the pleura, thoracoscopy, bronchoscopy or thoracotomy. There have been no prospective randomized studies that compare these approaches. However, there are some studies that provide data that are pertinent.

CT scan The author recommends that CT scan with a pulmonary embolus protocol be the first test obtained in the above situation.[72] Although there are no studies that have specifically evaluated the utility of the CT scan in this situation, recent reports have shown that CT will detect approximately 90% of pulmonary emboli that are evident on pulmonary arteriograms.[73] The other advantage of the CT scan is that it will demonstrate parenchymal disease or mediastinal pathology, which may influence decisions about subsequent procedures.[72]

Observation Observation is probably the best option if the patient is improving and there are no parenchymal infiltrates. No diagnosis is ever established in 10–15% of patients with pleural effusion. If the effusion is due to malignancy, spontaneous improvement is unlikely. If the effusion is due to tuberculous pleuritis, the pleural fluid marker for tuberculosis should be positive and, if the effusion is due to pulmonary embolus, the embolus should be demonstrated by the CT scan.

Needle biopsy of the pleura Over the past 40 years, needle biopsy of the pleura has been most commonly used to diagnose tuberculous pleuritis. However, at the present time, tests on pleural fluid, such as the ADA level, are as efficient as needle biopsy in establishing the diagnosis. The other diagnosis that is established with needle biopsy of the pleura is pleural malignancy. However, cytology is much more sensitive in establishing this diagnosis in most series.[4] If the patient has malignancy and the cytology of the fluid is negative, the needle biopsy of the pleura is usually also negative. In one series from the Mayo Clinic, the pleural biopsy was positive in 20 out of 118 (17%) patients with pleural malignancy and negative cytology.[74] Thoracoscopy is much more efficient in establishing the diagnosis of malignancy in this situation and is the preferred procedure.[75] If the patient has pleural thickening, CT-guided cutting needle biopsy of the pleura is very effective in establishing the diagnosis of pleural malignancy, including mesothelioma.[76]

Thoracoscopy Thoracoscopic procedures should be reserved for the diagnosis of pleural disease only when less invasive tests, such as thoracentesis with cytology and markers for tuberculosis, have not yielded a diagnosis. In one series of 620 patients with pleural effusions, only 48 (8%) remained without a diagnosis and were subjected to thoracoscopy.[77] Thoracoscopy is very efficient in establishing the diagnosis of pleural malignancy, being diagnostic in approximately 90% of cases.[78] Thoracoscopy is also effective in establishing the diagnosis of pleural tuberculosis. In one recent series, the diagnosis of tuberculous pleuritis was established in 42 out of 42 patients (100%) with thoracoscopy.[79] However, it should be emphasized that thoracoscopy does not establish diagnoses other than malignancy or tuberculosis. If thoracoscopy is performed for recurrent pleural effusion, a procedure such as the intrapleural injection of iodopovidone[80] or pleural abrasion should be performed to prevent recurrence of the pleural effusion.[4]

Bronchoscopy Bronchoscopy is useful in the diagnosis of a pleural effusion only if one or more of the following three conditions are present:[81] a pulmonary infiltrate on the chest radiograph or chest CT scan; haemoptysis, which suggests an endobronchial lesion; or a massive effusion (occupying more than three-quarters of the hemithorax). In the patient with positive pleural fluid cytology but an unknown primary, bronchoscopy is unlikely to be diagnostic if the patient does not have haemoptysis or a parenchymal infiltrate.[82]

Thoracotomy Open thoracotomy with direct biopsy of the pleura has been supplanted by VATS in many institutions. The main indication for open pleural biopsy (or for thoracoscopy) is progressive undiagnosed pleural disease. If both procedures are available, thoracoscopy is usually preferred because it is associated with less morbidity. Even open pleural biopsy does not always provide a diagnosis in a patient with an undiagnosed pleural effusion.[83] In one study from the Mayo Clinic, no diagnosis was established with open pleural biopsy in 51 patients during a 10-year period.[83] There was no recurrence of the effusion in 31 of the patients (61%), but 13 of the patients were eventually proven to have malignant disease.[83]

Management of various types of pleural effusions

Malignant pleural effusions

There are an estimated 200 000 cases of malignant pleural effusions in the United States each year.[4] Approximately 50% are large enough to produce symptoms. The presence of a pleural effusion indicates that the tumour has spread systemically and cannot be cured by surgery. As the median life expectancy of patients with malignant pleural effusion is about 120 days,[84] it is important to treat the effusion quickly and effectively. Although chemotherapy may improve the life expectancy of some patients with malignant pleural effusions, it will not be discussed in this chapter.

Treatment directed towards the effusion per se is indicated when the patient has shortness of breath that decreases the quality of his or her life and when the shortness of breath is relieved by a therapeutic thoracentesis. In many patients with malignant pleural effusions, shortness of breath is not relieved after a therapeutic thoracentesis.[85] Some advocate treatment of the effusion as soon as it is evident radiologically with the thought that earlier effusions are easier to treat. There are no studies evaluating whether patients have more good-quality days if they are treated as soon as the effusion is detected. As many patients with malignant pleural effusions never become symptomatic from their effusion, the author prefers to treat only symptomatic patients.

There are two primary approaches to managing symptomatic pleural effusions: drainage of the pleural space with an indwelling catheter and obliteration of the pleural space by the intrapleural injection of a sclerosing agent. There has only been one study comparing these two primary means of treatment. In a multicentre study, Putnam and coworkers[86] randomized 144 patients to receive an indwelling pleural catheter (Pleurx, Denver Biomaterials, Golden, CO, USA) or pleurodesis via a chest tube with doxycycline 500 mg. They reported that the degree of symptomatic improvement was similar in both groups, as was the life expectancy.[86] However, the median hospitalization time in the indwelling catheter group (1 day) was significantly less than the 6.5 days in the doxycycline group.[86]

Indwelling catheter The catheter that is most commonly used (Pleurx catheter) is a 15.5-Fr silicone rubber catheter that can be inserted on an outpatient basis[87,88] by pulmonologists, interventional radiologists or surgeons. The catheter is tunnelled and has a valve on the distal end that prevents fluid or air from passing in either direction through the catheter unless the catheter is accessed with the matched drainage line. The pleural fluid is drained at 24- to 48-hour intervals by inserting the access tip of the drainage line into the valve of the catheter and then draining the fluid via an external tube into vacuum bottles.[86] Interestingly, a spontaneous pleurodesis will occur in approximately 50% of patients in whom the catheter is inserted at a median of 25 days after insertion.[86] The biggest advantage of the indwelling catheter is that it can be inserted as an outpatient. Studies are presently under way to determine whether pleurodesis can be done as an outpatient by the injection of sclerosing agents through the catheter.

Pleurodesis Control of malignant effusions can be achieved if a pleurodesis is produced. By definition, pleurodesis is fusion of the visceral and parietal pleura. When a pleurodesis occurs, there is no space in which fluid can accumulate. It therefore prevents the accumulation of pleural fluid. Pleurodesis can be created by injecting an agent into the pleural space that will produce intense inflammation resulting in fibrosis and fusion of the visceral and parietal pleura.[89]

The ideal agent for producing a pleurodesis should be effective, inexpensive, widely available, not require a chest tube or hospitalization and cause no significant side-effects. Unfortunately, the ideal agent is yet to be discovered. The main agents to consider for the production of a pleurodesis are the tetracycline derivatives, talc, antineoplastics, silver nitrate and iodopovidone (betadine). No agent appears to be strikingly superior. Heffner and associates reviewed the results of pleurodesis in 433 patients and concluded that the agents used (talc, tetracycline derivatives, bleomycin and *Corynebacterium parvum*) in six different studies did not differ significantly in their effectiveness.[84] All were about 80% effective.[84]

The agent used most commonly for the production of a pleurodesis in English-speaking countries is talc.[90] Talc is used because it is effective, widely available and inexpensive. Talc can be administered either as a suspension (talc slurry) or aerosolized (insufflated). Both methods appear to be equally efficacious.[91,92] The primary problem with talc is that its intrapleural administration induces a fatal acute respiratory distress syndrome (ARDS) in about 1% of patients and non-fatal ARDS in another 5%.[93,94] The pathogenesis of the ARDS is not known, but it may be related to the size of the talc particles.[95–97] It has been suggested that talc preparations with particles smaller than 5 μm should not be used.[97] A joint committee of the ATS and the European Respiratory Society[98] recommends talc as the agent of choice. However, the BTS concluded that tetracycline derivatives are the agents of choice.[99] The author prefers not to use talc because it is no more efficacious than other agents and is associated with the development of ARDS.[17]

The agents used second most commonly for the production of a pleurodesis are the tetracycline derivatives.[90] In early animal studies on pleurodesis, tetracycline was found to be the most effective agent.[100] When parenteral tetracycline became unavailable, animal studies demonstrated that doxycycline[101] and minocycline[102] were equally effective. The primary side-effect of the tetracycline derivatives is severe chest pain. Patients receiving tetracycline derivatives intrapleurally should be under conscious sedation at the time of the injection.[4]

The agent used third most commonly for the production of a pleurodesis is bleomycin.[90] An older compilation of the literature suggested that bleomycin was less effective than talc or the tetracycline derivatives.[103] However, the more recent study by Heffner and associates showed that it was as effective as talc or the tetracycline derivatives. Bleomycin does not induce pleurodesis in rabbits.[100,104] One advantage of bleomycin is that it is associated with fewer side-effects than talc or tetracycline derivatives.[90] A disadvantage of bleomycin is that it is expensive, ~ $1000 per treatment. In animal studies, the most effective antineoplastic agent is nitrogen mustard,[105] which was the agent most commonly used for pleurodesis in the 1970s.

Three other agents that should be considered as pleurodesis agents should be mentioned: silver nitrate, iodopovidone and transforming growth factor β (TGF-β). It has been recently that 20 mL of 0.5% silver nitrate instilled through a chest tube is as effective as 5 g of talc in producing a pleurodesis in patients with malignant pleural effusion.[106] Another study[80] demonstrated that the administration of 100 mL of 2% iodopovidone resulted in pleurodesis in 50 out of 52 patients (96%). Additional studies are necessary to demonstrate the rightful place of these agents in the creation of a pleurodesis.

When any of the aforementioned agents is injected into the pleural space, the pleura is injured, and an intense inflammatory response develops. As a result of this inflammatory response, fibrosis sometimes results. The inflammatory response is mediated by cytokines, and it might be possible to produce a pleurodesis by injecting one or more of the cytokines into the pleural space. We have shown that the intrapleural injection of TGF-β in rabbits[107,108] or sheep[109] produces an excellent pleurodesis associated with pleural fluid that is much less inflammatory.[107] TGF-β has yet to be tried in humans for the production of a pleurodesis.

Tuberculous pleural effusions

The recommendations by the ATS for the treatment of tuberculous pleuritis are the same as for all other types of tuberculosis.[110] These recommendations may be somewhat intensive for isolated tuberculous pleuritis, as less invasive regimens appear to be effective, presumably because there is a small bacterial burden with tuberculous pleuritis. In one study, 130 patients were treated with 5 mg/kg isoniazid (INH) and 10 mg/kg rifampin daily for 6 months with no failures.[111] In another study, 198 patients were given 300 mg of INH plus 600 mg of rifampin daily for 1 month followed by 900 mg of INH plus 600 mg of rifampin twice a week for the next 6 months, and there was only one failure.[112]

There appears to be no advantage to draining the pleural fluid. A recent study[113] randomized 61 patients to have pigtail drainage of their pleural effusions or to have no drainage. Although the group that had the drainage had less dyspnoea in the first few days, thereafter there was no significant difference in the amount of symptoms or the degree of residual pleural thickening.[113] Additionally, two recent studies have failed to demonstrate any benefit from systemic corticosteroids in patients with tuberculous pleuritis.[114,115]

Pleural effusion post coronary artery bypass surgery

The incidence of pleural effusions occupying more than 25% of the hemithorax after coronary artery bypass graft (CABG) surgery is approximately 10%.[116] As more than 600 000 CABG operations are performed annually in the United States, these effusions are a significant problem. Although therapeutic thoracentesis, diuretics, non-steroidal anti-inflammatory agents and corticosteroids have been used for the treatment of these effusions, there are no randomized controlled studies evaluating any of these therapies. As most patients are cured with one to three therapeutic thoracenteses, this is the only treatment recommended for most patients. An occasional patient will still have recurrent pleural effusions after several thoracenteses. Such patients should be considered for thoracoscopy as they may have a membrane over their visceral pleura preventing the lung from re-expanding.[117]

Empyema and parapneumonic effusion

Pleural effusions secondary to pneumonia are the most common exudative pleural effusion in the United States.[4] Approximately 20–40% of hospitalized patients with bacterial pneumonia have an accompanying pleural effusion.[118,119] The morbidity and mortality rates for patients with pneumonia and pleural effusions are higher than for patients with pneumonia alone. In one study of patients with community-acquired pneumonia, patients with bilateral pleural effusions had a relative mortality risk 7.0 times higher than patients without a pleural effusion. Patients with a unilateral pleural effusion of moderate or greater size had a relative risk 3.4 times higher than patients without effusion.[120] It is possible that co-morbidity from diseases such as congestive heart failure might cause both the effusions and the excess mortality in this study. In assessing risks of patients with community-acquired pneumonia, the presence of a pleural effusion is given the same weight as a $P_{O2} < 60$ mmHg.[121]

Classification

An expert panel from the ACCP recently developed a new categorization of patients with parapneumonic effusions.[122] This new categorization is loosely modelled on the TMN classification of tumours and is based upon the anatomy of the effusion, the bacteriology of the pleural fluid and the chemistry of the pleural fluid (Table 1).

The category 1 effusion is a small (<10 mm thickness on decubitus radiograph, CT or ultrasound studies) free-flowing effusion. As the effusion is small, no thoracentesis is performed, and the bacteriology and chemistry of the fluid are unknown. The risk of a poor outcome with a category 1 effusion is very low.

The category 2 effusion is small to moderate in size (>10 mm thickness and <half the hemithorax) and is free flowing. The Gram stain and culture of the pleural fluid are negative, and the pleural fluid pH is above 7.20. It is important to emphasize that the pleural fluid pH must be measured with a blood gas machine. Neither a pH meter nor an indicator strip is sufficiently accurate.[53] If the pleural fluid pH is unavailable, the pleural fluid glucose must be more than 60 mg/dL. The risk of a poor outcome with a category 2 effusion is low.

The category 3 effusion meets at least one of the following criteria: (a) the effusion occupies more than half the hemithorax, is loculated or is associated with a thickened parietal pleura; (b) the Gram stain or culture is positive; or (c) the pleural fluid pH is <7.20 or the pleural fluid glucose is <60 mg/dL. The risk of a poor outcome with a category 3 effusion is moderate.

Table 1. Categorizing risk for poor outcome in patients with PPE.

	Pleural space anatomy			Pleural fluid bacteriology			Pleural fluid chemistry
A_0	Minimal, free-flowing effusion (<10 mm on lateral decubitus)	and	B_x	Culture and Gram stain results unknown	and	C_x	pH unknown
A_1	Small to moderate free-flowing effusion (>10 mm and < half hemithorax)	and	B_0	Negative culture and Gram stain	and	C_0	pH ≥ 7.20
A_2	Large, free-flowing effusion (≥half hemithorax) loculated effusion or effusion with thickened parietal pleura	or	B_1	Positive culture and Gram stain	or	C_1	pH < 7.20
			B_2	Pus			

From Colice *et al.*[122] with permission.

The category 4 effusion is characterized by pleural fluid that is pus. The risk of a poor outcome with a category 4 effusion is high.

Treatment

Treatment options available for parapneumonic effusions include observation, therapeutic thoracentesis, tube thoracostomy, intrapleural instillation of fibrinolytics, thoracoscopy with the breakdown of adhesions or decortication, thoracotomy with the breakdown of adhesions and decortication and open drainage procedures.

Observation

Observation is an acceptable option for category 1 pleural effusions as the risk of a poor outcome without drainage is very low.[118] In all other parapneumonic effusions, the pleural fluid must be examined in order to categorize the effusion properly.[122]

Although only about 10% of parapneumonic effusions require drainage, it is important not to delay drainage in those who require it. This is because an effusion that is free flowing and easy to drain can become loculated and difficult to drain over a period of 12–24 hours.[123,124]

In 1962, the American Thoracic Society recommended repeated thoracentesis for non-tuberculous empyemas that were in the early exudative phase.[125] Then, in 1968, Snider and Salleh recommended that patients with empyema be managed with two therapeutic thoracenteses but, if fluid accumulated again, then tube thoracostomy should be performed.[126] However, for the past several decades, therapeutic thoracentesis has not been used frequently for the treatment of parapneumonic effusion.

Recent studies in a rabbit model of empyema have shown that daily therapeutic thoracentesis starting 48 hours after empyema induction is at least as effective as tube thoracostomy initiated at the same time.[127] Moreover, Storm and coworkers.[128] reported that daily thoracentesis effected the resolution of empyema (purulent pleural fluid or positive microbiological studies on the pleural fluid) in 48 out of 51 patients (94%). Simmers and associates treated 29 patients with parapneumonic effusions that were pus, had positive

bacteriology or had positive chemistries with alternate-day, ultrasound-guided thoracenteses and reported that 24 (86%) were successfully treated.[129] A drawback to this study was that the patients underwent an average of 7.7 ± 3.5 thoracenteses and the average hospitalization was 31 days.[129] There have been no controlled studies comparing therapeutic thoracentesis with small tube thoracostomy in the treatment of patients with complicated non-loculated parapneumonic effusions.

Tube thoracostomy

The most common method by which parapneumonic effusions have been initially drained for the past several decades has been tube thoracostomy. The chest tube should be positioned in a dependent part of the pleural effusion. Although relatively large (28–36F) chest tubes have been recommended by most in the belief that smaller tubes would become obstructed with the thick fluid, such large tubes are probably not necessary. In one recent study, 103 patients with empyema were treated with 8–12F pigtail or 10–14F Malecot catheters inserted with the Seldinger technique under either ultrasound or CT guidance.[130] These small catheters served as the definitive treatment in 80 of the 103 patients (78%).[130] These results are at least as good as those reported in recent surgical series in which much larger tubes were used.[131,132] The correct positioning of the tube is probably more important than the size of the tube.[4] The small catheters were placed using either ultrasound or CT scans while no imaging was used to place the large catheters. The advantages of the smaller tube are that it is less painful to the patient and easier to insert.

Intrapleural fibrinolytics

If the pleural fluid becomes loculated, drainage of a parapneumonic effusion is difficult. More than 50 years ago, Tillett and associates[133] reported that the intrapleural injection of streptokinase (a fibrinolytic) and streptodornase (a DNase) facilitated pleural drainage in patients with empyemas. However, the use of intrapleural streptokinase and streptodornase was subsequently largely abandoned because their intrapleural injection was associated with systemic side-effects including febrile reactions, general malaise and leucocytosis. However, starting with the report of Bergh and colleagues in the late 1970s,[134] there have been at least five uncontrolled studies,[135–139] each with more than 20 patients, that concluded that fibrinolytics are useful in the management of patients with loculated parapneumonic effusions. Both streptokinase[135–138] and urokinase[135,138,139] have been reported to be effective. Both agents are administered intrapleurally in a total volume of 50–100 mL. The usual dose of urokinase is 100 000 IU, and the usual dose of streptokinase is 150 000 IU. The cost of one vial of streptokinase containing 250 000 IU is $127, and the cost of one vial of urokinase that contains 250 000 IU is $490.[4] The intrapleural injection of streptokinase has no effect on the systemic coagulation parameters.[140] At the present time, streptokinase is unavailable in the United States.

There have now been five controlled studies on the use of fibrinolytics for loculated parapneumonic effusions.[141–145] The first study was not randomized or blinded, in that the patients received no fibrinolytics for the first part of the study and then received streptokinase for the latter part of the study.[141] This study, which included 52 patients, concluded that there was no significant difference in the need for more invasive surgery or in the mortality rate in the two groups.[141] In a second study, 24 patients were randomized to receive streptokinase 250 000 IU/day or saline flushes as controls for up to 3 days.[142] The streptokinase group had a significantly greater reduction in the size of the pleural fluid collection and greater improvement in the chest radiograph.[142] In a third study, 31 patients were randomly assigned to receive either intrapleural urokinase or normal saline for 3 days.[143] Pleural fluid drainage was complete in 13 (86.5%) patients in the urokinase group but in only four (25%) in the control group. However, when urokinase was subsequently administered to the 12 patients with incomplete drainage in the saline control group, complete drainage of the effusion was observed in only six (50%).[143] In the fourth study, Tuncozgur and associates[144] randomly assigned 49 patients with parapneumonic empyema to receive intrapleural urokinase or normal saline daily for five consecutive days. Patients who received urokinase in this study had a shorter time for defervescence (7 ± 3 versus 13 ± 5 days, $P < 0.01$), a lower need for decortication (60% versus 29%, $P < 0.01$) and a shorter hospitalization (14 ± 4 versus 21 ± 4 days, $P < 0.01$).[144]

However, a recently completed multicentre study in the UK was unable to detect any benefit from intrapleural streptokinase.[145] In this randomized, double-blind study, 350 patients with loculated parapneumonic effusions were randomly assigned to receive either 250 000 IU streptokinase or saline daily for 3 days. The baseline characteristics of the two groups were nearly identical. There was no difference in the length of hospitalization, the need for additional surgery or the mortality in the two groups.[145]

From the above studies, giving the most weight to the multicentre study with 350 patients from the UK, one can conclude that the intrapleural administration of streptokinase to patients with loculated parapneumonic effusions does not have a great effect on the resolution of the effusion. It is likely that urokinase also does not have a great benefit in the treatment of these patients. There have been no studies on the utility of tissue plasminogen activator (TPA) in the treatment of parapneumonic effusions.

The original articles on enzymatic debridement for loculated parapneumonic effusions used Varidase, which consists of a fibrinolytic (streptokinase) and a DNase (streptodornase). It is unclear how much the DNase contributed to the efficacy of the preparation. We have shown that, when thick empyemic material from rabbits is incubated with either streptokinase or urokinase, there is no significant liquefaction of the fluid.[146] In contrast, when the fluid is incubated with Varidase, the fluid becomes completely liquefied over 4 hours. Although Varidase is presently not available in the United States, recombinant human DNase (Pulmozyme, Genentech, San Francisco, CA, USA) is available. Simpson and coworkers have recently demonstrated that recombinant DNase by itself is very effective in reducing the viscosity of human empyema fluid.[147] Although Simpson's group has also reported that DNase was useful in the treatment of one patient,[148] the usefulness of DNase with or without a fibrinolytic in the treatment of complicated parapneumonic effusions or empyema needs to be evaluated.

Thoracoscopy with lysis of adhesions

One option for the patient with an incompletely drained parapneumonic effusion is thoracoscopy. With thoracoscopy, the fibrin membranes creating the pleural loculations can be disrupted, the pleural space can be completely drained, and the chest tube can be optimally placed.[149] In addition, the pleural surfaces can be inspected to determine the necessity for further intervention such as decortication. If, at the time of thoracoscopy, the patient is found to have a very thick pleural peel with a large amount of debris and entrapment of the lung, the thoracoscopy incision can be enlarged to allow for decortication if the procedure cannot be accomplished via thoracoscopy.[149]

Thoracoscopy appears to be effective in the treatment of incompletely drained parapneumonic effusions. When four recent studies with a total of 232 patients are combined, thoracoscopy was the definitive procedure in 178 of the patients (77%).[150–153] The overall mortality was 3%, and the median time for chest tube drainage post procedure ranged from 3.3 to 7.1 days. The median hospital stay post thoracoscopy ranged from 5.3 to 12.3 days.[150–153]

It should be noted that the above four studies were uncontrolled. There was one small study that randomized 20 patients with parapneumonic effusions that were loculated or had a pleural fluid pH < 7.20 to receive either chest tube drainage plus streptokinase or thoracoscopy.[154] In this study, thoracoscopy was the definitive procedure in 10 out of 11 patients (91%) while streptokinase was definitive in four out of nine patients (44%).[154] Although the authors of this study concluded that, in patients with loculated parapneumonic effusions, a primary treatment strategy of VATS is associated with a higher efficacy, shorter hospital duration and less cost than a treatment strategy that utilizes catheter-directed fibrinolytic therapy,[154] larger randomized studies are necessary to validate this recommendation.

Decortication

Decortication involves the removal of all fibrous tissue from the visceral pleura and parietal pleura and the evacuation of all pus and debris from the pleural space.[155] Decortication eliminates the pleural sepsis and allows the underlying lung to expand. Decortication is a major thoracic operation usually requiring a full thoracotomy incision and should, therefore, not be performed on patients who are markedly debilitated.

Even though decortication is a major procedure, the postprocedure hospitalization is not long. The median postoperative stay reported in one study of 71 patients was only 7 days.[156] The mortality rate in this series was 10%, but all the patients who died had other serious medical problems.[156] The times for chest tube drainage and for hospitalization are shorter after thoracoscopy than after thoracotomy with decortication.[157]

When managing patients with pleural infections in the acute stages, decortication should only be considered for the control of pleural infection. Decortication should not be performed just to remove thickened pleura because such thickening usually resolves spontaneously over several months.[158] If, after 6 months, the pleura remains thickened and the patient's pulmonary function is sufficiently reduced to limit activities, decortication should be considered.

Recommended management of parapneumonic effusions

In their evidence-based guideline, the ACCP recommended drainage for category 3 or 4 parapneumonic effusions.[122] They also concluded that therapeutic thoracentesis or tube thoracostomy alone was insufficient for managing most patients with category 3 or 4 parapneumonic effusion[122] and concluded that fibrinolytics, VATS and surgery are acceptable approaches for managing patients with category 3 and category 4 effusions.[122] The ACCP consensus statement also acknowledged that the evidence for the above recommendations was only level C or D.[122]

The BTS guidelines for the management of pleural infections took a different tack and recommended a stepwise approach.[159] They recommended that all patients with class 3 or 4 parapneumonic effusions initially be treated with a chest tube. Then, if the chest tube did not drain the fluid or the patient remained septic, they recommended reassessment of the position of the chest tube and consideration of intrapleural fibrinolytics.[159] If the patient did not improve with these measures within 5–7 days, they recommended consultation with a thoracic surgeon for thoracoscopy or thoracotomy.[159]

When the author reviews the recommendations of the above two societies, he prefers the recommendations of the BTS even though he participated in the generation of the ACCP guidelines. He would suggest that, when the initial thoracentesis is performed, a therapeutic rather than a diagnostic thoracentesis be performed. If the fluid never returns after the initial therapeutic thoracentesis, one need not worry about the pleural fluid. This approach has never been assessed in a randomized study.

References

1 Seow A, Kazerooni EA, Pernicano PG et al. Comparison of upright inspiratory and expiratory chest radiographs for detecting pneumothoraces. AJR 1996; **166**:313–16.

2 Henry M, Arnold T, Harvey J. BTS guidelines for the management of spontaneous pneumothorax. Thorax 2003; 58(Suppl 2): II39–II52.

3 Baumann MH, Strange C, Heffner JE et al. Management of spontaneous pneumothorax: an American College of Chest Physicians Delphi Consensus Statement. Chest 2001; **119**:590–602.

4 Light RW. Pleural Diseases, 4th edn. Baltimore, Lippincott, Williams & Wilkins, 2001.

5 Noppen M, Alexander P, Driesen P et al. Quantification of the size of primary spontaneous pneumothorax: accuracy of the Light index. Respiration 2001; **68**:396–9.

6 Engdahl O, Toft T, Boe J. Chest radiograph – a poor method for determining the size of a pneumothorax. Chest 1993; **103**:26–9.

7 Sadikot RT, Greene T, Meadows K et al. Recurrence of primary spontaneous pneumothorax. Thorax 1997; **52**:805–9.

8 Smit HJ, Wienk MA, Schreurs AJ et al. Do bullae indicate a predisposition to recurrent pneumothorax? Br J Radiol 2000; **73**:356–9.

9 Janssen JP, Schramel FM, Sutedja TG et al. Videothoracoscopic appearance of first and recurrent pneumothorax. Chest 1995; **108**:330–4.

10 Gobbel WGJ, Rhea WGJ, Nelson IA et al. Spontaneous pneumothorax. J Thorac Cardiovasc Surg 1963; **46**:331–45.

11 Kircher LTJ, Swartzel RL. Spontaneous pneumothorax and its treatment. JAMA 1954; **155**:24–9.

12 Northfield TC. Oxygen therapy for spontaneous pneumothorax. BMJ 1971; **4**:86–8.

13 Noppen M, Alexander P, Driesen P et al. Manual aspiration versus chest tube drainage in first episodes of primary spontaneous pneumothorax: a multicenter, prospective, randomized pilot study. Am J Respir Crit Care Med 2002; **165**:1240–4.

14 Light RW. Manual aspiration. The preferred method for managing primary spontaneous pneumothorax? Am J Respir Crit Care Med 2002; **165**:1202–3.

15 Light RW, O'Hara VS, Moritz TE et al. Intrapleural tetracycline for the prevention of recurrent spontaneous pneumothorax. Results of a Department of Veterans Affairs cooperative study. JAMA 1990; **264**:2224–30.

16 Almind M, Lange P, Viskum K. Spontaneous pneumothorax: comparison of simple drainage, talc pleurodesis, and tetracycline pleurodesis. Thorax 1989; **44**:627–30.

17 Light RW. Talc should not be used for pleurodesis. Am J Respir Crit Care Med 2000; **162**:2024–6.

18 Margolis M, Gharagozloo F, Tempesta B et al. Video-assisted thoracic surgical treatment of initial spontaneous pneumothorax in young patients. Ann Thorac Surg 2003; **76**:1661–3.

19 Schramel FM, Sutedja TG, Braber JC et al. Cost-effectiveness of video-assisted thoracoscopic surgery versus conservative treatment for first time or recurrent spontaneous pneumothorax. Eur Respir J 1996; 9:1821–5.

20 Tschopp JM, Boutin C, Astoul P et al. Talcage by medical thoracoscopy for primary spontaneous pneumothorax is more cost-effective than drainage: a randomised study. Eur Respir J 2002; 20:1003–9.

21 Noppen M. Management of primary spontaneous pneumothorax. Curr Opin Pulm Med 2003; 9:272–5.

22 Nkere UU, Griffin SC, Fountain SW. Pleural abrasion: A new method of pleurodesis. Thorax 1991; 46:596–8.

23 Waller DA, Forty J, Morritt GN. Video-assisted thoracoscopic surgery versus thoracotomy for spontaneous pneumothorax. Ann Thorac Surg 1994; 58:372–6.

24 Weissberg D, Refaely Y. Pneumothorax. Chest 2000; 117:1279–85.

25 Phillips GD, Trotman-Dickenson B, Hodson ME et al. Role of CT in the management of pneumothorax in patients with complex cystic lung disease. Chest 1997; 112:275–8.

26 Lippert HL, Lund O, Blegvad S et al. Independent risk factors for cumulative recurrence rate after first spontaneous pneumothorax. Eur Respir J 1991; 4:324–31.

27 Ng AW, Chan KW, Lee SK. Simple aspiration of pneumothorax. Sing Med J 1994; 35:50–2.

28 Seaton D, Yoganathan K, Coady T et al. Spontaneous pneumothorax: marker gas technique for predicting outcome of manual aspiration. BMJ 1991; 302:262–5.

29 Dines DE, Clagett OT, Payne WS. Spontaneous pneumothorax in emphysema. Mayo Clin Proc 1970; 45:481–7.

30 Videm V, Pillgram-Larsen J, Ellingsen O et al. Spontaneous pneumothorax in chronic obstructive pulmonary disease: complications, treatment and recurrences. Eur J Respir Dis 1987; 71: 365–71.

31 Light RW. Pleural effusion. N Engl J Med 2002; 346:1971–7.

32 Romero-Candeira S, Hernandez L, Romero-Brufao S et al. Is it meaningful to use biochemical parameters to discriminate between transudative and exudative pleural effusions? Chest 2002; 122: 1524–9.

33 Light RW, MacGregor MI, Luchsinger PC et al. Pleural effusions: the diagnostic separation of transudates and exudates. Ann Intern Med 1972; 77:507–13.

34 Hamm H, Brohan U, Bohmer R et al. Cholesterol in pleural effusions: a diagnostic aid. Chest 1987; 92:296–302.

35 Valdes L, Pose A, Suarez J et al. Cholesterol: a useful parameter for distinguishing between pleural exudates and transudates. Chest 1991; 99:1097–102.

36 Costa M, Quiroga T, Cruz E. Measurement of pleural fluid cholesterol and lactate dehydrogenase. A simple and accurate set of indicators for separating exudates from transudates. Chest 1995; 108:1260–3.

37 Roth BJ, O'Meara TF, Cragun WH. The serum-effusion albumin gradient in the evaluation of pleural effusions. Chest 1990; 98:546–9.

38 Romero-Candeira S, Fernandez C, Martin C, Sanchez-Paya J, Hernandez L. Influence of diuretics on the concentration of proteins and other components of pleural transudates in patients with heart failure. Am J Med 2001; 110:681–6.

39 Meisel S, Shmiss A, Thaler M et al. Pleural fluid to serum bilirubin concentration ratio for the separation of transudates from exudates. Chest 1990; 98:141–4.

40 Garcia-Pachon E, Padilla-Navas I, Sanchez JF et al. Pleural fluid to serum cholinesterase ratio for the separation of transudates and exudates. Chest 1996; 110:97–101.

41 Romero S, Candela A, Martin C et al. Evaluation of different criteria for the separation of pleural transudates from exudates. Chest 1993; 104:399–404.

42 Burgess LJ, Maritz FJ, Taljaard JJ. Comparative analysis of the biochemical parameters used to distinguish between pleural transudates and exudates. Chest 1995; 107:1604–9.

43 Vives M, Porcel JM, De Vera MV et al. A study of Light's criteria and possible modifications for distinguishing exudative from transudative pleural effusions. Chest 1996; 109:1503–7.

44 Gazquez I, Porcel JM, Vives M et al. Comparative analysis of Light's criteria and other biochemical parameters for distinguishing transudates from exudates. Respir Med 1998; 92:762–5.

45 Vaz MA, Teixeira LR, Vargas FS et al. Relationship between pleural fluid and serum cholesterol levels. Chest 2001; 119:204–10.

46 Heffner JE, Brown LK, Barbieri CA. Diagnostic value of tests that discriminate between exudative and transudative pleural effusions. Chest 1997; 111:970–80.

47 Heffner JE, Sahn SA, Brown LK. Multilevel likelihood ratios for identifying exudative pleural effusions. Chest 2002; 121: 1916–20.

48 Heffner JE, Highland K, Brown LK. A Meta-analysis derivation of continuous likelihood ratios for diagnosing pleural fluid exudates. Am J Respir Crit Care Med 2003; 167:1591–9.

49 Peterman TA, Speicher CE. Evaluating pleural effusion: a two-stage laboratory approach. JAMA 1984; 252:1051–3.

50 Conner BD, Lee YC (Gary), Branca P et al. Variations in pleural fluid WBC count and differential counts with different sample containers and different methods. Chest 2003; 123:1181–7.

51 Xiol X, Castellvi JM, Guardiola J et al. Spontaneous bacterial empyema in cirrhotic patients: a prospective study. Hepatology 1996; 23:719–23.

52 Branca P, Rodrguez RM, Rogers JT et al. Routine measurement of pleural fluid amylase is not indicated. Arch Intern Med 2001; 161:228–32.

53 Cheng DS, Rodriguez RM, Rogers J et al. Comparison of pleural fluid pH values obtained using blood gas machine, pH meter, and pH indicator strip. Chest 1998; 114:1368–72.

54 Chandler TM, McCoskey EH, Byrd RP Jr et al. Comparison of the use and accuracy of methods for determining pleural fluid pH. South Med J 1999; 92:214–17.

55 Perez-Rodriguez E, Jimenez Castro D. The use of adenosine deaminase and adenosine deaminase isoenzymes in the diagnosis of tuberculous pleuritis. Curr Opin Pulm Med 2000; 6:259–66.

56 Valdés L, Alvarez D, San Jose E et al. Tuberculous pleurisy: a study of 254 cases. Arch Intern Med 1998; 158:2017–21.

57 Burgess LJ, Maritz FJ, Le Roux I et al. Combined use of pleural adenosine deaminase with lymphocyte/neutrophil ratio: increased specificity for the diagnosis of tuberculous pleuritis. Chest 1996; 109:414–19.

58 Riantawan P, Chaowalit P, Wongsangiem M et al. Diagnostic value of pleural fluid adenosine deaminase in tuberculous pleuritis with reference to HIV coinfection and a Bayesian analysis. Chest 1999; 116:97–103.

59 Ferrer JS, Munoz XG, Orriols RM et al. Evolution of idiopathic pleural effusion: a prospective, long-term follow-up study. Chest 1996; 109:1508–13.

60 Esteban C, Oribe M, Fernandez A et al. Increased adenosine deaminase activity in Q fever pneumonia with pleural effusion. Chest 1994; 105:648.

61 Dikensoy O, Namiduru M, Hocaoglu S et al. Increased pleural fluid adenosine deaminase in brucellosis is difficult to differentiate from tuberculosis. Respiration 2002; 69:556–9.

62 Lee YCG, Rogers JT, Rodriguez RM et al. Adenosine deaminase levels in nontuberculous lymphocytic pleural effusions. Chest 2001; 120:356–61.

63 Jimenez Castro D, Diaz Nuevo G, Perez-Rodriguez E *et al*. Diagnostic value of adenosine deaminase in nontuberculous lymphocytic pleural effusions. *Eur Respir J* 2003; **21**:220–4.

64 Villena V, Lopez-Encuentra A, Pozo F *et al*. Interferon gamma levels in pleural fluid for the diagnosis of tuberculosis. *Am J Med* 2003; **115**:365–70.

65 Villegas MV, Labrada LA, Saravia NG. Evaluation of polymerase chain reaction, adenosine deaminase, and interferon-gamma in pleural fluid for the differential diagnosis of pleural tuberculosis. *Chest* 2000; **118**:1355–64.

66 Querol JM, Minguez J, Garcia-Sanchez E *et al*. Rapid diagnosis of pleural tuberculosis by polymerase chain reaction. *Am J Respir Crit Care Med* 1995; **152**;1977–81.

67 Villena V, Rebollo J, Aguado JM *et al*. Polymerase chain reaction for the diagnosis of pleural tuberculosis in immunocompromised and immunocompetent patients. *Clin Infect Dis* 1998; **26**:212–14.

68 Moriarty AT, Wiersema L, Snyder W *et al*. Immunophenotyping of cytologic specimens by flow cytometry. *Diag Cytopathol* 1993; **9**:252–8.

69 Rodriguez de Castro F, Molero T, Acosta O *et al*. Value of DNA analysis in addition to cytological testing in the diagnosis of malignant pleural effusions. *Thorax* 1994; **49**:692–4.

70 Wick MR. Pleural fluid cytology, tumor markers and immunohistochemistry. In: Light RW, Lee YC (Gary), eds. *Textbook of Pleural Diseases*. London, Arnold Publishers, 2003:256–81.

71 Ordonez NG. The immunohistochemical diagnosis of mesothelioma: a comparative study of epithelioid mesothelioma and lung adenocarcinoma. *Am J Surg Pathol* 2003; **27**:1031–51.

72 Light RW. Effusions from vascular causes. In: Light RW, Lee YC (Gary), eds. *Textbook of Pleural Diseases*. London, Arnold Publishers, 2003:289–96.

73 Paterson DI, Schwartzman K. Strategies incorporating spiral CT for the diagnosis of acute pulmonary embolism: a cost-effectiveness analysis. *Chest* 2001; **119**:1791–800.

74 Prakash URS, Reiman HM. Comparison of needle biopsy with cytologic analysis for the evaluation of pleural effusion: analysis of 414 cases. *Mayo Clin Proc* 1985; **60**:158–64.

75 Light RW. Closed needle biopsy of the pleura is a valuable diagnostic procedure. Con closed needle biopsy. *J Bronchol* 1999; **5**:332–6.

76 Maskell N, Gleeson FV, Davies RJO. Standard pleural biopsy versus CT-guided cutting-needle biopsy for diagnosis of malignant disease in pleural effusions: a randomised controlled trial. *Lancet* 2003; **361**:1326–30.

77 Kendall SW, Bryan AJ, Large SR *et al*. Pleural effusions: is thoracoscopy a reliable investigation? A retrospective review. *Respir Med* 1992; **86**:437–440.

78 Hansen M, Faurschou P, Clementsen P. Medical thoracoscopy, results and complications in 146 patients: a retrospective study. *Respir Med* 1998; **92**:228–32.

79 Diacon AH, Van de Wal BW, Wyser C *et al*. Diagnostic tools in tuberculous pleurisy: a direct comparative study. *Eur Respir J* 2003; **22**:589–91.

80 Olivares-Torres CA, Laniado-Laborin R, Chavez-Garcia C *et al*. Iodopovidone pleurodesis for recurrent pleural effusion. *Chest* 2002; **122**:581–3.

81 Chang S-C, Perng RP. The role of fiberoptic bronchoscopy in evaluating the causes of pleural effusions. *Arch Intern Med* 1989; **149**:855–7.

82 Feinsilver SH, Barrows AA, Braman SS. Fiberoptic bronchoscopy and pleural effusion of unknown origin. *Chest* 1986; **90**:514–15.

83 Ryan CJ, Rodgers RF, Unni KK, Hepper NC. The outcome of patients with pleural effusion of indeterminate cause at thoracotomy. *Mayo Clin Proc* 1981; **56**:145–9.

84 Heffner JE, Nietert PJ, Barbieri C. Pleural fluid pH as a predictor of survival for patients with malignant pleural effusion. *Chest* 2000; **117**:79–86.

85 Shinto RA, Stansbury DW, Brown SE *et al*. Does therapeutic thoracentesis improve the exercise capacity of patients with pleural effusion. *Am Rev Respir Dis* 1987; **135**:A244.

86 Putnam JB, Light RW, Rodriguez MR *et al*. A randomized comparison of indwelling pleural catheter and doxycycline pleurodesis in the management of malignant pleural effusions. *Cancer* 1999; **86**:1992–9.

87 Pollak JS, Burdge CM, Rosenblatt M *et al*. Treatment of malignant pleural effusions with tunneled long-term drainage catheters. *J Vasc Interv Radiol* 2001; **12**:201–8.

88 Putnam JB Jr, Walsh GL, Swisher SG *et al*. Outpatient management of malignant pleural effusion by a chronic indwelling pleural catheter. *Ann Thorac Surg* 2000; **69**:369–75.

89 Light RW, Vargas FS. Pleural sclerosis for the treatment of pneumothorax and pleural effusion. *Lung* 1997; **175**:213–23.

90 Lee YC, Baumann MH, Maskell NA *et al*. Pleurodesis practice for malignant pleural effusions in five English-speaking countries: survey of pulmonologists. *Chest* 2003; **124**:2229–38.

91 Heffner JE, Nietert PJ, Barbieri C. Pleural fluid pH as a predictor of pleurodesis failure: analysis of primary data. *Chest* 2000; **117**:87–95.

92 Yim AP, Chan AT, Lee TW *et al*. Thoracoscopic talc insufflation versus talc slurry for symptomatic malignant pleural effusion. *Ann Thorac Surg* 1996; **62**:1655–8.

93 Milanez Campos JR, Werebe EC, Vargas FS *et al*. Respiratory failure due to insufflated talc. *Lancet* 1997; **349**:251–2.

94 Rehse DH, Aye RW, Florence MG. Respiratory failure following talc pleurodesis. *Am J Surg* 1999; **177**:437–40.

95 Ferrer J, Villarino MA, Tura JM *et al*. Talc preparations used for pleurodesis vary markedly from one preparation to another. *Chest* 2001; **119**:1901–5.

96 Ferrer J, Montes JF, Villarino MA *et al*. Influence of particle size on extrapleural talc dissemination after talc slurry pleurodesis. *Chest* 2002; **122**:108–27.

97 Rodriguez-Panadero, F. Effusions from malignancy. In: Light RW, Lee YC (Gary), eds. *Textbook of Pleural Diseases*. London, Arnold Publishers, 2003:297–309.

98 Antony VB, Loddenkemper R, Astoul P *et al*. Management of malignant pleural effusions. *Eur Respir J* 2001; **18**:402–19.

99 Antunes G, Neville E, Duffy J *et al*. BTS guidelines for the management of malignant pleural effusions. *Thorax* 2003; **58**(Suppl 2):II29–II38

100 Sahn SA, Good JT. The effect of common sclerosing agents on the rabbit pleural space. *Am Rev Respir Dis* 1981; **124**:65–67.

101 Wu W, Teixeira LR, Light RW. Doxycycline pleurodesis in rabbits. Comparison of results with and without chest tube. *Chest* 1998; **114**:563–8.

102 Light RW, Wang NS, Sassoon SCH *et al*. Comparison of the effectiveness of tetracycline and minocycline as pleural sclerosing agents in rabbits. *Chest* 1994; **106**:577–82.

103 Walker-Renard PB, Vaughan LM, Sahn SA. Chemical pleurodesis for malignant pleural effusions. *Ann Intern Med* 1994; **120**:56–64.

104 Vargas FS, Wang NS, Despars JA *et al*. Effectiveness of bleomycin in comparison to tetracycline as pleural sclerosing agent in rabbits. *Chest* 1993; **104**:1582–4.

105 Marchi E, Vargas FS, Teixeira LR *et al*. Comparison of nitrogen mustard, cytarabine and dacarbazine as pleural sclerosing agents in rabbits. *Eur Respir J* 1997; **10**:598–602.

106 Silveira Paschoalini M, Vargas FS, Marchi E *et al*. Prospective randomized trial of silver nitrate vs talc slurry in pleurodesis for symptomatic malignant pleural effusion. *Chest* 2005; in press.

107 Light RW, Cheng D-S, Lee YC *et al*. A single intrapleural injection of

transforming growth factor-β_2 produces excellent pleurodesis in rabbits. *Am J Respir Crit Care Med* 2000; **162**:98–104.

108 Lee YCG, Teixeira LR, Devin CJ *et al*. Transforming growth factor-$\beta(2)$ induces pleurodesis significantly faster than talc. *Am J Respir Crit Care Med* 2001; **163**:640–4.

109 Lee YC (Gary), Yasay JR, Johnson JE *et al*. Comparing transforming growth factor-β_2, talc, bleomycin as pleurodesing agents in sheep. *Respirology* 2002; **7**:209–16.

110 Bass JB Jr, Farer LS, Hopewell PC *et al*. Treatment of tuberculosis and tuberculosis infection in adults and children. *Am J Respir Crit Care Med* 1994; **149**:1359–74.

111 Canete C, Galarza I, Granados A *et al*. Tuberculous pleural effusion: experience with six months of treatment with isoniazid and rifampicin. *Thorax* 1994; **49**:1160–1.

112 Dutt AK, Moers D, Stead WW. Tuberculous pleural effusion: 6-month therapy with isoniazid and rifampin. *Am Rev Respir Dis* 1992; **145**:1429–32.

113 Lai YF, Chao TY, Wang YH *et al*. Pigtail drainage in the treatment of tuberculous pleural effusions: a randomized study. *Thorax* 2003; **58**:149–51.

114 Galarza I, Canete C, Granados A *et al*. Randomised trial of corticosteroids in the treatment of tuberculous pleurisy. *Thorax* 1995; **50**:1305–7.

115 Wyser C, Walzl G, Smedema JP *et al*. Corticosteroids in the treatment of tuberculous pleurisy. A double-blind, placebo-controlled, randomized study. *Chest* 1996; **110**:333–8.

116 Light RW, Rogers JT, Moyers JP *et al*. Prevalence and clinical course of pleural effusions at 30 days after coronary artery and cardiac surgery. *Am J Respir Crit Care Med* 2002; **166**:1563–6.

117 Lee YC (Gary), Vaz MAC, Ely KA *et al*. Symptomatic persistent post-coronary artery bypass graft pleural effusions requiring operative treatment. Clinical and histologic features. *Chest* 2001; **119**: 795–800.

118 Light RW, Girard WM, Jenkinson SG *et al*. Parapneumonic effusions. *Am J Med* 1980; **69**:507–11.

119 Musher DM, Alexandraki I, Graviss EA *et al*. Bacteremic and non-bacteremic pneumococcal pneumonia. A prospective study. *Medicine (Baltimore)* 2000; **79**:210–21.

120 Hasley PB, Albaum MN, Li Y-H *et al*. Do pulmonary radiographic findings at presentation predict mortality in patients with community-acquired pneumonia? *Arch Intern Med* 1996; **156**:2206–12.

121 Fine MJ, Auble TE, Yealy DM *et al*. A prediction rule to identify low-risk patients with community-acquired pneumonia. *JAMA* 1996; **275**:134–41.

122 Colice GL, Curtis A, Deslauriers J *et al*. Medical and surgical treatment of parapneumonic effusions: an evidence-based guideline. *Chest* 2000; **118**:1158–71.

123 Bartlett JG, Finegold SM. Anaerobic infections of the lung and pleural space. *Am Rev Respir Dis* 1974; **110**:56–77.

124 Cham CW, Haq SM, Rahamim J. Empyema thoracis: a problem with late referral? *Thorax* 1993; **48**:925–7.

125 Andrews NC, Parker EF, Shaw RR *et al*. Management of nontuberculous empyema. *Am Rev Respir Dis* 1962; **85**:935–6.

126 Snider GL, Saleh SS. Empyema of the thorax in adults: review of 105 cases. *Chest* 1968; **54**:12–17.

127 Sasse S, Nguyen T, Teixeira LR *et al*. The utility of daily therapeutic thoracentesis for the treatment of early empyema. *Chest* 1999; **116**:1703–8.

128 Storm HKR, Krasnik M, Bang K *et al*. Treatment of pleural empyema secondary to pneumonia: thoracocentesis regimen versus tube drainage. *Thorax* 1992; **47**:821–4.

129 Simmers TA, Jie C, Sie B. Minimally invasive treatment of thoracic empyema. *Thorac Cardiovasc Surg* 1999; **47**:77–81.

130 Shankar S, Gulati M, Kang M *et al*. Image-guided percutaneous drainage of thoracic empyema: can sonography predict the outcome? *Eur Radiol* 2000; **10**:495–9.

131 Ali I, Unruh H. Management of empyema thoracis. *Ann Thorac Surg* 1990; **50**:355–9.

132 Ashbaugh DG. Empyema thoracis. Factors influencing morbidity and mortality. *Chest* 1991; **99**:1162–5.

133 Tillett WS, Sherry S, Read CT. The use of streptokinase–streptodornase in the treatment of postpneumonic empyema. *J Thorac Surg* 1951; **21**:275–97.

134 Bergh NP, Ekroth R, Larsson S *et al*. Intrapleural streptokinase in the treatment of haemothorax and empyema. *Scand J Thorac Cardiovasc Surg* 1977; **11**:265–8.

135 Bouros D, Schiza S, Patsourakis G *et al*. Intrapleural streptokinase versus urokinase in the treatment of complicated parapneumonic effusions: a prospective, double-blind study. *Am J Respir Crit Care Med* 1997; **155**:291–5.

136 Jerjes-Sanchez C, Ramirez-Rivera A, Elizalde JJ *et al*. Intrapleural fibrinolysis with streptokinase as an adjunctive treatment in hemothorax and empyema: a multicenter trial. *Chest* 1996; **109**:1514–19.

137 Laisaar T, Puttsepp E, Laisaar V. Early administration of intrapleural streptokinase in the treatment of multiloculated pleural effusions and pleural empyemas. *Thorac Cardiovasc Surg* 1996; **44**:252–6.

138 Temes RT, Follis F, Kessler RM *et al*. Intrapleural fibrinolytics in management of empyema thoracis. *Chest* 1996; **110**:102–6.

139 Moulton JS, Moore PT, Mencini RA. Treatment of loculated pleural effusions with transcatheter intracavitary urokinase. *AJR* 1989; **153**:941–5.

140 Davies CW, Lok S, Davies RJ. The systemic fibrinolytic activity of intrapleural streptokinase. *Am J Respir Crit Care Med* 1998; **157**:328–30.

141 Chin NK, Lim TK. Controlled trial of intrapleural streptokinase in the treatment of pleural empyema and complicated parapneumonic effusions. *Chest* 1997; **111**:275–9.

142 Davies RJO, Traill ZC, Gleeson FV. Randomised controlled trial of intrapleural streptokinase in community acquired pleural infection. *Thorax* 1997; **52**:416–21.

143 Bouros D, Schiza S, Tzanakis N *et al*. Intrapleural urokinase versus normal saline in the treatment of complicated parapneumonic effusions and empyema. A randomized, double-blind study. *Am J Respir Crit Care Med* 1999; **159**:37–42.

144 Tuncozgur B, Ustunsoy H, Sivrikoz MC *et al*. Intrapleural urokinase in the management of parapneumonic empyema: a randomised controlled trial. *Int J Clin Pract* 2001; **55**:658–60.

145 Maskell NA, Davies CW, Nunn AJ *et al*. UK controlled trial of intrapleural streptokinase for pleural infection. *N Engl J Med* 2005; **352**:926–8.

146 Light RW, Nguyen T, Mulligan ME *et al*. The *in vitro* efficacy of varidase versus streptokinase or urokinase for liquefying thick purulent exudative material from loculated empyema. *Lung* 2000; **178**:13–18.

147 Simpson G, Roomes D, Heron M. Effects of streptokinase and deoxyribonuclease on viscosity of human surgical and empyema pus. *Chest* 2000; **117**:1728–33.

148 Simpson G, Roomes D, Reeves B. Successful treatment of empyema thoracis with human recombinant deoxyribonuclease. *Thorax* 2003; **58**:365–6.

149 Silen ML, Naunheim KS. Thoracoscopic approach to the management of empyema thoracis. Indications and results. *Chest Surg Clin N Am* 1996; **6**:491–9.

150 Landreneau RJ, Keenan RJ, Hazelrigg SR *et al*. Thoracoscopy for empyema and hemothorax. *Chest* 1995; **109**:18–24.

151 Cassina PC, Hauser M, Hillejan L *et al*. Video-assisted thoracoscopy in the treatment of pleural empyema: stage-based management and outcome. *J Thorac Cardiovasc Surg* 1999; **117**:234–8.

152 Lawrence DR, Ohri SK, Moxon RE *et al.* Thoracoscopic debridement of empyema thoracis. *Ann Thorac Surg* 1997; **64**: 1448–50.

153 Striffeler H, Gugger M, Im Hof V *et al.* Video-assisted thoracoscopic surgery for fibrinopurulent pleural empyema in 67 patients. *Ann Thorac Surg* 1998; **65**:319–23.

154 Wait MA, Sharma S, Hohn J *et al.* A randomized trial of empyema therapy. *Chest* 1997; **111**:1548–51.

155 Thurer RJ. Decortication in thoracic empyema. Indications and surgical technique. *Chest Surg Clin N Am* 1996; **6**:461–90.

156 Pothula V, Krellenstein DJ. Early aggressive surgical management of parapneumonic empyemas. *Chest* 1994; **105**:832–6.

157 Angelillo Mackinlay TA, Lyons GA, Chimondeguy DJ *et al.* VATS debridement versus thoracotomy in the treatment of loculated post-pneumonia empyema. *Ann Thorac Surg* 1996; **61**:1626–30.

158 Neff CC, VanSonnenberg E, Lawson DW *et al.* CT follow-up of empyemas: pleural peels resolve after percutaneous catheter drainage. *Radiology* 1990; **176**:195–7.

159 Davies CW, Gleeson FV, Davies RJ. BTS guidelines for the management of pleural infection. *Thorax* 2003; **58**(Suppl 2):II18–II28.

CHAPTER 6.3

Therapy of pulmonary thromboembolism: an evidence-based approach

Martin Riedel

Abstract

The first randomized trial of treatment of venous thromboembolism (deep venous thrombosis and pulmonary embolism) was done in 1960. Since then, impressive gains have been made in placing this treatment on a firm scientific footing. There are two phases in the therapy of patients with symptomatic pulmonary embolism: initial therapy usually consists of intravenous unfractionated heparin or subcutaneous low-molecular-weight heparin, whereas oral vitamin K antagonists are prescribed for secondary prophylaxis. This approach is highly effective in most patients. Conventional anticoagulant therapy reduces the risk of recurrent thromboembolism by 80–90%, but at an annual risk of bleeding of approximately 3%. Unfortunately, evidence-based recommendations on the duration of oral anticoagulant treatment are long on recommendations and short on evidence. Older trials indicated that longer therapy was superior to shorter therapy; data from recent trials have demonstrated that the benefit was maintained only while receiving therapy.

Within the last decade, the development of newer classes of antithrombotic agents has accelerated. Among these are heparin derivatives, direct thrombin inhibitors (parenteral and oral), selective inhibitors of factor Xa and of tissue factor VIIa, and others. These agents are able to target both free and clot-bound thrombin, and some of them might have the advantage of long-term oral administration without monitoring of anticoagulation or adjustments of dose.

Thrombolytic therapy can be life saving in patients with massive embolism, right heart failure and haemodynamic instability. Its use in patients without haemodynamically important embolism is not indicated, although it remains a controversial topic. Patients with right ventricular dysfunction observed on echocardiography who are treated with thrombolysis have more rapid return of right ventricular geometry and restoration of pulmonary perfusion, but these improvements have not translated to improved mortality in the absence of shock.

Urgent pulmonary embolectomy can only be considered in patients with acute massive embolism complicated by shock.

The only obvious and accepted indication for vena cava interruption are absolute contraindications to and documented failures of anticoagulant therapy in patients with acute venous thromboembolism. Other indications, such as 'prophylactic' or 'adjuvant' in patients who can receive anticoagulant therapy, remain a matter of debate. The presumed advantages of removable filters remain to be proven.

Introduction

Venous thromboembolism (VTE) is a common and potentially lethal disease that recurs frequently and is associated with long-term impairment and suffering. Patients with pulmonary embolism (PE) are at risk of death, recurrence of embolism or chronic morbidity.[1] Appropriate therapy can reduce the incidence of all. The mortality of PE can be up to 30% in untreated patients, more than 10 times the annual mortality for patients treated with anticoagulant drugs. Balanced against the danger of non-treatment are the risks of treatment. The short-term objectives for the treatment of VTE are to prevent extension of the thrombus, (fatal) PE and the early recurrence of the disease. Long-term aims are to prevent delayed recurrences and sequelae such as the post-thrombotic syndrome and pulmonary hypertension.

As the primary process leading to PE is deep venous thrombosis (DVT), antithrombotic regimens are the mainstay of therapy. These include drugs that inhibit blood coagulation (heparin, vitamin K antagonists, direct thrombin inhibitors) and thrombolytic drugs. Anticoagulation, by preventing clot propagation, allows endogenous fibrinolytic activity to dissolve existing thromboemboli. Anticoagulant therapy is essentially prophylactic, as these agents only interrupt progression of the thrombotic process; unlike thrombolytic agents, they do not actively resolve it. Direct mechanical resolution of the pulmonary vascular obstruction caused by PE can be performed by surgical embolectomy or catheter techniques.

Unfractionated heparin (UFH), low-molecular-weight heparin (LMWH), direct thrombin inhibitors and thrombolytic agents in appropriate doses, as well as surgical or catheter embolectomy, followed by vitamin K antagonists, are used to treat acute PE. Inferior vena caval procedures, physical techniques that counteract venous stasis, dextran and lower doses of UFH or LMWH are used for prevention, but these prophylactic regimens are not appropriate for treatment of acute disease.[1] Primary prevention of VTE is not dealt with in this chapter.

A general scheme for the therapy of PE is given in Figure 1. Given the high mortality rate of patients with acute PE if it is untreated, therapy should be initiated when PE is first seriously considered. When there is a suspicion of PE and no strong contraindication to heparin, it is wise to start therapy with a bolus of 5000–10 000 U while the diagnostic workup is pursued. If subsequent tests rule out the diagnosis, heparin can be stopped. With established diagnosis, the therapy depends on the circulatory state of the patient. With severely impaired circulation, i.e. hypotension or shock (present in less than 10% of patients in whom PE is diagnosed), the relief of pulmonary vascular obstruction must be as rapid as possible and, in these patients, immediate thrombolytic therapy, perhaps combined with mechanical fragmentation of the clot, is indicated.[2] If these measures fail or if thrombolysis is contraindicated, emergency embolectomy should be undertaken. If thrombolysis is successful, it is followed by heparin and oral anticoagulants. Patients with minor embolism, or even massive embolism but a stable circulation, are treated with heparin

followed by oral anticoagulants. If recurrent PE occurs during this therapy or if anticoagulation is contraindicated, venous interruption should be considered.

Patients with VTE who receive adequate anticoagulation generally do not die of recurrent disease.[3–7] However, patients who are treated for PE are almost four times more likely (1.5% versus 0.4%) to die of recurrent VTE in the next year than are patients who are treated for DVT.[4]

Bed rest is not mandatory in patients with PE once therapeutic levels of anticoagulation have been achieved. There are no data supporting the concern that early ambulation may dislodge thrombi in the lower extremities.[8–10]

Heparin

Unfractionated heparin is the mainstay of treatment after thrombolysis and for all patients who do not have severe circulatory embarrassment. It remains the reference therapy for initial anticoagulation. Heparin acts by catalysing the effect of antithrombin (AT), so that this inhibitor efficiently combines with and inactivates a number of serine proteases, notably thrombin (factor IIa), factor Xa and factor IXa. Of these three enzymes, thrombin is the most sensitive to inhibition by heparin–AT. Heparin also acts to inhibit activation of factors V and VIII by thrombin. In addition, heparin catalyses the inac-

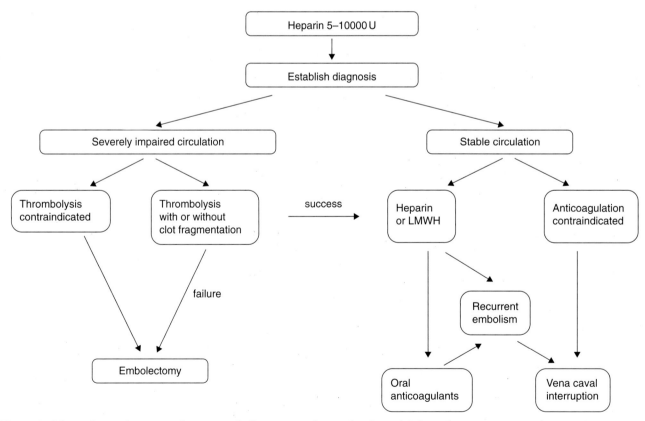

Figure 1. Scheme for treating acute pulmonary embolism. LMWH, low-molecular-weight heparin.

tivation of thrombin by another plasma cofactor, heparin cofactor II, which acts independently of AT.[11,12] All these actions prevent further fibrin deposition on the thrombus. This stops the formation and growth of thrombi and allows the patient's native fibrinolytic mechanisms to destroy both the emboli that have occurred already and thrombi that are potential further emboli. However, heparin does not directly dissolve thrombus that already exists. In PE, UFH also rapidly reduces mediator-induced pulmonary vasoconstriction and bronchoconstriction from thrombin activation and platelet aggregation.[13]

The evidence that an initial course of heparin is indeed warranted comes from two clinical trials. The first and only placebo-controlled, randomized trial of heparin in combination with an oral vitamin K antagonist in the treatment of PE was reported by Barritt and Jordan in 1960.[14] They randomized patients with a clinical diagnosis of acute PE into a group receiving heparin, 10 000 U intravenously (IV) q6h times six doses, with concurrent treatment with the oral anticoagulant nicoumalone for 14 days; the other group did not receive anticoagulant therapy. They reviewed the results after 35 patients had been randomized. Of 16 patients randomized to anticoagulant therapy, there were no deaths from PE and no non-fatal recurrences of PE. In the group not receiving anticoagulant therapy, there were five deaths from PE and five non-fatal recurrences of PE. As these results were highly statistically significant ($P = 0.0005$), they discontinued randomization and treated all additional patients with the anticoagulant regimen. A total of 54 patients had been treated with anticoagulants when the trial ended. In the treated group, there was one non-fatal recurrence of PE and no PE deaths. When these results were compared with the 19 untreated patients, the results were again highly significant.[14]

The second study evaluated the need for heparin therapy in patients presenting with DVT; this study demonstrated that combined use of heparin and oral anticoagulants is more effective than oral anticoagulants alone.[15] This study was also stopped prematurely after 120 patients had been randomized, because the patients who were not treated initially with heparin had an incidence of recurrent thromboembolism during the 3 months after randomization that was three times as high as that in the group that received heparin (20% versus 6.7%, $P = 0.058$).

In retrospect, the only randomized, placebo-controlled trial by Barritt and Jordan[14] of anticoagulation therapy for PE was underpowered, but the high rate of autopsy-confirmed fatal PE (25%) in the untreated patients remains persuasive. The diagnosis of the initial PE and recurrent PE was based entirely on clinical criteria and basic investigations, as lung scintigraphy and angiography were not available; therefore, most patients must have had moderate to severe PE. Because of the purely clinical diagnostic methods used in this study, the conclusions are of limited relevance to modern practice. Nevertheless, this influential study suggested that the mortality of

untreated patients with PE was 35%, a figure that is still quoted as representative and which causes many clinicians to use anticoagulation even when proof of VTE is lacking. Newer evidence suggests that untreated patients with either proven or probable smaller PE have a much lower recurrence rate.[16] In a series of almost 8000 hip replacements in which there were 83 postoperative deaths due to sudden PE, 308 patients who survived postoperative PE were not anticoagulated, with only 10 recurrences, none of which was fatal.[17] In one study of 627 patients with suspected PE who had indeterminate lung scans and no proximal DVT, a situation in which it can be estimated that 60–70 probably did have PE, anticoagulation was withheld and subsequent PE was rare.[18] A review of the PIOPED (Prospective Investigation of Pulmonary Embolism Diagnosis) pulmonary angiograms found that 20 patients were not anticoagulated because smaller PE had been overlooked; there were only two recurrences, one of which was fatal.[19] Thus, considering the risks of anticoagulation, it is possible that the benefit/risk ratio of this treatment of PE is less than previously assumed. It may be that patients with minor PE and no evidence of residual DVT do not necessarily require treatment, particularly if risk factors are only temporary. In the absence of further data, however, consensus opinion at this time is that any patient who has proven diagnosis of PE needs treatment unless there are extenuating circumstances such as terminal disease.

The study by Barritt and Jordan[14] had a major impact on clinical practice; the benefits of anticoagulants seen in PE were extrapolated to DVT. For both disorders, the standard of care became treatment with heparin followed by a vitamin K antagonist. With this treatment, the hospital mortality is quite low. Carson et al.[3] reported that, in the PIOPED study of 399 patients with angiographically documented acute PE, in whom 84% were treated with conventional anticoagulant therapy, the hospital mortality was 2.5%. Nine of the 10 deaths were due to recurrent PE, which occurred in 8.3% of all patients. Douketis et al.[4] reviewed 25 prospective studies of patients with well-documented acute PE who were treated with 5–10 days of heparin, followed by 3 months of oral anticoagulant therapy. The 2-week fatality rate was 2.3%. The majority of patients included in this review were enrolled in clinical trials; very few were in shock. In a recent trial of 1110 patients with haemodynamically stable PE treated with UFH and vitamin K antagonist, the total mortality after 3 months was 4.4%, with fatal PE in 1.4%.[20] The mortality of PE complicated by shock is in the range of 30–35%, despite treatment.[21–27]

Route of administration, dose and therapeutic range

UFH can be given by subcutaneous injection, by continuous infusion or as intermittent boluses 4-hourly. Haemorrhage is slightly more common with the bolus technique but, because patients receiving UFH in boluses usually receive greater doses of the drug, it is uncertain whether the difference noted in the rates of bleeding is related to the method of heparin administration or to the difference in the total dose of UFH given.[12,28]

Because UFH binds to several plasma, platelet and endothelial proteins (some of them are acute-phase reactants, the levels of which are elevated in sick patients), its plasma levels and anticoagulant response are unpredictable. This variability is independent of renal function and is seen even with weight-based dosing. Therefore, careful control of the level of anticoagulation and dose adjustments are mandatory to prevent complications and optimize therapeutic efficacy. In practice, this is easier to do when heparin is given by continuous infusion.

The most commonly used clotting test is the activated partial thromboplastin time (aPTT), which is a global coagulation test (sensitive to the inhibitory effects of heparin on thrombin and factors Xa and IXa). Different reagents and coagulation timers make the aPTT quite variable relative to a given heparin concentration.[29] The current recommendation is to give sufficient UFH to prolong the aPTT to a range that corresponds to a plasma heparin level of 0.2–0.4 U/mL by protamine titration, which in animal experiments is necessary to interrupt an ongoing thrombotic process. This relationship can be established a priori by a simultaneous comparison of aPTT and plasma heparin levels in 20–30 patients receiving heparin. Once the therapeutic range for the aPTT is known, monitoring of plasma heparin levels is seldom necessary. If the laboratory changes its coagulation timer or uses a different thromboplastin for the aPTT, the correlation between aPTT and plasma heparin levels should be re-established.[12,29]

The aPTT should be measured 4–6 hours after initiation of heparin therapy and repeated 6 hours after any change in dosage, and subsequently at least daily. The aPTT should be maintained at 1.5–2.5 times the patient pretreatment or the laboratory mean control value. Failure to achieve this range is associated with an increased risk of recurrent VTE. In contrast, there is only a weak association between supratherapeutic aPTT response and the risk of bleeding. A weight-based UFH dosing nomogram is useful in rapidly achieving therapeutic goals while avoiding prolonged periods of excessive anticoagulation (Table 1).[11,30–32] When the bolus method is used, close control is difficult because of the wide swings that occur in plasma heparin levels. The best that can be achieved is to prevent gross over- or underanticoagulation by ensuring that there is only a slight prolongation of clotting just before the next dose. If the aPTT is prolonged before UFH is started, the possibility of antiphospholipid antibodies should be considered and, in these circumstances, the concentration of heparin itself should be assayed.[33] A heparin dose greater than 45 000 U/day should not be administered unless a heparin level <0.2 U/mL is confirmed. True heparin resistance is mainly due to AT deficiency. Neither hepatic nor renal disease seems to interfere notably with the clearance of the drug at therapeutic concentrations.

The efficacy of heparin therapy depends on achieving a crit-

Table 1. Weight-based heparin dosing nomogram.

Initial dose	Bolus 80 U/kg, then 18 U/kg/h as an infusion
aPTT < 35 s (<1.2 × control)	Bolus 80 U/kg, increase infusion by 4 U/kg/h
aPTT 35–45 s (1.2–1.5 × control)	Bolus 40 U/kg, increase infusion by 2 U/kg/h
aPTT 46–70 s (1.5–2.5 × control)	No change
aPTT 71–90 s (2.5–3 × control)	Decrease infusion rate by 2 U/kg/h
aPTT > 90 s (>3 × control)	Hold infusion for 1 hour, then decrease rate by 3 U/kg/h

aPTT is measured 6 hours after change of dosage or at least once daily.
Modified from Raschke et al.[32]

ical therapeutic level of heparin within the first few hours of treatment. Two studies reported that the risk of recurrence was higher in patients with aPTT less than 1.5 times the control value early in treatment than in patients with aPTT greater than 1.5 times the control value.[34,35] A randomized trial comparing a standard starting heparin infusion rate of 1000 U/hour with a higher weight-adjusted dose clearly demonstrated the inadequacy of the standard dose; recurrent VTE was less common in patients who received the higher heparin dose.[32] Clinical recurrence is unusual as long as heparin is infused intravenously in a dose of at least 1250 U/hour. With subcutaneous injection, an adequate anticoagulant response is not achieved in the first 24 hours unless a starting dose of at least 17 500 U (or 250 U/kg) every 12 hours is used.[11] However, recurrent PE may occur during the first few days of heparin therapy before the clot becomes adherent to the endothelium, and this need not imply therapeutic failure.

Some clinical studies provide direct evidence that UFH therapy does not prevent thrombus progression in a large proportion of patients with DVT.[36] Possible reasons why UFH fails to arrest thrombus growth include the failure of UFH to inhibit the activity of clot-bound thrombin and the attainment of subtherapeutic levels during heparin infusion. Both thrombin and factor Xa bind to fibrin and retain their catalytic activities on this 'solid phase', resulting in continuous local conversion of fibrinogen to fibrin and continuous local activation of prothrombin to thrombin. UFH is relatively ineffective against clot-bound thrombin, consistent with steric interference imposed by the larger heparin–AT complex. On the contrary, direct thrombin inhibitors and direct and indirect factor Xa inhibitors (see below) effectively limit the activity of clot-bound thrombin; the degree to which this theoretical advantage actually translates into effective thrombus prevention and/or regression will only become apparent based on clinical trial findings.

Duration of heparin treatment

For many years, it was standard practice to administer heparin for about 10 days and to delay the initiation of oral anticoagulants for 3 or 4 days. This approach was supported by only meagre evidence and often delayed hospital discharge. Two randomized studies in the late 1980s reported that treatment with 4–5 days of heparin was as effective as the 9- to 10-day course.[37,38] In addition to reducing the length of hospital stay, the shorter heparin course also leads to reduction in the risk of heparin-induced thrombocytopenia (HIT) that usually requires at least 5 days of heparin exposure to manifest.[39,40] Thus, nowadays, the usual duration of heparin therapy for a major PE is about 1 week.[12,20] Vitamin K antagonists are started together with heparin therapy and should be administered jointly with heparin for at least 5 days; heparin may then be discontinued when the prothrombin time shows an international normalized ratio (INR) above 2.0 on two consecutive days.

Complications of heparin treatment

Haemorrhagic complications occur in up to 15% of patients on full-dose heparin, but are serious in less than 5%.[20,28,41] They are most likely if the patient has a potential source of bleeding such as an active peptic ulcer or any of a wide variety of risk factors, the most important of which are a pre-existing bleeding tendency, uraemia, advanced age, obesity, recent surgery or trauma, severe hypertension, previous gastrointestinal haemorrhage and concomitant antiplatelet therapy. Heparin therapy is absolutely contraindicated if the patient has had a recent haemorrhagic stroke.[28]

The management of bleeding on heparin treatment will depend on its location and severity, the risk of recurrent VTE and the aPTT. Heparin should be discontinued temporarily or permanently in such cases. Blood transfusion will correct massive blood loss, but protamine in a slow infusion (10–20 min) is the specific antidote. One milligram of protamine neutralizes about 100 U of UFH, but no more than 50 mg should be given with a single infusion unless a large overdose of heparin is known to have occurred. Generally, the effects of UFH wear off so rapidly that an antagonist is rarely required. Patients with recurrent VTE and bleeding while on heparin may be candidates for insertion of an inferior vena cava filter.

Occasionally, prolonged administration of high-dose heparin (over 2 months at > 15 000 U daily, which is used primarily during pregnancy) leads to osteoporosis.[42,43] No preventive therapy has been proved to be effective for heparin-induced osteopenia, although supplements of calcium and vitamin D are often given. Skin necrosis and hypersensitivity reactions to heparin are rare. Very rarely, continuous heparin infusion over a few days causes aldosterone depression by an unknown mechanism; this may cause clinically important hyperkalaemia in certain patients, e.g. those with renal failure or diabetes.[44]

UFH causes transient mild thrombocytopenia in about 5% of patients and severe thrombocytopenia in less than 2%.[11] The milder variety (HIT type I) occurs within the first 4 days of heparin administration and is the result of a direct aggregation effect of UFH on platelets. The platelet count is generally $100–150 \times 10^9$/L. The patient is usually asymptomatic, and thrombocytopenia resolves spontaneously in spite of continuation of heparin therapy.

The severe immunological type of heparin-induced thrombocytopenia (HIT type II) occurs 5+ days after starting heparin therapy (or sooner with re-exposure to heparin).[39,40] It is caused by heparin-dependent immunoglobulin (Ig)G antibodies that activate platelets leading to arterial or venous thrombus formation. It differs from other types of drug-induced thrombocytopenia as it gives rise to both arterial or venous thrombosis as well as haemorrhagic complications. The platelet count is below 100×10^9/L or less than half the pretreatment value. In established cases, heparin must be stopped immediately, and danaparoid (a heparinoid said to be free of contaminating heparin) or a direct thrombin inhibitor (lepirudin or argatroban) should be given for temporary anticoagulation.[45–47] Administering vitamin K antagonists in the acute phase of HIT may actually aggravate the thrombotic tendency, possibly by suppressing protein C synthesis. Adjunctive measures may include manoeuvres to salvage ischaemic limbs (thrombectomy or thrombolysis). Platelet transfusion may worsen the problem and should be avoided. The complications and morbidity related to the HIT can be prevented if thrombocytopenia is recognized and heparin stopped immediately. It is therefore essential to monitor the platelet count in all patients receiving heparin.[11,12,39]

Low-molecular-weight heparin

Low-molecular-weight heparin is formed by chemical or enzymatic depolymerization of UFH. LMWHs have ratios of anti-factor Xa to anti-factor IIa activity that vary between 8 : 1 and 2 : 1 (Table 2), depending on their molecular size distribution (UFH has a ratio of anti-factor Xa to anti-factor IIa of 1 : 1).[11] Owing to reduced non-specific binding to cationic proteins and cell surfaces,[48] the bioavailability of LMWH after subcutaneous injection is better and the half-life longer than that of UFH. Therefore, LMWH produces a more predictable anticoagulant response than UFH. The anticoagulant response of a given dose correlates with body weight, so that LMWH may be given in standard doses (anti-Xa U/kg body weight) once or twice daily subcutaneously without laboratory monitoring.[6] Monitoring is usually necessary only in the presence of renal failure (creatinine clearance < 30 mL/min)[49] or extreme obesity.

LMWH is progressively replacing standard UFH for therapy of VTE. The therapeutic index of LMWH (the potential for benefit versus the risk of bleeding) appears to be higher than that of standard UFH. The treatment is cost effective (despite the higher costs of LMWH) and convenient as it allows early

Table 2. Low-molecular-weight heparins.

LMWH	Trade name	Mean molecular weight (Da)	Ratio of anti-Xa to anti-IIa	Dosage in prophylaxis of VTE (subcutaneously)	Dosage in treatment of VTE (subcutaneously)
Ardeparin	Normiflo	6000	2.0	50 U/kg q12h	130 U/kg q12h
Bemiparin	Hibor, Ivor, Zivor	3600	8.0	2500–3500 U qd	115 U/kg qd
Certoparin	Mono-Embolex	5400	2.0	3000 U qd	8000 U q12h
Dalteparin	Fragmin	6000	2.6	2500–5000 U qd	120 U/kg q12h or 200 U/kg qd
Enoxaparin	Lovenox, Clexane	4200	3.0	2000–4000 U qd	100 U/kg q12h
Nadroparin	Fraxiparin, Selaprin	4500	3.4	40–60 U/kg qd	90 U/kg q12h
Parnaparin	Fluxum	4700	3.4	3200–6400 U qd	6400 U q12h
Reviparin	Clivarin	4000	4.0	1750 U qd	<60 kg: 4200 U q12h >60 kg: 6300 U q12h
Tinzaparin	Innohep, Logiparin	6500	1.9	3500 U qd or 50 U/kg qd	175 U/kg qd

U, international anti-factor-Xa units; VTE, venous thromboembolism.

mobilization and requires less nursing and laboratory supervision. Subcutaneous self-administration by the patient allows out-of-hospital treatment.[50] LMWH interacts with platelets and platelet factor-4 less readily, and the incidence of HIT is lower than with standard UFH.[51] The incidence of osteopenia during long-term use also appears to be less than with UFH.[43,52]

Body weight-adjusted LMWH once or twice daily subcutaneously has been shown to be as effective and safe as standard full-dose UFH in the treatment of proximal DVT[53–57] and acute haemodynamically stable PE.[5–7,58–60] In fact, LMWH regimens are more effective than UFH in reducing thrombus size on sequential venography, considered a surrogate marker for clot regression.[61] Furthermore, one randomized trial of one LMWH (reviparin) demonstrated its superiority over UFH in inhibiting *in vivo* thrombin generation in the initial treatment of acute VTE; these changes were associated with improved clinical response, as determined by a lower rate of recurrent VTE and a greater reduction in venographically assessed thrombus size.[62] Meta-analyses show that LMWH therapy results in slightly less recurrent VTE, less major bleeding and a slightly lower all-cause mortality over the ensuing 3 months.[56,59]

The accuracy of adjusting LMWH dosage on the basis of body weight is questionable, and the rationale for such practice has not been firmly established. A fixed-dose, body weight-independent LMWH (certoparin), administered twice daily for 8 days, has been shown to be at least as efficacious and safe as intravenous aPTT-adjusted UFH for 12 days for the initial treatment of acute DVT, with both regimens followed by oral anticoagulants for 6 months.[63] This treatment further simplifies the initial therapeutic approach to acute VTE.

As an alternative to vitamin K antagonists (which require laboratory monitoring) for long-term treatment, subcuta-

neous LMWH has been proposed and evaluated in randomized clinical trials, but they have all been small studies lacking the power to establish whether these two treatment modalities are equivalent in efficacy or safety. When all these studies were combined (a total of 1379 patients), a statistically nonsignificant reduction in the risk of recurrent VTE and in the risk of major bleeding in favour of LMWH treatment was found. No difference in total mortality was observed. The results of this meta-analysis indicate that a 3-month course of LMWH is as effective as a corresponding period of oral anticoagulant therapy,[64] and may thus be considered as a valuable alternative option for patients in whom oral anticoagulants appear to be contraindicated or problematic. This may be especially true in patients with cancer, who are at increased risk of recurrent VTE and anticoagulant-associated bleeding compared with non-cancer patients, and in whom oral anticoagulation can be problematic due to difficult venous access and unpredictable changes in the dose–response because of poor nutrition, infection, vomiting, concomitant medications and impaired hepatic function. One large randomized clinical trial has shown that 6 months of treatment with the LMWH dalteparin in place of 6 months of oral anticoagulant therapy significantly reduces the risk of recurrent VTE in cancer patients, without an increase in bleeding.[65] Lastly, the potential antineoplastic effects of LMWHs make these agents an attractive option in patients with cancer.[66,67]

Some unresolved issues remain to be addressed in specific trials before LMWHs can definitively replace UFH in the treatment of all forms of PE. Can LMWH alone be given from the onset or should a bolus of UFH (with a quicker onset of action) also be given at the same time? The therapeutic role of LMWH in patients with massive PE who are haemodynamically unstable remains to be determined. The safety of unmonitored out-of-hospital treatment of patients with stable PE (as is becoming routine in patients with DVT) also needs to be established. It is uncertain whether a weight-adjusted dosing regimen without laboratory monitoring should be used in very obese patients, those with renal insufficiency or pregnant women. The effectiveness of protamine as an antidote for LMWH is uncertain, because reversal of the anticoagulant effect of LMWH with protamine is limited to molecules larger than 4000 Da, and many LMWH chains are smaller than this. Different preparations of LMWH vary with respect to their mean molecular weights, ratios of anti-factor Xa to anti-factor IIa activity and degree of binding to plasma proteins (Table 2). Properties associated with one LMWH cannot be extrapolated to a different LMWH. For this reason, the findings of clinical trials apply only to the particular LMWH evaluated and should not be generalized to LMWHs at large.[11,12]

Synthetic pentasaccharide

The evolution of UFH has seemingly culminated in fondaparinux, a unique synthetic pentasaccharide (molecular weight 1726 Da) that represents the minimal AT-binding unit of heparin. To inhibit thrombin, UFH must bind not only to AT but also to thrombin itself, whereas fondaparinux binds only to AT and is thus a specific inhibitor of factor Xa. It inhibits thrombin generation without any direct inhibitory effect on the thrombin molecule. Fondaparinux is rapidly absorbed following subcutaneous administration and exhibits 100% bioavailability. It exhibits no non-specific binding to plasma or cellular proteins. These properties lead to a predictable dose–response effect and render the risk of HIT extremely unlikely. They allow for once-daily dosing, a rapid onset of action and a predictable duration of effect with no dose adjustment or dose monitoring required.

Several large-scale phase 2 and phase 3 trials have demonstrated the superiority of fondaparinux, compared with a LMWH, in reducing VTE risk following major orthopaedic surgery.[68–72] A meta-analysis of these trials indicates an overall significant 55% reduction in VTE risk, in favour of fondaparinux, with no difference in clinically relevant bleeding complications at the dosing regimens used. After these trials, fondaparinux was approved for the prevention of VTE in major hip and knee surgical procedures. One phase 2 trial demonstrated equivalent efficacy and safety of fondaparinux, compared with a LMWH, in the treatment of proximal DVT,[73] and one large controlled clinical trial found once-daily, subcutaneous administration of fondaparinux without monitoring at least as effective and safe as adjusted-dose, intravenous UFH in the initial treatment of haemodynamically stable patients with PE.[20]

Direct thrombin inhibitors

In contrast to all heparin products, which act indirectly via AT to inhibit both thrombin and factor Xa, direct thrombin inhibitors bind to thrombin specifically and inhibit its catalytic activity without the involvement of AT. Hirudin is a progenitor of this family of peptides. These peptides, particularly the low-molecular-weight analogues, more effectively inhibit fibrin deposition in the interstices of a thrombus than does the larger heparin–AT complex. They may therefore be more effective than heparin in inactivating thrombin bound to fibrin, which is a potent stimulus for thrombus growth. Their dose–response curve exhibits linearity over a range greater than that of UFH, and the aPTT test is well suited to monitoring their anticoagulant effect.

Drugs investigated so far include lepirudin (a recombinant hirudin), bivalirudin (semi-synthetic, formerly known as Hirulog), argatroban (a small synthetic arginine analogue that inhibits thrombin's active site by ionic binding), desirudin (a recombinant desulphato hirudin) and the dipeptide melagatran. Ximelagatran is an orally given prodrug that is rapidly metabolized to form melagatran, its active metabolite, which has been shown to have a shallower dose–response curve than warfarin in experimental models of thrombosis and, therefore, a better separation between efficacy and bleeding. Excess bleeding seen with hirudin is probably attributable to its irreversible binding to thrombin. Direct thrombin inhibitors that feature more reversible binding, such as argatroban, bivaluridin and melagatran, may be associated with less bleeding than seen with hirudin.

Clinical evaluation of direct thrombin inhibitors is just beginning. Lepirudin and argatroban are available for the treatment of HIT.[47,74] The half-life of lepirudin is relatively short (about 1.3 hours), which is helpful in patients who develop bleeding or who require surgery or invasive procedures. There is no known antidote. Administration of ximelagatran twice daily appears to require no patient monitoring or dose adjustment, based on clinical trials completed to date. Compared with vitamin K antagonists, oral direct thrombin inhibitors would offer enhanced convenience without diet or drug–drug interactions.

Direct thrombin inhibitors have been evaluated in trials of VTE prophylaxis in hip and knee arthroplasty, and were found to be as safe and effective as their respective comparator drugs, with proximal DVT and/or PE incidences of 2–10% reported.[75–80] Results from larger phase 3 clinical trials with the oral ximelagatran also failed to show any clear superiority to warfarin or enoxaparin in VTE prophylaxis after hip and knee surgery.[78,80,81] These disappointing findings call into question the concept that small direct thrombin inhibitors will inactivate clot-bound thrombin more effectively than AT-dependent drugs such as UFH and LMWH. Nevertheless, an oral drug that requires no monitoring of its anticoagulant effect is, in theory, of considerable interest.[82] Extended treatment with ximelagatran after completion of the 6 months of treatment with vitamin K antagonists effectively prevented VTE recurrences in patients with a relatively low risk of recurrence.[83] At present, there are no large controlled clinical trials evaluating direct thrombin inhibitors in the treatment of acute PE.

Oral anticoagulants (vitamin K antagonists)

Oral anticoagulants act in the liver by inhibiting the synthesis of four vitamin K-dependent coagulant proteins (factors II, VII, IX and X) and at least two vitamin K-dependent anticoagulant factors, proteins C and S. The three widely used drugs are warfarin, phenprocoumon and acenocoumon. Although these drugs are often referred to as oral anticoagulants, the term 'vitamin K antagonists' is preferable, as it distinguishes these drugs from selective coagulation factor inhibitors (such as oral inhibitors of factor Xa and oral thrombin inhibitors), which are currently in clinical trials but are not discussed here.

Vitamin K antagonists do not act immediately because time is required for coagulation factors already present in the plasma to be cleared. It is therefore essential to overlap them with heparin for at least 5 days, even if the prothrombin time reaches the target range sooner (the level of protein C declines quickly after initiation of oral anticoagulants, creating a thrombogenic potential).[12,84] Initial treatment with heparin and vitamin K antagonists simultaneously does not lead to more haemorrhages than does delayed initiation of the vitamin K antagonist, but it reduces the duration of treatment with heparin, thus decreasing the risk of HIT.

The evidence supporting the need for secondary prophylaxis with vitamin K antagonists is provided by two comparative studies. In one study, by Lagerstedt et al.,[85] patients with DVT who were initially treated with full-dose UFH were randomly assigned to receive no further treatment or vitamin K antagonists. In the other study, Hull and colleagues[86] compared vitamin K antagonists with a fixed low dose of subcutaneous UFH (5000 U twice a day) after initial treatment in patients with DVT. Both studies clearly indicated that the risk of recurrent VTE with no or inadequate secondary prophylaxis was higher than the risk among patients who received oral anticoagulant therapy (i.e. about 27% versus about 4% during the first 3 months of observation).[85–87] Therefore, vitamin K antagonists have become the standard for secondary prophylaxis for most patients with VTE. Two aspects of this therapy are frequently debated—the intensity and the duration of treatment.

Intensity of oral anticoagulant treatment

Because of multiple drug and dietary interactions with vitamin K antagonists, therapy must be frequently monitored and the dose of drug adjusted. The prothrombin time, used to adjust the dose of vitamin K antagonists, should be reported according to the international normalized ratio (INR), not the prothrombin time ratio or the prothrombin time expressed in seconds. The INR is essentially a 'corrected' prothrombin time that adjusts for the many different assays used.[84]

Effective therapy in VTE is achieved with an INR of 2.0 to 3.0. INR values falling below the therapeutic range are associated with an exponentially increasing risk of recurrent thrombosis with no advantage in terms of the risk of bleeding.[88] Values above the range place patients at a heightened risk of bleeding, without any benefit in the prevention of recurrent thrombotic episodes.[84,87,89,90] In addition, there is considerable evidence to suggest that increasing variability in a patient's INR values is also associated with a greater risk of haemorrhagic and thrombotic complications.[91] Therefore, every effort should be made to maintain the patient in the therapeutic range. This is facilitated by always aiming for an INR level that is in the mid-level of the INR range (i.e. 2.5). Patients with the antiphospholipid syndrome may require a higher INR (3.0 to 4.0),[33,92,93] but this recommendation is controversial, and one recent randomized study did not find any superiority of such a regimen over the standard intensity anticoagulation with an INR of 2.0–3.0.[94] The INR should be measured daily until it reaches the therapeutic range, then two to three times a week for 2 weeks and, later, in the presence of stable values, once every 2–4 weeks. In some settings, home self-testing with portable monitors of INR is convenient and cost-effective, and may ultimately improve anticoagulation control.[84,95]

Optimal duration of oral anticoagulant treatment

The duration of oral anticoagulation must be tailored to the individual patient. One should balance the risk of bleeding against the risk of recurrence when therapy is discontinued. The latter risk includes not only the likelihood of recurrence but also its potential clinical effect; patients with cardiopulmonary disease might tolerate recurrent PE poorly. For years, it was conventional to continue anticoagulation in patients with VTE for about 3 months. Some clinicians preferred 6 weeks of treatment, while others favoured 6 months. Patients with recurrent VTE or those with inherited or acquired thrombophilia were treated for longer periods. Early attempts to determine the optimal duration of treatment were unsuccessful because of methodological problems, including inadequate sample size, failure to use objective methods to confirm suspected recurrence and lack of blinded outcome assessment.[85,96] The results of these early studies suggested that the risk of recurrence after discontinuation of anticoagulant therapy was lower if the initial episode was associated with a reversible cause (such as postoperative DVT) than if it was idiopathic or associated with continuing risk factors (i.e. malignancy).[96]

In the first rigorously designed study, patients with a first episode of DVT were randomly assigned to 6 weeks or 6 months of oral anticoagulant therapy and were followed for recurrence.[97] The incidence of recurrence was significantly lower in the 6 months group; a subgroup analysis demonstrated that patients with reversible risk factors had a lower risk of recurrence than those with idiopathic DVT, confirming the results of previous studies. A second study from the same institution found that anticoagulation that was continued indefinitely after a second episode of VTE was associated with a much lower risk of recurrence during 4 years of follow-up than treatment for 6 months.[98] In a multicentre, double-blind, randomized trial, patients with idiopathic DVT were assigned to 3 months or 2 years of treatment with warfarin; the annual incidence of recurrence was 27% after 3 months of therapy and only 2% in patients who continued treatment.[99] The incidence of recurrence in all three studies was reduced by about 90% in patients assigned to long-term anticoagulation therapy.[97–99] A meta-analysis of 18 studies confirmed that the risk of recurrence decreases over time after cessation of anticoagulation, becoming quite low after 9 months.[100] Although it is widely held that recurrence of VTE is inversely related to duration of anticoagulation, being highest in the group that receives the shortest duration of anticoagulation, recent studies suggest that longer periods of anticoagulation only delay the time to recurrence until anticoagulant therapy is stopped.[101–103]

On the basis of the above-mentioned and many other studies, it is becoming increasingly clear that patients with VTE go through three phases, each associated with a different risk of recurrence. The first is a period of treatment with vitamin K antagonists, the second is the first 6–12 months after the discontinuation of this therapy, and the third reflects a more constant, long-term risk during the subsequent years. During therapy with vitamin K antagonists, the risk of recurrence is very effectively reduced—by approximately 90%—to 0.7 episodes per 100 person–years.[87,88] In the 6–12 months immediately after the discontinuation of treatment, a catch-up phenomenon occurs, resulting in an absolute incidence of VTE recurrence of 5–10%.[87,100,101] This phenomenon has been observed after 3, 6 and 12 months of oral anticoagulant therapy[100,101] and therefore suggests that prolonging this therapy simply delays recurrence until this therapy is stopped, rather than reducing the risk of recurrence. During the subsequent years, the risk of recurrence stabilizes, and the annual incidence of recurrence is 1–2%.

Most of the studies dealing with the duration of anticoagulant treatment for VTE included mainly patients presenting with DVT; only a limited proportion of patients presented with PE.[12,97,99,102–104] Although DVT and PE are generally considered to be two clinical manifestations of the same disease, patients presenting with PE are reported to have a higher incidence of fatal recurrent VTE than patients presenting with DVT.[3,4,103,105,106]

Besides the complex assessment of the risk of recurrent VTE, including consideration of the catch-up phenomenon, another element dominates the decision about how long to continue oral anticoagulant treatment. The benefit of long-term treatment is offset by major bleeding rates of 3–4% per year (with an annual case fatality rate of about 0.6%), which do not decrease over time.[28] The major determinants of oral anticoagulant-induced bleeding are the intensity of anticoagulant effect, the length of therapy, the patient's underlying disorder (past gastrointestinal bleeding, hypertension, cerebrovascular disease, renal insufficiency), advanced age and the concomitant use of drugs that interfere with haemostasis, above all aspirin. Approximately 20% of major bleeding episodes[99,107] and 5% of recurrences of VTE[4] are fatal. Therefore, patients who have a 10% estimated annual risk of recurrence and, consequently, a greater than 0.5% annual risk of fatal PE (e.g. those with an idiopathic event and those with ongoing risk factors), in association with a low risk of bleeding, should be considered for indefinite anticoagulation. In contrast, those with a very high risk of bleeding should receive anticoagulation for a limited period.

The following recommendations can be made on the basis of the above studies and the balance between the risk of recurrence and the risk of bleeding. For most patients with PE, provided there is no persisting risk factor, 6–12 months of treatment is indicated.[86,99,102,108] A recent study indicated that, after 6 months of anticoagulation to an INR of 2.0–3.0, subsequent anticoagulation to an INR of 1.5–2.0 results in a low incidence of recurrent VTE with a very low risk of bleeding.[109] However, another study seems to contradict this hypothesis; extended low-intensity anticoagulant therapy reduces the risk of recurrent events by only about 75%, whereas extended conventional intensity therapy reduces this risk by over 90%.[88]

In patients in whom risk factors can be removed, e.g. transient immobilization, surgery, trauma or oestrogen use, treatment may be shorter than 6 months.[96,97] The decision could be guided by a D-dimer assay after treatment.[110] Certain groups may require longer or indefinite treatment, including patients with active tumours,[111] homozygous or multiple thrombophilic disorders,[93,112] those with proven recurrence of VTE[98] and patients who have chronic thromboembolic pulmonary hypertension.[1] The single best predictor of an increased risk of VTE is a prior episode. Patients who have had one episode are at high risk of having another, whether or not they have a defined thrombophilic state.[84] Continuing anticoagulant therapy nearly eliminates the risk of recurrence, but other factors should be considered, including costs, possible effects on the quality of life, the risk of bleeding, numerous drug interactions, the need for frequent venepuncture for monitoring, the complex dose adjustments in patients undergoing surgery or biopsy procedures, the patient's compliance with therapy, any co-existing disease and the severity of the thromboembolic event. Ongoing therapy should be evaluated at least annually. After termination of the therapy with vitamin K antagonists, long-term treatment with oral direct thrombin inhibitors, without monitoring of coagulation or adjustments of the dose, may offer a clinically meaningful reduction in the incidence of further recurrent VTE.[83]

Available evidence indicates that the optimal long-term management of patients with VTE is unlikely to be defined by further studies comparing different durations of anticoagulant treatment. Rather, it indicates that strategies for risk stratification should be implemented to identify patients at high risk of recurrent VTE after anticoagulant treatment is discontinued. These patients are potential candidates for indefinite oral anticoagulation because it might result in more benefit than harm. The development of oral antithrombotic agents that have an improved safety profile and, as a consequence, do not require laboratory monitoring could pave the way towards extending anticoagulant therapy indefinitely.

The perioperative management of patients requiring vitamin K antagonists is problematic because the medication must be discontinued to prevent excessive bleeding. Substituting intravenous UFH or subcutaneous LMWH while oral anticoagulation is withheld can decrease the risk of VTE but may increase the risk of postoperative bleeding and, in the case of intravenous heparin, increase the hospitalization requirement. The optimal strategy is difficult to choose; no randomized controlled trials have been performed. However, this is a management dilemma that is too important to say there is no answer. Several 'bridging' strategies have been proposed.[113] It seems that most patients can safely undergo dental procedures, dermatological surgery, cataract surgery, arthrocentesis, injections or aspirations from soft tissues and diagnostic endoscopy or cardiac catheterization without a reduction in anticoagulation.[114]

Thrombolytic therapy

Thrombolytic therapy, by actively dissolving the clot, has several potential advantages over anticoagulation in the initial treatment of patients with massive PE. By relieving pulmonary artery obstruction, thrombolysis can quickly reduce the load on the right ventricle and reverse right heart failure and, consequently, has the potential to prevent death in the haemodynamically unstable patient who would not survive the many hours or days required for spontaneous fibrinolysis. Thrombolytic therapy is reserved for patients in whom there is evidence of a severely compromised circulation, e.g. right ventricular failure or hypotension with impaired peripheral circulation and metabolic acidosis.[1,2,27] In patients with PE who also have major proximal DVT, thrombolytic therapy reduces the late morbidity from the thrombosis, which is often considerable.[115,116] A further potential but unproven advantage of thrombolytic therapy over heparin in such patients is that it may reduce the chance of recurrent embolism by dissolving thrombus before it embolizes,[117] and may thus reduce the risk of chronic thromboembolic pulmonary hypertension developing subsequently.

Thrombolytic agents dissolve thrombi by activating plasminogen to plasmin. Plasmin, when in proximity to a thrombus or a haemostatic plug, degrades fibrin to soluble peptides. Circulating plasmin also degrades soluble fibrinogen and, to some extent, factors II, V and VIII. Moreover, elevated levels of fibrin and fibrinogen degradation products contribute to the coagulopathy by both inhibiting the conversion of fibrinogen to fibrin and interfering with fibrin polymerization.

Thrombolytic agents used in clinical practice or trials

The thrombolytic agents currently in use (Table 3) are streptokinase (SK), urokinase (UK), recombinant tissue plasminogen activator (rtPA, alteplase) and anisoylated plasminogen streptokinase activator complex (APSAC, anistreplase). SK is a purified bacterial protein; it binds to plasminogen non-covalently to form an activator complex, which converts other plasminogen molecules to plasmin. SK is antigenic and cannot be readministered for at least 6 months, as circulating antibodies may both inactivate the drug and produce allergic reactions. UK is isolated from human urine or cultured embryonic renal cells; unlike SK, UK is not antigenic and produces a lytic state by directly converting plasminogen to plasmin. Anistreplase has a longer half-life compared with SK, but the lack of any compelling advantages (other than bolus administration) and higher costs has relegated anistreplase to a very infrequently prescribed drug for PE. Alteplase is produced by recombinant DNA technology; like UK, it is non-antigenic and directly converts plasminogen to plasmin, but it is more fibrin specific (i.e. it produces less systemic plasminogen activation) than either SK or UK. Fibrin specificity is relative, however, and systemic fibrinogenolysis may occur after the administration of alteplase. Other thrombolytic agents are either not approved or only seldom used for the treatment of PE in most countries. Some new agents, notably mutants of tPA (reteplase,[118] tenekteplase, lanoteplase), staphylokinase and prourokinase (scuPA, saruplase)[119] are in clinical testing (Table 3).[120]

With the exception of one small study, which was terminated when all four patients given thrombolysis survived while all four given heparin died,[121] none of the trials comparing

Table 3. Thrombolytic regimens for massive pulmonary embolism.

Streptokinase (SK)	250 000 to 500 000 U as a loading dose over 15 min, followed by 100 000 U/h for 24 h or 1.5 million U over 60 min
Urokinase (UK)	4400 U/kg as a loading dose over 10 min, followed by 4400 U/kg/h for 12 h; or 1 million U in 10 min, followed by 2 million U over 2 h
Alteplase (rt-PA)	20 mg as an IV bolus, followed by 80 mg in a continuous infusion over 2 h
Anistreplase (APSAC)	30 mg in 5 min
Reteplase (r-PA)	Two IV bolus injections of 10 U, 30 min apart
Tenecteplase (TNK-tPA)	Bolus 0.5 mg (100 U)/kg. Maximum 50 mg
Lanoteplase (n-PA)	Bolus 120 U/kg
Saruplase (scu-PA)	Bolus 20 mg, followed by 60 mg over 1 h

Before treatment, stop heparin.

thrombolytic agents with UFH in PE detected any significant difference in the most important endpoint, i.e. mortality. Consequently, the degree of angiographic or scintigraphic resolution and changes in haemodynamics were used as surrogate measures. Accelerated early resolution of PE compared with UFH has been proved for all the tested agents (Table 4).[26,122–133] However, this benefit is short-lived, and there is no difference after several days. Many patients included in these studies did not have massive PE. Definite evidence that thrombolytic therapy as opposed to heparin reduces mortality in PE is lacking, and it is unlikely to be forthcoming because of the logistic problems involved in mounting such a study. The low mortality at 3 months (<5%) of patients treated with UFH and oral anticoagulants[3,4] precludes the identification of a mortality effect of thrombolytic therapy when a relatively small number of patients were studied. A further factor contributing to the lack of significant reduction in mortality despite impressive early acceleration of thrombus resolution is that patients who survive long enough to be entered into a clinical trial probably represent a group with a better prognosis as the most severely affected patients will have died before receiving therapy. Therefore, the numbers of patients required to demonstrate a difference in mortality far exceeds the numbers treated in the centres, and it is unlikely that robust evidence for reduced mortality with thrombolysis

will materialize.[120,131,132] In patients with right heart thrombus (in itself an ominous finding), mortality with thrombolysis is a third of that with heparin.[134]

There is only indirect evidence of better prognosis with thrombolysis. The rate of treatment failure (i.e. progression to another form of therapy such as heparin to thrombolysis or thrombolysis to embolectomy) in patients with severe PE is lower in those treated with thrombolytics than in those who receive UFH.[127,129,133] The rapid recovery of apparently moribund patients after massive PE treated with thrombolytics also supports their use in such patients.[121,135] Another indirect evidence comes from a non-randomized study (multicentre registry) of 719 patients without shock, in which 169 patients initially received thrombolytics and 550 were treated with heparin alone. In the group undergoing thrombolysis, mortality at 30 days was significantly lower (4.7% versus 11.1%) and recurrent PE significantly less frequent (7.7% versus 18.7%) than in the heparin-treated group.[117] Therefore, a more rapid resolution of PE seems to be desirable, because prolonged haemodynamic disturbance can only cause harm and, if further emboli develop, their haemodynamic effect will be lessened if previous emboli have been partially removed. This led some authorities to widen the indication of thrombolysis to patients with PE who have echocardiographic evidence of right ventricular dysfunction,[133,136] but this recommendation

Table 4. Thrombolysis versus heparin in acute PE — randomized trials.

Trial	PE	Therapy	n	Major bleeding (%)	Outcome with thrombolytics
UPET[26] 1970	All PE <5 days	UK 4400 U kg/h, 12 h	82	45	Accelerated resolution (A, S, H) at 24 h, no
		Heparin	78	27	difference at 7 days
Tibbutt[129] 1974	Massive PE only	SK 100 000 U/h, 72 h	13	8	Accelerated resolution (A, H) at 72 h
		Heparin	17	6	
Ly[125] 1978	Massive PE only, <5 days	SK 100 000 U/h, 72 h	14	24	Accelerated resolution (A) at 72 h
		Heparin	11	18	
Marini[142] 1988	Massive PE only	UK 800 000 U/12 h × 3	10	0	No difference at 1 day and 1 year (S), no
		UK 3 300 000 U/12 h	10	0	difference at 7 days (H)
		Heparin	10	0	
PIOPED[128] 1990	Submassive PE, <7 days	rtPA 40–80 mg + heparin	9	11	Accelerated resolution (H) at 2 h,
		Heparin alone	4	0	accelerated resolution (S) at 24 h
Dalla-Volta[122] 1992	MI > 11, <10 days	rtPA 100 mg/2 h	20	15	Accelerated resolution (A, H) at 2 h, no
		Heparin	16	13	difference at 7 days
Levine[124] 1990	All PE <14 days	rtPA 0.6 mg/kg/2 min + hep	33	0	Accelerated resolution (S) at 24 h, no
		Heparin	25	0	difference at 7 days
Goldhaber[123] 1993	Stable PE <14 days	rtPA 100 mg/2 h	46	7	Accelerated resolution (S), improved RV
		Heparin	55	4	function (Echo) at 24 h
Jerjes-Sanches[121] 1995	Massive PE only, <14 days	SK 1 500 000 U/1 h	4	0	Mortality 0%
		Heparin	4	0	Mortality 100% (P = 0.02)
Konstantinides[133] 2002	Submassive PE, <5 days	rtPA 100 mg/2 h + heparin	118	1	Escalation of therapy with rtPA needed less
		Heparin	138	4	often

A, angiography; S, scintigraphy; H, haemodynamics; Echo, echocardiography; MI, Miller index.

is derived from observational studies and subset analysis of studies not designed to investigate this proposal. Additional information is needed to determine whether right ventricular dysfunction by itself is an indication for thrombolysis.[24,27,137]

The report by Konstantinides *et al.*[133] of a randomized trial of alteplase plus heparin versus heparin alone in patients with PE complicated by right ventricular dysfunction, but without systemic hypotension or shock, indicated that, in these patients, the safest and most cost-effective therapy is heparin with the option of secondary thrombolysis. The mortality and incidence of documented recurrent PE were the same in the 118 patients randomized to receive alteplase plus heparin as in the 138 patients who were randomized to receive heparin alone, with the option of secondary thrombolysis if clinical conditions worsened. Thirty-two of the 138 patients randomized to heparin alone received secondary thrombolysis; the other 106 patients randomized to heparin avoided the increased cost and the potential bleeding complications associated with thrombolytic therapy.[133] As the risk of major haemorrhage is twice that with heparin,[131,132] the current majority view remains that thrombolysis should be reserved for those with clinically massive PE with systemic hypotension.

Several trials have compared different thrombolytics or different dosages of a given thrombolytic (Table 5). No clear-cut advantage of a given drug or a given dosage has been found.[118,138–142] Twelve hours of UK therapy had equivalent thrombolytic efficacy to 24 hours of SK therapy,[26] and these are the recommended infusion times for PE. Alteplase produces a faster improvement at 2–4 hours than UK but, at 12–24 h, there is no significant difference.[126,143–145] All thrombolytics appear to be equally effective and safe when equivalent doses are delivered. It probably matters little which agent is used; it is much more important to ensure that patients receive one of these drugs quickly.

In contrast to myocardial infarction, thrombolysis in acute massive PE appears to be effective for up to 10–14 days after the onset of symptoms.[146] Thrombolytics are equally effective given through a peripheral vein or via a catheter positioned in the pulmonary artery adjacent to the embolus.[141] Generally accepted fixed dosage regimens are given in Table 3. There is no need to obtain clotting tests during therapy as such tests are of no value in predicting complications or adjusting dosage. After the conclusion of therapy with SK or UK, measurements of aPTT and fibrinogen are mandatory in order to determine when heparin (without a bolus) should be instituted. If the post-thrombolysis aPTT exceeds twice the upper limit of normal or the fibrinogen level is under 1 g/L, these tests should be repeated every 4 hours until they reach these levels, at which heparin can be started (or resumed) safely. For alteplase or reteplase, concurrent use of heparin is optional. After the patient has been adequately heparinized, oral anticoagulation is initiated and, even if the prothrombin time quickly reaches the target range, they should overlap with heparin for at least 5 days.[1]

Table 5. Thrombolysis in acute PE — randomized trials

Trial	PE	Therapy	n	Major bleeding (%)	Outcome
USPET[138] 1974	All PE, <5 days	UK 4400 U/kg/h, 24 h	54	31	
		UK 4400 U/kg/h, 12 h	59	25	No difference at 24 h (A, H, S)
		SK 100 000 U/h, 24 h	54	22	
UKEP[140] 1987	All PE, <5 days	UK 2000 U/kg/h + Hep., 24 h	67	5	No difference at 48 h (A, H)
		UK 4400 U/kg/h, 12 h	62	3	
Verstraete[141] 1988	Massive PE, <5 days	rtPA into pulmonary artery	19	12	No difference at 2–18 h (A, H)
		rtPA IV	15	12	
Goldhaber[139] 1988	All PE, <14 days	rtPA 100 mg/2 h	22	18	Faster improvement with rtPA at 2 h (A, H),
		UK 4400 U/kg/h, 24 h	23	48	no difference at 24 h (S)
Meyer[126] 1992	Massive PE, <5 days	rtPA 100 mg/2 h	34	21	Faster improvement with rtPA at 2–4 h (H),
		UK 4400 U/kg/h, 12 h	29	28	no difference at 12 h (H, A)
Goldhaber[143] 1992	All PE, <14 days	rtPA 100 mg/2 h	42	11	No difference at 2 h (A),
		UK 3 million U/2 h	45	9	no difference at 24 h (S)
Meneveau[144] 1997	Massive PE, <5 days	rtPA 100 mg/2 h	25	16	Faster improvement with rtPA at 2–6 h (H),
		SK 100 000 U/h, 12 h	25	12	no difference at 12–24 h (H, A)
Meneveau[145] 1998	Massive PE, <5 days	rtPA 100 mg/2 h	23	20	Faster improvement with rtPA at 1 h (H),
		SK 1.5 million U/2 h	43	8	no difference at 2 and 48 h (H, S)
Tebbe[118] 1999	Massive PE, <5 days	Reteplase 2 × 10 U IV	23	4	No difference at 2–24 h (H)
		rtPA 100 mg/2 h	13	8	

A, angiography; S, scintigraphy; H, haemodynamics; IV, intravenously.

Bolus thrombolysis

Following experiments demonstrating that alteplase produces continuing thrombolysis after it is cleared from the circulation and that thrombolysis is both increased and accelerated and bleeding is reduced when the drug is administered over a short period, and after refinements of thrombolytic dosing strategies for myocardial infarction, interest was awakened in using very high doses over a short interval. The rationale supporting such therapy as opposed to prolonged infusion is that the initially high concentration of the drug overwhelms plasminogen activator inhibitor-1 and renders negligible any attenuating effects of this inhibitor on the drug activity. The higher peak plasma level results in a higher concentration of the activator on the surface and inside the thrombi. Further, the bolus is cleared rapidly from the circulation, thus preventing large amounts of degradation products from the lysed emboli interacting with continuously infused plasminogen activator, which converts circulating (rather than fibrin-bound) plasminogen to plasmin and, in turn, induces the systemic lytic state. However, all studies to date have failed to show any significant differences in the early resolution of PE or in bleeding complications (Table 6).[124,143,147,148] No trial has assessed large bolus doses of SK, which would probably be just as effective and considerably cheaper.[149]

Bolus thrombolysis may also be indicated during cardiopulmonary resuscitation, even without proof of fulminant embolism as the cause of cardiac arrest. In more than two-thirds of patients with cardiac arrest, either acute myocardial infarction or PE (i.e. intravasal thrombosis) are the cause of the arrest, and thrombolysis is an efficient strategy in both cases. An increasing number of clinical studies suggest that thrombolysis during cardiopulmonary resuscitation can contribute to haemodynamic stabilization and survival in patients with massive PE or acute myocardial infarction, when conventional resuscitation has been performed unsuccessfully.[150–152] Apart from the specific causal action of thrombolytics at the site of pulmonary emboli or coronary thrombosis, experimental data indicate that thrombolysis during resuscitation may improve microcirculatory reperfusion, which may be most important in the brain and may lead to a better neurological outcome for surviving patients. The benefit of this treatment might outweigh the risk of bleeding. However, one randomized study found no evidence of a beneficial effect of thrombolysis in patients with pulseless electrical activity of presumed cardiovascular cause; this study had limited statistical power, and it remains unknown whether there is a small treatment effect or whether selected subgroups may benefit.[153]

Complications of thrombolytic therapy

The main complication of thrombolytic therapy is bleeding. Thrombolytic therapy is accompanied by a significantly greater risk of major haemorrhage than is treatment with heparin alone. All thrombolytics are administered in dosing regimens that activate fibrinolysis systematically throughout the body. None of these agents will distinguish a pathological thrombus from a beneficial haemostatic plug. Although alteplase and anistreplase are somewhat more fibrin specific than SK and UK, all these agents have the potential to lyse a fresh platelet-fibrin plug anywhere and cause bleeding at this site. The two major factors that increase bleeding risk are prolonged administration of thrombolytics and the use of procedures that involve vessel puncture.

The reported incidence of haemorrhage has varied markedly. If major haemorrhage is arbitrarily defined as fatal bleeding, intracranial haemorrhage or bleeding that requires either surgery or transfusion, the average overall frequency of major haemorrhage with PE thrombolysis is about 10% and is similar among the thrombolytic agents used.[131,132,137]

The incidence of cerebral bleeding is about 0.5–2.0 % irrespective of the agent or ancillary therapy used.[120,154,155] The elderly, patients with uncontrolled hypertension and those with recent stroke or craniotomy appear to be at especially high risk of cerebral bleeding. Acute profuse gastrointestinal bleeding is usually the consequence of giving thrombolytics to a patient with unsuspected active peptic ulcer. Late bleeding

Table 6. Bolus thrombolysis in acute PE — randomized trials

Trial	PE	Therapy	n	Major bleeding (%)	Outcome
Levine[124] 1990	All PE, <14 days	rtPA 0.6 mg/kg/2 min + heparin	33	0	Faster improvement (S) at 24 h,
		Heparin alone	25	0	no difference after 7 days
Goldhaber[143] 1992	All PE, <14 days	UK 1 million U/10 min + 2 million U/2 h	45	13	No difference (A, H) at 2 h,
		rtPA 100 mg/2 h	42	18	no difference (S) after 24 h
Goldhaber[147] 1994	All PE, <14 days	rtPA 0.6 mg/kg/15 min (max. 50 mg)	61	13	No difference (A) at 2 h,
		rtPA 100 mg/2 h	29	22	no difference (S) after 24 h
Sors[148] 1994	Massive PE, <5 days	rtPA 0.6 mg/kg/15 min (max. 50 mg)	36	8	No difference (H) after 1–12 h,
		rtPA 100 mg/2 h	17	6	no difference (S) after 24 h

A, angiography; H, haemodynamics; S, scintigraphy.

(2–3 days) may be due to stress ulceration, particularly in gravely ill patients—thrombolysis is probably irrelevant but subsequent anticoagulation makes things worse. Rupture of the heart, liver or spleen during attempted resuscitation may lead to fatal bleeding. Arterial or venous puncture should be avoided if possible.

Pulmonary embolectomy

Embolectomy continues to be undertaken in emergency situations when more conservative measures have failed. Its only indication is to prevent death. Unfortunately, it is difficult to identify accurately those who will die without embolectomy. Certainly patients *in extremis* requiring prolonged resuscitation are indicated for embolectomy; there are only very few reports suggesting that such patients may survive with thrombolytic therapy.[121,135,150–152] Patients who deteriorate haemodynamically after the start of thrombolytic therapy and whose blood pressure remains below 90 mmHg in spite of vasopressors would also seem to be candidates for surgical intervention. Further, there are still patients in whom thrombolytic therapy is absolutely contraindicated (rarely an important consideration in a life-threatening situation) or would be too slow in producing benefit.[23,25,156,157] In all these patients, every attempt should be made to confirm the diagnosis of massive central PE before surgery, even if it requires partial cardiopulmonary bypass while definitive diagnostic procedures are being performed. The mortality rate of patients referred for embolectomy with an incorrect diagnosis approaches 100%.

With the inflow-occlusion technique, the venae cavae are occluded, and the pulmonary arteries are explored through an incision in the trunk. This can be done repeatedly with the occlusion limited to 2 min in normothermia. This method has the obvious advantage that it can be applied quickly and without special apparatus by a thoracic surgeon. Because of its simplicity, it can be performed during the early period after PE when the risk of death is greatest. Disadvantage is the limited time for exploration of the pulmonary arteries, so that residual emboli are common. The mortality of this procedure is in the range of 44–50%.[158,159]

Embolectomy done with cardiopulmonary bypass allows thorough examination of the right atrium, right ventricle and pulmonary arteries. These advantages are, however, negated if removal of the embolus is unduly delayed by the complex preparations required, and the operation can be carried out only in centres where cardiopulmonary bypass is immediately available.

Statistics regarding mortality following embolectomy are difficult to compare. Data are largely derived from retrospective reviews of historical series, often predating the advent of thrombolysis. In some series, considerable numbers of patients have been operated on more than 24 hours after embolism,[156,159,160] which throws doubt on the need for the procedure. The results depend greatly on the indications and the haemodynamic impairment (Table 7). Mortality will be high in those patients most in need of embolectomy and low in patients who would survive without it.[161] Until 1985, the overall mortality was 51% for those done without and 40% for those done with cardiopulmonary bypass.[162] These results have improved in recent years, mainly because of routine

Table 7. Pulmonary embolectomy.

Author	Period	n	Duration <24 h (%)	Shock (%)	Resuscitated (%)	Method applied	Mortality, overall, %	Mortality in resuscitated, %	Mortality in not resuscitated, %
Del Campo[162]*	?–1984	114	?	100?	NR	IO	51	NR	NR
Del Campo[162]*	?–1984	537	?	100?	NR	CPB	40	NR	NR
Clarke[158]	1960–86	55	100	100	35	IO	44	84	22
Lund[157]	1973–83	25	NR	92	28	CPB	20	43	11
Gray[156]	1964–86	71	65	NR	35	CPB	30	64	11
Bauer[164]	1978–90	44	?	64	34	CPB	20	47	7
Kieny[160]	1970–89	134	88	57	17	CPB >> IO	16	48	9
Meyer[23]	1968–88	96	NR	81	25	CPB	38	58	31
Meyns[168]	1973–91	30	?	80	40	CPB	20	50	0
Laas[166]	1975–92	34	NR	NR	56	CPB	44	53	33
Stulz[159]	1968–92	50	50	96	62	IO > CPB	46	61	21
Ullmann[169]	1989–97	40	NR	32	48	CPB	35	67	10
Doerge[165]	1979–98	41	NR	81	34	CPB	29	64	11
Aklog[161]	1999–01	29	NR	6	3	CPB	11	100	7
Own data	1976–01	24	50	38	29	CPB	17	29	12

*Literature review until 1985.
NR, not reported; IO, inflow occlusion; CPB, cardiopulmonary bypass.

administration of vasopressors before the induction of an-aesthesia and the use of partial (femoro-femoral) bypass in moribund patients in order to maintain the circulation while the patient and the equipment are prepared for full bypass.[163] There has been no randomized trial of embolectomy versus thrombolytic treatment, and it is unlikely that one of value will ever be performed because of the scarcity of these patients.

The main predictor of operative death is cardiac arrest with the need for resuscitation before the operation. Provided patients reach the operating room without requiring external cardiac massage, the mortality is in the range of 0–33%, but it is between 29% and 100% in those resuscitated.[23,156,158–161,164–169] Postoperative complications include ARDS, mediastinitis, acute renal failure and, of particular concern, severe neurological sequelae. Late morbidity of patients successfully operated on is principally neurological, and late mortality is low.[23,161,165,167,168,170]

Catheter transvenous embolectomy

An alternative technique in patients with massive PE who can still maintain their blood pressure with vasopressor support is catheter embolectomy employing a large steerable catheter with a suction cup on its tip, inserted via cutdown in the femoral or jugular vein. After localizing the embolus via pulmonary angiography, syringe suction captures the embolus in the cup and holds it there while the catheter and the embolus are withdrawn. Multiple retrievals of embolic material by the catheter are usually required before an improvement occurs in haemodynamics. However, this procedure is rarely undertaken. The results of the only two published studies show that embolus extraction is achieved in about two-thirds of the patients and the mortality in these studies was about 30%.[21,171]

An alternative manoeuvre of attempting to fragment the embolus is certainly much easier. If angiography shows massive emboli in the main pulmonary arteries, it may be possible to break these up using a pigtail catheter and a guidewire or an angiographic basket.[172–175] The rationale is that the cross-sectional area of the pulmonary vascular bed increases progressively from proximal to distal. Thus, the fragmented clot obstructs a smaller percentage of the whole cross-sectional area of the pulmonary vascular bed when displaced distally. The pulmonary vascular resistance will thus decrease, and the pulmonary blood flow will increase. A further advantage of this mechanical disruption of emboli would be enhanced clot exposure to lytic therapy by creation of multiple channels within the emboli.[176] However, the clinical benefit of catheter fragmentation has not been evaluated in a controlled study.

A number of rotational or hydraulic devices for percutaneous mechanical thrombolysis have been evaluated;[177] they work by high-speed clot fragmentation and aspiration. Embolectomy can also be accomplished with the use of a catheter that delivers high-velocity jets of saline that draw clot by a Ven-turi effect towards the side hole near the catheter tip and subsequently fragment it and suck the debris into the evacuation catheter.[178,179] None of these devices has been used extensively in patients to date; without control groups, the benefit of these techniques remains undefined.

Venous interruption

Venous interruption procedures are designed to prevent further emboli from reaching the lungs. They have no effect on the thrombotic process and do not prevent DVT. In the past, the main methods were ligation, plication or the application of clips to the outside of the inferior vena cava. These procedures carried an appreciable mortality and morbidity, of which lower limb swelling was the most troublesome. Nowadays, the method of choice is the pervenous placement of a filter in the inferior vena cava under fluoroscopic guidance. The design allows filtering to occur without occlusion of the venous return. Attention to detail, proper use of guidewires and preinsertion imaging are vital in preventing insertion-related complications. If necessary, for example in the intensive care unit, filters can be inserted at the bedside.[180]

There is no evidence that the filters have any advantages over anticoagulation for routine prophylaxis following an acute PE because the incidence of recurrence with anticoagulation alone is so low.[87,88,100,101] Their place is in the rare case in which intensive and prolonged anticoagulation alone fails or cannot be achieved because of strong contraindications (e.g. serious multiple injuries or during and after surgery).[181–184] Although caval filtration is probably effective in reducing PE rates in these indications, there is a remarkable lack of controlled studies to support its use. Even among the few larger prospective series,[180,185–189] the extreme heterogeneity of populations, indications for filter placement, evaluation criteria and follow-up preclude any relevant comparison and analysis. After 31 years of descriptive studies, the first and only randomized trial in 400 patients with proximal DVT has identified some of the limitations and benefits of vena caval interruption.[190] All patients received anticoagulants for at least 3 months. Filter placement significantly reduced new PE by day 12; this gives some credence to its use in patients at high risk of death in the event of anticoagulation failure. The incidence of death or major bleeding was not significantly different in those with or without the filter. However, the filter was associated with a doubled risk of recurrent DVT at 2 years, indicating thrombogenicity. The incidence of PE during the 2 years of follow-up was lower in those treated with a filter, 3.4% versus 6.3%, but the difference was not significant.[190] A large retrospective study also found that readmission for recurrent PE was unchanged and DVT was more common.[191] Until more relevant data become available, reviews about caval filters will remain narrative, and many if not most indications for filter placement will remain a matter of opinion.

Devices placed in the inferior vena cava may perforate the vessel wall or migrate within and outside the venous system. Thrombosis occurs frequently at the venous access site. Pulmonary emboli, either passing through or around the therapeutic obstruction or originating proximally, have been reported with all these measures.[181,190] Other late sequelae include caval thrombosis, filter fracture and leg oedema. Overall, the benefits of preventing PE may exceed the risks related to filter placement in properly selected patients. Because of the lack of controlled data regarding eventual outcome and the true incidence of complications, if a permanent filter is used, long-term clinical follow-up is appropriate.[181,187]

In many patients, the period of risk from anticoagulant therapy is relatively short; such patients do not require placement of a lifelong caval filter. Therefore, temporary retrievable filters have been developed to bridge the relatively short period of high risk of PE, especially in patients with extensive trauma.[192–195] Some filters are an integral part of an infusion system for the delivery of thrombolytics or heparin.[196–199] There are no controlled randomized studies on this topic. The indications remain unclear, and there are as yet few data about the complications and reliability of these filters.

General supportive measures in acute massive PE

Patients in pain should receive analgesia, but opiates should be used with caution in the hypotensive patient. When hypoxaemia is refractory to oxygen supplementation by face mask, intubation and mechanical ventilation may be necessary, but this may further deteriorate the haemodynamic situation by impeding venous return.[1,2,27] When the cardiac output is reduced, the dilated right ventricle is hypoxic and already near-maximally stimulated by the high level of endogenous catecholamines; it is unlikely to respond to inotropic agents, which may do no more than precipitate arrhythmias. When necessary because of a dangerous fall in systemic pressure, the judicious use of noradrenalin titrated against a moderate increase in blood pressure might be beneficial in improving right ventricular function and systemic haemodynamics.[2,200] There are, however, no randomized clinical trials comparing various vasoactive agents in acute massive PE; much of our understanding comes from animal models,[201] which are difficult to extrapolate to the treatment of patients.

The right atrial pressure should be maintained high (15 mmHg), as this filling pressure is necessary for the failing right ventricle to maintain its output;[202] if the right atrial pressure falls for any reason, administration of fluid is helpful. However, fluid loading might be detrimental if there is frank right ventricular distention and a high filling pressure, as it may augment ventricular interaction by both increasing pericardial pressure and shifting the ventricular septum leftwards, thus decreasing left ventricular preload and output. Vasodilators should be avoided at all times; an exception to this rule in

the future may be selective pulmonary vasodilatation by inhaled nitric oxide or prostacyclin.[13,203,204] The value of extracorporeal membrane oxygenation in cardiac arrest due to PE is unclear.[205]

Treatment of pulmonary embolism in pregnancy

The management of VTE during pregnancy remains controversial because of the lack of prospective trials. Current practice is based on extrapolation from results in non-pregnant populations and on observational studies. Unfractionated heparin and LMWH do not cross the placenta, and therefore do not have the potential to cause fetal bleeding or teratogenicity, although bleeding at the uteroplacental junction is possible. However, data are sparse for LMWH, with no reliable comparative trials or convincing dose assessment. In contrast to heparin, oral anticoagulants cross the placenta and may cause fetal developmental abnormalities, fetal bleeding, spontaneous abortions and stillbirth. Therefore, oral anticoagulants must not be administered in the first trimester of pregnancy (and, if possible, also throughout the entire pregnancy), and all women of childbearing potential taking vitamin K antagonists must avoid becoming pregnant.

Pregnant women with PE are best treated initially with continuous intravenous UFH or weight-adjusted doses of subcutaneous LMWH and should then be taught to self-administer LMWH once daily for the remainder of pregnancy until the onset of labour and further on in the puerperium.[206,207] If available, measurement of anti-Xa levels 4 hours after injection and adjustment to a level of approximately 0.5–1.2 U/mL should be performed.[208] A high index of suspicion for the development of osteopenia and a fortnightly assessment of the platelet count is important. Heparin should be discontinued 24 hours prior to elective induction of labour. If spontaneous labour occurs in women receiving adjusted-dose heparin, careful monitoring of the aPTT is required and, if it is prolonged near delivery, protamine may be required to reduce the risk of bleeding.[206]

Another acceptable approach is to give oral anticoagulants between the 13th and 36th week of gestation and switch to heparin during the last 2 weeks of pregnancy. If the mother is admitted in premature labour while still taking oral anticoagulants, she should be given fresh frozen plasma. Treatment with oral anticoagulants can be resumed immediately after delivery and continued for at least 6 weeks post partum. Their effect on the baby persists for 7–14 days after they are stopped and, therefore, the baby should be given vitamin K at delivery. Breast feeding is not contraindicated.[208]

Current evidence suggests that thrombolysis is appropriate treatment for massive PE with hypotension during pregnancy but not within 6 hours of delivery nor in the early post-partum period because of the high risk of bleeding complications.[209] Both SK and anteplase do not cross the placenta.

Summary and future

The practice of medicine has changed dramatically in the 45 years since Barritt and Jordan performed the first randomized trial involving the treatment of PE. Over the past decade, there has been an explosion of published research and development of new therapies relating to patients with VTE. Despite a great deal of effort, the incidence of VTE has not changed substantially in the last 20 years. Physicians are prepared to change their practice, but only when the recommended changes are based on properly designed trials using clinically relevant endpoints. Thanks to the evidence coming from such trials, we have abandoned some concepts that were previously considered to be 'logical' or 'good common sense' and had provided the rationale for what was in fact empirical treatment. The most important advances in the treatment of VTE have been the development of LMWH (which increased the convenience of initial treatment and has reduced the risks of some side-effects of heparin), the establishment of an optimal intensity for oral anticoagulant therapy (which improved its safety) and the establishment of thrombolytic therapy (which may be life saving in massive PE).

Despite the progress that has been made, several issues have yet to be resolved. A widespread use of LMWHs for the treatment of acute PE is certain, but comparative studies on the equivalency of various LMWHs are needed. Cost savings should prove substantial and will be directly proportional to the number of hospital days avoided. It is likely that heparin derivatives and specific thrombin inhibitors will replace UFH or LMWH for some indications, provided that their costs are not prohibitive. The development of synthetic thrombin inhibitors for oral use would open the possibility for long-term application. Better risk stratification will optimize the duration of anticoagulant therapy in different subgroups of patients with VTE. Much also remains unknown about the optimal treatment of VTE in pregnant women, patients with cancer and patients with antiphospholipid antibodies. Future research must determine whether thrombolytic therapy reduces mortality and morbidity in patients with a large clot burden and/or right ventricular dysfunction who do not have clinical signs of systemic hypoperfusion. The only way to determine the role of embolectomy in patients with massive PE complicated by shock is to perform an appropriately designed clinical trial. Inhalation of nitric oxide or prostacyclin might prove to be a useful adjunct in the therapy of acute massive PE.

Conflict of interest statement

The author has never been supported by any commercial company, has never taken part in any industry-funded study and has no financial interest in this article.

Conclusions
Unfractionated heparin in pulmonary embolism
- The risk of recurrence of thromboembolism is high in patients receiving inadequate initial heparin treatment (aPTT ratio < 1.5).
- The use of a heparin dosing nomogram ensures that all patients will achieve the therapeutic range for the aPTT.
- Heparin administered by the subcutaneous route cannot be recommended as the initial treatment of PE.
- Heparin should be given for at least 7 days; oral anticoagulants should overlap with heparin for at least 5 days. For massive PE, a longer duration of heparin therapy may be considered.
- Heparin can be discontinued if the INR > 2.0 for two consecutive days.
- Measurement of plasma heparin level is useful in patients with baseline elevated aPTT due to antiphospholipid antibodies and in those requiring large daily doses of heparin (>45 000 U).

Oral anticoagulants after pulmonary embolism
- Treatment with oral anticoagulants can be started together with UFH or LMWH once VTE has been reliably confirmed.
- Patients with reversible or time-limited risk factors should be treated for 3–6 months with an INR target range of 2.0–3.0.
- Patients with a first episode of idiopathic VTE should be treated for at least 6 months.
- Patients with recurrent VTE, active cancer, antiphospholipid syndrome, inhibitor deficiency states or homozygous factor V Leiden should probably be treated indefinitely, but the risk of bleeding should be balanced with that of further VTE.
- When oral anticoagulation is either contraindicated (pregnancy) or inconvenient, an adjusted dose of LMWH to prolong coagulation to a therapeutic level can be used.

References

1 Riedel M. Pulmonary embolic disease. In: Gibson GJ, Geddes DM, Costabel U et al., eds. Respiratory Medicine. London, Saunders, 2003:1711–58.
2 Wood KE. Major pulmonary embolism. Review of a pathophysiologic approach to the golden hour of hemodynamically significant pulmonary embolism. Chest 2002; 121:877–905.
3 Carson JL, Kelley MA, Duff A et al. The clinical course of pulmonary embolism. N Engl J Med 1992; 326:1240–5.
4 Douketis JD, Kearon C, Bates S et al. Risk of fatal pulmonary embolism in patients with treated venous thromboembolism. JAMA 1998; 279:458–62.
5 Hull RD, Raskob GE, Brant RF et al. Low-molecular-weight heparin vs heparin in the treatment of patients with pulmonary embolism. Arch Intern Med 2000; 160:229–36.
6 Simonneau G, Sors H, Charbonnier B et al. A comparison of low-molecular-weight heparin with unfractionated heparin for acute pulmonary embolism. The THESEE Study Group. N Engl J Med 1997; 337:663–9.
7 The Columbus Investigators. Low-molecular-weight heparin in the treatment of patients with venous thromboembolism. N Engl J Med 1997; 337:657–62.
8 Aschwanden M, Labs K-H, Engel H et al. Acute deep vein thrombosis: early mobilization does not increase the frequency of pulmonary embolism. Thromb Haemost 2001; 85:42–6.

9 Nielsen HK, Husted SE, Krusell LR *et al.* Anticoagulant therapy in deep venous thrombosis. A randomized controlled study. *Thromb Res* 1994; **73**:215–26.

10 Partsch H, Kechavarz B, Kohn H *et al.* The effect of mobilisation of patients during treatment of thromboembolic disorders with low-molecular-weight heparin. *Int Angiol* 1997; **16**:189–92.

11 Hirsh J, Warkentin TE, Shaughnessy SG *et al.* Heparin and low-molecular-weight heparin. Mechanisms of action, pharmacokinetics, dosing considerations, monitoring, efficacy, and safety. *Chest* 2001; **119**:64S–94S.

12 Hyers TM, Agnelli G, Hull RD *et al.* Antithrombotic therapy for venous thromboembolic disease. *Chest* 2001; **119**:176S–193S.

13 Smulders YM. Pathophysiology and treatment of haemodynamic instability in acute pulmonary embolism: the pivotal role of pulmonary vasoconstriction. *Cardiovasc Res* 2000; **48**:23–33.

14 Barritt PW, Jordan SC. Anticoagulant drugs in the treatment of pulmonary embolism — a controlled trial. *Lancet* 1960; **1**:1309–12.

15 Brandjes DP, Heijboer H, Büller HR *et al.* Acenocoumarol and heparin compared with acenocoumarol alone in the initial treatment of proximal-vein thrombosis. *N Engl J Med* 1992; **372**:1485–9.

16 Nielsen HK, Husted SE, Krusell LR *et al.* Silent pulmonary embolism in patients with deep venous thrombosis. Incidence and fate in a randomized, controlled trial of anticoagulation versus no anticoagulation. *J Intern Med* 1994; **235**:457–61.

17 Johnson R, Charnley J. Treatment of pulmonary embolism in total hip replacement. *Clin Orthop Rel Res* 1977; **124**:149–54.

18 Hull RD, Raskob GE, Ginsberg JS *et al.* A noninvasive strategy for the treatment of patients with suspected pulmonary embolism. *Arch Intern Med* 1994; **154**:289–97.

19 Stein PD, Henry JW, Relyea B. Untreated patients with pulmonary embolism. Outcome, clinical and laboratory assessment. *Chest* 1995; **107**:931–5.

20 The Matisse Investigators. Subcutaneous fondaparinux versus intravenous unfractionated heparin in the initial treatment of pulmonary embolism. *N Engl J Med* 2003; **249**:1695–702.

21 Greenfield LJ, Proctor MC, Williams DM *et al.* Long-term experience with transvenous catheter pulmonary embolectomy. *J Vasc Surg* 1993; **18**:450–7.

22 Gulba DC, Schmid C, Borst HG *et al.* Medical compared with surgical treatment for massive pulmonary embolism. *Lancet* 1994; **343**:576–7.

23 Meyer G, Tamisier D, Sors H *et al.* Pulmonary embolectomy: a 20-year experience at one center. *Ann Thorac Surg* 1991; **51**:232–6.

24 Grifoni S, Olivotto I, Cecchini P *et al.* Short-term clinical outcome of patients with acute pulmonary embolism, normal blood pressure, and echocardiographic right ventricular dysfunction. *Circulation* 2000; **101**:2817–22.

25 Miller GAH, Hall RJC, Paneth M. Pulmonary embolectomy, heparin and streptokinase: their place in the treatment of acute massive pulmonary embolism. *Am Heart J* 1977; **93**:568–74.

26 Urokinase Pulmonary Embolism Trial. A national cooperative study. *Circulation* 1973; **47 and 48**:1–108.

27 Vieillard-Baron A, Page B, Augarde R *et al.* Acute cor pulmonale in massive pulmonary embolism: incidence, echocardiographic pattern, clinical implications and recovery rate. *Intens Care Med* 2001; **27**:1481–6.

28 Levine MN, Raskob G, Landefeld S *et al.* Hemorrhagic complications of anticoagulant treatment. *Chest* 2001; **119**:108S–121S.

29 Raschke R, Hirsh J, Guidry JR. Suboptimal monitoring and dosing of unfractionated heparin in comparative studies with low-molecular-weight heparin. *Ann Intern Med* 2003; **138**:720–3.

30 Becker RC, Ball SP, Eisenberg P *et al.* A randomized, multicenter trial of weight-adjusted intravenous heparin dose titration and point-of-care coagulation monitoring in hospitalized patients with active thromboembolic disease. *Am Heart J* 1999; **137**:59–71.

31 Bernardi E, Piccioli A, Oliboni G *et al.* Nomograms for the administration of unfractionated heparin in the initial treatment of acute thromboembolism — an overview. *Thromb Haemost* 2000; **84**:22–6.

32 Raschke RA, Reilly BM, Guidry JR *et al.* The weight-based heparin dosing nomogram compared with a 'standard care' nomogram. *Ann Intern Med* 1993; **119**:874–81.

33 Greaves M. Antiphospholipid antibodies and thrombosis. *Lancet* 1999; **353**:1348–53.

34 Basu D, Gallus A, Hirsh J *et al.* A prospective study of the value of monitoring heparin treatment with the activated partial thromboplastin time. *N Engl J Med* 1972; **287**:324–7.

35 Hull RD, Raskob GE, Hirsh J *et al.* Continuous intravenous heparin compared with intermittent subcutaneous heparin in the initial treatment of proximal-vein thrombosis. *N Engl J Med* 1986; **315**:1109–14.

36 Harenberg J, Huisman MV, Tolle AR *et al.* Reduction in thrombus extension and clinical end points in patients after initial treatment for deep vein thrombosis with the fixed-dose body weight-independent low molecular weight heparin certoparin. *Semin Thromb Hemost* 2001; **27**:513–18.

37 Gallus A, Jackaman J, Tillett J *et al.* Safety and efficacy of warfarin started early after submassive venous thrombosis or pulmonary embolism. *Lancet* 1986; **2**:1293–6.

38 Hull RD, Raskob G, Rosenbloom D *et al.* Heparin for 5 days as compared with 10 days in the initial treatment of proximal venous thrombosis. *N Engl J Med* 1990; **322**:1260–4.

39 Lubenow N, Kempf R, Eichner A *et al.* Heparin-induced thrombocytopenia. Temporal pattern of thrombocytopenia in relation to initial use or reexposure to heparin. *Chest* 2002; **122**:37–42.

40 Warkentin TE, Kelton JG. Temporal aspects of heparin-induced thrombocytopenia. *N Engl J Med* 2001; **344**:1286–92.

41 Zidane M, Schram MT, Planken EW *et al.* Frequency of major hemorrhage in patients treated with unfractionated intravenous heparin for deep venous thrombosis or pulmonary embolism. *Arch Intern Med* 2000; **160**:2369–73.

42 Dahlman TC. Osteoporotic fractures and the recurrence of thromboembolism during pregnancy and the puerperium in 184 women undergoing thromboprophylaxis with heparin. *Am J Obstet Gynecol* 1993; **168**:1265–70.

43 Pettilä V, Leinonen P, Markkola A *et al.* Postpartum bone mineral density in women treated for thromboprophylaxis with unfractionated heparin or LMW heparin. *Thromb Haemost* 2002; **87**:182–6.

44 Siebels M, Andrassy K, Vecsei P *et al.* Dose dependent suppression of mineralocorticoid metabolism by different heparin fractions. *Thromb Res* 1992; **66**:467–73.

45 Chong BH, Gallus AS, Cade JF *et al.* Prospective randomised open-label comparison of danaparoid with dextran 70 in the treatment of heparin-induced thrombocytopaenia with thrombosis. A clinical outcome study. *Thromb Haemost* 2001; **86**:1170–5.

46 Farner B, Eichler P, Kroll H *et al.* A comparison of danaparoid and lepirudin in heparin-induced thrombocytopenia. *Thromb Haemost* 2001; **85**:950–7.

47 Lewis BE, Wallis DE, Berkowitz SD *et al.* Argatroban anticoagulant therapy in patients with heparin-induced thrombocytopenia. *Circulation* 2001; **103**:1838–43.

48 Young E, Prins M, Levine MN *et al.* Heparin binding to plasma proteins, an important mechanism for heparin resistance. *Thromb Haemost* 1992; **67**:639–43.

49 Chow SL, Zammit K, West K *et al.* Correlation of antifactor Xa concentrations with renal function in patients on enoxaparin. *J Clin Pharmacol* 2003; **43**:586–90.

50 Kovacs MJ, Anderson D, Morrow B *et al.* Outpatient treatment of pulmonary embolism with dalteparin. *Thromb Haemost* 2000; **83**:209–11.

51 Warkentin TE, Levine MN, Hirsh J et al. Heparin-induced thrombo-cytopenia in patients treated with low-molecular-weight heparin or unfractionated heparin. N Engl J Med 1995; **332**:1330–5.

52 Monreal M, Lafoz E, Olive A et al. Comparison of subcutaneous unfractionated heparin with a low molecular weight heparin (Fragmin) in patients with venous thromboembolism and contraindications to coumarin. Thromb Haemost 1994; **71**:7–11.

53 Hull RD, Raskob GE, Pineo GF et al. Subcutaneous low-molecular-weight heparin compared with continuous intravenous heparin in the treatment of proximal vein thrombosis. N Engl J Med 1992; **326**:975–82.

54 Koopman MM, Prandoni P, Piovella F et al. Treatment of venous thrombosis with intravenous unfractionated heparin administered in the hospital as compared with subcutaneous low-molecular-weight heparin administered at home. The Tasman Study Group. N Engl J Med 1996; **334**:682–7.

55 Prandoni P, Lensing AW, Buller HR et al. Comparison of subcuta-neous low-molecular-weight heparin with intravenous standard heparin in proximal deep-vein thrombosis. Lancet 1992; **339**:441–5.

56 Gould M, Dembitzer AD, Doyle RL et al. Low-molecular-weight he-parins compared with unfractionated heparin for treatment of acute deep venous thrombosis. A meta-analysis of randomized, con-trolled trials. Ann Intern Med 1999; **130**:800–9.

57 Merli G, Spiro TE, Olsson CG et al. Subcutaneous enoxaparin once or twice daily compared with intravenous unfractionated heparin for treatment of venous thromboembolic disease. Ann Intern Med 2001; **134**:191–202.

58 Thery C, Simonneau G, Meyer G et al. Randomized trial of subcuta-neous low-molecular-weight heparin CY 216 (Fraxiparine) com-pared with intravenous unfractionated heparin in the curative treatment of submassive pulmonary embolism. A dose-ranging study. Circulation 1992; **85**:1380–9.

59 Dolovich LR, Ginsberg JS, Douketis JD et al. A meta-analysis com-paring low-molecular-weight heparins with unfractionated he-parin in the treatment of venous thromboembolism. Arch Intern Med 2000; **160**:181–8.

60 Findik S, Erkan ML, Selcuk MB et al. Low-molecular-weight heparin versus unfractionated heparin in the treatment of patients with acute pulmonary thromboembolism. Respiration 2002; **69**:440–4.

61 Breddin HK, Hach-Wunderle V, Nakov R et al. Effects of a low-mo-lecular-weight heparin on thrombus regression and recurrent thromboembolism in patients with deep-vein thrombosis. N Engl J Med 2001; **344**:626–31.

62 Kakkar VV, Hoppenstead DA, Fareed J et al. Randomized trial of dif-ferent regimens of heparins and in vivo thrombin generation in acute deep vein thrombosis. Blood 2002; **99**:1965–70.

63 Harenberg J, Riess H, Buller HR et al. Comparison of six-month out-come of patients initially treated for acute deep vein thrombosis with a low molecular weight heparin at a fixed, body-weight-inde-pendent dosage or unfractionated heparin. Haematologica 2003; **88**:1157–62.

64 Iorio A, Guercini F, Pini M. Low-molecular-weight heparin for the long-term treatment of symptomatic venous thromboembolism: meta-analysis of the randomized comparisons with oral anticoagu-lants. J Thromb Haemost 2003; **1**:1906–13.

65 Lee AY, Levine MN, Baker RI et al. Low-molecular-weight heparin versus a coumarin for the prevention of recurrent venous throm-boembolism in patients with cancer. N Engl J Med 2003; **349**:146–53.

66 Hettiarachchi RJK, Smorenburg SM, Ginsberg J et al. Do heparins do more than just treat thrombosis? The influence of heparins on cancer spread. Thromb Haemost 1999; **82**:947–52.

67 Zacharski LR, Ornstein DL, Mamourian AC. Low-molecular-weight heparin and cancer. Semin Thromb Hemost 2000; **26**(Suppl. 1):69S–77S.

68 Bauer KA, Eriksson BI, Lassen MR et al. Fondaparinux compared with enoxaparin for the prevention of venous thromboembolism after elective major knee surgery. N Engl J Med 2001; **345**:1305–10.

69 Eriksson BI, Bauer KA, Lassen MR et al. Fondaparinux compared with enoxaparin for the prevention of venous thromboembolism after hip-fracture surgery. N Engl J Med 2001; **345**:1298–304.

70 Lassen MR, Bauer KA, Eriksson BI et al. Postoperative fondaparinux versus preoperative enoxaparin for prevention of venous throm-boembolism in elective hip-replacement surgery: a randomised double-blind comparison. Lancet 2002; **359**:1715–20.

71 Turpie AGG, Gallus AS, Hoek JA. A synthetic pentasaccharide for the prevention of deep-vein thrombosis after total hip replacement. N Engl J Med 2001; **344**:619–25.

72 Turpie AG, Bauer KA, Eriksson BI et al. Postoperative fondaparinux versus postoperative enoxaparin for prevention of venous throm-boembolism after elective hip-replacement surgery: a randomised double-blind trial. Lancet 2002; **359**:1721–6.

73 The Rembrandt Investigators. Treatment of proximal deep vein thrombosis with a novel synthetic compound (SR90107A/ORG31540) with pure anti-factor Xa activity. Circula-tion 2000; **102**:2726–31.

74 Greinacher A, Lubenow N. Recombinant hirudin in clinical prac-tice. Focus on lepirudin. Circulation 2001; **103**:1479–84.

75 Eriksson BI, Arfwidsson AC, Frison L et al. A dose-ranging study of the oral direct thrombin inhibitor, ximelagatran, and its subcuta-neous form, melagatran, compared with dalteparin in the prophy-laxis of thromboembolism after hip or knee replacement: METHRO I. Thromb Haemost 2002; **87**:231–7.

76 Eriksson BI, Bergqvist D, Kalebo P et al. Ximelagatran and melaga-tran compared with dalteparin for prevention of venous throm-boembolism after total hip or knee replacement: the METHRO II randomised trial. Lancet 2002; **360**:1441–7.

77 Ginsberg JS, Nurmohamed MT, Gent M et al. Use of Hirulog in the prevention of venous thrombosis after major hip or knee surgery. Circulation 1994; **90**:2385–9.

78 Francis CW, Davidson BL, Berkowitz SD et al. Ximelagatran versus warfarin for the prevention of venous thromboembolism after total knee arthroplasty. A randomized, double-blind trial. Ann Intern Med 2002; **137**:648–55.

79 Heit JA, Colwell CW, Francis CW et al. Comparison of the oral direct thrombin inhibitor ximelagatran with enoxaparin as prophylaxis against venous thromboembolism after total knee replacement: a phase 2 dose-finding study. Arch Intern Med 2001; **161**:2215–21.

80 Eriksson BI, Agnelli G, Cohen AT et al. Direct thrombin inhibitor melagatran followed by oral ximelagatran in comparison with enoxaparin for prevention of venous thromboembolism after total hip or knee replacement. Thromb Haemost 2003; **89**:288–96.

81 Francis CW, Berkowitz SD, Comp PC et al. Comparison of ximelaga-tran with warfarin for the prevention of venous thromboembolism after total knee replacement. N Engl J Med 2003; **349**:1703–12.

82 Wahlander K, Lapidus L, Olsson CG et al. Pharmacokinetics, pharmacodynamics and clinical effects of the oral direct thrombin inhibitor ximelagatran in acute treatment of patients with pul-monary embolism and deep vein thrombosis. Thromb Res 2002; **107**:93–9.

83 Schulman S, Wåhlander K, Lundström T et al. Secondary prevention of venous thromboembolism with the oral direct thrombin in-hibitor ximelagatran. N Engl J Med 2003; **349**:1713–21.

84 Hirsh J, Fuster V, Ansell J et al. American Heart Association/Ameri-can College of Cardiology Foundation guide to warfarin therapy. Circulation 2003; **107**:1692–711.

85 Lagerstedt CI, Olsson CG, Fagher BO et al. Need for long-term anti-coagulant therapy in symptomatic calf-vein thrombosis. Lancet 1985; **211**:515–18.

86 Hull R, Delmore T, Genton E et al. Warfarin sodium versus low-dose

heparin in the treatment of venous thrombosis. *N Engl J Med* 1979; **301**:855–8.

87 Prins MH, Hutten BA, Koopman MM *et al.* Long-term treatment of venous thromboembolic disease. *Thromb Haemost* 1999; **82**:892–8.

88 Kearon C, Ginsberg JS, Kovacs MJ *et al.* Comparison of low-intensity warfarin therapy with conventional-intensity warfarin therapy for long-term prevention of recurrent venous thromboembolism. *N Engl J Med* 2003; **349**:631–9.

89 Hylek EM, Chang Y, Skates SJ *et al.* Prospective study of the outcomes of ambulatory patients with excessive warfarin anticoagulation. *Arch Intern Med* 2000; **160**:1612–17.

90 Odén A, Fahlén M. Oral anticoagulation and risk of death: a medical record linkage study. *BMJ* 2002; **325**:1073–5.

91 Fihn SD, McDonell M, Martin D *et al.* Risk factors for complications of chronic anticoagulation. A multicenter study. Warfarin Optimized Outpatient Follow-up Study Group. *Ann Intern Med* 1993; **118**:511–20.

92 Ruiz-Irastorza G, Khamashta MA, Hunt BJ *et al.* Bleeding and recurrent thrombosis in definite antiphospholipid syndrome. Analysis of a series of 66 patients treated with oral anticoagulation to a target international normalized ratio of 3,5. *Arch Intern Med* 2002; **162**:1164–9.

93 Khamashta MA, Cuadrado MJ, Mujic F *et al.* The management of thrombosis in the antiphospholipid-antibody syndrome. *N Engl J Med* 1995; **332**:993–7.

94 Crowther M, Ginsberg JS, Julian J *et al.* A comparison of two intensities of warfarin for the prevention of recurrent thrombosis in patients with the antiphospholipid antibody syndrome. *N Engl J Med* 2003; **349**:1133–8.

95 Cromheecke ME, Levi M, Colly LP *et al.* Oral anticoagulation self-management and management by a specialist anticoagulation clinic: a randomised cross-over comparison. *Lancet* 2000; **356**:97–102.

96 Research Committee of the British Thoracic Society. Optimum duration of anticoagulation for deep-vein thrombosis and pulmonary embolism. *Lancet* 1992; **340**:873–6.

97 Schulman S, Rhedin AS, Lindmarker P *et al.* A comparison of six weeks with six months of oral anticoagulant therapy after a first episode of venous thromboembolism. *N Engl J Med* 1995; **332**:1661–5.

98 Schulman S, Granqvist S, Holmstrom M *et al.* The duration of oral anticoagulant therapy after a second episode of venous thromboembolism. The Duration of Anticoagulation Trial Study Group. *N Engl J Med* 1997; **336**:393–8.

99 Kearon C, Gent M, Hirsh J *et al.* A comparison of three months of anticoagulation with extended anticoagulation for a first episode of idiopathic venous thromboembolism. *N Engl J Med* 1999; **340**:901–7.

100 van Dongen CJ, Vink R, Hutten BA *et al.* The incidence of recurrent venous thromboembolism after treatment with vitamin K antagonists in relation to time since first event: a meta-analysis. *Arch Intern Med* 2003; **163**:1285–93.

101 Agnelli G, Prandoni P, Santamaria MG *et al.* Three months versus one year of oral anticoagulant therapy for idiopathic deep venous thrombosis. Warfarin Optimal Duration Italian Trial Investigators. *N Engl J Med* 2001; **345**:165–9.

102 Pinede L, Ninet J, Duhaut P *et al.* Comparison of 3 and 6 months of oral anticoagulant therapy after a first episode of proximal deep vein thrombosis or pulmonary embolism and comparison of 6 and 12 weeks of therapy after isolated calf deep vein thrombosis. *Circulation* 2001; **103**:2453–60.

103 Agnelli G, Prandoni P, Becattini C *et al.* Extended oral anticoagulant therapy after a first episode of pulmonary embolism. *Ann Intern Med* 2003; **139**:19–25.

104 Hansson P-O, Sörbo J, Eriksson H. Recurrent venous thromboembolism after deep vein thrombosis. Incidence and risk factors. *Arch Intern Med* 2000; **160**:769–74.

105 Heit JA, Silverstein MD, Mohr DN *et al.* Predictors of survival after deep vein thrombosis and pulmonary embolism: a population-based, cohort study. *Arch Intern Med* 1999; **159**:445–53.

106 Murin S, Romano PS, White RH. Comparison of outcomes after hospitalization for deep venous thrombosis or pulmonary embolism. *Thromb Haemost* 2002; **88**:407–14.

107 Palareti G, Leali N, Coccheri S *et al.* Bleeding complications of oral anticoagulant treatment: an inception-cohort, prospective collaborative study (ISCOAT). *Lancet* 1996; **348**:423–8.

108 Girard P, Mathieu M, Simonneau G *et al.* Recurrence of pulmonary embolism during anticoagulant treatment: a prospective study. *Thorax* 1987; **42**:481–6.

109 Ridker PM, Goldhaber SZ, Danielson E *et al.* Long-term, low-intensity warfarin therapy for the prevention of recurrent venous thromboembolism. *N Engl J Med* 2003; **348**:1425–34.

110 Palareti G, Legnani C, Cosmi B *et al.* Risk of venous thromboembolism recurrence: high negative predictive value of D-dimer performed after oral anticoagulation is stopped. *Thromb Haemost* 2002; **87**:7–12.

111 Hutten BA, Prins MH, Gent M *et al.* Incidence of recurrent thromboembolic and bleeding complications among patients with venous thromboembolism in relation to both malignancy and achieved international normalized ratio: a retrospective analysis. *J Clin Oncol* 2000; **18**:3078–83.

112 van den Belt AG, Hutten BA, Prins MH *et al.* Duration of oral anticoagulant treatment in patients with venous thromboembolism and a deficiency of antithrombin, protein C or protein S—a decision analysis. *Thromb Haemost* 2000; **84**:758–63.

113 Douketis JD. Perioperative anticoagulation management in patients who are receiving oral anticoagulant therapy: a practical guide for clinicians. *Thromb Res* 2003; **108**:3–13.

114 Dunn AS, Turpie AG. Perioperative management of patients receiving oral anticoagulants. *Arch Intern Med* 2003; **163**:901–8.

115 Schweizer J, Kirch W, Koch R *et al.* Short- and long-term results after thrombolytic treatment of deep venous thrombosis. *J Am Coll Cardiol* 2000; **36**:1336–43.

116 Wells PS, Forster AJ. Thrombolysis in deep vein thrombosis: is there still an indication? *Thromb Haemost* 2001; **86**:499–508.

117 Konstantinides S, Geibel A, Olschewski M *et al.* Association between thrombolytic treatment and the prognosis of hemodynamically stable patients with major pulmonary embolism: results of a multicenter registry. *Circulation* 1997; **96**:882–8.

118 Tebbe U, Graf A, Kamke W *et al.* Hemodynamic effects of double bolus reteplase versus alteplase infusion in massive pulmonary embolism. *Am Heart J* 1999; **138**:39–44.

119 Pacouret G, Barnes SJ, Hopkins G *et al.* Rapid haemodynamic improvement following saruplase in recent massive pulmonary embolism. *Thromb Haemost* 1998; **79**:264–7.

120 Arcasoy SM, Kreit JW. Thrombolytic therapy of pulmonary embolism. A comprehensive review of current evidence. *Chest* 1999; **115**:1695–707.

121 Jerjes-Sanchez C, Ramirez-Rivera A, Garcia M *et al.* Streptokinase and heparin versus heparin alone in massive pulmonary embolism: a randomized controlled trial. *J Thromb Thrombolysis* 1995; **2**:227–9.

122 Dalla-Volta S, Palla A, Santolicandro A *et al.* PAIMS 2: alteplase combined with heparin versus heparin in the treatment of acute pulmonary embolism. Plasminogen activator Italian multicenter study. *J Am Coll Cardiol* 1992; **20**:520–6.

123 Goldhaber SZ, Haire WD, Feldstein ML *et al.* Alteplase versus heparin in acute pulmonary embolism: randomised trial assessing right-ventricular function and pulmonary perfusion. *Lancet* 1993; **341**:507–11.

124 Levine M, Hirsh J, Weitz J *et al.* A randomized trial of a single bolus dosage regimen of recombinant tissue plasminogen activator in patients with acute pulmonary embolism. *Chest* 1990; **98**:1473–9.

125 Ly B, Arnesen H, Eie H *et al.* A controlled clinical trial of streptokinase and heparin in the treatment of major pulmonary embolism. *Acta Med Scand* 1978; **203**:465–70.

126 Meyer G, Sors H, Charbonnier B *et al.* Effects of intravenous urokinase versus alteplase on total pulmonary resistance in acute massive pulmonary embolism: a European multicenter double-blind trial. The European Cooperative Study Group for Pulmonary Embolism. *J Am Coll Cardiol* 1992; **19**:239–45.

127 Miller GAH, Sutton GC, Kerr IH *et al.* Comparison of streptokinase and heparin in treatment of isolated acute massive pulmonary embolism. *BMJ* 1971; **2**:681–5.

128 PIOPED Investigators. Tissue plasminogen activator for the treatment of acute pulmonary embolism. *Chest* 1990; **97**:528–33.

129 Tibbut DA, Davies JA, Anderson JA *et al.* Comparison by controlled clinical trial of streptokinase and heparin in treatment of life-threatening pulmonary embolism. *BMJ* 1974; **1**:343–7.

130 Vander Sande J, Bossaert L, Brochier M *et al.* Thrombolytic treatment of pulmonary embolism with APSAC. *Eur Respir J* 1988; **1**:721–5.

131 Agnelli G, Becattini C, Kirschstein T. Thrombolysis vs heparin in the treatment of pulmonary embolism: a clinical outcome-based meta-analysis. *Arch Intern Med* 2002; **162**:2537–41.

132 Thabut G, Thabut D, Myers RP *et al.* Thrombolytic therapy of pulmonary embolism: A meta-analysis. *J Am Coll Cardiol* 2002; **40**:1660–7.

133 Konstantinides S, Geibel A, Heusel G *et al.* Heparin plus alteplase compared with heparin alone in patients with submassive pulmonary embolism. *N Engl J Med* 2002; **347**:1143–50.

134 Rose PS, Punjabi NM, Pearse DB. Treatment of right heart thromboemboli. *Chest* 2002; **121**:806–14.

135 Gonzalez-Juanatey J, Valdes L, Amaro A *et al.* Treatment of massive pulmonary thromboembolism with low intrapulmonary dosages of urokinase. Short-term angiographic and hemodynamic evolution. *Chest* 1992; **102**:341–6.

136 Goldhaber SZ, Simons GR, Elliott CG *et al.* Quantitative plasma D-dimer levels among patients undergoing pulmonary angiography for suspected pulmonary embolism. *JAMA* 1993; **270**:2819–22.

137 Hamel E, Pacouret G, Vincentelli D *et al.* Thrombolysis or heparin therapy in massive pulmonary embolism with right ventricular dilation: results from a 128-patient monocenter registry. *Chest* 2001; **120**:120–5.

138 Bell WR, Simon TL, Stengle JM *et al.* The urokinase-streptokinase pulmonary embolism trial (phase II) results. *Circulation* 1974; **50**:1070–1.

139 Goldhaber SZ, Kessler CM, Heit J *et al.* Randomised controlled trial of recombinant tissue plasminogen activator versus urokinase in the treatment of acute pulmonary embolism. *Lancet* 1988; **2**:293–8.

140 The UKEP Study Research Group. The UKEP Study: multicentre clinical trial on two local regimens of urokinase in massive pulmonary embolism. *Eur Heart J* 1987; **8**:2–10.

141 Verstraete M, Miller GA, Bounameaux H *et al.* Intravenous and intrapulmonary recombinant tissue-type plasminogen activator in the treatment of acute massive pulmonary embolism. *Circulation* 1988; **77**:353–60.

142 Marini C, Di RG, Rossi G *et al.* Fibrinolytic effects of urokinase and heparin in acute pulmonary embolism: a randomized clinical trial. *Respiration* 1988; **54**:162–73.

143 Goldhaber SZ, Kessler CM, Heit JA *et al.* Recombinant tissue-type plasminogen activator versus a novel dosing regimen of urokinase in acute pulmonary embolism: a randomized controlled multicenter trial. *J Am Coll Cardiol* 1992; **20**:24–30.

144 Meneveau N, Schiele F, Vuillemenot A *et al.* Streptokinase vs alteplase in massive pulmonary embolism. A randomized trial assessing right heart haemodynamic and pulmonary vascular obstruction. *Eur Heart J* 1997; **18**:1141–8.

145 Meneveau N, Schiele F, Metz D *et al.* Comparative efficacy of a two-hour regimen of streptokinase versus alteplase in acute massive pulmonary embolism: immediate clinical and hemodynamic outcome and one-year follow-up. *J Am Coll Cardiol* 1998; **31**:1057–63.

146 Daniels LB, Parker JA, Patel SR *et al.* Relation of duration of symptoms with response to thrombolytic therapy in pulmonary embolism. *Am J Cardiol* 1997; **80**:184–8.

147 Goldhaber SZ, Agnelli G, Levine MN. Reduced dose bolus alteplase vs conventional alteplase infusion for pulmonary embolism thrombolysis. An international multicenter randomized trial. The Bolus Alteplase Pulmonary Embolism Group. *Chest* 1994; **106**:718–24.

148 Sors H, Pacouret G, Azarian R *et al.* Hemodynamic effects of bolus vs 2-h infusion of alteplase in acute massive pulmonary embolism. A randomized controlled multicenter trial. *Chest* 1994; **106**:712–17.

149 Jerjes-Sanches C, Ramirez-Rivera A, Arriaga-Nava R *et al.* High dose and short-term streptokinase infusion in patients with pulmonary embolism: prospective with seven-year follow-up trial. *J Thromb Thrombolysis* 2001; **12**:237–47.

150 Bailen MR, Cuadra JA, Aguayo De Hoyos E. Thrombolysis during cardiopulmonary resuscitation in fulminant pulmonary embolism: a review. *Crit Care Med* 2001; **29**:2211–19.

151 Böttiger BW, Bode C, Kern S *et al.* Efficacy and safety of thrombolytic therapy after initially unsuccessful cardiopulmonary resuscitation: a prospective clinical trial. *Lancet* 2001; **357**:1583–5.

152 Janata K, Holzer M, Kurkciyan I *et al.* Major bleeding complications in cardiopulmonary resuscitation: the place of thrombolytic therapy in cardiac arrest due to massive pulmonary embolism. *Resuscitation* 2003; **57**:49–55.

153 Abu-Laban RB, Christenson JM, Innes GD *et al.* Tissue plasminogen activator in cardiac arrest with pulseless electrical activity. *N Engl J Med* 2002; **346**:1522–8.

154 Kanter DS, Mikkola KM, Patel SR *et al.* Thrombolytic therapy for pulmonary embolism. Frequency of intracranial hemorrhage and associated risk factors. *Chest* 1997; **111**:1241–5.

155 Mehta SR, Eikelboom JW, Yusuf S. Risk of intracranial haemorrhage with bolus versus infusion thrombolytic therapy: a meta-analysis. *Lancet* 2000; **356**:449–54.

156 Gray HH, Morgan JM, Paneth M *et al.* Pulmonary embolectomy for acute massive pulmonary embolism: an analysis of 71 cases. *Br Heart J* 1988; **60**:196–200.

157 Lund O, Nielsen TT, Schifter S *et al.* Treatment of pulmonary embolism with full-dose heparin, streptokinase or embolectomy—results and indications. *Thorac Cardiovasc Surg* 1986; **34**:240–6.

158 Clarke DB, Abrams LD. Pulmonary embolectomy: a 25 year experience. *J Thorac Cardiovasc Surg* 1986; **92**:442–5.

159 Stulz P, Schläpfer R, Feer R *et al.* Decision making in the surgical treatment of massive pulmonary embolism. *Eur J Cardiothorac Surg* 1994; **8**:188–93.

160 Kieny R, Charpentier A, Kieny MT. What is the place of pulmonary embolectomy today? *J Cardiovasc Surg Torino* 1991; **32**:549–54.

161 Aklog L, Williams CS, Byrne JG *et al.* Acute pulmonary embolectomy: a contemporary approach. *Circulation* 2002; **105**:1416–19.

162 Del Campo C. Pulmonary embolectomy: a review. *Can J Surg* 1985; **28**:111–13.

163 Ohteki H, Norita H, Sakai M *et al.* Emergency pulmonary embolectomy with percutaneous cardiopulmonary bypass. *Ann Thorac Surg* 1997; **63**:1584–6.

164 Bauer EP, Laske A, von Segesser L *et al.* Early and late results after surgery for massive pulmonary embolism. *Thorac Cardiovasc Surg* 1991; **39**:353–6.

165 Doerge H, Schoendube FA, Voß M *et al.* Surgical therapy of fulmi-

nant pulmonary embolism: early and late results. *Thorac Cardiovasc Surg* 1999; **47**:9–13.

166 Laas J, Schmid C, Albes JM *et al.* Chirurgische Aspekte zur fulminanten Lungenembolie. *Z Kardiol* 1993; **2**:25–8.

167 Lund O, Nielsen TT, Ronne K *et al.* Pulmonary embolism: long-term follow-up after treatment with full-dose heparin, streptokinase or embolectomy. *Acta Med Scand* 1987; **221**:61–71.

168 Meyns B, Sergeant P, Flameng W *et al.* Surgery for massive pulmonary embolism. *Acta Cardiol* 1992; **47**:487–93.

169 Ullmann M, Hemmer W, Hannekum A. The urgent pulmonary embolectomy: mechanical resuscitation in the operating theatre determines the outcome. *Thorac Cardiovasc Surg* 1999; **47**:5–8.

170 Habicht JM, Hammerli R, Perruchoud A *et al.* Long-term follow-up in pulmonary embolectomy: is NYHA (dyspnea) classification reliable? *Eur J Cardiothorac Surg* 1996; **10**:32–7.

171 Timsit JF, Reynaud P, Meyer G *et al.* Pulmonary embolectomy by catheter device in massive pulmonary embolism. *Chest* 1991; **100**:655–8.

172 Brady AJ, Crake T, Oakley CM. Percutaneous catheter fragmentation and distal dispersion of proximal pulmonary embolus. *Lancet* 1991; **338**:1186–9.

173 Hiramatsu S, Ogihara A, Kitano Y *et al.* Clinical outcome of catheter fragmentation and aspiration therapy in patients with acute pulmonary embolism. *J Cardiol* 1999; **34**:71–8.

174 Horstkotte D, Heintzen MP, Strauer BE. Kombinierte mechanische und thrombolytische Wiedereröffnung der Lungenstrombahn bei massiver Lungenarterienembolie mit kardiogenem Schock. *Intensivmedizin* 1990; **27**:124–32.

175 Schmitz-Rode T, Janssens U, Schild HH *et al.* Fragmentation of massive pulmonary embolism using a pigtail rotation catheter. *Chest* 1998; **114**:1427–36.

176 Essop MR, Middlemost S, Skoularigis J *et al.* Simultaneous mechanical clot fragmentation and pharmacologic thrombolysis in acute massive pulmonary embolism. *Am J Cardiol* 1992; **69**:427–30.

177 Müller-Hülsbeck S, Brossmann J, Jahnke T *et al.* Mechanical thrombectomy of major and massive pulmonary embolism with use of the Amplatz thrombectomy device. *Invest Radiol* 2001; **36**:317–22.

178 Fava M, Loyola S, Huete I. Massive pulmonary embolism: treatment with the hydrolyser thrombectomy catheter. *J Vasc Interv Radiol* 2000; **11**:1159–64.

179 Reekers JA, Baarslag HJ, Koolen MG *et al.* Mechanical thrombectomy for early treatment of massive pulmonary embolism. *Cardiovasc Interv Radiol* 2003; **26**:246–50.

180 Sing RF, Jacobs DG, Heniford BT. Bedside insertion of inferior vena cava filters in the intensive care unit. *J Am Coll Surg* 2001; **192**:570–5.

181 Athanasoulis CA, Kaufman JA, Halpern EF *et al.* Inferior vena caval filters: review of a 26-year single-center clinical experience. *Radiology* 2000; **216**:54–66.

182 Carlin AM, Tyburski JG, Wilson RF *et al.* Prophylactic and therapeutic inferior vena cava filters to prevent pulmonary emboli in trauma patients. *Arch Surg* 2002; **137**:521–7.

183 Greenfield LJ, Proctor MC, Michaels AJ *et al.* Prophylactic vena caval filters in trauma: the rest of the story. *J Vasc Surg* 2000; **32**:490–5.

184 Headrick JR Jr, Barker DE, Pate LM *et al.* The role of ultrasonography and inferior vena cava filter placement in high-risk trauma patients. *Am Surg* 1997; **63**:1–8.

185 Aswad MA, Sandager GP, Pais SO *et al.* Early duplex scan evaluation of four vena caval interruption devices. *J Vasc Surg* 1996; **24**:809–18.

186 Crochet DP, Brunel P, Trogrlic S *et al.* Long-term follow-up of Vena Tech-LGM filter: predictors and frequency of caval occlusion. *J Vasc Interv Radiol* 1999; **10**:137–42.

187 Greenfield LJ, Proctor MC. The percutaneous Greenfield filter: outcomes and practice patterns. *J Vasc Surg* 2000; **32**:888–93.

188 Roehm JO, Johnsrude IS, Barth MH *et al.* The bird's nest inferior vena cava filter: progress report. *Radiology* 1988; **168**:745–9.

189 Schleich JM, Morla O, Laurent M *et al.* Long-term follow-up of percutaneous vena cava filters: a prospective study in 100 consecutive patients. *Eur J Vasc Endovasc Surg* 2001; **21**:450–7.

190 Decousus H, Leizorovicz A, Parent F *et al.* A clinical trial of vena caval filters in the prevention of pulmonary embolism in patients with proximal deep-vein thrombosis. *N Engl J Med* 1998; **338**:409–15.

191 White RH, Zhou H, Kim J *et al.* A population-based study of the effectiveness of inferior vena cava filter use among patients with venous thromboembolism. *Arch Intern Med* 2000; **160**:2033–41.

192 Asch MR. Initial experience in humans with a new retrievable inferior vena cava filter. *Radiology* 2002; **225**:835–44.

193 De Gregorio MA, Gamboa P, Gimeno MJ *et al.* The Gunther Tulip retrievable filter: prolonged temporary filtration by repositioning within the inferior vena cava. *J Vasc Interv Radiol* 2003; **14**:1259–65.

194 Millward SF, Oliva VL, Bell SD *et al.* Gunther Tulip retrievable vena cava filter: results from the Registry of the Canadian Interventional Radiology Association. *J Vasc Interv Radiol* 2001; **12**:1053–8.

195 Offner PJ, Hawkes A, Madayag R *et al.* The role of temporary inferior vena cava filters in critically ill surgical patients. *Arch Surg* 2003; **138**:591–5.

196 Lorch H, Zwaan M, Siemens HJ *et al.* Temporary vena cava filters and ultrahigh streptokinase thrombolysis therapy: a clinical study. *Cardiovasc Interv Radiol* 2000; **23**:273–8.

197 Noguchi M, Eishi K, Sakamoto I *et al.* Thrombus removal with a temporary vena caval filter in patients with acute proximal deep vein thrombosis. *Heart Vessels* 2003; **18**:197–201.

198 Scholz KH, Just M, Buchwald AB *et al.* Erfahrungen mit temporären Vena-cava-Filtern bei 114 Risiko-Patienten mit Thrombosen oder Thromboembolien. *Dtsch Med Wochenschr* 1999; **124**:307–13.

199 Vos LD, Tielbeek AV, Bom EP *et al.* The Günther temporary inferior vena cava filter for short-term protection against pulmonary embolism. *Cardiovasc Interv Radiol* 1997; **20**:91–7.

200 Hirsch LJ, Rooney MW, Wat SS *et al.* Norepinephrine and phenylephrine effects on right ventricular function in experimental canine pulmonary embolism. *Chest* 1991; **100**:796–801.

201 Layish DT, Tapson VF. Pharmacologic hemodynamic support in massive pulmonary embolism. *Chest* 1997; **111**:218–24.

202 Mercat A, Diehl J-L, Meyer G *et al.* Hemodynamic effects of fluid loading in acute massive pulmonary embolism. *Crit Care Med* 1999; **27**:540–4.

203 Bhorade S, Christenson J, O'Connor M *et al.* Response to inhaled nitric oxide in patients with acute right heart syndrome. *Am J Respir Crit Care Med* 1999; **159**:571–9.

204 Capellier G, Jacques T, Balvay P *et al.* Inhaled nitric oxide in patients with pulmonary embolism. *Intens Care Med* 1997; **23**:1089–92.

205 Kawahito K, Murata S, Adachi H *et al.* Resuscitation and circulatory support using extracorporeal membrane oxygenation for fulminant pulmonary embolism. *Artif Organs* 2000; **24**:427–30.

206 Bates SM, Ginsberg JS. How we manage venous thromboembolism during pregnancy. *Blood* 2002; **100**:3470–8.

207 Laurent P, Dussarat GV, Bonal J *et al.* Low molecular weight heparins: a guide to their optimum use in pregnancy. *Drugs* 2002; **62**:463–77.

208 Ginsberg JS, Greer IA, Hirsh J. Use of antithrombotic agents during pregnancy. *Chest* 2001; **119**:122S–131S.

209 Ahearn GS, Hadjiliadis D, Govert JA *et al.* Massive pulmonary embolism during pregnancy successfully treated with recombinant tissue plasminogen activator: a case report and review of treatment options. *Arch Intern Med* 2002; **162**:1221–7.

CHAPTER 6.4

Pulmonary hypertension

Horst Olschewski

There is new hope for patients with pulmonary hypertension as new treatment strategies have been developed and their efficacy has been shown in randomized controlled studies. But with this development, new questions came up, including the right indication for a drug, the right drug for an indication, the right dose, the right time for changes in the therapy regimen and combination therapies. None of these questions can currently be answered based on the strict criteria of evidence-based medicine.

This chapter will mainly focus on those issues with sufficient evidence in the literature. Because pulmonary hypertension belongs to the orphan diseases and many important questions cannot be addressed by means of controlled studies, expert opinions will also be included in this chapter. The author participated in the second (Evian, 1998) and third world conferences (Venice, 2003) on pulmonary hypertension and is a member of the Task Force on Pulmonary Hypertension of the European Society of Cardiology, of the scientific leadership counsel of the Pulmonary Hypertension Association and of a German expert group of cardiologists, pulmonologists and paediatric cardiologists who have been working on consensus papers on diagnosis and therapy of pulmonary hypertension. Unfortunately, none of these papers has been published yet, except the executive summary of the Evian conference.[1] When a 'consensus among experts' is claimed in this chapter, this refers to the discussions in all these expert groups. The literature search has been performed by means of PubMed and updated until November 2003.

Classification of pulmonary hypertension

After the first world conference on pulmonary hypertension in 1973, the disease was classified into primary and secondary pulmonary hypertension. During the second world conference on pulmonary hypertension in Evian, 1998, this classification was revised. Five types of pulmonary hypertension were defined (Table 1). During the third world conference on pulmonary hypertension in Venice, 2003, these disease groups remained unchanged; however, there were some minor changes. Pulmonary veno-occlusive disease (PVOD), which had been assigned to pulmonary venous hypertension, and pulmonary capillary haemangiomatosis, previously assigned to the fifth group, were now assigned to pulmonary arterial

hypertension, and the term primary pulmonary hypertension was changed to idiopathic pulmonary hypertension.

Identification of patients with pulmonary hypertension

Before a physician can take responsibility for any therapy decision in a patient with pulmonary hypertension, he or she must achieve a precise diagnosis, including the disease severity and presence or absence of associated and unrelated diseases and risk factors associated with available therapies. The first step, however, is the identification of patients with pulmonary hypertension.

Symptoms

The typical complaint is shortness of breath during exercise. One of the achievements of the National Institutes of Health (NIH) registry on primary pulmonary hypertension was to quantify the patients' complaints.[2] In the majority of patients (60%), dyspnoea on exertion is among the first symptoms. At the time of diagnosis, nearly every patient (98%) suffers from dyspnoea on exertion. Another frequent, yet unspecific complaint is fatigue, being present in 20% of patients among the first symptoms and in 73% at the time of diagnosis. In contrast, peripheral oedema is very rarely among the first symptoms (3%) and, even at the time of diagnosis, is present in only 33% of patients. Patients with pulmonary hypertension may experience thoracic pain during exertion (47% at time of diagnosis), which has similar characteristics to that in coronary artery disease. About the same number of patients (41%) have had syncope or near syncope at the time of diagnosis, and this sign is among the first symptoms in 12% of all patients, especially in patients of younger age.

Physical examination

The physical examination detects a loud second heart sound in the majority of patients, often so loud that it can be palpated over the left anterior thorax. If there is significant tricuspid regurgitation, there is a long systolic murmur with its punctum maximum at the left fourth intercostal space. If there is pulmonary valve insufficiency, there is a diastolic murmur, very similar to aortic insufficiency (Graham-Steell murmur), best heard at the third left intercostal space. Often, there is a jugular

Table 1. Nomenclature and classification of pulmonary hypertension according to the WHO Symposium, in Evian, 1998.

1   Pulmonary arterial hypertension
1.1 Primary pulmonary hypertension
    a) Sporadic
    b) Familial
1.2 Related to:
    a) Collagen vascular disease
    b) Congenital systemic-to-pulmonary shunt defects
    c) Portal hypertension
    d) HIV infection
    e) Drugs/toxins
       1) Anorectics
       2) Other
    f) Persistent pulmonary hypertension of the newborn
    g) Other

2   Pulmonary venous hypertension
2.1 Left-sided atrial or ventricular heart disease
2.2 Left-sided valvular heart disease
2.3 Extrinsic compression of the central pulmonary veins
    a) Fibrosing mediastinitis
    b) Adenopathy/tumours
2.4 Pulmonary veno-occlusive disease
2.5 Other

3   Pulmonary hypertension associated with disorders of the respiratory system and/or hypoxaemia
3.1 Chronic obstructive pulmonary disease
3.2 Interstitial lung disease
3.3 Sleep apnoea
3.4 Alveolar hypoventilation disorders
3.5 Chronic exposure to high altitude
3.6 Neonatal lung disease
3.7 Alveolar-capillary dysplasia
3.8 Other

4   Pulmonary hypertension due to chronic thrombotic and/or embolic disease
4.1 Thromboembolic obstruction of proximal pulmonary arteries
4.2 Obstruction of distal pulmonary arteries
    a) Pulmonary embolism (thrombus, tumour, parasites, foreign bodies)
    b) *In situ* thrombosis
    c) Sickle cell anaemia

5   Pulmonary hypertension due to disorders directly affecting the pulmonary vasculature
5.1 Inflammatory
    a) Schistosomiasis
    b) Sarcoidosis
    c) Other
5.2 Pulmonary capillary haemangiomatosis

double pulse. If the jugular veins are overfilled, this points to right ventricular decompensation, which is severe if pulsations of the liver can be detected.[3]

Laboratory methods for detection of pulmonary hypertension

According to a study in 61 patients with primary pulmonary hypertension and collagen vascular disease-associated pulmonary hypertension, being treated in a centre for pulmonary hypertension, the electrocardiogram (ECG) shows pathological findings in 83% of patients.[4] Typically, there is a right axis deviation with a negative main vector in lead I, incomplete or complete right bundle branch block and characteristic ST-T changes in lead V2-4.

In many cases, the chest radiograph shows enlarged central pulmonary arteries and an enlarged right ventricle, which can be best seen in the lateral view. Typically, but not always, the descending right pulmonary artery is enlarged.

There is consensus among experts that echocardiography is the most sensitive and specific method for non-invasive diagnosis of pulmonary hypertension. In most patients, there is some tricuspid regurgitation, which allows the assessment of systolic pulmonary artery pressure from the maximum velocity of the regurgitant jet during systole.[5,6] While this pressure is very important for diagnosis of pulmonary hypertension, it is not so important for the assessment of prognosis and response to therapy, as shown in an echo substudy of the Bosentan trial in pulmonary arterial hypertension.[7] Prognostic parameters are being evaluated. There are few data in the literature indicating that the Tei index,[8] the left ventricular eccentricity index and pericardial effusion[5,9,10] and the right ventricular acceleration time in the outflow tract[11] might have prognostic value.

Spiroergometry allows the assessment of peak oxygen consumption, oxygen pulse and many other parameters that are associated with a lowered cardiac output and a low stroke volume. All these are considerably altered in severe pulmonary hypertension.[12] In primary pulmonary hypertension (PPH) patients who were candidates for lung transplantation, it was shown that both a low peak oxygen consumption and a low peak systemic artery systolic pressure, and particularly a combination of these factors, are associated with an unfavourable prognosis.[13] However, in mild or even moderate disease, these parameters may be normal or nearly normal and do not allow the exclusion of significant pulmonary hypertension. According to the German expert group, the method can be recommended for assessment of prognosis and for the decision either to perform a complete workup including catheter investigation or to end without further investigations of the circulation. This applies especially to patients in whom it is difficult to decide whether cardiorespiratory, peripheral (muscular) or mental factors cause dyspnoea.

In highly experienced centres, stress echocardiography has been shown to be suitable for assessing pulmonary artery systolic pressure during exercise. Healthy relatives of PPH patients who shared the genetic risk haplotype showed an abnormal pulmonary pressure increase during exercise, compared with those relatives who did not share the risk haplotype.[14] This method could be suitable for the detection of patients with mild disease or even those with an increased risk of developing pulmonary hypertension. Currently, this is a hypothesis and an issue of ongoing studies.

Natriuretic peptides have been shown to be increased in patients with left and right ventricular impairment.[15] In PPH patients, left ventricular strain is lower than normal, but the right atrium and the right ventricle are the major sources of increased natriuretic peptide levels. Atrial natriuretic peptide (ANP) was the first peptide to be discovered.[16,17] It is correlated with pulmonary haemodynamics and responds instantly to haemodynamic changes during pharmacological testing.[18] Highly elevated plasma brain natriuretic peptide (BNP) levels have been suggested as an indicator of a poor prognosis in PPH, particularly if they persist during therapy.[19] In comparison with ANP levels, BNP levels are associated with ventricular strain[20] rather than atrial strain, and BNP is released steadily, while ANP is secreted from granules in response to a secretion stimulus. Currently, the diagnostic value of natriuretic peptides for pulmonary hypertension has not been defined. The levels may reflect right ventricular strain rather than pulmonary pressure.

Diagnosis

Pulmonary hypertension has been defined as an increase in mean pulmonary artery pressure >25 mmHg at rest or >30 mmHg during exercise in the US literature. In many European countries, a different definition is used. This was based on the range of pulmonary pressures in healthy adults.[21] According to this, pulmonary hypertension was defined as a mean pulmonary artery pressure >20 mmHg at rest. If this pressure was normal but exceeded 28 mmHg during exercise, this was called 'latent' pulmonary hypertension. Currently, there is a tendency for European centres to adopt the American definition.

Catheter investigation is still considered the gold standard for diagnosis of pulmonary hypertension and for assessment of response to therapy, although there is consensus that non-invasive techniques may allow important therapy decisions without a catheter investigation. The main value of the catheter investigation is the determination of cardiac output, pulmonary artery mean pressure and pulmonary artery occlusion (wedge) pressure, allowing the calculation of pulmonary vascular resistance. It was recommended at the Evian and Venice conferences to combine this diagnostic investigation with pharmacological testing, at least if the patient suffers from PPH. If the catheter investigation is combined with exercise, it allows the diagnosis of 'latent' pulmonary hypertension and the decision as to whether this is caused by an increase in pulmonary venous pressure. It is important to note that occlusion of small pulmonary veins (pulmonary veno-occlusive disease) does not normally result in increased pulmonary artery wedge pressures.[22]

Pharmacological testing is used to identify patients with a major acute pulmonary vasodilatation upon short-acting vasodilators. Such a response allows the identification of patients who may profit from high-dose calcium channel blockers.[23] In Europe, the most established test is inhalation with nitric oxide (NO), whereas in the US, intravenous adenosine or prostacyclin is being used. According to expert opinion, the application of calcium channel blockers as an acute test is no longer recommended because of the risk of right ventricular decompensation in non-responders, as described by the French group.[24] The major advantage with the use of NO is the lack of systemic side-effects during the test and its predictive value for an acute response to calcium channel blockers.[24,25] As an alternative, inhaled iloprost has been used in experienced centres, particularly in Germany. The acute responses to inhaled NO and inhaled iloprost are correlated in individual patients but, among PPH patients, the rate of responders to iloprost is higher than the rate of NO responders.[26]

Assessment of severity of disease

For assessment of functional impairment, a modified New York Heart Association (NYHA) classification has been recommended by the World Health Organization (WHO) conference on pulmonary hypertension in Evian.[1] In the literature, this classification has been referred to as the 'WHO functional classification' (Table 2). Functional impairment has a major impact on prognosis.[2,27] Improvement to class I or II during therapy is associated with a favourable prognosis

Table 2. Functional assessment of pulmonary hypertension according to the WHO symposium in Evian, 1998.

Class 1	Patients with pulmonary hypertension without limitation of physical activity. Ordinary physical activity does not cause increased dyspnoea or fatigue, chest pain or near syncope.
Class 2	Patients with pulmonary hypertension resulting in slight limitation of physical activity. No discomfort at rest. Normal physical activity causes increased dyspnoea or fatigue, chest pain or near syncope.
Class 3	Patients with pulmonary hypertension resulting in marked limitation of physical activity. There is no discomfort at rest. Less than ordinary activity causes increased dyspnoea or fatigue, chest pain or near syncope.
Class 4	Patients with pulmonary hypertension with inability to carry out any physical activity without discomfort. Indications of manifest right heart failure. Dyspnoea and/or fatigue may even be present at rest. Discomfort is increased by the least physical activity.

during intravenous prostacyclin therapy.[28,29] Therefore, improvement of functional class is one of the major goals with any therapy approach for pulmonary hypertension.

The 6-min walk test has evolved as a major parameter to assess the efficacy of drugs for pulmonary hypertension (see section on Therapy). In most of the studies, the change in 6-min walk distance from baseline has been used as an indicator of improvement. In contrast, the analysis of data that were measured during long-term therapy with epoprostenol suggested that it was not the change in 6-min walk but the absolute value during therapy that was indicative of the prognosis.[27,29,30] The 6-min walk should be performed according to the American Thoracic Society (ATS) guidelines as an unencouraged walk at a comfortable speed.[31]

Differential diagnosis

Once the diagnosis of pulmonary hypertension has been established, it is most important to search for underlying diseases as this might have a major impact on the treatment strategy.

Pulmonary venous hypertension is normally easy to diagnose by means of echocardiography. There may be left ventricular systolic impairment or diastolic impairment or mitral valve diseases that are detected by this method. As a hallmark of this type of pulmonary hypertension, the left atrium is dilated. However, diagnosis may be difficult based on echocardiography alone, particularly in patients with amyloidosis or pericardial disease and in patients with both left ventricular impairment and severely increased pulmonary vascular resistance. In these cases, it may be necessary to use catheter investigations to decide on the assignment to a disease group and the correct therapy.

Pulmonary hypertension associated with disorders of the respiratory system and/or hypoxaemia is ruled out by arterial blood gas analysis, chest radiograph and pulmonary function test. Lung function is generally normal or near normal in patients with PPH, although quite often there is some degree of peripheral airway obstruction.[32] However, some patients with pulmonary disease causing pulmonary hypertension present with a normal pulmonary function test. These patients typically show a severely reduced carbon monoxide (CO) diffusion capacity and/or changes in high-resolution computerized tomography (HRCT). Therefore, the expert groups also recommend measurement of CO diffusion capacity and/or HRCT to rule out pulmonary diseases causing pulmonary hypertension.

Pulmonary hypertension due to chronic thromboembolic and/or embolic disease (CTEPH) can be excluded by perfusion scintigraphy. This shows a homogeneous perfusion or a speckled pattern in patients with pulmonary arterial hypertension,[33–35] whereas in CTEPH, in nearly all cases, typical peripheral perfusion defects are detected. One of the differential diagnoses then is PVOD according to a small observational study.[36] If CTEPH was not excluded by scintigraphy, spiral CT and/or pulmonary angiography is recommended. If the patient is a candidate for pulmonary endarterectomy, a pulmonary angiogram with consecutive contrast injections to both lungs and radiography in at least two views is recommended.

Pulmonary hypertension due to disorders directly affecting the pulmonary vasculature can normally be excluded by chest CT combined with HRCT, which shows characteristic changes in most of these diseases.

Pulmonary arterial hypertension (PAH) is an inhomogeneous group of diseases, characterized by severe narrowing of precapillary pulmonary arteries that is not caused by increased pulmonary capillary pressure, hypoxic pulmonary vasoconstriction, thromboembolic obstruction and diseases directly affecting the pulmonary vessels.

Congenital left-to-right shunt can normally be excluded by transthoracic echocardiography. Sometimes, transoesophageal echocardiography[37] or injection of contrast media is helpful. In case of aberrant pulmonary veins and other rare diseases, diagnosis may be difficult, even with catheter investigations and magnetic resonance tomography of the heart.

Collagen vascular diseases most often belong to the scleroderma group of diseases and are easily diagnosed by the typical skin changes. A hallmark of this type of underlying disease is a thickening of the tongue frenulum. Sometimes, clinical signs are quite discrete. Therefore, assessment of antinuclear antibodies and, if positive, of extractable nuclear antibodies is recommended in patients with PAH.

HIV infection can be ruled out by laboratory methods. This test is recommended together with tests for hepatitis B and C in PAH patients.

Portopulmonary hypertension is diagnosed by signs of portal hypertension or liver cirrhosis. However, these signs may be discrete and easily overlooked. Oesophagogastroscopy seems to be the most reliable method to check for portal hypertension.

PVOD and pulmonary capillary haemangiomatosis can be suspected from HRCT of the lungs.[38] Open lung biopsy is diagnostic but associated with a considerable risk in patients with severe pulmonary hypertension. Bronchoalveolar lavage may be indicative of this disease by an increased number of iron-laden macrophages but, most importantly, it is recommended that patients with suspicious HRCT be very carefully monitored during therapy with vasodilators as these may induce lung oedema and death in PVOD.[39]

Therapy

Supportive therapy and anticoagulation

There are no controlled studies on the use of supportive therapy, but there is consensus among experts about the importance of these measures.

Diuretics are recommended once the central venous pressure exceeds 8 mmHg (German expert group), as this is associated with adverse prognosis.[13] Long-term oxygen therapy is recommended in pulmonary hypertension (PH) patients with an arterial P_{O_2} below 55–60 mmHg and low cardiac output in order to prevent peripheral organ hypoxia combined with low perfusion. According to the world conferences and the expert groups, anticoagulation has been recommended for PAH patients as a result of positive experience with PPH patients.[23,40] This recommendation is less clear for patients with portopulmonary hypertension and Eisenmenger syndrome, as they have an increased incidence of gastro-oesophageal and pulmonary haemorrhage. For PAH patients, an international normalized ratio (INR) of 1.5–2.0 has been recommended; in CTEPH and other forms with a history of pulmonary embolism or specific risk factors, the target INR is 2.5–3.5.

Medications with no use

There is no indication for nitrates, β-blockers, angiotensin-converting enzyme (ACE) inhibitors and AT-1 antagonists for treatment of pulmonary arterial hypertension. The same applies to calcium channel blockers (CCB) in patients who do not respond favourably to short-acting vasodilators. ACE inhibitors and AT-1 antagonists as well as CCB can be useful if there is a significant comorbidity with systemic arterial hypertension.

Therapy of pulmonary venous hypertension

Pulmonary venous hypertension (PVH) is characterized by increased pulmonal arterial pressure due to increased pressures in the pulmonary veins. In addition to a 'passive' pressure increase, there may be precapillary vasoconstriction and remodelling, which may add considerably to the pulmonary arterial pressure increase. For left heart failure and valve diseases, there are recommendations for state of the art treatment that should also be followed in patients with unusually severe pulmonary arterial pressure increase resulting from PVH. There are no good data indicating that therapy approaches aiming at lowering the pulmonary vascular resistance are beneficial for PVH patients. This has been thoroughly investigated for the endothelin receptor antagonist bosentan[41] and for epoprostenol. Indeed, the randomized controlled study with epoprostenol (FIRST) showed increased mortality in the epoprostenol group compared with the control group.[42]

Therapy of pulmonary hypertension associated with respiratory diseases

In patients with chronic obstructive pulmonary disease (COPD) and in patients with pulmonary fibrosis, cor pulmonale is quite common, although pulmonary pressure at rest is mostly in the high normal range or only slightly elevated.[43] Even small increases in resting pulmonary pressure may have a

prognostic impact.[44] Long-term oxygen therapy improves the overall prognosis of chronic hypoxic patients with COPD and may also improve the natural course of pulmonary hypertension.[45] Currently, there are no controlled data that show a significant long-term benefit of medications targeted to pulmonary vascular resistance in chronic lung diseases.

Chronic thromboembolic disease

It is imperative that the possibility of pulmonary endarterectomy (PEA) be considered following a definite diagnosis of chronic proximal pulmonary embolism. This operation is technically difficult, requiring that the patient be in circulatory arrest under hypothermic conditions on a heart–lung machine. Such a procedure is performed with a high success rate in few centres worldwide. The leading centre is San Diego, CA, USA, where more than 1500 of these operations have been performed.[46,47]

With proper indication, the haemodynamic and clinical improvements are impressive. It is not possible to operate if no organized embolic material is present in the proximal arteries. A recent embolism should not be operated on within the first 3–6 months because of the possibility of spontaneous recanalization during this time and because the material to be removed is not yet sufficiently organized. In this case, prevention of relapse via anticoagulation has first priority. If chronic embolism proves inoperable, then an attempt at treatment with vasodilators may be justified,[48,49] although there are no controlled data demonstrating the efficacy of such an approach.

Targeted drugs for pulmonary arterial hypertension

Recently, drugs have been approved in the indication of pulmonary arterial hypertension, although some of the diseases belonging to this group were excluded from all the relevant studies.

Bosentan

Bosentan is an endothelin antagonist blocking both the ETA and the ETB receptor. It has been shown that bosentan effectively antagonizes pulmonary arterial remodelling in chronic hypoxic models of pulmonary hypertension.[50,51] Given at relatively high doses in patients with pulmonary hypertension, bosentan acutely reduced both pulmonary and systemic vascular resistance.[52] At lower doses (250–500 mg/day), bosentan has only minor if any acute vasodilatory effects. During long-term application, however, there is a significant decrease in pulmonary vascular resistance.[53,54] In a 3-month pilot study, bosentan improved the 6-min walk distance in idiopathic and collagen vascular disease-associated pulmonary hypertension by 72 m. These results were confirmed in a pivotal study (BREATHE-1) (Table 3). In this double-blind, placebo-controlled study,[55] 213 patients with PAH (primary or

Table 3. Synopsis of the pivotal trials in pulmonary hypertension.

Drug	Epoprostenol	Epoprostenol	Treprostenil	Beraprost	Iloprost	Bosentan
Reference	63	76	81	87	48	55
Mode of application	Cont. IV	Cont. IV	Cont. SC	Oral	Inhaled	Oral
Subjects (n)						
PPH	81	—	270	63	111	150
CTD	—	111	90	13	35	63
CHD	—	—	109	24	—	—
CTEPH	—	—	—	—	57	—
Other	—	—	—	30	—	—
Design	RCT	RCT	RCT	RCT	RCT	RCT
Intervention	12-week OL	12-week OL	12-week DB	12-week DB	12-week DB	16-week DB
Outcome						
P, PEP	<0.003	<0.001	0.006	0.035	0.007	<0.001
delta 6-mw all	47	108	16	25	36	44
delta 6-mw PPH	47	NA	NA	46	59	50

PPH, primary pulmonary hypertension; CTD, connective tissue disease; CHD, congenital heart disease; CTEPH, chronic thromboembolic pulmonary hypertension; RCT, randomized controlled trial; OL, open label; DB, double blind; P, probability of error; PEP, primary endpoint; delta 6-mw, change in 6-min walk distance with the active drug, compared with control; NA, not available.

associated with connective tissue disease) received placebo or 62.5 mg of bosentan twice daily for 4 weeks followed by either of two doses of bosentan (125 or 250 mg twice daily) for a minimum of 12 weeks. The primary endpoint was the degree of change in exercise capacity. Secondary endpoints included the change in the Borg dyspnoea index, the change in the WHO functional class and the time to clinical worsening. At week 16, patients treated with bosentan had an improved 6-min walking distance; the mean difference between the placebo group and the combined bosentan groups was 44 m [95% confidence interval (CI) 21–67; P < 0.001]. Bosentan also improved the Borg dyspnoea index and WHO functional class and increased the time to clinical worsening.[55] As an adverse effect, in about 10% of patients, there were significant increases in liver function tests within 16 weeks of therapy and, in about half these patients, therapy was discontinued. This effect appeared to be less frequent in the 125 mg bid group compared with the 250 mg bid group. Bosentan received approval in the indication PAH in NYHA class III and IV in the US and Canada and in the indication PAH NYHA class III in Europe. A 1-year follow-up study of 29 out of 32 patients who had participated in a double-blind 3-month study with bosentan showed sustained benefits on exercise capacity and haemodynamics over 1 year. About 10% of patients developed increases in liver aminotransferase levels but did not warrant discontinuation of bosentan treatment. One patient needed additional treatment with intravenous epoprostenol and no patient died.[54]

The advantage of bosentan, compared with other treatments of pulmonary hypertension, is simple dosing with just two tablets per day, few side-effects and no tachyphylaxis. The major disadvantage is hepatotoxicity, the rate of which has not been finally evaluated during long-term treatment. Another potential problem is teratogenicity, which has been documented in animal models. Therefore, safe contraception is very important in patients of childbearing age. Bosentan is metabolized by cytochrome P450 isoenzymes. It can cause significant drug–drug interactions due to both blocking and induction of these enzymes. This is particularly important for oral anticoagulants, oral contraceptives, glyburide and cyclosporin A. In Europe, there is the practical disadvantage that bosentan has only been approved for NYHA class III patients. For NYHA class IV patients, the European authorities recommended the use of intravenous epoprostenol, although this has not been approved in most European countries.

Epoprostenol

In 1976, prostacyclin was discovered as an endogenous, endothelium-derived, vasodilative and anti-aggregatory substance.[56] Epoprostenol is a synthetic analogue with a very short half-life of 2–3 min. It has been used as a pulmonary vasodilator since 1980.[57] The first publication describing acute effects in adults with idiopathic PAH appeared 2 years later.[58] The first therapeutic application of prostacyclin via continuous intravenous infusion was published in 1984.[59] In 1990, the first randomized short-term trial was published,[60] and open-label, long-term treatment in a cohort of PPH patients was published in 1993 from the UK[61] and in 1994 from the US.[62] In

1996, the first controlled open-label trial with intravenous prostacyclin showed improved physical capacity, haemodynamics and survival compared with the control group.[63] These studies, together with various other observations and reports, were instrumental in the approval of continuous intravenous epoprostenol (Flolan®) in the USA in the indication PPH NYHA class III and IV. In the following years, this therapy was also approved in several European countries. There are multiple studies reporting beneficial long-term effects of intravenous prostacyclin that are clearly superior to the acute and short-term effects.[64] A recent long-term study from Chicago included 162 patients over a median period of 31 months. Observed survival with epoprostenol therapy at 1, 2 and 3 years was 87.8%, 76.3% and 62.8%, which was significantly greater than expected survival of 58.9%, 46.3% and 35.4%.[28] These results were similar to a previous report from the US[65] and a recent study in France.[29]

Owing to the short half-life, epoprostenol can only be applied as a continuous intravenous infusion by means of an implanted intravenous catheter and a mobile minipump. The starting dose is 4–8 ng/kg/min, which is increased by about 2–4 ng/kg/min every 2 weeks until a dose of about 50 ng/kg/min is reached. This mode of dosing is commonly used in the US whereas, in European countries, the doses are frequently lower than this. Much higher doses, up to 200 ng/kg/min, have been used in the US, but this increased the side-effects without adding considerable therapeutic benefit and has increasingly been abandoned.[66]

Prostacyclin has also been used in conditions with pulmonary hypertension other than idiopathic PAH. Several of the early studies included chronic thromboembolic pulmonary hypertension.[61] This therapy has also been applied successfully in children with idiopathic PAH,[62,67] HIV-associated pulmonary hypertension,[68–72] portopulmonary hypertension[64,73,74] and Eisenmenger's syndrome,[75] which indicates that intravenous prostacyclin might be as effective in all these groups of patients as in PPH. However, the only controlled study in patients other than PPH enrolled patients with PAH associated with scleroderma. It showed significant improvement in physical capacity and haemodynamics after 3 months[76] but no improved survival.

The advantage of intravenous epoprostenol is the well-documented efficacy in PPH, including improvement in prognosis, and similar beneficial effects in many other forms of PAH particularly in NYHA class III and IV.

The disadvantages originate from the mode of application and the systemic side-effects. Even short interruptions in the therapy carry the risk of right ventricular failure.[62,77] With intravenous iloprost, because of the longer half-life, this seems to be less problematic. More or less frequent local infections at the entry point of the catheter require antibiotic treatment. Sepsis is quite rare (at experienced centres 0.5/patient/year) but has a potentially fatal outcome. Hickman line infections are seen more frequently in the absence of sepsis. The true incidence is not known. Infections often necessitate the removal of the catheter. Side-effects of this therapy are common and include jaw pain, leg and foot pain (similar to Sudeck's syndrome), headache, diarrhoea, ascites and red skin.[78] Moreover, in a small group of patients, there is unexplained weight loss after long treatment periods.[79] The high cost of therapy is mostly explained by the price of the agent itself, which is considerably lower in North America than in the rest of the world.

Treprostinil

Treprostinil is another synthetic prostacyclin analogue with a plasma half-life of more than 30 min.[80] It was clinically developed as a continuous subcutaneous infusion (Remodulin®) in order to avoid the risk of intravenous drug application, such as catheter-related infections and temporary interruption of the infusion due to malfunction of the pump or dislodgement of the central venous catheter.

There have been three pilot studies assessing the safety and efficacy of treprostinil.[80] Additionally, a large randomized multicentre study showed the efficacy of continuous subcutaneous infusion of treprostinil in patients with PPH and other forms of PAH (Table 3).[81] Improvement in exercise capacity was greater in the sicker patients and was dose related but independent of the underlying disease. At low tolerated doses up to 8.2 ng/kg/min, there was no improvement in the 6-min walk test, whereas at 8.2–13.8 ng/kg/min, the increase was 20 m and, in patients tolerating more than 13.8 ng/kg/min, it was 36 m. Most patients (85%) reported infusion site pain mostly associated with skin reactions at the infusion site (83%) and 8% discontinued their study medication because of intolerable abdominal infusion site pain. There were small but significant improvements in pulmonary haemodynamics and an improvement in the Borg Dyspnoea Score.

In current practice, the target dose is about 30 ng/kg/min. If this is tolerated, there are comparable haemodynamic and clinical effects to those with intravenous prostacyclin. After these studies, treprostinil was approved by the Federal Drug Administration (FDA) and by the Canadian authorities, but approval is still pending by the European authorities.

The main advantages, compared with intravenous epoprostenol, are the independence of a central venous line and the lower price, particularly in Europe. As major disadvantages, there are local complications at the infusion site. Most of the patients experience pain at the infusion site, and there is a risk of abscess formation. Compared with oral therapies, patients are still dependent on technical equipment such as the infusion pump. Another drawback for European patients is the lack of approval.

Beraprost

Beraprost was developed in Japan as a synthetic prostacyclin analogue for oral use.[82] Beraprost is readily absorbable from the small intestine, and excretion in the urine and faeces is rapid and almost complete after both oral and intravenous dosing. In 1994, the drug was approved in Japan for primary and secondary pulmonary hypertension. There were several uncontrolled studies from Japan reporting favourable effects of beraprost in PPH and secondary pulmonary hypertension, including reports on haemodynamic improvement[83,84] and improved survival compared with historical controls.[85,86]

A European, controlled, double-blind, multicentre study (ALPHABET), enrolling NYHA class II and III patients, showed significant effects only in PPH patients (Table 3).[87] The dose of beraprost was given in four doses per day and up-titrated by 80 µg every week to a maximum tolerated dose or a maximum of 480 µg. The mean dose per day after the titration period was 320 µg. Adverse events were common during the first 6 weeks of therapy and included headache (67%), flushing (54%), jaw pain (28%) and diarrhoea (26%). These incidences were markedly reduced during weeks 7–12. Some 9% of the beraprost group withdrew prematurely from the study because of adverse events.

A 1-year, double-blind, controlled, randomized study in moderate pulmonary hypertension was performed in the US. The daily dose of beraprost was 80 µg qid. The 6-min walk was increased after 3 months; however, after 9 months and 1 year, there was no advantage in the beraprost compared with the placebo group.[88]

The advantage of beraprost is that the drug is available as an oral medication and that this medication is relatively cheap. The disadvantages are systemic side-effects, comparable to intravenous prostacyclin, gaps between drug applications due to short half-life and no convincing long-term efficacy. Beraprost has not been approved in the US or Europe.

Iloprost

Iloprost is another synthetic prostacyclin analogue. It has been approved as intravenous infusion for primary and secondary pulmonary hypertension in New Zealand. While iloprost is approved and available as an infusion solution in the indication peripheral arterial occlusive disease in most European countries, it is not marketed in the US. The long-term doses used for continuous intravenous therapy range between 1 and 10 ng/kg/min, whereas the doses used with continuous prostacyclin range between 10 and 50 ng/kg/min. The reasons for this huge difference are not clear but probably result from both a higher potency of iloprost and a different dosing practice in Europe compared with the US.

In order to achieve pulmonary selectivity, iloprost was inhaled as an aerosol over a period of 8–12 min. By means of modern inhalers, inhalation times could be reduced to 4 min.[89] In patients with severe pulmonary hypertension, both primary and secondary, inhalation of aerosolized iloprost resulted in a substantial acute decrease in pulmonary artery pressure and resistance, concomitant with an increase in cardiac output, in the absence of significant systemic artery pressure drop and ventilation–perfusion mismatch.[90,91] This observation was consistent with previous findings in mechanically ventilated patients with acute respiratory failure.[92–96] In severe lung fibrosis, an increase in the pulmonary shunt blood flow may limit the use of intravenous prostacyclin, whereas inhaled iloprost can be administered safely if the dose per inhalation is not too high.[91] In uncontrolled studies with inhaled iloprost in severe primary and secondary pulmonary hypertension, a significant clinical and haemodynamic improvement was demonstrated together with an improved physical capacity.[97,98]

A large, randomized, double-blind, placebo-controlled, European, multicentre study (AIR) with inhaled iloprost showed the efficacy of this approach (Table 3).[48] Patients in NYHA class III or IV were enrolled. The primary endpoint was defined as an improvement in NYHA class, combined with at least 10% improvement in the 6-min walking test and no prior deterioration or death (combined clinical endpoint). Treatment effects did not differ between subgroups. In addition, there was a significant treatment effect on NYHA functional class, quality of life assessments by means of the EuroQoL visual analogue scale and on the Mahler Dyspnoea Transition Index. Haemodynamics deteriorated significantly in the placebo group, whereas in the iloprost group, preinhalation values were unchanged compared with baseline, and post-inhalation values were significantly improved. Importantly, the number of patients remaining on study medication was significantly higher in the iloprost group than in the placebo group. Overall, the therapy was well tolerated. Cough occurred more frequently in the iloprost group compared with the placebo group (38.6% versus 25.5%) as well as headache (29.7% versus 19.6%) and flush (26.7% versus 8.8%). These adverse events were mild and mostly transient. Syncope occurring in the iloprost group was more often rated as serious than in the placebo group, but was commonly not associated with clinical deterioration.

A long-term study with inhaled iloprost over 2 years with an initial 3-month controlled randomized phase (AIR-2) enrolled 63 patients with primary (PPH, $n = 40$) and secondary pulmonary hypertension (SPH, $n = 23$) and suggested long-term efficacy and tolerability without toxic effects and significant tachyphylaxis.[99]

As a conclusion of these studies, inhalation of iloprost was considered as an effective and safe therapy for primary and non-primary pulmonary hypertension in NYHA functional class III and IV. However, inhaled iloprost has been approved by the European authorities (EMEA) only in the indication PPH NYHA class III. It will be marketed as Ventavis® in most European countries in 2004.

The advantages of inhaled iloprost include potent acute pulmonary vasodilatation without systemic side-effects and risk of catheter complications. Owing to pulmonary selectivity and intrapulmonary selectivity, it can be used safely in patients with pre-existent ventilation–perfusion mismatch. The most important drawback is the fact that the haemodynamic effect of inhaled iloprost levels off within 30–90 min, that six to nine inhalations per day are necessary and a special inhalation device is needed.

Phosphodiesterase inhibitors

As potent phosphodiesterase (PDE) inhibitors are available, it has been shown that these substances have pulmonary vasodilative effects and that they can augment the effects of prostanoids even if they are applied at very low doses without haemodynamic effects of their own.[100–104]

Sildenafil, a potent PDE5+6 inhibitor has been used to treat severe pulmonary hypertension.[49,105–109] PDE5 is predominantly expressed in the genital and pulmonary circulation. Its action, counteracting the vasodilatation induced by local NO production, is blocked by sildenafil. Only in the lung is there continuous NO production at a high level. Hence, sildenafil causes a pulmonary selective vasodilatation. In patients with inoperable chronic thromboembolic disease, treatment with sildenafil had beneficial long-term effects[49] and, in patients with pulmonary fibrosis, sildenafil achieved pulmonary vasodilation without increasing intrapulmonary right-to-left shunt blood flow, corresponding to intrapulmonary selectivity to the ventilated areas.[102]

An intercontinental, controlled, randomized, double-blind study with sildenafil has been performed in patients with PPH, scleroderma-associated and corrected left-to-right shunt-associated pulmonary arterial hypertension. The results are not yet available.

The advantage of phosphodiesterase inhibitors is that they are orally available, pulmonary selective and intrapulmonary selective and have very few side-effects in adults. Unfortunately, the data from the placebo-controlled randomized trial are not yet available, and there is no approval in the indication pulmonary hypertension worldwide.

Calcium channel blockers

Calcium channel blockers have been used for more than 30 years in patients with PPH. Their lifelong use at high doses leads to a favourable prognosis in a small subset (about 10%) of patients.[110] All these PPH patients respond to short-acting vasodilators such as inhaled NO, intravenous adenosine or intravenous prostacyclin with a major acute vasodilatation. In other forms of pulmonary hypertension, the rate of clinical responders is much lower than 10% if there is any.[110] Currently, the criteria for a favourable acute vasodilative response are being discussed. Most experts agree that three criteria should be fulfilled: a decrease in pulmonary arterial mean pressure and pulmonary vascular resistance by more than 20% and a pulmonary arterial mean pressure below 40 mmHg during vasodilator application.[110]

Treatment costs

All current therapies of pulmonary hypertension are very expensive. Bosentan costs about €45 000/year, continuous intravenous epoprostenol costs about €500 000/year and inhaled iloprost, using six inhalations/day, will be around €65 000/year.

Therapy decisions for patients with pulmonary arterial hypertension

Among all expert groups, there was consensus that patients on optimized supportive therapy should be assessed for NYHA class. Patients in class I–III should be subjected to pharmacological testing, especially if they suffer from PPH. Responders to short-acting vasodilators are treated with doses of calcium channel blockers increasing every week with repeated controls of physical capacity. As long as this increases, the dose can be increased until an average maximum daily dose for nifedipin of 120–160 mg, for diltiazem 480–720 mg and for amlodipin 15–25 mg is reached or there are side-effects. If patients improve and achieve NYHA class I or II, this therapy is continued lifelong. Non-responders in NYHA class I and II continue to receive supportive therapy and are controlled every 3–6 months. Non-responders in NYHA class III are treated with prostaglandins or endothelin receptor blockers. If they profit sufficiently from this therapy, this therapy is continued lifelong. If not, a change in therapy and/or combination therapy must be considered. If this is not sufficient, lung transplantation should be considered. As a method of improving survival on the waiting list for lung transplantation, balloon atrial septostomy should be considered.[111–113] There is no consensus as to whether patients in NYHA class IV who respond to vasodilators should be treated with calcium channel blockers. There is consensus that patients who present with severe right ventricular decompensation need intensive care medicine including intravenous diuretics and eventually catecholamines. According to the German expert group, this should be performed in parallel with starting treatments that rapidly release the pulmonary vascular resistance, such as intravenous epoprostenol or inhaled iloprost. Combinations may be necessary to achieve sufficient effects. After recompensation, these patients can be treated as the other patients.

Summary for clinicians

Pulmonary hypertension (PH) has become a treatable disease. Yet, therapy is difficult and the prognosis is not ideal, even with the most advanced therapy regimens. Since the WHO conference in Evian, 1998, there is a new classification of PH into five classes: pulmonary arterial hypertension (PAH), pulmonary venous hypertension, PH associated with disorders of the respiratory system and/or hypoxaemia, PH due to chronic thrombotic and/or embolic disease and PH due to disorders directly affecting the pulmonary vasculature. In idiopathic PAH (formerly PPH), in most cases, diagnosis is settled at late stages, although increased awareness and the availability of Doppler echocardiography has improved the detection rate.

It is very important to perform a complete diagnostic workup before starting long-term therapy, e.g. chronic thromboembolic PH can be operated on with a high success rate and moderate risk in the few highly experienced centres, in contrast to all other forms of PH. The disease-targeted therapy for PAH may not be suitable and even contraindicated for other forms of PH, particularly pulmonary venous hypertension.

Currently, only oral bosentan (PAH, NYHA III) and inhaled iloprost (PPH, NYHA III) have been approved by the European authorities (EMEA) and, in several European countries, continuous intravenous epoprostenol has been approved for PAH, NYHA III–IV. New therapies (phosphodiesterase inhibitors, new endothelin receptor antagonists) are being developed.

Expert centres for pulmonary hypertension have developed in most European countries. It is important that these centres get involved in the long-term therapy decisions in patients with severe PH in order to optimize both individual results and future recommendations.

References

1 Rich S. Primary pulmonary hypertension. [WWW document] URL http://www.who.int/ncd/cvd/pph.html, 1998.

2 Rich S, Dantzker DR, Ayres SM et al. Primary pulmonary hypertension. A national prospective study. *Ann Intern Med* 1987; **107**:216–23.

3 Olschewski H, Seeger W. *Pulmonary Hypertension – Pathophysiology, Diagnosis, Treatment, and Development of a Pulmonary-selective Therapy*, 1st edn. Bremen, Germany, UNI-MED, 2002.

4 Ahearn GS, Tapson VF, Rebeiz A, Greenfield JC Jr. Electrocardiography to define clinical status in primary pulmonary hypertension and pulmonary arterial hypertension secondary to collagen vascular disease. *Chest* 2002; **122**:524–7.

5 Hinderliter AL, Willis PW, Barst RJ et al. Effects of long-term infusion of prostacyclin (epoprostenol) on echocardiographic measures of right ventricular structure and function in primary pulmonary hypertension. Primary Pulmonary Hypertension Study Group. *Circulation* 1997; **95**:1479–86.

6 Yock PG, Linker DT, White NW et al. Clinical applications of intravascular ultrasound imaging in atherectomy. *Int J Cardiol Imaging* 1989; **4**:117–25.

7 Galie N, Hinderliter AL, Torbicki A et al. Effects of the oral endothelin-receptor antagonist bosentan on echocardiographic and doppler measures in patients with pulmonary arterial hypertension. *J Am Coll Cardiol* 2003; **41**:1380–6.

8 Yeo TC, Dujardin KS, Tei C, Mahoney DW, McGoon MD, Seward JB. Value of a Doppler-derived index combining systolic and diastolic time intervals in predicting outcome in primary pulmonary hypertension. *Am J Cardiol* 1998; **81**:1157–61.

9 Hinderliter AL, Willis PW, Long W et al. Frequency and prognostic significance of pericardial effusion in primary pulmonary hypertension. PPH Study Group. Primary pulmonary hypertension. *Am J Cardiol* 1999; **84**:481–4, A10.

10 Raymond RJ, Hinderliter AL, Willis PW et al. Echocardiographic predictors of adverse outcomes in primary pulmonary hypertension. *J Am Coll Cardiol* 2002; **39**:1214–19.

11 Eysmann SB, Palevsky HI, Reichek N, Hackney K, Douglas PS. Two-dimensional and Doppler-echocardiographic and cardiac catheter-ization correlates of survival in primary pulmonary hypertension. *Circulation* 1989; **80**:353–60.

12 Sun XG, Hansen JE, Oudiz RJ, Wasserman K. Exercise pathophysiology in patients with primary pulmonary hypertension. *Circulation* 2001; **104**:429–35.

13 Wensel R, Opitz CF, Anker SD et al. Assessment of survival in patients with primary pulmonary hypertension: importance of cardiopulmonary exercise testing. *Circulation* 2002; **106**:319–24.

14 Grunig E, Janssen B, Mereles D et al. Abnormal pulmonary artery pressure response in asymptomatic carriers of primary pulmonary hypertension gene. *Circulation* 2000; **102**:1145–50.

15 Levin ER, Gardner DG, Samson WK. Natriuretic peptides. *N Engl J Med* 1998; **339**:321–8.

16 de Bold AJ. Atrial natriuretic factor: a hormone produced by the heart. *Science* 1985; **230**:767–70.

17 Flynn TG, Davies PL, Kennedy BP, de Bold ML, de Bold AJ. Alignment of rat cardionatrin sequences with the preprocardionatrin sequence from complementary DNA. *Science* 1985; **228**:323–5.

18 Wiedemann R, Ghofrani HA, Weissmann N et al. Atrial natriuretic peptide in severe primary and nonprimary pulmonary hypertension: response to iloprost inhalation. *J Am Coll Cardiol* 2001; **38**:1130–6.

19 Nagaya N, Nishikimi T, Uematsu M et al. Plasma brain natriuretic peptide as a prognostic indicator in patients with primary pulmonary hypertension. *Circulation* 2000; **102**:865–70.

20 Nagaya N, Nishikimi T, Okano Y et al. Plasma brain natriuretic peptide levels increase in proportion to the extent of right ventricular dysfunction in pulmonary hypertension. *J Am Coll Cardiol* 1998; **31**:202–8.

21 Keller R, Kopp C, Zutter W, Mlzoch J, Herzog H. Der Lungenkreislauf als leistungsbegrenzender Faktor bei Patienten. *Verh Dtsch Ges Lungen Atmungsforsch* 1976; **5**:27–40.

22 Mandel J, Mark EJ, Hales CA. Pulmonary veno-occlusive disease. *Am J Respir Crit Care Med* 2000; **162**:1964–73.

23 Rich S, Kaufmann E, Levy PS. The effect of high doses of calcium-channel blockers on survival in primary pulmonary hypertension. *N Engl J Med* 1992; **327**:76–81.

24 Sitbon O, Humbert M, Jagot JL et al. Inhaled nitric oxide as a screening agent for safely identifying responders to oral calcium-channel blockers in primary pulmonary hypertension. *Eur Respir J* 1998; **12**:265–70.

25 Sitbon O, Brenot F, Denjean A et al. Inhaled nitric oxide as a screening vasodilator agent in primary pulmonary hypertension. A dose–response study and comparison with prostacyclin. *Am J Respir Crit Care Med* 1995; **151**(2 Pt 1):384–9.

26 Hoeper MM, Olschewski H, Ghofrani HA et al. A comparison of the acute hemodynamic effects of inhaled nitric oxide and aerosolized iloprost in primary pulmonary hypertension. German PPH study group. *J Am Coll Cardiol* 2000; **35**:176–82.

27 Miyamoto S, Nagaya N, Satoh T et al. Clinical correlates and prognostic significance of six-minute walk test in patients with primary pulmonary hypertension. Comparison with cardiopulmonary exercise testing. *Am J Respir Crit Care Med* 2000; **161**(2 Pt 1): 487–92.

28 McLaughlin VV, Shillington A, Rich S. Survival in primary pulmonary hypertension: the impact of epoprostenol therapy. *Circulation* 2002; **106**:1477–82.

29 Sitbon O, Humbert M, Nunes H et al. Long-term intravenous epoprostenol infusion in primary pulmonary hypertension: prognostic factors and survival. *J Am Coll Cardiol* 2002; **40**:780–8.

30 Humbert M, Sitbon O, Simmoneau G. Treatment of pulmonary arterial hypertension. *N Engl J Med* 2004; **351**:1425–36.

31 ATS statement: guidelines for the six-minute walk test. *Am J Respir Crit Care Med* 2002; **166**:111–17.

32 Meyer FJ, Ewert R, Hoeper MM et al. Peripheral airway obstruction in primary pulmonary hypertension. *Thorax* 2002; **57**:473–6.

33 Ogawa Y, Nishimura T, Hayashida K, Uehara T, Shimonagata T. Perfusion lung scintigraphy in primary pulmonary hypertension. *Br J Radiol* 1993; **66**:677–80.

34 Powe JE, Palevsky HI, McCarthy KE, Alavi A. Pulmonary arterial hypertension: value of perfusion scintigraphy. *Radiology* 1987; **164**:727–30.

35 Rush C, Langleben D, Schlesinger RD, Stern J, Wang NS, Lamoureux E. Lung scintigraphy in pulmonary capillary hemangiomatosis. A rare disorder causing primary pulmonary hypertension. *Clin Nucl Med* 1991; **16**:913–17.

36 Bailey CL, Channick RN, Auger WR et al. 'High probability' perfusion lung scans in pulmonary venoocclusive disease. *Am J Respir Crit Care Med* 2000; **162**:1974–8.

37 Chen WJ, Chen JJ, Lin SC, Hwang JJ, Lien WP. Detection of cardiovascular shunts by transesophageal echocardiography in patients with pulmonary hypertension of unexplained cause. *Chest* 1995; **107**:8–13.

38 Resten A, Maitre S, Humbert M et al. Pulmonary arterial hypertension: thin-section CT predictors of epoprostenol therapy failure. *Radiology* 2002; **222**:782–8.

39 Humbert M, Maitre S, Capron F, Rain B, Musset D, Simonneau G. Pulmonary edema complicating continuous intravenous prostacyclin in pulmonary capillary hemangiomatosis. *Am J Respir Crit Care Med* 1998; **157**(5 Pt 1):1681–5.

40 Fuster V, Steele PM, Edwards WD, Gersh BJ, McGoon MD, Frye RL. Primary pulmonary hypertension: natural history and the importance of thrombosis. *Circulation* 1984; **70**:580–7.

41 Kalra PR, Moon JC, Coats AJ. Do results of the ENABLE (endothelin antagonist bosentan for lowering cardiac events in heart failure) study spell the end for non-selective endothelin antagonism in heart failure? *Int J Cardiol* 2002; **85**:195–7.

42 Califf RM, Adams KF, McKenna WJ et al. A randomized controlled trial of epoprostenol therapy for severe congestive heart failure: the Flolan International Randomized Survival Trial (FIRST). *Am Heart J* 1997; **134**:44–54.

43 Scharf SM, Iqbal M, Keller C, Criner G, Lee S, Fessler HE. Hemodynamic characterization of patients with severe emphysema. *Am J Respir Crit Care Med* 2002; **166**:314–22.

44 Weitzenblum E. Prognosis of pulmonary hypertension in chronic obstructive pulmonary disease. *Cor Vasa* 1980; **22**:418–27.

45 Weitzenblum E, Sautegeau A, Ehrhart M, Mammosser M, Pelletier A. Long-term oxygen therapy can reverse the progression of pulmonary hypertension in patients with chronic obstructive pulmonary disease. *Am Rev Respir Dis* 1985; **131**:493–8.

46 Jamieson SW, Kapelanski DP, Sakakibara N et al. Pulmonary endarterectomy: experience and lessons learned in 1,500 cases. *Ann Thorac Surg* 2003; **76**:1457–62.

47 Fedullo PF, Auger WR, Kerr KM, Rubin LJ. Chronic thromboembolic pulmonary hypertension. *N Engl J Med* 2001; **345**:1465–72.

48 Olschewski H, Simonneau G, Galie N et al. Inhaled iloprost for severe pulmonary hypertension. *N Engl J Med* 2002; **347**:322–9.

49 Ghofrani HA, Schermuly RT, Rose F et al. Sildenafil for long-term treatment of nonoperable chronic thromboembolic pulmonary hypertension. *Am J Respir Crit Care Med* 2003; **167**:1139–41.

50 Chen SJ, Chen YF, Meng QC, Durand J, DiCarlo VS, Oparil S. Endothelin-receptor antagonist bosentan prevents and reverses hypoxic pulmonary hypertension in rats. *J Appl Physiol* 1995; **79**:2122–31.

51 Eddahibi S, Raffestin B, Clozel M, Levame M, Adnot S. Protection from pulmonary hypertension with an orally active endothelin receptor antagonist in hypoxic rats. *Am J Physiol* 1995; **268**(2 Pt 2):H828–H835.

52 Williamson DJ, Wallman LL, Jones R et al. Hemodynamic effects of bosentan, an endothelin receptor antagonist, in patients with pulmonary hypertension. *Circulation* 2000; **102**:411–18.

53 Channick R, Badesch DB, Tapson VF et al. Effects of the dual endothelin receptor antagonist bosentan in patients with pulmonary hypertension: a placebo-controlled study. *J Heart Lung Transplant* 2001; **20**:262–3.

54 Sitbon O, Badesch DB, Channick RN et al. Effects of the dual endothelin receptor antagonist bosentan in patients with pulmonary arterial hypertension: a 1-year follow-up study. *Chest* 2003; **124**:247–54.

55 Rubin LJ, Badesch DB, Barst RJ et al. Bosentan therapy for pulmonary arterial hypertension. *N Engl J Med* 2002; **346**:896–903.

56 Whittaker N, Bunting S, Salmon J et al. The chemical structure of prostaglandin X (prostacyclin). *Prostaglandins* 1976; **12**:915–28.

57 Watkins WD, Peterson MB, Crone RK, Shannon DC, Levine L. Prostacyclin and prostaglandin E1 for severe idiopathic pulmonary artery hypertension. *Lancet* 1980; **1**:1083.

58 Rubin LJ, Groves BM, Reeves JT, Frosolono M, Handel F, Cato AE. Prostacyclin-induced acute pulmonary vasodilation in primary pulmonary hypertension. *Circulation* 1982; **66**:334–8.

59 Higenbottam T, Wheeldon D, Wells F, Wallwork J. Long-term treatment of primary pulmonary hypertension with continuous intravenous epoprostenol (prostacyclin). *Lancet* 1984; **1**:1046–7.

60 Rubin LJ, Mendoza J, Hood M et al. Treatment of primary pulmonary hypertension with continuous intravenous prostacyclin (epoprostenol). Results of a randomized trial. *Ann Intern Med* 1990; **112**:485–91.

61 Higenbottam TW, Spiegelhalter D, Scott JP et al. Prostacyclin (epoprostenol) and heart–lung transplantation as treatments for severe pulmonary hypertension. *Br Heart J* 1993; **70**:366–70.

62 Barst RJ, Rubin LJ, McGoon MD, Caldwell EJ, Long WA, Levy PS. Survival in primary pulmonary hypertension with long-term continuous intravenous prostacyclin. *Ann Intern Med* 1994; **121**:409–15.

63 Barst RJ, Rubin LJ, Long WA et al. A comparison of continuous intravenous epoprostenol (prostacyclin) with conventional therapy for primary pulmonary hypertension. The Primary Pulmonary Hypertension Study Group. *N Engl J Med* 1996; **334**:296–302.

64 McLaughlin VV, Genthner DE, Panella MM, Hess DM, Rich S. Compassionate use of continuous prostacyclin in the management of secondary pulmonary hypertension: a case series. *Ann Intern Med* 1999; **130**:740–3.

65 Shapiro SM, Oudiz RJ, Cao T et al. Primary pulmonary hypertension: improved long-term effects and survival with continuous intravenous epoprostenol infusion. *J Am Coll Cardiol* 1997; **30**:343–9.

66 McLaughlin VV, Genthner DE, Panella MM, Rich S. Reduction in pulmonary vascular resistance with long-term epoprostenol (prostacyclin) therapy in primary pulmonary hypertension. *N Engl J Med* 1998; **338**:273–7.

67 Barst RJ, Maislin G, Fishman AP. Vasodilator therapy for primary pulmonary hypertension in children. *Circulation* 1999; **99**:1197–208.

68 Petitpretz P, Brenot F, Azarian R et al. Pulmonary hypertension in patients with human immunodeficiency virus infection. Comparison with primary pulmonary hypertension. *Circulation* 1994; **89**:2722–7.

69 Speich R, Jenni R, Opravil M, Jaccard R. Regression of HIV-associated pulmonary arterial hypertension and long-term survival during antiretroviral therapy. *Swiss Med Wkly* 2001; **131**:663–5.

70 Opravil M, Pechere M, Speich R et al. HIV-associated primary pulmonary hypertension. A case control study. Swiss HIV Cohort Study. *Am J Respir Crit Care Med* 1997; **155**:990–5.

71 Speich R, Jenni R, Opravil M, Pfab M, Russi EW. Primary pulmonary hypertension in HIV infection. *Chest* 1991; **100**:1268–71.

72 Nunes H, Humbert M, Sitbon O *et al*. Prognostic factors for survival in HIV-associated pulmonary arterial hypertension. *Am J Respir Crit Care Med* 2003; **167**:1433–9.

73 Kuo PC, Plotkin JS, Gaine S *et al*. Portopulmonary hypertension and the liver transplant candidate. *Transplantation* 1999; **67**:1087–93.

74 Plotkin JS, Kuo PC, Rubin LJ *et al*. Successful use of chronic epoprostenol as a bridge to liver transplantation in severe portopulmonary hypertension. *Transplantation* 1998; **65**:457–9.

75 Rosenzweig EB, Kerstein D, Barst RJ. Long-term prostacyclin for pulmonary hypertension with associated congenital heart defects. *Circulation* 1999; **99**:1858–65.

76 Badesch DB, Tapson VF, McGoon MD *et al*. Continuous intravenous epoprostenol for pulmonary hypertension due to the scleroderma spectrum of disease. A randomized, controlled trial. *Ann Intern Med* 2000; **132**:425–34.

77 Cremona G, Higenbottam T. Role of prostacyclin in the treatment of primary pulmonary hypertension. *Am J Cardiol* 1995; **75**:67A–71A.

78 Ahearn GS, Selim MA, Tapson VF. Severe erythroderma as a complication of continuous epoprostenol therapy. *Chest* 2002; **122**:378–80.

79 Brundage BH. Medical treatment of pulmonary hypertension with prostacyclin. In: Rich S, ed. *1998 World Symposium on Primary Pulmonary Hypertension*. Chicago, The Rush Heart Institute Center for Pulmonary Heart Disease, 1998.

80 McLaughlin VV, Gaine SP, Barst RJ *et al*. Efficacy and safety of treprostinil: an epoprostenol analog for primary pulmonary hypertension. *J Cardiovasc Pharmacol* 2003; **41**:293–9.

81 Simonneau G, Barst RJ, Galie N *et al*. Continuous subcutaneous infusion of treprostinil, a prostacyclin analogue, in patients with pulmonary arterial hypertension. A double-blind, randomized, placebo-controlled trial. *Am J Respir Crit Care Med* 2002; **165**:800–4.

82 Nishio S, Matsuura H, Kanai N *et al*. The *in vitro* and *ex vivo* antiplatelet effect of TRK-100, a stable prostacyclin analog, in several species. *Jpn J Pharmacol* 1988; **47**:1–10.

83 Saji T, Ozawa Y, Ishikita T, Matsuura H, Matsuo N. Short-term hemodynamic effect of a new oral PGI2 analogue, beraprost, in primary and secondary pulmonary hypertension. *Am J Cardiol* 1996; **78**:244–7.

84 Okano Y, Yoshioka T, Shimouchi A, Satoh T, Kunieda T. Orally active prostacyclin analogue in primary pulmonary hypertension. *Lancet* 1997; **349**:1365.

85 Nagaya N, Uematsu M, Okano Y *et al*. Effect of orally active prostacyclin analogue on survival of outpatients with primary pulmonary hypertension. *J Am Coll Cardiol* 1999; **34**:1188–92.

86 Nagaya N, Shimizu Y, Satoh T *et al*. Oral beraprost sodium improves exercise capacity and ventilatory efficiency in patients with primary or thromboembolic pulmonary hypertension. *Heart* 2002; **87**: 340–5.

87 Galie N, Humbert M, Vachiery JL *et al*. Effects of beraprost sodium, an oral prostacyclin analogue, in patients with pulmonary arterial hypertension: a randomized, double-blind, placebo-controlled trial. *J Am Coll Cardiol* 2002; **39**:1496–502.

88 Barst RJ, McGoon M, McLaughlin V *et al*. Beraprost therapy for pulmonary arterial hypertension. *J Am Coll Cardiol* 2003; **41**:2119–25.

89 Gessler T, Schmehl T, Hoeper MM *et al*. Ultrasonic versus jet nebulization of iloprost in severe pulmonary hypertension. *Eur Respir J* 2001; **17**:14–19.

90 Olschewski H, Walmrath D, Schermuly R, Ghofrani A, Grimminger F, Seeger W. Aerosolized prostacyclin and iloprost in severe pulmonary hypertension. *Ann Intern Med* 1996; **124**:820–4.

91 Olschewski H, Ghofrani HA, Walmrath D *et al*. Inhaled prostacyclin and iloprost in severe pulmonary hypertension secondary to lung fibrosis. *Am J Respir Crit Care Med* 1999; **160**:600–7.

92 Walmrath D, Schneider T, Pilch J, Grimminger F, Seeger W. Aerosolised prostacyclin in adult respiratory distress syndrome. *Lancet* 1993; **342**:961–2.

93 Walmrath D, Schneider T, Pilch J, Schermuly R, Grimminger F, Seeger W. Effects of aerosolized prostacyclin in severe pneumonia. Impact of fibrosis. *Am J Respir Crit Care Med* 1995; **151**(3 Pt 1):724–30.

94 Walmrath D, Schneider T, Schermuly R, Olschewski H, Grimminger F, Seeger W. Direct comparison of inhaled nitric oxide and aerosolized prostacyclin in acute respiratory distress syndrome. *Am J Respir Crit Care Med* 1996; **153**:991–6.

95 Zwissler B, Kemming G, Habler O *et al*. Inhaled prostacyclin (PGI2) versus inhaled nitric oxide in adult respiratory distress syndrome. *Am J Respir Crit Care Med* 1996; **154**(6 Pt 1):1671–7.

96 De Jaegere AP, van den Anker JN. Endotracheal instillation of prostacyclin in preterm infants with persistent pulmonary hypertension. *Eur Respir J* 1998; **12**:932–4.

97 Hoeper MM, Schwarze M, Ehlerding S *et al*. Long-term treatment of primary pulmonary hypertension with aerosolized iloprost, a prostacyclin analogue. *N Engl J Med* 2000; **342**:1866–70.

98 Olschewski H, Ghofrani HA, Schmehl T *et al*. Inhaled iloprost to treat severe pulmonary hypertension. An uncontrolled trial. German PPH Study Group. *Ann Intern Med* 2000; **132**:435–43.

99 Olschewski H, Nikkho S., Behr J *et al*. Long-term survival in patients with pulmonary hypertension inhaling iloprost. *Eur Heart J* 2003; **24**:482.

100 Schermuly RT, Krupnik E, Tenor H *et al*. Coaerosolization of phosphodiesterase inhibitors markedly enhances the pulmonary vasodilatory response to inhaled iloprost in experimental pulmonary hypertension. Maintenance of lung selectivity. *Am J Respir Crit Care Med* 2001; **164**:1694–700.

101 Schermuly RT, Roehl A, Weissmann N *et al*. Combination of nonspecific PDE inhibitors with inhaled prostacyclin in experimental pulmonary hypertension. *Am J Physiol Lung Cell Mol Physiol* 2001; **281**:L1361–8.

102 Ghofrani H, Wiedemann R, Rose F *et al*. Sildenafil for treatment of lung fibrosis and pulmonary hypertension: a randomised controlled trial. *Lancet* 2002; **360**:895.

103 Wilkens H, Guth A, Konig J *et al*. Effect of inhaled iloprost plus oral sildenafil in patients with primary pulmonary hypertension. *Circulation* 2001; **104**:1218–22.

104 Ghofrani HA, Wiedemann R, Rose F *et al*. Combination therapy with oral sildenafil and inhaled iloprost for severe pulmonary hypertension. *Ann Intern Med* 2002; **136**:515–22.

105 Abrams D, Schulze-Neick I, Magee AG. Sildenafil as a selective pulmonary vasodilator in childhood primary pulmonary hypertension. *Heart* 2000; **84**:E4.

106 Carlsen J, Kjeldsen K, Gerstoft J. Sildenafil as a successful treatment of otherwise fatal HIV-related pulmonary hypertension. *AIDS* 2002; **16**:1568–9.

107 Jackson G, Chambers J. Sildenafil for primary pulmonary hypertension: short and long-term symptomatic benefit. *Int J Clin Pract* 2002; **56**:397–8.

108 Prasad S, Wilkinson J, Gatzoulis MA. Sildenafil in primary pulmonary hypertension. *N Engl J Med* 2000; **343**:1342.

109 Zimmermann AT, Calvert AF, Veitch EM. Sildenafil improves right-ventricular parameters and quality of life in primary pulmonary hypertension. *Intern Med J* 2002; **32**:424–6.

110 Sitbon O, Humbert M, Ioos V *et al*. Who does benefit from long-term calcium-channel blocker (CCB) therapy in primary pulmonary hypertension (PPH)? *Am J Respir Crit Care Med* 2003; **167**:A440.

111 Rothman A, Beltran D, Kriett JM, Smith C, Wolf P, Jamieson SW. Graded balloon dilation atrial septostomy as a bridge to lung

transplantation in pulmonary hypertension. *Am Heart J* 1993; **125**:1763–6.

112 Rothman A, Sklansky MS, Lucas VW *et al*. Atrial septostomy as a bridge to lung transplantation in patients with severe pulmonary hypertension. *Am J Cardiol* 1999; **84**:682–6.

113 Sandoval J, Gaspar J, Pulido T *et al*. Graded balloon dilation atrial septostomy in severe primary pulmonary hypertension. A therapeutic alternative for patients nonresponsive to vasodilator treatment. *J Am Coll Cardiol* 1998; **32**:297–304.

Index

Note: numbers in bold type refer to figures; figures on CD-ROM are cited in index as CD-ROMFig.1 etc.